The Consult Manual of Internal Medicine
Harry Rosen, M.D.
Academic Hospitalist
harry.rosen@gmail.com

S0-ABB-625

Cover design: Niraj Naveri
Cover photography: Rick Chou
Indexer: WordCo
Printer: Victor Graphics
Printed in the USA

Library of Congress Control Number: 2005928868

DISCLAIMER & LIMITATION OF LIABILITY

INTERPRETATION OF MEDICATION TABLES

M=metabolism†
- B=bile
- C=cellular
- E=erythrocytes
- F=fecal excretion
- K=kidney
- L=liver
- M=monocytes/ macrophages
- P=plasma
- Ø=not metabolized
- ?=uncertain

♀=safety in pregnancy
- S=safe
- P=presumed safe
- ?=uncertain safety
- U=unsafe

---

†If more than one organ is responsible for a medications metabolism, they are listed in order of primacy

DEDICATION

•Maya, for your love, understanding, intelligence, & sense of humor.
•Eden, for giving new meaning to life and love.

TABLE OF CONTENTS

CARDIOPULMONARY RESUSCITATION–CPR

•The #1 cause of cardiorespiratory arrest in adults is the acute coronary syndrome, usually via ventricular fibrillation

"CHAIN OF SURVIVAL"

1. CHECK FOR CONSCIOUSNESS

•Assessed by tapping on the patient, & shouting for the patient to wake up
 ◦If unresponsive, initiate an emergency medical response
  –Hospital: Have someone call a "code blue" to activate the in–house code teams
  –Community: Have someone call 911, & obtain an automated external defibrillator–AED†
Note: If no one is nearby, initiate the emergency medical response yourself & return to the patient to initiate CPR

---

†Automated external defibrillators–AEDs are becoming increasingly available in public locations

2. PERFORM THE ABCs OF SURVIVAL
A=AIRWAY
•Assessed for patency by viewing the oral cavity
 ◦Remove a possible obstruction via a finger sweep or suction device
•Tilt the head backwards (except if cervical spine injury is suspected) & thrust the mandible forward w/ your 3rd–5th digits under the bilateral mandibular rami→
 ◦**Open airway**. This position must be maintained for adequate ventilation until the patient is intubated

B=BREATHING
•Assessed by looking, listening, & feeling for both:
 ◦A rising & falling chest & abdominal wall
 ◦Nasal or oral exhalation
 …X 3–5seconds
  •If the patient is breathing, a pulse must be present
  •**If the patient is not breathing, give 2 slow positive pressure ventilations,** each over 2 seconds† via:
   ◦Mouth to mouth (while pinching the nose closed)
   ◦Mouth to nose
   ◦Bag–valve mask
   …while looking & feeling for the corresponding rise & fall of the chest & abdominal wall

C=CIRCULATION
•Assessed by **palpating for a carotid pulse** X 5–10seconds
 ◦A palpable carotid artery pulse indicates a systolic blood pressure >60mmHg
 ◦A palpable femoral artery pulse indicates a systolic blood pressure >70mmHg
 ◦A palpable radial artery pulse indicates a systolic blood pressure > 80mmHg

---

†In order to ↓gastric distention

3. PERFORM BASIC LIFE SUPPORT–BLS
IF NO PULSE IS PALPATED
•**Initiate chest compressions**
 ◦**If not intubated:** 15 chest compressions, interrupted by 2 slow ventilations, each over 2seconds
 ◦**If intubated:** 100 chest compressions/ min. without interruption, w/ ventilation @ 10–12 slow/ min.

IF A PULSE IS PALPATED, BUT THE PATIENT IS NOT BREATHING
•**Give 1 slow positive pressure ventilation q5seconds**

4. PERFORM ADVANCED CARDIAC LIFE SUPORT–ACLS
•Electrical cardioversion or defibrillation as indicated
•Intravenous, intrapulmonary, or intraosseous medications as indicated
•Search for, & attempt to treat the etiology

1

GOAL OF CARDIOPULMONARY RESUSCITATION–CPR
•**Organized electrocardiographic–ECG activity**→
  ◦**Tissue perfusion, as inferred from a palpable pulse, not consciousness**
•The most powerful predictors of successful resuscitation are:
  ◦Early initiation of CPR
  ◦Defibrillation as indicated

TEAMWORK CPR
•**One person should assume a leadership role** (usually a senior physician knowledgeable about cardiac resuscitation if in a hospital) & immediately assign resuscitation tasks to the others involved=the team, as well as make clinical decisions (while inviting suggestions from team members) without directly performing procedures
•The decision to terminate resuscitative efforts should be agreed upon by all team members
•Regardless of the outcome, the code leader should debrief the team so that all may learn from the experience

PROPER TECHNIQUES
HOW TO PROPERLY VENTILATE A PATIENT
1. W/ the head tilted back & mandible thrust forward, insert a plastic oral airway (which serves to keep the tongue forward) & place a bag–valve mask on the patient
2. Use your 3rd–5th digits to maintain the head position while placing your thumbs & index fingers around the mask in a 'C' like shape, maintaining a strong skin–mask seal
   •You may use both hands while another person ventilates, or maintain position & seal w/ your dominant hand alone
3. During intubation attempts, CPR should not be held for >20seconds, after which time the laryngoscope should be withdrawn, & CPR continued until the next intubation attempt
4. Once the patient is intubated (as evidenced by carbon dioxide detection), detach the bag device from the mask, attach it to the endotracheal tube, & **continue ventilations @ 10–12 slow breaths/ min.** without interruption

HOW TO PROPERLY PERFORM CHEST COMPRESSIONS
1. Place yourself at the patient's side w/ knees to the floor, or to the bed, depending on where the patient is found
2. When possible, move the patient to a bed or gurney for easier patient access & management by the code team
   •If cervical spine injury is suspected, place on a flatboard & position a cervical spine collar prior to movement
3. Place the heel of 1 hand over the lower half of the sternum, 2 finger widths above the xiphoid process, w/ the other hand atop the first
4. Maintain shoulder position directly above your hands & lock your elbows
5. Use your entire upper body as a pendulum to intermittently **compress directly downward 1.5–2"** **@ 100/ min.**, without ever lifting your hands off position
   •If this action does not produce a palpable carotid pulse, ↑chest compression force

Closed vs. open chest compression:
•Closed chest compressions→
  ◦Near–equivalent rise in both arterial & right atrial pressures→
    –↓Arteriovenous pressure gradient→systemic blood flow <25% normal levels
•Emergent thoracotomy, w/ direct ventricular massage→
  ◦↑Arterial pressure w/ ↓right atrial pressure→
    –↑Arteriovenous pressure gradient→ ≥ normal systemic blood flow

MEDICATION ADMINISTRATION
•It is preferable to administer intravenous medications via a central venous line→
  ◦↓Systemic distribution time by ≥ 2min.
•If a central venous line is unavailable, medication may be given via either:
  ◦A peripheral intravenous line, followed by a 20mL saline flush, w/ limb elevation X 10–20seconds
  ◦Endotracheal tube @ 2–3X† the intravenous dosage, until an intravenous line is placed
•Intravenous access below the diaphragm (ex. femoral vein) should not be used, as there is minimal subdiaphragmatic venous blood flow during cardiac arrest

2

Proper administration of medication via an endotracheal tube:
1. Place a catheter into the endotracheal tube which is long enough to extend beyond its distal end
2. Interrupt chest compressions, & inject a mixture of the medication in 10mL normal saline or distilled water into the lungs, w/ several subsequent bag–mask valve ventilations prior to resuming chest compressions→
   •Medication nebulization to the alveoli→
     ○↑Absorption
Medications which can be administered via endotracheal tube:
•Naloxone, Atropine, Vasopressin, Epinephrine, Lidocaine=NAVEL
Contraindications:
•Never give sodium bicarbonate via an endotracheal tube

Rational for administering epinephrine or vasopressin:
•Epinephrine & vasopressin→systemic vasoconstriction→
  ○↑Peripheral vascular resistance→
    –↑Aortic diastolic blood pressure→↑coronary perfusion pressure
  ○Relatively ↑external carotid artery vasoconstriction→
    –Internal carotid artery shunting of blood→↑cerebral perfusion pressure
  ○Epinephrine is used in asystole due to its pro–dysrhythmic potential→
    –↑Chance of conversion to a shockable, & thereby more potentially treatable rhythm

†Except vasopressin, which is administered in the same 40unit dosage

MONITORING ORGAN PERFUSION STATUS DURING CPR ▬▬▬▬
END TIDAL PCO$_2$
•End tidal or end–expiratory CO_2 is usually <10mmHg† in cardiac arrest patients, being measured in real time, on a breath by breath basis via nasal cannula or endotracheal tube
  ○A value ≤10mmHg after 20min. of CPR indicates unlikely successful resuscitation

Pathophysiology:
•↑Systemic perfusion pressure→
  ○↑Pulmonary CO_2 delivery→
    –↑End tidal CO_2, indicating ↑organ perfusion & better prognosis

VENOUS BLOOD GAS ANALYSIS
•Venous blood more accurately represents peripheral tissue oxygenation & acid/ base status than arterial blood

†Normal is 40–45mmHg, being nearly equivalent to the arterial PCO$_2$

CPR LENGTH ▬▬▬▬
•Length of cardiac arrest prior to the initiation of CPR, the presence of asystole, & etiology are the determinative factors
  ○**If asystole, continue CPR for 10min.†**
  ○**For all other dysrhythmias:**
    –**If <6min. prior to CPR initiation, continue CPR for 30min.†**
    –**If >6min. prior to CPR initiation, continue CPR for 15min.†**
  ...as prolonged CPR→
    •Ischemia & nutrient paucity mediated neuronal cell dysfunction ± death=anoxic encephalopathy→
      ○Neurologic impairment. Even within the parameters listed, neurologic impairment is common, & may be transient or permanent

•**The following requirements must be met prior to the termination of any cardiac resuscitation attempt:**
  ○**Basic life support–BLS**
  ○**Endotracheal tube ventilation**
  ○**Intravenous medication administration X 2 rounds**
  ○**Normothermia ≥97°F**

†Satisfactory neurologic recovery has occurred several hours after beginning resuscitation, if due to, or accompanied by:
•Barbiturate overdose
•Childhood
•Drowning
•Electrocution
•Hypothermia

3

ONCE RESUSCITATED

•The patient should be monitored in an intensive care unit
•Most successfully resuscitated patients do not immediately regain consciousness, due to anoxic encephalopathy. Comatose patients may need mechanical ventilation if they lack either:
  ◦Spontaneous respiration
  ◦Adequate ventilation, as per arterial blood gas values
  …w/ ischemia & nutrient paucity mediated neuronal cell dysfunction ± death=anoxic encephalopathy→
    •↑Time needed to heal to the point of regaining consciousness, the length of which is inversely proportional to the prognosis for a favorable neurologic recovery
      ◦If **>24hours, only 10%** will successfully recover most of their neurologic function, w/ concomitant absence of the pupillary light reflex indicating a very low probability of any neurologic recovery
      ◦If **>1week, only 5%** will successfully recover most of their neurologic function
      ◦If **>2weeks, no** neurologic recovery occurs
•Once conscious, the patient may manifest:
  ◦Behavioral disturbances
  ◦Post-arrest amnesia
  ◦Other neurologic impairment, which may be severe

Neurologic assessment via brainstem reflexes
•**Dolls eye maneuver**
  ◦Elicited by rotating the patients head from side to side†
    −An intact brainstem is indicated by an intact vestibulo-ocular reflex attempting to stabilize the eyes in space in order to maintain a steady retinal image, w/ both eyes deviating away from the direction of rotation, resembling the fixed forward gaze of a doll's eye
    −A dysfunctional brainstem is indicated by no eye deviation

•**Ice water calorics**, being a stronger stimulus than the dolls eye maneuver
  ◦Elicited by injecting 50mL of ice cold water into the external auditory canal‡ of a supine patient whose head is at a 30° angle, which orients the lateral semicircular canals in the most vertical plane
    −An intact brainstem is indicated by both eyes deviating towards the irrigated ear, as the cold inactivates the ipsilateral vestibular input to the eye movement center. This typically begins @ 20-30seconds, lasting ~1min. If the patient is not in a coma, contralateral saccades also appear, being a corrective fast phase beat away from the cold stimulus. The eyes should be observed for one minute after irrigation is completed, repeating the test on the other side after 5min.
    −A dysfunctional brainstem is indicated by no eye deviation

•**Corneal reflex**
  ◦Elicited by using either a wisp of cotton to lightly touch the cornea, or a straw or syringe to squirt air at the cornea (not the scleral conjunctiva which is less sensitive)
    −An intact brainstem is indicated by a bilateral blink reflex
    −A dysfunctional brainstem is indicated by no blink reflex

---

†If the patient has suffered trauma, ensure that the cervical spine is stable via x ray prior to performing this test
‡View the tympanic membrane to rule out perforation prior to performing this test

VENTRICULAR FIBRILLATION/ PULSELESS VENTRICULAR TACHYCARDIA

1. A **precordial thump** is recommended only w/ a witnessed cardiac arrest, being equivalent to the administration of 20–40joules

2. Perform **BASIC LIFE SUPPORT** throughout, except when defibrillating

3. Once the defibrillator is placed, confirm the rhythm, then:
- **DEFIBRILLATE X 3**, checking the rhythm & vital signs after each defibrillation

Defibrillation types:
- **Monophasic**, in which the current flows from one electrode to the other
- **Biphasic**, in which the current flows from one electrode to the other & back, within the same time as in monophasic defibrillation→
  - ○↓Joule requirement→
    - –↓Myocardial cell death

Monophasic defibrillation	Biphasic defibrillation
200 joules, then	150 joules, then
300 joules, then	200 joules, then
360 joules	200 joules

Outcomes:
- ↑Delay in initiating defibrillation→
  - ○↓Survival
    - –A 5min. delay→40% ↓survival, w/ a 10%↓ q5min. thereafter

4. If the rhythm does not respond to defibrillation, continue **BASIC LIFE SUPPORT** while **promptly intubating & obtaining intravenous access for the following medications:**

A. Epinephrine 1mg IV push OR Vasopressin 40units IV push (half life=20min.)
↓

B. Chest compressions X 30–60seconds, w/ subsequent defibrillation at maximal energy
↻

C. Epinephrine† 1mg IV push q3min. + anti–dysrhythmics ± sodium bicarbonate ± CaCl

---

†The epinephrine dosing protocol may be initiated 10 min. after vasopressin administration. However, if epinephrine is used initially, do not use vasopressin
- If the rhythm does not respond to initial epinephrine dosing attempts, consider the following regimens:
  - ○Intermediate dosing @ 2–5mg q3min.
  - ○Escalating dosing @ 1mg, 3mg, then 5mg q3min.
  - ○High dosing @ 0.1mg/ kg q3min.

ANTI–DYSRHYTHMICS		
Generic	**Dose**	**Max**
FIRST LINE		
Amiodarone	300mg IV push, then	
	150mg IV push q10min. prn	
Maintenance infusion:		
	1mg/ min. X 6hours, then	
	0.5mg/ min. X 18–72h	2.2g IV/ 24hour
Lidocaine	1mg/ kg IV push, then	
	0.5mg/ kg IV push q5–10min. prn	3mg/ kg total
Maintenance infusion:		
	Rebolus 75mg IV push, then	
	1–4mg/ min. IV infusion	
SECOND LINE		
Magnesium sulfate	2g IV slow push q5–10min. prn	8g
Indications:		
•**Torsades de pointes**		
•Suspected hypomagnesemia		
•Suspected Digoxin toxicity		
•Ventricular fibrillation refractory to first line treatment medications		
Procainamide	20mg–50mg/ min. IV infusion	
Maintenance infusion:		
	1–4mg/ min. IV infusion	17mg/ kg total

- Upon cardioversion, a maintenance intravenous infusion of 1 of the above should be administered for ≥24h. The loading dose is as above if not already given during the resuscitative effort

Lidocaine specific dose adjustment:
- •If cardiac failure, liver disease, or elderly: 1-2mg/ min. IV maintenance infusion

Procainamide specific dose adjustment:
- •If cardiac or renal failure: 1-2mg/ min. IV maintenance infusion (max: 12mg/ kg total)
- •Discontinue infusion temporarily if either:
  - ∘Hypotension
  - ∘QRS widens >50%

Amiodarone specific immediate side effects:
- •Dose dependent hypotension
- •Dose dependent ↑QT interval→
  - ∘Torsades de pointes

Procainamide specific immediate side effects:
- •↑QT interval→
  - ∘Torsades de pointes

BICARBONATE

Indications:
- •**Hyperkalemia**
- •**Acidemia**
- •**Medication/ drug overdose**
  - ∘Aspirin
  - ∘Diphenhydramine
  - ∘Tricyclic antidepressant
  - ∘Cocaine
  - ...→urine alkalinization
- •**Empirically after 5-10min.† if acidemic & not responding to resuscitative efforts**
- •**Upon return of spontaneous circulation, after a prolonged resuscitation, w/ effective ventilation via intubation‡**

†As the initial acidemia is likely pulmonary in etiology
‡Sodium bicarbonate is metabolized to CO_2→
- •Worsening acidemia in inadequately ventilated patients

Generic	M ♀	Dose
Sodium bicarbonate	K ?	1mEq/ kg IV push (1 ampule = ~50mEq), then 0.5mEq/ kg IV q10min. prn

Onset: 15-30min., Duration: 1-2hours

Side effects:
- •May exacerbate volume overload due to sodium content

CALCIUM

Indications:
- •**Hyperkalemia**

Generic	Dose	Max
10% Calcium chloride†	10mL (1 ampule) IV slow push over 3min. q5min. prn until electrocardiographic changes resolve	
•Continuous infusion	0.3mEq/ hour	0.7mEq/ hour

Onset: 1-2 min., Duration: 30-60 min.

- •Use cautiously in patients taking Digoxin, as hypercalcemia→
  - ∘Digoxin cardiotoxicity
†Preferred to calcium gluconate, as it contains 3X more elemental calcium

Mechanism:
- •Calcium→
  - ∘↑Action potential threshold→
    - -↓Hyperkalemia mediated membrane depolarization

Contraindications:
- •Digoxin toxicity

6

PULSELESS ELECTRICAL ACTIVITY-PEA

•**Organized cardiac electrical activity w/ ineffective perfusion**, also termed electromechanical dissociation

1. Perform **BASIC LIFE SUPPORT** throughout, while **promptly intubating & obtaining intravenous access for the following medications:**

> Epinephrine 1mg IV push q3min. **+ volume repletion† ± sodium bicarbonate ± CaCl**
> **±**
> **If bradycardic**
> Atropine 1mg IV push q3min. (max ~3mg→complete parasympathetic blockade)

...while searching for & treating the underlying etiology:

If suspect	Attempt
•Hypovolemia†	Volume repletion (should be occurring)
•Hypoxemia	Ventilation (should be occurring)
•Hypothermia	Rewarming to >97°F
•Hypokalemia‡	Potassium repletion
•Hyperkalemia	Calcium chloride, glucose, & insulin
•Acidemia	Sodium bicarbonate
•Pericardial tamponade	Pericardiocentesis
•Tension pneumothorax	Needle decompression
•Massive pulmonary embolism	Embolectomy or thrombolytic medication
•Massive myocardial infarction	
•Medication overdose:	
∘β receptor blocker	Glucagon or calcium chloride
∘Calcium channel blocker	Calcium chloride or glucagon
∘Digitalis	Digoxin-immune Fab 20 vials IV over 15min. prn
∘Opiates	Naloxone hydrochloride 2mg IV q2min. prn.
∘Tricyclic antidepressant	Sodium bicarbonate

†Hypovolemia is the #1 correctable cause, & ↑venous return in obstructive causes
‡Hypokalemia alone will not cause serious ventricular dysrhythmias unless accompanied by another pro-dysrhythmic risk factor, such as:
  •Heart disease
  •Hypomagnesemia
  •Digitalis administration
•If the rhythm does not respond to initial epinephrine dosing attempts, consider the following regimens:
  ∘Intermediate dosing @ 2-5mg q3min.
  ∘Escalating dosing @ 1mg, 3mg, then 5mg q3min.
  ∘High dosing @ 0.1mg/ kg q3min.

BICARBONATE

Indications:
  •**Hyperkalemia**
  •**Acidemia**
  •**Medication/ drug overdose**
    ∘Aspirin
    ∘Diphenhydramine
    ∘Tricyclic antidepressant
    ∘Cocaine
    ...→urine alkalinization
  •**Empirically after 5-10min.† if acidemic & not responding to resuscitative efforts**
  •**Upon return of spontaneous circulation, after a prolonged resuscitation, w/ effective ventilation via intubation‡**

†As the initial acidemia is likely pulmonary in etiology
‡Sodium bicarbonate is metabolized to CO_2→
  •Worsening acidemia in inadequately ventilated patients

Generic	M ♀	Dose
Sodium bicarbonate	K ?	1mEq/ kg IV push (1 ampule = ~50mEq), then 0.5mEq/ kg IV q10min. prn

Onset: 15-30min., Duration: 1-2hours

Side effects:
  •May exacerbate volume overload due to sodium content

7

CALCIUM		
Indications:		
•**Hyperkalemia**		
Generic	**Dose**	**Max**
10% Calcium chloride†	10mL (1 ampule) IV slow push over 3min., q5min. prn until electrocardiographic changes resolve	
•Continuous infusion	0.3mEq/ hour	0.7mEq/ hour
Onset: 1–2 min., Duration: 30–60 min.		

•Use cautiously in patients taking Digoxin, as hypercalcemia→
 ∘↑Digoxin cardiotoxicity risk
†Preferred to calcium gluconate, as it contains 3X more elemental calcium

Mechanism:
 •Calcium→
  ∘↑Action potential threshold→
   −↓Hyperkalemia mediated membrane depolarization

Contraindications:
 •Digoxin toxicity

GLUCAGON
Dose
3mg IV slow push over 1min., then
5mg IV slow push over 1 min. if needed
Continuous infusion: 5mg/ hour

PROGNOSIS
•Only 1/ 150 patients are successfully resuscitated

ASYSTOLE

1. **Confirm asystole in >1 lead**
   - There is little harm or benefit in mistakenly defibrillating asystole thought to be "fine" ventricular fibrillation
2. Perform **BASIC LIFE SUPPORT** throughout, while **promptly intubating & obtaining intravenous access for the following medications**
3. **Transcutaneous pacing**
   - Start at 200milliamps–mA
   - If capture occurs–<18%, ↓voltage until capture is lost, then
   - ↑Voltage until capture occurs + 2mA, w/ a goal of 60–70bpm, as you do not want to overwork the diseased myocardium

   Note: **Milliamps allow safety when touching the patent**

   &

   Epinephrine 1mg IV push q3min. ± sodium bicarbonate ± CaCl
   ↻ spaced apart by 30seconds
   Atropine 1mg IV push q3min. (max ~3mg→complete parasympathetic blockade)

...while searching for & treating the underlying etiology:

If suspect	Attempt
•**Hypovolemia**	Volume repletion
•**Hypoxemia**	Ventilation (should be occurring)
•**Hypothermia**	Rewarming to >97°F
•**Hypokalemia**†	Potassium repletion
•**Hyperkalemia**	Calcium chloride, glucose, & insulin
•**Acidemia**	Sodium bicarbonate
•**Pericardial tamponade**	Pericardiocentesis
•**Tension pneumothorax**	Needle decompression
•**Massive pulmonary embolism**	Embolectomy or thrombolytic medication
•**Massive myocardial infarction**	
•**Medication overdose:**	
∘β receptor blocker	Glucagon or calcium chloride
∘Calcium channel blocker	Calcium chloride or glucagon
∘Digitalis	Digoxin–immune Fab 20 vials IV over 15min. prn
∘Opiates	Naloxone hydrochloride 2mg IV q2min. prn.
∘Tricyclic antidepressant	Sodium bicarbonate

‡Hypokalemia alone will not cause serious ventricular dysrhythmias unless accompanied by another pro–dysrhythmic risk factor, such as:
   - Heart disease
   - Hypomagnesemia
   - Digitalis administration
- If the rhythm does not respond to initial epinephrine dosing attempts, consider the following regimens:
   - ∘Intermediate dosing @ 2–5mg q3min.
   - ∘Escalating dosing @ 1mg, 3mg, then 5mg q3min.
   - ∘High dosing @ 0.1mg/ kg q3min.

BICARBONATE

Indications:
- •**Hyperkalemia**
- •**Acidemia**
- •**Medication/ drug overdose**
   - ∘Aspirin
   - ∘Diphenhydramine
   - ∘Tricyclic antidepressant
   - ∘Cocaine
   - ...→urine alkalinization
- •**Empirically after 5–10min.† if acidemic & not responding to resuscitative efforts**
- •**Upon return of spontaneous circulation, after a prolonged resuscitation, w/ effective ventilation via intubation‡**

---

†As the initial acidemia is likely pulmonary in etiology
‡Sodium bicarbonate is metabolized to CO_2→
   - •Worsening acidemia in inadequately ventilated patients

Generic	M	♀	Dose
Sodium bicarbonate	K	?	1mEq/ kg IV push (1 ampule = ~50mEq), then
			0.5mEq/ kg IV q10min. prn

Onset: 15–30min., Duration: 1–2hours

Side effects:
•May exacerbate volume overload due to sodium content

CALCIUM

Indications:
•**Hyperkalemia**

Generic	Dose	Max
10% Calcium chloride†	10mL (1 ampule) IV slow push over 3min., q5min. prn	
	until electrocardiographic changes resolve	
•Continuous infusion	0.3mEq/ hour	0.7mEq/ hour

Onset: 1–2 min., Duration: 30–60 min.

•Use cautiously in patients taking Digoxin, as hypercalcemia→
  ∘Digoxin cardiotoxicity
†Preferred to calcium gluconate, as it contains 3X more elemental calcium

Mechanism:
•Calcium→
  ∘↑Action potential threshold→
    −↓Hyperkalemia mediated membrane depolarization

Contraindications:
•Digoxin toxicity

GLUCAGON

Dose

3mg IV slow push over 1min., then
5mg IV slow push over 1 min. if needed
Continuous infusion: 5mg/ hour

PROGNOSIS
•Only 1/ 150 patients are successfully resuscitated

BRADYCARDIA
•Pulse <60bpm

ASYMPTOMATIC
•No immediate treatment necessary
•Observe & have atropine & transcutaneous pacing readily available at bedside in case the patient becomes symptomatic

SYMPTOMATIC
•↓Cardiac output→either:
  ○Altered mental status
  ○Heart failure
  ○Hypotension
  ○Myocardial ischemic syndrome

Atropine 1mg IV push q3min. (max ~3mg→complete parasympathetic blockade)
Indications:
  •Sinus bradycardia
  •First degree atrioventricular block
  •Second degree atrioventricular block–Mobitz type 1
⬇

Indications to skip atropine treatment:
  •Second degree atrioventricular block–Mobitz type 2
  •Third degree atrioventricular block
  •Status post–cardiac transplant
  …as either:
    ○The disease is below the atrioventricular node, & thus beyond the level of atropine action
    ○The myocardium is not under the effect of the Vagus nerve, as in transplant patients

Transcutaneous pacing as a bridge, until a transvenous pacer is placed
⬇
Dopamine start 5µg/kg/min. infusion & titrate prn (max 20µg/kg/min.)
⬇
Epinephrine start 2µg/ min. infusion & titrate prn (max 10µg/ min.)
⬇
Aminophylline 250mg IV push over 1–2min. q5min. X 2 doses

INDICATIONS FOR PACEMAKER PLACEMENT
Permanent:
  •Symptomatic bradycardia not otherwise controlled
  •Second degree atrioventricular block–Mobitz type 2
  •Third degree atrioventricular block
  •Pulse <40bpm while awake
  •Pauses ≥3seconds while awake
  •Carotid sinus syndrome→
    ○Pre–syncope/ syncope
  •Medical management for possible tachydysrhythmia of sick sinus syndrome

Temporary:
  •As a bridge to permanent pacemaker placement
  •After an acute myocardial infarction→
    ○Left bundle branch block
    ○Bifascicular bundle branch block
      −Right bundle branch block & left anterior incomplete block
    ○Trifascicular bundle branch block
      −Bifascicular bundle branch block & first degree atrioventricular block

11

PHYSIOLOGIC SINUS BRADYCARDIA

Risk factors:
- **•Athlete**
- **•Sleep**
- **•↓Myocardial metabolism**
  - ◦Elderly
  - ◦Hypothermia
  - ◦Hypothyroidism
- **•↑Autonomic parasympathetic tone,** via the Vagus nerve
  - ◦Carotid sinus stimulation
  - ◦↑Intracranial pressure
  - ◦Vasodepressor pre–syncope/ syncope
- **•Medications**
  - ◦**↓Autonomic sympathetic tone**
    - –Amiodarone, β–receptor blockers, non–dihydropyridine calcium channel blockers, Clonidine, Digoxin, Methyldopa, Sotalol

HEART BLOCK
- •Normally, the PR interval (measured from the beginning of the P wave to the beginning of the QRS complex) is normally ~0.16seconds, shortening & lengthening w/ ↑ & ↓ pulse respectively, but not exceeding 0.2seconds (1 big block on the ECG)
- •Heart block is defined as a PR interval >0.2seconds
  - ◦Any block may progress in severity, esp.:
    - –Second degree heart block–Mobitz type 2
    - –Third degree heart block

Risk factors:
- **•Conduction tissue ischemia ± infarction,** esp. that affecting the inferior or septal myocardium
- **•Conduction tissue inflammation**=myocarditis
- **•Conduction tissue compression** via fibrotic &/or calcified tissue
- **•Conduction tissue degeneration**
  - ◦↑Age
- **•Structural cardiac alteration**
  - ◦Cardiomyopathy
  - ◦Congenital defects
- **•↑Autonomic parasympathetic tone,** via the Vagus nerve
  - ◦Carotid sinus stimulation
  - ◦↑Intracranial pressure
  - ◦Vasodepressor pre–syncope/ syncope
- **•Medications**
  - ◦**↓Autonomic sympathetic tone**
    - –Amiodarone, β–receptor blockers, non–dihydropyridine calcium channel blockers, Clonidine, Digoxin, Methyldopa, Sotalol

FIRST DEGREE ATRIOVENTRICULAR BLOCK
- •Delayed atrioventricular conduction→
  - ◦**A PR interval >0.20seconds**
  - ◦A PR interval >0.35seconds may→
    - –Complete heart block

SECOND DEGREE ATRIOVENTRICULAR BLOCK
- •Altered atrioventricular or distal fiber conduction→
  - ◦**A PR interval >0.20seconds, w/ conduction of only some of the P waves**

Mobitz type 1–95%
- •Delayed atrioventricular conduction→
  - ◦**Wenckebach's phenomenon,** being progressively ↑PR intervals→
    - –Eventual loss of the conduction of a P wave, w/ the loss of the corresponding QRS complex, w/ the process subsequently starting anew
    - –The degree of Wenckebach is described as P wave to QRS complex ratios of 3:2, 4:3, 5:4, etc...
  - ◦**The QRS complexes are typically narrow,** as the conduction delay is supraventricular

12

Mobitz type 2–5%
- •**Delayed conduction distal to the atrioventricular node→**
  - ◦Loss of conduction of a ≥1 P† wave, without previously ↑PR intervals
    - –May occur intermittently, or in a fixed ratio
    - –Described as P wave to QRS complex ratios of 2:1, 3:1, 4:1, etc…(careful as a 2:1 ratio may be Mobitz type 1)
  - ◦**The QRS complexes are typically wide,** due to a concomitant bundle branch block
  - ◦**May rapidly progress to third degree atrioventricular block or asystole**

---

†Mobitz type 1 will only allow loss of one QRS complex at time, whereas Mobitz type 2 may allow loss of ≥1 QRS complex at a time, being termed **high grade atrioventricular block** if successive P waves are not conducted

THIRD DEGREE ATRIOVENTRICULAR BLOCK=COMPLETE HEART BLOCK
- •**Complete loss of P wave conduction to the ventricles→**
  - ◦Ventricular escape rhythm→
    - –Slow & regular QRS complexes, dissociated from the intervening P waves (which outnumber the QRS complexes)=complete atrioventricular dissociation
    - –May conduct retrograde to the atria→retrograde P waves buried in the QRS complex, or which distort its terminal portion→pseudo S waves in the inferior leads (II, III, aVF) & pseudo R' waves in lead V1
  - ◦Occurs at the level of either the:
    - –Atrioventricular node→narrow QRS complexes @ a rate of 40–60/ min.
    - –Distal to the atrioventricular node→widened QRS complex @ a rate of 20–40/ min.

SICK SINUS SYNDROME
- •The sinoatrial node impulse is either:
  - ◦Blocked prior to spreading to the atrial myocardium→
    - –Atrial standstill→loss of P wave, w/ a distal escape rhythm
  - ◦Delayed→
    - –Sinus &/or inappropriate bradycardia

Risk factors:
- •**Conduction tissue degeneration**
  - ◦↑Age
    - –Typically associated w/ diffuse conduction system abnormalities→varying degrees of concomitant atrioventricular &/or interventricular block→symptomatic bradycardia

TACHYCARDIA/ BRADYCARDIA SYNDROME
- •A variant of the sick sinus syndrome, in which the patient experiences the sick sinus syndrome before &/or after a supraventricular tachydysrhythmia

13

•Pulse >100bpm

SYMPTOMATIC ▬▬▬▬▬▬▬▬▬▬▬▬▬▬▬▬▬▬▬▬▬▬▬▬▬▬▬▬▬▬▬▬▬▬▬▬▬▬▬
•↓Cardiac output, usually occurring @ ≥150bpm→either:
- ◦Altered mental status
- ◦Heart failure
- ◦Hypotension
- ◦Myocardial ischemic syndrome
•Rule out sinus tachycardia, for which you must treat the underlying cause

IMMEDIATE SYNCHRONIZED CARDIOVERSION†
•If the patient is conscious & time permits, administer sedation ± analgesia

Monophasic cardioversion
100 joules, then
200 joules, then
300 joules, then
360 joules

Rational for synchronized rather than non-synchronized cardioversion=defibrillation
•The end of each cardiac cycle (being the terminal portion of the T wave) is referred to as the vulnerable period for the initiation of ventricular fibrillation, as the dispersion of both areas of refractory & non-refractory myocardium are greatest during this time. An electrical impulse administered during this time may→
- ◦Ventricular fibrillation. Synchronized cardioversion ensures delivery of the electrical impulse at some other specific time in the cardiac cycle, such as the R wave upstroke or S wave downslope

---

†Although listed below are some tachydysrythmias for which cardioversion may not be ideally indicated, you should not be faulted for attempting cardioversion of a symptomatic tachydysrhythmia

SINUS TACHYCARDIA ▬▬▬▬▬▬▬▬▬▬▬▬▬▬▬▬▬▬▬▬▬▬▬▬▬▬▬▬▬▬▬▬▬▬▬▬
•Determine & treat the underlying cause

NARROW COMPLEX SUPRAVENTRICULAR TACHYCARDIA ▬▬▬▬▬▬▬▬▬▬▬
•If Atrial flutter or fibrillation, see corresponding chapter

Vagal stimulation
&/ OR

ADENOSINE (Adenocard)		
Indications: •To ↓ventricular rate in order to determine the rhythm •To terminate a micro-reentrant paroxysmal supraventricular tachycardia–PSVT		
M ♀ **Dose**		
P ? 6mg IV rapid push over 1–3seconds, & immediate flush w/ 20mL saline & limb elevation If unresponsive @ 2min., repeat w/ 12mg IV rapid push q2min. prn X 2 doses		
Dose adjustment: •↓Dose by 50% ◦When administering via a central line, as full dose may→ –Asystole ◦In patients receiving β–receptor blockers, non–dihydropyridine calcium channel blockers, or Dipyridamole		
Mechanism: •↓Atrioventricular node conduction •Vascular adenosine receptor activation→ ◦Coronary artery dilation		
Outcomes: •Will terminate micro–reentrant paroxysmal supraventricular tachycardias–PSVT in 95% of cases		
Transient side effects: **Cardiovascular** •Atrioventricular block→ ◦**Sinus bradycardia–50%**, possibly being marked •↓Blood flow to coronary atherosclerotic regions which are less able to dilate=intracoronary steal syndrome→ ◦Myocardial ischemia–20% in the presence of significant epicardial stenosis, being ≥50%		

Gastrointestinal
•Nausea ± vomiting
Mucocutaneous
•Facial flushing–50%
Neurologic
•Dizziness
•Headache
Pulmonary
•Bronchoconstriction→
∘**Dyspnea–35%**
Contraindications:
•**Asthma or COPD w/ a bronchoconstricting component**

PAROXYSMAL SUPRAVENTRICULAR TACHYCARDIA–PSVT†
•**Symptomatic**
  ∘First line: Cardioversion
  ∘Second line: Digoxin
  ∘Third line: Amiodarone
  ∘Fourth line: Diltiazem
•**Asymptomatic**
  ∘First line: β1 selective receptor or non–dihydropyridine calcium channel blocker
  ∘Second line: Cardioversion
  ∘Third line: Amiodarone or Procainamide

JUNCTIONAL TACHYCARDIA
•**Symptomatic:** Amiodarone (no cardioversion)
•**Asymptomatic**
  ∘First line: β1 selective receptor or non–dihydropyridine calcium channel blocker
  ∘Second line: Amiodarone

ECTOPIC OR MULTIFOCAL ATRIAL TACHYCARDIA–MFAT
•**Symptomatic**
  ∘First line: Amiodarone (no cardioversion)
  ∘Second line: Diltiazem
•**Asymptomatic**
  ∘First line: β1 selective receptor or non–dihydropyridine calcium channel blocker→
  ∘Second line: Amiodarone

Cure:
•**Atrioventricular node ablation**
  Procedure:
  •Radiofrequency catheter mediated ablation of the atrioventricular node→
    ∘Complete heart block
  Outcomes:
  •Requires the implantation of a permanent pacemaker
•**Myocardial ablation**
  Indications:
  •**Paroxysmal supraventricular tachycardia–PSVT**
  Procedure:
  •Electrophysiologic study to define the precise location of the responsible tract for subsequent
    radiofrequency catheter or surgical ablation (ex. left ventricular aneurysm)

---

†If you suspect atrial fibrillation in patients w/ Wolf Parkinson White–WPW syndrome, do not treat w/ vagal maneuvers or atrioventricular node depressant medications (adenosine, β receptor blockers, non–dihydropyridine calcium channel blockers), as **atrial fibrillation may→**
  •**Ventricular fibrillation via the accessory pathway.** Use Procainamide if stable, or cardioversion if unstable

15

WIDE COMPLEX TACHYCARDIA
•**If unstable, assume ventricular tachycardia→**
  ◦**Synchronized cardioversion**
•If supraventricular tachycardia w/ aberrant conduction or bundle branch block, treat as for narrow complex tachycardia

FREQUENT PREMATURE VENTRICULAR CONTRACTIONS (>10/ min.)
•**Cardiac disease or R on T phenomenon:** Lidocaine
•**No cardiac disease:** β1 selective receptor blocker

ASYMPTOMATIC VENTRICULAR TACHYCARDIA
•**Monomorphic**
  ◦First line: Amiodarone, Procainamide, or Lidocaine
  ◦Second line: Cardioversion
•**Polymorphic:** Cardioversion

Cure:
•**Myocardial ablation**
  Procedure:
    •Electrophysiologic study to define the precise location of the responsible tract for subsequent radiofrequency catheter or surgical ablation (ex. left ventricular aneurysm)

β1 SELECTIVE RECEPTOR BLOCKERS				
Generic (Trade)	**M**	♀	**Start**	**Max**
Atenolol (Tenormin)	K	U		
•IV form			5mg slow IV push (1mg/ min.) q5min. X 2 prn, then	
•PO form			25–50mg PO q24hours	200mg/ 24h
Metoprolol (Lopressor)	L	?		
•IV form			5mg slow IV push (1mg/ min.) q5min. X 3 prn, then	
•PO form			25mg PO q12hours, then	100mg q12h
◦XR form (Toprol XL)			As per PO requirement	400mg q24h
Esmolol (Brevibloc)	K	?	0.5mg=500µg/ kg IV loading bolus (over 1 min.), then	
			0.05mg=50µg/kg/min. continuous IV infusion w/ titration prn†	
			Max: 0.3mg=300µg/kg/min.	

Onset: 1–2 min., Duration: 10 min.

†Titrate q4 min. via re–administration of the loading bolus & an additional 50µg/kg/min. IV infusion

α1 & NONSELECTIVE β RECEPTOR BLOCKERS				
Generic (Trade)	**M**	♀	**Start**	**Max**
Carvedilol (Coreg)	L	?	6.25mg PO q12hours	25mg q12h
Labetalol (Normodyne)	LK	?	20mg IV push over 2min., then	
			40mg IV push q10min. prn goal blood pressure, then	300mg total
•PO form			100mg PO q12hours	1200mg q12h
•IV form			0.5–2mg/ min. IV infusion	

Onset: 5–10min., Duration: 3–6hours

Mechanism:
•Competitive antagonist of the β1 ± β2 receptor→
  ◦↓Sinoatrial & atrioventricular node conduction (β1)→
    –↓Pulse
  ◦Anti–dysrhythmic via nodal effects (β1)
  ◦↓Cardiac muscle contractile strength (β1)
  ◦↓Juxtaglomerular cell renin release (β1)→
    –↓Angiotensin 1, angiotensin 2, & aldosterone formation
  ◦↓Cardiovascular remodeling
  ◦↑Vascular/ organ smooth muscle contraction (β2)→
    –Vasoconstriction
    –Bronchoconstriction
    –Uterine contraction
  ◦↓Tremor (β2)
  ◦↓Hepatocyte glycogenolysis (β2)
•↓Extrathyroidal tetraiodothyronine–T4 (also termed thyroxine) conversion to the more metabolically active triiodothyronine–T3 form

Side effects:
General
- •Fatigue
- •Malaise

Cardiovascular
- •Bradycardia ± heart block
- •Hypotension
  - ◦Orthostatic hypotension
  - ◦Pelvic hypotension→
    - −Impotence, being the inability to achieve &/or maintain an erection
- •Initial worsening of systolic heart failure
- •Worsening symptoms of peripheral vascular disease
  - ◦Intermittent claudication
  - ◦Raynaud's phenomenon

Pulmonary
- •Bronchoconstriction

Endocrine
- •↑Risk of developing diabetes mellitus
- •May block catecholamine mediated:
  - ◦Physiologic reversal of hypoglycemia via:
    - −↓Hepatocyte gluconeogenesis
  - ◦↓Hypoglycemic symptoms, termed hypoglycemic unawareness→
    - −↓Tachycardia as a warning sign

Gastrointestinal
- •Diarrhea
- •Nausea ± vomiting
- •Gastroesophageal reflux

Mucocutaneous
- •Hair thinning

Neurologic
- •Sedation
- •Sleep alterations
- •↓Libido→
  - ◦Impotence

Psychiatric
- •Depression

Hematologic
- •↓High density lipoprotein−HDL levels

- •Most patients w/ chronic obstructive pulmonary disease−COPD (including asthma), diabetes, &/or peripheral vascular disease can be safely treated w/ **cardioselective β1 receptor blockers**, as they have ↓peripheral effects

Contraindications:
Cardiovascular
- •**Acutely decompensated heart failure**
- •Hypotension
- •Pulse <50bpm
- •Atrioventricular heart block of any degree

Pulmonary
- •Moderate to severe chronic obstructive pulmonary disease−COPD, including asthma

Hyper−catacholamine state
- •Amphetamine use
- •**Cocaine use†**
- •Clonidine withdrawal
- •Monoamine oxidase inhibitor−MAOi mediated tyramine effect
- •Pheochromocytoma
  - ...→relatively ↑vascular α1 receptor stimulation="unopposed α effect"→
    - •Vasoconstriction→
      - ◦Myocardial ischemic syndrome
      - ◦Cerebrovascular accident syndrome
      - ◦Peripheral vascular ischemic syndrome
  - Note: **Carvedilol** & **Labetalol** may be used due to their α1 blocking property

---

†Cocaine use→
- •Varying ischemic syndrome onset per administration route, & may occur @ min. to days (usually within 3hours)

ANTIDOTES

Generic	M	♀	Dose		Max
Glucagon	LK	P	3mg IV slow push over 1min., then		
			5mg IV slow push over 1 min. if needed		
•Continuous infusion			5mg/ hour		
10% Calcium chloride†			10mL (1 ampule) IV slow push over 3min., q5min. prn		
•Continuous infusion			0.3mEq/ hour		0.7mEq/ h
Onset: 1–2 min., Duration: 30–60 min.					

†Use cautiously in patients taking Digoxin, as hypercalcemia→
•Digoxin cardiotoxicity

CALCIUM CHANNEL BLOCKERS: Non–dihydropyridines

Generic	M	♀	Start	Max
Diltiazem	L	?		
•IV form			5–20mg slow IV push over 2 min., then	
			25mg slow IV push over 2 min., 15 min. later, then	
			5mg/ hour IV infusion	15mg/ hour
•PO form			30mg PO q8hours	120mg q8hours
•XR form			As per daily requirement	
QD–XR form				540mg q24hours
BID–XR form				180mg q12hours
Verapamil	L	U		
•IV form			2.5–5mg slow IV push over 2min., then	
			5–10mg slow IV push over 2min., 15min. later, then	
•PO form			40mg PO q8hours	160mg q8hours
∘XR form			As per daily requirement	
–Calan XR form				480mg/ 24hours
–Veleran XR form				400mg qhs
–Covera XR form				480mg qhs

Mechanism:
•Block voltage dependent calcium ion channels in smooth & cardiac muscle→
  ∘↓Calcium influx→
    –↓Sinoatrial & atrioventricular node conduction (non–dihydropyridines)→↓pulse
    –Anti–dysrhythmic via nodal effects (mainly non–dihydropyridines)
    –↓Cardiac muscle contractile strength (mainly non–dihydropyridines)
    –Vasodilation: Arterial > venous (mainly dihydropyridines)

Side effects:
Cardiovascular
  •Bradycardia ± heart block
  •Edema
  •Flushing
  •Hypotension
Gastrointestinal
  •Constipation
  •Nausea ± vomiting
Neurologic
  •Dizziness
  •Headache

ANTIDOTES

Generic	M	♀	Dose	Max
Glucagon	LK	P	3mg IV slow push over 1min., then	
			5mg IV slow push over 1 min. if needed	
•Continuous infusion			5mg/ hour	
10% Calcium chloride†			10mL (1 ampule) IV slow push over 3min., then	
			repeat @5min. if needed	
•Continuous infusion			Start 0.3mEq/ hour	0.7mEq/ hour
Onset: 1–2 min., Duration: 30–60 min.				
Magnesium sulfate	K	S	2g MgSO$_4$ in 50mL saline infused over 15min., then	
			6g MgSO$_4$ in 500mL saline infused over 6hours	

†Use cautiously in patients taking Digoxin, as hypercalcemia→
•Digoxin cardiotoxicity

18

DIGITALIS GLYCOSIDES			
Generic (Trade)	**M**	**♀**	**Dose**
Digoxin (Lanoxin)	KL	?	0.5mg IV loading dose, then
			0.25mg IV q2–6h X 2→total loading dose of 1mg, then
•Age <60 years:			0.25mg PO/ IV q24hours
•Age >60years or renal failure:			0.25mg PO/ IV q48hours vs. 0.125mg PO/ IV q24hours

Onset: 4–6hours, Half life: 40hours

Dose adjustment:
- •Adjust dose based on clinical response & plasma levels (therapeutic 0.8–1.8ng/ mL) w/ toxicity typically occurring @ >1.8ng/ mL, but may occur @ therapeutic levels
- •Amiodarone & Verapamil→
  - ∘↑Digoxin levels (↓Digoxin dose by 50%)
- •Quinidine mediated displacement of Digoxin from tissue binding sites→
  - ∘↓Clearance

Mechanism:
- •↓Cell membrane Na^+/K^+ ATPase function→
  - ∘↑Intracellular sodium→
    - −↓Na^+/Ca^{+2} anti–transporter function→↑intracellular calcium→↑myocardial inotropy

Side effects†:
- •**General**
  - ∘↓Appetite
  - ∘Fatigue
  - ∘Headache
  - ∘Malaise
  - ∘Weakness
- •**Cardiac**
  - ∘The sequential occurrence of electrocardiographic–ECG changes:
    - −Atrioventricular block (1°,2°,3°)→↑PR interval
    - −T wave flattening
    - −**ST segment depression**
    - −↓QT interval
    - −T wave inversion
    - −**Supraventricular &/or ventricular dysrhythmias**
    - −**U wave**
- •**Gastrointestinal**
  - ∘Abdominal pain
  - ∘Diarrhea
  - ∘Nausea ± vomiting
- •**Genitourinary/ cutaneous**
  - ∘Digoxin's structural similarity to estrogen→
    - −Gynecomastia, being the ↑development of male mammary glands
    - −Impotence, being the inability to achieve &/or maintain an erection
    - −↓Libido
- •**Neurologic**
  - ∘Altered mental status
  - ∘Dizziness
  - ∘Paresthesias
  - ∘Psychosis
  - ∘**Visual changes 50–95%**
    - −Altered pupil size
    - −Photophobia
    - −Ocular muscle palsies
    - −Yellow–green halos around bright lights
- **Hematologic**
  - •↓Cell membrane Na^+/K^+ ATPase function→
    - ∘↑Extracellular potassium→
      - −Hyperkalemia

††Risk w/ electrolyte abnormalities:
- •Hypercalcemia
- •Hypokalemia

•Hypomagnesemia
...even w/ therapeutic Digoxin levels

ANTIDOTE

Indications:
•Ingested Digoxin dose >10mg
•Plasma Digoxin level >6ng/ mL
•≥2° atrioventricular block
•Supraventricular &/or ventricular dysrhythmias
•Plasma potassium >5.5mEq/ L, being refractory to conventional treatment modalities

Generic (Trade)	M ♀	Vials
Digoxin–immune Fab (Digibind) K	?	Administered via IV fluids over 15–30min., w/ repeat if toxicity persists (range: 2–20 vials)
•Acute ingestion of unknown quantity		20vials
•Acute ingestion of known quantity		[Ingested Digoxin (mg) X 0.8] / 0.6
•Chronic ingestion mediated overdose		[Plasma Digoxin level (ng/ mL) X weight (kg)] / 100

Mechanism:
•Each vial being 40mg & binding ~0.5mg Digoxin

•Plasma Digoxin levels will be falsely ↑for several days after administration

ANTI-DYSRHYTHMICS

Generic	Dose	Max
Amiodarone	300mg IV push, then 150mg IV push q10min. prn	
Maintenance infusion:	1mg/ min. X 6hours, then 0.5mg/ min. X 18–72hours	2.2g IV/ 24hours
Lidocaine	1mg/ kg IV push, then 0.5mg/ kg IV push q5–10min. prn	3mg/ kg total
Maintenance infusion:	Rebolus 75mg IV push, then 1–4mg/ min. IV infusion	
Procainamide	20mg–50mg/ min. IV infusion	
Maintenance infusion:	1–4mg/ min. IV infusion	17mg/ kg total

•Upon cardioversion, a maintenance intravenous infusion of 1 of the above should be administered for ≥24h. The loading dose is as above if not already given during the resuscitative effort

Lidocaine specific dose adjustment:
•If cardiac failure, liver disease, or elderly: 1–2mg/ min. IV maintenance infusion

Procainamide specific dose adjustment:
•If cardiac or renal failure: 1–2mg/ min. IV maintenance infusion (max: 12mg/ kg total)
•Discontinue infusion temporarily if either:
 ◦Hypotension
 ◦QRS widens >50%

Amiodarone specific immediate side effects:
•Dose dependent hypotension
•Dose dependent ↑QT interval→
 ◦Torsades de pointes

Procainamide specific immediate side effects:
•↑QT interval→
 ◦Torsades de pointes

PHYSIOLOGIC SINUS TACHYCARDIA ━━━
•Atrial & ventricular rate of 100–180bpm, usually being <150bpm

Risk factors:
•↑**Myocardial metabolism**
  ∘Anemia
  ∘Exercise
  ∘Fever
  ∘Hyperthyroidism
  ∘Pregnancy
•↑**Autonomic sympathetic tone**
  ∘↓Cardiac output (stroke volume X heart rate)
  ∘Anxiety
  ∘Excitement
  ∘Pain
  ∘Caffeine
  ∘Nicotine
  ∘Adrenergic medications
    –Catecholamines
    –β1 receptor agonists
    –Ephedrine
    –Phenylpropanolamine
    –Yohimbine
  ∘Autonomic neuropathy via ↓parasympathetic tone
  ∘Illicit drugs
    –Amphetamines
    –Cocaine
    –Ecstasy

PREMATURE CONTRACTIONS ━━━━━━━━━━━
•Contraction of a cardiac chamber prior to that normally expected, due to an ectopic focus of tissue below the sinoatrial node→
  ∘Myocardial depolarization

Risk factors:
•**Conduction tissue ischemia ± infarction**, esp. that affecting the inferior or septal myocardium
•**Conduction tissue inflammation**=myocarditis
•**Conduction tissue compression** via fibrotic &/or calcified tissue
•**Conduction tissue degeneration**
  ∘↑Age
•**Structural cardiac alteration**
  ∘Cardiomyopathy
  ∘Congenital defects
•**Myocardial irritants**
  ∘Alcohol
  ∘Lack of sleep
•↑**Autonomic sympathetic tone**
  ∘↓Cardiac output (stroke volume X heart rate)
  ∘Anxiety
  ∘Excitement
  ∘Pain
  ∘Caffeine
  ∘Nicotine
  ∘Adrenergic medications
    –Catecholamines
    –β1 receptor agonists
    –Ephedrine
    –Phenylpropanolamine
    –Yohimbine
  ∘Illicit drugs
    –Amphetamines
    –Cocaine
    –Ecstasy

PREMATURE ATRIAL CONTRACTIONS-PACs
Electrocardiographic findings:
- •The electrical impulse spreads predominantly through slowly conducting muscle tissue→
  - ◦Morphologically abnormal **P wave, typically being retrograde** (negatively deflected in the inferior leads-II, III, & aVF) due to altered directional flow, which may precede, follow, or be hidden in the QRS complex
- •The electrical impulse typically resets the sinoatrial node→
  - ◦↑**RR interval=compensatory pause**, comprised of the premature & subsequent QRS complex
- •If it occurs during the previous cycle's absolute refractory period, it will be blocked→
  - ◦A slight distortion (notching) of the terminal T wave
  - ◦Compensatory pause
- •If it occurs during the previous cycle's relative refractory period, it will be aberrantly conducted→
  - ◦A distortion (notching) of the terminal T wave
  - ◦Prolonged QRS complex
Physical findings
- •The premature contraction→
  - ◦↓Ventricular diastole→
    - -↓Ventricular filling→↓cardiac output→weakened to non-palpable pulse relative to the auscultated pulse=**pulse deficit**
- •If the pulse is palpable, it is appreciated in close succession to the previous pulse, followed by a prolonged diastolic interval
  - ◦Repetitive occurrence→
    - -2 different pulses close together=**bigeminal pulse**
  - ◦Frequent occurrence→
    - -**Irregularly irregular rhythm**, which may not be discernable via palpation or auscultation if tachycardic

PREMATURE VENTRICULAR CONTRACTIONS-PVCs
Electrocardiographic findings:
- •The electrical impulse spreads predominantly through slowly conducting muscle tissue→
  - ◦Morphologically abnormal **QRS complex, being widened (>0.12seconds)**
  - ◦↑**Voltage** due to non-simultaneous ventricular spread, as simultaneous ventricular spread→
    - -Partial neutralization
  - ◦**Retrograde T waves**, as repolarization tends to occur along the same route
- •The electrical impulse usually does not travel into the atria to reset the sinoatrial node. Therefore, the RR interval, comprised of the premature & subsequent QRS complex is normal
- •Premature ventricular contractions occurring during the terminal portion of the previous T wave (the R on T phenomenon) may→
  - ◦Ventricular fibrillation, much like ill-timed non-synchronized cardioversion. However, most R on T premature ventricular contractions do not cause ventricular fibrillation
Physical findings
- •The premature contraction→
  - ◦↓Ventricular diastole→
    - -↓Ventricular filling→↓cardiac output→weakened to non-palpable pulse relative to the auscultated pulse=**pulse deficit**
- •If the pulse is palpable, it is appreciated in close succession to the previous pulse, followed by a prolonged diastolic interval
  - ◦Repetitive occurrence→
    - -2 different pulses close together=**bigeminal pulse**
  - ◦Frequent occurrence→
    - -**Irregularly irregular rhythm**, which may not be discernable via palpation or auscultation if tachycardic

ECTOPIC ATRIAL TACHYCARDIA ▬▬▬▬▬▬▬▬▬▬▬▬▬▬▬▬▬▬▬▬▬▬▬▬
Electrocardiographic findings:
- •Persistent **premature atrial contractions originating from 1 ectopic focus**
Atrial & ventricular rate:
- •110-200bpm
Major risk factors:
- •**Conduction tissue inflammation**=myocarditis
- •**Age** <18years

MULTIFOCAL ATRIAL TACHYCARDIA-MFAT ▬▬▬▬▬▬▬▬▬▬▬▬
Electrocardiographic findings:
- •Persistent **premature atrial contractions originating alternately from ≥3 ectopic foci**→
  - ∘Several P wave variants
Atrial & ventricular rate:
- •>100bpm
Major risk factors:
- •**Serious illness, esp. heart or lung disease**

PAROXYSMAL SUPRAVENTRICULAR TACHYCARDIA-PSVT ▬▬▬▬▬▬▬▬▬▬▬
- •Due to the circus movement of an electrical impulse which abruptly starts & stops, lasting from several seconds to several weeks, & occurring several times/ day to several times/ lifetime

MICRO-REENTRANT=AV NODAL REENTRANT TACHYCARDIA-75%
Electrocardiographic findings:
- •A reentrant **circuit within the atrioventricular node**, containing both a slow & fast pathway→
  - ∘Circus movement→
    - −Narrow QRS complex
    - −Retrograde P waves buried in the QRS complex, or distorting its terminal portion→pseudo S waves in the inferior leads (II, III, aVF) & pseudo R' waves in lead V1
Atrial & ventricular rate:
- •120−220bpm

MACRO-REENTRANT=AV RECIPROCATING TACHYCARDIA-20%
Electrocardiographic findings:
- •A reentrant **circuit utilizing the atrioventricular node, as well as a bypass tract from a ventricle to an atrium**, composed of myocardium crossing their fibrous separation=Bundle of Kent→
  - ∘Circus movement→
    - −Narrow QRS complex
    - −Retrograde P waves just following the QRS complex, or buried in the T wave
    - −The QRS axis may shift slightly from beat to beat=electrical alternans
Note: The bypass tract may also serve as an opposite pathway from the atria to the ventricles, bypassing the physiologic refractoriness of the atrioventricular node→
- •Ventricular pre−excitation=**Wolf−Parkinson−White−WPW syndrome**→
  - ∘The rapid conduction velocity of the Bundle of Kent→
    - −↓**PR interval**
  - ∘A QRS complex composed of an initial characteristic **delta wave (only during sinus rhythm)**, as the impulse spreads through the slowly conducting myocardium until it reaches the bundle of His→
    - −Rapid ventricular depolarization
Atrial & ventricular rate:
- •140−220
Caution:
- •If you suspect atrial fibrillation in patients w/ Wolf Parkinson White−WPW syndrome, do not treat w/ vagal maneuvers or atrioventricular node depressant medications (adenosine, β receptor blockers, non−dihydropyridine calcium channel blockers), as **atrial fibrillation may**→
  - ∘**Ventricular fibrillation via the accessory pathway.** Use Procainamide if stable, or cardioversion if unstable

VENTRICULAR TACHYCARDIA ▬▬▬▬▬▬▬▬▬▬▬▬▬▬▬▬▬▬▬▬
Electrocardiographic findings:
- •**≥3 premature ventricular contractions, w/ a pulse ≥100bpm**
Atrial rate: 60−140bpm
Ventricular rate: 140−280bpm
Risk factors:
- •**Conduction tissue ischemia ± infarction**, esp. that affecting the inferior or septal myocardium
- •**Conduction tissue inflammation**=myocarditis
- •**Conduction tissue compression**, via fibrotic &/or calcified tissue
- •**Conduction tissue degeneration**
  - ∘↑Age
- •**Structural cardiac alteration**
  - ∘Cardiomyopathy
  - ∘Congenital defects
- •**Medications**
  - ∘Digoxin
- •**Electrolytes**
  - ∘Hypo or hyperkalemia

Morphologic classification:
- **Monomorphic:** Having 1 form
- **Polymorphic:** Having beat to beat variations in form

Severity based classification:
- **Non-sustained:** Persisting <30seconds
- **Sustained:** Persisting for ≥30seconds, or requiring termination due to symptoms
  - ∘**Sustained polymorphic ventricular tachycardia** Is unstable, often→
    - -Ventricular fibrillation
  - ∘**Sustained monomorphic ventricular tachycardia** is relatively more stable

TORSADES DE POINTES
Electrocardiographic findings:
- •A form of polymorphic ventricular tachycardia **developing from a prolonged QT interval** (usually ≥0.5seconds)→
  - ∘**The QRS complex is repeatedly inverting & reverting**→
    - -Twisting about the isoelectric line

Atrial rate: 40-140bpm
Ventricular rate: 200-300bpm
Risk factors:
- **Bradycardia**
- **Congenital**
- **Medications**
  - ∘Type 1a anti-dysrhythmics
    - -Disopyramide
    - -Procainamide
    - -Quinidine
  - ∘Type 3 anti-dysrhythmics
    - -Amiodarone
    - -Sotalol
  - ∘Pentamidine
  - ∘Tricyclic antidepressants
  - ∘Erythromycin
  - ∘Gemfibrozil
- **Electrolyte alterations**
  - ∘Hypocalcemia
  - ∘Hypomagnesemia
  - ∘Although hypo or hyperkalemia do not ↑QT interval, they do predispose to dysrhythmias in general
- **Myocardial inflammation**=myocarditis
- **Mitral valve prolapse**

VENTRICULAR FIBRILLATION ▬▬▬▬▬▬▬▬▬▬▬▬▬▬▬▬▬▬▬▬▬▬▬▬▬▬
•The end of each cardiac cycle (being the terminal portion of the T wave) is referred to as the vulnerable period for the initiation of ventricular fibrillation, as the dispersion of both areas of refractory & non-refractory myocardium are greatest during this time. An electrical impulse occurring during this time may→
  - ∘Ventricular fibrillation, as electrical wave fronts are divided by refractory areas→
    - -**Incoordinate ventricular fibrillatory contractions, which appear as low voltage, irregular waves**

Ventricular rate: >300bpm

24

Indications:
- Primary prevention
  - Coronary artery disease, left ventricular dysfunction, & induceable ventricular tachycardia
  - Coronary artery disease & ejection fraction–EF ≤30%
  - ↑Risk inherited or acquired disease syndromes
    - Brugada's syndrome
    - Hypertrophic cardiomyopathy
    - Long QT syndrome
- Secondary prevention
  - Cardiac arrest due to ventricular fibrillation or ventricular tachycardia, except w/:
    - Idiopathic ventricular tachycardia, which has an excellent prognosis
    - Reversible causes such as acid–base/ electrolyte disturbances, myocardial ischemia, or atrial fibrillation in patients w/ Wolff–Parkinson–White syndrome
  - Sustained ventricular tachycardia (persisting for ≥30 seconds or requiring termination due to symptoms)
  - Symptomatic, non–sustained ventricular tachycardia
  - Unexplained syncope w/ either:
    - Advanced structural heart disease
    - Inducible, sustained ventricular fibrillation or tachycardia

- **Internal cardioverter–defibrillator–ICD**
  Composed of 3 parts:
  - **Generator**
    - Placed in the pectoral area, rather than older models which were placed in the abdomen
  - **Transvenous defibrillating leads**
    - Inserted into the subclavian vein, & advanced to the right ventricular apex
  - **Electrodes**
    - In the lead tips, capable of sensing, cardioverting, defibrillating, &
      - Anti–tachycardia pacing, being painless, & used to terminate monomorphic tachycardias
  Complications:
  - Infection–2%, necessitating device removal
  - Lead malfunction→
    - False signals→
      - Inappropriate shock administration
  Limitations:
  - Anti–tachycardia pacing may:
    - Accelerate ventricular tachycardia
    - Induce a ventricular dysrhythmia if applied during a supraventricular rhythm
    …necessitating cardioversion or defibrillation if ineffective
                                 &
- Only **β receptor blockers** (as above) & **Amiodarone** medically→
  - ↓**Cardiac arrest risk in patients w/ systolic dysfunction**

ANTI-DYSRHYTHMIC MEDICATIONS			
Generic (Trade)	M	♀	Dose
Amiodarone (Cordarone)	L	U	
•IV form			150mg IV slow push over 10 min., then
			1mg/ min. IV infusion X 6hours, then
			0.5mg/ min. IV infusion
•PO form			800–1600mg PO loading q24hours X 1–3weeks, then
			when controlled or adverse effects,
			400–800mg q24hours X 1month, then
			Titrate to the lowest effective dose (usually 200–400mg q24hours)

Dose adjustment:
- Amiodarone→↓hepatocyte cytochrome P450 function→
  - ↓Hepatic metabolism, necessitating concomitant ↓medication dose
    - **↓Digoxin & Warfarin dose by 50%**

Side effects:
  Cardiovascular
  - Dose dependent ↑**QT interval**→
    - **Torsades de pointes**
  - Dose dependent **hypotension**

Cutaneous
- Microcrystalline skin deposits→
  - Blue-gray tinted skin
- Photosensitivity

Endocrine
- Thyroid dysfunction (**hypothyroidism or hyperthyroidism**) due to its iodine moiety

Gastrointestinal
- Hepatitis

Opthalmologic
- Microcrystalline corneal deposits→
  - Blurred vision

Pulmonary
- Pulmonary deposition→
  - Pulmonary fibrosis

Contraindications:
- QTc >0.44seconds

MYOCARDIAL ISCHEMIC SYNDROMES

•Caused by any disease→
  ◦↓**Epicardial blood flow**, being either:
    −Absolute
    −Relative to the myocardium's metabolic demands
    ...→**myocardial ischemia**
Statistics:
  •**#1 cause of death in the U.S.**, responsible for the death of 35% of the adult population via either:
    ◦Dysrhythmia due to any ischemic syndrome
    ◦Heart failure post−myocardial infarction
  •**2 million people in the U.S.** are admitted to a hospital every year for the evaluation of acute chest
  pain, 30% of whom are found to have an acute coronary syndrome, being either:
    ◦Unstable angina
    ◦Myocardial infarction
    ...w/ ~5% of patients w/ an acute myocardial infarction being inappropriately discharged from
    emergency departments

RISK FACTORS

•**Age:** ♂ ≥45years, ♀ ≥menopause=~50years (esp. @ ≥65years)
•**Gender:** ♂ > ♀ due to the protective effects of estrogens &/or possible atherogenic effects of
androgens
•**Genetic**
  ◦Significant family history of myocardial ischemic syndrome or sudden death in a first degree relative
    −♂ **<55years**
    −♀ **<65years**
  ◦Homocystinemia
  ◦Genetic lipid diseases
•↑**Atherosclerosis**
  ◦**Endothelial stress/ damage**
    −**Cigarette smoking, being the #1 risk factor**
    −**Hypertension**
    −Homocystinemia
  ◦**Hyperlipidemia**
    −Total cholesterol ≥200mg/ dL in adults
    −Low density lipoprotein−LDL cholesterol† ≥130mg/ dL
    −Triglycerides ≥150mg/ dL
  ◦**Known peripheral or cerebrovascular disease**
  ◦↑**Hepatocyte lipoprotein formation**
    −High fat diet
    −Genetic disposition
    −Nephrotic syndrome
  ◦↓**Hepatocyte lipoprotein removal**
    −**Diabetes mellitus**
    −Estrogen containing medications (oral contraceptives−OCPs, hormone replacement therapy−HRT)
    −Genetic disposition
    −Hypothyroidism
  ◦↓**Vascular cholesterol removal**
    −↓High density lipoprotein−HDL level (<40mg/ dL)
  ◦**HIV infected patients** treated w/ combination antiretroviral regimens experience ↑**atherosclerosis**
  via:
    ◦HIV &/or antiretroviral mediated endothelial inflammation
    ◦HIV &/or antiretroviral mediated dyslipidemia
    ◦Antiretroviral mediated insulin resistance
•**Hematologic disease**
  ◦Hypercoagulable state
  ◦Sickle cell anemia
•**Type A aortic dissection**→
  ◦Coronary artery ostial occlusion
•**Personality**
  ◦Poor stress management, w/ a tendency to react to various situations w/ anger &/or frustration
•**Sedentary lifestyle**
•**Illicit drug use**
  ◦Amphetamines→
    −↑Release of presynaptic catecholamines
  ◦Cocaine→
    −↓Presynaptic reuptake of released catecholamines

•**Inflammation**
  ∘↑**C reactive protein−CRP** (normal: <2mg/ L), being an acute phase reactant used as a marker of systemic inflammation, being directly proportionate to severity. Elevation indicates ↑vascular disease risk via:
   −Atherosclerotic plaque mediated inflammation
   −C−reactive protein mediated compliment & endothelial cell activation, as well as tissue damage
   ...↔↑atherosclerotic plaque formation & instability (a vicious cycle)
   Outcomes:
     •↑C reactive protein→
    ∘↑All cause mortality in the elderly
•**Obesity**, specifically referring to excess total body fat
  Body mass index−BMI‡ classification:
    •<18.5: Underweight
    •18.5−24.9: Normal
    •25−29.9: Overweight
    •30−34.9: Mild obesity
    •35−39.9: Moderate obesity
    •≥40: Severe, termed morbid obesity, being ≥2X the upper limit of normal body weight
  Waist circumference based obesity classification:
    •As body fat distribution affects health risks, meeting the following criteria indicate the need for weight loss regardless of BMI
     ∘>**40 inches** indicates ↑cardiovascular risk in ♂s
     ∘>**35 inches** indicates ↑cardiovascular risk in ♀s

---

†LDL=total cholesterol − HDL − (triglycerides/ 5)
‡BMI= Weight (kg)   or   Weight (lbs)
         Height (m)^2 Height (in)^2 X 703.1

PROTECTIVE FACTORS
•**High density lipoprotein−HDL** >60mg/ dL

CLASSIFICATION
•**Demand angina, termed stable angina**
  Mechanism:
    •**Stable coronary artery atherosclerotic plaque**→
     ∘Stenosis (usually being ≥70%), w/ ↑myocardial O_2 demand→relative ischemia→myocardial anaerobic metabolism→myocardial lactic acidemia→**thoracic discomfort, relieved via:**
      −↓Myocardial O_2 demand, via **relaxation**
      −↑Myocardial O_2 supply via **nitroglycerin**
      ...**within 5 min.**
  Cardiovascular society classification of stable angina
    •**Class 1:** Asymptomatic @ ordinary physical activity
    •**Class 2:** Symptomatic upon walking >2 blocks
    •**Class 3:** Symptomatic upon walking <2 blocks
    •**Class 4:** Symptomatic @ rest

•**Supply angina, termed unstable angina**
  Mechanism:
    •**Acute coronary artery stenosis**→
     ∘Absolute myocardial ischemia→myocardial anaerobic metabolism→myocardial lactic acidemia→
      thoracic discomfort, usually lasting <15 min., being unreliably relieved
  Diagnosis:
    •Consider the diagnosis if thoracic discomfort is:
     ∘**New**, occurring at rest or exertion
     ∘**Changed**, as in a patient w/ known stable angina, either:
      −Occurring w/ ↓exertion than typically required
      −Being longer lasting
      −Being less responsive to rest or medications which typically relieve symptoms
  Etiologies:
    •**Thromboembolic−97%**
    •**Coronary artery vasospasm−2%**
    •**Collagen vascular disease** via arteritis
    •**Endocardial thrombus or vegetation** via embolism
    •**Stanford type A dissecting aortic aneurysm** via coronary artery ostial occlusion

28

•Myocardial infarction
Mechanism:
- •**Myocardial ischemia ≥30min.**→
  - ∘Myocardial necrosis, being either:
    - −Transmural, via proximal coronary artery stenosis
    - −Subendocardial, via distal coronary artery stenosis
    - …which may be asymptomatic, termed **silent**, w/ 80% of symptomatic patients having silent ischemic episodes

SUBCLASSIFICATION
- •**Angina equivalent**
  - Mechanism:
    - •Myocardial ischemia→
      - ∘Dyspnea
      - ∘Syncope
    - …or other symptom of myocardial ischemia, without thoracic discomfort
- •**Stunned myocardium**
  - Mechanism:
    - •Myocardial ischemia→
      - ∘Altered myocardial contraction &/or mitral valve function, persisting transiently despite the resolution of ischemia
- •**Hibernating myocardium**
  - Mechanism:
    - •Chronic, stable, low grade myocardial ischemia→
      - ∘Reversible, altered myocardial contraction &/or mitral valve function
- •**Angina decubitus**
  - Mechanism:
    - •Supine position→
      - ∘↑Venous return→
        - −↑Myocardial contraction→↑O_2 demand

PATHOPHYSIOLOGY OF ATHEROSCLEROSIS
- •A disease of lipoprotein (composed of cholesterol & other lipids) deposition, being limited to arteries & arterioles throughout the body, w/ resultant intermittent localized:
  - ∘Smooth muscle cell hyperplasia, w/ concomitant intimal migration, termed neointimal hyperplasia
  - ∘Fibroblast deposition of connective tissue=fibrosis
  - ∘Calcium salt deposition→
    - −Bone hard calcifications
  - …→atherosclerotic plaque formation→
    - •Luminal bulging→
      - ∘**Vascular luminal narrowing**
- •The atherosclerotic plaque is considered stable unless it protrudes through the covering endothelium, w/ **instability having little to do w/ the degree of vascular luminal narrowing, but rather w/ intermittent periods of intense biologic activity or endothelial damage†**→
  - ∘Exposure of subendothelial collagen & atherosclerotic plaque→
    - −Platelet adhesion & activation
    - −Fibrin deposition
  - …→**thrombus formation & vasospasm**
- •A common site for atherosclerotic lesions are the first several centimeters of the major coronary arteries, as these areas are exposed to the greatest shear forces→
  - ∘Endothelial damage
- •As the intimal atherosclerotic plaque enlarges, medial smooth muscle cells are lost→
  - ∘Vascular wall weakening→dilation, **termed aneurysm**→
    - −↑Rupture risk
    - −Altered blood flow
  - …→thrombus formation

---

†65% of myocardial infarctions are due to an underlying "non−significant" atherosclerotic plaque, causing <50% coronary artery stenosis

Cardiovascular
- Myocardial ischemia→myocardial anaerobic metabolism→cellular production & release of lactic acid & proteolytic enzymes→
  ○ **Pain**, gripping pressure, heaviness, &/or other discomfort anywhere above the waist, usually being substernal or precordial ± radiation to the head, neck, shoulder, upper extremities, &/or epigastrium
  ○ Altered myocardial contraction, **dysrhythmia**, &/or mitral valve dysfunction→
    –Heart failure
  ○ Eventual myocardial necrosis
    –Although often thought of as indicating noncardiac disease, up to 15% of patients w/ a myocardial infarction have reproducible chest pain to palpation
Gastrointestinal
- Nausea ± vomiting, esp. w/ inferior myocardial ischemia
Hematologic
- Myocardial infarction→
  ○ Cell death mediated plasma myocardial protein release

Proteins indicating myocardial necrosis:
- Total creatine kinase–CK >270 IU/ L
  ○ Rising @ 3–12hours for 0.5–1day
- Creatine kinase–CK MB isoenzyme >5% of total CK (see below)
  ○ Rising @ 3–12hours for 1–1.5days
- **Creatine kinase–CK MB isoenzyme relative mass >5%†**, having a 90% sensitivity @ ≥6hours after syndrome onset
- **Cardiac troponin I–CTnI >0.1ng/ mL**, having a 100% sensitivity @ ≥6hours after syndrome onset
  ○ Rising @ 3–12hours for 7–10days
- **Cardiac troponin T–CTnT >0.2ng/ mL**, having a 95% sensitivity @ ≥6hours after syndrome onset
  ○ Rising @ 3–12hours for 10–14days
- Myoglobin >105
  ○ Rising @ 1–4hours for 18–24hours
- Aspartate aminotransferase–AST >35 U/ L
  ○ Rising @ 6–10hours for 3–4days
- Lactate dehydrogenase–LDH1/ LDH2 >1
  ○ Occurring @ 1–3days for 2weeks

- Renal failure→
  ○ †Of all the above enzymes, except for aspartate aminotransferase–AST which may be ↓
†Creatine kinase–CK occurs as 3 isoenzymes, each being a dimer variably composed of 2 polypeptides termed M & B subunits:
- CK–BB
- CK–MM
- CK–MB
…w/ **CK–MB constituting 6–15% of myocardial creatine kinase & <4% of skeletal muscle creatine kinase,** w/ the percentages termed the enzymes relative index. Thus, an ↑creatine kinase w/ an MB isoenzyme level >5% is considered evidence of myocardial necrosis, whereas an isoenzyme level <4% is considered evidence of skeletal muscle necrosis. Levels of 4–5% are indeterminate

- Myocardial ischemia→
  ○ **Dysrhythmias–80%,** w/ **ventricular fibrillation** usually occurring within the first several hours
  ○ Altered myocardial contraction &/or dysrhythmia→
    –Altered chamber blood flow→**mural thrombus ± embolization**
  ○ Papillary muscle dysfunction→
    –Mitral regurgitation→heart failure
  ○ Sinoatrial &/or atrioventricular node dysfunction→bradycardia ± heart block, having a:
    –Good prognosis if accompanied by inferior ischemia, usually indicating right coronary artery occlusion, w/ resolution usually within 10 days
    –Very poor prognosis if accompanied by anterior ischemia, indicating left main or left anterior descending coronary artery occlusion
- Inferior myocardial ischemia→
  ○ **Mitral regurgitation**
  ○ Reflex ↑autonomic parasympathetic tone via the vagus nerve→
    –Bradycardia
    –Hypotension
  ○ **Right ventricular ischemia–35%†→**
    –Right heart failure→cardiogenic shock

30

- Myocardial infarction→
  - Inflammatory cytokine release→**fever** &/or **leukocytosis**, esp. w/ a large infarct
  - Myocyte release of cellular molecules→
    - **-Autoimmune serositis <5%**, termed **Dressler's syndrome**→pericarditis, pleuritis, &/or systemic inflammatory syndrome @ 2weeks–6months
  - Myocardial fibrosis→
    - -Abnormal conduction pathways around the fibrotic area→dysrhythmias
    - -Myocardial thinning, dilation, & weakness=**dilated cardiomyopathy**→↓ventricular contractile strength→↓cardiac output→systolic heart failure
- Transmural infarction→
  - **Pericarditis within 5 days post–myocardial infarction**
  - Ventricular wall weakening & **rupture @ 2–5 days**→
    - -Pericardial tamponade→heart failure
    - …w/ anterior or inferior left ventricular infarction→
      - Septal infarction & rupture

---

†Being that the right ventricle is predominantly preload dependent, these patients are extremely sensitive to the effects of vasodilators such as nitroglycerin & morphine, which may→
- Hypotension

ELECTRICAL STUDIES
- **Electrocardiogram–ECG**
  Lead placement:
  - **Precordial leads**
    - **V1** @ the right parasternal 4th intercostal space
    - **V2** @ the left parasternal 4th intercostal space
    - **V3** @ midway between V2 & V4
    - **V4** @ the left midclavicular 5th intercostal space
      - **-V4R†** @ right midclavicular 5th intercostal space
    - **V5** @ the left anterior axillary 5th intercostal space
    - **V6** @ the left midaxillary 5th intercostal space
  - **Limb leads**
    - **aVR** on the right arm
    - **aVL** on the left arm
    - **aVF** on the left leg
  Interpretation:
  - **Septal wall:** V1 & V2 via a septal branch of the left anterior descending–LAD artery
  - **Anterior wall:** V3 & V4 via a diagonal branch of the left anterior descending–LAD artery
  - **Lateral wall:** V5–V6, I, & aVL via the circumflex artery
  - **Inferior wall:** II, III, & aVF ± reciprocal ↓ST segments in leads V1–V3 if transmural, via the posterior descending artery–PDA, branching off either the:
    - Right coronary artery–80%
    - Circumflex artery
  - **Right ventricle:** V4R via the proximal branches of the right coronary artery–RCA
  - **Posterior ventricle:** ↓ST segments in leads V1–V4 via either the:
    - Right coronary artery–80%
    - Circumflex artery
    - Posterior descending artery–PDA
  Findings:
  - Subendocardial ischemia→
    - **Downsloping or horizontal ↓ST segment**
    - ↓**T wave**
    …w/ persistence ≥30min.→
      - Myocardial infarction (subendocardial–90% > transmural)
  - Transmural ischemia→
    - ↑**ST segment**, having an upward convexity
    - ↑**T wave**
    …w/ persistence ≥30min.→
      - Myocardial ischemia (transmural–90% > subendocardial), w/ **transmural infarction**→
        - A series of electrocardiographic changes over 3–15hours
          1. **Q wave formation**, being permanent & deepening over the following days, w/ subsequent ↓**R wave**
          2. **ST segment** gradually returning to baseline, or remaining permanently elevated, w/ subsequent ↓**T wave**, beginning at its terminal portion, being upright days to weeks later, or remaining permanently inverted

31

•A normal electrocardiogram in an emergency department chest pain patient has the following prognosis w/ respect to final hospital diagnosis:
  ◦**Noncardiac chest pain–95%**
  ◦**Unstable angina–4%**
  ◦**Myocardial infarction–1%**

•Because either subendocardial or transmural myocardial ischemia may or may not lead to q wave formation, it is best to refer to:
  ◦Suspected subendocardial infarction as non–ST segment elevation myocardial infarction–NSTEMI
  ◦Suspected transmural infarction as ST segment elevation myocardial infarction–STEMI
  …for the first 24hours, after which, distinction via Q wave formation may be used
†35% of inferior left ventricular wall infarcts are accompanied by right ventricular infarction, w/ standard limb & precordial leads not able to detect right ventricular ischemia. You must either reverse the precordial lead placement, or simply reverse V4 placement=V4R
‡Absence of:
  •Nonspecific ST segment & T wave changes
  •Atrioventricular block of any degree
  •Intraventricular conduction delay
  •Repolarization changes
  •Non–sinus rhythms

Criteria for pathologic Q waves: Either:
  •**≥0.04seconds=1small box**
  •**>25% the R wave height of that complex**
  Exceptions:
  •Small septal Q waves may normally be found in leads I, aVL, V5, & V6
  •Isolated Q waves may be found in leads III, aVR (may be large), & V1
  •Certain forms of primary hypertrophic cardiomyopathy→
    ◦Septal hypertrophy→
      –Deep Q waves, termed pseudo–Q waves, in leads II, III, & aVF
  •Left bundle branch block may→
    ◦ECG changes resembling ischemia ± infarction, including Q waves & ST segment deviation. Thus, **you cannot diagnose an acute coronary syndrome w/ a concomitant left bundle branch block**

Differential diagnosis of ↑ST segments:
  •**Transmural myocardial ischemia ± infarction**, having an upward convexity
  •**Prior transmural myocardial infarction** w/ persistently ↑ST segments, having an upward convexity
  •**Pericarditis**, being diffuse, w/ an upward concavity being possible in all leads ± accompanying ↓PR segments in the precordial leads
  •**Normal early repolarization**, having an upward concavity, usually in leads V1–V5, w/ the following characteristics:
    ◦J point ↑1–4mv
    ◦Downstroke notch of the R wave
    ◦Large T waves
    ◦ST segment elevation being <25% of T wave amplitude
  •**Repolarization abnormaility** associated w/ either:
    ◦Left bundle branch block
    ◦Left ventricular hypertrophy
    …usually in leads V1 & V2
  •**Myocarditis**
  •**Cardiomyopathies**
  •**Left ventricular aneurysm**, usually being a result of previous transmural myocardial infarction, w/ blunt trauma, Sarcoidosis, or Chagas' disease being other etiologies
  •**Hyperkalemia**
  •**Ventricular paced rhythms**

Differential diagnosis of ↓ST segments:
  •**Subendocardial ischemia ± infarction**
  •**Repolarization abnormality** associated w/ either:
    ◦Left bundle branch block
    ◦Left ventricular hypertrophy
    …usually in leads V5, V6, 1, & aVL
    ◦**Hypokalemia**
    ◦**Digitalis effect**, poorly correlating w/ plasma levels
    ◦**Rate related**

Indications:
- To establish the diagnosis of stable angina
- To assess the effectiveness of anti-ischemic treatment (medical &/or surgical)
- To evaluate patients w/ a change in clinical status or degree of exercise capacity

Contraindications:
- Myocardial infarction within 48hours
- Unstable angina
- Acute myocarditis or pericarditis
- Acute pulmonary embolism
- Acute aortic dissection
- Uncontrolled dysrhythmia
- Decompensated heart failure
- Uncontrolled, severe hypertension
- Known left main coronary artery stenosis
- Severe valvular disease, esp. aortic or mitral stenosis
- Severe primary hypertrophic cardiomyopathy

EXERCISE STRESS TESTING

Procedure:
- A 12-lead ECG is placed on the patient who then either:
  - Runs on a treadmill
  - Rotates a hand pedal operated bicycle, being useful in patients w/ lower extremity:
    - Amputation
    - Arthritis
    - Claudication
    ...@ work loads that ↑progressively by ↑device speed &/or inclination, w/ the duration of the test determined by the time required to reach a predetermined pulse, being 90% of an age determined maximum (220-age), usually attained within 15min. In the elderly, a lesser pulse approximating the patients workload during a chest pain producing activity may also be useful, as the patient may tire or have comorbid conditions preventing the patient from attaining the goal heart rate

Exercise protocols:
- Bruce protocol
- Modified Bruce protocol
- Naughton protocol
- Symptom limited protocol
  ...w/ data reported in terms of **metabolic equivalents-METs** achieved prior to test discontinuation, which allows for counseling the patient regarding safe activity levels

Metabolic equivalents-METs:
- ≤3 being equivalent to very light exertion, such as activities of daily living
- 3-5 being equivalent to light exertion, such as household & light yard chores
- 5-7 being equivalent to moderate exertion, such as slow stair climbing
- 7-9 being equivalent to heavy exertion, such as stair climbing
- ≥9 being equivalent to very heavy exertion, such as quick stair climbing

Note: Sexual activity approximates 3 METs during foreplay & 5 METs @ climax w/ a usual partner, which is equivalent to the oxygen demands of climbing 1 flight of stairs or a brisk walk around 1 block

ELECTROCARDIOGRAPHIC MONITORING

Mechanism:
- Exercise→
  - ↑Autonomic sympathetic tone→
    - ↑Cardiac O_2 & nutrient demand
    - Coronary artery dilation→↓blood flow to atherosclerotic regions which are less able to dilate= intracoronary steal syndrome
    ...→myocardial ischemia in the presence of significant epicardial stenosis, being ≥50%

Findings suggesting left main or 3 vessel disease:
- Low workload (<6 METs) induced ischemia
- Global (≥ 5 leads) ischemia
- Hypotension
- Persistence of ischemia ≥6min. into recovery

Indications to stop an exercise stress test:
- Exhaustion or danger of falling
- ↓ST segment >2mm
- Ventricular dysrhythmia, not including premature ventricular contractions
- Hypotension

33

Outcomes:
- **A negative study is strongly suggestive against stable angina**, w/ sensitivity & specificity being ↑by concomitant echocardiography &/or radioisotope imaging

Limitations:
- False positive:
  - Baseline ST segment abnormality
  - Baseline dysrhythmia
  - Left or right bundle branch block
  - Left ventricular hypertrophy
  - Mitral valve prolapse
  - Any medication which alters hemodynamics (anti–hypertensives, Digoxin)
    - When possible, these medications should be temporarily discontinued 4–5 half lives (~2days) prior to exercise testing

Complications:
- Myocardial infarction &/or death in 1/ 2500 tests

PHARMACOLOGIC STRESS TESTING ▬▬▬▬▬▬▬▬▬▬▬▬▬▬▬▬▬▬▬▬▬▬▬▬

Indications:
- Patients unable to adequately exercise

Procedure:
- Pharmacologic agents are administered in order to partly replicate the physiology of exercise induced ↑myocardial O_2 & nutrient demand

Agents used:
- **Adenosine (♀?)**
- **Dipyridamole** (Persantine–♀P)
- **Dobutamine (♀U)**: Dobutamine does not ↑myocardial blood flow as much as adenosine or Dipyridamole. It is therefore indicated when:
  - There are contraindications to the use of Adenosine or Dipyridamole
  - When echocardiographic monitoring will be used, due to ↑sensitivity compared to Adenosine or Dipyridamole

Adenosine & Dipyridamole specific mechanism:
- Vascular adenosine receptor activation, being either direct (via Adenosine) or indirect (via Dipyridamole mediated inhibition of cellular uptake of adenosine)→
  - Coronary artery dilation→
    - ↓Blood flow to atherosclerotic regions which are less able to dilate=intracoronary steal syndrome→myocardial ischemia in the presence of significant epicardial stenosis, being ≥50%

Dobutamine specific mechanism:
- A sympathomimetic agent (β1 > β2)→
  - ↑Autonomic sympathetic tone→
    - ↑Myocardial O_2 & nutrient demand

Adenosine & Dipyridamole specific side effects:
- **Cardiovascular**
  - Atrioventricular block→
    - **Sinus bradycardia–50%**, possibly marked
- **Gastrointestinal**
  - Nausea ± vomiting
- **Mucocutaneous**
  - Facial flushing–50%
- **Neurologic**
  - Dizziness
  - Headache
- **Pulmonary**
  - Bronchoconstriction→
    - **Dyspnea–35%**

Adenosine & Dipyridamole specific contraindications:
- **Asthma or COPD w/ a bronchoconstricting component**

Adenosine & Dipyridamole specific antidote:
- Aminophylline

34

MONITORING

•Transthoracic echocardiography–TTE (exercise or pharmacologic)
<u>Procedure:</u>
- •A 2 dimensional ultrasonographic image, allowing real time visualization of:
  - ◦Ventricular wall thickness
  - ◦Cavity size (both atrial & ventricular)
  - ◦Myocardial & valve function, allowing ejection fraction–EF estimation (% of end diastolic volume ejected during ventricular systole)
  - ◦The pericardial space
- •Doppler ultrasonography uses Doppler shift to detect vessel flow velocity→
  - ◦Valve regurgitation visualization
  - ◦Estimation of valve pressure gradients

<u>Findings:</u>
- •New or worsened wall motion abnormalities via hypokinetic &/or akinetic myocardium

<u>Outcomes:</u>
- •Sensitivity: 85% & specificity: 80% in detecting significant (≥50%) stenosis

<u>Limitations:</u>
- •↓Visualization in obese or emphysematous patients
- •May not allow adequate:
  - ◦Visualization of the anterior aspect of a prosthetic aortic valve
  - ◦Functional assessment of a prosthetic aortic valve
- •Transesophageal echocardiography–TEE is more sensitive in detecting:
  - ◦Thrombotic ± infectious vegetations
  - ◦Abscesses
  - ◦Valve damage
  - …esp. in a patient w/ a prosthetic heart valve. However, transthoracic echocardiography is the initial test of choice due to its noninvasive nature, as transesophageal echocardiography may→
    - •Pharyngeal swallow receptor mediated reflex:
      - ◦Bradycardia
      - ◦Hypotension

•Radioisotope imaging (exercise or pharmacologic) via:
- ◦Single photon emission computerized tomographic–SPECT scanning
- ◦Positron emission tomographic–PET scanning

<u>Indications:</u>
- •To assess both myocardial perfusion & metabolism

<u>Procedure:</u>
- •A radioactive agent=tracer is injected intravenously @ maximal stress, w/ subsequent scintigraphic imaging & re–imaging after a 2nd intravenous injection 3hours later during relaxation. Tracer distribution is proportional to myocardial blood flow

<u>Tracers used in SPECT:</u>
- •[201]thallium, being a biological substitute for potassium
- •[99m]technitium–Tc (99mTc–sestamibi, 99mTc–teboroxime, 99mTc–tetrofosmin)

<u>Tracers used in PET:</u>
- •Carbon–11
- •Fluorine–18
- •Nitrogen–13
- •Oxygen–15
- •Rubidium–82

<u>Outcomes:</u>
- •SPECT: Sensitivity: 85% & specificity: 80% in detecting significant (≥50%) stenosis
- •PET: Sensitivity: 85% & specificity: 65% in detecting significant (≥50%) stenosis

TEST RESULTS

Pathology	@ Maximal stress	@ Relaxation	Term
Normal	▬▬▬▬ Diffuse equivalent uptake ▬▬▬▬		Normal uptake
Myocardial ischemia	Regional ↓relative uptake	Diffuse equivalent uptake†	Reversible defect
Myocardial fibrosis	▬▬▬▬▬▬ No uptake ▬▬▬▬▬		Fixed defect

†May be persistently ↓w/ hibernating myocardium

•**Smoking cessation** via smoking cessation clinic
  ◦Cigarette smoking contributes to 20% of deaths in the U.S., & is the #1 modifiable cause of premature death
•**Exercise**
  ◦An enjoyable form of aerobic exercise on a regular basis (≥3X/ week) for 20–30min., preceded by stretching
•**Emotional stress management**
  ◦Psychological therapy
  ◦Regular exercise
  ◦Biofeedback
  ◦Yoga
  ◦Listening to music
  ◦Gardening
•**Dietician consultation**
•**Glycemic control if hyperglycemic**
•**Hypertension control**
  ◦Systolic blood pressure <120mmHg & diastolic blood pressure <80mmHg
•↓**Sodium intake**
  ◦≤100mmol sodium/ 24hours=2g elemental sodium or 6g salt/ 24h, which can usually be achieved w/ a no-added salt diet. Patients w/ poorly compensated heart failure should only consume 0.5–1g elemental sodium or 1.5–3g salt/ 24hours
  ◦→↓Renal potassium loss if taking a diuretic
•↓**Alcohol consumption**
  ◦Only 1drink q24hours (8–12 ounces of beer, 3–5 ounces of wine, or 1 ounce of liquor) in patients without a history of drug abuse
  ◦≥2 drinks/ 24hours→
    –Hypertension
    –Hepatitis ($♀ > ♂$)
    –↑Abuse risk
  ◦If alcohol is suspected to be causative, total abstinence is required

PLATELET INHIBITING MEDICATIONS			
Efficacy: Glycoprotein 2b/ 3a inhibitors > thienopyridines > Aspirin			
Generic	M	♀	Dose
Acetylsalicylic acid–ASA=Aspirin	K	U	81mg PO q24hours

Mechanism:
•Aspirin is the only nonsteroidal anti–inflammatory drug–NSAID→
  ◦Irreversible inhibition of both cyclooxygenase–COX enzymes (COX1 & COX2), w/ COX1 being responsible for the production of both thromboxane A_2† & prostacyclin‡→
    –**Near complete inhibition of platelet thromboxane A_2 production within 15 min.**, w/ endothelial & vascular smooth muscle cells producing new enzymes in several hours→ relatively ↑prostacyclin
•Being that platelets lack the enzymatic machinery for protein synthesis, only newly formed platelets (platelet half life=10 days) have the functional enzyme
…this shift in the balance of cytokine production→
    •↓**Thrombus formation**

In Brief:
•**Cyclooxygenase–COX1 enzymes** are found in most cells of the body, being responsible for normal physiologic processes
•**Cyclooxygenase–COX 2 enzymes** are responsible for the production of inflammatory cell prostaglandins

---

•Concomitant NSAID administration→
  ◦Competition for the cyclooxygenase–COX 1 enzyme binding site, w/:
    –Unbound Aspirin being rapidly cleared from plasma
    –Bound NSAID action being reversible & short lived
    …→↓overall antiplatelet effect, requiring either:
      •Aspirin to be taken @ ≥1hour prior to other NSAIDs
      •Switch to thienopyridine derivative for the antiplatelet effect
†Platelet mediated **thromboxane A_2** release at the site of vascular injury→
  •Platelet aggregation
  •Vasoconstriction
  …w/ both processes→
    •Thrombus formation

‡Endothelial & vascular smooth muscle cell mediated **prostacyclin** release in the surrounding area→
•Inhibition of platelet aggregation
•Vasodilation
...w/ both processes→
•↓Thrombus formation

Outcomes:
•↓Morbidity & mortality

Side effects:
Gastrointestinal
•Inhibition of the cyclooxygenase–COX1 enzyme→↑peptic inflammatory disease risk→↑**upper gastrointestinal hemorrhage risk** via:
○↓Gastric mucosal prostaglandin synthesis→
  –↓Epithelial cell proliferation
  –↓Mucosal blood flow→↓bicarbonate delivery to the mucosa
  –↓Mucus & bicarbonate secretion from gastric mucosal cells

Indications for peptic inflammatory disease prophylaxis:
•Prophylax w/ proton pump inhibitors–PPI's, histamine 2 selective receptor blockers, or Misoprostol in patients w/ any of the following:
○Age >60 years w/ a history of peptic inflammatory disease
○Anticipated therapy >3 months
○Concurrent glucocorticoid use
○Moderate to high dose NSAID use
Note: Newer NSAIDs (Etodolac, Nabumetone, Salsalate)→
•↓Risk of NSAID induced peptic inflammation/ ulcer

Genitourinary
•Patients w/ pre–existing bilateral ↓renal perfusion, not necessarily failure:
○Heart failure
○Bilateral renal artery stenosis
○Hypovolemia
○Renal failure
...rely more on the compensatory production of vasodilatory prostaglandins→
•Afferent arteriole dilation→
○Maintained glomerular filtration rate–GFR, whereas NSAIDs→
  –↓Prostaglandin production, which may→renal failure
Pulmonary
•Inhibition of both cyclooxygenase enzymes (COX 1 & COX2)→
○↑Lipoxygenase activity→
  –↑Leukotriene synthesis→symptomatic asthma within 2hours of ingestion in 5% of asthmatics
Rheumatologic
•Acetylsalicylic acid competes w/ uric acid secretion in the renal tubules→
○↑Uric acid levels→
  –↑Risk of uric acid precipitation in the tissues=gout
Pediatric
•**Reye's syndrome**
○A life threatening fulminant hepatitis→
  –Hepatic encephalopathy in children age ≤16 years w/ a viral infection (esp. Influenza or Varicella–zoster virus–VZV)

Overdose:
Pulmonary
•Direct brainstem respiratory center mediated stimulation of pulmonary ventilation→
○Hyperventilation→
  –**Initial respiratory alkalemia, w/ the subsequent development of an anion gap metabolic acidemia**
•Pulmonary edema
Neurologic
•Altered mental status
•Aseptic meningitis
•Depression
•Hallucinations
•Hyperactivity
•Hyperthermia
•Lightheadedness

- •Seizures
- •Tinnitus
- **Gastrointestinal**
  - •Nausea ± vomiting
- **Mucocutaneous**
  - •Pharyngitis

THIENOPYRIDINE DERIVATIVE

Indications:
- •Intolerance to Aspirin

Generic (Trade)	M	♀	Dose
Clopidogrel (Plavix)	LK	P	75mg PO q24hours

Mechanism:
- •Inhibits adenosine diphosphate−ADP mediated activation of the glycoprotein 2b/ 3a complex→
  - ◦↓Platelet activation

- •A 300mg loading dose may be used, as maximal effect occurs @ 5hours rather than 5days w/ initiation of the standard 75mg dosage

Side effects:
- **Gastrointestinal**
  - •Diarrhea
- **Mucocutaneous**
  - •Dermatitis
- **Hematologic**
  - •**Thrombotic thrombocytopenic purpura−TTP** within several weeks of initiation

β1 SELECTIVE RECEPTOR BLOCKERS

Generic (Trade)	M	♀	Start	Max
Atenolol (Tenormin)	K	U	25mg PO q24hours	100mg/ 24hours
Metoprolol (Lopressor)	L	?	25mg PO q12hours	225mg q12hours
•XR form (Toprol XL)			50mg PO q24hours	400mg q24hours

α1 & NONSELECTIVE β RECEPTOR BLOCKERS

Generic (Trade)	M	♀	Start	Max
Carvedilol (Coreg)	L	?	6.25mg PO q12hours	25mg q12hours
Labetalol (Normodyne)	LK	?	100mg PO q12hours	1200mg q12hours

Mechanism:
- •Competitive antagonist of the β1 ± β2 receptor→
  - ◦↓Sinoatrial & atrioventricular node conduction (β1)→
    - −↓Pulse
  - ◦Anti−dysrhythmic via nodal effects (β1)
  - ◦↓Cardiac muscle contractile strength (β1)
  - ◦↓Juxtaglomerular cell renin release (β1)→
    - −↓Angiotensin 1, angiotensin 2, & aldosterone formation
  - ◦↓Cardiovascular remodeling
  - ◦↑Vascular/ organ smooth muscle contraction (β2)→
    - −Vasoconstriction
    - −Bronchoconstriction
    - −Uterine contraction
  - ◦↓Tremor (β2)
  - ◦↓Hepatocyte glycogenolysis (β2)
- •↓Extrathyroidal tetraiodothyronine−T4 (also termed thyroxine) conversion to the more metabolically active triiodothyronine−T3 form

Outcomes:
- •↓Morbidity & mortality

Side effects:
- **General**
  - •Fatigue
  - •Malaise
- **Cardiovascular**
  - •Bradycardia ± heart block
  - •Hypotension
    - ◦Orthostatic hypotension
    - ◦Pelvic hypotension→
      - −Impotence, being the inability to achieve &/or maintain an erection
  - •Initial worsening of systolic heart failure

- •Worsening symptoms of peripheral vascular disease
  - ◦Intermittent claudication
  - ◦Raynaud's phenomenon

Pulmonary
- •Bronchoconstriction

Endocrine
- •↑Risk of developing diabetes mellitus
- •May block catecholamine mediated:
  - ◦Physiologic reversal of hypoglycemia via:
    - −↓Hepatocyte gluconeogenesis
  - ◦↓Hypoglycemic symptoms, termed hypoglycemic unawareness→
    - −↓Tachycardia as a warning sign

Gastrointestinal
- •Diarrhea
- •Nausea ± vomiting
- •Gastroesophageal reflux

Mucocutaneous
- •Hair thinning

Neurologic
- •Sedation
- •Sleep alterations
- •↓Libido→
  - ◦Impotence

Psychiatric
- •Depression

Hematologic
- •↓High density lipoprotein−HDL levels

- •Most patients w/ chronic obstructive pulmonary disease−COPD (including asthma), diabetes, &/or peripheral vascular disease can be safely treated w/ **cardioselective β1 receptor blockers**, as they have ↓peripheral effects

---

Contraindications:

Cardiovascular
- •**Acutely decompensated heart failure**
- •Hypotension
- •Pulse <50bpm
- •Atrioventricular heart block of any degree

Pulmonary
- •Moderate to severe chronic obstructive pulmonary disease−COPD, including asthma

Hyper−catacholamine state
- •Amphetamine use
- •**Cocaine use†**
- •Clonidine withdrawal
- •Monoamine oxidase inhibitor−MAOi mediated tyramine effect
- •Pheochromocytoma
  - …→relatively ↑vascular α1 receptor stimulation="unopposed α effect"→
    - •Vasoconstriction→
      - ◦Myocardial ischemic syndrome
      - ◦Cerebrovascular accident syndrome
      - ◦Peripheral vascular ischemic syndrome

  Note: **Carvedilol** & **Labetalol** may be used due to their α1 blocking property

---

†Cocaine use→
- •Varying ischemic syndrome onset per administration route, & may occur @ min. to days (usually within 3hours)

ANTIDOTES

Generic	M	♀	Dose	Max
Glucagon	LK	P	3mg IV slow push over 1min., then 5mg IV slow push over 1 min. if needed	
•Continuous infusion			5mg/ hour	
10% Calcium chloride†			10mL (1 ampule) IV slow push over 3min., q5min. prn	
•Continuous infusion			0.3mEq/ hour	0.7mEq/ h
Onset: 1−2 min., Duration: 30−60 min.				

---

†Use cautiously in patients taking Digoxin, as hypercalcemia→
- •Digoxin cardiotoxicity

ANGIOTENSIN CONVERTING ENZYME INHIBITORS-ACEi				
Generic (Trade)	M	♀	Start	Max
Benazepril (Lotensin)	LK	U	10mg PO q24hours	40mg/ 24hours
Captopril (Capoten)	LK	U	12.5mg PO q12hours	450mg/ 24hours
Enalapril (Vasotec)	LK	U	5mg PO q24hours	40mg/ 24hours
Fosinopril (Monopril)	LK	U	10mg PO q24hours	40mg/ 24hours
Lisinopril (Prinivil, Zestril)	K	U	10mg PO q24hours	40mg q24hours

Dose adjustment:
- ↓Initial dose by 50% if:
  - ○Elderly
  - ○Concomitant diuretic use
  - ○Renal disease

Mechanism:
- •Reversibly inhibits angiotensin converting enzyme-ACE→
  - ○↓Bradykinin degradation→
    - -Vasodilation
  - ○↓Angiotensin 2 formation→
    - -Vasodilation (**arterial** > venous)
    - -↓Renal NaCl & water retention
    - -↓Adrenal cortex aldosterone release→↓renal NaCl & water retention
    - -↓Facilitation of adrenal medullary & presynaptic norepinephrine release→vasodilation
    - -Glomerular efferent arteriole vasodilation→↓intraglomerular hydrostatic pressure→↓filtration→ ↓proteinuria in patients w/ nephropathy
  - ○↓Cardiovascular remodeling

Side effects:
Cardiovascular
- •Hypotension

Gastrointestinal
- •Altered gustatory sense=dysguesia-3%

Genitourinary
- •Acute interstitial nephritis
- •Patients w/ pre-existing bilateral ↓renal perfusion, not necessarily failure:
  - ○Heart failure
  - ○Bilateral renal artery stenosis
  - ○Hypovolemia
  - ○Renal failure
  - …rely more on the compensatory production of angiotensin 2→
    - •Efferent arteriole constriction→
      - ○Maintained glomerular filtration rate-GFR, whereas either:
        - -Angiotensin converting enzyme inhibition
        - -Angiotensin 2 receptor blockade
      - …→↓angiotensin 2 production & action respectively, which may→
        - •**Pre-renal renal failure**

Mucocutaneous
- •↓Bradykinin & substance P degradation→↑levels→hypersensitivity-like syndrome→
  - ○**Angioedema-0.4%**, usually within 2weeks of treatment, but may manifest @ months to years→
    - -Soft tissue edema of the epiglottis, face, lips, oropharynx, &/or tongue
  - ○**Dermatitis-10%**

Pulmonary
- •↑Bradykinin levels→
  - ○**Chronic cough-20%**, usually being dry & involuntary

Materno-fetal
- •**Fetal & neonatal morbidity & mortality**

Hematologic
- •↓Aldosterone production ± renal failure→
  - ○**Hyperkalemia**
- •Neutropenia

Monitoring:
- •Check creatinine & potassium @ 3-10days after initiation or dose↑, then
  - ○Q3-6months

Contraindications:
Genitourinary
- •Acute renal failure
- •Bilateral renal artery stenosis

•Unilateral renal artery stenosis of a solitary functioning kidney
Mucocutaneous
•Angiotensin converting enzyme inhibitor induced angioedema or dermatitis
Materno–fetal
•Breast feeding
•**Pregnancy**
Hematologic
•**Potassium >5mEq/ L**

LIPID LOWERING MEDICATIONS
•≥20% of Americans have a plasma lipid abnormality→
 ◦↑Cardiovascular, cerebrovascular, & peripheral vascular disease risk

Indications:
•↓Plasma LDL cholesterol to a goal of <70mg/ dL→
 ◦↓Atherosclerotic disease progression, w/ some degree of regression

Note: Total & HDL cholesterol levels are more accurate in the non–fasting state, whereas triglyceride levels should only be measured in the fasting state, as they are elevated after a meal. Thus, being as ↑triglycerides→↓calculated LDL level, the LDL cholesterol level may be falsely ↓in the non–fasting state. LDL values cannot be accurately calculated w/ a triglyceride level >400mg/ dL

Relative lipid effects:
•**HMG Co–A reductase inhibitors** correct all lipids, esp. Atorvastatin, Rosuvastatin & Simvastatin
•**Selective cholesterol absorption inhibitors** correct all lipids to half the extent of HMG Co–A reductase inhibitors
•**Niacin** primarily ↓triglyceride levels
•**Fibric acid medications** primarily ↓triglyceride levels
•**Bile acid sequestrants** primarily ↓LDL cholesterol levels
•**Omega–3 fatty acids** primarily ↓VLDL levels
•**Significant dietary lipid restriction** ↓total cholesterol by ~10%

HMG Co–A REDUCTASE INHIBITORS

Generic (Trade)	M ♀	Start	Max
Atorvastatin (Lipitor)	L U	10mg PO qhs	80mg qhs
Fluvastatin (Lescol)	L U	40mg PO qhs	80mg qhs
Lovastatin (Mevacor)	L U	20mg PO qhs	80mg qhs
Pravastatin (Pravachol)	L U	40mg PO qhs	80mg qhs
Rosuvastatin (Crestor)	L U	10mg PO qhs	40mg qhs
Simvastatin (Zocor)	L U	20mg PO qhs	80mg qhs

•These medications are maximally effective if administered in the evening, when the majority of cholesterol synthesis occurs

Mechanisms:
•Inhibit hydroxymethylglutaryl coenzyme A reductase function, being the hepatocyte rate limiting enzyme in cholesterol formation→
 ◦↓Hepatic cholesterol formation→
  –Feedback ↑hepatocyte LDL receptor formation→↑**plasma LDL cholesterol removal**
•Anti–inflammatory effects→
 ◦↓Atherosclerotic plaque formation, w/ ↑stability

Outcomes:
•↓Morbidity & mortality

Side effects:
Gastrointestinal
•**Hepatitis–1.5%**, usually starting within 3months of initial or ↑dose, being:
 ◦Dose related
 ◦Gradual in onset
 ◦Usually benign
•Nausea ± vomiting

Musculoskeletal
- **Myositis-3%**, being:
  - ○Dose related
  - ○Possibly sudden in onset
  - …→muscle pain &/or weakness which progress to **rhabdomyolysis <0.5%**, diagnosed via ↑creatine kinase-CK levels
  - Risk factors:
    - •↑Age
    - •Hypothyroidism
    - •Renal failure
    - •Small body frame
    - •Concomitant administration of:
      - ○Fibric acid medications
      - ○Bile acid sequestrants
      - ○Niacin

Neurologic
- •Headaches
- •Sleep disturbances

Ophthalmologic
- •Minor lens opacities

Interactions
- **Garlic & St. Johns wort→**
  - ○↑Hepatocyte cytochrome P450 system activity→
    - -↑HMG-CoA reductase inhibitor degradation→↓plasma levels (except Pravastatin)
- **Diltiazem & protease inhibitors→**
  - ○↓Hepatocyte cytochrome P450 system activity→
    - -↓HMG-CoA reductase inhibitor degradation→↑plasma levels (except Pravastatin)

Monitoring:
- •Baseline:
  - ○**Liver function tests**, then
    - -3months after dose↑, then periodically thereafter, w/ treatment to be withdrawn @ plasma values >3X the upper limit of normal
  - ○**Creatine kinase** (as an asymptomatic ↑ may be present), then
    - -Prior to dose↑ or adding an interacting medication, in order to compare future possible values, to be obtained if symptomatic, w/ treatment to be discontinued @ either plasma values >10X the upper limit of normal, or lower if class switching fails to relieve the syndrome

---

SELECTIVE CHOLESTEROL ABSORPTION INHIBITORS: Relatively safe to use in combination w/ HMG-CoA reductase inhibitors

Generic (Trade)	M	♀	Dose
Ezetimibe (Zetia)	L	?	10mg PO q24hours

Mechanism:
- •Acts on the small intestinal brush border membrane enzymes→
  - ○Selectively ↓cholesterol absorption↑→
    - -↓Hepatic cholesterol stores→feedback ↑hepatocyte LDL receptor formation→↑**plasma LDL cholesterol removal**

---

†No significant effects on lipid soluble vitamin absorption (A, D, E, K)

Side effects:
- **Gastrointestinal**
  - •Combination treatment w/ HMG Co-A reductase inhibitors→
    - ○↑**Hepatitis** risk, but **no** ↑**myositis risk**, which makes it the medication of choice for combination treatment

Monitoring:
- •Liver function tests as per concomitant HMG Co-A reductase inhibitor

FIBRIC ACID MEDICATIONS

Generic (Trade)	M	♀	Start	Max
Fenofibrate (Tricor)	LK	?	67mg PO q24hours, w/ a meal	200mg q24hours
Gemfibrozil (Lopid)	LK	?	600mg PO q12hours, prior to meals	1500mg/ 24hours

Side effects:
- **Gastrointestinal**
  - •Nausea

NIACIN

Generic	M	♀	Start		Max
Niacin	K	?	50mg PO q12hours, w/ meals		6g/ 24hours
•XR form			500mg qhs w/ a low fat snack		2g qhs

Mechanism:
- •Inhibits hepatocyte VLDL synthesis & release

Side effects:
- **Gastrointestinal**
  - •Epigastric pain
  - •Hepatitis, esp. w/ the XR form
  - •Nausea
- **Mucocutaneous**
  - •**Cutaneous flushing reaction**, being ↓ w/ NSAID administration 30 min. prior
- **Neurologic**
  - •Headache
- **Hematologic**
  - •**Hyperglycemia**
  - •↑Uric acid

BILE ACID SEQUESTRANTS

Generic (Trade)	M	♀	Start	Max
Cholestyramine (Questran)	F	?	4g PO q24hours prior to meals	12g q12hours
Colesevelam (Welchol)	Ø	P	3.75g=6tabs q24hours w/ a meal	5.625g=7tabs/ 24hours

Mechanism:
- •Bind to intestinal bile acids→
  - ◦↓Bile acid absorption→
    - −Feedback ↑hepatic conversion of cholesterol to bile acids→↓hepatic cholesterol stores→
    feedback ↑hepatocyte LDL receptor formation→↑plasma LDL cholesterol removal

Side effects:
- **Gastrointestinal**
  - •↓Absorption of concomitantly administered medications. Other medications should be taken 1hour prior to, or 5hours after taking a bile acid sequestrant
  - •Bloating
  - •Constipation
  - •Nausea
  - •High doses→
    - ◦Lipid soluble vitamin deficiencies (A, D, E, K)
    - ◦↑Stool fat, termed steatorrhea

COMBINATION MEDICATIONS

Generic (Trade)	M	♀	Start	Max
Lovastatin & Niacin (Advicor)	LK	U	20mg/ 500mg qhs w/ a low fat snack	20mg/ 1g

DIETARY

Generic (Trade)	M	♀	Dose
Omega 3–fatty acids (Fish oil)	L	?	A combination dose of EPA + DHA†
•Cardioprotection			1g PO q24hours
•Hypertriglyceridemia			2–4g PO q24hours

†Eicosapentanoic acid–EPA & docosahexanoic acid–DHA
- •There are only 2 types of polyunsaturated fatty acids
  - ◦Omega 3–fatty acids, mainly from:
    - −Fish or fish oils, esp. herring, mackerel, salmon, sardines, trout, & tuna
    - −Beans, esp. soybeans
    - −Green leafy vegetables
    - −Nuts, esp. walnuts
    - −Plant seeds, esp. canola oil & flaxseed
  - ◦Omega 6–fatty acids, mainly from:
    - −Grains
    - −Meats
    - −Nuts, esp. peanuts
    - −Plant seeds, esp. borage oil, corn oil, cottonseed oil, grape seed oil, primrose oil, safflower oil, sesame oil, soybean oil, & sunflower oil
- •The Western diet is abundant in omega 6–fatty acids (which are prothrombotic & proinflammatory), w/ humans lacking the necessary enzymes to convert them to omega 3–fatty acids, which therefore need to be obtained from separate dietary sources. However, significant amounts of methylmercury

& other environmental toxins may be concentrated in certain fish species (w/ high quality fish oil supplements usually lacking contaminants):
- •King Mackerel
- •Shark
- •Swordfish
- •Tilefish, aka golden bass or golden snapper
- ...which are to be avoided by:
  - •♀ who may become or are pregnant
  - •♀ who are breastfeeding
  - •Young children

Mechanism:
- •Vasodilation→
  - ∘↓Blood pressure, being dose dependent, w/ a minimal effect of 4/ 2 mmHg w/ doses of 3–6g q24h
- •↓Lipid, esp. triglycerides
- •Anti–dysrhythmic
- •Anti–inflammatory
- •↓Platelet activity

Outcomes:
- •In patients w/ coronary artery disease:
  - ∘↓All cause mortality
  - ∘↓Dysrhythmia mediated sudden death

Side effects:
Cardiovascular
- •↑Bleeding time→
  - ∘Excessive hemorrhage

Gastrointestinal
- •Belching
- •Bloating
- •Fishy aftertaste
- •Nausea ± vomiting

Hematologic
- •Hyperglycemia

Interactions
- •None known, making it safe for use in combination w/ other:
  - ∘Anticoagulant medications
  - ∘Antiplatelet medications
  - ∘Lipid lowering medications

POTASSIUM
•Always measure the magnesium level concomitantly

Indications:
- •Ensure a potassium of 4–5mEq/ L

Generic
- •Potassium chloride–KCL
- •Potassium bicarbonate
- •Potassium citrate
- •Potassium acetate
- •Potassium gluconate
- •Potassium phosphate

POTASSIUM DOSAGE ADJUSTMENT SCALE†_____

Plasma K^+ (mEq/ L)	K^+ repletion (mEq)
≥3.9	None
3.7–3.8	20
3.5–3.6	40
3.3–3.4	60
3.1–3.2	80
≤3	100

†Half all above doses @ a glomerular filtration rate–GFR ≤30mL/ min.

Outcomes:
- •Anti–dysrhythmic
- •↑Cardiac contractility in heart failure
- •Modest hypotensive effect in some patients
- •↓Cerebrovascular disease risk, apart from its possible blood pressure lowering effects

44

DIETARY			
Generic (Trade)	**M ♀**	**Dose**	
Garlic (Allium sativum)	? U	600–900mg PO q24hours	

Mechanism:
- ↓Blood pressure
- ↓Lipids
- ↓Platelet activity

ALTERNATIVE/ ADDITIVE MEDICATIONS ■■■■■■

NITROVASODILATORS: Long acting

Indications:
- Syndrome refractory to maximal tolerated doses of the above medications

Generic	M ♀	Start	Max
Isosorbide dinitrate (Isordil, Sorbitrate)	L ?	5–20mg PO q8hours	40mg PO q8hours
•XR form (Isordil Tembids, Dilatrate SR)		40mg PO q12hours	80mg PO q12hours
Isosorbide mononitrate (ISMO, Monoket)	L ?	20mg PO q12hours	40mg PO q12hours
•XR form (Imdur)		30mg PO q24hours	240mg q24hours
Nitroglycerin–transdermal	L ?	Lowest dose, applied to non–hairy skin for 14hours/ day	

Trade	Available doses (mg/ hour)
Deponit	0.2, 0.4
Minitran	0.1, 0.2, 0.4, 0.6
Nitrodisc	0.2, 0.3, 0.4
Nitro–Dur	0.1, 0.2, 0.3, 0.4, 0.6, 0.8
Transderm–Nitro	0.1, 0.2, 0.4, 0.6, 0.8

Mechanism:
- Vasodilation (**venous** > arterial)→
  - ↓Preload→
    - –↓Myocardial contractile strength→↓O_2 & nutrient demand
  - ↑Coronary artery dilation→↑perfusion

Side effects:
Cardiovascular
- Systemic vasodilation→
  - Reflex tachycardia
  - Orthostatic hypotension
  - Facial flushing
- Meningeal arterial dilation→
  - Headache

Pharmacokinetics/ pharmacodynamics
- Tolerance to medication effects

Contraindications:
Cardiovascular
- Hypotension

Neurologic
- **Hypertensive encephalopathy**, as it ↑ intracranial pressure

Interactions
- **Sildenafil** (Viagra) **is contraindicated** in patients taking concomitant nitrates, as the combination within 24hours may→severe hypotension→
  - ↓Myocardial perfusion→
    - –Stable angina mediated acute coronary syndrome
  - ↓Cerebral perfusion→
    - –Pre–syncope/ syncope
    - –Cerebrovascular accident syndrome

CALCIUM CHANNEL BLOCKERS: Non–dihydropyridines				

Indications:
•Intolerance to, or inadequately controlled by β receptor blockers

Generic	M ♀	Start	Max
Diltiazem	L ?	30mg PO q8hours	120mg q8hours
•XR form		As per daily requirement	
∘QDXR form		120mg PO q12hours	540mg q24hours
∘BIDXR form		60mg PO q12hours	180mg q12hours
Verapamil	L ?	40mg PO q8hours	160mg q8hours
•XR form		As per daily requirement	
∘Calan XR form		120mg PO q24hours	480mg/ 24hours
∘Veleran XR form		100mg PO q24hours	400mg q24hours
∘Covera XR form		180mg PO q24hours	480mg qhs

Mechanism:
•Block voltage dependent calcium ion channels in smooth & cardiac muscle→
  ∘↓Calcium influx→
    –↓Sinoatrial & atrioventricular node conduction (non–dihydropyridines)→↓pulse
    –Anti–dysrhythmic via nodal effects (mainly non–dihydropyridines)
    –↓Cardiac muscle contractile strength (mainly non–dihydropyridines)
    –Vasodilation: Arterial > venous (mainly dihydropyridines)

Side effects:
Cardiovascular
•Bradycardia ± heart block
•Edema
•Flushing
•Hypotension
Gastrointestinal
•Constipation
•Nausea ± vomiting
Neurologic
•Dizziness
•Headache

ANTIDOTES				

Generic	M ♀	Dose		Max
Glucagon	LK P	3mg IV slow push over 1min., then		
		5mg IV slow push over 1 min. if needed		
•Continuous infusion		5mg/ hour		
10% Calcium chloride†		10mL (1 ampule) IV slow push over 3min., then		
		repeat @5min. if needed		
•Continuous infusion		Start 0.3mEq/ hour		0.7mEq/ hour
Onset: 1–2 min., Duration: 30–60 min.				
Magnesium sulfate	K S	2g $MgSO_4$ in 50mL saline infused over 15min., then		
		6g $MgSO_4$ in 500mL saline infused over 6hours		

†Use cautiously in patients taking Digoxin, as hypercalcemia→
  •Digoxin cardiotoxicity

ANGIOTENSIN 2 RECEPTOR BLOCKERS–ARBs				

Indications:
•Intolerance of, hypersensitivity to, or contraindication to angiotensin converting enzyme
  inhibitors–ACEi

Generic (Trade)	M ♀	Start	Max
Candesartan (Atacand)	K ?	16mg PO q24hours	32mg q24hours
Eprosartan (Teveten)	F U	600mg PO q24hours	800mg/ 24hours
Irbesartan (Avapro)	L U	150mg PO q24hours	300mg q24hours
Olmisartan (Benicar)	K U	20mg PO q24hours	40mg q24hours
Losartan (Cozaar)	L U	50mg PO q24hours	100mg/ 24hours
Telmisartan (Micardis)	L U	40mg PO q24hours	80mg q24hours
Valsartan (Diovan)	L U	80mg PO q24hours	320mg q24hours

Dose adjustment:
•↓Initial dose by 50% if:
  ∘Elderly
  ∘Concomitant diuretic use
  ∘Renal disease

Losartan specific:
•Starting dose is halved if concomitant hepatic disease

Mechanism:
•Angiotensin 2 receptor blockade→
 ∘↓Angiotensin 2 action→
  –Vasodilation (**arterial** > venous)
  –↓Renal NaCl & water retention
  –↓Adrenal cortex aldosterone release→↓renal NaCl & water retention
  –↓Facilitation of adrenal medullary & presynaptic norepinephrine release→vasodilation
  –Glomerular efferent arteriole vasodilation→↓intraglomerular hydrostatic pressure→↓filtration→
   ↓proteinuria in patients w/ nephropathy
 ∘↓Cardiovascular remodeling

Side effects†:
Cardiovascular
•Hypotension
Gastrointestinal
•Altered gustatory sense=dysguesia–3%
Genitourinary
•Acute interstitial nephritis
•Patients w/ preexisting bilateral ↓renal perfusion, not necessarily failure:
 ∘Heart failure
 ∘Bilateral renal artery stenosis
 ∘Hypovolemia
 ∘Renal failure
 ...rely more on the compensatory production of angiotensin 2→
  •Efferent arteriole constriction→
   ∘Maintained glomerular filtration rate–GFR, whereas either:
    –Angiotensin converting enzyme inhibition
    –Angiotensin 2 receptor blockade
    ...→↓angiotensin 2 production & action respectively, which may→
     •**Pre-renal renal failure**
Materno-fetal
•**Fetal & neonatal morbidity & mortality**
Hematologic
•↓Aldosterone production ± renal failure→
 ∘**Hyperkalemia**
•Neutropenia

†Do not cause the hypersensitivity-like syndrome associated w/ ACE inhibitors, due to lack of bradykinin & substance P elevation

Monitoring:
•Check creatinine & potassium @ 3–10days after initiation or dose↑, then
 ∘Q3–6months

Contraindications:
Genitourinary
•Acute renal failure
•Bilateral renal artery stenosis
•Unilateral renal artery stenosis of a solitary functioning kidney
Materno-fetal
•Breast feeding
•**Pregnancy**
Hematologic
•**Potassium >5mEq/ L**

EXACERBATION ▮▮▮▮▮▮▮▮▮▮▮▮▮▮▮▮▮▮

NITROVASODILATORS: Short acting			
Generic	M ♀	Start	
Nitroglycerin, sublingual (Nitrostat)	L ?	0.4mg sublingual q5min. X3prn	
Nitroglycerin, spray (Nitrolingual)	L ?	1 sublingual spray=0.4mg q5min. X3prn	

•All patients w/ angina pectoris should carry a fast-acting nitrate. Those w/ stable angina may also use the medication prophylactically within 10min. prior to initiating a typically exacerbatory activity

Mechanism:
•Vasodilation (**venous** >> arterial)→
  ◦↓Preload→↓myocardial contractile strength
    −↓Cardiac output→↓blood pressure
    −↓Myocardial O_2 & nutrient demand
    −↓Pulmonary congestion if present
  ◦↑Coronary artery dilation→↑perfusion

Side effects:
Cardiovascular
  •Systemic vasodilation→
    ◦Reflex tachycardia
    ◦Orthostatic hypotension
    ◦Facial flushing
  •Meningeal arterial dilation→
    ◦Headache
Pharmacokinetics/ pharmacodynamics
  •Tolerance to medication effects

Contraindications:
Cardiovascular
  •Hypotension
Neurologic
  •**Hypertensive encephalopathy**, as it ↑intracranial pressure
Interactions
  •**Sildenafil** (Viagra) **is contraindicated** in patients taking concomitant nitrates, as the combination within 24hours may→severe hypotension→
    ◦↓Myocardial perfusion→
      −Stable angina mediated acute coronary syndrome
    ◦↓Cerebral perfusion→
      −Pre-syncope/ syncope
      −Cerebrovascular accident syndrome

▮▮▮▮▮▮▮▮▮▮▮▮ **INVASIVE PROCEDURES** ▮▮▮▮▮▮▮▮▮▮▮▮

•**Coronary angiography**
  Indications:
    •All patients suspected of having coronary artery disease
    •Acute coronary syndrome, being either:
      ◦Unstable angina
      ◦Myocardial infarction
    •Inadequate symptom control despite medical treatment to its tolerable limits

•**Percutaneous coronary intervention–PCI**
  ◦**Percutaneous transluminal coronary angioplasty–PTCA**
    Indications:
      •≥1 discrete, anatomically approachable (proximal), noncalcified coronary stenosis, being ≤10mm in length, not meeting the criteria for coronary artery bypass–CABG surgery
    Outcomes:
      •85% of patients have complete syndrome relief
  ◦**Intracoronary stent placement**
    Procedure:
      •Once the stenotic lesion has undergone PTCA, a flexible coil or tube composed of stainless steel alloys is placed via expandable balloon or may self expand→
        ◦Circumferential apposition of the diseased endothelial segment→
          −↑Luminal diameter
          −↓Vascular recoil
          −Intimal flap seal

48

Complications:
- **Procedural mortality is 1%**, as stent deployment may→
  - ∘Intimal dissection ± epicardial hemorrhage into the pericardial space→pericardial tamponade
  - ∘Thromboembolism→coronary artery stenosis→acute coronary syndrome
  - ...both of which may require **emergent thoracotomy** ± coronary artery bypass grafting–CABG, which is why **all patients should be surgical candidates**
- **Acute in–stent restenosis rate is ≤3% within 1month**, usually occurring within 10 days
  Pathophysiology:
  - The result of thrombus formation ± embolism
  Restenosis rate reduction:
  - **Peri–procedural glycoprotein 2b/ 3a inhibitor** or direct thrombin inhibitor infusion
- **Chronic restenosis rate is 40% within 1year**, usually occurring within 6 months
  Pathophysiology:
  - The result of continued atherosclerosis, w/ ingrowth of tissue through the struts of the stent, in part exacerbated via procedural mediated vascular injury→
    - ∘↑Localized inflammation
  Restenosis rate reduction:
  - **Chronic thienopyridine administration**
  - **Drug eluting stent**
    - ∘Sirolimus: An anti–fungal isolated from Streptomyces hygroscopicus→cell cycle arrest→
      - –↓Lymphocyte & plasma cell proliferation→↓localized inflammatory mediators→↓lesion biologic activity
      - –↓Smooth muscle cell proliferation & intimal migration
    Note: The stent is coated w/ a mixture of Sirolimus blended w/ synthetic polymers which serve as a medication reservoir, allowing for the gradual elution of Sirolimus over ~1month. This allows for localized action via a small quantity of the medication, thus avoiding systemic side effects of immunosuppression, hyperlipidemia, &/or thrombocytopenia

GLYCOPROTEIN 2b/ 3a INHIBITORS				
Generic (Trade)	M ♀	Start		Max
Abciximab (ReoPro)	P ?	0.25µg/ kg IV bolus loading over 1min., given within 1 hour prior to PCI, then 0.125µg/kg/min. IV infusion X 12hours after PCI		10µg/min.
Epifibatide (Integrilin)	K P	180µg/ kg IV bolus loading dose just prior to PCI, then 2µg/kg/min. IV infusion X 18–24hours after PCI		22.6mg
Tirofiban (Aggrastat)	K P	0.4µg/kg/min. IV loading infusion over 30min., just prior to PCI, then 0.1µg/kg/min. X 12–24hours after PCI		

Eptifibatide specific dose adjustment:
- ↓IV infusion to 1µg/kg/min. in patients w/ renal failure

Mechanism:
- Glycoprotein 2b/ 3a receptors bind platelet aggregation inducing cytokines, thus affecting the final common pathway of platelet activation

DIRECT THROMBIN INHIBITORS		
Generic (Trade)	M ♀	Dose
Bivalirudin (Angiomax)	K P	1mg/ kg IV bolus just prior to PCI, then 2.5mg/kg/hour IV infusion X 4hours, then 0.2mg/kg/hour IV infusion X 20hours

Monitoring:
- Obtain the aPTT @baseline, 2hours after starting the infusion, & 2hours after any adjustment until the goal value of 1.5–2.5 X baseline (50–80seconds) is obtained

THIENOPYRIDINE DERIVATIVE		
Generic (Trade)	M ♀	Dose
Clopidogrel (Plavix)	LK P	300mg PO loading dose X 1 @ ≥4hours prior to procedure, then 75mg PO q24hours X 1year

Mechanism:
- Inhibits adenosine diphosphate–ADP mediated activation of the glycoprotein 2b/ 3a complex→
  - ∘↓Platelet activation

- A 300mg loading dose is used, as maximal effect occurs @ 5hours rather than 5days w/ initiation of the standard 75mg dosage

49

> Side effects:
> **Gastrointestinal**
> •Diarrhea
> **Mucocutaneous**
> •Dermatitis
> **Hematologic**
> •**Thrombotic thrombocytopenic purpura–TTP** within several weeks of initiation

•**Coronary artery bypass grafting–CABG**
   Indications:
      •Patients w/ diabetes mellitus & coronary artery disease
      •Left main coronary artery stenosis ≥50%
      •Proximal left anterior descending–LAD coronary artery stenosis ≥70%
      •Triple vessel disease† w/ left ventricular systolic dysfunction via ejection fraction–EF <50%
      •Less severe coronary artery disease w/ either:
         ∘The concomitant need for valve or aneurysm repair
         ∘Inadequate symptom control despite PTCA & medical treatment to its tolerable limits
   Mechanism:
      •Uses either a **saphenous vein** &/or **internal mammary artery** graft to bypass the stenotic vasculature
   Outcomes:
      •70% of patients have complete or near-complete syndrome relief
      •20% have partial syndrome relief
      •50% of patients develop recurrent angina within 5years
      •Internal mammary artery grafts→
         ∘10%↓ mortality rate by 10years compared to saphenous vein grafts
   Complications:
      •Aortic cross-clamping may→
         ∘Cerebral hypoperfusion of watershed area(s)→
            –Cerebrovascular accident
      •Perioperative myocardial infarction

---

†Left anterior descending, circumflex, & right coronary arteries

•25% of persons experiencing a myocardial infarction do not seek medical attention while symptomatic

•**Oxygen** to maintain PaO_2 >60mmHg or SaO_2 >92%, usually accomplished via nasal cannula @ 2-4L/min.
  Mechanism:
    •Oxygenation if required
    •Calming effect→
      ∘↓Autonomic sympathetic tone→
        -↓Myocardial O_2 & nutrient demand
  Duration:
    •24-48hours, or longer if needed for oxygenation
•**Antipyretics** if febrile, as fever→
  ∘↑Cellular O_2 & nutrient demand
•**Hyperglycemic control** in diabetic patients, as hyperglycemia→
  ∘↑Ischemic cellular anaerobic glycolysis→
    -Myocardial lactic acidemia→myocyte dysfunction ± death

NITROVASODILATORS: Short acting			
Generic	**M** ♀	**Start**	
Nitroglycerin, sublingual (Nitrostat)	L ?	0.4mg sublingual q5min. X3prn	
Nitroglycerin, spray (Nitrolingual)	L ?	1 sublingual spray=0.4mg q5min. X3prn	

PLATELET INHIBITING MEDICATIONS		
Efficacy: Glycoprotein 2b/ 3a inhibitors > thienopyridines > Aspirin		
Generic	**M** ♀	**Dose**
Acetylsalicylic acid–ASA=Aspirin	K U	325mg crushed or chewed PO X1 or PR if unable to timely administer PO, then 81mg PO q24hours lifelong

THIENOPYRIDINE DERIVATIVE		
Generic (Trade)	**M** ♀	**Dose**
Clopidogrel (Plavix)	LK P	300mg PO loading dose, then 75mg PO q24hours

β1 SELECTIVE RECEPTOR BLOCKERS			
Generic (Trade)	**M** ♀	**Start**	**Max**
Atenolol (Tenormin)	K U		
•IV form		5mg slow IV push (1mg/ min.) q5min. X 2 prn, then	
•PO form		25-50mg PO q24hours	200mg/ 24h
Metoprolol (Lopressor)	L ?		
•IV form		5mg slow IV push (1mg/ min.) q5min. X 3 prn, then	
•PO form		25mg PO q12hours, then	100mg q12h
∘XR form (Toprol XL)		As per PO requirement	400mg q24h
Esmolol (Brevibloc)	K ?	0.5mg=500µg/ kg IV loading bolus (over 1 min.), then 0.05mg=50µg/kg/min. continuous IV infusion w/ titration prn† Max: 0.3mg=300µg/kg/min.	
Onset: 1-2 min., Duration: 10 min.			

†Titrate q4 min. via re-administration of the loading bolus & an additional 50µg/kg/min. IV infusion

α1 & NONSELECTIVE β RECEPTOR BLOCKERS			
Generic (Trade)	**M** ♀	**Start**	**Max**
Carvedilol (Coreg)	L ?	6.25mg PO q12hours	25mg q12h
Labetalol (Normodyne)	LK ?	20mg IV push over 2min., then 40mg IV push q10min. prn goal blood pressure, then	300mg total
•PO form		100mg PO q12hours	1200mg q12h
•IV form		0.5-2mg/ min. IV infusion	
Onset: 5-10min., Duration: 3-6hours			

Goal parameters:
  •Target pulse of 50-60/ min. w/ normotension
Outcomes:
  •↓Morbidity & mortality

ANGIOTENSIN CONVERTING ENZYME INHIBITORS–ACEi

Generic (Trade)	M	♀	Start	Max
Benazepril (Lotensin)	LK	U	10mg PO q24hours	40mg/ 24hours
Captopril (Capoten)	LK	U	12.5mg PO q12hours	450mg/ 24hours
Enalapril (Vasotec)	LK	U	5mg PO q24hours	40mg/ 24hours
Fosinopril (Monopril)	LK	U	10mg PO q24hours	40mg/ 24hours
Lisinopril (Prinivil, Zestril)	K	U	10mg PO q24hours	40mg q24hours

•In order to rapidly titrate the dosage in ACEi naïve patients, start w/ low dose Captopril & double the dose q8h, if tolerated, until the 50mg dosage is reached. At that point, you can simply switch to the max dose of any of the others listed for ↓dosing frequency

Dose adjustment:
•↓Initial dose by 50% if:
  ◦Elderly
  ◦Concomitant diuretic use
  ◦Renal disease

Outcomes:
•↓Morbidity & mortality w/ myocardial infarction if started within 24hours

LIPID LOWERING MEDICATIONS

Indications:
•All patients w/ atherosclerotic mediated acute coronary syndromes should receive an HMG Co–A reductase inhibitor during hospitalization, & indefinitely regardless of baseline LDL, unless intolerant due to side effects

HMG Co–A REDUCTASE INHIBITORS

Generic (Trade)	M	♀	Start @ Max
Atorvastatin (Lipitor)	L	U	80mg qhs
Fluvastatin (Lescol)	L	U	80mg qhs
Lovastatin (Mevacor)	L	U	80mg qhs
Pravastatin (Pravachol)	L	U	80mg qhs
Rosuvastatin (Crestor)	L	U	40mg qhs
Simvastatin (Zocor)	L	U	80mg qhs

•These medications are maximally effective if administered in the evening, when the majority of cholesterol synthesis occurs

Outcomes:
•↓Morbidity & mortality

HIGH MOLECULAR WEIGHT HEPARIN

Indications:
•Started promptly & continued until the patient has been chest pain free ≥48hours, or coronary intervention is performed (whichever is soonest)

M	♀	Start
M	?	60units/ kg IV bolus (or 5000units empirically)
		12units/kg/hour infusion (or 1000units/ hour empirically)

•Titrated by 2.5units/kg/hour to achieve an activated partial thromboplastin time–aPTT of 1.5–2X control value or **50–70seconds**

aPTT (seconds)	Action	Obtain next aPTT
<40	Bolus 5000units & ↑infusion rate by 100units/ hour	6hours
40–49	↑Infusion rate by 50units/ hour	6hours
50–70 (or 1.5–2Xcontrol)	**NO ACTION**	**24hours**
71–85	↓Infusion rate by 50units/ hour	6hours
86–100	Hold infusion 30min., then ↓infusion rate by 100units/ hour	6hours
101–150	Hold infusion 60min., then ↓infusion rate by 150units/ hour	6hours
>150	Hold infusion 60min., then ↓infusion rate by 300units/ hour	6hours

Monitoring:
•Complete blood count q24hours to monitor for side effects

LOW MOLECULAR WEIGHT HEPARIN

Generic (Trade)	M	♀	Start	Max
Enoxaparin (Lovenox)	KL	P	1.5mg kg SC q24hours or 1mg/ kg SC q12hours	180mg/ 24hours
Dalteparin (Fragmin)	KL	P	200 anti–factor Xa units/ kg SC q24hours or 100 anti–factor Xa units/ kg SC q12hours	18,000units q24hours

<u>Dose adjustment:</u>
- •Obesity
  - ∘Most manufacturers recommend a maximum dose of that for a 90kg patient

<u>Monitoring:</u>
- •Monitoring of anti−Xa levels is recommended in patients w/:
  - ∘Abnormal coagulation/ hemorrhage
  - ∘Obesity
  - ∘Renal failure
  - ∘Underweight
- •Check 4hours after 2nd SC dose. Further monitoring is not necessary once the correct dose is established in obese patients

Administration frequency	Therapeutic anti−Xa levels
Q12hours	0.6−1 units/ mL
Q24hours	1−2 units/ mL

<u>Mechanism:</u>
- •Heparin combines w/ plasma antithrombin 3→
  - ∘↑Antithrombin 3 activity in removing thrombin & activated factors 9, 10, 11,& 12→
    - −↓Coagulation→↓vascular & mural thrombus formation &/or propagation
- •Heparin is metabolized by the plasma enzyme heparinase

<u>Outcomes:</u>
- •↓Morbidity & mortality

<u>Side effects:</u>
Cardiovascular
- •**Hemorrhage**
- •**Heparin induced thrombocytopenia−HIT 10%**, esp. w/ high molecular weight Heparin
  <u>Mechanism:</u>
  - •Heparin mediated platelet agglutination→
    - ∘Monocyte/ macrophage mediated extravascular removal via the splenic trabecular network=red pulp, & hepatic sinusoids→
      - −**Thrombocytopenia**
  <u>Outcomes:</u>
  - •Benign, as it resolves spontaneously, even w/ continued exposure
- •**Heparin induced thrombocytopenia ± thrombosis−HITT ≤3%**, esp. w/ high molecular weight Heparin
  <u>Mechanism:</u>
  - •Heparin mediated platelet agglutination→
    - ∘Monocyte/ macrophage mediated extravascular removal via the splenic trabecular network=red pulp, & hepatic sinusoids→
      - −**Thrombocytopenia**
    - ∘Platelet release of Heparin neutralizing factor=platelet factor 4−PF4, which complexes w/ Heparin→
      - −Production of anti−complex antibodies→↑platelet activation↔↑platelet factor 4 release→ a vicious cycle of **platelet mediated arterial &/or venous thrombus formation, termed the "white clot syndrome,"** being as the clot is relatively devoid of erythrocytes
  <u>Outcomes:</u>
  - •Must discontinue treatment as **20% develop thromboembolic complications**. Being that both Heparins may cross−react w/ the etiologic antibodies, their further use is contraindicated. Consider continued treatment w/ direct thrombin inhibitors
    - ∘Antibody cross−reactivity:
      - −Low molecular weight Heparin−85%
      - −Heparinoids−5%

Mucocutaneous
- •Skin necrosis−rarely occurring w/ high molecular weight Heparins, & not being associated w/ anticoagulant deficiency

Musculoskeletal
- •Osteoporosis, esp. w/ high molecular weight Heparin
  - ∘Usually @ use ≥1month

Hematologic
- •↓Aldosterone production→
  - ∘**Hyperkalemia−8%**

CHARACTERISTICS OF HEPARIN INDUCED THROMBOCYTOPENIC SYNDROMES		
	HIT	HITT
Onset	<2days	4-10 days
Re-exposure	<2days	Earlier if re-exposed within 3 months
Platelet count	↓, being <150,000 or ≥50%	
Platelet median nadir	~90,000	~60,000

- ^{14}C-Serotonin release assay
  Indications:
  - Suspected HITT
  Procedure:
  - Normal donor platelets are radiolabeled w/ ^{14}C-serotonin. They are then washed & combined w/ patient serum & therapeutic Heparin concentrations (0.1 U/ mL). Induction of ^{14}C-serotonin release from platelets constitutes a positive test
  Limitations:
  - Expense, due to the use of radioactive material
  Outcomes:
  - Considered the gold standard in the detection of HITT
- Enzyme linked immunosorbent assay-ELISA
  Indications:
  - Suspected HITT
  Procedure:
  - Heparin-PF4 complexes affixed to a plastic plate are incubated w/ the patient's serum. If the patient has produced antibodies, then the addition of enzymatically (horseradish peroxidase) labeled anti-human IgG allows for color visualization via spectrophotometer
  Limitations:
  - Many antibody positive patients do not develop clinical HITT
  - 30% false positive

Contraindications:
- Active hemorrhage
- Severe bleeding diathesis
- Severe thrombocytopenia (platelet count ≤20,000/ μL)
- Recent significant trauma
- Neurosurgery, ocular surgery, or intracranial hemorrhage within 10days

ANTIDOTE				
Generic	M	♀	Amount IV over 10min.	Max
Protamine	P	?	1mg/ 100units of HMWH	50mg
			1mg/ 100units Dalteparin	"
			1mg/ 1mg Enoxaparin	"

Mechanism:
- Protamine combines electrostatically w/ Heparin→
  - Inability to bind to antithrombin 3

POTASSIUM
•Always measure the magnesium level concomitantly

Indications:
- Ensure a potassium of 4-5mEq/ L

Generic

If concomitant alkalemia:
- Potassium chloride-KCL
If concomitant acidemia:
- Potassium bicarbonate
- Potassium citrate
- Potassium acetate
- Potassium gluconate
- Potassium phosphate
  - Preferred in diabetic ketoacidemia-DKA due to concomitant phosphate depletion
Monitoring:
- Q4hours until goal of 4-5mEq/ L X 2 consecutive readings, then q6hours

POTASSIUM DOSAGE ADJUSTMENT SCALE†

Plasma K$^+$ (mEq/ L)	K$^+$ repletion (mEq)
≥3.9	None
3.7–3.8	20
3.5–3.6	40
3.3–3.4	60
3.1–3.2	80
≤3	100

†Half all above doses @ a glomerular filtration rate–GFR ≤30mL/ min.

Intravenous repletion guidelines:
- •Use dextrose–free solutions for the initial, repletion as dextrose→
  - ◦↑Insulin secretion→
    - –↑Potassium transcellular shift
- •The hyperosmolar infusion→
  - ◦Vascular irritation/ inflammation. Add 1% Lidocaine to the bag to ↓pain
- •**Do not administer >20mEq potassium IV/ hour**
  - ◦≤10mEq/ hour prn via peripheral line. May give via 2 peripheral lines=20mEq/ hour total
  - ◦≤20mEq/ hour prn via central line
  - ...as more→
    - •Transient right sided heart hyperkalemia→
      - ◦Dysrhythmias

Outcomes:
- •Anti–dysrhythmic
- •↑Cardiac contractility in heart failure
- •Modest hypotensive effect in some patients
- •↓Cerebrovascular disease risk, apart from its possible blood pressure lowering effects

MAGNESIUM SULFATE

M ♀	Dose
K S	Every 1g IV→0.1mEq/ L ↑in plasma magnesium

Mechanism:
- •↓Magnesium→
  - ◦↓Renal tubular potassium reabsorption

BENZODIAZEPINES

Generic (Trade)	M ♀	Dose	Max
Lorazepam (Ativan)	LK U		
•PO form		0.5–1mg q8hours prn	10mg/ 24hours
•IM/ IV form		0.05mg/ kg q8hours prn	4mg/ dose

Mechanism:
- •Sedation→
  - ◦↓Autonomic sympathetic tone→
    - –↓Myocardial O_2 & nutrient demand

STOOL SOFTENERS

Generic (Trade)	M ♀	Dose
Docusate calcium (Surfak)	L S	240mg PO q24hours
Docusate sodium (Colace)	L S	100mg q12hours

Mechanism:
- •↓Defecation effort→
  - ◦↓Autonomic sympathetic tone→
    - –↓Myocardial O_2 & nutrient demand

ALTERNATIVE/ ADDITIONAL TREATMENTS ▬▬▬

NITROVASODILATORS: Short acting

Indications:
- •Angina syndrome despite the above treatment

Generic	M	♀	Start
Nitroglycerin–IV infusion	L	?	10μg/ min.

OPIOID RECEPTOR AGONISTS

Indications:
- •Angina syndrome despite the above treatment

Generic	M	♀	Start
Morphine sulfate	LK	?	2–4mg IV slow push (1mg/ min.) q5min. prn

Mechanism:
- •Vasodilation (**venous** >> arterial)→
  - ∘↓Preload→↓myocardial contractile strength
    - –↓Cardiac output→↓blood pressure
    - –↓Myocardial O_2 & nutrient demand
    - –↓Pulmonary congestion if present
- •↓Pain ± dyspnea→
  - ∘↓Autonomic sympathetic tone→
    - –↓Myocardial O_2 & nutrient demand

OPIOID RECEPTOR AGONIST/ ANTAGONIST

Indications:
- •Hypotension w/ angina syndrome

Generic (Trade)	M	♀	Start	Max
Nalbuphine (Nubain)	LK	P	10–20mg IV q3h prn	160mg/ 24hours

GLYCOPROTEIN 2b/ 3a INHIBITORS

Generic (Trade)	M	♀	Start	Max
Abciximab (ReoPro)	P	?	0.25μg/ kg IV bolus loading over 1min., given within 1 hour prior to PCI, then 0.125μg/kg/min. IV infusion X 12hours after PCI	10μg/min.
Epifibatide (Integrilin)	K	P	180μg/ kg IV bolus loading dose just prior to PCI, then 2μg/kg/min. IV infusion X 18–24hours after PCI	22.6mg
Tirofiban (Aggrastat)	K	P	0.4μg/kg/min. IV loading infusion over 30min., just prior to PCI, then 0.1μg/kg/min. X 12–24hours after PCI	

Eptifibatide specific dose adjustment:
- •↓IV infusion to 1μg/kg/min. in patients w/ renal failure

Mechanism:
- •Glycoprotein 2b/ 3a receptors bind platelet aggregation inducing cytokines, thus affecting the final common pathway of platelet activation

CALCIUM CHANNEL BLOCKERS: Non–dihydropyridines

Indications:
- •Intolerance of, hypersensitivity to, or contraindication to β receptor blockers

Generic	M	♀	Start	Max
Diltiazem	L	?		
•IV form			5–20mg slow IV push over 2 min., then 25mg slow IV push over 2 min., 15 min. later, then 5mg/ hour IV infusion	15mg/ hour
•PO form			30mg PO q8hours	120mg q8hours
•XR form			As per daily requirement	
QD–XR form				540mg q24hours
BID–XR form				180mg q12hours
Verapamil	L	U		
•IV form			2.5–5mg slow IV push over 2min., then 5–10mg slow IV push over 2min., 15min. later, then	
•PO form			40mg PO q8hours	160mg q8hours
∘XR form			As per daily requirement	
–Calan XR form				480mg/ 24hours
–Veleran XR form				400mg qhs

ANGIOTENSIN 2 RECEPTOR BLOCKERS–ARBs

Indications:
- •Intolerance of, hypersensitivity to, or contraindication to angiotensin converting enzyme inhibitors–ACEi

Generic (Trade)	M	♀	Start	Max
Candesartan (Atacand)	K	?	16mg PO q24hours	32mg q24hours
Eprosartan (Teveten)	F	U	600mg PO q24hours	800mg/ 24hours
Irbesartan (Avapro)	L	U	150mg PO q24hours	300mg q24hours
Olmisartan (Benicar)	K	U	20mg PO q24hours	40mg q24hours
Losartan (Cozaar)	L	U	50mg PO q24hours	100mg/ 24hours
Telmisartan (Micardis)	L	U	40mg PO q24hours	80mg q24hours
Valsartan (Diovan)	L	U	80mg PO q24hours	320mg q24hours

Dose adjustment:
- •↓Initial dose by 50% if:
  - ∘Elderly
  - ∘Concomitant diuretic use
  - ∘Renal disease

Losartan specific:
- •Starting dose is halved if concomitant hepatic disease

RESCUE PROCEDURES ━━━━━━━━━━━━━━━

•**Rescue percutaneous transluminal coronary angioplasty–PTCA**

Indications:
- •Angina syndrome in:
  - ∘**All patients if performed within 2hours of presentation**
  - ∘Patients w/ absolute contraindications to thrombolytic treatment
  - ∘Patients unresponsive to thrombolytic treatment @ 90min. after administration

Outcomes:
- •↓Mortality or nonfatal myocardial re–infarction by 20% if performed by a skilled operator within 2hours of presentation

Advantages:
- •Normalization of blood flow in 90% of patients, without the ↑intracranial hemorrhage risk of thrombolytic treatment
- •When compared to thrombolytic treatment, it is superior in terms of:
  - ∘↓Short–term mortality
  - ∘↓Nonfatal myocardial re–infarction
  - ∘↓Cerebrovascular accident syndrome
  - …even when on site thrombolytic treatment is compared to delayed PTCA due to timely patient transfer to a medical center capable of performing the procedure

Limitations:
- •Takes longer to implement than thrombolytic treatment
- •Requires the 24hour availability of a catheterization laboratory

THROMBOLYTIC MEDICATIONS

Indications:
- •Patients who cannot undergo primary percutaneous transluminal coronary angioplasty within 2 hours of presentation, & who meet both the following syndromal & electrocardiographic criteria:
  - ∘**Syndromal criteria:** Either
    - –Myocardial ischemic syndrome being >30min., up to 24hours
  - ∘**Electrocardiographic criteria:** Either
    - –↑ST segments ≥1mv in ≥2 contiguous limb leads (I, II, III, aVR, aVL, aVF)
    - –↑ST segments ≥2mv in ≥2 precordial leads (V1–V6)
    - –New left bundle branch block
    - –↓ST segment & R waves in leads V1–V3, indicating a posterior infarction

Generic (trade)	M	♀	Dose	Max
Alteplase (Tissue plasminogen activator–tPA)	L	?	15mg IV push, then	
			0.75mg/kg IV infusion over 30min., then	50mg
			0.5mg/kg IV infusion over 1hour	35mg
Anistreplase (Eminase)	L	?	30mg IV slow push over 2min.	
Reteplase (Retavase)	L	?	10mg IV slow push over 2 min., then	
			repeat dose in 30min.	
Streptokinase (Kabikinase, Streptase)	L	?	1.5million units IV infusion over 1hour	

Tenecteplase (TNKase)	L	?	Single IV push over 5seconds

Body weight	Dosage
<60kg= <132 lbs	30mg
60–69kg=132–153 lbs	35mg
70–79kg=154–175 lbs	40mg
80–89kg=176–197 lbs	45mg
≥90kg= ≥198 lbs	50mg

•Aspirin & IV Heparin therapy (X 48hours) must be administered concomitantly→
  ◦↓Re–occlusion rate

Mechanism:
•Fibrinolysis→
  ◦↑Blood flow to the ischemic myocardium→
    –Salvaged myocardium
    –Stronger necrotic area scar formation
    ...both being ↑ w/ earlier administration

Outcomes:
•**Effective thrombolysis occurs in 80% of patients†**, w/ normalization of blood flow in 50% of patients within 2hours
•**≥ 50% ↓mortality w/ administration within 3hours**. 50% of patients treated @ >3hours have no salvaged myocardium, w/ the main mechanism of benefit being stronger scar formation
•**10% ↓mortality up to 12hours**

†Rescue PTCA should be considered in patients unresponsive to thrombolytic treatment @ 90min. after administration

Complications:
Cardiovascular
  •**Hemorrhage**
    ◦Most important being **intracranial hemorrhage**
      –Streptokinase–0.5%
      –Alteplase–0.7%
      –Lanetoplase, Reteplase or Tenecteplase–1%
    ...→**cerebrovascular accident syndrome** having a 65% overall mortality, being 95% @ age
        >75years
  Risk factors:
    •Elderly
    •Hypertension
    •History of cerebrovascular accident

Absolute contraindications:
  •Lifetime history of hemorrhagic stroke
  •Ischemic stroke within 1year
  •Suspected aortic dissection
  •Acute pericarditis
  •Active internal hemorrhage, not including menses
  •Intracranial or spinal:
    ◦Aneurysm
    ◦Arteriovenous malformation–AVM
    ◦Neoplasm

Relative contraindications:
  •≥Severe hypertension refractory to medical treatment, via either:
    ◦Systolic blood pressure ≥180mmHg
    ◦Diastolic blood pressure ≥110mmHg
  •History of ischemic stroke @ >1year
  •Significant trauma or surgery within 1month
  •Prolonged (>10min.) or traumatic CPR, or traumatic intubation
  •Noncompressible vascular punctures
  •Active peptic ulcer
  •Internal hemorrhage within 1month
  •Known bleeding diathesis
  •Current anticoagulation treatment w/ INR ≥2
  •Pregnancy
  •Liver failure
  •Diabetic hemorrhagic retinopathy
  •Hypersensitivity reaction to Streptokinase or Anistreplase, which contains Streptokinase. Also, patients should not receive Streptokinase if it was administered within 2years

<u>Monitoring:</u>
- Vital signs & neurologic examination q15min. during any infusion, then:
  - Q30min. X 6hours, then
    - -Q1hour X 16hours

- If severe headache, acute hypertension, altered mental status, nausea, or vomiting occur, discontinue the infusion, if still running, give cryoprecipitate, & obtain an emergent non-contrast computed tomography-CT scan to rule out intracranial hemorrhage

PROGNOSIS OF MYOCARDIAL INFARCTION
- Q wave formation, having an overall 1month mortality of 12%
- Non-Q wave formation, having an overall 1month mortality of 5%
- Overall 2 year mortality being 30%

<u>Killip class 30 day mortality</u>
- Based on hemodynamic compromise
  - **Class 1-85%:** No heart failure, having a 30 day mortality of 5%
  - **Class 2-13%:** Basilar crackles, ↑jugular venous distention, or S3, having a 30 day mortality of 14%
  - **Class 3-1%:** Crackles >50% of lung fields, having a 30 day mortality of 30%
  - **Class 4-1%:** Cardiogenic shock, having a 30 day mortality of 60%

HYPERTENSION

•A degenerative disease caused by any process→
 ◦**Persistently elevated systolic &/or diastolic arterial blood pressure**
•Arterial blood pressure = cardiac output (usually 4–7L/ min.) X peripheral vascular resistance
 ◦↑Of either→
  –↑Blood pressure, w/ ↑peripheral vascular resistance being necessary for it to be persistent
<u>Statistics:</u>
•One of the most preventable causes of premature death worldwide

CLASSIFICATION/ RISK FACTORS

ESSENTIAL HYPERTENSION >95% ▬▬▬▬▬▬▬▬▬▬▬▬▬▬▬▬▬▬▬▬▬▬▬▬▬▬▬▬▬▬▬▬
•Actually a misnomer, as hypertension is not essential to aging in order to ensure adequate blood flow through atherosclerotic arteries

•↑**Age**, affecting ≥50% of persons age >65years
 ◦Isolated systolic hypertension is the #1 form of hypertension @ age >60years
<u>Mechanism:</u>
 •↓Arterial capacitance→
  ◦↑Peripheral vascular resistance→
   –↑Systolic blood pressure relative to diastolic blood pressure→widened pulse pressure
    (systolic – diastolic blood pressure)
•↑**Dietary sodium**
•↓**Physical activity**
•**Obesity**
•**Skin color:** Blacks > whites
•**Insulin resistance→**
 ◦Diabetes mellitus type 2→
  –↑Insulin→renal NaCl & water reabsorption
•**Altered cytokine production**
 ◦↓Vasodilators: Nitric oxide, prostacyclin, &/or bradykinin
 ◦↑Vasoconstrictors: Angiotensin 2 &/or endothelin 1
•**Autonomic nervous system dysregulation**
 ◦↑Sympathetic nervous system activity

SECONDARY HYPERTENSION <5% ▬▬▬▬▬▬▬▬▬▬▬▬▬▬▬▬▬▬▬▬▬▬▬▬▬▬▬▬▬▬▬▬
•Is meant to include etiologic diseases & medications

•**Renal disease**
 ◦Parenchymal disease
 ◦**Renal artery stenosis–1%**→renin–angiotensin–aldosterone system mediated ↑renal retention of
  NaCl & water→hypertension via:
  –Atherosclerotic disease–65%, usually @ age >60years (♂ > ♀)
  –Fibromuscular dysplasia–35%, usually @ age 30–50 years (♀ > ♂), being rare in blacks
•**Medications**
 ◦Abrupt discontinuation of:
  –Chronic antihypertensive use, esp. Clonidine
  –Chronic opioid analgesic use
 ◦Estrogen containing oral contraceptives
 ◦Glucocorticoids via ↑renal retention of NaCl & water
 ◦Mineralocorticoids via ↑renal retention of NaCl & water
 ◦Monoamine oxidase inhibitors–MAOIs
<u>Mechanism:</u>
  •Tyramine, a byproduct of tyrosine metabolism in the body & in foods, is metabolized by the
   enzyme monoamine oxidase–MAO→
   ◦Suppression of its indirect sympathomimetic effect via its causing the release of presynaptic
    catecholamine granules. However, patients who take an MAOI (esp. type A inhibitors) lose the
    ability to metabolize large amounts of ingested tyramine found in certain foods:
    –Alcoholic beverages (ale, beer, chianti, cognac, red wine, sherry, vermouth), broad & fava
     beans, canned figs, cheeses (except cottage & cream cheese), chocolate, fish (anchovies,
     herring, sardines, shrimp paste, smoked or pickled fish), liver of all types, overripe fruits,
     processed meat, sauerkraut, sausage, soy sauce, yeast→hypertension
•**Sympathomimetic medications**
 ◦Decongestants

- **Illicit drug use, or abrupt discontinuation after chronic use**
  - ∘Amphetamines→
    - –↑Release of presynaptic catecholamines
  - ∘Cocaine→
    - –↓Presynaptic reuptake of released catecholamines
- **Dietary**
  - ∘**Alcohol**, causing 8% of hypertension in ♂s @ ≥2 drinks/ day
  - ∘**Chewing tobacco**
  - ∘↓**Potassium diet**
  - ∘**Licorice**
- **Endocrine**
  - ∘**Acromegally**
  - ∘**Hyperparathyroidism**
  - ∘**Hyperthyroidism**→
    - –↑Cardiac output→systolic hypertension
  - ∘**Hypothyroidism**→
    - –↑Peripheral vascular resistance→diastolic hypertension
  - ∘**Insulinoma**→↑insulin→
    - –↑Renal retention of NaCl & water
    - –↑Sympathetic nervous system activity
  - ∘**Glucocorticoid or mineralocorticoid excess**→↑renal retention of NaCl & water→hypertension
    - –Cushing's disease or syndrome
    - –Hyperaldosteronism, being either primary=Conn's syndrome, or secondary
  - ∘**Pheochromocytoma–0.2%**
- **•↑Intracranial pressure**, termed the Cushing reaction, via:
  - ∘Vascular compression→↓cerebral blood flow→ischemia→central nervous system vasomotor center mediated reflex hypertension→↑cerebral arterial pressure relative to intracerebral pressure→ ↑cerebral blood flow
    - –However, intracerebral pressure which cannot be overcome→vasomotor center dysfunction→ hypotension→distributive shock→death
- **Anatomic abnormality**
  - ∘Coarctation of the aorta
- **Gestational hypertension syndromes**
  - ∘Pre–eclampsia/ eclampsia

BLOOD PRESSURE CLASSIFICATION: Based on the average of 2 measurements			
Class	**Systolic** (mmHg)		**Diastolic** (mmHg)
Hypotensive	<90	or	<60
Normotensive	90–119	&	60–79
Pre–hypertension	120–139	or	80–89
Stage 1 hypertension	140–159	or	90–99
Stage 2 hypertension	160–209	or	100–119
Hypertensive urgency	≥210	or	≥120 being asymptomatic†
Hypertensive emergency	≥180	or	≥110 being symptomatic

†Requires reduction within 24hours

DIAGNOSIS

Cardiovascular
- •Hypertension→
  - ∘**Atherosclerosis** mediated macrovascular disease→
    - –**Coronary artery disease**→myocardial ischemic syndromes
    - –**Cerebrovascular disease**→cerebrovascular accident syndromes
    - –**Peripheral vascular disease**→renal artery stenosis, intermittent claudication, & thromboembolic disease
  - ∘↑Cardiac work to pump blood against the ↑systemic vascular resistance, termed the afterload→
    - –Myocardial hypertrophy, termed **secondary hypertrophic cardiomyopathy ± heart failure**→
    ↑Myocardial O$_2$ & nutrient demand, w/ concomitant ↓relative myocardial vascularity→myocardial ischemia→eventual **dilated cardiomyopathy ± heart failure**

How to properly measure arterial blood pressure†:
  1. Place the cuff snuggly around the biceps, in direct skin contact, as clothing→
     - •Lateral displacement of the generated pressure→
       - ∘Falsely ↑pressure readings
  2. Have the arm supported @ the level of the heart

3. Place the bell of the stethoscope lightly (but w/ skin contact over its entire circumference) over the brachial arterial pulse, just distal to the cuff
4. One hand should palpate the ipsilateral radial arterial pulse, while the other hand inflates the cuff quickly to a pressure ~10mmHg above the point at which the radial pulse disappears
   •A calcified radial artery may be palpable in the absence of a pulse, termed Osler's sign
5. To obtain the **systolic arterial blood pressure**, slowly deflate the cuff @1-3mmHg/ second or heart beat, until you auscultate the first Korotkoff sounds, being the episodic jet-like sounds of blood being forced through the narrowed artery during ventricular systole
6. To obtain the **diastolic blood pressure**, continue slowly deflating the cuff until the Korotkoff sounds disappear, indicating equalization of cuff pressure to arterial blood pressure during ventricular diastole

---

•One way to help patients understand the dangers of hypertension & the importance of treatment is by explaining that the discomfort they feel during the systolic arterial blood pressure measurement is the pressure being exerted on their arteries all day long
†Perform bilaterally at initial visit for possible significant differences due to atherosclerosis mediated peripheral vascular disease, w/ the higher result being the actual arterial blood pressure

Genitourinary
•Hypertension↔
  ◦Microvascular disease, including the glomerulus→renal disease, termed **nephropathy**, via:
   −Albuminuria↔renal failure

Categorization of albuminuria via urinary albumin (µg) ÷ urinary creatinine (mg)†:
  •<30: Normal
  •30-299: Microalbuminuria
  •≥300: Macroalbuminuria
  Limitations:
    •The following ↑urinary albumin excretion:
    ◦Heart failure
    ◦Exercise within 24hours
    ◦Fever
    ◦Infection
    ◦Severe hyperglycemia

---

†Via spot or 24hour urine collection. The measurement of urinary albumin without the concomitant measurement of urinary creatinine→
  •Falsely ↑ or ↓determinations as a result of variation of urine concentration

Opthalmologic
•Hypertension→
  ◦Microvascular disease, including the retinal vasculature→
   −Retinal disease, termed **retinopathy** (visible in the macula via opthalmoscopic examination), which may be asymptomatic despite the presence of severe disease
Hematologic
•Nephropathy→
  ◦Intra-renal renal failure→
   −↑Blood urea nitrogen−BUN & creatinine
•Severe hypertension→
  ◦Microangiopathic hemolytic anemia

TREATMENT
Outcomes:
  ◦↓**Left ventricular hypertrophy**
  ◦↓**Cardiovascular mortality**
  ◦**40%↓incidence of heart failure**
  …w/ most patients requiring ≥2 medications to reach their goal blood pressure

•**Smoking cessation** via smoking cessation clinic
  ◦Cigarette smoking contributes to 20% of deaths in the U.S., & is the #1 modifiable cause of premature death
•**Exercise**
  ◦An enjoyable form of aerobic exercise on a regular basis (≥3X/ week) for 20-30min., preceded by stretching

- **Emotional stress management**
  - Biofeedback
  - Gardening
  - Listening to music
  - Psychological therapy
  - Regular exercise
  - Yoga
- **Dietician consultation**
- **Glycemic control if hyperglycemic**
- **Weight loss if overweight/ obese†, via goal daily caloric requirement**
  - The caloric total needed to reach & maintain a goal weight depends on physical activity level
  - 10 calories/ lb of goal weight +
    - −33% if sedentary
    - −50% if moderately physically active
    - −75% if very physically active
  - 3500 calories are roughly equivalent to 1 lb of body fat
    - −Consuming 500calories less/ day X 1week→1 lb weight loss
    - −Exercising 500calories/ day X 1week→1 lb weight loss
  - …w/ the average human body being able to lose 3.5 lbs/ week maximum, aside from a diuretic effect
- **↓Sodium intake**
  - ≤100mmol sodium/ 24hours=2g elemental sodium or 6g salt/ 24hours, which can usually be achieved w/ a no-added salt diet. Patients w/ poorly compensated heart failure should only consume 0.5–1g elemental sodium or 1.5–3g salt/ 24hours
  - →↓Renal potassium loss if taking a diuretic
- **↓Alcohol consumption**
  - Only 1drink q24hours (8–12 ounces of beer, 3–5 ounces of wine, or 1 ounce of liquor) in patients without a history of drug abuse
  - ≥2 drinks/ 24hours→
    - −Hypertension
    - −Hepatitis (♀ > ♂)
    - −↑Abuse risk
  - If alcohol is suspected to be causative, total abstinence is required
- **↓Saturated & total fat consumption**
- **↑Fruit & vegetable consumption**

β1 SELECTIVE RECEPTOR BLOCKERS				
Generic (Trade)	M	♀	**Start**	**Max**
Atenolol (Tenormin)	K	U	25mg PO q24hours	100mg/ 24hours
Metoprolol (Lopressor)	L	?	25mg PO q12hours	225mg q12hours
•XR form (Toprol XL)			50mg PO q24hours	400mg q24hours
α1 & NONSELECTIVE β RECEPTOR BLOCKERS				
Generic (Trade)	M	♀	**Start**	**Max**
Carvedilol (Coreg)	L	?	6.25mg PO q12hours	25mg q12hours
Labetalol (Normodyne)	LK	?	100mg PO q12hours	1200mg q12hours

Mechanism:
- Competitive antagonist of the β1 ± β2 receptor→
  - ↓Sinoatrial & atrioventricular node conduction (β1)→
    - −↓Pulse
  - Anti-dysrhythmic via nodal effects (β1)
  - ↓Cardiac muscle contractile strength (β1)
  - ↓Juxtaglomerular cell renin release (β1)→
    - −↓Angiotensin 1, angiotensin 2, & aldosterone formation
  - ↓Cardiovascular remodeling
  - ↑Vascular/ organ smooth muscle contraction (β2)→
    - −Vasoconstriction
    - −Bronchoconstriction
    - −Uterine contraction
  - ↓Tremor (β2)
  - ↓Hepatocyte glycogenolysis (β2)
- ↓Extrathyroidal tetraiodothyronine−T4 (also termed thyroxine) conversion to the more metabolically active triiodothyronine−T3 form

Side effects:
General
- Fatigue
- Malaise

Cardiovascular
- Bradycardia ± heart block
- Hypotension
  - Orthostatic hypotension
  - Pelvic hypotension→
    - −Impotence, being the inability to achieve &/or maintain an erection
- Initial worsening of systolic heart failure
- Worsening symptoms of peripheral vascular disease
  - Intermittent claudication
  - Raynaud's phenomenon

Pulmonary
- Bronchoconstriction

Endocrine
- ↑Risk of developing diabetes mellitus
- May block catecholamine mediated:
  - Physiologic reversal of hypoglycemia via:
    - −↓Hepatocyte gluconeogenesis
  - ↓Hypoglycemic symptoms, termed hypoglycemic unawareness→
    - −↓Tachycardia as a warning sign

Gastrointestinal
- Diarrhea
- Nausea ± vomiting
- Gastroesophageal reflux

Mucocutaneous
- Hair thinning

Neurologic
- Sedation
- Sleep alterations
- ↓Libido→
  - Impotence

Psychiatric
- Depression

Hematologic
- ↓High density lipoprotein−HDL levels

- Most patients w/ chronic obstructive pulmonary disease−COPD (including asthma), diabetes, &/or peripheral vascular disease can be safely treated w/ **cardioselective β1 receptor blockers**, as they have ↓peripheral effects

Contraindications:
Cardiovascular
- **Acutely decompensated heart failure**
- Hypotension
- Pulse <50bpm
- Atrioventricular heart block of any degree

Pulmonary
- Moderate to severe chronic obstructive pulmonary disease−COPD, including asthma

Hyper−catacholamine state
- Amphetamine use
- **Cocaine use†**
- Clonidine withdrawal
- Monoamine oxidase inhibitor−MAOi mediated tyramine effect
- Pheochromocytoma
  ...→relatively ↑vascular α1 receptor stimulation="unopposed α effect"→
      - Vasoconstriction→
        - Myocardial ischemic syndrome
        - Cerebrovascular accident syndrome
        - Peripheral vascular ischemic syndrome
  Note: **Carvedilol** & **Labetalol** may be used due to their α1 blocking property

---

†Cocaine use→
- Varying ischemic syndrome onset per administration route, & may occur @ min. to days (usually within 3hours)

64

ANGIOTENSIN CONVERTING ENZYME INHIBITORS–ACEi				
Generic (Trade)	**M**	**♀**	**Start**	**Max**
Benazepril (Lotensin)	LK	U	10mg PO q24hours	40mg/ 24hours
Captopril (Capoten)	LK	U	12.5mg PO q12hours	450mg/ 24hours
Enalapril (Vasotec)	LK	U	5mg PO q24hours	40mg/ 24hour
Fosinopril (Monopril)	LK	U	10mg PO q24hours	40mg/ 24hours
Lisinopril (Prinivil, Zestril)	K	U	10mg PO q24hours	40mg q24hours

Dose adjustment:
- ↓Initial dose by 50% if:
  - ∘Elderly
  - ∘Concomitant diuretic use
  - ∘Renal disease

Mechanism:
- •Reversibly inhibits angiotensin converting enzyme–ACE→
  - ∘↓Bradykinin degradation→
    - –Vasodilation
  - ∘↓Angiotensin 2 formation→
    - –Vasodilation (**arterial** > venous)
    - –↓Renal NaCl & water retention
    - –↓Adrenal cortex aldosterone release→↓renal NaCl & water retention
    - –↓Facilitation of adrenal medullary & presynaptic norepinephrine release→vasodilation
    - –Glomerular efferent arteriole vasodilation→↓intraglomerular hydrostatic pressure→↓filtration→ ↓proteinuria in patients w/ nephropathy
  - ∘↓Cardiovascular remodeling

Side effects:
Cardiovascular
- •Hypotension
Gastrointestinal
- •Altered gustatory sense=dysguesia–3%
Genitourinary
- •Acute interstitial nephritis
- •Patients w/ pre–existing bilateral ↓renal perfusion, not necessarily failure:
  - ∘Heart failure
  - ∘Bilateral renal artery stenosis
  - ∘Hypovolemia
  - ∘Renal failure
  - …rely more on the compensatory production of angiotensin 2→
    - •Efferent arteriole constriction→
      - ∘Maintained glomerular filtration rate–GFR, whereas either:
        - –Angiotensin converting enzyme inhibition
        - –Angiotensin 2 receptor blockade
        - …→↓angiotensin 2 production & action respectively, which may→
          - •Pre–renal renal failure
Mucocutaneous
- •↓Bradykinin & substance P degradation→↑levels→hypersensitivity–like syndrome→
  - ∘**Angioedema–0.4%**, usually within 2weeks of treatment, but may manifest @ months to years→
    - –Soft tissue edema of the epiglottis, face, lips, oropharynx, &/or tongue
  - ∘**Dermatitis–10%**
Pulmonary
- •↑Bradykinin levels→
  - ∘**Chronic cough–20%**, usually being dry & involuntary
Materno–fetal
- •**Fetal & neonatal morbidity & mortality**
Hematologic
- •↓Aldosterone production ± renal failure→
  - ∘**Hyperkalemia**
- •Neutropenia

Monitoring:
- •Check creatinine & potassium @ 3–10days after initiation or dose↑, then
  - ∘Q3–6months

Contraindications:
Genitourinary
- •Acute renal failure
- •Bilateral renal artery stenosis
- •Unilateral renal artery stenosis of a solitary functioning kidney

Mucocutaneous
- •Angiotensin converting enzyme inhibitor induced angioedema or dermatitis

Materno-fetal
- •Breast feeding
- •**Pregnancy**

Hematologic
- •**Potassium >5mEq/ L**

ANGIOTENSIN 2 RECEPTOR BLOCKERS-ARBs

Generic (Trade)	M	♀	Start	Max
Candesartan (Atacand)	K	?	16mg PO q24hours	32mg q24hours
Eprosartan (Teveten)	F	U	600mg PO q24hours	800mg/ 24hours
Irbesartan (Avapro)	L	U	150mg PO q24hours	300mg q24hours
Olmisartan (Benicar)	K	U	20mg PO q24hours	40mg q24hours
Losartan (Cozaar)	L	U	50mg PO q24hours	100mg/ 24hours
Telmisartan (Micardis)	L	U	40mg PO q24hours	80mg q24hours
Valsartan (Diovan)	L	U	80mg PO q24hours	320mg q24hours

Dose adjustment:
- •↓Initial dose by 50% if:
  - ◦Elderly
  - ◦Concomitant diuretic use
  - ◦Renal disease

Losartan specific:
- •Starting dose is halved if concomitant hepatic disease

Mechanism:
- •Angiotensin 2 receptor blockade→
  - ◦↓Angiotensin 2 action→
    - −Vasodilation (**arterial** > venous)
    - −↓Renal NaCl & water retention
    - −↓Adrenal cortex aldosterone release→↓renal NaCl & water retention
    - −↓Facilitation of adrenal medullary & presynaptic norepinephrine release→vasodilation
    - −Glomerular efferent arteriole vasodilation→↓intraglomerular hydrostatic pressure→↓filtration→
      ↓proteinuria in patients w/ nephropathy
  - ◦↓Cardiovascular remodeling

Side effects†:
Cardiovascular
- •Hypotension

Gastrointestinal
- •Altered gustatory sense=dysguesia−3%

Genitourinary
- •Acute interstitial nephritis
- •Patients w/ preexisting bilateral ↓renal perfusion, not necessarily failure:
  - ◦Heart failure
  - ◦Bilateral renal artery stenosis
  - ◦Hypovolemia
  - ◦Renal failure
  - …rely more on the compensatory production of angiotensin 2→
    - •Efferent arteriole constriction→
      - ◦Maintained glomerular filtration rate−GFR, whereas either:
        - −Angiotensin converting enzyme inhibition
        - −Angiotensin 2 receptor blockade
        - …→↓angiotensin 2 production & action respectively, which may→
          - •**Pre-renal renal failure**

Materno-fetal
- •**Fetal & neonatal morbidity & mortality**

Hematologic
- •↓Aldosterone production ± renal failure→
  - ◦**Hyperkalemia**
- •Neutropenia

66

†Do not cause the hypersensitivity–like syndrome associated w/ ACE inhibitors, due to lack of bradykinin & substance P elevation

Monitoring:
- Check creatinine & potassium @ 3–10days after initiation or dose†, then
  - Q3–6months

Contraindications:
  Genitourinary
  - Acute renal failure
  - Bilateral renal artery stenosis
  - Unilateral renal artery stenosis of a solitary functioning kidney
  Materno–fetal
  - Breast feeding
  - **Pregnancy**
  Hematologic
  - **Potassium >5mEq/ L**

CALCIUM CHANNEL BLOCKERS: Dihydropyridines

Generic (Trade)	M	♀	Start	Max
Amlodipine (Norvasc)	L	?	2.5mg PO q24hours	10mg q24hours
Felodipine (Plendil)	L	?	2.5mg PO q24hours	10mg q24hours
Isradipine (DynaCirc)	L	?	2.5mg PO q12hours	10mg q12hours
•XR form			5mg PO q24hours	20mg q24hours
Nicardipine (Cardene)	L	?		
•XR form			30mg PO q12hours	60mg q12hours
Nifedipine (Procardia)	L	?		
•XR form			30mg PO q24hours	120mg PO q24hours
Nisoldipine (Sular)	L	?	20mg PO q24hours	60mg q24hours

Dose adjustment:
- **Isradipine:** Maximal dose is halved in the elderly
- **Nisoldipine:** Starting dose is halved in the elderly or hepatic disease

CALCIUM CHANNEL BLOCKERS: Non–dihydropyridines

Generic	M	♀	Start	Max
Diltiazem	L	?	30mg PO q8hours	120mg q8hours
•XR form			As per daily requirement	
◦QDXR form			120mg PO q12hours	540mg q24hours
◦BIDXR form			60mg PO q12hours	180mg q12hours
Verapamil	L	?	40mg PO q8hours	160mg q8hours
•XR form			As per daily requirement	
◦Calan XR form			120mg PO q24hours	480mg/ 24hours
◦Veleran XR form			100mg PO q24hours	400mg q24hours
◦Covera XR form			180mg PO q24hours	480mg qhs

Mechanism:
- Block voltage dependent calcium ion channels in smooth & cardiac muscle→
  - ↓Calcium influx→
    - ↓Sinoatrial & atrioventricular node conduction (non–dihydropyridines)→↓pulse
    - Anti–dysrhythmic via nodal effects (mainly non–dihydropyridines)
    - ↓Cardiac muscle contractile strength (mainly non–dihydropyridines)
    - Vasodilation: Arterial > venous (mainly dihydropyridines)

Side effects:
  Cardiovascular
  - Bradycardia ± heart block
  - Edema
  - Flushing
  - Hypotension
  Gastrointestinal
  - Constipation
  - Nausea ± vomiting
  Neurologic
  - Dizziness
  - Headache

ANTIDOTES				
Generic	**M**	**♀**	**Dose**	**Max**
Glucagon	LK	P	3mg IV slow push over 1min., then	
			5mg IV slow push over 1 min. if needed	
•Continuous infusion			5mg/ hour	
10% Calcium chloride†			10mL (1 ampule) IV slow push over 3min., then	
			repeat @5min. if needed	
•Continuous infusion			Start 0.3mEq/ hour	0.7mEq/ hour
Onset: 1–2 min., Duration: 30–60 min.				
Magnesium sulfate	K	S	2g MgSO$_4$ in 50mL saline infused over 15min., then	
			6g MgSO$_4$ in 500mL saline infused over 6hours	

†Use cautiously in patients taking Digoxin, as hypercalcemia→
  •Digoxin cardiotoxicity

THIAZIDE DIURETICS				
Generic (Trade)	**M**	**♀**	**Start**	**Max**
Hydrochlorothiazide	L	U	12.5mg PO q24hours	50mg q24hours
Metolazone (Zaroxolyn)	L	U	5mg PO q24hours	10mg q24hours
Duration: 6–12hours				

•There is synergistic efficacy of combination treatment w/ a loop diuretic

Mechanism:
  •Inhibits NaCl reabsorption in the early distal convoluted tubule→
    ∘↑Urination→
      −↓Intravascular volume→↓cardiac preload→↓cardiac output→eventual compensatory
       intravascular volume repletion to near pre-treatment levels, but w/ peripheral vascular
       resistance falling below pre-treatment baseline being responsible for the chronic hypotensive
       effect

Limitations:
  •↓Efficacy in patients w/ a glomerular filtration rate <30mL/ min.

Side effects:
  Genitourinary
    •Acute interstitial nephritis
  Neurologic
    •**Ototoxicity**
  Hematologic
    •Acid base disturbances
      ∘Hypochloremic metabolic alkalemia
    •Dyslipidemia
      ∘↑Cholesterol & triglycerides
    •Electrolyte disturbances
      ∘**Hypokalemia**
      ∘Hypomagnesemia
      ∘Hyponatremia
      ∘Hypercalcemia
    •Hyperglycemia
    •Hyperuricemia

Contraindications:
  •**Sulfa allergy**, as all thiazide & loop diuretics (except Ethacrynic acid) contain a sulfa component

LOOP DIURETICS

Generic (Trade)	M	♀	Start	Max
Furosemide (Lasix)	K	?	20mg q24–12hours PO	600mg/ 24hours

Onset: 1hour, Duration: 6hours (La**six** lasts **six** hours)

•There is synergistic efficacy of combination treatment w/ a thiazide diuretic
•Administer 2nd dose in the mid–afternoon to avoid nocturia

Mechanism:
 •Inhibits $Na^+/K^+/2Cl^-$ reabsorption in the thick ascending limb of the loop of Henle→
  ∘↑Urination→
   –↓Intravascular volume→↓cardiac preload→↓cardiac output→eventual compensatory
    intravascular volume repletion to near pre–treatment levels, but w/ peripheral vascular
    resistance falling below pre–treatment baseline being responsible for the chronic hypotensive
    effect

Limitations:
 •↓Efficacy in patients w/ a glomerular filtration rate <10mL/ min.

Side effects:
 Genitourinary
  •Acute interstitial nephritis
 Neurologic
  •**Ototoxicity**
 Hematologic
  •Acid base disturbances
   ∘Hypochloremic metabolic alkalemia
  •Dyslipidemia
   ∘↑Cholesterol & triglycerides
  •Electrolyte disturbances
   ∘**Hypokalemia**
   ∘Hypomagnesemia
   ∘Hyponatremia
   ∘Hypercalcemia
  •Hyperglycemia
  •Hyperuricemia

Contraindications:
 •**Sulfa allergy**, as all thiazide & loop diuretics (except Ethacrynic acid) contain a sulfa component

DIETARY

Generic (Trade)	M	♀	Dose
Omega 3–fatty acids (Fish oil)	L	?	A combination dose of EPA + DHA†
•Cardioprotection			1g PO q24hours
•Hypertriglyceridemia			2–4g PO q24hours

---

†Eicosapentanoic acid–EPA & docosahexanoic acid–DHA
•There are only 2 types of polyunsaturated fatty acids
 ∘Omega 3–fatty acids, mainly from:
  –**Fish or fish oils**, esp. herring, mackerel, salmon, sardines, trout, & tuna
  –Beans, esp. soybeans
  –Green leafy vegetables
  –Nuts, esp. walnuts
  –Plant seeds, esp. canola oil & flaxseed
 ∘Omega 6–fatty acids, mainly from:
  –Grains
  –Meats
  –Nuts, esp. peanuts
  –Plant seeds, esp. borage oil, corn oil, cottonseed oil, grape seed oil, primrose oil, safflower oil,
   sesame oil, soybean oil, & sunflower oil
•The Western diet is abundant in omega 6–fatty acids (which are prothrombotic & proinflammatory),
 w/ humans lacking the necessary enzymes to convert them to omega 3–fatty acids, which therefore
 need to be obtained from separate dietary sources. However, significant amounts of methylmercury
 & other environmental toxins may be concentrated in certain fish species (w/ high quality fish oil
 supplements usually lacking contaminants):
  •King Mackerel
  •Shark
  •Swordfish
  •Tilefish, aka golden bass or golden snapper

...which are to be avoided by:
- •♀ who may become or are pregnant
- •♀ who are breastfeeding
- •Young children

Mechanism:
- •Vasodilation→
  - ∘↓Blood pressure, being dose dependent, w/ a minimal effect of 4/ 2 mmHg w/ doses of 3–6g q24h
- •↓Lipid, esp. triglycerides
- •Anti–dysrhythmic
- •Anti–inflammatory
- •↓Platelet activity

Outcomes:
- •In patients w/ coronary artery disease:
  - ∘↓All cause mortality
  - ∘↓Dysrhythmia mediated sudden death

Side effects:
Cardiovascular
- •↑Bleeding time→
  - ∘Excessive hemorrhage
Gastrointestinal
- •Belching
- •Bloating
- •Fishy aftertaste
- •Nausea ± vomiting
Hematologic
- •Hyperglycemia
Interactions
- •None known, making it safe for use in combination w/ other:
  - ∘Anticoagulant medications
  - ∘Antiplatelet medications
  - ∘Lipid lowering medications

POTASSIUM
- **•Always measure the magnesium level concomitantly**

Indications:
- •Ensure a potassium of 4–5mEq/ L

Generic
- •Potassium chloride–KCL
- •Potassium bicarbonate
- •Potassium citrate
- •Potassium acetate
- •Potassium gluconate
- •Potassium phosphate

POTASSIUM DOSAGE ADJUSTMENT SCALE†_____

Plasma K^+ (mEq/ L)	K^+ repletion (mEq)
≥3.9	None
3.7–3.8	20
3.5–3.6	40
3.3–3.4	60
3.1–3.2	80
≤3	100

†Half all above doses @ a glomerular filtration rate–GFR ≤30mL/ min.

Outcomes:
- •Anti–dysrhythmic
- •↑Cardiac contractility in heart failure
- •Modest hypotensive effect in some patients
- •↓Cerebrovascular disease risk, apart from its possible blood pressure lowering effects

70

DIETARY			
Generic (Trade)	M ♀	Dose	
Garlic (Allium sativum)	? U	600–900mg PO q24hours	

Mechanism:
- ↓Blood pressure
- ↓Lipids
- ↓Platelet activity

SECOND LINE TREATMENT

POTASSIUM SPARING DIURETICS: Although these medications are weak antihypertensive agents when used alone, they provide an additive hypotensive effect when used in combination w/ other diuretic types, as well as ↓potassium & magnesium loss

Generic (Trade)	M	♀	Start	Target
Amiloride (Midamor)	LK	P	5mg PO q24hours	20mg q24hours
Eplerenone (Inspra)	L	P	50mg PO q24hours	50mg q12hours
Spironolactone (Aldactone)	LK	U	50mg PO q24hours	100mg/ 24hours
Triamterene (Dyrenium)	LK	P	25mg PO q24hours	100mg q24hours

Duration:
- Amiloride & Triamterene: 12–24hours
- Spironolactone: 24–72hours

Titration:
- Based on plasma potassium
- A urinary sodium/ potassium ratio >1 indicates effective aldosterone antagonism

Amiloride & Triamterene specific mechanism:
- Terminal distal convoluted tubule & collecting duct membrane sodium channel blockade→
  ∘↓Sodium reabsorption→
    –↓Compensatory potassium & hydrogen excretion for the maintenance of electroneutrality, regardless of the presence of aldosterone

Eplerenone & Spironolactone specific mechanism:
- Structurally similar to aldosterone→
  ∘Competitive inhibition of the intracellular aldosterone receptor in the distal convoluted tubule & collecting duct

...all→↑urination→
- ↓Intravascular volume→
  ∘↓Cardiac preload→↓cardiac output→
    –↓Blood pressure, w/ eventual compensatory intravascular volume repletion to near pre-treatment levels, but w/ peripheral vascular resistance falling below pre-treatment baseline being responsible for the chronic hypotensive effect

Side effects:
  Hematologic
- Acid base disturbances
  ∘Non-anion gap hypochloremic metabolic acidemia
- Electrolyte disturbances
  ∘**Hyperkalemia**
  ∘Hyponatremia
- Hyperuricemia

Spironolactone specific:
  Endocrine
- Anti-androgenic effects→
  ∘**Gynecomastia**, being the ↑development of male mammary glands

Monitoring:
- Monitor creatinine & potassium @ baseline, then
  ∘@ 1week, then
  ∘@ 1, 2, & 3months, then
  ∘Q3months for the remainder of the 1st year, then
  ∘Q6months thereafter

Contraindications:
- Potassium >5 mEq/ L

α2 SELECTIVE RECEPTOR AGONIST

Generic	M ♀	Start	Max
Clonidine	KL ?	0.1mg PO q12hours to q8hours	2.4mg/ 24hours
•Transdermal form		0.1mg q24hours patch qweek	0.6mg q24hours

Mechanisms:
- •Presynaptic cholinergic & adrenergic α2 receptor agonism→
  - ∘↑Presynaptic negative feedback→
    - −↓Catecholamine & acetylcholine release→↓autonomic sympathetic function relative to autonomic parasympathetic function

Side effects:
Cardiovascular
- •Bradycardia
- •Sexual dysfunction

Gastrointestinal
- •Constipation

Mucocutaneous
- •Dry mouth

Neurologic
- •Sedation

Other
- •Sudden discontinuation→
  - ∘Severe **rebound hypertension**

α1 SELECTIVE RECEPTOR BLOCKERS

Generic (Trade)	M ♀	Start	Max
Alfuzosin (UroXatral)	KL P	10mg PO qhs	10mg qhs
Doxazosin (Cardura)	L ?	1mg PO qhs	8mg qhs
Terazosin (Hytrin)	LK ?	1mg PO qhs	20mg qhs

Mechanism:
- •Reversible α1 receptor antagonist→
  - ∘Vasodilation (arterial=venous)

Side effects:
Cardiovascular
- •**Orthostatic hypotension**→
  - ∘Pre-syncope/ syncope, being ↓by:
    - −Low starting dose w/ gradual titration. If treatment is interrupted X several days, restart @ low dose w/ gradual titration
    - −Bedtime administration
    - −Continued use
- •Sexual dysfunction

Mucocutaneous
- •Dry mouth

Neurologic
- •Headache
- •Lethargy
- •Nightmares

VASODILATORS

Generic (Trade)	M ♀	Start	Max
Hydralazine (Apresoline)	LK ?	10mg PO q12hours X 2–4days, then 25mg PO q12hours	200mg q12hours
Minoxidil (Loniten)	K ?	2.5mg PO q24hours	100mg q24hours

Mechanism:
- •Vasodilation (**arterial** >> venous)

Side effects:
Cardiovascular
- •Systemic vasodilation→
  - ∘Edema
  - ∘Reflex tachycardia
  - ∘Orthostatic hypotension
- •Meningeal arterial dilation→
  - ∘Headache

72

Pulmonary
•Pulmonary vasodilation→
  ◦Exacerbation of ventilation/ perfusion mismatches

Hydralazine specific:
Autoimmune
•**Systemic lupus erythematosis–SLE like syndrome–10%,** being reversible upon discontinuation of the medication

Minoxidil specific:
Cardiovascular
•Pericardial lesions
Mucocutaneous
•Hirsutism

Contraindications:
Cardiovascular
•Hypotension
•Severe aortic or mitral stenosis

Hydralazine specific:
Autoimmune
•Systemic lupus erythematosis–SLE

VASCULAR PROTECTION

PLATELET INHIBITING MEDICATIONS
Efficacy: Glycoprotein 2b/ 3a inhibitors > thienopyridines > Aspirin

Generic	M	♀	Dose
Acetylsalicylic acid–ASA=Aspirin	K	U	81mg PO q24hours

Mechanism:
•Aspirin is the only nonsteroidal anti–inflammatory drug–NSAID→
  ◦Irreversible inhibition of both cyclooxygenase–COX enzymes (COX1 & COX2), w/ COX1 being responsible for the production of both thromboxane A_2† & prostacyclin‡→
    –**Near complete inhibition of platelet thromboxane A_2 production within 15 min.,** w/ endothelial & vascular smooth muscle cells producing new enzymes in several hours→ relatively ↑prostacyclin
•Being that platelets lack the enzymatic machinery for protein synthesis, only newly formed platelets (platelet half life=10 days) have the functional enzyme
…this shift in the balance of cytokine production→
  •↓**Thrombus formation**

In Brief:
•**Cyclooxygenase–COX1 enzymes** are found in most cells of the body, being responsible for normal physiologic processes
•**Cyclooxygenase–COX 2 enzymes** are responsible for the production of inflammatory cell prostaglandins

---

•Concomitant NSAID administration→
  ◦Competition for the cyclooxygenase–COX 1 enzyme binding site, w/:
    –Unbound Aspirin being rapidly cleared from plasma
    –Bound NSAID action being reversible & short lived
    …→↓overall antiplatelet effect, requiring either:
      •Aspirin to be taken @ ≥1hour prior to other NSAIDs
      •Switch to thienopyridine derivative for the antiplatelet effect
†Platelet mediated **thromboxane A_2** release at the site of vascular injury→
  •Platelet aggregation
  •Vasoconstriction
  …w/ both processes→
    •Thrombus formation
‡Endothelial & vascular smooth muscle cell mediated **prostacyclin** release in the surrounding area→
  •Inhibition of platelet aggregation
  •Vasodilation
  …w/ both processes→
    •↓Thrombus formation

<u>Side effects:</u>
Gastrointestinal
- Inhibition of the cyclooxygenase–COX1 enzyme→↑peptic inflammatory disease risk→↑**upper gastrointestinal hemorrhage risk** via:
  - ↓Gastric mucosal prostaglandin synthesis→
    - –↓Epithelial cell proliferation
    - –↓Mucosal blood flow→↓bicarbonate delivery to the mucosa
    - –↓Mucus & bicarbonate secretion from gastric mucosal cells

<u>Indications for peptic inflammatory disease prophylaxis:</u>
- Prophylax w/ proton pump inhibitors–PPI's, histamine 2 selective receptor blockers, or Misoprostol in patients w/ any of the following:
  - Age >60 years w/ a history of peptic inflammatory disease
  - Anticipated therapy >3 months
  - Concurrent glucocorticoid use
  - Moderate to high dose NSAID use
  <u>Note:</u> Newer NSAIDs (Etodolac, Nabumetone, Salsalate)→
    - ↓Risk of NSAID induced peptic inflammation/ ulcer

Genitourinary
- Patients w/ pre-existing bilateral ↓renal perfusion, not necessarily failure:
  - Heart failure
  - Bilateral renal artery stenosis
  - Hypovolemia
  - Renal failure
  …rely more on the compensatory production of vasodilatory prostaglandins→
    - Afferent arteriole dilation→
      - Maintained glomerular filtration rate–GFR, whereas NSAIDs→
        - –↓Prostaglandin production, which may→renal failure
Pulmonary
- Inhibition of both cyclooxygenase enzymes (COX 1 & COX2)→
  - ↑Lipoxygenase activity→
    - –↑Leukotriene synthesis→symptomatic asthma within 2hours of ingestion in 5% of asthmatics
Rheumatologic
- Acetylsalicylic acid competes w/ uric acid secretion in the renal tubules→
  - ↑Uric acid levels→
    - –↑Risk of uric acid precipitation in the tissues=gout
Pediatric
- **Reye's syndrome**
  - A life threatening fulminant hepatitis→
    - –Hepatic encephalopathy in children age ≤16 years w/ a viral infection (esp. Influenza or Varicella–zoster virus–VZV)

<u>Overdose:</u>
Pulmonary
- Direct brainstem respiratory center mediated stimulation of pulmonary ventilation→
  - Hyperventilation→
    - –**Initial respiratory alkalemia, w/ the subsequent development of an anion gap metabolic acidemia**
- Pulmonary edema
Neurologic
- Altered mental status
- Aseptic meningitis
- Depression
- Hallucinations
- Hyperactivity
- Hyperthermia
- Lightheadedness
- Seizures
- Tinnitus
Gastrointestinal
- Nausea ± vomiting
Mucocutaneous
- Pharyngitis

74

THIENOPYRIDINE DERIVATIVE			
Indications:			
•Intolerance to Aspirin			
Generic (Trade)	**M**	♀	**Dose**
Clopidogrel (Plavix)	LK	P	75mg PO q24hours

Mechanism:
  •Inhibits adenosine diphosphate–ADP mediated activation of the glycoprotein 2b/ 3a complex→
    ∘↓Platelet activation

•A 300mg loading dose may be used, as maximal effect occurs @ 5hours rather than 5days w/ initiation of the standard 75mg dosage

Side effects:
  Gastrointestinal
    •Diarrhea
  Mucocutaneous
    •Dermatitis
  Hematologic
    •**Thrombotic thrombocytopenic purpura–TTP** within several weeks of initiation

75

TREATMENT OF HYPERTENSIVE EMERGENCY

- •This is a **medical emergency**, indicative of altered **vascular autoregulation**→
  - ∘The inability to compensate for acutely ↓blood pressure→
    - –↓Renal perfusion→acute pre–renal renal failure→acute tubular necrosis→intra–renal renal failure
    - –↓Cerebral perfusion→pre–syncope/ syncope &/or cerebrovascular accident
    - –↓Myocardial perfusion→stable angina mediated acute coronary syndrome
- •The patient must be admitted to the hospital where intravenous medications can be administered in order to initially
  - ∘↓**Systolic blood pressure to 150–160** X several days, in order for the systemic vasculature to regain its autoregulating ability, after which the blood pressure may be normalized. **However, the treatment of ischemic cerebrovascular accidents differs** (see section)

- •Blood pressure should be monitored in real time via an arterial line

---

β1 SELECTIVE RECEPTOR BLOCKERS

Generic (Trade)	M	♀	Start
Esmolol (Brevibloc)	K	?	0.5mg=500µg/ kg IV loading bolus (over 1 min.), then
			0.05mg=50µg/kg/min. continuous IV infusion w/ titration prn†
			Max: 0.3mg=300µg/kg/min.

Onset: 1–2 min., Duration: 10 min.

---

†Titrate q4 min. via re–administration of the loading bolus & an additional 50µg/kg/min. IV infusion

α1 & NONSELECTIVE β RECEPTOR BLOCKERS

Generic (Trade)	M	♀	Start	Max
Labetalol (Normodyne)	LK	?	20mg IV push over 2min., then	
			40mg IV push q10min. prn goal blood pressure, then	300mg total
			0.5–2mg/ min. IV infusion	

Onset: 5–10min., Duration: 3–6hours

CALCIUM CHANNEL BLOCKERS: Dihydropyridines

Generic	M	♀	Start	Max
Nicardipine	L	?	5mg/ hour IV infusion	15mg/ hour

CALCIUM CHANNEL BLOCKERS: Non–dihydropyridines

Generic	M	♀	Start	Max
Diltiazem	L	?	5mg/ hour infusion	15mg/ hour

NITROVASODILATORS

Generic	M	♀	Start	Max
Nitroglycerin		L	?	10µg/ min. IV infusion	100µg/ min.
Nitroprusside sodium (Nipride, Nitropress)	E	?	0.3µg/kg/min. IV infusion	8µg/kg/min.

Onset: 2–5min., w/ tolerance typically within 24–48hours, Duration: ≤5min. after discontinuation

---

- •Nitroglycerin binds to soft plastics such as polyvinylchloride–PVC, which is a common constituent of plastic bags & infusion tubing→
  - ∘≤80% absorptive loss, being avoided via the use of glass bottles & hard/ stiff plastics
- •Protect the Nitroprusside bottle from light

Mechanism:
- •Vasodilation (**venous** >> arterial)→
  - ∘↓Preload→
    - –↓Cardiac output→↓blood pressure
    - –↓Myocardial O$_2$ demand
    - –↓Pulmonary congestion if present
- •Platelet inhibiting activity

Side effects:
- **Cardiovascular**
  - •Hypotension
  - •Systemic vasodilation→
    - ∘Reflex tachycardia
    - ∘Orthostatic hypotension
    - ∘Facial flushing
  - •Meningeal arterial dilation→
    - ∘Headache

Pulmonary
- •Pulmonary vasodilation→
  - ∘Exacerbation of ventilation/ perfusion mismatches
Hematologic
Nitroglycerin specific:
- •Nitroglycerin metabolism→
  - ∘Inorganic nitrites→oxidation of heme bound iron (Fe^{+2}) to the ferric form (Fe^{+3}), creating **methemoglobin,** which does not carry O_2 effectively→
    - −Hypoxemia, being unreliably detected by pulse oximeters, requiring the use of co−oximeters
    - −Brown colored blood due to the brown color of methemoglobin
    - …usually occurring only at ↑↑doses, w/ levels (fraction of total hemoglobin):
      - •>3% being abnormal
      - •>40% possibly causing hypoxemia→
        - ∘Lactic acidemia
      - •>70% being lethal
      - …requiring discontinuation of infusion in all cases. If hypoxemia exists, administer Methylene blue (a reducing agent) @ 2mg/ kg IV over 10min.†→
        - •Conversion of iron to the normal ferrous form (Fe^{+2})
- •Being as nitroglycerin does not readily dissolve in aqueous solutions, nonpolar solvents such as ethanol & propylene glycol are required to keep the medication in solution, & can accumulate→
  - ∘Ethanol intoxication
  - ∘Propylene glycol toxicity→
    - −Altered mental status
    - −Anion gap metabolic acidemia
    - −Dysrhythmias
    - −Hemolysis
    - −Hyperosmolarity
    - −Acute tubular necrosis→renal failure
    - …→↑plasma levels & osmolar gap

Pharmacokinetics/ pharmacodynamics
- •Tolerance to medication effects
Nitroprusside specific:
- •Nitroprusside metabolism releases 5 cyanide ions (CN) along w/ nitric oxide→
  - ∘**Potential cyanide &/or thiocyanate toxicity**
    - −Cyanide−CN + thiosulfate−S_2O_3 (a sulfur donor source)→thiocyanate−SCN‡ + sulfate−SO_3
Cyanide toxicity
- •The body stores of thiosulfate are readily depleted→
  - ∘↑Cyanide, which is why 500mg of thiosulfate must be added to each infusion solution
Thiocyanate toxicity
- •Renal failure→
  - −↑Thiocyanate toxicity risk→anorexia, hallucinations, nausea ± vomiting, &/or seizures

---

†Intravenous administration of methylene blue→
- •Spuriously ↓SaO_2, up to 65%
‡Thiocyanate is renally cleared

Contraindications:
Cardiovascular
- •Hypotension
Neurologic
- •**Hypertensive encephalopathy,** as it ↑intracranial pressure
Interactions
- •**Sildenafil** (Viagra) **is contraindicated** in patients taking concomitant nitrates, as the combination within 24hours may→severe hypotension→
  - ∘↓Myocardial perfusion→
    - −Stable angina mediated acute coronary syndrome
  - ∘↓Cerebral perfusion→
    - −Pre−syncope/ syncope
    - −Cerebrovascular accident syndrome

Monitoring:
- •Thiocyanate levels frequently (should be <10mg/ dL)

ATRIAL FIBRILLATION

•Caused by **chaotic atrial myocardial depolarization**→
  ◦Multiple, irregularly occurring, segmental areas of contraction, w/ concurrent areas of relaxation, being termed fibrillation→uncoordinated myocardial contraction→
    −Inefficient atrial contraction
    −Irregularly conducted atrioventricular impulses
•Atrial flutter is an uncommon, transient dysrhythmia, often→
  ◦Atrial fibrillation
Statistics:
  •#1 cause of ischemic cerebrovascular accidents in patients age ≥70years

RISK FACTORS

•**Age ≥50 years**, as it affects:
  ◦0.5% of persons age >50 years
  ◦10% of persons age >80 years
•**Gender:** ♂1.5 X ♀
•**Atrial distention**
  ◦**Any cause of heart failure**→
    −Atrial hypertension→atrial distention
•**Cardiopulmonary bypass surgery**
  ◦30% develop atrial flutter &/or fibrillation @ postoperative days 2−4
•**Chronic obstructive pulmonary disease−COPD**
  ◦Asthma
  ◦Emphysema
  ◦Chronic bronchitis
•**Drugs**
  ◦**Recent large alcohol consumption**, termed "holiday heart"
•**Dysrhythmia**
  ◦Wolff−Parkinson−White WPW syndrome
•**Electrolyte alterations**
  ◦Calcium
  ◦Potassium
  ◦Sodium
•**Inflammation**
  ◦**Any intrathoracic inflammation**
  ◦Systemic inflammatory response syndrome−SIRS
    ...→inflammatory cytokine mediated myocardial interstitial changes
•**Neoplasm**
  ◦Atrial myxoma→
    −Atrial irritation
•**Pulmonary embolism**
•↑**Sympathetic autonomic nervous system tone**
  ◦Anemia
  ◦Autonomic neuropathy via ↓parasympathetic tone
  ◦Exercise
  ◦Fever
  ◦Heart failure
  ◦Hyperthyroidism
  ◦**Hypovolemia**
  ◦Inflammation
  ◦Postoperative, via tissue damage ± related fever &/or pain
  ◦Pregnancy
  ◦Adrenergic medications
    −Catecholamines
    −β1 receptor agonists
    −Ephedrine
    −Phenylpropanolamine
    −Theophylline
    −Yohimbine
  ◦Illicit drug use, or abrupt discontinuation after chronic use
    −Amphetamines→↑release of presynaptic catecholamines
    −Cocaine→↓presynaptic reuptake of released catecholamines
    −Ecstasy
•**An ectopic electrical focus in a pulmonary vein** may mimic atrial fibrillation &/or degenerate into true atrial fibrillation

78

Symptom based classification:
•**Unstable atrial fibrillation**→
　◦↓Cardiac output, usually occurring @ ≥150bpm→either:
　　−Altered mental status, being termed cardiac arrest if loss of consciousness occurs
　　−Heart failure
　　−Hypotension
　　−Myocardial ischemic syndrome
　　...considered **a medical emergency requiring immediate synchronized cardioversion**
•**Stable atrial fibrillation**
　◦Rapid ventricular response: ≥120 beats/ min.
　◦Moderate ventricular response: 60−119 beats/ min.
　◦Slow ventricular response: <60 beats/ min.†

Duration based classification:
•**Paroxysmal atrial fibrillation**
　◦Recurrent, episodic, atrial fibrillation
•**Chronic atrial fibrillation**
　◦Continuous atrial fibrillation ≥2weeks

Etiology based classification:
•**Non−lone atrial fibrillation−97%**
　◦Due to **known or suspected cardiac disease**
•**Lone atrial fibrillation−3%**
　◦Atrial fibrillation in a patient **without known or suspected cardiac disease,** perhaps being due to either:
　　−Idiopathic fibrotic myocardial areas
　　−Focal atrial myocarditis
　　−↑Responsiveness to autonomic sympathetic stimulation, as w/ hyperthyroidism
　Exclusionary criteria for lone atrial fibrillation:
　•**Age >75 years**
　•**Diabetes mellitus**
　•**Hypertension,** including that being currently treated
　•**Coronary artery disease**
　•**Cerebrovascular disease**
　•**Peripheral vascular disease**
　•**Valvular heart disease,** including mitral annular calcification
　•**Left ventricular dysfunction**
　•**Left atrial enlargement**

---

†In the absence of atrioventricular nodal depressant medications, such as:
•Amiodarone
•β receptor blockers
•Calcium channel blockers
•Digoxin
...a slow ventricular response may occur in patients w/ either:
　•Conduction system disease
　•↑Vagal tone, such as athletes

•Atrial fibrillation may be intermittently symptomatic

Cardiovascular
•**Irregularly irregular ventricular rhythm**†, which may not be discernable via palpation or auscultation if sufficiently tachycardic→
　◦Subjective awareness of a forceful &/or accelerated heart beat, termed **palpitations−30%**
　◦Lack of coordinated atrial contraction→
　　−25% ↓ventricular preload, w/ 75% flowing into the left ventricle during atrial diastole→↓**cardiac output**
　　−Atrial blood stasis→↑risk of **atrial mural thrombus ± embolization**→distal vascular occlusion→ischemia ± infarction ± reperfusion hemorrhage, especially **cerebrovascular accidents‡** which account for 80% of symptomatic thromboembolic events

∘**Ventricular tachycardia**°→↓ventricular diastolic time→↓**cardiac output**→
　　–Beat to beat blood pressure variation
　　–Heart failure, esp. w/ underlying cardiomyopathy
　　–Cardiac apex:radial artery **pulse deficit** via simultaneous auscultation of the cardiac apex
　　ventricular rate & palpation of the radial artery pulse→radial pulse < ventricular contraction rate
　　(except @ <50bpm). Occurring due to ↓↓ventricular preload→stroke volume insufficient to
　　transmit a palpable pressure wave to the radial artery
•Vagus nerve stimulation via either the:
　∘Carotid sinus massage
　∘Diving reflex, via face or body water immersion, esp. in cold water
　∘Valsalva's maneuver
　…→↑autonomic parasympathetic tone & ↓sympathetic tone→
　　•↑Atrioventricular node refractoriness→
　　　∘↓Heart rate

How to properly perform a carotid sinus massage:
　1. Tilt the supine patients head back & to the side, allowing for easier palpation of the carotid sinus,
　　being located just below the angle of the jaw at the level of the superior thyroid notch
　2. Apply vigorous pressure medio–posteriorly X ≤5seconds→
　　•Sinus compression against the vertebral spine
　3. Repeat if necessary after several seconds, until ↓heart rate & blood pressure occur, being more
　　pronounced in patients w/ concomitant cardiovascular disease
Contraindications:
　•Age ≥75 years, indicating known or likely cerebrovascular disease, as it may further ↓cerebral
　　blood supply→
　　∘Cerebrovascular accident
　•Simultaneous bilateral carotid artery massage, as it may further ↓cerebral blood supply→
　　∘Cerebrovascular accident
　•Common carotid artery bruit (either side)
　　∘Auscultate each common carotid artery prior to initiating sinus massage

---

†Also occurring w/:
　•Frequent premature atrial or ventricular contractions
　•Multifocal atrial tachycardia–MFAT
‡Other associated syndromes:
　•Mesenteric ischemic syndromes
　•Non–mesenteric, intra–abdominal organ ischemic syndromes
　•Pulmonary thromboembolic syndrome, as atrial fibrillation affects both atria concomitantly
°Which if chronic→
　•Tachycardia mediated myocarditis→
　　∘Dilated cardiomyopathy

ELECTRICAL STUDIES

•**Electrocardiogram–ECG**
　Findings:
　　•Multiple chaotic, small atrial myocardial depolarization waves, many being of opposite polarity at
　　any given time→
　　　∘**Near electrical neutralization**→
　　　　–High frequency, low voltage, dissimilar p wave recordings→waveline effect, being termed
　　　　fibrillatory waves
　　•Atrial myocardial depolarization waves arrive at the atrioventricular node† rapidly & irregularly→
　　　∘**Irregularly irregular ventricular contractions**→
　　　　–Correspondingly spaced narrow QRS complexes, being ≤ 0.12seconds=3 small boxes wide.
　　　　However, the depolarization wave may travel into a partially refractory atrioventricular node or
　　　　bundle branch→wide QRS complex (>0.12seconds), termed aberrant conduction
　　　–**Irregularly irregular RR interval**

---

†Normally having a refractory period of 0.35seconds, within which no atrial impulses pass through

•**Chest x ray**
Indications:
  •All patients, in order to look for signs of possible:
    ◦Emphysema
    ◦Dilated cardiomyopathy
    ◦Heart failure
    ◦Pneumonia
    ◦Pulmonary embolism

•**Transthoracic echocardiography–TTE**
Procedure:
  •A 2 dimensional ultrasonographic image, allowing real time visualization of:
    ◦Ventricular wall thickness
    ◦Cavity size (both atrial & ventricular)
    ◦Myocardial & valve function, allowing ejection fraction–EF estimation (% of end diastolic volume ejected during ventricular systole)
    ◦The pericardial space
  •Doppler ultrasonography uses Doppler shift to detect vessel flow velocity→
    ◦Valve regurgitation visualization
    ◦Estimation of valve pressure gradients
Outcomes:
  •Atrial cavitary size ≥5cm indicates:
    ◦↑Cerebrovascular accident risk
    ◦↓Likelihood of cardioversion to sinus rhythm
Limitations:
  •↓Visualization in obese or emphysematous patients
  •May not allow adequate:
    ◦Visualization of the anterior aspect of a prosthetic aortic valve
    ◦Functional assessment of a prosthetic aortic valve
  •Transesophageal echocardiography–TEE is more sensitive in detecting:
    ◦Thrombotic ± infectious vegetations
    ◦Abscesses
    ◦Valve damage
    …esp. in a patient w/ a prosthetic heart valve. However, transthoracic echocardiography is the initial test of choice due to its noninvasive nature, as transesophageal echocardiography may→
      •Pharyngeal swallow receptor mediated reflex:
        ◦Bradycardia
        ◦Hypotension

•**Unstable atrial fibrillation**
  ◦**Emergent synchronized cardioversion protocol**, converting 85% of patients w/ recent onset atrial fibrillation
    –**Biphasic defibrillation: 100joules→200joules→300joules→360joules**
  ◦**Post–cardioversion protocol†:**
    –Cardioversion→atrial myocardial mechanical stunning→reversible ↓myocardial contraction, requiring anticoagulation prophylaxis X 1month, to allow for normalization of function

•**Stable atrial fibrillation**
  ◦**Elective electrical or synchronized cardioversion protocol**, to be considered w/ either:
    –Transesophageal echocardiograph showing lack of an atrial mural thrombus. If a mural thrombus is visualized, anticoagulate X 1month & repeat a transesophageal echocardiogram to ensure either thrombus lysis or endothelial organization & incorporation prior to cardioversion
    –Adequate anticoagulation, being either initiated within 48hours after onset, or for 1 month prior to elective cardioversion
    –**Spontaneous cardioversion is common within 24hours after onset in 60% of persons**, w/ subsequent ↓likelihood, being rare @ >1week
  ◦**Post–cardioversion protocol†:**
    –Cardioversion→atrial myocardial mechanical stunning→reversible ↓myocardial contraction, requiring anticoagulation prophylaxis X 1month, to allow for normalization of function

Admission criteria:
  •Unstable atrial fibrillation
  •Early cardioversion is being considered
  Note: In the absence of a myocardial ischemic syndrome, there is no need to admit the patient in order to rule out myocardial infarction, as ischemia rarely presents solely w/ atrial fibrillation

81

Thromboembolic risk in non−anticoagulated persons (paroxysmal or chronic):
- **Non−lone atrial fibrillation**
  - **Rheumatic heart disease** @ any age→
    - −15−20%/ year risk
  - **Other** @ age:
    - −<75 years→5%/ year risk
    - −≥75 years→8%/ year risk
- **Lone atrial fibrillation** @ age:
  - <60 years→
    - −No risk
  - >60 years→
    - −2%/ year risk
- **Cardioversion (electrical or chemical)** @
  - >48hours after onset, without either:
    - −Transesophageal echocardiograph showing lack of an atrial mural thrombus
    - −Adequate anticoagulation, being either initiated within 48hours after onset, or for 1 month prior to elective cardioversion
    - …→2−5% immediate risk. Whereas, **w/ either, it is rare**

Rational for synchronized rather than non−synchronized cardioversion
- The end of each cardiac cycle (being the terminal portion of the T wave) is referred to as the vulnerable period for the initiation of ventricular fibrillation, as the dispersion of both areas of refractory & non−refractory myocardium are greatest during this time. An electrical impulse administered during this time may→
  - **Ventricular fibrillation**. Synchronized cardioversion ensures delivery of the electrical impulse at some other specific time in the cardiac cycle, such as the R wave upstroke or S wave downslope
- †Recurrences usually occur within 3months after initial cardioversion

ACUTE RATE CONTROL ▄▄▄▄▄▄▄▄▄▄▄▄▄▄▄▄▄▄▄▄▄▄
- **Pulse is considered controlled if both:**
  - A resting ventricular rate <100
  - Ventricular rate <150 after modest exercise
  …are attained, without a pulse deficit, which, if present, indicates a significantly impaired stroke volume
  Caution: If you suspect atrial fibrillation in patients w/ Wolf Parkinson White−WPW syndrome, do not treat w/ vagal maneuvers or atrioventricular node depressant medications (adenosine, β receptor blockers, non−dihydropyridine calcium channel blockers), as **atrial fibrillation may→**
  - **Ventricular fibrillation via the accessory pathway.** Use Procainamide if stable, or cardioversion if unstable

β1 SELECTIVE RECEPTOR BLOCKERS				
Generic (Trade)	M	♀	**Start**	**Max**
Atenolol (Tenormin)	K	U		
•IV form			5mg slow IV push (1mg/ min.) q5min. X 2 prn, then	
•PO form			25−50mg PO q24hours	200mg/ 24h
Metoprolol (Lopressor)	L	?		
•IV form			5mg slow IV push (1mg/ min.) q5min. X 3 prn, then	
•PO form			25mg PO q12hours, then	100mg q12h
◦XR form (Toprol XL)			As per PO requirement	400mg q24h
Esmolol (Brevibloc)	K	?	0.5mg=500µg/ kg IV loading bolus (over 1 min.), then	
			0.05mg=50µg/kg/min. continuous IV infusion w/ titration prn†	
			Max: 0.3mg=300µg/kg/min.	
Onset: 1−2 min., Duration: 10 min.				

†Titrate q4 min. via re−administration of the loading bolus & an additional 50µg/kg/min. IV infusion

α1 & NONSELECTIVE β RECEPTOR BLOCKERS				
Generic (Trade)	M	♀	**Start**	**Max**
Carvedilol (Coreg)	L	?	6.25mg PO q12hours	25mg q12h
Labetalol (Normodyne)	LK	?	20mg IV push over 2min., then	
			40mg IV push q10min. prn goal blood pressure, then	300mg total
•PO form			100mg PO q12hours	1200mg q12h
•IV form			0.5−2mg/ min. IV infusion	
Onset: 5−10min., Duration: 3−6hours				

•Competitive antagonist of the β1 ± β2 receptor→
  ∘↓Sinoatrial & atrioventricular node conduction (β1)→
    –↓Pulse
  ∘Anti–dysrhythmic via nodal effects (β1)
  ∘↓Cardiac muscle contractile strength (β1)
  ∘↓Juxtaglomerular cell renin release (β1)→
    –↓Angiotensin 1, angiotensin 2, & aldosterone formation
  ∘↓Cardiovascular remodeling
  ∘↑Vascular/ organ smooth muscle contraction (β2)→
    –Vasoconstriction
    –Bronchoconstriction
    –Uterine contraction
  ∘↓Tremor (β2)
  ∘↓Hepatocyte glycogenolysis (β2)
•↓Extrathyroidal tetraiodothyronine–T4 (also termed thyroxine) conversion to the more metabolically active triiodothyronine–T3 form

Side effects:
General
•Fatigue
•Malaise
Cardiovascular
•Bradycardia ± heart block
•Hypotension
  ∘Orthostatic hypotension
  ∘Pelvic hypotension→
    –Impotence, being the inability to achieve &/or maintain an erection
•Initial worsening of systolic heart failure
•Worsening symptoms of peripheral vascular disease
  ∘Intermittent claudication
  ∘Raynaud's phenomenon
Pulmonary
•Bronchoconstriction
Endocrine
•↑Risk of developing diabetes mellitus
•May block catecholamine mediated:
  ∘Physiologic reversal of hypoglycemia via:
    –↓Hepatocyte gluconeogenesis
  ∘↓Hypoglycemic symptoms, termed hypoglycemic unawareness→
    –↓Tachycardia as a warning sign
Gastrointestinal
•Diarrhea
•Nausea ± vomiting
•Gastroesophageal reflux
Mucocutaneous
•Hair thinning
Neurologic
•Sedation
•Sleep alterations
•↓Libido→
  ∘Impotence
Psychiatric
•Depression
Hematologic
•↓High density lipoprotein–HDL levels

•Most patients w/ chronic obstructive pulmonary disease–COPD (including asthma), diabetes, &/or peripheral vascular disease can be safely treated w/ **cardioselective β1 receptor blockers**, as they have ↓peripheral effects

Contraindications:
Cardiovascular
•**Acutely decompensated heart failure**
•Hypotension
•Pulse <50bpm
•Atrioventricular heart block of any degree

Pulmonary
•Moderate to severe chronic obstructive pulmonary disease–COPD, including asthma
Hyper–catacholamine state
•Amphetamine use
•**Cocaine use**†
•Clonidine withdrawal
•Monoamine oxidase inhibitor–MAOi mediated tyramine effect
•Pheochromocytoma
...→relatively ↑vascular α1 receptor stimulation="unopposed α effect"→
•Vasoconstriction→
◦Myocardial ischemic syndrome
◦Cerebrovascular accident syndrome
◦Peripheral vascular ischemic syndrome
Note: **Carvedilol** & **Labetalol** may be used due to their α1 blocking property

---

†Cocaine use→
•Varying ischemic syndrome onset per administration route, & may occur @ min. to days
(usually within 3hours)

ANTIDOTES

Generic	M	♀	Dose	Max
Glucagon	LK	P	3mg IV slow push over 1min., then	
			5mg IV slow push over 1 min. if needed	
•Continuous infusion			5mg/ hour	
10% Calcium chloride†			10mL (1 ampule) IV slow push over 3min., q5min. prn	
•Continuous infusion			0.3mEq/ hour	0.7mEq/ h

Onset: 1–2 min., Duration: 30–60 min.

---

†Use cautiously in patients taking Digoxin, as hypercalcemia→
•Digoxin cardiotoxicity

CALCIUM CHANNEL BLOCKERS: Non–dihydropyridines

Generic	M ♀	Start	Max
Diltiazem	L ?		
•IV form		5–20mg slow IV push over 2 min., then	
		25mg slow IV push over 2 min., 15 min. later, then	
		5mg/ hour IV infusion	15mg/ hour
•PO form		30mg PO q8hours	120mg q8hours
•XR form		As per daily requirement	
QD–XR form			540mg q24hours
BID–XR form			180mg q12hours
Verapamil	L U		
•IV form		2.5–5mg slow IV push over 2min., then	
		5–10mg slow IV push over 2min., 15min. later, then	
•PO form		40mg PO q8hours	160mg q8hours
◦XR form		As per daily requirement	
–Calan XR form			480mg/ 24hours
–Veleran XR form			400mg qhs
–Covera XR form			480mg qhs

Mechanism:
•Block voltage dependent calcium ion channels in smooth & cardiac muscle→
◦↓Calcium influx→
–↓Sinoatrial & atrioventricular node conduction (non–dihydropyridines)→↓pulse
–Anti–dysrhythmic via nodal effects (mainly non–dihydropyridines)
–↓Cardiac muscle contractile strength (mainly non–dihydropyridines)
–Vasodilation: Arterial > venous (mainly dihydropyridines)

Side effects:
Cardiovascular
•Bradycardia ± heart block
•Edema
•Flushing
•Hypotension
Gastrointestinal
•Constipation
•Nausea ± vomiting

84

Neurologic			
•Dizziness			
•Headache			

ANTIDOTES

Generic	M ♀	Dose	Max
Glucagon	LK P	3mg IV slow push over 1min., then	
		5mg IV slow push over 1 min. if needed	
•Continuous infusion		5mg/ hour	
10% Calcium chloride†		10mL (1 ampule) IV slow push over 3min., then	
		repeat @5min. if needed	
•Continuous infusion		Start 0.3mEq/ hour	0.7mEq/ hour
Onset: 1–2 min., Duration: 30–60 min.			
Magnesium sulfate	K S	2g MgSO₄ in 50mL saline infused over 15min., then	
		6g MgSO₄ in 500mL saline infused over 6hours	

†Use cautiously in patients taking Digoxin, as hypercalcemia→
  •Digoxin cardiotoxicity

CHRONIC RATE CONTROL ▬▬▬▬
•Either:
  ∘β1 selective receptor blockers
  ∘Non–dihydropyridine calcium channel blocker
  …as above

DIGITALIS GLYCOSIDES

Indications:
  •Ejection fraction–EF ≤35%
  •Cardiothoracic ratio of ≥0.5=50%
  •Chronic atrial fibrillation† w/ ventricular systolic dysfunction→
    ∘Heart failure

†Effective in ↓resting rate, **but not exertional or paroxysmal rate**

Generic (Trade)	M ♀	Dose	Max
Digoxin (Lanoxin)	KL ?	0.125mg PO q48–24hours	0.25mg q24hours

Onset: 4–6hours, Half life: 40hours

Dose adjustment:
  •Adjust dose based on clinical response & plasma levels (therapeutic 0.8–1.8ng/ mL) w/ toxicity
   typically occurring @ >1.8ng/ mL, but may occur @ therapeutic levels
  •Amiodarone & Verapamil→
    ∘↑Digoxin levels (↓Digoxin dose by 50%)
  •Quinidine mediated displacement of digoxin from tissue binding sites→
    ∘↓Clearance

Mechanism:
  •↓Cell membrane Na⁺/K⁺ ATPase function→
    ∘↑Intracellular sodium→
      –↓Na⁺/Ca⁺² anti–transporter function→↑intracellular calcium→↑myocardial inotropy

Side effects†:
  •**General**
    ∘↓Appetite
    ∘Fatigue
    ∘Headache
    ∘Malaise
    ∘Weakness
  •**Cardiac**
    ∘The sequential occurrence of electrocardiographic–ECG changes:
      –Atrioventricular block (1°,2°,3°)→↑PR interval
      –T wave flattening
          ↓
      –**ST segment depression**
      –↓QT interval
      –T wave inversion
          ↓

-Supraventricular &/or ventricular dysrhythmias
-U wave
•Gastrointestinal
  ◦Abdominal pain
  ◦Diarrhea
  ◦Nausea ± vomiting
•Genitourinary/ cutaneous
  ◦Digoxin's structural similarity to estrogen→
    -Gynecomastia, being the ↑development of male mammary glands
    -Impotence, being the inability to achieve &/or maintain an erection
    -↓Libido
•Neurologic
  ◦Altered mental status
  ◦Dizziness
  ◦Paresthesias
  ◦Psychosis
  ◦Visual changes 50–95%
    -Altered pupil size
    -Photophobia
    -Ocular muscle palsies
    -Yellow–green halos around bright lights
Hematologic
  •↓Cell membrane Na^+/K^+ ATPase function→
    ◦↑Extracellular potassium→
      -Hyperkalemia

↑↑Risk w/ electrolyte abnormalities:
•Hypercalcemia
•Hypokalemia
•Hypomagnesemia
…even w/ therapeutic Digoxin levels

ANTIDOTE
Indications:
•Ingested Digoxin dose >10mg
•Plasma Digoxin level >6ng/ mL
•≥2° atrioventricular block
•Supraventricular &/or ventricular dysrhythmias
•Plasma potassium >5.5mEq/ L, being refractory to conventional treatment modalities

Generic (Trade)	M ♀	Vials
Digoxin–immune Fab (Digibind)	K ?	Administered via IV fluids over 15–30min., w/ repeat if toxicity persists (range: 2–20 vials)
•Acute ingestion of unknown quantity		20vials
•Acute ingestion of known quantity		[Ingested Digoxin (mg) X 0.8] / 0.6
•Chronic ingestion mediated overdose		[Plasma Digoxin level (ng/ mL) X weight (kg)] / 100

Mechanism:
•Each vial being 40mg & binding ~0.5mg Digoxin

•Plasma Digoxin levels will be falsely ↑for several days after administration

ANTI-DYSRHYTHMIC MEDICATIONS
Indications:
•**Chemical cardioversion**, being successful in 10–30% of persons
•**Paroxysmal atrial fibrillation prophylaxis**

•Failure of a medication to convert the rhythm does not mean that it will not be effective maintenance treatment

Generic (Trade)	M ♀	Dose
Amiodarone (Cordarone)	L U	
•IV form		150mg IV slow push over 10 min., then 1mg/ min. IV infusion X 6hours, then 0.5mg/ min. IV infusion

•PO form	800–1600mg PO loading q24hours X 1–3weeks, then
	when controlled or adverse effects,
	400–800mg q24h X 1month, then
	Titrate to the lowest effective dose (usually 200–400mg q24hours)

Dose adjustment:
- •Amiodarone→↓hepatocyte cytochrome P450 function→
  - ∘↓Hepatic metabolism, necessitating concomitant ↓medication dose
  - −↓**Digoxin & Warfarin dose by 50%**

Mechanism:
- •↑Interval between paroxysms
- •↓Duration of paroxysms
- •Converts what would have otherwise been symptomatic episodes to asymptomatic ones

Outcomes:
- •There is **no evidence** to indicate that ↓paroxysms of atrial fibrillation (total or symptomatic)→
  - ∘↓Cerebrovascular accident risk or ↓mortality
- •↓Symptoms, but also ↑dysrhythmia risk

Side effects:
Cardiovascular
- •Dose dependent ↑**QT interval**→
  - ∘**Torsades de pointes**
- •Dose dependent **hypotension**

Cutaneous
- •Microcrystalline skin deposits→
  - ∘Blue–gray tinted skin
- •Photosensitivity

Endocrine
- •Thyroid dysfunction **(hypothyroidism or hyperthyroidism)** due to its iodine moiety

Gastrointestinal
- •Hepatitis

Opthalmologic
- •Microcrystalline corneal deposits→
  - ∘Blurred vision

Pulmonary
- •Pulmonary deposition→
  - ∘Pulmonary fibrosis

Contraindications:
- •QTc >0.44seconds

Treatment algorithm:
- **Non–lone atrial fibrillation:**
  - ∘Warfarin→
    - −70%↓risk
  - ∘Aspirin, being used w/ contraindication or adverse reaction to Warfarin→
    - −20%↓risk
- **Lone atrial fibrillation**
  - ∘Age <60 years: Aspirin vs. no treatment
  - ∘Age 60–75 years: Warfarin vs. Aspirin

ANTICOAGULANTS: High molecular weight Heparin

Indications:
- •Atrial fibrillation
- •Ejection fraction <30%
- •Large ventricular akinetic segment
- •Mural thrombus

M	♀	Start
M	?	60units/ kg IV bolus (or 5000units empirically)
		12units/kg/hour infusion (or 1000units/ hour empirically)

•Titrated by 2.5units/kg/hour to achieve an activated partial thromboplastin time–aPTT of 1.5–2X control value or **50–70seconds**

aPTT (seconds)	Action	Obtain next aPTT
<40	Bolus 5000units & ↑infusion rate by 100units/ hour	6hours
40–49	↑Infusion rate by 50units/ hour	6hours
50–70 (or 1.5–2Xcontrol)	NO ACTION	24hours
71–85	↓Infusion rate by 50units/ hour	6hours
86–100	Hold infusion 30min., then ↓infusion rate by 100units/ hour	6hours
101–150	Hold infusion 60min., then ↓infusion rate by 150units/ hour	6hours
>150	Hold infusion 60min., then ↓infusion rate by 300units/ hour	6hours

Monitoring:
- •Complete blood count q24hours to monitor for side effects

ANTICOAGULANTS: Low molecular weight Heparin

Generic (Trade)	M	♀	Start	Max
Enoxaparin (Lovenox)	KL	P	1.5mg/ kg SC q24hours or	180mg/ 24hours
			1mg/ kg SC q12hours	
Dalteparin (Fragmin)	KL	P	200 anti–factor Xa units/ kg SC q24hours or	18,000units q24h
			100 anti–factor Xa units/ kg SC q12hours	

Dose adjustment:
- •Obesity
  - ∘Most manufacturers recommend a maximum dose of that for a 90kg patient

Monitoring:
- •Monitoring of anti–Xa levels is recommended in patients w/:
  - ∘Abnormal coagulation/ hemorrhage
  - ∘Obesity
  - ∘Renal failure
  - ∘Underweight
- •Check 4h after 2nd SC dose. Further monitoring is not necessary once the correct dose is established in obese patients

Administration frequency	Therapeutic anti–Xa levels
Q12hours	0.6–1 units/ mL
Q24hours	1–2 units/ mL

Mechanism:
- •Heparin combines w/ plasma antithrombin 3→
  - ∘↑Antithrombin 3 activity in removing thrombin & activated factors 9, 10, 11,& 12→
    - −↓Coagulation→↓vascular & mural thrombus formation &/or propagation
- •Heparin is metabolized by the plasma enzyme heparinase

Outcomes:
- •↓Morbidity & mortality

Side effects:
- **Cardiovascular**
  - •Hemorrhage

•**Heparin induced thrombocytopenia–HIT** 10%, esp. w/ high molecular weight Heparin
  Mechanism:
    •Heparin mediated platelet agglutination→
      ∘Monocyte/ macrophage mediated extravascular removal via the splenic trabecular
      network=red pulp, & hepatic sinusoids→
        –**Thrombocytopenia**
  Outcomes:
    •Benign, as it resolves spontaneously, even w/ continued exposure
•**Heparin induced thrombocytopenia ± thrombosis–HITT** ≤3%, esp. w/ high molecular weight
  Heparin
  Mechanism:
    •Heparin mediated platelet agglutination→
      ∘Monocyte/ macrophage mediated extravascular removal via the splenic trabecular
      network=red pulp, & hepatic sinusoids→
        –**Thrombocytopenia**
      ∘Platelet release of Heparin neutralizing factor=platelet factor 4–PF4, which complexes w/
      Heparin→
        –Production of anti–complex antibodies→↑platelet activation↔↑platelet factor 4 release→
        a vicious cycle of **platelet mediated arterial &/or venous thrombus formation, termed
        the "white clot syndrome,"** being as the clot is relatively devoid of erythrocytes
  Outcomes:
    •Must discontinue treatment as **20% develop thromboembolic complications**. Being that
    both Heparins may cross–react w/ the etiologic antibodies, their further use is contraindicated.
    Consider continued treatment w/ direct thrombin inhibitors
      ∘Antibody cross–reactivity:
        –Low molecular weight Heparins–85%
        –Heparinoids–5%
Mucocutaneous
  •Skin necrosis–rarely occurring w/ high molecular weight Heparins, & not being associated w/
  anticoagulant deficiency
Musculoskeletal
  •Osteoporosis, esp. w/ high molecular weight Heparin
    ∘Usually @ use ≥1month
Hematologic
  •↓Aldosterone production→
    ∘Hyperkalemia–8%

CHARACTERISTICS OF HEPARIN INDUCED THROMBOCYTOPENIC SYNDROMES

	HIT	HITT
Onset	<2days	4–10 days
Re-exposure	<2days	Earlier if re–exposed within 3 months
Platelet count	↓, being <150,000 or ≥50%	
Platelet median nadir	~90,000	~60,000

•**^{14}C–Serotonin release assay**
  Indications:
    •Suspected HITT
  Procedure:
    •Normal donor platelets are radiolabeled w/ ^{14}C–serotonin. They are then washed & combined w/
    patient serum & therapeutic Heparin concentrations (0.1 U/ mL). Induction of ^{14}C–serotonin
    release from platelets constitutes a positive test
  Limitations:
    •Expense, due to the use of radioactive material
  Outcomes:
    •Considered the gold standard in the detection of HITT
•**Enzyme linked immunosorbent assay–ELISA**
  Indications:
    •Suspected HITT
  Procedure:
    •Heparin–PF4 complexes affixed to a plastic plate are incubated w/ the patient's serum. If the
    patient has produced antibodies, then the addition of enzymatically (horseradish peroxidase)
    labeled anti–human IgG allows for color visualization via spectrophotometer
  Limitations:
    •Many antibody positive patients do not develop clinical HITT
    •30% false positive

Contraindications:
•Active hemorrhage
•Severe bleeding diathesis
•Severe thrombocytopenia (platelet count ≤20,000/ μL)
•Recent significant trauma
•Neurosurgery, ocular surgery, or intracranial hemorrhage within 10days

ANTIDOTE

Generic	M	♀	Amount IV over 10min.	Max
Protamine	P	?	1mg/ 100units of HMWH	50mg
			1mg/ 100units Dalteparin	"
			1mg/ 1mg Enoxaparin	"

Mechanism:
•Protamine combines electrostatically w/ Heparin→
 ◦Inability to bind to antithrombin 3

FOLLOWED BY

ANTICOAGULANTS

Generic	M	♀	Start

Warfarin (Coumadin) L U 5mg PO q24hours
•Because the anticoagulant proteins↓ relatively faster than the procoagulant proteins, an initial transient hypercoagulable state develops. Due to this, Warfarin is started once the patient is therapeutic on Heparin, via either:
 ◦Goal aPTT w/ high molecular weight Heparin
 ◦Evening of initiation of low molecular weight Heparin
 …requiring ~7days (corresponding to 2 half lives of factor 2, or a 75% reduction) to reach a true therapeutic level of an **international normalized ratio–INR of 2–3**

INR	Action	Obtain next INR
<1.5	↑Weekly dose by 15%	1 week
1.5–1.9	↑Weekly dose by 10%	2 weeks
2–3	NO ACTION	1 month if stable
3.1–3.9	↓Weekly dose by 10%	2 weeks
4–5	Skip 1 day, then ↓weekly dose by 15%	1 week
>5	DISCONTINUE WARFARIN	Q day until ≤3, then ↓weekly dose by 50%

Mechanism:
•Competitively inhibits hepatocyte enzymatic vitamin K reactive sites→
 ◦↓Formation of both:
  –Procoagulant proteins 2, 7, 9, & 10
  –Anticoagulant proteins C & S
  …w/ the anticoagulant effect requiring several days, as it must await the metabolism of the pre–existing plasma procoagulant proteins, w/ normal coagulation returning within several days of discontinuation

Side effects:
Cardiovascular
 •**Hemorrhage**
  ◦Fatal: 0.6%/ year
  ◦Major: 3%/ year
  ◦Minor: 7%/ year
Cutaneous
 •Tissue necrosis w/ protein C or S deficiency or dysfunction

Contraindications:
•Active hemorrhage
•Severe bleeding diathesis
•Severe thrombocytopenia (platelet count ≤20,000/ μL)
•Recent significant trauma
•Neurosurgery, ocular surgery, or intracranial hemorrhage within 10days
•Injury risk (including falls & sports) or compliance risk via:
 ◦Alcoholism
 ◦Altered mental status
 ◦Illicit drug abuse
 ◦Orthostatic hypotension
 ◦Poor compliance
 ◦Seizure disease
 ◦Syncope
 ◦Unstable gait

Special considerations:
- **If undergoing elective surgery during treatment**
  - ○Stop Warfarin 5 days prior to surgery, & begin Heparin
- **Anticoagulation during pregnancy**
  - ○Substitute low molecular weight Heparin for Warfarin, followed by Warfarin treatment postpartum if necessary

ANTIDOTES
- **Gastric lavage & activated charcoal** if recently administered; forced emesis at home

VITAMIN K=Phytonadione
Indications:
- To correct the international normalized ration–INR or prothrombin time–PT

Dose

10mg SC/ IV slow push @ 1mg/ min. in order to ↓anaphylactoid reaction risk

Mechanism:
- Requires several hours to days for effect

Side effects:
- Avoid intramuscular administration which may→
  - ○Intramuscular hemorrhage

FRESH FROZEN PLASMA–FFP
Indications:
- To correct the international normalized ration–INR or prothrombin time–PT under the following conditions:
  - ○**INR >20**
  - ○**Severe hemorrhage**
  - ○**Other need for rapid reversal, such as an emergent procedure**

Dose†

15mL/ kg IV (w/ ~200mL FFP/ unit) q4hours prn ↑INR

Mechanism:
- Contains clotting factors 2, 7, 9–13, & heat labile 5 & 7→
  - ○Immediate onset of action
- Each unit→
  - ○8% ↑coagulation factors
  - ○4% ↑blood volume

PLATELET INHIBITING MEDICATIONS
Efficacy: Glycoprotein 2b/ 3a inhibitors > thienopyridines > Aspirin

Generic	M	♀	Dose
Acetylsalicylic acid–ASA=Aspirin	K	U	81mg PO q24hours

Mechanism:
- Aspirin is the only nonsteroidal anti–inflammatory drug–NSAID→
  - ○Irreversible inhibition of both cyclooxygenase–COX enzymes (COX1 & COX2), w/ COX1 being responsible for the production of both thromboxane A_2† & prostacyclin‡→
    - –**Near complete inhibition of platelet thromboxane A_2 production within 15 min.**, w/ endothelial & vascular smooth muscle cells producing new enzymes in several hours→ relatively ↑prostacyclin
- Being that platelets lack the enzymatic machinery for protein synthesis, only newly formed platelets (platelet half life=10 days) have the functional enzyme
...this shift in the balance of cytokine production→
  - •↓**Thrombus formation**

In Brief:
- **Cyclooxygenase–COX1 enzymes** are found in most cells of the body, being responsible for normal physiologic processes
- **Cyclooxygenase–COX 2 enzymes** are responsible for the production of inflammatory cell prostaglandins

---

- Concomitant NSAID administration→
  - ○Competition for the cyclooxygenase–COX 1 enzyme binding site, w/:
    - –Unbound Aspirin being rapidly cleared from plasma
    - –Bound NSAID action being reversible & short lived
    ...→↓overall antiplatelet effect, requiring either:
      - •Aspirin to be taken @ ≥1hour prior to other NSAIDs
      - •Switch to thienopyridine derivative for the antiplatelet effect

†Platelet mediated **thromboxane A$_2$** release at the site of vascular injury→
- •Platelet aggregation
- •Vasoconstriction
- ...w/ both processes→
  - •Thrombus formation
‡Endothelial & vascular smooth muscle cell mediated **prostacyclin** release in the surrounding area→
- •Inhibition of platelet aggregation
- •Vasodilation
- ...w/ both processes→
  - •↓Thrombus formation

Side effects:
Gastrointestinal
- •Inhibition of the cyclooxygenase–COX1 enzyme→↑peptic inflammatory disease risk→↑**upper gastrointestinal hemorrhage risk** via:
  - ○↓Gastric mucosal prostaglandin synthesis→
    - –↓Epithelial cell proliferation
    - –↓Mucosal blood flow→↓bicarbonate delivery to the mucosa
    - –↓Mucus & bicarbonate secretion from gastric mucosal cells

Indications for peptic inflammatory disease prophylaxis:
- •Prophylax w/ proton pump inhibitors–PPI's, histamine 2 selective receptor blockers, or Misoprostol in patients w/ any of the following:
  - ○Age >60 years w/ a history of peptic inflammatory disease
  - ○Anticipated therapy >3 months
  - ○Concurrent glucocorticoid use
  - ○Moderate to high dose NSAID use
Note: Newer NSAIDs (Etodolac, Nabumetone, Salsalate)→
  - •↓Risk of NSAID induced peptic inflammation/ ulcer

Genitourinary
- •Patients w/ pre–existing bilateral ↓renal perfusion, not necessarily failure:
  - ○Heart failure
  - ○Bilateral renal artery stenosis
  - ○Hypovolemia
  - ○Renal failure
  - ...rely more on the compensatory production of vasodilatory prostaglandins→
    - •Afferent arteriole dilation→
      - ○Maintained glomerular filtration rate–GFR, whereas NSAIDs→
        - –↓Prostaglandin production, which may→renal failure
Pulmonary
- •Inhibition of both cyclooxygenase enzymes (COX 1 & COX2)→
  - ○↑Lipoxygenase activity→
    - –↑Leukotriene synthesis→symptomatic asthma within 2hours of ingestion in 5% of asthmatics
Rheumatologic
- •Acetylsalicylic acid competes w/ uric acid secretion in the renal tubules→
  - ○↑Uric acid levels→
    - –↑Risk of uric acid precipitation in the tissues=gout
Pediatric
- •**Reye's syndrome**
  - ○A life threatening fulminant hepatitis→
    - –Hepatic encephalopathy in children age ≤16 years w/ a viral infection (esp. influenza or Varicella–zoster virus–VZV)

Overdose:
Pulmonary
- •Direct brainstem respiratory center mediated stimulation of pulmonary ventilation→
  - ○Hyperventilation→
    - –**Initial respiratory alkalemia, w/ the subsequent development of an anion gap metabolic acidemia**
- •Pulmonary edema
Neurologic
- •Altered mental status
- •Aseptic meningitis
- •Depression
- •Hallucinations

- •Hyperactivity
- •Hyperthermia
- •Lightheadedness
- •Seizures
- •Tinnitus

Gastrointestinal
- •Nausea ± vomiting

Mucocutaneous
- •Pharyngitis

THIENOPYRIDINE DERIVATIVE

Indications:
- •Intolerance to Aspirin

Generic (Trade)	M	♀	Dose
Clopidogrel (Plavix)	LK	P	75mg PO q24hours

Mechanism:
- •Inhibits adenosine diphosphate–ADP mediated activation of the glycoprotein 2b/ 3a complex→
  - ∘↓Platelet activation

- •A 300mg loading dose may be used, as maximal effect occurs @ 5hours rather than 5days w/ initiation of the standard 75mg dosage

Side effects:
Gastrointestinal
- •Diarrhea

Mucocutaneous
- •Dermatitis

Hematologic
- •**Thrombotic thrombocytopenic purpura–TTP** within several weeks of initiation

INVASIVE PROCEDURES

Indications:
- •Chronic or paroxysmal atrial fibrillation refractory to conservative treatment

•Atrioventricular node ablation
Procedure:
- •Radiofrequency catheter mediated ablation of the atrioventricular node→
  - ∘Complete heart block

Outcomes:
- •Requires both:
  - ∘The implantation of a permanent pacemaker
  - ∘Continuation of anticoagulation, as the atria continue to fibrillate

•Atrioventricular node modification
Procedure:
- •Radiofrequency catheter mediated partial ablation of the atrioventricular node→
  - ∘↓Nodal conduction→
    - –1st or 2nd degree atrioventricular block

Outcomes:
- •Although not meant to require implantation of a permanent pacemaker, 25% or persons require subsequent permanent pacemaker placement due to unintentional complete ablation
- •Requires continued anticoagulation, as the atria continue to fibrillate

•Focal ectopic locus ablation
- ∘In some patients, atrial fibrillation is mediated via a rapidly firing focus of tissue in the pulmonary veins

Procedure, being either:
- •Radiofrequency catheter mediated ablation of the ectopic pulmonary vein focus
- •Electrical isolation of the pulmonary veins

•Atrial corridor procedure
Procedure:
- •The atrial appendages, termed auricles are excised, &
- •The pulmonary veins are electrically isolated, &
- •Carefully placed incisions→
  - ∘Formation of a narrow tortuous path or "corridor" of right atrial myocardial tissue, which connects the sinoatrial node to the atrioventricular node (w/ no area being wide enough to sustain multiple reentrant circuits), being electrically isolated form the rest of the atria, thus preserving the physiologic pacing of the sinoatrial node

Outcomes:
- •As the corridor involves a significant portion of the right atrium, it usually→
  - ∘Preserved right atrial contraction, but requires continued anticoagulation as the left atrium continues to fibrillate

•Maze procedure
Procedure:
- •Basically, an atrial corridor procedure w/ the addition of several "dead-end" branches from the corridor, creating "maze-like" pathways involving both atria→
  - ∘Synchronous depolarization of all atrial tissue, thus eliminating atrial fibrillation

HEART FAILURE

•Caused by any disease→
◦↓**Cardiac output** (stroke volume X heart rate), being either:
 −Absolute
 −Relative to the body's metabolic demands
 ...→retrograde vascular congestion
Statistics:
 •Affects 5million persons in the U.S., being the **#1 cause of hospitalization**, accounting for ≥20% of hospital admissions @ age >65years

CLASSIFICATION

Syndromal classification:
•**Cardiac dysfunction:** ↓Ventricular function without correlating syndrome
 Classification:
 •**Systolic dysfunction−50%:** Impaired ventricular myocardial contraction
 •**Diastolic dysfunction−50%:** Impaired ventricular myocardial relaxation or passive elasticity
•**Cardiac failure:** ↓Ventricular function w/ correlating syndrome
 New York Heart Association Classification
 •**Class 1:** Asymptomatic @ ordinary physical activity
 •**Class 2:** Symptomatic @ ordinary physical activity
 •**Class 3:** Symptomatic @ < ordinary physical activity
 •**Class 4:** Symptomatic @ rest
 ...w/ patients alternating among classes via exacerbations & improvements

Anatomic classification:
•**Left sided failure**→pulmonary vascular congestion
•**Right sided failure**→systemic venous congestion, w/ the #1 cause being left sided heart failure

Cardiac output classification:
•**Low output failure:** Absolute low cardiac output
 ◦Cardiomyopathy
 −Dilated−95%
 −Hypertrophic−4%
 −Restrictive−1%
 ◦Valvular disease
 −Regurgitation
 −Stenosis
 ◦Pericardial disease
 −Pericardial tamponade
 −Constrictive pericarditis
 ◦Pulmonary embolus
 ◦Renal failure
•**High output failure:** ↑Cardiac output, still being unable to meet the body's ↑metabolic demands, being due to chronic exacerbating factors causing ↑venous return in patients w/ underlying heart disease

EXACERBATORY FACTORS

•**Medical noncompliance w/ heart failure medications**
•↑**Venous return**
 ◦↑Autonomic sympathetic tone
 −Anemia
 −Autonomic neuropathy→↓parasympathetic tone
 −↓Cardiac output
 −Caffeine
 −Exercise
 −Illicit drugs: Amphetamines, cocaine, ecstasy
 −Inflammation
 −Fever
 −Hyperthyroidism
 −Nicotine
 −Pain
 −Stress
 −Adrenergic medications: Catecholamines, β1 receptor agonists, Ephedrine, Phenylpropanolamine
 −Yohimbine
 ◦Supine position

○↑Extracellular volume
  −Pregnancy
  −Renal failure
  −↑Sodium intake
○Arteriovenous fistulas
  −Paget's disease→multiple bone arteriovenous fistulas
  −Pregnancy, wherein the placenta acts as an arteriovenous fistula
  −Renal dialysis
○Thiamine deficiency→peripheral vasodilation, termed wet beriberi
•↓**Cardiac output**
  ○Hypertension, being either pulmonary &/or systemic
  ○Dysrhythmia, being either tachydysrhythmia or bradydysrhythmia
  ○Infectious endocarditis
  ○Medications:
    −β receptor blockers
    −Calcium channel blockers
  ○Myocardial ischemia
  ○Sinus tachycardia

DIAGNOSIS

LEFT SIDED HEART FAILURE ▬▬▬▬▬▬▬▬▬▬▬▬▬▬▬▬▬▬

Cardiovascular
•Certain etiologies†→
  ○3rd &/or 4th heart sounds, w/ both→
    −Gallop rhythm
•↓Cardiac output→
  ○Hypotension→↓perfusion mediated organ failure→
    −Pre−renal renal failure
    −Cerebral failure→altered mental status
    −Lactic acidemia
    ...termed cardiogenic shock.

Pulmonary
•↑Left atrial volume→↑left atrial hydrostatic pressure→
  ○Pulmonary vascular congestion→↑pulmonary vascular hydrostatic pressure→transudation of
  intravascular fluid to the interstitium & alveoli, forming **interstitial & pulmonary edema**
  respectively→
    −↑Alveolar−capillary diffusion distance
    −Cough ± frothy sputum, which may be blood tinged due to alveolar hemorrhage
    −Expiratory alveolar collapse, w/ subsequent inspiratory opening→crackling sound, termed
    crackles or rhales
    −↑Lung turgor
    −↓Bronchiolar caliber ± bronchospasm→wheezing, termed cardiac asthma
    −Diaphragm flattening, being the most reliable sign of pulmonary edema
    ...→
        •↓Inhalation ability→↓thoracic & abdominal expansion upon inhalation→
          ○↑Respiratory effort→difficulty breathing=**dyspnea**→
            −Respiratory rate >16/ min.=**tachypnea**
            −Accessory muscle usage (sternocleidomastoid muscles for inspiration & abdominal
            muscles for expiration)
            −Speech frequently interrupted by inspiration=telegraphic speech
            −Pursed lip breathing &/or grunting expirations→positive end−expiratory pressure−PEEP
            −Paradoxical abdominal motion: Negative intrathoracic pressure→fatigued diaphragm
            being pulled into the thorax→inspiratory inward motion of the anterior abdominal wall,
            rather than expected outward motion due to diaphragmatic contraction
        •↑Alveolar−capillary diffusion distance→
          ○Ventilation/ perfusion mismatch via:
            −↑Alveolar dead space: Alveolar ventilation through relatively underperfused capillaries
            −↑Vascular shunting‡: Capillary blood flow through relatively underventilated alveoli.
            usually occurring, or exacerbated via ↑venous return
            ...→↓diffusion of O_2 & CO_2→

•Hypoxemia ($SaO_2 \leq 91\%$ or $PaO_2 \leq 60mmHg°$) on room air, w/ subsequent
hypercapnia ($PaCO_2 \geq 45mmHg$) due to either:
  ◦Respiratory muscle fatigue
  ◦Alveolar hypoventilation
  …as CO_2 clearance is unimpaired (& may be ↑in the dyspneic patient) as long as
  adequate ventilation (including lack of diffuse severe ventilation/ perfusion
  mismatching) is maintained, as:
    •CO_2 diffuses 20X as rapidly as O_2
    •Hypercapnia→
      ◦Immediate brain stem respiratory center mediated stimulation of pulmonary
      ventilation, which may correct the hypercapnia, but not necessarily the
      hypoxia
  ◦↑Pulmonary artery pressure^→
    –Right ventricular heave→a palpable lift over the left sternal border
    –Tricuspid regurgitation murmur
    –↑Pulmonic component of the 2nd heart sound
    –Right sided heart failure

---

†3rd heart sounds are heard only w/:
  •Dilated cardiomyopathy
  •Restrictive cardiomyopathy
  •Constrictive pericarditis
  …whereas 4th heart sounds may be heard w/ any cardiomyopathy having ↑atrial contribution
‡Being exacerbated by the supine position→
  •↑Systemic venous return→
    ◦↑Vascular shunting→↑dyspnea, being termed:
      –**Orthopnea**, if persistent
      –**Paroxysmal nocturnal dyspnea** if intermittent
    …causing the patient to either use multiple pillows or sleep in a chair
°Age adjusted normal $PaO_2 = 101 − (0.43 X age)$
^Indicates limited cardiopulmonary reserve via either:
  •Underlying heart failure
  •Underlying chronic obstructive pulmonary disease–COPD
  •Massive or recurrent pulmonary embolism→
    ◦Cor pulmonale

COMPARATIVE THORACIC EXAMINATION FINDINGS			
Physical examination	Consolidation/ empyema	Pleural effusion	Pneumothorax†
Chest expansion	⬇	⬇	⬇‡
Auscultation	⬇Breath sounds w/ crackles, rhonchi, wheezes, &/or egophony°	⬇	⬇Breath sounds
Percussion	⬇	⬇	⬆^
Tactile or auscultatory fremitus	⬆n	⬇	⬇

Note: Outlining lung compression by all 3 etiologies→
        •Atelectasis→
          ◦Signs of consolidation
†If via bronchopleural fistula, may be accompanied by:
  •Hemothorax (a pleural effusion)
  •Pyothorax=empyema
‡Loss of intrapleural negative pressure→
  •Ipsilateral chest wall expansion→
    ◦↑Anteroposterior diameter→
      –↓Respiratory movement
°A patients verbalization of the sound 'E' is heard as 'A'
^Best detected over the midclavicle w/ the patient sitting or standing. The ipsilateral ↓breath sounds
should guide you, as otherwise, you may be fooled by the contralateral side being relatively dull to
percussion, assuming it to be the diseased lung
nUnless accompanied by a concomitant pleural effusion

Cutaneous
- •Severe heart failure→
  - ∘Reflex mediated peripheral arteriole vasoconstriction in order to maintain central organ perfusion, w/ ↓mucocutaneous blood flow→
    - −Pale skin & mucus membranes, w/ progression to ↑relative mucocutaneous O_2 extraction→bluish color=cyanosis
    - −↓Peripheral vascular heat dissipation→cool skin w/ perspiration

Musculoskeletal
- •↓Cardiac output→
  - ∘↓Tissue O_2 & nutrient supply→
    - −↓Skeletal muscle metabolic capability→fatigue

Neurologic
- •Severe heart failure→
  - ∘Delayed transport of pulmonary venous blood to the medullary respiratory center→delayed respiratory response to pulmonary venous blood gases→
    - −Cyclic, alternating hyperventilation & hypoventilation due to conflicting extracellular CO_2 & O_2 in the brain as opposed to the lung. This cycle repeats every 40−60seconds, & occurs episodically, termed **Cheyne−Stokes breathing**, being the #1 form of periodic breathing
    <u>Limitations:</u>
    - •Also occurs w/ brain damage

RIGHT SIDED HEART FAILURE ■■■

Cardiovascular
- •↑Right atrial volume→↑right atrial hydrostatic pressure→systemic vascular congestion→
  - ∘↑Jugular venous hydrostatic pressure→
    - −Jugular venous dilation
  - ∘↓Lymphatic return→
    - −↑Lymphatic hydrostatic pressure→pleural effusion, usually beginning on the right lung due to ↑pleural surface area
  - ∘Systemic fluid transudation→interstitial edema→
    - −↑Weight (1L fluid=1kg=2.2 lbs)
    - −**Pitting edema**, requiring ≥3L of fluid, usually beginning in the most dependent body part (feet & ankles=pedal edema &/or sacral edema in bed−bound patients)→eventual generalized edema= **anasarca**

Gastrointestinal
- •↑Right atrial volume→↑right atrial hydrostatic pressure→systemic vascular congestion→
  - ∘Hepatic congestion→hepatomegally→
    - −Liver capsule (Glisson's capsule) distention ± right upper quadrant abdominal pain
    - −Congestive hepatitis, which if chronic→cirrhosis=cardiac cirrhosis
  - ∘Congested gastrointestinal vasculature→
    - −↓Nutrient absorption→↓dry weight (careful, as weight loss may be offset by fluid gain)
    - −Hepatojugular reflux via abdominal pressure, w/ the patient supine @ a 45° angle→↑venous return→↑jugular venous pressure→jugular venous distention as long as the pressure is applied

Genitourinary
- •↓Cardiac output→↓arterial perfusion→
  - −**Pre−renal renal failure**
  - −Reflex ↑autonomic sympathetic tone
  - ...→↑juxtaglomerular cell renin release→
    - •↑Angiotensin 2 formation→
      - ∘Efferent glomerular arteriole constriction→
        - −↑Glomerular filtrate→↓distal peritubular capillary hydrostatic pressure & osmolarity→ ↑NaCl & water reabsorption
      - ∘↑Adrenal cortical aldosterone release→
        - −Distal convoluted tubule NaCl & water reabsorption
      - ∘↑Posterior pituitary antidiuretic hormone−ADH release→
        - −↑Late distal convoluted tubule & collecting duct H_2O reabsorption→**hypervolemic hyponatremia**
    - ...→circulatory congestion (extracellular volume may ↑>200%) & ↑peripheral vascular resistance→
      - •↑Afterload

98

•Supine position→
  ◦↓Systemic venous hydrostatic pressure→
    −↑Venous return
    −Osmosis of interstitial edematous fluid to the intravascular space→↑venous return
    ...→↑cardiac output→
      •↑Renal perfusion→
        ◦Nocturnal diuresis=**nocturia**

GENERAL ▬▬▬▬▬▬▬▬
Hematologic
•↓Cardiac output→↓arterial perfusion→
  ◦↑Creatinine & blood urea nitrogen−BUN, indicating pre−renal renal failure
•↑**B−type natriuretic peptide−BNP**
  ◦>100pg/ mL indicates likely heart failure
  ◦A level ≥50% above baseline, adequately diuresed weight, indicates decompensated heart failure
Mechanism:
  •↑Atrial, ventricular, & vascular hydrostatic pressure→reflex ↑A−type, B−type, & C−type natriuretic
  peptides release respectively, w:
    ◦ANP produced by the atrial myocardium
    ◦BNP produced by the ventricular myocardium
    ◦CNP produced by the vascular endothelium
    ...→
        •**Suppression of the renin−angiotension−aldosterone system**
        •**Directly mediated ↓renal retention of NaCl & water**
        •↓**Vascular endothelin release**
        ...→diuresis & vasodilation→
          •↓Ventricular preload & afterload. However, the overwhelming neuroendocrine
          response to heart failure is toward the upregulation of the renin−angiotensin−
          aldosterone system, as well as the renal retention of NaCl & water, thus giving the
          natriuretic peptide response little clinical significance except in the fact that
          measurement of B−type natriuretic peptide can be used to:
            ◦**Confirm a suspected diagnosis of heart failure**
            ◦**Quantify its severity**
            ◦**Evaluate treatment efficacy**
Limitations:
  •Glomerular filtration rate <60mL/ min. or dialysis dependence→
    ◦↓Renal tubular enzymatic mediated B−type natriuretic peptide degradation
  •Predominant atrial hypertension via:
    ◦Acute mitral regurgitation
    ◦Flash pulmonary edema
    ◦Mitral stenosis
    ...→lower than expected heart failure mediated BNP levels, based on the syndrome

INDICATIONS FOR HOSPITALIZATION
•Hypotension
•Pulmonary edema
•Hypoxemia (SaO$_2$ ≤ 91% or PaO$_2$ ≤ 60mmHg)
•Symptoms refractory to outpatient therapy
•Myocardial ischemic syndrome

ELECTRICAL STUDIES
•**Electrocardiogram−ECG**
Findings:
  •↓Voltage w/ dilated or restrictive cardiomyopathy, w/ diagnostic criteria being either:
    ◦Peak to peak QRS <5mm in the limb leads (I, II, III, aVR, aVL, aVF)
    ◦Peak to peak QRS <10mm in the precordial leads (V1−V6)
    ...due to either:
      •↓Myocardial mass (ex. dilated cardiomyopathy)
      •Interposing tissue (ex. obesity, restrictive cardiomyopathy), fluid (ex. pericardial or pleural
      effusion), &/or gas (ex. emphysema, pneumothorax) between the electrical impulse & the
      electrodes
  •Criteria for left ventricular hypertrophy−LVH
    ◦Lead V1−V6 progressively ↑R waves
    ◦Tall V5 & V6 R waves & deep V1 & V2 S waves
    ◦Lead aVL R wave >11mm
    ◦Lead aVL R wave + lead V3 S wave being ♂>28mm or ♀>20mm
    ◦Lead V1 S wave + lead V5 R wave being >35mm

- Criteria for right ventricular hypertrophy–RVH
  - Lead V1–V6 progressively ↓R waves
  - Lead V1 R wave > S wave
  - Lead V6 S wave > R wave
  - Lead V1 R wave >6mm
  - Lead V5 & V6 S waves
- Atrial dilation, occurring in all forms of chronic heart failure
  - Criteria for left atrial dilation:
    - Negative terminal P wave deflection in lead V1, being > 1X1mm
    - Notched P wave in lead II, being >3mm in length
  - Criteria for right atrial dilation:
    - ↑P wave in lead II, being ≥2.5mm in height
    - Biphasic P wave in lead V1, w/ a larger initial portion being ≥2mm in height

IMAGING

Chest x ray

Findings:
- ↑Pulmonary vascular hydrostatic pressure→
  - Pulmonary arterial flow redistribution to the apices, as they are areas of less vascular resistance→
    - **Prominence of the upper lobe vasculature, termed cephalization of the vasculature**
  - Transudation of intravascular fluid to the interstitium & alveoli, forming **interstitial & pulmonary edema** respectively→
    - Diffuse "ground–glass" infiltrate
    - Diaphragm flattening, being the most reliable sign of pulmonary edema
    - Fluid infiltrate surrounding the bronchi=**air bronchogram**
- Right heart failure→
  - Lymphatic congestion→
    - Linear opacities perpendicular to the pleura, termed **Kerley lines**
    - ↓Pleural fluid absorption→**pleural effusion**, usually beginning on the right lung due to ↑pleural surface area
- An enlarged heart, termed cardiomegally, indicates a dilated cardiomyopathy

•Transthoracic echocardiography–TTE

Procedure:
- A 2 dimensional ultrasonographic image, allowing real time visualization of:
  - Ventricular wall thickness
  - Cavity size (both atrial & ventricular)
  - Myocardial & valve function, allowing ejection fraction–EF estimation (% of end diastolic volume ejected during ventricular systole)
  - The pericardial space
- Doppler ultrasonography uses Doppler shift to detect vessel flow velocity→
  - Valve regurgitation visualization
  - Estimation of valve pressure gradients

Limitations:
- ↓Visualization in obese or emphysematous patients
- May not allow adequate:
  - Visualization of the anterior aspect of a prosthetic aortic valve
  - Functional assessment of a prosthetic aortic valve
- Transesophageal echocardiography–TEE is more sensitive in detecting:
  - Thrombotic ± infectious vegetations
  - Abscesses
  - Valve damage
  …esp. in a patient w/ a prosthetic heart valve. However, transthoracic echocardiography is the initial test of choice due to its noninvasive nature, as transesophageal echocardiography may→
    - Pharyngeal swallow receptor mediated reflex:
      - Bradycardia
      - Hypotension

•Radionuclide ventriculography

Procedure:
- Requires the harvesting, radioactive labeling, & reinjecting of the patients erythrocytes, allowing the visualization of:
  - Cavity size (both atrial & ventricular)
  - Myocardial & valve function, allowing ejection fraction–EF estimation (% of end diastolic volume ejected during ventricular systole)

Advantages:
- Equally well visualized in obese or emphysematous patients

100

•**Endomyocardial biopsy**
Indications:
  •Histologic diagnosis of suspected &/or unknown etiologies

•**Central venous pressure–CVP monitoring**
  ○The pressure obtained from the large central veins (venae cavae, common iliac veins) or right atrium (normal 1–6mm Hg†), w/ spontaneous intravascular variation usually being ≤4mmHg, but as high as 7mmHg), being equivalent to the right ventricular end diastolic pressure when there is no obstruction between the right atrium & ventricle
  ○A calibrated transducer is connected to the catheter, & placed at the zero reference point for central venous pressure, being the midaxillary 4th intercostal space, corresponding to the position of the atria in the supine position
  ○Intravascular pressure is the pressure in the vessel lumen relative to atmospheric pressure (zero). However, respiratory mediated intrathoracic & intra–abdominal pressure changes are transmitted into the lumen of the vasculature, w/ extravascular pressure being close to zero at the end of a spontaneous expiration‡. Thus, the intravascular pressure is the:
    –Highest pressure recorded during spontaneous respiration
    –Lowest pressure recorded during positive pressure ventilation
  ○An ↑value indicates heart failure, whereas a normal pressure in the setting of hypotension indicates either hypovolemic or distributive hypotension (septic or anaphylactic), w/ shock defined as hypotension **refractory to intravenous fluid bolus infusion w/ ↓perfusion mediated organ failure**, such as:
    –Cardiovascular system→hypotension, lactic acidemia, disseminated intravascular coagulation
    –Central nervous system→altered mental status
    –Kidneys→renal failure
    –Lungs→respiratory failure

---

†CVP in mmHg X 1.36 = CVP in cm H_2O
‡Unless either:
  •Positive end expiratory pressure–PEEP, which should be subtracted from the end expiratory pressure value
  •↑intra–abdominal pressure
  …are being produced

•**Cardiovascular remodeling**
Inciting conditions:
  •**Cardiomyopathy**
  •**Hypertension**, being systemic, pulmonary, &/or cardiac chamber
  •**Myocardial infarction**
Mechanism:
  •The **renin–angiotensin–aldosterone** & **catecholamine** (norepinephrine, epinephrine) neuroendocrine systems evolved as adaptive mechanisms to:
    ○Regulate circulatory integrity, intravascular volume, & organ perfusion pressure
    ○Promote an adaptive & reparative response to tissue injury via complex tissue based molecular signaling pathways, w/ localized tissue dysfunction→
      –Localized neurohormonal paracrine & autocrine effects, whereas systemic, or progressively increasing localized dysfunction→systemic endocrine mediated effects, w/ chronic neurohormonal activation→cardiovascular endothelial, muscle, & connective tissue dysfunction ↔tissue remodeling via inappropriate hyperplasia, hypertrophy, & fibrosis (a vicious cycle)→ altered organ size, shape, & function
Prophylaxis:
  •These chronic maladaptive effects are reduced ± reversed w/ the administration of medications interfering w/ the neurohormonal pathways:
    ○**β receptor blockers**
    ○**Angiotensin converting enzyme inhibitors–ACEi**
    ○**Aldosterone receptor blockers–ARBs**

•The following treatments should be used w/ dysfunction or heart failure due to any cardiomyopathy

•**Smoking cessation** via smoking cessation clinic
  ◦Cigarette smoking contributes to 20% of deaths in the U.S., & is the #1 modifiable cause of premature death
•**Exercise**
  ◦An enjoyable form of aerobic exercise on a regular basis (≥3X/ week) for 20–30min., preceded by stretching
•**Emotional stress management**
  ◦Psychological therapy
  ◦Regular exercise
  ◦Biofeedback
  ◦Yoga
  ◦Listening to music
  ◦Gardening
•**Dietician consultation**
•**Glycemic control if hyperglycemic**
•**Air conditioning**
  ◦Used during hot days→
    −↓Myocardial O_2 & nutrient demand
•**Daily weights** to monitor for fluid retention (edema &/or effusion)→
  ◦↑Weight (1L fluid=1kg=2.2 lbs)
•**Hypertension control**
  ◦Systolic blood pressure <120mmHg & diastolic blood pressure <80mmHg
•**↓Sodium intake**
  ◦≤100mmol sodium/ 24hours=2g elemental sodium or 6g salt/ 24hours, which can usually be achieved w/ a no-added salt diet. Patients w/ poorly compensated heart failure should only consume 0.5–1g elemental sodium or 1.5–3g salt/ 24hours
  ◦→↓Renal potassium loss if taking a diuretic
•**↓Alcohol consumption**
  ◦Only 1drink q24hours (8–12 ounces of beer, 3–5 ounces of wine, or 1 ounce of liquor) in patients without a history of drug abuse
  ◦≥2 drinks/ 24hours→
    −Hypertension
    −Hepatitis (♀ > ♂)
    −↑Abuse risk
  ◦If alcohol is suspected to be causative, total abstinence is required
•**Fluid restriction**
  ◦Patients w/ poorly compensated heart failure should restrict fluid intake to ≤1.5L/ 24hours (~6 cups)
  Guide:
    •1oz = 30mL
    •1cup = 8oz = 240mL
    •4cups = 32oz = ~1L
•**Medication restriction**
  ◦↑**Hypertension risk**
    −Estrogen containing oral contraceptives
    −Glucocorticoids
    −Mineralocorticoids
    −Sympathomimetic drugs, such as decongestants
  ◦Calcium channel blockers should be avoided in patients w/ systolic dysfunction as they→
    −↓Left ventricular function
•**Medication caution**
  ◦**Nonsteroidal anti-inflammatory drugs–NSAIDs**, including Aspirin
  ◦**Angiotensin converting enzyme inhibitors** or **angiotensin 2 receptor blockers**
  Mechanism:
    •Patients w/ pre-existing bilateral ↓renal perfusion, not necessarily failure:
      ◦Heart failure
      ◦Bilateral renal artery stenosis
      ◦Hypovolemia
      ◦Renal failure
    …rely more on the compensatory production of:
      •Prostaglandin→
        ◦Afferent arteriole dilation→maintained glomerular filtration rate, whereas NSAIDs→
          −↓Prostaglandin production→pre-renal renal failure

102

- •Angiotensin 2→
  - ∘Efferent arteriole constriction→maintained glomerular filtration rate, whereas either:
    - –Angiotensin converting enzyme inhibition
    - –Angiotensin 2 receptor blockade
    - …→↓angiotensin 2 production & action respectively→
    - •Pre–renal renal failure
- •**Coronary revascularization**

Indications:
- •Patients in whom myocardial ischemia is thought to be at least partially responsible, w/ confirmation via radioisotope imaging

Procedure:
- •Via percutaneous transluminal angioplasty–PTCA or coronary artery bypass grafting–CABG

β1 SELECTIVE RECEPTOR BLOCKERS				
Generic (Trade)	M ♀	**Start**	**Max**	
Metoprolol (Lopressor)	L ?	6.25mg PO q12hours	100mg q12hours	
•XR form (Toprol XL)		12.5mg PO q24hours	400mg q24hours	

α1 & NONSELECTIVE β RECEPTOR BLOCKERS				
Generic (Trade)	M ♀	**Start**	**Max**	
Carvedilol (Coreg)	L ?	3.1.25mg PO q12hours	25mg q12hours if <85kg	
			50mg q12hours if >85kg	

Mechanism:
- •Competitive antagonist of the β1 ± β2 receptor→
  - ∘↓Sinoatrial & atrioventricular node conduction (β1)→
    - –↓Pulse
  - ∘Anti–dysrhythmic via nodal effects (β1)
  - ∘↓Cardiac muscle contractile strength (β1)
  - ∘↓Juxtaglomerular cell renin release (β1)→
    - –↓Angiotensin 1, angiotensin 2, & aldosterone formation
  - ∘↓Cardiovascular remodeling
  - ∘↑Vascular/ organ smooth muscle contraction (β2)→
    - –Vasoconstriction
    - –Bronchoconstriction
    - –Uterine contraction
  - ∘↓Tremor (β2)
  - ∘↓Hepatocyte glycogenolysis (β2)
- •↓Extrathyroidal tetraiodothyronine–T4 (also termed thyroxine) conversion to the more metabolically active triiodothyronine–T3 form

Outcomes:
- •↓Morbidity & mortality
- •↑Ejection fraction, after initial transient ↓

Side effects:
General
- •Fatigue
- •Malaise

Cardiovascular
- •Bradycardia ± heart block
- •Hypotension
  - ∘Orthostatic hypotension
  - ∘Pelvic hypotension→
    - –Impotence, being the inability to achieve &/or maintain an erection
- •Initial worsening of systolic heart failure
- •Worsening symptoms of peripheral vascular disease
  - ∘Intermittent claudication
  - ∘Raynaud's phenomenon

Pulmonary
- •Bronchoconstriction

Endocrine
- •↑Risk of developing diabetes mellitus
- •May block catecholamine mediated:
  - ∘Physiologic reversal of hypoglycemia via:
    - –↓Hepatocyte gluconeogenesis
  - ∘↓Hypoglycemic symptoms, termed hypoglycemic unawareness→
    - –↓Tachycardia as a warning sign

Gastrointestinal
- Diarrhea
- Nausea ± vomiting
- Gastroesophageal reflux

Mucocutaneous
- Hair thinning

Neurologic
- Sedation
- Sleep alterations
- ↓Libido→
  - Impotence

Psychiatric
- Depression

Hematologic
- ↓High density lipoprotein–HDL levels

- Most patients w/ chronic obstructive pulmonary disease–COPD (including asthma), diabetes, &/or peripheral vascular disease can be safely treated w/ **cardioselective β1 receptor blockers**, as they have ↓peripheral effects

Contraindications:
Cardiovascular
- **Acutely decompensated heart failure**
- Hypotension
- Pulse <50bpm
- Atrioventricular heart block of any degree

Pulmonary
- Moderate to severe chronic obstructive pulmonary disease–COPD, including asthma

Hyper–catacholamine state
- Amphetamine use
- **Cocaine use†**
- Clonidine withdrawal
- Monoamine oxidase inhibitor–MAOi mediated tyramine effect
- Pheochromocytoma

...→relatively ↑vascular α1 receptor stimulation="unopposed α effect"→
- Vasoconstriction→
  - Myocardial ischemic syndrome
  - Cerebrovascular accident syndrome
  - Peripheral vascular ischemic syndrome

Note: **Carvedilol** & **Labetalol** may be used due to their α1 blocking property

---

†Cocaine use→
- Varying ischemic syndrome onset per administration route, & may occur @ min. to days (usually within 3hours)

ANGIOTENSIN CONVERTING ENZYME INHIBITORS–ACEi				
Generic (Trade)	M	♀	Start	Max
Benazepril (Lotensin)	LK	U	10mg PO q24hours	40mg/ 24hours
Captopril (Capoten)	LK	U	12.5mg PO q12hours	450mg/ 24hours
Enalapril (Vasotec)	LK	U	5mg PO q24hours	40mg/ 24hours
Fosinopril (Monopril)	LK	U	10mg PO q24hours	40mg/ 24hours
Lisinopril (Prinivil, Zestril)	K	U	10mg PO q24hours	40mg q24hours

Dose adjustment:
- ↓Initial dose by 50% if:
  - Elderly
  - Concomitant diuretic use
  - Renal disease

Mechanism:
- Reversibly inhibits angiotensin converting enzyme–ACE→
  - ↓Bradykinin degradation→
    - –Vasodilation
  - ↓Angiotensin 2 formation→
    - –Vasodilation (**arterial** > venous)
    - –↓Renal NaCl & water retention
    - –↓Adrenal cortex aldosterone release→↓renal NaCl & water retention
    - –↓Facilitation of adrenal medullary & presynaptic norepinephrine release→vasodilation

104

−Glomerular efferent arteriole vasodilation→↓intraglomerular hydrostatic pressure→↓filtration→
    ↓proteinuria in patients w/ nephropathy
   ◦↓Cardiovascular remodeling

Outcomes:
- ↓Morbidity & mortality

Side effects:

Cardiovascular
- Hypotension

Gastrointestinal
- Altered gustatory sense=dysguesia−3%

Genitourinary
- Acute interstitial nephritis
- Patients w/ pre−existing bilateral ↓renal perfusion, not necessarily failure:
  - Heart failure
  - Bilateral renal artery stenosis
  - Hypovolemia
  - Renal failure
  …rely more on the compensatory production of angiotensin 2→
  - Efferent arteriole constriction→
    - Maintained glomerular filtration rate−GFR, whereas either:
      - −Angiotensin converting enzyme inhibition
      - −Angiotensin 2 receptor blockade
        …→↓angiotensin 2 production & action respectively, which may→
        - **Pre−renal renal failure**

Mucocutaneous
- ↓Bradykinin & substance P degradation→↑levels→hypersensitivity−like syndrome→
  - **Angioedema−0.4%**, usually within 2weeks of treatment, but may manifest @ months to years→
    - −Soft tissue edema of the epiglottis, face, lips, oropharynx, &/or tongue
  - **Dermatitis−10%**

Pulmonary
- ↑Bradykinin levels→
  - **Chronic cough−20%**, usually being dry & involuntary

Materno−fetal
- **Fetal & neonatal morbidity & mortality**

Hematologic
- ↓Aldosterone production ± renal failure→
  - **Hyperkalemia**
- Neutropenia

Monitoring:
- Check creatinine & potassium @ 3−10days after initiation or dose↑, then
  - Q3−6months

Contraindications:

Genitourinary
- Acute renal failure
- Bilateral renal artery stenosis
- Unilateral renal artery stenosis of a solitary functioning kidney

Mucocutaneous
- Angiotensin converting enzyme inhibitor induced angioedema or dermatitis

Materno−fetal
- **Breast feeding**
- **Pregnancy**

Hematologic
- **Potassium >5mEq/ L**

ANGIOTENSIN 2 RECEPTOR BLOCKERS–ARBs				
Generic (Trade)	M	♀	Start	Max
Candesartan (Atacand)	K	?	16mg PO q24hours	32mg q24hours
Eprosartan (Teveten)	F	U	600mg PO q24hours	800mg/ 24hours
Irbesartan (Avapro)	L	U	150mg PO q24hours	300mg q24hours
Olmisartan (Benicar)	K	U	20mg PO q24hours	40mg q24hours
Losartan (Cozaar)	L	U	50mg PO q24hours	100mg/ 24hours
Telmisartan (Micardis)	L	U	40mg PO q24hours	80mg q24hours
Valsartan (Diovan)	L	U	80mg PO q24hours	320mg q24hours

Dose adjustment:
- ↓Initial dose by 50% if:
  - Elderly
  - Concomitant diuretic use
  - Renal disease

Losartan specific:
- Starting dose is halved if concomitant hepatic disease

Mechanism:
- Angiotensin 2 receptor blockade→
  - ↓Angiotensin 2 action→
    - –Vasodilation (**arterial** > venous)
    - –↓Renal NaCl & water retention
    - –↓Adrenal cortex aldosterone release→↓renal NaCl & water retention
    - –↓Facilitation of adrenal medullary & presynaptic norepinephrine release→vasodilation
    - –Glomerular efferent arteriole vasodilation→↓intraglomerular hydrostatic pressure→↓filtration→
      - ↓proteinuria in patients w/ nephropathy
  - ↓Cardiovascular remodeling

Side effects†:
Cardiovascular
- Hypotension
Gastrointestinal
- Altered gustatory sense=dysguesia–3%
Genitourinary
- Acute interstitial nephritis
- Patients w/ preexisting bilateral ↓renal perfusion, not necessarily failure:
  - Heart failure
  - Bilateral renal artery stenosis
  - Hypovolemia
  - Renal failure
  - …rely more on the compensatory production of angiotensin 2→
    - Efferent arteriole constriction→
      - Maintained glomerular filtration rate–GFR, whereas either:
        - –Angiotensin converting enzyme inhibition
        - –Angiotensin 2 receptor blockade
        - …→↓angiotensin 2 production & action respectively, which may→
          - **Pre-renal renal failure**
Materno–fetal
- **Fetal & neonatal morbidity & mortality**
Hematologic
- ↓Aldosterone production ± renal failure→
  - **Hyperkalemia**
- Neutropenia

†Do not cause the hypersensitivity–like syndrome associated w/ ACE inhibitors, due to lack of bradykinin & substance P elevation

Monitoring:
- Check creatinine & potassium @ 3–10days after initiation or dose†, then
  - Q3–6months

Contraindications:
Genitourinary
- Acute renal failure
- Bilateral renal artery stenosis
- Unilateral renal artery stenosis of a solitary functioning kidney
Materno–fetal
- Breast feeding
- **Pregnancy**

DIETARY

Generic (Trade)	M ♀	Dose
Omega 3–fatty acids (Fish oil)	L ?	A combination dose of EPA + DHA†
•Cardioprotection		1g PO q24hours
•Hypertriglyceridemia		2–4g PO q24hours

†Eicosapentanoic acid–EPA & docosahexanoic acid–DHA
•There are only 2 types of polyunsaturated fatty acids
  ∘Omega 3–fatty acids, mainly from:
    –**Fish or fish oils**, esp. herring, mackerel, salmon, sardines, trout, & tuna
    –Beans, esp. soybeans
    –Green leafy vegetables
    –Nuts, esp. walnuts
    –Plant seeds, esp. canola oil & flaxseed
  ∘Omega 6–fatty acids, mainly from:
    –Grains
    –Meats
    –Nuts, esp. peanuts
    –Plant seeds, esp. borage oil, corn oil, cottonseed oil, grape seed oil, primrose oil, safflower oil, sesame oil, soybean oil, & sunflower oil
•The Western diet is abundant in omega 6–fatty acids (which are prothrombotic & proinflammatory), w/ humans lacking the necessary enzymes to convert them to omega 3–fatty acids, which therefore need to be obtained from separate dietary sources. However, significant amounts of methylmercury & other environmental toxins may be concentrated in certain fish species (w/ high quality fish oil supplements usually lacking contaminants):
  •King Mackerel
  •Shark
  •Swordfish
  •Tilefish, aka golden bass or golden snapper
  …which are to be avoided by:
    •♀ who may become or are pregnant
    •♀ who are breastfeeding
    •Young children

Mechanism:
•Vasodilation→
  ∘↓Blood pressure, being dose dependent, w/ a minimal effect of 4/ 2 mmHg w/ doses of 3–6g q24hours
•↓Lipid, esp. triglycerides
•Anti–dysrhythmic
•Anti–inflammatory
•↓Platelet activity

Outcomes:
•In patients w/ coronary artery disease:
  ∘↓All cause mortality
  ∘↓Dysrhythmia mediated sudden death

Side effects:
Cardiovascular
  •↑Bleeding time→
    ∘Excessive hemorrhage
Gastrointestinal
  •Belching
  •Bloating
  •Fishy aftertaste
  •Nausea ± vomiting
Hematologic
  •Hyperglycemia
Interactions
  •None known, making it safe for use in combination w/ other:
    ∘Anticoagulant medications
    ∘Antiplatelet medications
    ∘Lipid lowering medications

POTASSIUM
•**Always measure the magnesium level concomitantly**

Indications:
•Ensure a potassium of 4–5mEq/ L

Generic
•Potassium chloride–KCL
•Potassium bicarbonate
•Potassium citrate
•Potassium acetate
•Potassium gluconate
•Potassium phosphate

POTASSIUM DOSAGE ADJUSTMENT SCALE†_____

Plasma K^+ (mEq/ L)	K^+ repletion (mEq)
≥3.9	None
3.7–3.8	20
3.5–3.6	40
3.3–3.4	60
3.1–3.2	80
≤3	100

†Half all above doses @ a glomerular filtration rate–GFR ≤30mL/ min.

Outcomes:
•Anti–dysrhythmic
•↑Cardiac contractility in heart failure
•Modest hypotensive effect in some patients
•↓Cerebrovascular disease risk, apart from its possible blood pressure lowering effects

ALTERNATIVE TREATMENTS ▬▬▬▬

Indications:
•Symptomatic heart failure in a patient, w/ intolerance of, hypersensitivity to, or contraindication to
angiotensin converting enzyme inhibitors–ACEi & aldosterone receptor blockers–ARBs
Outcomes:
•The combination of Hydralazine & Isosorbide dinitrate→
  ◦↓Mortality in symptomatic patients, but not as good as either ACEi or ARB

VASODILATORS

Generic (Trade)	M	♀	Start	Target	Max
Hydralazine (Apresoline)	LK	?	10mg PO q8hours	75mg q8hours	100mg q8hours

Mechanism:
•Vasodilation (**arterial** >> venous)

Side effects:
Cardiovascular
•Systemic vasodilation→
  ◦Edema
  ◦Reflex tachycardia
  ◦Orthostatic hypotension
•Meningeal arterial dilation→
  ◦Headache
Pulmonary
•Pulmonary vasodilation→
  ◦Exacerbation of ventilation/ perfusion mismatches
Autoimmune
•**Systemic lupus erythematosis–SLE like syndrome–10%**, being reversible upon
discontinuation of the medication

Contraindications:
Cardiovascular
•Hypotension
•Severe aortic or mitral stenosis
Autoimmune
•Systemic lupus erythematosis–SLE

&

108

NITROVASODILATORS: Long acting					
Generic	**M ♀**	**Start**		**Target**	**Max**
Isosorbide dinitrate (Isordil)	L ?	10mg PO q8hours (7am, noon, 5pm)		40mg q8h	80mg q8h

Mechanism:
- Vasodilation (**venous** > arterial)→
  - ↓Preload→
    - −↓Myocardial contractile strength→↓O_2 & nutrient demand
  - ↑Coronary artery dilation→↑perfusion

Side effects:
Cardiovascular
- Systemic vasodilation→
  - Reflex tachycardia
  - Orthostatic hypotension
  - Facial flushing
- Meningeal arterial dilation→
  - Headache

Pharmacokinetics/ pharmacodynamics
- Tolerance to medication effects

Contraindications:
Cardiovascular
- Hypotension

Neurologic
- **Hypertensive encephalopathy**, as it ↑ intracranial pressure

Interactions
- **Sildenafil** (Viagra) **is contraindicated** in patients taking concomitant nitrates, as the combination within 24hours may→severe hypotension→
  - ↓Myocardial perfusion→
    - −Stable angina mediated acute coronary syndrome
  - ↓Cerebral perfusion→
    - −Pre−syncope/ syncope
    - −Cerebrovascular accident syndrome

THIAZIDE DIURETICS

Generic (Trade)	M	♀	Start	Max
Hydrochlorothiazide	L	U	12.5mg PO q24hours	50mg q24hours
Metolazone (Zaroxolyn)	L	U	5mg PO q24hours	10mg q24hours

Duration: 6–12hours

•There is synergistic efficacy of combination treatment w/ a loop diuretic

Dose adjustment:
•Once organ edema has resolved, consider maintenance dosing @ half dose q24hours w/ titration

Mechanism:
•Inhibits NaCl reabsorption in the early distal convoluted tubule→
  ∘↑Urination→
    −↓Intravascular volume→↓cardiac preload→↓cardiac output→eventual compensatory intravascular volume repletion to near pre−treatment levels, but w/ peripheral vascular resistance falling below pre−treatment baseline being responsible for the chronic hypotensive effect

Outcomes:
•↓Symptoms, but **no effect on mortality**

Limitations:
•↓Efficacy in patients w/ a glomerular filtration rate <30mL/ min.

Side effects:
  Genitourinary
    •Acute interstitial nephritis
  Neurologic
    •**Ototoxicity**
  Hematologic
    •Acid base disturbances
      ∘Hypochloremic metabolic alkalemia
    •Dyslipidemia
      ∘↑Cholesterol & triglycerides
    •Electrolyte disturbances
      ∘**Hypokalemia**
      ∘Hypomagnesemia
      ∘Hyponatremia
      ∘Hypercalcemia
    •Hyperglycemia
    •Hyperuricemia

Contraindications:
•**Sulfa allergy**, as all thiazide & loop diuretics (except Ethacrynic acid) contain a sulfa component

LOOP DIURETICS

Generic (Trade)	M	♀	Start	Max
Furosemide (Lasix)	K	?	20mg q24−12hours PO	600mg/ 24hours

Onset: 1hour, Duration: 6hours (**Lasix** lasts **six** hours)

•There is synergistic efficacy of combination treatment w/ a thiazide diuretic
•Administer 2nd dose in the mid−afternoon to avoid nocturia

Mechanism:
•Inhibits $Na^+/K^+/2Cl^-$ reabsorption in the thick ascending limb of the loop of Henle→
  ∘↑Urination→
    −↓Intravascular volume→↓cardiac preload→↓cardiac output→eventual compensatory intravascular volume repletion to near pre−treatment levels, but w/ peripheral vascular resistance falling below pre−treatment baseline being responsible for the chronic hypotensive effect

Outcomes:
•↓Symptoms, but **no effect on mortality**

Limitations:
•↓Efficacy in patients w/ a glomerular filtration rate <10mL/ min.

Side effects:
  Genitourinary
    •Acute interstitial nephritis

Neurologic
- **Ototoxicity**

Hematologic
- Acid base disturbances
  - ○Hypochloremic metabolic alkalemia
- Dyslipidemia
  - ○↑Cholesterol & triglycerides
- Electrolyte disturbances
  - ○**Hypokalemia**
  - ○Hypomagnesemia
  - ○Hyponatremia
  - ○Hypercalcemia
- Hyperglycemia
- Hyperuricemia

<u>Contraindications:</u>
- **Sulfa allergy**, as all thiazide & loop diuretics (except Ethacrynic acid) contain a sulfa component

111

POTASSIUM SPARING DIURETICS: ↓Potassium & magnesium loss when used in combination w/ other diuretic types

Generic (Trade)	M	♀	Start	Target
Spironolactone (Aldactone)	LK	U	12.5mg PO q24hours	After 5 days to 25mg q24hours

Duration: 24–72hours

Titration:
•Based on plasma potassium
•A urinary sodium/ potassium ratio >1 indicates effective aldosterone antagonism

Mechanism:
•Structurally similar to aldosterone→
  ∘Competitive inhibition of the intracellular aldosterone receptor in the distal convoluted tubule & collecting duct→
    −↑Urination→↓intravascular volume→↓cardiac preload→↓cardiac output→↓blood pressure, w/ eventual compensatory intravascular volume repletion to near pre−treatment levels, but w/ peripheral vascular resistance falling below pre−treatment baseline being responsible for the chronic hypotensive effect

Outcomes:
•↓Mortality in NYHA classes 3 & 4

Side effects:
Endocrine
  •Anti−androgenic effects→
    ∘**Gynecomastia**, being the ↑development of male mammary glands
Hematologic
  •Acid base disturbances
    ∘Non−anion gap hypochloremic metabolic acidemia
  •Electrolyte disturbances
    ∘**Hyperkalemia**
    ∘Hyponatremia
  •Hyperuricemia

Monitoring:
•Monitor creatinine & potassium @ baseline, then
  ∘@ 1week, then
  ∘@ 1, 2, & 3months, then
  ∘Q3months for the remainder of the 1st year, then
  ∘Q6months thereafter

Contraindications:
•Potassium >5 mEq/ L

DIGITALIS GLYCOSIDES

Indications:
•Ejection fraction−EF ≤35%
•Cardiothoracic ratio of ≥0.5=50%
•Chronic atrial fibrillation† w/ ventricular systolic dysfunction→
  ∘Heart failure

†Effective in ↓resting rate, **but not exertional or paroxysmal rate**

Generic (Trade)	M	♀	Dose	Max
Digoxin (Lanoxin)	KL	?	0.125mg PO q48−q24hours	0.25mg q24hours

Onset: 4−6hours, Half life: 40hours

Dose adjustment:
•Adjust dose based on clinical response & plasma levels (therapeutic 0.8−1.8ng/ mL) w/ toxicity typically occurring @ >1.8ng/ mL, but may occur @ therapeutic levels
•Amiodarone & Verapamil→
  ∘↑Digoxin levels (↓Digoxin dose by 50%)
•Quinidine mediated displacement of Digoxin from tissue binding sites→
  ∘↓Clearance

Mechanism:
•↓Cell membrane Na^+/K^+ ATPase function→
  ∘↑Intracellular sodium→
    −↓Na^+/Ca^{+2} anti−transporter function→↑intracellular calcium→↑myocardial inotropy

112

Outcomes:
•↓Symptoms, but **no effect on mortality**

Side effects†:
- **General**
  - ◦↓Appetite
  - ◦Fatigue
  - ◦Headache
  - ◦Malaise
  - ◦Weakness
- **Cardiac**
  - ◦The sequential occurrence of electrocardiographic–ECG changes:
    - –Atrioventricular block (1°,2°,3°)→↑PR interval
    - –T wave flattening
    ⬇
    - –**ST segment depression**
    - –↓QT interval
    - –T wave inversion
    ⬇
    - –**Supraventricular &/or ventricular dysrhythmias**
    - –**U wave**
- **Gastrointestinal**
  - ◦Abdominal pain
  - ◦Diarrhea
  - ◦Nausea ± vomiting
- **Genitourinary/ cutaneous**
  - ◦Digoxin's structural similarity to estrogen→
    - –Gynecomastia, being the ↑development of male mammary glands
    - –Impotence, being the inability to achieve &/or maintain an erection
    - –↓Libido
- **Neurologic**
  - ◦Altered mental status
  - ◦Dizziness
  - ◦Paresthesias
  - ◦Psychosis
  - ◦**Visual changes 50–95%**
    - –Altered pupil size
    - –Photophobia
    - –Ocular muscle palsies
    - –Yellow–green halos around bright lights
- **Hematologic**
  - •↓Cell membrane Na^+/K^+ ATPase function→
    - ◦↑Extracellular potassium→
      - –Hyperkalemia

---

††Risk w/ electrolyte abnormalities:
- •Hypercalcemia
- •Hypokalemia
- •Hypomagnesemia
- …even w/ therapeutic Digoxin levels

ANTIDOTE

Indications:
- •Ingested Digoxin dose >10mg
- •Plasma Digoxin level >6ng/ mL
- •≥2° atrioventricular block
- •Supraventricular &/or ventricular dysrhythmias
- •Plasma potassium >5.5mEq/ L, being refractory to conventional treatment modalities

Generic (Trade)	M ♀	Vials
Digoxin-immune Fab (Digibind)	K ?	Administered via IV fluids over 15–30min., w/ repeat if toxicity persists (range: 2–20 vials)
•Acute ingestion of unknown quantity		20vials
•Acute ingestion of known quantity		[Ingested Digoxin (mg) X 0.8] / 0.6
•Chronic ingestion mediated overdose		[Plasma Digoxin level (ng/ mL) X weight (kg)] / 100

Mechanism:
•Each vial being 40mg & binding ~0.5mg Digoxin

•Plasma Digoxin levels will be falsely ↑for several days after administration

•**Cardiac resynchronization therapy**
 Indications being both:
  •Symptomatic heart failure ≥ NYHA class 3, being refractory to medical treatment
  •Interventricular conduction defects†, esp. left bundle branch block→
   ∘Wide QRS complex, being >0.12seconds
 Procedure:
  •A percutaneous 3-lead biventricular pacemaker system is utilized, w/ a lead placed in the:
   ∘Right atrium
   ∘Right ventricle
   ∘Cardiac vein on the lateral wall of the left ventricle, via passing the lead progressively through
    the right atrium & coronary sinus
 Outcomes:
  •Biventricular electromechanical coordination→
   ∘↑Ventricular synchrony→ reduced ± reversed ventricular remodeling→↑ejection fraction→
    −↓Morbidity & mortality
    −↑Exercise tolerance & quality of life
 Limitations:
  •Inability to implant the left ventricular lead appropriately, usually due to unfavorable coronary
   venous anatomy
 Complications:
  •Lead dislodgement–10%
  •Coronary sinus dissection
  •Cardiac perforation

†30% of patients w/ heart failure have some form of interventricular conduction delay→
 •↑QRS duration, which is associated w/ a worse prognosis

114

•**Oxygen** to maintain PaO_2 >60mmHg or SaO_2 >92%, usually accomplished via nasal cannula @ 2–4L/ min.
  Indications:
    •Hypoxemia (SaO_2 ≤ 91% or PaO_2 ≤ 60mmHg)
  Dose adjustment:
    •As hypoxemia may worsen during air travel, a general recommendation is to ↑oxygen flow rate by 2L/ min. during flight
  Mechanism:
    •Continuous† (≥18h/ day) low flow oxygen treatment via nasal cannula→
    ∘↓Formation or progression of cor pulmonale

---

†Patients must understand that the medication is not used to treat dyspnea, & thus is not to be reserved for symptomatic treatment

•**Ventricular assist device–VAD**
  Mechanism:
    •A non–pulsatile pump placed intraoperatively in parallel w/ the right ventricle–RVAD, left ventricle–LVAD, or both ventricles–BiVAD
  Complications:
    •Hemorrhage
    •Thromboembolism

•**Orthotopic cardiac transplantation**
  Indications:
    •A candidate must meet all of the following criteria†:
    ∘Age <60years
    ∘Free of complicating, irreversible, extracardiac organ dysfunction, as this may ↓recovery & ↑post–transplantation complications
    ∘Prepared to undergo the post–transplantation regimen
      –Post–transplant immunosuppressive therapy includes glucocorticoids & Azathioprine &/or Cyclosporine
    ∘Adequate psychosocial support system
  Outcomes:
    •1year survival rate: 85%
    •5year survival rate: 70%

---

†Even when a candidate meets these criteria, a compatible heart may not become available until after the patient has already died

ANTICOAGULANTS: High molecular weight Heparin

Indications:
- •Atrial fibrillation
- •Ejection fraction <30%
- •Large ventricular akinetic segment
- •Mural thrombus
- •Restrictive cardiomyopathy

M	♀	Start
M	?	60units/ kg IV bolus (or 5000units empirically)
		12units/kg/hour infusion (or 1000units/ hour empirically)

•Titrated by 2.5units/kg/hour to achieve an activated partial thromboplastin time–aPTT of 1.5–2X control value or **50–70seconds**

aPTT (seconds)	Action	Obtain next aPTT
<40	Bolus 5000units & ↑infusion rate by 100units/ hour	6hours
40–49	↑Infusion rate by 50units/ hour	6hours
50–70 (or 1.5–2Xcontrol)	NO ACTION	24hours
71–85	↓Infusion rate by 50units/ hour	6hours
86–100	Hold infusion 30min., then ↓infusion rate by 100units/ hour	6hours
101–150	Hold infusion 60min., then ↓infusion rate by 150units/ hour	6hours
>150	Hold infusion 60min., then ↓infusion rate by 300units/ hour	6hours

Monitoring:
- •Complete blood count q24hours to monitor for side effects

ANTICOAGULANTS: Low molecular weight Heparin

Generic (Trade)	M	♀	Start	Max
Enoxaparin (Lovenox)	KL	P	1.5mg/ kg SC q24hours or	180mg/ 24hours
			1mg/ kg SC q12hours	
Dalteparin (Fragmin)	KL	P	200 anti–factor Xa units/ kg SC q24hours or	18,000units q24hours
			100 anti–factor Xa units/ kg SC q12hours	

Dose adjustment:
- •Obesity
  - ◦Most manufacturers recommend a maximum dose of that for a 90kg patient

Monitoring:
- •Monitoring of anti–Xa levels is recommended in patients w/:
  - ◦Abnormal coagulation/ hemorrhage
  - ◦Obesity
  - ◦Renal failure
  - ◦Underweight
- •Check 4h after 2nd SC dose. Further monitoring is not necessary once the correct dose is established in obese patients

Administration frequency	Therapeutic anti–Xa levels
Q12hours	0.6–1 units/ mL
Q24hours	1–2 units/ mL

Mechanism:
- •Heparin combines w/ plasma antithrombin 3→
  - ◦↑Antithrombin 3 activity in removing thrombin & activated factors 9, 10, 11,& 12→
    - –↓Coagulation→↓vascular & mural thrombus formation &/or propagation
- •Heparin is metabolized by the plasma enzyme Heparinase

Outcomes:
- •↓Morbidity & mortality

Side effects:
Cardiovascular
- •**Hemorrhage**
- •**Heparin induced thrombocytopenia–HIT 10%**, esp. w/ high molecular weight Heparin
  - Mechanism:
    - •Heparin mediated platelet agglutination→
      - ◦Monocyte/ macrophage mediated extravascular removal via the splenic trabecular network=red pulp, & hepatic sinusoids→
        - –**Thrombocytopenia**
  - Outcomes:
    - •Benign, as it resolves spontaneously, even w/ continued exposure

•**Heparin induced thrombocytopenia ± thrombosis–HITT ≤3%**, esp. w/ high molecular weight Heparin
   Mechanism:
   •Heparin mediated platelet agglutination→
      ◦Monocyte/ macrophage mediated extravascular removal via the splenic trabecular network=red pulp, & hepatic sinusoids→
      –**Thrombocytopenia**
      ◦Platelet release of Heparin neutralizing factor=platelet factor 4–PF4, which complexes w/ Heparin→
         –Production of anti–complex antibodies→↑platelet activation↔↑platelet factor 4 release→ a vicious cycle of **platelet mediated arterial &/or venous thrombus formation, termed the "white clot syndrome,"** being as the clot is relatively devoid of erythrocytes
   Outcomes:
   •Must discontinue treatment as **20% develop thromboembolic complications**. Being that both Heparins may cross–react w/ the etiologic antibodies, their further use is contraindicated. Consider continued treatment w/ direct thrombin inhibitors
      ◦Antibody cross–reactivity:
         –Low molecular weight Heparins–85%
         –Heparinoids–5%
Mucocutaneous
   •Skin necrosis–rarely occurring w/ high molecular weight Heparins, & not being associated w/ anticoagulant deficiency
Musculoskeletal
   •Osteoporosis, esp. w/ high molecular weight Heparin
      ◦Usually @ use ≥1month
Hematologic
   •↓Aldosterone production→
      ◦**Hyperkalemia–8%**

CHARACTERISTICS OF HEPARIN INDUCED THROMBOCYTOPENIC SYNDROMES

	HIT	HITT
Onset	<2days	4–10 days
Re-exposure	<2days	Earlier if re-exposed within 3 months
Platelet count	↓, being <150,000 or ≥50%	
Platelet median nadir	~90,000	~60,000

•**^{14}C–Serotonin release assay**
   Indications:
   •Suspected HITT
   Procedure:
   •Normal donor platelets are radiolabeled w/ ^{14}C–serotonin. They are then washed & combined w/ patient serum & therapeutic Heparin concentrations (0.1 U/ mL). Induction of ^{14}C–serotonin release from platelets constitutes a positive test
   Limitations:
   •Expense, due to the use of radioactive material
   Outcomes:
   •Considered the gold standard in the detection of HITT
•**Enzyme linked immunosorbent assay–ELISA**
   Indications:
   •Suspected HITT
   Procedure:
   •Heparin–PF4 complexes affixed to a plastic plate are incubated w/ the patient's serum. If the patient has produced antibodies, then the addition of enzymatically (horseradish peroxidase) labeled anti–human IgG allows for color visualization via spectrophotometer
   Limitations:
   •Many antibody positive patients do not develop clinical HITT
   •30% false positive
Contraindications:
•Active hemorrhage
•Severe bleeding diathesis
•Severe thrombocytopenia (platelet count ≤20,000/ µL)
•Recent significant trauma
•Neurosurgery, ocular surgery, or intracranial hemorrhage within 10days

117

ANTIDOTE			
Generic	M ♀	Amount IV over 10min.	Max
Protamine	P ?	1mg/ 100units of HMWH	50mg
		1mg/ 100units Dalteparin	"
		1mg/ 1mg Enoxaparin	"

Mechanism:
- •Protamine combines electrostatically w/ Heparin→
  - ◦Inability to bind to antithrombin 3

FOLLOWED BY

ANTICOAGULANTS		
Generic	M ♀	Start
Warfarin (Coumadin)	L U	5mg PO q24hours

- •Because the anticoagulant proteins↓ relatively faster than the procoagulant proteins, an initial transient hypercoagulable state develops. Due to this, Warfarin is started once the patient is therapeutic on Heparin, via either:
  - ◦Goal aPTT w/ high molecular weight Heparin
  - ◦Evening of initiation of low molecular weight Heparin
  ...requiring ~7days (corresponding to 2 half lives of factor 2, or a 75% reduction) to reach a true therapeutic level of an **international normalized ratio–INR of 2–3**

INR	Action	Obtain next INR
<1.5	↑Weekly dose by 15%	1 week
1.5–1.9	↑Weekly dose by 10%	2 weeks
2–3	NO ACTION	1 month if stable
3.1–3.9	↓Weekly dose by 10%	2 weeks
4–5	Skip 1 day, then ↓weekly dose by 15%	1 week
>5	DISCONTINUE WARFARIN	Q day until ≤3, then ↓weekly dose by 50%

Mechanism:
- •Competitively inhibits hepatocyte enzymatic vitamin K reactive sites→
  - ◦↓Formation of both:
    - –Procoagulant proteins 2, 7, 9, & 10
    - –Anticoagulant proteins C & S
    ...w/ the anticoagulant effect requiring several days, as it must await the metabolism of the pre–existing plasma procoagulant proteins, w/ normal coagulation returning within several days of discontinuation

Side effects:
Cardiovascular
- •**Hemorrhage**
  - ◦Fatal: 0.6%/ year
  - ◦Major: 3%/ year
  - ◦Minor: 7%/ year
Cutaneous
- •Tissue necrosis w/ protein C or S deficiency or dysfunction

Contraindications:
- •Active hemorrhage
- •Severe bleeding diathesis
- •Severe thrombocytopenia (platelet count ≤20,000/ μL)
- •Recent significant trauma
- •Neurosurgery, ocular surgery, or intracranial hemorrhage within 10days
- •Injury risk (including falls & sports) or compliance risk via:
  - ◦Alcoholism
  - ◦Altered mental status
  - ◦Illicit drug abuse
  - ◦Orthostatic hypotension
  - ◦Poor compliance
  - ◦Seizure disease
  - ◦Syncope
  - ◦Unstable gait

Special considerations:
- •**If undergoing elective surgery during treatment**
  - ◦Stop Warfarin 5 days prior to surgery, & begin Heparin
- •**Anticoagulation during pregnancy**
  - ◦Substitute low molecular weight Heparin for Warfarin, followed by Warfarin treatment postpartum if necessary

118

ANTIDOTES
•**Gastric lavage & activated charcoal** if recently administered; forced emesis at home

VITAMIN K=Phytonadione
Indications:
•To correct the international normalized ration–INR or prothrombin time–PT

Dose
10mg SC/ IV slow push @ 1mg/ min. in order to ↓anaphylactoid reaction risk

Mechanism:
•Requires several hours to days for effect

Side effects:
•Avoid intramuscular administration which may→
  ◦Intramuscular hemorrhage

FRESH FROZEN PLASMA–FFP
Indications:
•To correct the international normalized ration–INR or prothrombin time–PT under the following conditions:
  ◦**INR >20**
  ◦**Severe hemorrhage**
  ◦**Other need for rapid reversal, such as an emergent procedure**

Dose†
15mL/ kg IV (w/ ~200mL FFP/ unit) q4hours prn ↑INR

Mechanism:
•Contains clotting factors 2, 7, 9–13, & heat labile 5 & 7→
  ◦Immediate onset of action
•Each unit→
  ◦8% ↑coagulation factors
  ◦4% ↑blood volume

VENTRICULAR DYSRHYTHMIA PROPHYLAXIS
Indications:
•Primary prevention
  ◦Coronary artery disease, left ventricular dysfunction, & induceable ventricular tachycardia
  ◦Coronary artery disease & ejection fraction–EF ≤30%
  ◦↑Risk inherited or acquired disease syndromes
    –Brugada's syndrome
    –Hypertrophic cardiomyopathy
    –Long QT syndrome
•Secondary prevention
  ◦Cardiac arrest due to ventricular fibrillation or ventricular tachycardia, except w/:
    –Idiopathic ventricular tachycardia, which has an excellent prognosis
    –Reversible causes such as acid–base/ electrolyte disturbances, myocardial ischemia, or atrial fibrillation in patients w/ Wolff–Parkinson–White syndrome
  ◦Sustained ventricular tachycardia (persisting for ≥30seconds or requiring termination due to symptoms)
  ◦Symptomatic, non–sustained ventricular tachycardia
  ◦Unexplained syncope w/ either:
    –Advanced structural heart disease
    –Inducible, sustained ventricular fibrillation or tachycardia

•**Internal cardioverter–defibrillator–ICD**
  Composed of 3 parts:
  •**Generator**
    ◦Placed in the pectoral area, rather than older models which were placed in the abdomen
  •**Transvenous defibrillating leads**
    ◦Inserted into the subclavian vein, & advanced to the right ventricular apex
  •**Electrodes**
    ◦In the lead tips, capable of sensing, cardioverting, defibrillating, &
      –Anti–tachycardia pacing, being painless, & used to terminate monomorphic tachycardias
  Complications:
  •Infection–2%, necessitating device removal
  •Lead malfunction→
    ◦False signals→
      –Inappropriate shock administration

Limitations:
- Anti-tachycardia pacing may:
  - Accelerate ventricular tachycardia
  - Induce a ventricular dysrhythmia if applied during a supraventricular rhythm
  - ...necessitating cardioversion or defibrillation if ineffective

  &
- Only β receptor blockers (as above) & Amiodarone medically→
  - ↓Cardiac arrest risk in patients w/ systolic dysfunction

ANTI-DYSRHYTHMIC MEDICATIONS		
Generic (Trade)	M ♀	Dose
Amiodarone (Cordarone) L U		
•IV form		150mg IV slow push over 10 min., then
		1mg/ min. IV infusion X 6hours, then
		0.5mg/ min. IV infusion
•PO form		800–1600mg PO loading q24hours X 1–3weeks, then
		when controlled or adverse effects,
		400–800mg q24hours X 1month, then
		Titrate to the lowest effective dose (usually 200–400mg q24hours)
Dose adjustment:		
•Amiodarone→↓hepatocyte cytochrome P45O function→		
↓Hepatic metabolism, necessitating concomitant ↓medication dose		
−↓Digoxin & Warfarin dose by 50%		
Side effects:		
Cardiovascular		
•Dose dependent ↑QT interval→		
◦Torsades de pointes		
•Dose dependent hypotension		
Cutaneous		
•Microcrystalline skin deposits→		
◦Blue–gray tinted skin		
•Photosensitivity		
Endocrine		
•Thyroid dysfunction (hypothyroidism or hyperthyroidism) due to its iodine moiety		
Gastrointestinal		
•Hepatitis		
Opthalmologic		
•Microcrystalline corneal deposits→		
◦Blurred vision		
Pulmonary		
•Pulmonary deposition→		
◦Pulmonary fibrosis		
Contraindications:		
•QTc >0.44seconds		

PULMONARY EDEMA ▬▬▬▬▬▬
- **Position**
  - ○Sitting upright w/ legs dependent
- **Oxygen** to maintain PaO_2 >60mmHg or SaO_2 >92%, usually accomplished via nasal cannula @ 2–4L/ min.
  - Mechanism:
    - •Oxygenation if required
    - •Calming effect→
      - ○↓Autonomic sympathetic tone→
        - −↓Myocardial O_2 & nutrient demand
  - Duration:
    - •24–48hours, or longer if needed for oxygenation
- **↓Sodium intake**
  - ○Patients w/ poorly compensated heart failure should only consume 0.5–1g elemental sodium or 1.5–3g salt/ 24hours
  - ○→↓Renal potassium loss if taking a diuretic
- **Fluid restriction**
  - ○Restrict fluid intake to ≤1.5L/ 24hours (~6 cups)
    - Guide:
      - •1oz = 30mL
      - •1cup = 8oz = 240mL
      - •4cups = 32oz = ~1L

OPIOID RECEPTOR AGONISTS				
Generic	M	♀	Start	Max
Morphine sulfate	LK	?	2–4mg IV slow push (1mg/ min.) q10min. prn dyspnea	15mg total

Mechanism:
- •Vasodilation (**venous** >> arterial)→
  - ○↓Preload→↓myocardial contractile strength
    - −↓Blood pressure
    - −↓Myocardial O_2 & nutrient demand
    - −↓Pulmonary congestion if present
- •↓Pain ± dyspnea→
  - ○↓Autonomic sympathetic tone→
    - −↓Myocardial O_2 & nutrient demand

- **Diuretic treatment**
  - Titration:
    - •Diurese 1L/ day (1L fluid=1kg=2.2 lbs) during decompensated heart failure, as this is the usual maximum that the body can reabsorb from the interstitial tissue

LOOP DIURETICS				
Generic (Trade)	M	♀	Start	Max
Furosemide (Lasix)	K	?	20mg q24–12hours PO/ IM/ IV	600mg/ 24hours
•IV infusion†:			0.05mg/kg/hour	160mg/ hour

Onset: 1hour, Duration: 6hours (La**six** lasts **six** hours)

- •There is synergistic efficacy of combination treatment w/ a thiazide diuretic
- •Intravenous administration may be preferred, as intestinal edema→
  - ○↓Absorption
- •Administer 2nd dose in the mid-afternoon to avoid nocturia
- †Furosemide→
  - •↑Juxtaglomerular cell renin secretion→
    - −↑Angiotensin 2 & aldosterone levels→vasoconstriction→↑afterload→↓cardiac output, which may→clinical deterioration during acute decompensated heart failure. Being that the diuretic effect is related predominantly to its renal tubular secretion rate (as it is not filtered by the glomerulus), while its vasoconstricting effects are related to its plasma concentration, some advocate the **administration of continuous intravenous Furosemide** when >80mg IV is needed for adequate diuresis, thus providing a means for ↑diuretic effectiveness

Dose adjustment:
•For patients currently on chronic loop diuretic treatment, starting dose=current dose + above starting dose
•Once organ edema has resolved, consider maintenance dosing @ same dose q24h w/ titration

Conversion equivalents
40mg PO = 20mg IV

THIAZIDE DIURETICS

Generic (Trade)	M	♀	Start	Max
Hydrochlorothiazide	L	U	12.5mg PO q24hours	50mg q24hours
Metolazone (Zaroxolyn)	L	U	5mg PO q24hours	10mg q24hours

Duration: 6–12hours

•There is synergistic efficacy of combination treatment w/ a loop diuretic

ANGIOTENSIN CONVERTING ENZYME INHIBITORS–ACEi

Generic (Trade)	M	♀	Start	Max
Benazepril (Lotensin)	LK	U	10mg PO q24hours	40mg/ 24hours
Captopril (Capoten)	LK	U	12.5mg PO q12hours	450mg/ 24hours
Enalapril (Vasotec)	LK	U	5mg PO q24hours	40mg/ 24hours
Fosinopril (Monopril)	LK	U	10mg PO q24hours	40mg/ 24hours
Lisinopril (Prinivil, Zestril)	K	U	10mg PO q24hours	40mg q24hours

•In order to rapidly titrate the dosage in ACEi naïve patients, start w/ low dose Captopril & double the dose q8h, if tolerated, until the 50mg dosage is reached. At that point, you can simply switch to the max dose of any of the others listed for ↓dosing frequency

Dose adjustment:
•↓Initial dose by 50% if:
  ◦Elderly
  ◦Concomitant diuretic use
  ◦Renal disease

Caution:
•Although the medication→↓afterload→↑cardiac output→↑renal perfusion pressure, patients w/ heart failure rely more on the compensatory production of angiotensin 2→
  ◦Efferent arteriole constriction→maintained glomerular filtration rate–GFR, whereas either:
    –Angiotensin converting enzyme inhibition
    –Angiotensin 2 receptor blockade
    …→↓angiotensin 2 production & action respectively, which may→
      •Pre–renal renal failure

POTASSIUM
•Always measure the magnesium level concomitantly

Indications:
•Ensure potassium 4–5mEq/ L

Generic

If concomitant alkalemia:
•Potassium chloride–KCL
If concomitant acidemia:
•Potassium bicarbonate
•Potassium citrate
•Potassium acetate
•Potassium gluconate
•Potassium phosphate
  ◦Preferred in diabetic ketoacidosis–DKA due to concomitant phosphate depletion

Monitoring:
•Q4hours until goal of 4–5mEq/ L X 2 consecutive readings, then q6hours

POTASSIUM DOSAGE ADJUSTMENT SCALE†

Plasma K⁺ (mEq/ L)	K⁺ repletion (mEq)
≥3.9	None
3.7–3.8	20
3.5–3.6	40
3.3–3.4	60
3.1–3.2	80
≤3	100

†Half all above doses @ glomerular filtration rate–GFR ≤30mL/ min.

Intravenous repletion guidelines:
- •Use dextrose–free solutions for the initial repletion, as dextrose→
  - ∘↑Insulin secretion→
    - –↑Potassium transcellular shift
- •The hyperosmolar infusion→
  - ∘Vascular irritation/ inflammation. Add 1% Lidocaine to the bag to ↓pain
- **•Do not administer >20mEq potassium IV/ hour**
  - ∘≤10mEq/ hour prn via peripheral line. May give via 2 peripheral lines=20mEq/ hour total
  - ∘≤20mEq/ hour prn via central line
  - …as more→
    - •Transient right sided heart hyperkalemia→
      - ∘Dysrhythmias

Outcomes:
- •Anti–dysrhythmic
- •↑Cardiac contractility in heart failure
- •Modest hypotensive effect in some patients
- •↓Cerebrovascular disease risk, apart from its possible blood pressure lowering effects

MAGNESIUM SULFATE

M ♀	Dose
K S	Every 1g IV→0.1mEq/ L ↑in plasma magnesium

Mechanism:
- •↓Magnesium→
  - ∘↓Renal tubular potassium reabsorption

SEVERE HEART FAILURE W/ NORMOTENSON

RECOMBINANT HUMAN VENTRICULAR NATRIURETIC PEPTIDE–BNP

Generic (Trade)	M	♀	Dose	Titrate
Nesiritide (Natrecor)	KP	?	2µg/ kg IV slow push, then 0.01µg/kg/min. IV infusion	q3hours prn by 0.005µg/kg/min., preceded by 1µg/ kg IV slow push Max: 0.03µg/kg/min.

Dose adjustment:
- •If hypotension occurs, discontinue the infusion
  - ∘May restart w/ normotension @ 30% lower dose without a bolus

Mechanism:
- •B–type natriuretic peptide→
  - ∘Suppression of the renin–angiotension–aldosterone system
  - ∘Directly mediated ↓renal retention of NaCl & water
  - ∘↓Vascular endothelin release
  - …→diuresis & vasodilation→
    - •↓Ventricular preload & afterload

Note: Plasma BNP level may be measured @ >6hours after discontinuation of infusion

Side effects:
Cardiovascular
•Hypotension

OR

Generic	M	♀	Start	Max
Nitroglycerin	L	?	10µg/ min. IV infusion	100µg/ min.
Nitroprusside sodium (Nipride, Nitropress)	E	?	0.3µg/kg/min. IV infusion	8µg/kg/min.

Onset: 2–5min., w/ tolerance typically within 24–48hours, Duration: ≤5min. after discontinuation

•Nitroglycerin binds to soft plastics such as polyvinylchloride–PVC, which is a common constituent of plastic bags & infusion tubing→
 ○≤80% absorptive loss, being avoided via the use of glass bottles & hard/ stiff plastics
•Protect the Nitroprusside bottle from light

Mechanism:
•Vasodilation (**venous** >> arterial)→
 ○↓Preload→
  –↓Cardiac output→↓blood pressure
  –↓Myocardial O_2 demand
  –↓Pulmonary congestion if present
•Platelet inhibiting activity

Side effects:
Cardiovascular
•Hypotension
•Systemic vasodilation→
 ○Reflex tachycardia
 ○Orthostatic hypotension
 ○Facial flushing
•Meningeal arterial dilation→
 ○Headache
Pulmonary
•Pulmonary vasodilation→
 ○Exacerbation of ventilation/ perfusion mismatches
Hematologic
Nitroglycerin specific:
•Nitroglycerin metabolism→
 ○Inorganic nitrites→oxidation of heme bound iron (Fe^{+2}) to the ferric form (Fe^{+3}), creating **methemoglobin**, which does not carry O_2 effectively→
  –Hypoxemia, being unreliably detected by pulse oximeters, requiring the use of co–oximeters
  –Brown colored blood due to the brown color of methemoglobin
  …usually occurring only at ↑↑doses, w/ levels (fraction of total hemoglobin):
   •>3% being abnormal
   •>40% possibly causing hypoxemia→
    ○Lactic acidemia
   •>70% being lethal
    …requiring discontinuation of infusion in all cases. If hypoxemia exists, administer methylene blue (a reducing agent) @ 2mg/ kg IV over 10min.†→
     •Conversion of iron to the normal ferrous form (Fe^{+2})
•Being as nitroglycerin does not readily dissolve in aqueous solutions, nonpolar solvents such as ethanol & propylene glycol are required to keep the medication in solution, & can accumulate→
 ○Ethanol intoxication
 ○Propylene glycol toxicity→
  –Altered mental status
  –Anion gap metabolic acidemia
  –Dysrhythmias
  –Hemolysis
  –Hyperosmolarity
  –Acute tubular necrosis→renal failure
 …→↑plasma levels & osmolar gap
Pharmacokinetics/ pharmacodynamics
•Tolerance to medication effects
Nitroprusside specific:
•Nitroprusside metabolism releases 5 cyanide ions (CN) along w/ nitric oxide→
 ○**Potential cyanide &/or thiocyanate toxicity**
  –Cyanide–CN + thiosulfate–S_2O_3 (a sulfur donor source)→thiocyanate–SCN‡ + sulfate–SO_3
Cyanide toxicity
 •The body stores of thiosulfate are readily depleted→
  ○↑Cyanide, which is why 500mg of thiosulfate must be added to each infusion solution

124

•Renal failure→
  −↑Thiocyanate toxicity risk→anorexia, hallucinations, nausea ± vomiting, &/or seizures

†Intravenous administration of methylene blue→
•Spuriously ↓SaO$_2$, up to 65%
‡Thiocyanate is renally cleared

Contraindications:
Cardiovascular
•Hypotension
Neurologic
•**Hypertensive encephalopathy**, as it ↑intracranial pressure
Interactions
•**Sildenafil** (Viagra) **is contraindicated** in patients taking concomitant nitrates, as the combination within 24hours may→severe hypotension→
  ◦↓Myocardial perfusion→
    −Stable angina mediated acute coronary syndrome
  ◦↓Cerebral perfusion→
    −Pre−syncope/ syncope
    −Cerebrovascular accident syndrome

Monitoring:
•Thiocyanate levels frequently (should be <10mg/ dL)

CARDIOGENIC HYPOTENSION

INOTROPIC & PRESSOR MEDICATIONS: The following medications must be administered via a central line, & should be titrated based on blood pressure response to keep the systolic blood pressure >90mmHg

Medication	Mechanism	Clinical effects†
Dobutamine	β1 > β2 > α1agonism	•↑Chronotropy, inotropy, &
Start @ 2μg/kg/min. (max 20μg/kg/min.)		vasodilation
Milrinone	Intracellular phosphodiesterase inhibition→ ↓cAMP degradation→↑cAMP	•↑Inotropy & vasodilation
Start @ 50μg/ kg slow push over 10min., then 0.375μg/kg/min. (max 0.75μg/kg/min.)		

†Chronotropy=rate of contraction; inotropy=strength of muscular contractility

IF UNRESPONSIVE TO THE ABOVE
•**CPAP or assisted ventilation**
  Mechanism:
  •Positive end expiratory pressure−PEEP→↑mean intrathoracic pressure, being determined by:
    ◦Airways resistance
    ◦Thoracic compliance
    ◦Added PEEP
    ...→↑atrial & thoracic venous pressure→
      •↓**Venous return**→
        ◦↓Pulmonary congestion→
          −↓Dyspnea→↓autonomic sympathetic tone
        ◦↓Myocardial contractile strength
          ...→↓myocardial O$_2$ & nutrient demand
      •↓Transmural aortic pressure→
        ◦↓**Afterload**
      ...→**improved heart failure syndrome**

•**Phlebotomy**
  ◦Removal of 250−500mL→
    −↓Preload

•**Intra-aortic balloon pump–IABP**
  Mechanism:
    •A large bore catheter w/ an inflatable 30cm polyurethane balloon at its tip, is percutaneously
     inserted into the femoral artery & advanced up the aorta until the tip is just distal to the left
     subclavian artery, w/ subsequent alternating balloon inflations & deflations during ventricular
     diastole
      ∘**Inflation**→
        –↑Peak diastolic blood pressure→↑proximal (ex. carotid, coronary) & distal (peripheral) arterial
         blood pressure→↑organ perfusion
      ∘**Deflation**→
        –↓End diastolic blood pressure→↓afterload→↑cardiac output→↑arterial blood pressure→↑organ
         perfusion
  Complications:
    •Lower extremity ischemia, being ipsilateral &/or contralateral to the canulated femoral artery
    •Sepsis
  Contraindications:
    •Aortic dissection
    •Aortic regurgitation
    •Prosthetic thoracic aortic graft placed within 1year
  Weaning parameters, either via gradually (over 1–24hours):
    •↓Balloon inflation frequency per cardiac cycle (1:2, 1:3,...)
    •↓Balloon inflation volume to a goal of 10% the original volume

•**Ventricular assist device–VAD**
  Mechanism:
    •A non–pulsatile pump placed intraoperatively in parallel w/ the right ventricle–RVAD, left ventricle-
     LVAD, or both ventricles–BiVAD
  Complications:
    •Hemorrhage
    •Thromboembolism

•**Orthotopic cardiac transplantation**
  Indications:
    •A candidate must meet all of the following criteria†:
      ∘Age <60years
      ∘Free of complicating, irreversible, extracardiac organ dysfunction, as this may ↓recovery & ↑post-
       transplantation complications
      ∘Prepared to undergo the post–transplantation regimen
        –Post–transplant immunosuppressive therapy includes glucocorticoids & Azathioprine &/or
         Cyclosporine
      ∘Adequate psychosocial support system
  Outcomes:
    •1year survival rate: 85%
    •5year survival rate: 70%

•Caused by any disease→
  ◦Myocardial inflammation=myocarditis→
    −**Myocardial fibrosis**→myocardial thinning, dilation, & weakness→↓ventricular contractile
      strength→↓cardiac output→systolic heart failure
Statistics:
  •**Comprises 95% of all cardiomyopathies**

RISK FACTORS

•**Idiopathic−50%**
  ◦Genetic disposition−5%
  ◦Previous viral myocarditis
•**Ischemia**
  ◦Myocardial infarction
•**Ethanol**
•**Collagen vascular disease**, esp.:
  ◦Polyarteritis nodosa
  ◦Progressive systemic sclerosis
  ◦Rheumatoid arthritis
  ◦Scleroderma
  ◦Systemic lupus erythematosus−SLE
  ◦Wegener's granulomatosus
•**Endocrine**
  ◦Pheochromocytoma→
    −↑Catecholamines (epinephrine &/or norepinephrine)
  ◦Thyroid dysfunction
    −Hypothyroidism
    −Hyperthyroidism
•**Infectious**
  ◦Bacterial
    −Streptococcus pyogenes→rheumatic fever→rheumatic heart disease
  ◦Spirochetal
    −Borrelia burgdorferi
  ◦Viral, esp. Coxsackievirus group B→either:
    −Myocardial infection
    −Molecular mimicry mediated autoimmune disease via anti−myocardial β receptor, calcium channel,
      mitochondrial, &/or sarcolemma antibodies
•**Medications**
  ◦α interferon
  ◦Methylodopa
  ◦Penicillin
  ◦Phenylbutazone
  ◦Sulfa−containing medications
  ◦Tetracycline
  ◦Tuberculosis medications→
    −Hypersensitivity myocarditis→eosinophilic myocarditis
  ◦Chemotherapeutic medications
    −Daunorubicin
    −Doxorubicin=Adriamycin
    −Mitoxantrone
    −5−fluorouracil
•**Peripartum**
  ◦Last month of pregnancy to 5 months postpartum
•**Radiation therapy**
  ◦Radiation field containing the heart
•**Sarcoidosis**
•**Sympathomimetic drugs**
  ◦Amphetamines→
    −↑Release of presynaptic catecholamines
  ◦Cocaine→
    −↓Presynaptic reuptake of released catecholamines
•**Chronic tachycardia**, possibly due to ischemia
•**Any cause of hypertrophic or restrictive cardiomyopathy**→
  ◦Mixed cardiomyopathy→
    −End stage dilated cardiomyopathy

Cardiovascular
- Dilated cardiomyopathy→
  - Ventricular dilation→
    - Valvular annulus dilation & downwardly displaced papillary muscles→mitral &/or tricuspid regurgitation
  - Laterally displaced & weak point of maximal impulse-PMI
    - Normally found @ the intersection of the left 5th intercostal space & an imaginary midclavicular line
  - 3rd &/or 4th heart sounds†, w/ both→
    - Gallop rhythm

---

†3rd heart sounds are heard only w/:
- Dilated cardiomyopathy
- Restrictive cardiomyopathy
- Constrictive pericarditis
...whereas 4th heart sounds may be heard w/ any cardiomyopathy having ↑atrial contribution

•Electrocardiogram-ECG
Findings:
- Nonspecific ST segment &/or T wave changes
- Q waves, indicating previous myocardial infarction
- ↓Voltage, w/ diagnostic criteria being either:
  - Peak to peak QRS <5mm in the limb leads (I, II, III, aVR, aVL, aVF)
  - Peak to peak QRS <10mm in the precordial leads (V1-V6)
  ...due to either:
    - ↓Myocardial mass (ex. dilated cardiomyopathy)
    - Interposing tissue (ex. obesity, restrictive cardiomyopathy), fluid (ex. pericardial or pleural effusion), &/or gas (ex. emphysema, pneumothorax) between the electrical impulse & the electrodes
- Atrial dilation, occurring in all forms of chronic heart failure
  - Criteria for left atrial dilation:
    - Negative terminal P wave deflection in lead V1, being > 1X1mm
    - Notched P wave in lead II, being >3mm in length
  - Criteria for right atrial dilation:
    - ↑P wave in lead II, being ≥2.5mm in height
    - Biphasic P wave in lead V1, w/ a larger initial portion being ≥2mm in height

•Chest x-ray
Findings:
- **Cardiomegally**

•Transthoracic echocardiography-TTE
Procedure:
- A 2 dimensional ultrasonographic image, allowing real time visualization of:
  - Ventricular wall thickness
  - Cavity size (both atrial & ventricular)
  - Myocardial & valve function, allowing ejection fraction-EF estimation (% of end diastolic volume ejected during ventricular systole)
  - The pericardial space
- Doppler ultrasonography uses Doppler shift to detect vessel flow velocity→
  - Valve regurgitation visualization
  - Estimation of valve pressure gradients
Findings:
- **↓Ejection fraction-EF** (normal 50-70%)
- **Ventricular chamber dilation**
- ↓Ventricular myocardial thickness
- Regional or global myocardial hypo/ akinesis
- Shortened ventricular relaxation time, w/ normal ventricular filling
Limitations:
- ↓Visualization in obese or emphysematous patients
- May not allow adequate:
  - Visualization of the anterior aspect of a prosthetic aortic valve
  - Functional assessment of a prosthetic aortic valve

•Transesophageal echocardiography–TEE is more sensitive in detecting:
  ◦Thrombotic ± infectious vegetations
  ◦Abscesses
  ◦Valve damage
  …esp. in a patient w/ a prosthetic heart valve. However, transthoracic echocardiography is the
    initial test of choice due to its noninvasive nature, as transesophageal echocardiography may→
    •Pharyngeal swallow receptor mediated reflex:
      ◦Bradycardia
      ◦Hypotension

•**Radioisotope imaging** (exercise or pharmacologic) via:
  ◦Single photon emission computerized tomographic–SPECT scanning
  ◦Positron emission tomographic–PET scanning
  Indications:
    •To assess both myocardial perfusion & metabolism
  Procedure:
    •A radioactive agent=tracer is injected intravenously @ maximal stress, w/ subsequent scintigraphic
      imaging & re-imaging after a 2nd intravenous injection 3hours later during relaxation. Tracer
      distribution is proportional to myocardial blood flow
  Tracers used in SPECT:
    •^{201}**thallium**, being a biological substitute for potassium
    •^{99m}**technitium–Tc** (99mTc–sestamibi, 99mTc–teboroxime, 99mTc–tetrofosmin)
  Tracers used in PET:
    •Carbon–11
    •Fluorine–18
    •Nitrogen–13
    •Oxygen–15
    •Rubidium–82
  Outcomes:
    •SPECT: Sensitivity: 85% & specificity: 80% in detecting significant (≥50%) stenosis
    •PET: Sensitivity: 85% & specificity: 65% in detecting significant (≥50%) stenosis

TEST RESULTS			
Pathology	@ Maximal stress	@ Relaxation	Term
Normal	Diffuse equivalent uptake		Normal uptake
Myocardial ischemia	Regional ↓relative uptake	Diffuse equivalent uptake†	Reversible defect
Myocardial fibrosis	No uptake		Fixed defect

†May be persistently ↓w/ hibernating myocardium

INVASIVE PROCEDURES
•**Coronary angiography**
  Indications:
    •In order to view the epicardial anatomy for possible causative atherosclerotic disease

PROGNOSIS
•1year survival: 70%, 5 year survival: 20%, w/ death due to:
  ◦Dysrhythmia–50%, esp. ventricular tachycardia, ventricular fibrillation, or bradydysrhythmia→
    –Cardiac arrest
  ◦Progressive left ventricular dysfunction
  ◦Thromboembolic disease
    –15% of patients not receiving anticoagulation have symptomatic thromboembolism
•Patients w/ NYHA class 4 heart failure have an annual mortality rate of 50%
•45% of discharged patients are readmitted within 1year

•Caused by any disease→
　◦**Myocardial hypertrophy**→
　　−↓**Ventricular relaxation**→↓end diastolic volume→↓cardiac output→**diastolic heart failure**
Statistics:
•Comprises 4% of all cardiomyopathies

RISK FACTORS/ CLASSIFICATION

•**Primary hypertrophic cardiomyopathy**
Mechanism:
　•Inheritance or acquisition of mutated sarcomere protein genes, being **autosomal dominant**, w/
　100% penetrance→
　　◦Myocyte hypertrophy & disarray
Statistics:
　•Affects 1/ 500 persons
Risk factors:
　•Familial−50%
　•Sporadic=idiopathic−50%

Mutated sarcomere protein	Chromosome	Presenting age (years)
Cardiac β myosin heavy chain protein−35%	14	20−40
Troponin−T−15%	1	20−40
Myosin−binding protein C−15%	11	>50
A−tropomyosin protein <5%	15	20−40

•**Secondary hypertrophic cardiomyopathy**
Mechanism:
　•A compensatory reaction attempting to maintain adequate cardiac output via replication of
　sarcomeres in parallel→
　　◦↑Contractile strength
Risk factors:
　•**Hypertension**
　•**Valvular disease**
　　◦Stenosis (esp. aortic stenosis) &/or regurgitation

DIAGNOSIS

Cardiovascular
•Hypertrophic cardiomyopathy→
　◦Sustained & forceful point of maximal impulse−PMI ± displacement
　　−Normally found @ the intersection of the 5th intercostal space & an imaginary midclavicular line
　◦↑Atrial contribution to ventricular preload→
　　−**4th heart sound**† (3rd heart sound is never heard)
　◦Misaligned &/or separated valve leaflets→
　　−Regurgitation
　◦↓Ventricular diastolic filling→
　　−Poorly tolerated tachycardia, as it further ↓ventricular diastole→↓cardiac output
•Ventricular systole→
　◦Formation of a myocardial pressure gradient, as the outer layers place additive pressure on the
　inner layers, w/ pressure being greatest on the subendocardium→
　　−Subendocardial vascular compression→↓systolic myocardial blood flow→subendocardial
　　reliance on diastolic flow for O$_2$ & nutrient supply. Being that hypertrophic cardiomyopathy→
　　delayed & incomplete diastole, its blood supply is progressively diminished→compensatory
　　↑subendocardial vascular anastomoses, which eventually become unable to compensate for the
　　progressively hypertrophied myocardial demand→subendocardial ischemia, esp. in patients w/
　　compromised supply (coronary artery disease, hypotension) &/or ↑demand (tachycardia)

Subsyndromes:
•**Septal hypertrophy**, occurring in certain forms of primary hypertrophic cardiomyopathy→
　◦Functional subaortic stenosis via mid to end systolic mid−chamber wall contact, termed cavitary
　obliteration→↑left ventricular outflow velocity→
　　−Turbulent blood flow against the aortic walls→aortic wall vibration→intra−systolic ejection
　　murmur=**diamond shaped murmur** (↑, then ↓), beginning after the 1st heart sound & ending
　　before the 2nd heart sound, w/ radiation to the carotid arteries &/or palpable flow mediated
　　vibrations=thrill over the upper chest &/or lower neck, w/ ↑severity→**progressively delayed
　　murmur peak intensity**, w/ a weak & delayed arterial pulse, termed pulsus parvus et
　　tardus, indicating severe disease

130

○Delayed aortic component of the 2nd heart sound→

   –**Paradoxical 2nd heart sound splitting‡ on expiration (P2 prior to A2)**, which may become unified upon inspiration. The 2nd heart sound may become single as the aortic closing component is lost

---

†3rd heart sounds are heard only w/:
- Dilated cardiomyopathy
- Restrictive cardiomyopathy
- Constrictive pericarditis

...whereas 4th heart sounds may be heard w/ any cardiomyopathy having ↑atrial contribution
‡A physiologic splitting of the 2nd heart sound (A2 prior to P2) may occur normally during inspiration, and become nearly unified on expiration

ELECTRICAL STUDIES

- **Electrocardiogram–ECG**
  Findings:
  - Nonspecific ST segment &/or T wave changes
  - Axis deviation toward the side of the hypertrophied ventricle
  - ↑QRS complex voltage & duration
  - Septal hypertrophy→
    ○ Deep Q waves, termed pseudo–Q waves, in leads II, III, & aVF (inferior leads)
  - Criteria for left ventricular hypertrophy–LVH
    ○ Lead V1–V6 progressively ↑R waves
    ○ Tall V5 & V6 R waves & deep V1 & V2 S waves
    ○ Lead aVL R wave >11mm
    ○ Lead aVL R wave + lead V3 S wave being ♂>28mm or ♀>20mm
    ○ Lead V1 S wave + lead V5 R wave being >35mm
  - Criteria for right ventricular hypertrophy–RVH
    ○ Lead V1–V6 progressively ↓R waves
    ○ Lead V1 R wave > S wave
    ○ Lead V6 S wave > R wave
    ○ Lead V1 R wave >6mm
    ○ Lead V5 & V6 S waves
  - Atrial dilation, occurring in all forms of chronic heart failure
    ○ Criteria for left atrial dilation:
      –Negative terminal P wave deflection in lead V1, being > 1X1mm
      –Notched P wave in lead II, being >3mm in length
    ○ Criteria for right atrial dilation:
      –↑P wave in lead II, being ≥2.5mm in height
      –Biphasic P wave in lead V1, w/ a larger initial portion being ≥2mm in height

IMAGING STUDIES

- **Transthoracic echocardiography–TTE**
  Procedure:
  - A 2 dimensional ultrasonographic image, allowing real time visualization of:
    ○ Ventricular wall thickness
    ○ Cavity size (both atrial & ventricular)
    ○ Myocardial & valve function, allowing ejection fraction–EF estimation (% of end diastolic volume ejected during ventricular systole)
    ○ The pericardial space
  - Doppler ultrasonography uses Doppler shift to detect vessel flow velocity→
    ○ Valve regurgitation visualization
    ○ Estimation of valve pressure gradients
  Findings:
  - Normal to ↑ejection fraction (normal 50–70%), as systolic function is enhanced
  - **↓Ventricular chamber size**
  - **Prolonged ventricular relaxation time→**
    ○ Delayed mitral valve opening
    ○ ↓Early diastolic filling→
      –Delayed increase in cavity size
      –↓E wave & ↑late diastolic filling due to atrial systole→↑A wave, termed **reversal of the E:A ratio**, being absent in patients w/ atrial fibrillation
  - Ventricular systole→
    ○ Redundant chordea tendineae→
      –Valvular regurgitation

131

◦Mid to end systolic mid–chamber wall contact→intraventricular pressure gradient→
  –↑Left ventricular outflow velocity
  –Residual peri–mitral valve ventricular base area ± small apical area
Septal hypertrophy specific:
  •Rapid outflow through a narrowed ventricular outflow tract→
  ◦Venturi effect→
    –Anterior mitral valve leaflet movement into the outflow tract, termed **systolic anterior movement**
Limitations:
  •↓Visualization in obese or emphysematous patients
  •May not allow adequate:
  ◦Visualization of the anterior aspect of a prosthetic aortic valve
  ◦Functional assessment of a prosthetic aortic valve

INVASIVE PROCEDURES

•**Cardiac catheterization**
Indications:
  •Septal hypertrophy
Procedure:
  •Measures the intraventricular pressure gradient, via catheterization of the left ventricular apex & either the ventricular outflow tract or the aorta
Findings:
  •After ventricular chamber obliteration, the apex continues to contract→
  ◦Apical pressure > systolic blood pressure, w/ the difference being the pressure gradient

TREATMENT

•The treatment for secondary hypertrophic cardiomyopathy is to treat the etiologic disease.

PRIMARY HYPERTROPHIC CARDIOMYOPATHY ▅▅▅▅▅▅▅▅▅▅▅▅▅▅▅▅▅▅▅▅▅▅▅
•**Avoid dehydration**
•**Avoid undue vigorous physical exertion** such as competitive sports & weight lifting, even if asymptomatic, due to ↑**sudden death risk**
•**Medication restriction**
  ◦Avoid or use caution w/ medications→
    –↑Ventricular contractility (digoxin, vasodilators)
    –↓Ventricular diastole (β receptor agonists)
    –↓Ventricular preload (diuretics, vasodilators)
    ...as all→
      •↓Ventricular end–diastolic volume, which may→
      ◦Hypotension
                                              &
•Treatment goal is palliation, as treatment (medical or surgical) has not been reliably shown to prevent sudden death. W/ that in mind, there has been much debate about the treatment of asymptomatic patients in order to potentially ↓disease progression→
  ◦Delayed symptom onset, also being unproven

Indications:
  •Symptomatic disease
  •Asymptomatic patients who have either:
  ◦Massive hypertrophy, via a maximal ventricular wall thickness ≥35mm, being extremely rare @ age >50years
  ◦Obstructive Pathophysiology, via an intraventricular pressure gradient of ≥50mmHg

β1 SELECTIVE RECEPTOR BLOCKERS			
Generic (Trade)	M ♀	Start	Max
Metoprolol (Lopressor) L ?		6.25mg PO q12hours	100mg q12hours
•XR form (Toprol XL)		12.5mg PO q24hours	400mg q24hours
α1 & NONSELECTIVE β RECEPTOR BLOCKERS			
Generic (Trade)	M ♀	Start	Max
Carvedilol (Coreg) L ?		3.125mg PO q12hours	25mg q12hours if <85kg
			50mg q12hours if >85kg
Mechanism:			
•Competitive antagonist of the β1 ± β2 receptor→ ◦↓Sinoatrial & atrioventricular node conduction (β1)→ –↓Pulse ◦Anti–dysrhythmic via nodal effects (β1)			

132

- ○↓Cardiac muscle contractile strength (β1)
- ○↓Juxtaglomerular cell renin release (β1)→
  - −↓Angiotensin 1, angiotensin 2, & aldosterone formation
- ○↓Cardiovascular remodeling
- ○↑Vascular/ organ smooth muscle contraction (β2)→
  - −Vasoconstriction
  - −Bronchoconstriction
  - −Uterine contraction
- ○↓Tremor (β2)
- ○↓Hepatocyte glycogenolysis (β2)
- •↓Extrathyroidal tetraiodothyronine−T4 (also termed thyroxine) conversion to the more metabolically active triiodothyronine−T3 form

Side effects:
General
- •Fatigue
- •Malaise

Cardiovascular
- •Bradycardia ± heart block
- •Hypotension
  - ○Orthostatic hypotension
  - ○Pelvic hypotension→
    - −Impotence, being the inability to achieve &/or maintain an erection
- •Initial worsening of systolic heart failure
- •Worsening symptoms of peripheral vascular disease
  - ○Intermittent claudication
  - ○Raynaud's phenomenon

Pulmonary
- •Bronchoconstriction

Endocrine
- •↑Risk of developing diabetes mellitus
- •May block catecholamine mediated:
  - ○Physiologic reversal of hypoglycemia via:
    - −↓Hepatocyte gluconeogenesis
  - ○↓Hypoglycemic symptoms, termed hypoglycemic unawareness→
    - −↓Tachycardia as a warning sign

Gastrointestinal
- •Diarrhea
- •Nausea ± vomiting
- •Gastroesophageal reflux

Mucocutaneous
- •Hair thinning

Neurologic
- •Sedation
- •Sleep alterations
- •↓Libido→
  - ○Impotence

Psychiatric
- •Depression

Hematologic
- •↓High density lipoprotein−HDL levels

•Most patients w/ chronic obstructive pulmonary disease−COPD (including asthma), diabetes, &/or peripheral vascular disease can be safely treated w/ **cardioselective β1 receptor blockers**, as they have ↓peripheral effects

Contraindications:
Cardiovascular
- •**Acutely decompensated heart failure**
- •Hypotension
- •Pulse <50bpm
- •Atrioventricular heart block of any degree

Pulmonary
- •Moderate to severe chronic obstructive pulmonary disease−COPD, including asthma

Hyper-catacholamine state
- Amphetamine use
- **Cocaine use**†
- Clonidine withdrawal
- Monoamine oxidase inhibitor-MAOi mediated tyramine effect
- Pheochromocytoma
  - ...:→relatively ↑vascular α1 receptor stimulation="unopposed α effect"→
    - Vasoconstriction→
      - ∘Myocardial ischemic syndrome
      - ∘Cerebrovascular accident syndrome
      - ∘Peripheral vascular ischemic syndrome

Note: **Carvedilol** & **Labetalol** may be used due to their α1 blocking property

---

†Cocaine use→
- Varying ischemic syndrome onset per administration route, & may occur @ min. to days (usually within 3hours)

CALCIUM CHANNEL BLOCKERS: Non-dihydropyridines

Generic	M ♀	Start	Max
Diltiazem	L ?	30mg PO q8hours	120mg q8hours
•XR form		As per daily requirement	
∘QDXR form		120mg PO q12hours	540mg q24hours
∘BIDXR form		60mg PO q12hours	180mg q12hours
Verapamil	L ?	40mg PO q8hours	160mg q8hours
•XR form		As per daily requirement	
∘Calan XR form		120mg PO q24hours	480mg/ 24hours
∘Veleran XR form		100mg PO q24hours	400mg q24hours
∘Covera XR form		180mg PO q24hours	480mg qhs

Mechanism:
- Block voltage dependent calcium ion channels in smooth & cardiac muscle→
  - ∘↓Calcium influx→
    - −↓Sinoatrial & atrioventricular node conduction (non-dihydropyridines)→↓pulse
    - −Anti-dysrhythmic via nodal effects (mainly non-dihydropyridines)
    - −↓Cardiac muscle contractile strength (mainly non-dihydropyridines)
    - −Vasodilation: Arterial > venous (mainly dihydropyridines)

Side effects:
Cardiovascular
- Bradycardia ± heart block
- Edema
- Flushing
- Hypotension

Gastrointestinal
- Constipation
- Nausea ± vomiting

Neurologic
- Dizziness
- Headache

ANTIDOTES

Generic	M ♀	Dose	Max
Glucagon	LK P	3mg IV slow push over 1min., then 5mg IV slow push over 1 min. if needed	
•Continuous infusion		5mg/ hour	
10% Calcium chloride†		10mL (1 ampule) IV slow push over 3min., then repeat @5min. if needed	
•Continuous infusion		Start 0.3mEq/ hour	0.7mEq/ hour

Onset: 1-2 min., Duration: 30-60 min.

Magnesium sulfate	K S	2g $MgSO_4$ in 50mL saline infused over 15min., then 6g $MgSO_4$ in 500mL saline infused over 6hours	

---

†Use cautiously in patients taking Digoxin, as hypercalcemia→
- Digoxin cardiotoxicity

134

SECOND LINE TREATMENT

ANTI-DYSRHYTHMIC MEDICATIONS			
Generic (Trade)	M	♀	Dose
Disopyramide (Norpace)	KL	?	
•XR form			200–400mg PO q12hours

Mechanism:
- •Sodium channel blockade→
  - ◦↓Myocardial inotropy

Side effects:
Cardiovascular
- •↑Atrioventricular conduction in the event of a supraventricular tachycardia, requiring the concomitant use of the above medications

THIRD LINE TREATMENT

Obstructive Pathophysiology:
- •**Alcohol septal ablation**
  - Mechanism:
    - •100% ethanol infusion into the 1st septal perforator artery→
      - ◦Occlusion→
        - –Localized myocardial infarction
  - Complications:
    - •Complete heart block or left bundle branch block

- •**Septal myectomy**
  - Mechanism:
    - •Surgical removal of a portion of the basal septum through the aortic valve→
      - ◦↑Outflow tract
  - Complications:
    - •**Death**, being <2% @ experienced centers
    - •Aortic regurgitation
    - •Complete heart block or left bundle branch block
    - •Ventricular septal defect

- •**Mitral valve replacement**
  - Mechanism:
    - •↓Systolic anterior motion

- •**Permanent pacemaker placement**
  - Mechanism:
    - •Placement @ the right ventricular apex→
      - ◦Functional left bundle branch block→delayed left ventricular activation→
        - –↑Left ventricular diastole
        - –Relatively delayed septal depolarization, as the current travels from the left ventricular apex to the base→↑left ventricular end systolic cavity size
        - …→↑cardiac output
  - Outcomes:
    - •It is now thought that perhaps most of the symptomatic improvement is due to placebo effect

Nonobstructive pathophysiology:
- •**Orthotopic cardiac transplantation**
  - Indications:
    - •A candidate must meet all of the following criteria†:
      - ◦Age <60years
      - ◦Free of complicating, irreversible, extracardiac organ dysfunction, as this may ↓recovery & ↑post-transplantation complications
      - ◦Prepared to undergo the post–transplantation regimen
        - –Post–transplant immunosuppressive therapy includes glucocorticoids & Azathioprine &/or Cyclosporine
      - ◦Adequate psychosocial support system
  - Outcomes:
    - •1year survival rate: 85%
    - •5year survival rate: 70%

---

†Even when a candidate meets these criteria, a compatible heart may not become available until after the patient has already died

Indications: Primary hypertrophic cardiomyopathy w/:
- •**History of significant dysrhythmia**
  - ∘Personal of family history of cardiac arrest
  - ∘Sustained ventricular tachycardia (persisting for ≥30seconds or requiring termination due to symptoms)
  - ∘Non–sustained ventricular tachycardia, being either:
    - –Symptomatic
    - –Multiple (>5)
    - –Prolonged (≥10beats)
    - …via 24–48hour Holter monitor
  - ∘Unexplained syncope
- •**Significant family history of sudden death** via ≥2 young family members
- •**Younger age,** as achievement of advanced age indicates a relatively benign form of the disease
- •**High risk mutation**
  - ∘Arg403Gln mutation of the β–myosin heavy chain gene, as 50% die @ age ≤45years
  - ∘Cardiac troponin T mutation

- •**Internal cardioverter–defibrillator–ICD**
  Composed of 3 parts:
  - •**Generator**
    - ∘Placed in the pectoral area, rather than older models which were placed in the abdomen
  - •**Transvenous defibrillating leads**
    - ∘Inserted into the subclavian vein, & advanced to the right ventricular apex
  - •**Electrodes**
    - ∘In the lead tips, capable of sensing, cardioverting, defibrillating, &
      - –Anti–tachycardia pacing, being painless, & used to terminate monomorphic tachycardias
  Complications:
  - •Infection–2%, necessitating device removal
  - •Lead malfunction→
    - ∘False signals→
      - –Inappropriate shock administration
  Limitations:
  - •Anti–tachycardia pacing may:
    - ∘Accelerate ventricular tachycardia
    - ∘Induce a ventricular dysrhythmia if applied during a supraventricular rhythm
    - …necessitating cardioversion or defibrillation if ineffective
  - •Only β receptor blockers (as above) & **Amiodarone** medically→
    - ∘↓Cardiac arrest risk in patients w/ systolic dysfunction

ANTI–DYSRHYTHMIC MEDICATIONS			
Generic (Trade)	M	♀	Dose
Amiodarone (Cordarone)	L	U	
•IV form			150mg IV slow push over 10 min., then
			1mg/ min. IV infusion X 6hours, then
			0.5mg/ min. IV infusion
•PO form			800–1600mg PO loading q24hours X 1–3weeks, then
			when controlled or adverse effects,
			400–800mg q24hours X 1month, then
			titrate to the lowest effective dose (usually 200–400mg q24hours)

Dose adjustment:
•Amiodarone→↓hepatocyte cytochrome P45O function→
∘↓Hepatic metabolism, necessitating concomitant ↓medication dose
–↓Digoxin & Warfarin dose by 50%

Side effects:
Cardiovascular
•Dose dependent ↑QT interval→
∘**Torsades de pointes**
•Dose dependent **hypotension**
Cutaneous
•Microcrystalline skin deposits→
∘Blue–gray tinted skin
•Photosensitivity
Endocrine
•Thyroid dysfunction **(hypothyroidism or hyperthyroidism)** due to its iodine moiety

136

Gastrointestinal
- Hepatitis

Opthalmologic
- Microcrystalline corneal deposits→
  - Blurred vision

Pulmonary
- Pulmonary deposition→
  - Pulmonary fibrosis

Contraindications:
- QTc >0.44seconds

PROGNOSIS

- **Primary hypertrophic cardiomyopathy**
  - **Sudden death risk: 2.5%/ year**
    - Although dysrhythmias are often assumed to be the cause of sudden death in these patients, in the few patients who have died while under electrocardiographic monitoring, primary dysrhythmias were often not the terminal event preceding asystole. In fact, the etiology of sudden death is multifactorial, w/ dysrhythmias being one component. This may be why **anti-dysrhythmic treatment does not ↓mortality**

137

•Caused by myocardial infiltrative disease (usually as a consequence of a systemic disease)→
  ◦Myocardial thickening→
    −↓Ventricular elasticity→↓end diastolic volume→↓cardiac output→diastolic heart failure
Statistics:
  •Comprises 1% of all cardiomyopathies

•Collagen vascular disease
  ◦Pseudoxanthoma elasticum
  ◦Scleroderma
•Endocardial disease
  ◦Endocardial fibroelastosis, being a disease of infancy
  ◦Endomyocardial fibrosis
  ◦Loeffler's eosinophilic endocarditis−extremely rare
  ◦Medications
    −Anthracycline
    −Busulfan
    −Mercurial agents
    −Methysergide
    −Serotonin: Carcinoid syndrome, ergot alkaloids, serotonin agonists
•Endocrine
  ◦Diabetes mellitus
•Familial−rare
•Friedreich's ataxia, being an autosomal recessive disease→
  ◦Interstitial myocarditis→
    −Interstitial fibrosis
•Idiopathic
•Infiltrative disease
  ◦Amyloidosis
  ◦Iron storage disease
    −Hemochromatosis, w/ cardiac disease following hepatic & pancreatic disease→diabetes mellitus
    −Transfusion siderosis, esp. @ >50 cumulative lifetime units of packed red blood cells
    −Hemolytic anemias
  ◦Sarcoidosis
•Neoplastic
  ◦Metastatic malignancy
•Radiation therapy
  ◦Radiation field containing the heart
•Storage diseases
  ◦Fabry's disease
  ◦Gaucher's disease
  ◦Glycogen storage diseases
  ◦Hurler's disease

Cardiovascular
  •Restrictive cardiomyopathy→
    ◦Predominantly right sided heart failure
    ◦3rd &/or 4th heart sounds†, w/ both→
      −Gallop rhythm
    ◦Kussmaul's sign, being inspiration→
      −Diaphragm contraction→↑systemic venous return→↑jugular venous pressure as the restrictive
        myocardium & inter−atrial septal rightward bulging do not allow for accommodation of ↑preload
    ◦Misaligned &/or separated valve leaflets→
      −Regurgitation
    ◦↓Ventricular diastolic filling→
      −Poorly tolerated tachycardia, as it further ↓ventricular diastole→↓cardiac output
  •Ventricular systole→
    ◦Formation of a myocardial pressure gradient, as the outer layers place additive pressure on the
      inner layers, w/ pressure being greatest on the subendocardium→
      −Subendocardial vascular compression→↓systolic myocardial blood flow→subendocardial
        reliance on diastolic flow for O_2 & nutrient supply. Being that restrictive cardiomyopathy→
        incomplete diastole, its blood supply is progressively diminished. This is however, offset by
        infiltrative disease mediated myocyte death→↓demand. Ischemia, esp. subendocardial, only
        occurs in association w/ amyloidosis

†3rd heart sounds are heard only w/:
- Dilated cardiomyopathy
- Restrictive cardiomyopathy
- Constrictive pericarditis

...whereas 4th heart sounds may be heard w/ any cardiomyopathy having ↑atrial contribution

ELECTRICAL STUDIES

- **Electrocardiogram–ECG**
  Findings:
  - Nonspecific ST segment &/or T wave changes
  - Q waves, indicating previous myocardial infarction or representing a pseudoinfarct pattern
  - ↓**Voltage**, w/ diagnostic criteria being either:
    ○ Peak to peak QRS <5mm in the limb leads (I, II, III, aVR, aVL, aVF)
    ○ Peak to peak QRS <10mm in the precordial leads (V1–V6)
    ...due to either:
      - ↓Myocardial mass (ex. dilated cardiomyopathy)
      - Interposing tissue (ex. obesity, restrictive cardiomyopathy), fluid (ex. pericardial or pleural effusion), &/or gas (ex. emphysema, pneumothorax) between the electrical impulse & the electrodes
  - Atrial dilation, occurring in all forms of chronic heart failure
    ○ Criteria for left atrial dilation:
      - Negative terminal P wave deflection in lead V1, being > 1X1mm
      - Notched P wave in lead II, being >3mm in length
    ○ Criteria for right atrial dilation:
      - ↑P wave in lead II, being ≥2.5mm in height
      - Biphasic P wave in lead V1, w/ a larger initial portion being ≥2mm in height

IMAGING STUDIES

- **Transthoracic echocardiography–TTE**
  Procedure:
  - A 2 dimensional ultrasonographic image, allowing real time visualization of:
    ○ Ventricular wall thickness
    ○ Cavity size (both atrial & ventricular)
    ○ Myocardial & valve function, allowing ejection fraction–EF estimation (% of end diastolic volume ejected during ventricular systole)
    ○ The pericardial space
  - Doppler ultrasonography uses Doppler shift to detect vessel flow velocity→
    ○ Valve regurgitation visualization
    ○ Estimation of valve pressure gradients
  Findings:
  - ↓, ↑, or normal ejection fraction (normal 50–70%)
  - ↓ to normal ventricular chamber size
  - Thickened ventricular myocardium, but not hypercontractile
  - **Incomplete ventricular relaxation**, w/ abrupt cessation due to ↓compliance→
    ○ Delayed mitral valve opening
    ○ ↓Early diastolic filling→
      - Delayed increase in cavity size
      - ↓E wave & ↑late diastolic filling due to atrial systole→↑A wave, termed **reversal of the E:A ratio**, being absent in patients w/ atrial fibrillation
  - Amyloidosis→
    - Glittery appearance
  Limitations:
  - ↓Visualization in obese or emphysematous patients
  - May not allow adequate:
    ○ Visualization of the anterior aspect of a prosthetic aortic valve
    ○ Functional assessment of a prosthetic aortic valve

INVASIVE PROCEDURES

- **Cardiac catheterization**
  Findings:
  - Rapidly ↓early diastolic ventricular pressure→
    ○ Diastolic steep fall, w/ subsequent rapidly ↑diastolic ventricular pressure→
      - Rise w/ plateau, termed the "square root sign"
  - ↑Atrial pressure, w/ M or W shaped wave forms indicating prominent x & y descents

•Treat the underlying disease
•**Medication restriction**
  ◦Avoid or use caution w/ medications→
    −↑Ventricular contractility (Digoxin, vasodilators)
    −↓Ventricular diastole (β receptor agonists)
    −↓Ventricular preload (diuretics, vasodilators)
    ...as all→
      •↓Ventricular end−diastolic volume which may→
      ◦Hypotension

THROMBOEMBOLIC PROPHYLAXIS

ANTICOAGULANTS: High molecular weight Heparin

M	♀	Start
M	?	60units/ kg IV bolus (or 5000units empirically)
		12units/kg/hour infusion (or 1000units/ hour empirically)

•Titrated by 2.5units/kg/hour to achieve an activated partial thromboplastin time−aPTT of 1.5−2X control value or **50−70seconds**

aPTT (seconds)	Action	Obtain next aPTT
<40	Bolus 5000units & ↑infusion rate by 100units/ hour	6hours
40−49	↑Infusion rate by 50units/ hour	6hours
50−70 (or 1.5−2Xcontrol)	NO ACTION	24hours
71−85	↓Infusion rate by 50units/ hour	6hours
86−100	Hold infusion 30min., then ↓infusion rate by 100units/ hour	6hours
101−150	Hold infusion 60min., then ↓infusion rate by 150units/ hour	6hours
>150	Hold infusion 60min., then ↓infusion rate by 300units/ hour	6hours

Monitoring:
•Complete blood count q24hours to monitor for side effects

ANTICOAGULANTS: Low molecular weight Heparin

Generic (Trade)	M	♀	Start	Max
Enoxaparin (Lovenox)	KL	P	1.5mg/ kg SC q24hours or	180mg/ 24hours
			1mg/ kg SC q12hours	
Dalteparin (Fragmin)	KL	P	200 anti−factor Xa units/ kg SC q24hours or	18,000units q24hours
			100 anti−factor Xa units/ kg SC q12hours	

Dose adjustment:
•Obesity
  ◦Most manufacturers recommend a maximum dose of that for a 90kg patient

Monitoring:
•Monitoring of anti−Xa levels is recommended in patients w/:
  ◦Abnormal coagulation/ hemorrhage
  ◦Obesity
  ◦Renal failure
  ◦Underweight
•Check 4h after 2nd SC dose. Further monitoring is not necessary once the correct dose is established in obese patients

Administration frequency	Therapeutic anti−Xa levels
Q12hours	0.6−1 units/ mL
Q24hours	1−2 units/ mL

Mechanism:
•Heparin combines w/ plasma antithrombin 3→
  ◦↑Antithrombin 3 activity in removing thrombin & activated factors 9, 10, 11,& 12→
    −↓Coagulation→↓vascular & mural thrombus formation &/or propagation
•Heparin is metabolized by the plasma enzyme heparinase

Outcomes:
•↓Morbidity & mortality

Side effects:
  Cardiovascular
    •**Hemorrhage**
    •**Heparin induced thrombocytopenia−HIT 10%,** esp. w/ high molecular weight Heparin
      Mechanism:
        •Heparin mediated platelet agglutination→
          ◦Monocyte/ macrophage mediated extravascular removal via the splenic trabecular network=red pulp, & hepatic sinusoids→
            −**Thrombocytopenia**

140

Outcomes:
 •Benign, as it resolves spontaneously, even w/ continued exposure
•**Heparin induced thrombocytopenia ± thrombosis–HITT ≤3%**, esp. w/ high molecular weight
 Heparin
 Mechanism:
  •Heparin mediated platelet agglutination→
   ◦Monocyte/ macrophage mediated extravascular removal via the splenic trabecular
   network=red pulp, & hepatic sinusoids→
    –**Thrombocytopenia**
   ◦Platelet release of Heparin neutralizing factor=platelet factor 4–PF4, which complexes w/
   Heparin→
    –Production of anti-complex antibodies→↑platelet activation↔↑platelet factor 4 release→
    a vicious cycle of **platelet mediated arterial &/or venous thrombus formation, termed
    the "white clot syndrome,"** being as the clot is relatively devoid of erythrocytes
 Outcomes:
  •Must discontinue treatment as **20% develop thromboembolic complications**. Being that
  both Heparins may cross-react w/ the etiologic antibodies, their further use is contraindicated.
  Consider continued treatment w/ direct thrombin inhibitors
   ◦Antibody cross-reactivity:
    –Low molecular weight Heparins–85%
    –Heparinoids–5%
Mucocutaneous
 •Skin necrosis–rarely occurring w/ high molecular weight Heparins, & not being associated w/
 anticoagulant deficiency
Musculoskeletal
 •Osteoporosis, esp. w/ high molecular weight Heparin
  ◦Usually @ use ≥1month
Hematologic
 •↓Aldosterone production→
  ◦**Hyperkalemia–8%**

CHARACTERISTICS OF HEPARIN INDUCED THROMBOCYTOPENIC SYNDROMES		
	HIT	HITT
Onset	<2days	4–10 days
Re-exposure	<2days	Earlier if re-exposed within 3 months
Platelet count	↓, being <150,000 or ≥50%	
Platelet median nadir	~90,000	~60,000

•**^{14}C–Serotonin release assay**
 Indications:
  •Suspected HITT
 Procedure:
  •Normal donor platelets are radiolabeled w/ ^{14}C–serotonin. They are then washed & combined w/
  patient serum & therapeutic Heparin concentrations (0.1 U/ mL). Induction of ^{14}C–serotonin
  release from platelets constitutes a positive test
 Limitations:
  •Expense, due to the use of radioactive material
 Outcomes:
  •Considered the gold standard in the detection of HITT
•**Enzyme linked immunosorbent assay–ELISA**
 Indications:
  •Suspected HITT
 Procedure:
  •Heparin–PF4 complexes affixed to a plastic plate are incubated w/ the patient's serum. If the
  patient has produced antibodies, then the addition of enzymatically (horseradish peroxidase)
  labeled anti-human IgG allows for color visualization via spectrophotometer
 Limitations:
  •Many antibody positive patients do not develop clinical HITT
  •30% false positive

Contraindications:
 •Active hemorrhage
 •Severe bleeding diathesis
 •Severe thrombocytopenia (platelet count ≤20,000/ μL)
 •Recent significant trauma
 •Neurosurgery, ocular surgery, or intracranial hemorrhage within 10days

ANTIDOTE				
Generic	M ♀	Amount IV over 10min.	Max	
Protamine	P ?	1mg/ 100units of HMWH	50mg	
		1mg/ 100units Dalteparin	"	
		1mg/ 1mg Enoxaparin	"	

Mechanism:
- Protamine combines electrostatically w/ Heparin→
  - Inability to bind to antithrombin 3

FOLLOWED BY

ANTICOAGULANTS		
Generic	M ♀	Start

Warfarin (Coumadin) L U 5mg PO q24hours
- Because the anticoagulant proteins↓ relatively faster than the procoagulant proteins, an initial transient hypercoagulable state develops. Due to this, Warfarin is started once the patient is therapeutic on Heparin, via either:
  - Goal aPTT w/ high molecular weight Heparin
  - Evening of initiation of low molecular weight Heparin
  …requiring ~7days (corresponding to 2 half lives of factor 2, or a 75% reduction) to reach a true therapeutic level of an **international normalized ratio–INR of 2—3**

INR	Action	Obtain next INR
<1.5	↑Weekly dose by 15%	1 week
1.5–1.9	↑Weekly dose by 10%	2 weeks
2–3	NO ACTION	1 month if stable
3.1–3.9	↓Weekly dose by 10%	2 weeks
4–5	Skip 1 day, then ↓weekly dose by 15%	1 week
>5	DISCONTINUE WARFARIN	Q day until ≤3, then ↓weekly dose by 50%

Mechanism:
- Competitively inhibits hepatocyte enzymatic vitamin K reactive sites→
  - ↓Formation of both:
    - −Procoagulant proteins 2, 7, 9, & 10
    - −Anticoagulant proteins C & S
    …w/ the anticoagulant effect requiring several days, as it must await the metabolism of the pre−existing plasma procoagulant proteins, w/ normal coagulation returning within several days of discontinuation

Side effects:
Cardiovascular
- **Hemorrhage**
  - Fatal: 0.6%/ year
  - Major: 3%/ year
  - Minor: 7%/ year
Cutaneous
- Tissue necrosis w/ protein C or S deficiency or dysfunction

Contraindications:
- Active hemorrhage
- Severe bleeding diathesis
- Severe thrombocytopenia (platelet count ≤20,000/ μL)
- Recent significant trauma
- Neurosurgery, ocular surgery, or intracranial hemorrhage within 10days
- Injury risk (including falls & sports) or compliance risk via:
  - Alcoholism
  - Altered mental status
  - Illicit drug abuse
  - Orthostatic hypotension
  - Poor compliance
  - Seizure disease
  - Syncope
  - Unstable gait

Special considerations:
- **If undergoing elective surgery during treatment**
  - Stop Warfarin 5 days prior to surgery, & begin Heparin
- **Anticoagulation during pregnancy**
  - Substitute low molecular weight Heparin for Warfarin, followed by Warfarin treatment postpartum if necessary

142

ANTIDOTES
•**Gastric lavage & activated charcoal** if recently administered; forced emesis at home

VITAMIN K=Phytonadione
Indications:
•To correct the international normalized ration–INR or prothrombin time–PT
Dose
10mg SC/ IV slow push @ 1mg/ min. in order to ↓anaphylactoid reaction risk
Mechanism:
•Requires several hours to days for effect
Side effects:
•Avoid intramuscular–IM administration which may→   ∘Intramuscular hemorrhage

FRESH FROZEN PLASMA–FFP
Indications:

•To correct the international normalized ration–INR or prothrombin time–PT under the following conditions:
  ∘**INR >20**
  ∘**Severe hemorrhage**
  ∘**Other need for rapid reversal, such as an emergent procedure**

Dose†
15mL/ kg IV (w/ ~200mL FFP/ unit) q4hours prn ↑INR
Mechanism:

•Contains clotting factors 2, 7, 9–13, & heat labile 5 & 7→
  ∘Immediate onset of action
•Each unit→
  ∘8% ↑coagulation factors
  ∘4% ↑blood volume

143

•Caused by either:
  ◦Pericardial inflammation=pericarditis→
    −Exudative effusion
  ◦Systemic transudative effusive process

EXUDATIVE EFFUSIVE PROCESSES ▬▬▬▬▬▬▬▬▬▬▬▬▬▬▬▬▬▬▬▬▬▬▬▬▬▬
Infectious:
•**Bacterial pericarditis**
  ◦Francisella tularensis
  ◦Mycobacteria sp.
  ◦Mycoplasma pneumoneae
  ◦Neisseria sp.
  ◦Rickettsiae sp.
  ◦Staphylococcus aureus
  ◦Streptococcus pneumoneae
•**Fungal pericarditis**
  ◦Blastomyces dermatitides
  ◦Candida albicans
  ◦Coccidiodes immitis
  ◦Histoplasma capsulatum
•**Viral pericarditis**
  ◦**Coxsackievirus group A or B**
  ◦**Echovirus type B**
  ◦Adenovirus
  ◦Epstein−Barr virus−EBV
  ◦Herpes simplex virus−HSV type 1 or 2
  ◦Human immune deficiency virus−HIV
  ◦Influenza virus
  ◦Mumps virus
  ◦Varicella−zoster virus−VZV

Noninfectious:
•**Idiopathic, being the most common**
  ◦Most, likely being unrecognized viral infections
•**Myocardial injury**
  Mechanisms:
    •Transmural infarction→
      ◦**Pericarditis within 5 days post−myocardial infarction**
    •Myocardial injury via infarction or heart surgery→
      ◦Myocyte release of cellular molecules→
        −**Autoimmune serositis <5%†**→pericarditis, pleuritis, &/or systemic inflammatory syndrome
          @ 2weeks−6months post−myocardial injury
•**Neoplastic**
  ◦Metastasized malignancy, esp.:
    −Breast cancer
    −Leukemia
    −Lung cancer
    −Lymphoma
    −Renal cancer
  ◦Radiation induced @ >4000cGy
•**Rheumatologic disease**
  ◦Polyarteritis nodosa
  ◦Rheumatic fever
  ◦Rheumatoid arthritis, including the subsyndrome of systemic juvenile rheumatoid arthritis
  ◦Scleroderma
  ◦Systemic lupus erythematosus−SLE
  ◦Wegener's granulomatosis

- **Medications**
  - Drug induced lupus
    - Chlorpromazine
    - **Hydralazine**–10% of patients, usually @ >200mg/ 24h
    - Isoniazid–INH
    - Methyldopa
    - Minocycline
    - **Procainamide**–30% of patients taking for >1year
    - Quinidine
    - Sulfasalazine
  - Doxorubicin
  - Penicillin
  - Phenylbutazone
  - Phenytoin
- **Uremia**→
  - Pericarditis, esp. @ a blood urea nitrogen >100mg/ dL
- **Chest trauma**
- **Any cardiac procedure**

---

†Being termed **Dressler's syndrome** if post–myocardial infarction or **Post–cardiotomy syndrome**

TRANSUDATIVE EFFUSIVE PROCESSES ▬▬▬▬▬▬▬
- **↑Lymphatic hydrostatic pressure**
  - Heart failure, esp. w/ biventricular failure, as right ventricular failure→
    - ↑Lymphatic hydrostatic pressure
- **↓Vascular oncotic pressure**
  - Liver cirrhosis
  - Malnutrition
  - Nephrotic syndrome
  - ...→↓plasma albumin
- **↑Interstitial fluid oncotic pressure**
  - Hypothyroidism→
    - ↑Interstitial fluid albumin

DIAGNOSIS
Cardiovascular
- Pericardial inflammation=pericarditis→
  - **Sharp** &/or burning pain > gripping pressure, heaviness, &/or other discomfort anywhere above the waist, usually being substernal w/:
    - Radiation to the back, neck, or shoulder, due to diaphragmatic &/or phrenic nerve inflammation
    - Pleurisy, being thoracic pain exacerbated by either deep inhalation (including coughing & sneezing), supine position, or thoracic palpation, & being **relieved by leaning forward**
  - Exudative effusion–10%→**pericardial friction rub**, usually being intermittent, without correlation to effusion size, & unusual w/ transudative effusions→
    - High pitched scratching sound (like rubbing hair together) w/ 2 to 3 components, being due to ventricular systole & either rapid ventricular filling during early diastole &/or atrial systole, best heard during inspiration @ the left lower sternal border, w/ the patient sitting forward

Indicators of a large pericardial effusion:
- ↓Heart sounds
- Left lower lung compression atelectasis→
  - Inspiratory crackles
  - ↓Breath sounds
  - Dullness to percussion
  - ↑Tactile fremitus
  - Egophony: A patients verbalization of the sound 'E' is heard as 'A'
- Motion dampening effect→
  - Non–observable/ non–palpable point of maximal impulse–PMI, being ironic as the patient has an ↑cardiac silhouette on imaging

Eponymomous signs of a large pericardial effusion:
- **Ewart's/ Conner's signs:** Large pericardial effusion→
  - Lower posterior lung compression atelectasis→
    - Dullness to percussion, best heard beneath the angle of the left &/or right scapula, termed Ewart's & Conner's sign respectively
- **Bamberger's sign:** If either the above signs disappear as the patient leans forward
- **Dressler's sign**: Absolute dullness to percussion of the lower 2/3 to 1/2 of the sternum

Pulmonary
- Pleurisy→attempts to ↓thoracic movement→
  ◦ Small volume inhalations→
    –Atelectasis
    –Difficulty breathing=dyspnea
    –Respiratory rate >16/ min.=tachypnea

Hematologic
- Myopericarditis→
  ◦ Cell death mediated plasma myocardial protein release

Proteins indicating myocardial necrosis:
- Total creatine kinase–CK >170 U/ L
  ◦ Rising @ 3–12hours for 0.5–1day
- Creatine kinase–CK MB isoenzyme >5ng/ mL
  ◦ Rising @ 3–12hours for 1–1.5days
- **Creatine kinase–CK MB isoenzyme relative mass >5%†**, being very specific
- **Cardiac troponin I–CTnl >0.1ng/ mL**, being very specific
  ◦ Rising @ 3–12hours for 7–10days
- **Cardiac troponin T–CTnT >0.2ng/ mL**, being very specific
  ◦ Rising @ 3–12hours for 10–14days
- Myoglobin >106
  ◦ Rising @ 1–4hours for 18–24hours
- Aspartate aminotransferase–AST >59 U/ L
  ◦ Rising @ 6–10hours for 3–4days
- Lactate dehydrogenase–LDH1/ LDH2 >1
  ◦ Occurring @ 1–3days for 2weeks

- Renal failure→
  ◦ ↑Of all the above enzymes, except for aspartate aminotransferase–AST, which may be ↓

†Creatine kinase–CK occurs as 3 isoenzymes, each being a dimer variably composed of 2 polypeptides termed M & B subunits:
- CK–BB
- CK–MM
- CK–MB
  …w/ **CK–MB constituting 6–15% of myocardial creatine kinase & <4% of skeletal muscle creatine kinase,** w/ the percentages termed the enzymes relative index. Thus, an ↑creatine kinase w/ an MB isoenzyme level >5% is considered evidenced of myocardial necrosis, whereas an isoenzyme level <4% is considered evidence of skeletal muscle necrosis. Levels of 4–5% are indeterminate

ELECTRICAL STUDIES

- **Electrocardiogram–ECG**

Findings:
- Ventricular pericardial inflammation→
  ◦ **Diffuse, concave upward ST segment elevation, possible in all leads**
- Atrial pericardial inflammation→
  ◦ **Diffuse PR segment depression in the precordial leads**
- Pericardial effusion→
  ◦ ↓**Voltage,** w/ diagnostic criteria being either:
    –Peak to peak QRS <5mm in the limb leads (I, II, III, aVR, aVL, aVF)
    –Peak to peak QRS <10mm in the precordial leads (V1–V6)
    …due to either:
      - ↓Myocardial mass (ex. dilated cardiomyopathy)
      - Interposing tissue (ex. obesity, restrictive cardiomyopathy), fluid (ex. pericardial or pleural effusion), &/or gas (ex. emphysema, pneumothorax) between the electrical impulse & the electrodes
- Large pericardial effusion→
  ◦ **Alternating QRS height, termed electrical alternans, indicating** ↑**pericardial tamponade risk**

STAGES OF PERICARDITIS MEDIATED ECG CHANGES

Time frame	PR interval	ST segment	T wave
Hours	↓	Concave ↑	Upright
Days	Isoelectric	Isoelectric	Flat†, then inverted‡, then upright

---

†In a myocardial infarction, the T wave begins flattening prior to the ST segment becoming isoelectric
‡Rarely may remain permanently inverted

146

•**Chest x ray**
Findings:
  •Pericardial effusion→
    ○↑**Cardiac silhouette**, being very sharp, due to ↓epicardial motion→
    –Wide diaphragmatic & narrow upper mediastinal surfaces, termed a "water bottle" shape
    –Radiolucent space between the pericardial layers on lateral view, termed the "oreo cookie" sign

•**Transthoracic echocardiography–TTE**
Procedure:
  •A 2 dimensional ultrasonographic image, allowing real time visualization of:
    ○Ventricular wall thickness
    ○Cavity size (both atrial & ventricular)
    ○Myocardial & valve function, allowing ejection fraction–EF estimation (% of end diastolic volume ejected during ventricular systole)
    ○The pericardial space
  •Doppler ultrasonography uses Doppler shift to detect vessel flow velocity→
    ○Valve regurgitation visualization
    ○Estimation of valve pressure gradients
Findings:
  •Pericardial effusion→
    ○Echo–free space between the pericardial layers
    ○Stranding, indicating an exudative effusion
Progressive effusion growth mediated visualization:
  1. Visualized posteriorly during systole, w/ separation of the parietal & visceral pericardium
  2. Visualized anteriorly & posteriorly throughout the cardiac cycle
  3. Exaggerated swinging cardiac motion within the pericardial sac
Limitations:
  •↓Visualization in obese or emphysematous patients

•**Pericardiocentesis**
Procedure:
  •Ultrasound guided percutaneous needle mediated pericardial fluid removal
Indications:
  •Fluid analysis
  •Symptom relief
Contraindications:
  •Coagulopathy (INR >1.3 &/or aPTT >35seconds) &/or thrombocytopenia (<150,000/ μL)→
    ○↑Hemothorax risk
  •Ventilator dependent patient, continuous cough &/or hiccups, &/or uncooperative patient→↑risk of:
    ○Air embolism
    ○Hemothorax
    ○Organ perforation, esp. the liver or spleen depending on side
    ○Pneumothorax
  •Overlying skin infection→
    ○↑Deep tissue infection risk
Lab studies:
  •**Tube 1:** Protein, lactate dehydrogenase–LDH, & glucose
  •**Tube 2:** Cell count & differential
  •**Tube 3:** Gram stain & culture
  •**Tube 4:** Other studies as clinically indicated

PERICARDIAL FLUID STUDIES

Studies†	Transudate	Exudate
Gross appearance	Serous=clear straw colored	•**Serous**=clear straw colored •**Turbid:** Leukocytes, lipid, organisms •**Purulent:** Empyema •**Bloody:** Malignancy, mycobacterial infection, trauma (including traumatic tap), coagulopathy, aortic dissection, post–coronary artery bypass
Smell	None	Foul odor=anaerobic infection
Protein level (1–1.5g/dL)	<3g/ dL (CHF may ≥3g/ dL)	≥3g/ dL
Pericardial/ serum protein level	<0.50=50%	≥0.50=50%‡
LDH level	<200 IU	≥200 IU or ≥2/3rds upper normal serum limit‡
Pericardial/ serum LDH level	<0.60=60%	≥0.60=60%‡
Serum–effusion albumin	>1.1	≤1.1
Cholesterol	<45mg/ dL	>55mg/ dL
Glucose level	Same as serum	<60mg/ dL <20mg/ dL: Empyema or rheumatoid arthritis
Leukocytes	<1000/ µL	≥1,000/ µL° >30,000/ µL: Empyema
Differential	Mononuclear predominant	•**Mononuclear^:** Malignancy, mycobacterial or viral pericarditis, rheumatoid arthritis, vasculitides •**Eosinophils >10%:** Asbestos, Churg–Strauss syndrome, medication mediated, paragonomiasis •**Neutrophil predominant:** All others
Erythrocytes (0–5/ µL)	<1,000/µL (CHF <10,000/ µL)	≥1000/ µL >50% plasma hematocrit: hemopericardium
Amylase	60–130 U/ L	>2X serum level: Esophageal rupture, pancreatitis, malignancy
pH	7.38–7.44	<7.2: Empyema
Adenosine deaminase–ADA		Positive in granulomatous disease >70: Poss. mycobacterial pericarditis <40: Excludes mycobacterial pericarditis
Fibrinogen	Negative	Positive
Specific gravity	<1.016	≥1.016
Triglyceride		>110mg/ dL: Chylopericardium
Sudan III staining	Negative	Positive: Chylopericardium
Microscopy	–	•AFB stain positive: Mycobacterial pericarditis Sensitivity: 10%. •Cytology positive: Malignancy Sensitivity: 55% w/ 1 sample 80% w/ 3 samples •Gram stain positive: Bacterial
Culture (aerobic & anaerobic)	–	±

†Consider transudative values to be normal
‡The presence of any of these, termed **Light's criteria**, indicate an exudative effusion
°To correct for the neutrophil count in a traumatic tap, subtract 1 neutrophil for every 250 erythrocytes
^Lymphocyte & monocyte

148

•**Antimicrobial medications if infectious**
•**Anti-inflammatory treatment duration:** Until the patient is asymptomatic X 1week, w/ subsequent taper if taking glucocorticoids ≥2weeks

NONSTEROIDAL ANTI-INFLAMMATORY DRUGS-NSAIDs

Generic	M ♀		Start	Max
Ibuprofen	L	P in 1st & 2nd, U in 3rd trimester	600mg PO q8hours	3.2g/ 24hours
Indomethacin	L	P in 1st & 2nd, U in 3rd trimester	50mg PO/ PR q8hours	
Naproxen	L	P in 1st & 2nd, U in 3rd trimester	375mg PO q12hours	
•XR form			750mg PO q24hours	

•One cannot predict which NSAID a patient will respond to
•Attempt to eventually ↓dosage &/or limit use to exacerbations in order to ↓side effect risk

Mechanism:
•Aspirin & other anti-inflammatory medications→
  ◦Respectively to irreversible & reversible inhibition of both cyclooxygenase enzymes (COX-1 & COX-2), being responsible for the production of neural & inflammatory cell prostaglandins respectively→
    −↓Pain
    −↓Temperature (antipyretic)
    −↓Inflammation

Background pathophysiology:
•Inflammatory cell mediated prostaglandins are released at sites of inflammation (in addition to other inflammatory cytokines)→
  ◦Leukocyte migration→↑inflammation via:
    −Vasodilation→↑blood flow→erythema, edema, warmth, &/or tenderness/ pain via enhanced neuronal sensitivity
•Interleukin−IL1→
  ◦↑Hypothalamic prostaglandin production→
    −Fever

In Brief:
•**Cyclooxygenase-COX1 enzymes** are found in most cells of the body, being responsible for normal physiologic processes
•**Cyclooxygenase-COX 2 enzymes** are responsible for the production of inflammatory cell prostaglandins

Side effects:
Gastrointestinal
  •Inhibition of the cyclooxygenase−COX1 enzyme→↑peptic inflammatory disease risk→↑**upper gastrointestinal hemorrhage risk** via:
    ◦↓Gastric mucosal prostaglandin synthesis→
      −↓Epithelial cell proliferation
      −↓Mucosal blood flow→↓bicarbonate delivery to the mucosa
      −↓Mucus & bicarbonate secretion from gastric mucosal cells

Indications for peptic inflammatory disease prophylaxis:
  •Prophylax w/ proton pump inhibitors−PPI's, histamine 2 selective receptor blockers, or Misoprostol in patients w/ any of the following:
    ◦Age >60 years w/ a history of peptic inflammatory disease
    ◦Anticipated therapy >3 months
    ◦Concurrent glucocorticoid use
    ◦Moderate to high dose NSAID use
  Note: Newer NSAIDs (Etodolac, Nabumetone, Salsalate)→
      •↓Risk of NSAID induced peptic inflammation/ ulcer

Genitourinary
- •Patients w/ pre-existing bilateral ↓renal perfusion, not necessarily failure:
  - ◦Heart failure
  - ◦Bilateral renal artery stenosis
  - ◦Hypovolemia
  - ◦Renal failure
  - …rely more on the compensatory production of vasodilatory prostaglandins→
    - •Afferent arteriole dilation→
      - ◦Maintained glomerular filtration rate–GFR, whereas NSAIDs→
        - –↓Prostaglandin production, which may→renal failure

Pulmonary
- •Inhibition of both cyclooxygenase enzymes (COX 1 & COX2)→
  - ◦↑Lipoxygenase activity→
    - –↑Leukotriene synthesis→symptomatic asthma within 2hours of ingestion in 5% of asthmatics

SECOND LINE TREATMENT

SYSTEMIC GLUCOCORTICOID TREATMENT: Only once active infection has been excluded

Generic	M ♀	Dose
Methylprednisolone	L ?	30–60mg PO q24hours
Prednisolone	L ?	30–60mg PO q24hours
Prednisone	L ?	30–60mg PO q24hours

- •Once disease control is achieved, taper to the lowest effective maintenance dose in order to minimize serious side effects, w/ the goal of discontinuation if possible, w/ attention to relapse syndrome

Glucocorticoids	Relative potencies Anti–inflammatory	Mineralocorticoid	Duration	Dose equiv.
Cortisol (physiologic†)	1	1	10hours	20mg
Cortisone (PO)	0.7	2	10hours	25mg
Hydrocortisone (PO, IM, IV)	1	2	10hours	20mg
Methylprednisolone (PO, IM, IA, IV)	5	0.5	15–35hours	5mg
Prednisone (PO)	5	0.5	15–35hours	5mg
Prednisolone (PO, IM, IV)	5	0.8	15–35hours	5mg
Triamcinolone (PO, IM)	5	~0	15–35hours	5mg
Betamethasone (PO, IM, IA)	25	~0	35–70hours	0.75mg
Dexamethasone (PO)	25	~0	35–70hours	0.75mg
Fludrocortisone (PO)	10	125	10hours	

†The physiologic rate of adrenal cortical cortisol production is 20–30mg/ 24hours

Side effects of chronic use:
General
- •Anorexia→
  - ◦Cachexia
- •↑Perspiration

Cardiovascular
- •Mineralocorticoid effects→
  - ◦↑Renal tubular NaCl & water retention as well as potassium secretion→
    - –**Hypertension**
    - –**Edema**
    - –**Hypokalemia**
- •Counter–regulatory=anti–insulin effects→
  - ◦↑Plasma glucose→
    - –**Secondary diabetes mellitus**, which may→ketoacidemia
  - ◦Hyperlipidemia→↑atherosclerosis→
    - –**Coronary artery disease**
    - –Cerebrovascular disease
    - –Peripheral vascular disease

Cutaneous/ subcutaneous
- •↓Fibroblast function→
  - ◦↓Intercellular matrix production→
    - –↑Bruisability→ecchymoses
    - –Poor wound healing
    - –Skin striae

- •Androgenic effects→
  - ◦Acne
  - ◦↑Facial hair
  - ◦Thinning scalp hair
- •Fat redistribution from the extremities to the:
  - ◦Abdomen→
    - −Truncal obesity
  - ◦Shoulders→
    - −Supraclavicular fat pads
  - ◦Upper back→
    - −Buffalo hump
  - ◦Face→
    - −Moon facies
  - …w/ concomitant thinning of the arms & legs

Endocrine
- •**Adrenal failure** upon abrupt discontinuation after 2weeks

Gastrointestinal
- •Inhibition of phospholipase A$_2$ mediated conversion of cell membrane lipids to arachidonic acid, which is the precursor for both cyclooxygenase−COX enzymes, w/ the cyclooxygenase−COX1 enzyme found in most cells of the body, responsible for normal physiologic function. Inhibition of the cyclooxygenase−COX1 enzyme→↑peptic inflammatory disease risk→↑**upper gastrointestinal hemorrhage risk** via:
  - ◦↓Gastric mucosal prostaglandin synthesis→
    - −↓Epithelial cell proliferation
    - −↓Mucosal blood flow→↓bicarbonate delivery to the mucosa
    - −↓Mucus & bicarbonate secretion from gastric mucosal cells

Musculoskeletal
- •**Avascular necrosis of bone**
- •**Osteoporosis**
- •Proximal muscle weakness

Neurologic
- •Anxiety
- •Insomnia
- •Psychosis

Opthalmologic
- •**Cataracts**

Immunologic
- •Inhibition of phospholipase A$_2$ mediated conversion of cell membrane lipids to arachidonic acid, which is the precursor for both cyclooxygenase−COX enzymes (COX1 & COX2) being responsible for the production of neuronal & inflammatory cell prostaglandins respectively→
    - −↓Pain
    - −↓Temperature (antipyretic)
    - −↓**Inflammation**
- •Stabilization of lisosomal & cell membranes→
  - ◦↓Cytokine & proteolytic enzyme release
- •↓Lymphocyte & eosinophil production
  - …all→
    - •**Immunosuppression**→
      - −↑**Infection** &/or neoplasm risk

Hematologic
- •↑Erythrocyte production→
  - ◦Polycythemia
- •↑Neutrophil demargination→
  - ◦Neutrophilia→
    - −**Leukocytosis**

COLCHICINE		
M ♀	**Start**	
L ?	0.6mg PO q12hours	

- •Although available, intravenous administration is discouraged due to:
  - ◦Possible lethal side effects
  - ◦Teratogenicity

Dose adjustment:
- •Adjust according to renal function, w/ further dose↓ by 50% in patients age ≥70years

Creatinine clearance	Dose
35–49ml/ min.	0.6mg q24hours
10–34ml/ min.	0.6mg q2–3days

Mechanism:
- •Binds to tubulin (a microtubular protein)→
  - ○↓Mitotic spindle & microtubular formation→
    - ─↓Inflammatory cell division, chemotaxis, & phagocytosis→↓inflammation

Limitations:
- •Most effective if administered within 48hours of syndrome onset. Not effective if administered once the inflammatory process if fully established

Side effects:
  Gastrointestinal
  - •**Diarrhea**
  - •Nausea ± vomiting
  Mucocutaneous
  - •Alopecia

Overdose (IV >> PO):
  Gastrointestinal
  - •Hemorrhagic gastroenteritis
  - •Hepatitis
  Genitourinary
  - •**Renal failure**
  Musculoskeletal
  - •Myopathy, being limited to patients age >60years w/ a plasma creatinine >2mg/ dL→
    - ○Weakness &/or rhabdomyolysis
  Hematologic
  - •Hypocalcemia
  - •**Myelosuppression**

Contraindications:
- •**PO form**
  - ○Glomerular filtration rate–GFR <10mL/ min. or hemodialysis, as the medication is not dialyzed
- •**IV form**
  - ○Hepatitis
  - ○Renal failure
  - ○Infusion extravasation mediated inflammation

Monitoring:
- •Regular complete blood count for possible myelosuppression

INVASIVE PROCEDURES ▬▬▬▬▬
•**Pericardiocentesis**
  Indications:
  - •Fluid analysis
  - •Symptom relief

•**Pericardial window**
  Indications:
  - •Recurrent or likely recurrent (as w/ malignancy) pericardial effusion

152

RISK FACTORS
•**Any cause of pericardial effusion**, esp.:
- ○**Malignancy, being most common**
- ○Idiopathic
- ○Hemorrhage s/p cardiac surgery
- ○Ventricular wall rupture
- ○Pericardial rupture
- ○Proximal aortic dissection→
  - −Pericardial space rupture
- ○Uremia

CLASSIFICATION
•**Acute pericardial tamponade**
- ○Rapidly forming effusion, thus not allowing for pericardial compensatory stretching→
  - −Tamponade w/ **≤200mL** of fluid
•**Chronic pericardial tamponade**
- ○Slowly forming effusion, allowing for pericardial compensatory stretching, capable of holding up to **2L** of fluid→
  - −Tamponade

DIAGNOSIS
Cardiovascular
•↑Pericardial space hydrostatic pressure→
- ○↑Atrial hydrostatic pressure→
  - −↓Systemic & pulmonary venous return→**biventricular heart failure**
- ○"Tight" unyielding pericardium→
  - −Intraventricular pressure being increasingly transferred to the interventricular septum, w/ inhalation→↑venous return→↑right ventricular preload→↑right ventricular hydrostatic pressure→ ↑diastolic leftward bulging of the interventricular septum→↓left ventricular size→↓left ventricular preload (also due to inspiration mediated ↑pulmonary blood volume)→↓systemic cardiac output→ **pulsus paradoxus–75%†** **via inspiratory arterial systolic blood pressure fall >10mmHg**
...w/ eventual:
  - •**Hypotension**, being refractory to intravenous fluid infusion→
    - ○Cerebral failure→
      - −Altered mental status
    - ○Pre–renal renal failure
    - ○Lactic acidemia
    - ...termed **cardiogenic shock**

Eponymous signs:
•**Beck's triad**, composed of:
- ○↓Blood pressure
- ○Distant cardiac sounds
- ○↑Jugular venous pressure

Cutaneous
•Severe heart failure→
- ○Reflex mediated peripheral arteriole vasoconstriction in order to maintain central organ perfusion, w/ ↓mucocutaneous blood flow→
  - −Pale skin & mucus membranes, w/ progression to ↑relative mucocutaneous O_2 extraction→bluish color=cyanosis
  - −↓Peripheral vascular heat dissipation→cool skin w/ perspiration

---

†A normal phenomenon, exaggerated in certain diseases. A quick test to check for the presence of pulsus paradoxus consists of palpating the pulse w/ attention to possible respiratory variation, which, if absent, rules out significant pulsus paradoxus

IMAGING

•**Transthoracic echocardiography–TEE**
  Findings:
    •Pericardial effusion→
      ◦Echo–free space between the pericardial layers, w/ **right atrial & ventricular compression**
      ◦Inhalation→
        −Leftward septal shift
        −Transvalvular velocity changes, being ↑across the tricuspid valve & ↓across the mitral valve

TREATMENT

•**Intravenous fluid**, w/ attention to:
  ◦**Intravascular volume expansion via Normal saline** (0.9% NaCl) or **lactated Ringer's solution**

•**Therapeutic pericardiocentesis**
  Contraindications:
    •Aortic or myocardial rupture

CONSTRICTIVE PERICARDITIS
A PERICARDIAL COMPRESSIVE SYNDROME

•Pericardial inflammation=pericarditis→
  ◦Visceral & parietal pericardial thickening & fibrosis→
    −Membrane fusion, w/ subsequent calcification (generalized > localized)→noncompliant pericardium
•Termed effusive−constrictive pericarditis if a concomitant pericardial effusion exists, being a stage in the progression to sole constrictive pericarditis

RISK FACTORS
•**Any cause of chronic pericarditis**, esp.:
  ◦**Idiopathic, being the most common**
  ◦Tuberculosis
  ◦Mediastinal radiation
  ◦Previous cardiac surgery
  ◦Post−viral
  ◦Uremia

DIAGNOSIS
Cardiovascular
•Pericardial fibrosis→a rigid pericardium→
  ◦↑Atrial hydrostatic pressure→
    −↓Systemic & pulmonary venous return→**biventricular diastolic heart failure (right > left sided)**
  ◦Abrupt cessation of early diastolic ventricular filling, as the expanding ventricular chambers reach the noncompliant pericardium→
    −A high pitched 3rd heart sound†, termed a pericardial knock, being ↑ w/ ↑venous return
  ◦↓Accommodation for excessive preload, as inhalation→
    −↑Venous return→↑jugular venous pressure, termed **Kussmaul's sign**
  ◦Motion dampening effect→
    −Non−observable/ non−palpable point of maximal impulse−PMI
Gastrointestinal
•Pericardial fibrosis→right sided heart failure→
  ◦Hepatic congestion→**hepatomegally−100%**→
    −Liver capsule (Glisson's capsule) distention ± right upper quadrant abdominal pain
    −Congestive hepatitis, which if chronic→cirrhosis=cardiac cirrhosis
  ◦Congested gastrointestinal vasculature→
    −↓Nutrient absorption→↓dry weight (careful, as weight loss may be offset by fluid gain)
    −Hepatojugular reflux via abdominal pressure, w/ the patient supine @ a 45° angle→↑venous return→↑jugular venous pressure→jugular venous distention as long as the pressure is applied
  ◦↑Portal venous pressure→
    −Peritoneal transudative effusion, termed ascites
    −Splenomegally
    ...→↑abdominal girth & weight‡ (1L fluid=1kg=2.2 lbs)

---

†3rd heart sounds are heard only w/:
  •Dilated cardiomyopathy
  •Restrictive cardiomyopathy
  •Constrictive pericarditis
  ...whereas 4th heart sounds may be heard w/ any cardiomyopathy having ↑atrial contribution
‡However, the congested gastrointestinal vasculature→
  •↓Nutrient absorption→
    ◦↓Dry weight (careful, as weight loss may be offset by fluid gain)

ELECTRICAL STUDIES
•**Electrocardiogram−ECG**
  Findings:
    •Diffuse nonspecific T wave abnormalities
    •Distended atria→
      ◦**Atrial fibrillation−50%**

IMAGING
•**Chest x ray**
  ◦**Pericardial calcification**, best visualized on lateral view, having an "egg−shell" appearance

155

- **Transthoracic echocardiography–TTE**
  - Findings:
    - •Thickened, calcified pericardium w/ a normal ejection fraction–EF (50–70%)
    - •Little to no pericardial effusion
    - •Rapid early diastolic filling→
      - ○Abrupt leftward displacement of the interventricular septum, termed "septal bounce"

INVASIVE PROCEDURES

- **Cardiac catheterization**
  - Procedure:
    - •Simultaneous, bilateral heart catheterization for concomitant pressure recordings
  - Findings:
    - •Generalized noncompliant pericardium→
      - ○**Near equalization of ↑right & left atrial & ventricular diastolic pressures,** usually having ≤5mmHg difference

TREATMENT

- **Pericardiectomy**

VALVULAR HEART DISEASE

• Caused by valvular &/or paravalvular disease→
  ◦ Valve dysfunction

CLASSIFICATION/ RISK FACTORS

• **Valvular stenosis** (mitral or aortic)
  ◦ ↑**Age**→
    – Chronic valvular degenerative disease→calcific leaflet stenosis. 35% of persons age ≥60years & 50% of persons age ≥80years have an aortic systolic murmur, being due to either aortic stenosis or sclerosis
  ◦ **Congenital heart disease**
    – Leaflet aplasia
    – Paravalvular membrane
    ...→chronic valvular degenerative disease
  ◦ **Leaflet inflammation†**
    – Endocarditis
    – Rheumatic heart disease
    – Vasculitis
    ...→leaflet scarring after months to years
  ◦ **Myxoma** mediated blockage

Aortic sclerosis
  • A roughening of the aortic valve→
    ◦ A murmur nearly indistinguishable from aortic stenosis, occurring **without stenosis**, which may eventually→
      – Aortic stenosis

• **Valvular regurgitation** (mitral or aortic)
  ◦ **Leaflet inflammation†**
    – Endocarditis
    – Rheumatic heart disease
    – Vasculitis
    ...→perforation
  ◦ **Ventricular cardiomyopathy**
    – Dilated
    – Hypertrophic
    – Restrictive
    ...→misaligned &/or separated leaflets
  ◦ **Connective tissue disease**
    – Ehlers–Danlos syndrome
    – Marfan's syndrome
    ...→valve structure weakening

Mitral valve regurgitation, affecting 3% of the population
  • **Myxomatous degeneration→**
    ◦ **Mitral valve prolapse, being the #1 cause**
  • **Myocardial ischemia→**
    ◦ Papillary muscle dysfunction &/or rupture
  • **Ruptured chordae tendinae**

---

†Infective endocarditis & rheumatic heart disease affect the **mitral valve** > aortic valve > tricuspid valve > pulmonic valve. However, intravenous drug use→
  • Tricuspid valve infective endocarditis in 50% of cases

DIAGNOSIS

Cardiovascular
  • Valvular heart disease→
    ◦ Abnormal cardiac blood flow sounds, termed **murmurs**, during diastole &/or systole, w/ ↑intensity over the valve auscultation area:
      – Mitral valve: Left 5th midclavicular intercostal space ≈ cardiac apex
      – Aortic valve: Right 2nd parasternal intercostal space ≈ cardiac base
      – Tricuspid valve: Left 5th parasternal intercostal space
      – Pulmonic valve: Left 2nd parasternal intercostal space
    ...w/ valvular stenosis & regurgitation often coexisting

Murmur intensity:
- **Grade 1:** Barely audible
- **Grade 2:** Audible
- **Grade 3:** Loud
- **Grade 4:** Loud w/ a palpable thrill
- **Grade 5:** Audible w/ chest piece rim to skin
- **Grade 6:** Audible w/ chest piece just off skin

Murmur intensity variation:
- Squatting or passive leg elevation→
  - ↑Venous return→
    - −↑**Murmur intensity across all stenotic & regurgitant valves**
- Rapid standing/ sitting, or the Valsalva maneuver†→
  - ↓Venous return→
    - −↓**Murmur intensity across all stenotic & regurgitant valves**
- Inspiration or the Muller maneuver‡→
  - ↑Right sided venous return→
    - −↑**Intensity across all right sided valves**
  - ↓Left sided venous return due to pooling in the lungs→
    - −↓**Intensity across all left sided valves**
  - …w/ **expiration** doing the opposite
- Handgrip→
  - ↑Peripheral vascular resistance→↑afterload→
    - −↑**Intensity across all left sided regurgitant valves**
    - −↓**Intensity across all left sided stenotic valves**
- Ventricular dysfunction (systolic &/or diastolic)→
  - ↓Murmur intensity, whereas high output states may→
    - −↑Murmur intensity

---

†**Valsalva maneuver:** Have the patient deeply inspire, followed by forceful expiration against a closed glottis X 10–20seconds. Place the palm of your hand on the abdominal wall (which should be contracted) in order to assess for the degree & duration of effort
‡**Muller maneuver:** Have the patient close their mouth & nostrils followed by a deep inspiratory effort X 10seconds

MITRAL/ TRICUSPID STENOSIS ▬▬▬▬▬▬▬▬▬▬▬▬▬▬▬▬▬▬▬▬▬▬

Murmur:
- Stenotic flow against the contracted, non–taut ventricular walls→
  - No murmur during the 1st third of diastole, w/ subsequent ventricular tautness→low frequency, **mid–diastolic rumbling, ↑in late diastole due to atrial contraction**

Mitral stenosis specific:
- **Best heard w/ the patient in the left lateral decubitus position, w/ the bell of the stethoscope.** Palpable murmur mediated vibrations, termed thrills, may be present over the cardiac apex, even in the absence of an auscultable murmur, which is usually beneath the low frequency end of human hearing

Other sounds:
- **Fibrotic, mobile, as yet noncalcified, stenosed valve→**
  - **Opening snap**
  - ↑**Heart sound**
  - …both of which disappear as calcification develops→
    - ↓Valvular mobility

MITRAL/ TRICUSPID REGURGITATION ▬▬▬▬▬▬▬▬▬▬▬▬▬▬▬▬▬▬

Murmur:
- Regurgitant flow against the atrium→
  - Chronic: **High frequency, holosystolic murmur**
  - Acute: Systolic murmur, ↓in late systole as atrial pressure equilibrates w/ ventricular pressure

Mitral regurgitation specific:
- **Best heard at the apex, w/ radiation to the axilla**

158

AORTIC/ PULMONIC STENOSIS ━━━━━━━━━━━━━━
Murmur:
• Stenotic flow against the great vessels→
   ◦ intra-systolic **diamond shaped murmur**†, beginning after the 1st heart sound, & ending before the
      2nd heart sound, w/ ↑severity→**progressively delayed peak murmur intensity**
Aortic stenosis specific:
• Radiation to the carotid arteries
• Palpable murmur mediated vibrations, termed thrills, over the upper chest &/or lower neck
Pulmonic stenosis specific:
• Radiation to the back
Other sounds:
• **Fibrotic, mobile, as yet noncalcified, stenosed valve**→
   ◦ **Opening snap**
   ◦ ↑**Heart sound**
   …both of which disappear as calcification develops→
      • ↓Valvular mobility
Aortic stenosis specific:
• Weak & delayed arterial pulse, indicating severe disease

━━━

†Only the shape of the murmur can reliably distinguish it from mitral regurgitation, as it may sound
holosystolic over the cardiac apex, termed the **Gallavardin effect**

AORTIC/ PULMONIC REGURGITATION ━━━━━━━━━━━━━━
Murmur:
• Regurgitant flow against the ventricular blood→
   ◦ Chronic: **High frequency, decrescendo, early diastolic murmur**, beginning upon valve closure
   ◦ Acute: **Low frequency, early diastolic murmur**, beginning upon valve closure, & ending in
      mid-diastole as ventricular pressure quickly equilibrates w/ vascular pressure
   ◦ ↑Ventricular volume (indicating severe disease)→
      −Systolic turbulent flow→**systolic ejection murmur** in the absence of aortic/ pulmonic stenosis
      −Early mitral/ tricuspid leaflet closure→↓component of the 1st heart sound & a **mid to late
         diastolic murmur**, termed the Austin Flint murmur
Chronic aortic regurgitation specific:
• Regurgitant flow→
   ◦ ↑Left ventricular preload→
      −↑Cardiac output→↑systolic blood pressure & ↓diastolic blood pressure→↑**pulse pressure** (SBP
       − DBP)→a strong pulse, being swift to rise & fall→**hyperkinetic circulatory signs**, all of which
         are lost w/ atrial fibrillation, as it→variable cardiac output→beat to beat systolic blood pressure
         variation
Acute aortic regurgitation specific:
• ↓Diastolic regurgitant flow into a small left ventricle→
   ◦ Little to no ↓in diastolic blood pressure→
      −Normal pulse pressure→**lack of hyperkinetic circulatory signs**

HYPERKINTEIC SIGNS OF CHRONIC AORTIC REGURGITATION	
Eponymous sign	**Physical findings**
Becker's sign	• Pulsating retinal vessels, synchronous w/ the pulse
Water-Hammer pulse	• Strong peripheral arterial pulsation, followed by vessel collapse per palpation
De Musset's sign	• Head bobbing, synchronous w/ the pulse
Hills sign	• Supine lower extremity > upper extremity systolic blood pressure by ≥30mmHg (≤20mmHg being normal)
Muller's sign	• Pulsating uvula, synchronous w/ the pulse
Pulses bisferiens	• Palpable central arterial double systolic impulse
Quincke's pulse	• Subungual capillary pulsations seen w/ nail free edge pressure which is >diastolic but <systolic pressure
Rosenbach's sign	• Palpable hepatic pulsation, synchronous w/ the pulse

ALL EXCEPT TRICUSPID DISEASE ━━━━━━━━━━━━━━━
• Eventual right ventricular hypertension→
   ◦ Right ventricular hypertrophy→
      −**Systolic parasternal lift**, as the ventricle is moved forward in the thorax due to the pulmonary
         artery pressure, termed afterload, it is attempting to overcome

LEFT SIDED DISEASE
- •Eventual **pulmonary hypertension**→
  - ∘↑Pulmonic component of the 2nd heart sound

COMPLICATIONS
- •**Heart failure**
  - Pathophysiology:
    - •Valvular stenosis→
      - ∘Proximal hypertension→
        - −Ventricular hypertrophy &/or atrial dilation→heart failure
    - •Chronic regurgitation→
      - ∘Proximal & distal hypertension→
        - −Ventricular hypertrophy & atrial dilation→heart failure
    - •Acute regurgitation
      - ∘Proximal hypertension without time for chamber adaptation→
        - −Heart failure
- •Valve disease &/or cardiomyopathy→
  - ∘↑Risk of microbial colonization→
    - −**Infective endocarditis**
- •Chronic valve disease→
  - ∘**Hypertrophic cardiomyopathy**
- •Chamber dilation &/or hypertrophy→
  - ∘**Dysrhythmia**→
    - −Cardiac arrest
    - −Heart failure
    - −Palpitations
    - −Pre−syncope/ syncope
- •Altered vascular flow &/or cardiomyopathy→
  - ∘**Thromboembolic syndrome**
- •Severe stenotic flow, in the setting of a fixed cardiac output→
  - ∘Vascular steal syndrome via:
    - −Exertion
    - −Heat
    - −Upright positioning
    - −Vasodilating medication
    - ...→↓cerebral perfusion pressure→
      - •**Pre−syncope/ syncope**
- •Atrial enlargement→
  - ∘Recurrent laryngeal nerve compression→
    - −**Hoarseness, termed Ortner's syndrome**
- •Mitral or pulmonic stenosis→
  - ∘**Malar flush**, due to dilated facial capillaries w/ sluggish flow→
    - −Facial redness→eventual bluish color=cyanosis, which blanches to palpation

ELECTRICAL STUDIES
- •**Electrocardiogram−ECG**
  - Findings:
    - •Nonspecific ST segment &/or T wave changes
    - •Criteria for left ventricular hypertrophy−LVH
      - ∘Lead V1−V6 progressively ↑R waves
      - ∘Tall V5 & V6 R waves & deep V1 & V2 S waves
      - ∘Lead aVL R wave >11mm
      - ∘Lead aVL R wave + lead V3 S wave being ♂>28mm or ♀>20mm
      - ∘Lead V1 S wave + lead V5 R wave being >35mm
    - •Criteria for right ventricular hypertrophy−RVH
      - ∘Lead V1−V6 progressively ↓R waves
      - ∘Lead V1 R wave > S wave
      - ∘Lead V6 S wave > R wave
      - ∘Lead V1 R wave >6mm
      - ∘Lead V5 & V6 S waves
    - •Atrial dilation, occurring in all forms of chronic heart failure
      - ∘Criteria for left atrial dilation:
        - −Negative terminal P wave deflection in lead V1, being > 1X1mm
        - −Notched P wave in lead II, being >3mm in length
      - ∘Criteria for right atrial dilation:
        - −↑P wave in lead II, being ≥2.5mm in height
        - −Biphasic P wave in lead V1, w/ a larger initial portion being ≥2mm in height

160

•**Transthoracic echocardiography–TTE**
Procedure:
•A 2 dimensional ultrasonographic image, allowing real time visualization of:
  ◦Ventricular wall thickness
  ◦Cavity size (both atrial & ventricular)
  ◦Myocardial & valve function, allowing ejection fraction–EF estimation (% of end diastolic volume ejected during ventricular systole)
  ◦The pericardial space
•Doppler ultrasonography uses Doppler shift to detect vessel flow velocity→
  ◦Valve regurgitation visualization
  ◦Estimation of valve pressure gradients
Limitations:
•↓Visualization in obese or emphysematous patients
•May not allow adequate:
  ◦Visualization of the anterior aspect of a prosthetic aortic valve
  ◦Functional assessment of a prosthetic aortic valve
•Transesophageal echocardiography–TEE is more sensitive in detecting:
  ◦Thrombotic ± infectious vegetations
  ◦Abscesses
  ◦Valve damage
  …esp. in a patient w/ a prosthetic heart valve. However, transthoracic echocardiography is the initial test of choice due to its noninvasive nature, as transesophageal echocardiography may→
  •Pharyngeal swallow receptor mediated reflex:
    ◦Bradycardia
    ◦Hypotension

VALVULAR STENOSIS SEVERITY			
Severity	**Aortic valve area (cm^2)→Mean pressure gradient**		**Left ventricular EF**
Normal	3–4	0mmHg	Normal (50–70%)
Mild	1.6–2.5	<20mmHg	"
Moderate	1–1.5	20–40mmHg	"
Severe	<1.0	>40mmHg	"
Severe decompensated	<1.0	Variable	↓

Severity	**Mitral valve area (cm^2)→Mean pressure gradient**	
Normal	4–6	0mmHg
Mild	1.6–2.5	1–6mmHg
Moderate	1–1.5	7–12mmHg
Severe	<1.0	>12mmHg

•**Valve commissurotomy**
Indications:
•**Fibrotic, mobile, as yet noncalcified, stenosed valves**
Procedure:
•Mechanical splitting of the fused valve leaflet commissures via:
  ◦**Open commissurotomy**, performed under direct vision, via thoracotomy, w/ the patient on cardiopulmonary bypass
  ◦**Closed commissurotomy**. performed under direct vision, via thoracotomy, by introducing a dilator through the left ventricular apex, being guided by a finger in the left atrial appendage= auricle
  ◦**Valvuloplasty**, being a nonsurgical procedure performed by guiding a percutaneously inserted inflatable balloon to the diseased valve, w/ subsequent dilation

•**Valve replacement**
Indications:
•**Symptomatic disease**
•**Asymptomatic aortic valve disease**, w/ either:
  ◦↓Left ventricular ejection fraction (normal 50–70%)
  ◦Mean stenotic transvalvular pressure gradient >30mmHg
Prosthetic valve characteristics:
•**Mechanical valves†**
  ◦Composed of metal or carbon alloys, having crisp, high pitched opening & closing clicks
  ◦Lifespan of 20–30years

- **Bioprosthetic valves**
  - ○Being human cadaveric, porcine aortic, or fabricated of bovine pericardium
  - ○Lifespan of 10–15years
  - Indications:
    - •Persons participating in activities placing them at risk for injury
    - •♀planning future pregnancy
    - •Persons w/ a contraindication to anticoagulation:
      - ○Active hemorrhage
      - ○Severe bleeding diathesis
      - ○Severe thrombocytopenia (platelet count ≤20,000/ μL)
      - ○Recent significant trauma
      - ○Injury risk (including falls & sports) or compliance risk via:
        - –Alcoholism
        - –Altered mental status
        - –Illicit drug abuse
        - –Orthostatic hypotension
        - –Poor compliance
        - –Seizure disease
        - –Syncope
        - –Unstable gait

---

†**Magnetic resonance imaging–MRI** can be safely performed in patients w/ mechanical prosthetic heart valves other than the:
- •Pre6000 Starr–Edwards caged–ball prosthesis, which was available from 1960–1964

PROSTHETIC VALVE COMPLICATIONS
•All prosthetic valve recipients should undergo transthoracic echocardiography–TTE prior to hospital discharge, in order to obtain baseline imaging with which to compare to future echocardiographic imaging performed if prosthetic valvular dysfunction is suspected

Indicators of prosthetic malfunction:
- •Altered timing or quality of heart sounds
- •New regurgitant murmur
- •Heart failure
- •Myocardial ischemic syndrome
- •↑Intravascular hemolysis
- •Syncope
- •Thromboembolic event despite adequate anticoagulation

- **Thromboembolic syndrome**
  - ○The majority of thromboemboli manifest as **cerebrovascular accident syndromes**
  - ↑Risk factors:
    - •Inadequate anticoagulation
    - •Mitral valve prosthesis
    - •Pregnancy
  - Mechanical prosthetic valve cerebrovascular accident risk:
    - •No prophylaxis: 4%/ year
    - •Antiplatelet treatment: 2%/ year
    - •Adequate anticoagulation: 1%/ year
  - Note: Anticoagulation treatment should be discontinued in patients w/ cerebral thromboembolization, w/ reinstitution @ 72hours if there is no evidence of intracerebral hemorrhage

- **Prosthetic valve endocarditis–5%**, having a similar risk for both bioprosthetic & adequately anticoagulated mechanical valves
  - ○**Early:** <2months after surgery, indicating acquisition @ implantation
    - Outcomes:
      - •Mortality: 40–80%
  - ○**Late:** >2months after surgery, indicating hematogenous acquisition
    - Outcomes:
      - •Mortality: 20–40%
  - …w/ prophylaxis being required for all procedures involving mucous membranes

- **Paravalvular leakage**→
  - ○Regurgitation

•**Valvular dehiscence**
  Bioprosthetic valve specific:
  •**Eventual valve thickening & calcification**→
    ∘Leaflet stenosis
    ∘Leaflet retraction→
    –Regurgitation
  Mechanical prosthetic valve specific:
  •**Faulty valve struts or disc**, esp. w/ single tilting disk valves
  •**Intravascular hemolysis**
    ∘Occurs w/ all mechanical valves, usually being mild & readily compensated by ↑erythrocyte
     production. However, chronic intravascular hemolysis→
      –Urinary iron loss which may→iron deficiency anemia
    ∘Severe hemolysis usually indicates prosthesis dysfunction
  •**Tissue ingrowth into the prosthetic orifice**

THROMBOEMBOLIC PROPHYLAXIS

Indications:
  •All mechanical valves† (listed below in order of ↓thrombogenicity) to an INR of:
    ∘**Caged Ball valve:** 4–5
      –Starr–Edwards
    ∘**Single tilting disk valve:** 3–4
      –Bjork–Shiley
      –Medtronic–Hall
      –Omnicarbon
    ∘**Bileaflet tilting disk valve:** 2.5–2.9
      –Edwards–Duromedics
      –St. Jude Medical
    …w/ those @ high risk‡ achieving 3–4.5 w/ Aspirin 80–160mg q24hours
  •Certain bioprosthetic valves to an INR of:
    ∘Porcine or bovine valves, termed **heterografts:** 2–3 X 3months ± subsequent Aspirin 325mg q24h
      –Carpentier–Edwards
      –Hancock
      –Ionescu–Shiley
    ∘Human valves, termed **homografts:** No anticoagulation necessary
    …w/ those @ high risk‡ achieving 2–3 indefinitely

---

†Adequate anticoagulation of mechanical valves nullifies their thrombogenic differences & allows for
equivalence to bioprosthetic valves
‡High risk factors:
  •Atrial fibrillation
  •History of a thromboembolic event
  •↓↓Left ventricular ejection fraction
  •Dilated atrium
  •Mural thrombus
  •>1 prosthetic valves

ANTICOAGULANTS: High molecular weight Heparin

M ♀	Start
M ?	60units/ kg IV bolus (or 5000units empirically)
	12units/kg/hour infusion (or 1000units/ hour empirically)

•Titrated by 2.5units/kg/hour to achieve an activated partial thromboplastin time–aPTT of 1.5–2X
control value or **50–70seconds**

aPTT (seconds)	Action	Obtain next aPTT
<40	Bolus 5000units & ↑infusion rate by 100units/ hour	6hours
40–49	↑Infusion rate by 50units/ hour	6hours
50–70 (or 1.5–2Xcontrol)	NO ACTION	24hours
71–85	↓Infusion rate by 50units/ hour	6hours
86–100	Hold infusion 30min., then ↓infusion rate by 100units/ hour	6hours
101–150	Hold infusion 60min., then ↓infusion rate by 150units/ hour	6hours
>150	Hold infusion 60min., then ↓infusion rate by 300units/ hour	6hours

Monitoring:
  •Complete blood count q24hours to monitor for side effects

ANTICOAGULANTS: Low molecular weight Heparin				
Generic (Trade)	M	♀	Start	Max
Enoxaparin (Lovenox)	KL	P	1.5mg/ kg SC q24hours or 1mg/ kg SC q12hours	180mg/ 24hours
Dalteparin (Fragmin)	KL	P	200 anti-factor Xa units/ kg SC q24hours or 100 anti-factor Xa units/ kg SC q12hours	18,000units q24hours

Dose adjustment:
- •Obesity
  - ◦Most manufacturers recommend a maximum dose of that for a 90kg patient

Monitoring:
- •Monitoring of anti-Xa levels is recommended in patients w/:
  - ◦Abnormal coagulation/ hemorrhage
  - ◦Obesity
  - ◦Renal failure
  - ◦Underweight
- •Check 4h after 2nd SC dose. Further monitoring is not necessary once the correct dose is established in obese patients

Administration frequency	Therapeutic anti-Xa levels
Q12hours	0.6-1 units/ mL
Q24hours	1-2 units/ mL

Mechanism:
- •Heparin combines w/ plasma antithrombin 3→
  - ◦↑Antithrombin 3 activity in removing thrombin & activated factors 9, 10, 11,& 12→
    - -↓Coagulation→↓vascular & mural thrombus formation &/or propagation
- •Heparin is metabolized by the plasma enzyme heparinase

Outcomes:
- •↓Morbidity & mortality

Side effects:
Cardiovascular
- •**Hemorrhage**
- •**Heparin induced thrombocytopenia-HIT 10%**, esp. w/ high molecular weight Heparin

  Mechanism:
  - •Heparin mediated platelet agglutination→
    - ◦Monocyte/ macrophage mediated extravascular removal via the splenic trabecular network=red pulp, & hepatic sinusoids→
      - -**Thrombocytopenia**

  Outcomes:
  - •Benign, as it resolves spontaneously, even w/ continued exposure
- •**Heparin induced thrombocytopenia ± thrombosis-HITT ≤3%**, esp. w/ high molecular weight Heparin

  Mechanism:
  - •Heparin mediated platelet agglutination→
    - ◦Monocyte/ macrophage mediated extravascular removal via the splenic trabecular network=red pulp, & hepatic sinusoids→
      - -**Thrombocytopenia**
    - ◦Platelet release of Heparin neutralizing factor=platelet factor 4-PF4, which complexes w/ Heparin→
      - -Production of anti-complex antibodies→↑platelet activation↔↑platelet factor 4 release→ a vicious cycle of **platelet mediated arterial &/or venous thrombus formation, termed the "white clot syndrome,"** being as the clot is relatively devoid of erythrocytes

  Outcomes:
  - •Must discontinue treatment as **20% develop thromboembolic complications**. Being that both Heparins may cross-react w/ the etiologic antibodies, their further use is contraindicated. Consider continued treatment w/ direct thrombin inhibitors
    - ◦Antibody cross-reactivity:
      - -Low molecular weight Heparins-85%
      - -Heparinoids-5%

Mucocutaneous
- •Skin necrosis-rarely occurring w/ high molecular weight Heparins, & not being associated w/ anticoagulant deficiency

Musculoskeletal
- •Osteoporosis, esp. w/ high molecular weight Heparin
  - ◦Usually @ use ≥1month

Hematologic
- ↓Aldosterone production→
  - ∘Hyperkalemia-8%

CHARACTERISTICS OF HEPARIN INDUCED THROMBOCYTOPENIC SYNDROMES

	HIT	HITT
Onset	<2days	4-10 days
Re-exposure	<2days	Earlier if re-exposed within 3 months
Platelet count	↓, being <150,000 or ≥50%	
Platelet median nadir	~90,000	~60,000

- ^{14}C-Serotonin release assay
  Indications:
  - Suspected HITT
  Procedure:
  - Normal donor platelets are radiolabeled w/ ^{14}C-serotonin. They are then washed & combined w/ patient serum & therapeutic Heparin concentrations (0.1 U/ mL). Induction of ^{14}C-serotonin release from platelets constitutes a positive test
  Limitations:
  - Expense, due to the use of radioactive material
  Outcomes:
  - Considered the gold standard in the detection of HITT
- **Enzyme linked immunosorbent assay-ELISA**
  Indications:
  - Suspected HITT
  Procedure:
  - Heparin-PF4 complexes affixed to a plastic plate are incubated w/ the patient's serum. If the patient has produced antibodies, then the addition of enzymatically (horseradish peroxidase) labeled anti-human IgG allows for color visualization via spectrophotometer
  Limitations:
  - Many antibody positive patients do not develop clinical HITT
  - 30% false positive

Contraindications:
- Active hemorrhage
- Severe bleeding diathesis
- Severe thrombocytopenia (platelet count ≤20,000/ μL)
- Recent significant trauma
- Neurosurgery, ocular surgery, or intracranial hemorrhage within 10days

ANTIDOTE

Generic	M	♀	Amount IV over 10min.	Max
Protamine	P	?	1mg/ 100units of HMWH	50mg
			1mg/ 100units Dalteparin	"
			1mg/ 1mg Enoxaparin	"

Mechanism:
- Protamine combines electrostatically w/ Heparin→
  - ∘Inability to bind to antithrombin 3

FOLLOWED BY

ANTICOAGULANTS

Generic	M	♀	Start
Warfarin (Coumadin)	L	U	5mg PO q24hours

- Because the anticoagulant proteins↓ relatively faster than the procoagulant proteins, an initial transient hypercoagulable state develops. Due to this, warfarin is started once the patient is therapeutic on Heparin, via either:
  - ∘Goal aPTT w/ high molecular weight Heparin
  - ∘Evening of initiation of low molecular weight Heparin
  ...requiring ~7days (corresponding to 2 half lives of factor 2, or a 75% reduction) to reach a true therapeutic level of an **international normalized ratio-INR of 2-3**

INR	Action	Obtain next INR
<1.5	↑Weekly dose by 15%	1 week
1.5-1.9	↑Weekly dose by 10%	2 weeks
2-3	NO ACTION	1 month if stable
3.1-3.9	↓Weekly dose by 10%	2 weeks
4-5	Skip 1 day, then ↓weekly dose by 15%	1 week
>5	DISCONTINUE WARFARIN	Q day until ≤3, then ↓weekly dose by 50%

Mechanism:
•Competitively inhibits hepatocyte enzymatic vitamin K reactive sites→
∘↓Formation of both:
−Procoagulant proteins 2, 7, 9, & 10
−Anticoagulant proteins C & S
…w/ the anticoagulant effect requiring several days, as it must await the metabolism of the pre−existing plasma procoagulant proteins, w/ normal coagulation returning within several days of discontinuation

Side effects:
Cardiovascular
•**Hemorrhage**
∘Fatal: 0.6%/ year
∘Major: 3%/ year
∘Minor: 7%/ year
Cutaneous
•Tissue necrosis w/ protein C or S deficiency or dysfunction

Contraindications:
•Active hemorrhage
•Severe bleeding diathesis
•Severe thrombocytopenia (platelet count ≤20,000/ μL)
•Recent significant trauma
•Neurosurgery, ocular surgery, or intracranial hemorrhage within 10days
•Injury risk (including falls & sports) or compliance risk via:
∘Alcoholism
∘Altered mental status
∘Illicit drug abuse
∘Orthostatic hypotension
∘Poor compliance
∘Seizure disease
∘Syncope
∘Unstable gait

Special considerations:
•**If undergoing elective surgery during treatment**
∘Stop warfarin 5 days prior to surgery, & begin Heparin
•**Anticoagulation during pregnancy**
∘Substitute low molecular weight Heparin for warfarin, followed by warfarin treatment postpartum if necessary

ANTIDOTES
•**Gastric lavage & activated charcoal** if recently administered; forced emesis at home

VITAMIN K=Phytonadione
Indications:
•To correct the international normalized ration−INR or prothrombin time−PT
Dose
10mg SC/ IV slow push @ 1mg/ min. in order to ↓anaphylactoid reaction risk
Mechanism:
•Requires several hours to days for effect
Side effects:
•Avoid intramuscular administration which may→
∘Intramuscular hemorrhage

FRESH FROZEN PLASMA−FFP
Indications:
•To correct the international normalized ration−INR or prothrombin time−PT under the following conditions:
∘**INR >20**
∘**Severe hemorrhage**
∘**Other need for rapid reversal, such as an emergent procedure**
Dose†
15mL/ kg IV (w/ ~200mL FFP/ unit) q4hours prn ↑INR
Mechanism:
•Contains clotting factors 2, 7, 9−13, & heat labile 5 & 7→
∘Immediate onset of action
•Each unit→
∘8% ↑coagulation factors
∘4% ↑blood volume

166

AORTIC DISSECTION

•A transverse aortic intimal tear→
  ∘Pulsatile blood dissection into the media→
    −Longitudinal propagation (distal > proximal) ± a luminal re−entry tear
•**A medical emergency**

RISK FACTORS

•**Hypertension−75%**
•↑**Age:** >50years
•**Gender:** ♂ 2X ♀
•**Aortic disease**
  ∘Aortic aneurysm, esp. >6cm diameter
  ∘Aortic stenosis
  ∘Bicuspid aortic valve
  ∘Coarctation of the aorta, being associated w/ Turner's syndrome
•**Connective tissue disease**
  ∘Cystic medial fibrosis
  ∘Ehler's−Danlos syndrome
  ∘Marfan's syndrome
•**Pregnancy, comprising 50% of all ♀dissections @ age <40years**
  ∘↑Aortic & coronary artery dissection risk, esp. @:
    −3rd trimester
    −Labor
    −Postpartum
•**Iatrogenic**
  ∘Aortic cannulation for cardiopulmonary bypass
  ∘Intra−aortic balloon pump
•**Infectious**
  ∘Cardiovascular syphilis
•**Blunt trauma**

CLASSIFICATION

Stanford anatomic classification:
•**Type A dissection−55%:** Involving the ascending aorta
  ∘Intimal tear usually occurring several cm above the aortic valve, esp. on the right lateral wall of the ascending aorta, which is the point of maximal shear stress
•**Type B dissection−45%:** Not involving the ascending aorta
  ∘Intimal tear occurring:
    −Just distal to the left subclavian artery−30%
    −Aortic arch−12%
    −Abdominal aorta−3%

Duration based classification:
•**Acute aortic dissection:** <2weeks
•**Chronic aortic dissection:** >2weeks

DIAGNOSIS

Cardiovascular
•**Hypertension−75%**, esp. w/ Stanford type B dissections
•Aortic medial dissection→
  ∘**Sudden severe, ripping, tearing, or stabbing pain**, usually lacking the pressure or squeezing quality of a myocardial ischemic syndrome
    −Ascending aorta involvement→anterior thoracic pain−90%
    −Descending aorta involvement→posterior thoracic pain−96%
    ...w/ propagation (distal > proximal)→
      •Adjacent organ compression
      •**Vascular ostium occlusion**→vascular bruit &/or ischemia ± infarction
Hematologic
•↑Smooth muscle myosin heavy−chain protein
  Outcomes:
    •Sensitivity−90%, specificity−98%

Rupture/ fistula syndromes:
- •Aorto-pericardial rupture, being the **#1 cause of death**→
  - ◦Pericardial hemorrhage→
    - **-Pericardial tamponade**→cardiogenic shock
- •Aorto-pleural rupture, being the **#2 cause of death**→
  - ◦Pleural hemorrhage=hemothorax→
    - **-Tension hemothorax**→cardiogenic shock
- •Aorto-esophageal fistula→
  - ◦Gastrointestinal hemorrhage→
    - -Vomiting blood=**hematemesis**
- •Aorto-tracheal fistula (Type A only)→
  - ◦Pulmonary hemorrhage→
    - -Coughing blood=hemoptysis

Vascular obstructive syndromes:
- •Coronary artery ostial occlusion (Type A only)→
  - ◦**Myocardial ischemia ± infarction**
- •Right carotid artery ostial occlusion (Type A only)→
  - ◦Weak & delayed carotid arterial pulse, termed pulsus parvus et tardus
  - ◦**Cerebrovascular accident-35%**
- •Aortic luminal occlusion→
  - ◦↑Proximal perfusion pressure→**upper extremity hypertension**
    - **-Type B-55%**, affecting the right ± left upper extremity
    - -Type A-10%, affecting the right upper extremity
  - ◦↓Distal perfusion pressure→**distal hypotension**→
    - -↓Palpable pulse
    - -Vascular bruit
    - -Weak & delayed arterial pulse, termed pulsus parvus et tardus
    - -Limb ischemia→cool skin w/ perspiration, being either pale or bluish color=cyanosis
- •Celiac trunk, superior &/or inferior mesenteric artery occlusion→
  - ◦Gastrointestinal ischemia ± infarction
- •Posterior intercostal &/or lumbar sacral artery ostial occlusion→
  - ◦Spinal neuron ischemia ± infarction→
    - **-Neurologic deficits**
- •Renal artery ostial occlusion→
  - ◦↓Renal perfusion pressure→
    - -Pre-renal renal failure (if bilateral or having only 1 functional kidney) ± renal ischemia→acute tubular necrosis

Organ compressive syndromes:
- •Esophageal compression→
  - ◦Difficulty swallowing=**dysphagia**
- •Left recurrent laryngeal nerve compression (Type A only)→
  - ◦Hoarseness
- •**Superior vena cava compression** (Type A only)→
  - ◦↑Proximal hydrostatic pressure→
    - -Dilation of bilateral arm, neck, & head vasculature→facial erythema, edema, &/or bluish color=cyanosis
    - -↑Collateral blood flow→dilated abdominal collateral vessels w/ downward flow
  - Note: Considered a medical emergency if the patient develops altered mental status
- •**Horner's syndrome:** Cervical sympathetic ganglion compression (Type A only)→↓ipsilateral facial autonomic sympathetic tone→
  - ◦↓Iris radial smooth muscle contraction→
    - -Pupil constriction=**myosis**
  - ◦↓Levator palpebrae smooth muscle contraction→
    - -Drooping eyelid=**ptosis**
  - ◦↓Sweat gland activation→
    - -↓Facial sweat=**anhidrosis**→facial dryness
  - ◦↓Ciliary epithelium aqueous humor formation→
    - -Retracted eyeball

Other:
•Ascending aortic dissection→
 ∘Aortic valve cusp malalignment→
  −**Aortic regurgitation−70%**→heart failure
•Aortic wall inflammation→
 ∘Left pleural exudative effusion

INVASIVE PROCEDURES

•**Transesophageal echocardiography−TEE**
 Indications:
 •**Diagnostic test of choice if high clinical suspicion**
 Procedure:
 •A 2 dimensional ultrasonographic image, allowing real time visualization of:
  ∘A possible **aortic intimal flap** separating the true lumen (which expands during systole) from the false lumen
  ∘The thoracic aorta (ascending, arch, & descending segments)
  ∘The proximal coronary arteries & ostia
  ∘Myocardial & valve function, allowing ejection fraction−EF estimation (% of end diastolic volume ejected during ventricular systole)
  ∘The pericardial space
  •Doppler ultrasonography uses Doppler shift to detect vessel flow velocity→
  ∘Valve regurgitation visualization
  ∘Estimation of valve pressure gradients
 Outcomes:
 •**Sensitivity−99.5%, specificity−98%**
 Limitations:
 •Invasive, requiring esophageal intubation
 Complications:
 •Pharyngeal swallow receptor mediated reflex:
  ∘Bradycardia
  ∘Hypotension

IMAGING

•**Chest x ray**
 Findings:
 •**Widened mediastinal shadow−85%**
 •Aorto−pericardial rupture→
  ∘Pericardial hemorrhage→
   −Cardiomegally
 •Aorto−pleural rupture→
  ∘Pleural hemorrhage=hemothorax
 •Heart failure→
  ∘Interstitial ± pulmonary edema

•**Thoracic computed tomographic−CT scan**
 Indications:
 •**Diagnostic test of choice if either:**
  ∘**Low clinical suspicion in a stable patient**
  ∘Transesophageal echocardiography−TEE is not readily available
 •**Serial follow−up of stable patients**
 Advantages:
 •Noninvasive
 Limitations:
 •The scanner is usually distant from the intensive care unit & operating rooms
 •**Cannot assess branch vessels**
 •**Cannot quantify regurgitation**
 Outcomes:
 •Sensitivity: 90%, specificity: 85−100%

•**Thoracic magnetic resonance imaging−MRI scan**
 Indications:
 •**Serial follow−up of stable patients**
 Advantages:
 •Noninvasive
 Limitations:
 •The scanner is usually distant from the intensive care unit & operating rooms
 •Time consuming

169

Outcomes:
- Sensitivity~99%, specificity~100%

•**Retrograde aortography**
Limitations:
- Invasive, time consuming procedure
- Requires a radiocontrast agent
- Cannot detect a pericardial effusion
- The patient must remain supine w/ leg extension X 6hours following the procedure, in order to allow adequate healing of the common femoral artery catheter entry site
Outcomes:
- Sensitivity~90%, specificity~95%

TREATMENT OF ACUTE AORTIC DISSECTION

•This is a **medical emergency** for which the patient must be admitted to the hospital where intravenous medications can be administered in order to initially:
- ↓**Systolic blood pressure to 100–120 & pulse to 50–60/ min.**, first by the administration of an atrioventricular node blocking medication, followed by a vasodilator, w/ this sequence meant to prevent vasodilator mediated reflex tachycardia

•Blood pressure should be monitored in real time via an arterial line

•**Type & cross match blood** for 10units of packed red blood cells for possible surgery &/or rupture

OPIOID RECEPTOR AGONISTS			
Generic	M	♀	Start
Morphine sulfate	LK	?	2–4mg IV slow push (1mg/ min.) q5min. prn

Mechanism:
- Vasodilation (**venous** >> arterial)→
  - ↓Preload→↓myocardial contractile strength
    - –↓Blood pressure
    - –↓Myocardial O_2 & nutrient demand
    - –↓Pulmonary congestion if present
- ↓Pain ± dyspnea→
  - ↓Autonomic sympathetic tone→
    - –↓Myocardial O_2 & nutrient demand

ATRIOVENTRICULAR NODE BLOCKING MEDICATIONS ▬▬▬

β1 SELECTIVE RECEPTOR BLOCKERS			
Generic (Trade)	M	♀	Start
Esmolol (Brevibloc)	K	?	0.5mg=500µg/ kg IV loading bolus (over 1 min.), then 0.05mg=50µg/kg/min. continuous IV infusion w/ titration prn† Max: 0.3mg=300µg/kg/min.

Onset: 1–2 min., Duration: 10 min.

†Titrate q4 min. via re–administration of the loading bolus & an additional 50µg/kg/min. IV infusion

α1 & NONSELECTIVE β RECEPTOR BLOCKERS: May be used as **monotherapy** due to their concomitant cardiac & vascular effects

Generic (Trade)	M	♀	Start	Max
Labetalol (Normodyne)	LK	?	20mg IV push over 2min., then 40mg IV push q10min. prn goal blood pressure, then 0.5–2mg/ min. IV infusion	300mg total

Onset: 5–10min., Duration: 3–6hours

Mechanism:
- Competitive antagonist of the β1 ± β2 receptor→
  - ↓Sinoatrial & atrioventricular node conduction (β1)→
    - –↓Pulse
  - Anti–dysrhythmic via nodal effects (β1)
  - ↓Cardiac muscle contractile strength (β1)
  - ↓Juxtaglomerular cell renin release (β1)→
    - –↓Angiotensin 1, angiotensin 2, & aldosterone formation
  - ↓Cardiovascular remodeling

170

∘↑Vascular/ organ smooth muscle contraction (β2)→
  −Vasoconstriction
  −Bronchoconstriction
  −Uterine contraction
∘↓Tremor (β2)
∘↓Hepatocyte glycogenolysis (β2)
•↓Extrathyroidal tetraiodothyronine−T4 (also termed thyroxine) conversion to the more metabolically active triiodothyronine−T3 form

Side effects:
General
- Fatigue
- Malaise

Cardiovascular
- Bradycardia ± heart block
- Hypotension
  - ∘Orthostatic hypotension
  - ∘Pelvic hypotension→
    - −Impotence, being the inability to achieve &/or maintain an erection
- Initial worsening of systolic heart failure
- Worsening symptoms of peripheral vascular disease
  - ∘Intermittent claudication
  - ∘Raynaud's phenomenon

Pulmonary
- Bronchoconstriction

Endocrine
- ↑Risk of developing diabetes mellitus
- May block catecholamine mediated:
  - ∘Physiologic reversal of hypoglycemia via:
    - −↓Hepatocyte gluconeogenesis
  - ∘↓Hypoglycemic symptoms, termed hypoglycemic unawareness→
    - −↓Tachycardia as a warning sign

Gastrointestinal
- Diarrhea
- Nausea ± vomiting
- Gastroesophageal reflux

Mucocutaneous
- Hair thinning

Neurologic
- Sedation
- Sleep alterations
- ↓Libido→
  - ∘Impotence

Psychiatric
- Depression

Hematologic
- ↓High density lipoprotein−HDL levels

•Most patients w/ chronic obstructive pulmonary disease−COPD (including asthma), diabetes, &/or peripheral vascular disease can be safely treated w/ **cardioselective β1 receptor blockers,** as they have ↓peripheral effects

Contraindications:
Cardiovascular
- **Acutely decompensated heart failure**
- Hypotension
- Pulse <50bpm
- Atrioventricular heart block of any degree

Pulmonary
- Moderate to severe chronic obstructive pulmonary disease−COPD, including asthma

Hyper−catacholamine state
- Amphetamine use
- **Cocaine use†**
- Clonidine withdrawal
- Monoamine oxidase inhibitor−MAOi mediated tyramine effect
- Pheochromocytoma

171

...→relatively ↑vascular α1 receptor stimulation="unopposed α effect"→
- •Vasoconstriction→
  - ◦Myocardial ischemic syndrome
  - ◦Cerebrovascular accident syndrome
  - ◦Peripheral vascular ischemic syndrome
<u>Note:</u> **Carvedilol** & **Labetalol** may be used due to their α1 blocking property

---

†Cocaine use→
- •Varying ischemic syndrome onset per administration route, & may occur @ min. to days (usually within 3hours)

ANTIDOTES

Generic	M ♀	Dose	Max
Glucagon	LK P	3mg IV slow push over 1min., then 5mg IV slow push over 1 min. if needed	
•Continuous infusion		5mg/ hour	
10% Calcium chloride†		10mL (1 ampule) IV slow push over 3min., q5min. prn	
•Continuous infusion		0.3mEq/ hour	0.7mEq/ h
<u>Onset:</u> 1–2 min., <u>Duration:</u> 30–60 min.			

---

†Use cautiously in patients taking Digoxin, as hypercalcemia→
- •Digoxin cardiotoxicity

CALCIUM CHANNEL BLOCKERS: Non-dihydropyridines

Generic	M ♀	Start	Max
Diltiazem	L ?	5mg/ hour infusion	15mg/ hour

<u>Mechanism:</u>
- •Block voltage dependent calcium ion channels in smooth & cardiac muscle→
  - ◦↓Calcium influx→
    - −↓Sinoatrial & atrioventricular node conduction (non–dihydropyridines)→↓pulse
    - −Anti–dysrhythmic via nodal effects (mainly non–dihydropyridines)
    - −↓Cardiac muscle contractile strength (mainly non–dihydropyridines)
    - −Vasodilation: Arterial > venous (mainly dihydropyridines)

<u>Side effects:</u>
Cardiovascular
- •Bradycardia ± heart block
- •Edema
- •Flushing
- •Hypotension

Gastrointestinal
- •Constipation
- •Nausea ± vomiting

Neurologic
- •Dizziness
- •Headache

ANTIDOTES

Generic	M ♀	Dose	Max
Glucagon	LK P	3mg IV slow push over 1min., then 5mg IV slow push over 1 min. if needed	
•Continuous infusion		5mg/ hour	
10% Calcium chloride†		10mL (1 ampule) IV slow push over 3min., then repeat @5min. if needed	
•Continuous infusion		Start 0.3mEq/ hour	0.7mEq/ hour
<u>Onset:</u> 1–2 min., <u>Duration:</u> 30–60 min.			
Magnesium sulfate	K S	2g MgSO$_4$ in 50mL saline infused over 15min., then 6g MgSO$_4$ in 500mL saline infused over 6hours	

---

†Use cautiously in patients taking Digoxin, as hypercalcemia→
- •Digoxin cardiotoxicity

CALCIUM CHANNEL BLOCKERS: Dihydropyridines			
Generic	M ♀	Start	Max
Nicardipine	L ?	5mg/ hour IV infusion	15mg/ hour

NITROVASODILATORS			
Generic	M ♀	Start	Max
Nitroglycerin	L ?	10µg/ min. IV infusion	100µg/ min.
Nitroprusside sodium (Nipride, Nitropress)	E ?	0.3µg/kg/min. IV infusion	8µg/kg/min.

Onset: 2–5min., w/ tolerance typically within 24–48hours, Duration: ≤5min. after discontinuation

---

•Nitroglycerin binds to soft plastics such as polyvinylchloride–PVC, which is a common constituent of plastic bags & infusion tubing→
  ∘≤80% absorptive loss, being avoided via the use of glass bottles & hard/ stiff plastics
•Protect the nitroprusside bottle from light

Mechanism:
•Vasodilation (venous >> arterial)→
  ∘↓Preload→
    −↓Blood pressure
    −↓Myocardial O_2 demand
    −↓Pulmonary congestion if present
•Platelet inhibiting activity

Side effects:
Cardiovascular
•Hypotension
•Systemic vasodilation→
  ∘Reflex tachycardia
  ∘Orthostatic hypotension
  ∘Facial flushing
•Meningeal arterial dilation→
  ∘Headache
Pulmonary
•Pulmonary vasodilation→
  ∘Exacerbation of ventilation/ perfusion mismatches
Hematologic
Nitroglycerin specific:
•Nitroglycerin metabolism→
  ∘Inorganic nitrites→oxidation of heme bound iron (Fe^{+2}) to the ferric form (Fe^{+3}), creating
  methemoglobin, which does not carry O_2 effectively→
    −Hypoxemia, being unreliably detected by pulse oximeters, requiring the use of co–oximeters
    −Brown colored blood due to the brown color of methemoglobin
    ...usually occurring only at ↑↑doses, w/ levels (fraction of total hemoglobin):
      •>3% being abnormal
      •>40% possibly causing hypoxemia→
        ∘Lactic acidemia
      •>70% being lethal
      ...requiring discontinuation of infusion in all cases. If hypoxemia exists, administer
      methylene blue (a reducing agent) @ 2mg/ kg IV over 10min.†→
      •Conversion of iron to the normal ferrous form (Fe^{+2})
•Being as nitroglycerin does not readily dissolve in aqueous solutions, nonpolar solvents such as ethanol & propylene glycol are required to keep the medication in solution, & can accumulate→
  ∘Ethanol intoxication
  ∘Propylene glycol toxicity→
    −Altered mental status
    −Anion gap metabolic acidemia
    −Dysrhythmias
    −Hemolysis
    −Hyperosmolarity
    −Acute tubular necrosis→renal failure
    ...→↑plasma levels & osmolar gap

Pharmacokinetics/ pharmacodynamics
•Tolerance to medication effects
Nitroprusside specific:
  •Nitroprusside metabolism releases 5 cyanide ions (CN) along w/ nitric oxide→
    ∘**Potential cyanide &/or thiocyanate toxicity**
      −Cyanide−CN + thiosulfate−S_2O_3 (a sulfur donor source)→thiocyanate−SCN‡ + sulfate−SO_3
  Cyanide toxicity
    •The body stores of thiosulfate are readily depleted→
      ∘↑Cyanide, which is why 500mg of thiosulfate must be added to each infusion solution
  Thiocyanate toxicity
    •Renal failure→
      −↑Thiocyanate toxicity risk→anorexia, hallucinations, nausea ± vomiting, &/or seizures

---

†Intravenous administration of methylene blue→
•Spuriously ↓SaO_2, up to 65%
‡Thiocyanate is renally cleared

Contraindications:
Cardiovascular
  •Hypotension
Neurologic
  •**Hypertensive encephalopathy**, as it ↑intracranial pressure
Interactions
  •**Sildenafil** (Viagra) **is contraindicated** in patients taking concomitant nitrates, as the combination within 24hours may→severe hypotension→
    ∘↓Myocardial perfusion→
      −Stable angina mediated acute coronary syndrome
    ∘↓Cerebral perfusion→
      −Pre−syncope/ syncope
      −Cerebrovascular accident syndrome

Monitoring:
•Thiocyanate levels frequently (should be <10mg/ dL)

SUBSEQUENT TREATMENT
•**Type A dissection**
  ∘**Prompt cardiothoracic surgical consultation**
  Procedure:
    •Excision & replacement of the dissection origin (not the entire dissected segment) within hours via a Dacron graft being inserted, w/ the coronary arteries &/or the brachiocephalic artery being either re−implanted or bypassed
    •An aortic valve prosthesis is placed for severe aortic regurgitation

•**Type B dissection**
  ∘**Continue hypertensive medical treatment indefinitely**

Indications for prompt cardiothoracic surgical consultation:
  •**Significant branch artery involvement**
  •**Refractory to medical therapy**
    ∘Refractory pain
    ∘Refractory hypertension
    ∘Continued dissection
    ∘Enlarging aortic silhouette via imaging
    ∘Aortic rupture

PROGNOSIS
ACUTE MORTALITY PRIOR TO HOSPITAL DISCHARGE

Dissection type	Medical treatment	Surgical treatment
Type A	1%/ hour X 48hours; 80%/ 1st week	25%
Type B	15%	25%

•**Surgical mortality in chronic dissection (Type A or B) is 15%**

174

<u>Morbidity & mortality after hospital discharge:</u>
- •30% of patients will experience either a new dissection, or a complication of their original dissection within 5years, w/ the highest risk during the first 2 years
- **•50% 10year survival w/ appropriate treatment (Type A or B)**

FOLLOW UP SURVEILANCE

•Being that progressive false lumen expansion usually occurs without symptoms, perform a **thoracic &/or abdominal magnetic resonance imaging scan q6months X 2years, then q1year indefinitely,** provided that the anatomy is stable

•Forms of **positive pressure assisted ventilation** meant as temporary support measures while treating the underlying cause of respiratory failure

•**Severe hypoxemic respiratory failure**
  ◦PaO_2 <55mmHg (normal >60mmHg) on 100% O_2 via a non–rebreathing mask
•**Severe hypercapnic respiratory failure**
  ◦$PaCO_2$ >55mmHg (normal 35–45mmHg)→
    –Respiratory acidemia
•**Respiratory distress** (respiratory rate >35/ min., accessory muscle use, or paradoxical abdominal motion) or **shock**
  ◦In order to ↓breathing work, which can account for 50% of total O_2 consumption
•**Airways protection**
  ◦Patients w/ a condition that predisposes to aspiration via ↓cough reflex:
    –Altered mental status
    –Dysphagia
    –Neurologic deficîts
•**Pulmonary toilet**
  ◦Prevention &/or reversal of atelectasis
•**Pulmonary procedure**
  ◦Allows for sedation or neuromuscular blockade
•↑**Intracranial pressure**
  ◦Hyperventilation→
    –↓Cerebral blood flow
•**Thoracic stabilization**
  ◦Massive flail chest†

---

†Flail chest occurs when >1 rib segment is separated from the thoracic cage, requiring ≥2 fractures/ rib→
  •Thoracic instability, as the involved segment is unable to contribute to lung expansion, w/ physical examination showing segmental paradoxical motion (inwards during inspiration & outwards during expiration) during spontaneous respirations→
    ◦↓Pulmonary ventilation
    ◦↑Work of breathing
    …which if severe, requires mechanical ventilation

Flow rate:
  •**Inspiratory to expiratory–I:E ratio**
    ◦1–2 to 1–4, accomplished by adjusting the inspiratory flow rate
  •**Inspiratory flow rate**
    ◦↑Flow rate→
      –↑Tidal volume delivery rate→↓inspiratory time→↑expiratory time, allowing for I:E ratio adjustment

Pressure:
  •**Peak inspiratory (airways) pressure–PIP**
    ◦**Measurement of airways pressure during inspiration**, being determined by both:
      –Airways resistance, 90% being due to the large airways
      –Thoracic compliance
  •**Plateau (alveolar) pressure–Pplat**
    ◦**Measurement of airways pressure at end–inspiration, prior to expiration, when there is no airflow**, being determined by thoracic compliance alone (↓thoracic compliance→↑Pplat) as airways resistance is not a factor due to lack of airflow

•Positive end-expiratory pressure–PEEP
Indications:
•↑Gas exchange to achieve an **SaO$_2$ ≥91%** of adequate hemoglobin (≥ 10g/ dL), in order to achieve the use of nontoxic O$_2$ concentrations **(FiO$_2$ <60%)**, while minimally ↓cardiac output
Mechanism:
•Normal exhalation→
  ∘Pressure equivalence of alveolar & atmospheric pressure→some amount of end-expiratory alveolar collapse, termed atelectasis, being ↑ w/ all pulmonary diseases→
    –↓Gas exchange
    –↓Thoracic compliance
  ...w/ positive end-expiratory pressure→
    •↓End expiratory alveolar collapse→
      ∘↑Gas exchange
      ∘↑Thoracic compliance
      ∘↓Phasic bronchoalveolar collapse mediated pneumonitis
      ...→↓required FiO$_2$
Subclassification:
•Extrinsic PEEP
  ∘Accomplished via a pressure-limiting valve in the exhalation port exerting a back pressure, allowing exhalation to occur until the back pressure is reached→
    –Valve closure
Settings:
  •Start @ 5cm H$_2$O (max 15cm H$_2$O)
Measurement:
  •Via end expiratory pressure prior to inhalation, when there is no airflow, which normally should be 0mmHg
  •Positive end-expiratory pressure→
    ∘Upwardly displaced pressure waveform, w/ ↑mean intrathoracic pressure
      –To adjust for this, subtract the PEEP value from the waveform value to obtain the actual peak inspiratory pressure & plateau pressure
•Intrinsic PEEP
  ∘Inadequate exhalation time afforded by the mechanical ventilator→premature ventilation→↑end expiratory pressure↔"breath stacking"→
    –↓Cardiac output→hypotension
    –↑Breathing effort, as the patient must overcome progressive ventilator mediated lung expansion to initiate a breath

NONINVASIVE OXYGENATION

•**Room air**, having an FiO$_2$† of 21%
•**Nasal cannula**, having an FiO$_2$ of 22–45%, via an oxygen flow rate of 1–6L/ min.
•**Face mask**, having an FiO$_2$ of 40–60%, via an oxygen flow rate of 5–10L/ min.
•**Mask–reservoir bag**
  ∘Partial rebreather, having an FiO$_2$ of 35–75%
  ∘Non-rebreather, having an FiO$_2$ of 40–100%
•**High flow**, allowing for more precise FiO$_2$ titration, up to 100%
•**Continuous positive airways pressure–CPAP**
Indications:
  •**Sole hypoxemic respiratory failure**, as it provides a positive end-expiratory pressure→
    ∘↑Gas exchange to achieve an **SaO$_2$ ≥91%** of adequate hemoglobin (≥ 10g/ dL), in order to achieve the use of nontoxic O$_2$ concentrations **(FiO$_2$ <60%)**, while minimally ↓cardiac output
Mechanism:
  •Provides a preset, continuous positive airways pressure in order to produce extrinsic PEEP
Settings:
  •Start w/:
    ∘A positive airways pressure of 5cm H$_2$O (max 15cm H$_2$O)
    ∘2L O$_2$/ min.
    ...then titrate the pressure by 2cm H$_2$O q20min., & O$_2$ prn, as tolerated, to reach goal parameters. Most patients cannot tolerate an expiratory positive airways pressure–EPAP >10cm H$_2$O

---

†Fraction of inspired air that is oxygen–FiO$_2$

•**Bilevel positive airways pressure–BiPAP**
Indications:
  •**Hypercapnic respiratory failure**
Mechanism:
  •A ventilator is connected to a tight fitting mask, providing variable preset positive airways inspiratory
   & expiratory pressures, in order to produce both extrinsic PEEP as well as provide pressure
   supported ventilation (inspiratory – expiratory pressure)
Outcomes:
  •↓Intubation need
  •↓Length of hospital stay
  •↓In–hospital mortality in patients w/ COPD exacerbations
Settings:
  •Start w/:
    ∘An inspiratory pressure of 10cm H_2O (max: 25cm H_2O)
    ∘An expiratory pressure of 5cm H_2O (max: 15cm H_2O)
    ∘2L O_2/ min.
    …then titrate either pressure by 2cm H_2O q20min., & O_2 prn, as tolerated, to reach goal
      parameters. Most patients cannot tolerate an expiratory positive airways pressure–EPAP >10cm
      H_2O
  •Administer BiPAP in 2–3hour blocks, w/ 30–60min. breaks in order to allow the patient to eat,
   speak, & rest. If the patient is unable to tolerate intermittent discontinuation of noninvasive
   ventilation, consider intubation
Goal Parameters:
  •IPAP to a goal volume of 5–10mL/ kg (as w/ invasive mechanical ventilation)
  •EPAP & O_2 to achieve an **SaO_2 ≥91%** of adequate hemoglobin (≥ 10g/ dL), in order to achieve the
   use of nontoxic O_2 concentrations **(FiO_2 <60%)**, while minimally ↓cardiac output
Indications for endotracheal intubation:
  •Worsening, or lack of improvement within 1 hour
Contraindications:
  •**Apnea**
  •**Hemodynamic instability**
    ∘Hypotension
  •**Inability to tolerate the mask**
  •**↓Ability to protect the airway**
    ∘Absent gag reflex
    ∘Altered mental status
    ∘Status epilepticus
    ∘Unconsciousness
    ∘Uncontrollable vomiting
  •↑**Need for suctioning**
    ∘Secretions >50mL/ hour
  •↓**Skin–mask air seal**
    ∘Abnormal facial anatomy
    ∘Beard (which should be shaved)

•**Volume targeted ventilation**
  ∘**Assist Control–AC ventilation**
    Mechanism:
    •Delivers a **preset lung inflation volume** at a **preset minimal rate**, the timing of which can be
     altered if the patient is able to initiate inhalation→
      ∘Opening of a one–way pressure activated valve via a preset amount, termed the trigger
       sensitivity→
        –Volume delivery, being termed assisted ventilation. Spontaneous respiratory efforts beyond
         the preset value will also→preset volume delivery
    •If the patient dose not initiate the minimal preset respiratory rate, the ventilator will automatically
     deliver them, being termed controlled ventilation
  ∘**Synchronized intermittent mandatory ventilation–SIMV**
    Mechanism:
    •As for assist control ventilation, without volume delivery during excess spontaneous respiratory
     efforts

178

•Pressure targeted ventilation
∘Pressure support ventilation–PSV
Mechanism:
- •Augmenting the patients respiratory efforts by providing a preset positive pressure upon spontaneous inhalatory efforts→
  - ∘Opening of a one–way pressure activated valve via a preset amount, termed the trigger sensitivity. Once the patient's inspiratory flow rate falls below a preset threshold level, gas flow terminates. It may be combined w/ SIMV to assist spontaneous inspiration, by at least overcoming the resistance of the ventilator tubing & endotracheal tube

Settings:
- •Start @5cm H_2O (max 20cm H_2O)

∘Pressure control ventilation–PCV
Mechanism:
- •As for assist control ventilation, using a **preset lung inflation pressure** rather than volume

VENTILATION SETTINGS				
Setting	Normal	Ventilator	↑O_2	↓CO_2
Inflation Volume	5–7mL/ kg	5–10mL/ kg† (max 15mL/ kg)		↑
Respiratory rate	12/ min.	12/ min. (max 20/ min.), ↓w/ COPD/ asthma‡		↑
		18–24/ min. for therapeutic hyperventilation°		
Pressure support		Start @ 5cm H_2O^ & titrate prn (max 20cm H_2O)		↑
FiO_2	20%	Start @ 100%, w/ taper to <60%	↑	
I:E ratio	1:2	1:2; 1:3–4 w/ COPD/ asthma‡	↑	
PEEP		Start @ 5cm H_2O & titrate prn (max 15cm H_2O)	↑	
		Use caution w/ COPD/ asthma‡		
Trigger sensitivity		Minimal (–2cm H_2O)		
Peak inspiratory pressure–PIP		<35cm H_2O		
Plateau pressure–Pplat		<35cm H_2O		
Arterial blood gas		Normal to usual $PaCO_2$, w/ a pH of 7.36–7.44, or		
		permissive hypercapnia[n] w/ a pH ≥7.2		

†Patients w/ acute respiratory distress syndrome–ARDS should be started at an initial tidal volume of 5–8mL/ kg, as lower tidal volumes→
- •↓Mortality

‡Due to the prolonged expiratory phase needed to adequately empty the lungs in patients w/ chronic obstructive pulmonary disease→
- •↑Gas trapping→
  - ∘↑Intrinsic–PEEP risk

Limitations:
- •↑Inspiratory flow rates→
  - ∘↑Peak inspiratory pressures, which may exceed ventilator safety limits

°To a goal $PaCO_2$ of 25mmHg→
- •↓Intracranial pressure

^5cm H_2O is needed to overcome the resistance of the endotracheal tube

[n]In order to achieve a safe peak inspiratory pressure &/or plateau pressure. Tidal volume may need to be decreased to <5mL/ kg, a ventilatory strategy of intentional hypoventilation termed **permissive hypercapnia**, allowing for:
- •$PaCO_2$ <80mmHg
- •pH >7.2, w/ some infusing bicarbonate to minimize acidemia

Contraindications:
- •Cerebrovascular disease
- •Hemodynamic instability
- •Pulmonary hypertension
- •Renal failure

APPROACH TO ACUTE VENTILATORY DETERIORATION			
PIP	Pplat	Pathology	Causes
↔			•Extrathoracic process •Pulmonary embolus
↓		↓Airways resistance	•Circuit leakage (tracheal tube or ventilator tubing) •Hyperventilation
↑	↔	↑Airways resistance	•Chronic obstructive pulmonary disease–COPD/ asthma •Secretions ± airways plugging •Ventilator tubing obstruction ∘Patient biting tube
↑	↑	↓Thoracic compliance	•Abdominal distention •Atelectasis •Asynchronous breathing •Intrinsic PEEP •Mainstem bronchus intubation •Pneumonia •Pneumothorax •Pulmonary edema

COMPLICATIONS

•**Alveolar rupture–15%** w/ invasive ventilation
  ∘↑Volume or pressure mediated ventilation or ↑positive end expiratory pressure–PEEP→
  ↑bronchoalveolar pressure→rupture→
    –Pneumothorax
    –Pneumomediastinum
    –Pneumoperitoneum, via passage through diaphragmatic rents
    –Subcutaneous emphysema, via gaseous dissection into the neck→skin distention→
    "puffy" appearance & palpation of air bubbles ± crackling sound=crepitus

•**Deep venous thrombosis ± pulmonary thromboembolism**
  ∘Due to immobilization→
    –Altered vascular flow

•**Laryngeal dysfunction**
  ∘Endotracheal tube mediated laryngeal inflammation→
    –Edema
    –Fibrosis
    –Granuloma formation
    –Ulceration
    …→vocal cord paralysis risk

•**Oxygen toxicity**
  ∘Occurring @ **an FiO$_2$ >60%**, being directly proportional to the degree & duration of treatment

•**Respiratory muscle atrophy**

•**Sinusitis** via nasal & oral tubes

•**Tracheal necrosis**
  ∘Due to endotracheal tube cuff pressure being > tracheal mucosal systolic pressure (normal
  20–25mmHg, being lower in those w/ hypotension)→
    –Tracheal vascular congestion→ischemia→necrosis

•**↓Venous return/ cardiac output**
  ∘Positive end expiratory pressure–PEEP→↑mean intrathoracic pressure, being determined by:
    –Airways resistance
    –Thoracic compliance
    –Added PEEP
    …→↑atrial & vena caval pressure→
      •↓Systemic & pulmonary venous return→
        ∘↓Ventricular preload→
          –↓Cardiac output→**heart failure**→hypotension→obstructive shock (hypotension + organ
          failure unresponsive to fluid resuscitation)

Advantages:
- ↓**Venous return**→
  - ○↓Pulmonary congestion→
    - −↓Dyspnea→↓autonomic sympathetic tone
  - ○↓Myocardial contractile strength
    - ...→↓myocardial O_2 & nutrient demand
- ↓**Transmural aortic pressure**→
  - ○↓**Afterload**
  - ...→**improved heart failure syndrome**

HOSPITAL ACQUIRED PNEUMONIA

Prophylaxis:
- •Staff hand washing
- •Adequate nutritional support
- •Early removal of nasal & oral tubes
- •**Severe illness induced gastric inflammation/ ulceration prophylaxis**
  Mechanism:
  - •↓Mucosal blood flow→
    - ○↓Bicarbonate delivery to the mucosa
    - ○↓Mucus & bicarbonate secretion from gastric mucosal cells
    - ○↓Epithelial proliferation
  Indications:
  - •Emergent or major surgery
  - •**Severe illness**
  - •Severe trauma, esp. head injury
  Prophylaxis:
  - •Proton pump inhibitors, histamine 2 selective receptor blockers, antacids, or pernicious anemia→
    - ○Loss of the protective gastic acid coating→gastroesophageal colonization by oropharyngeal organisms→
      - −↑**Hospital acquired pneumonia risk via aspiration**
      - −↑**Stress erosion/ ulceration mediated organism translocation risk**→bacteremia
      - ...all being ↓risk w/ the use of **sucralfate**, which typically does not ↑gastric pH
- •**Selective digestive decontamination**
  - ○Moderate to severe illness–induced loss of the protective fibronectin coating of the oropharynx→
    - −Oropharyngeal colonization by the organisms typically responsible for hospital acquired pneumonia

MUCOSAL COATING MEDICATIONS			
Generic (Trade)	M	♀	Dose
Sucralfate (Carafate)	Ø	P	2g PO q12hours (1hour prior to meals &/or qhs)

•Do not administer concomitantly w/ other acid suppressing medications, as ↑gastric pH→
  ○↓Efficacy, as this medication requires an acidic environment

Mechanism:
- •An aluminum hydroxide complex of sucrose that:
  - ○Forms a protective coating over the inflammatory/ ulcerated area
  - ○↑Prostaglandin synthesis
  - ○Binds to bile salts
  - ...and does not ↑gastric pH

Side effects:
Gastrointestinal
- •Constipation

Genitourinary
- •Aluminum toxicity, in the presence of renal failure

Hematologic
- •Aluminum binding to intestinal phosphate→
  - ○↓Intestinal phosphate absorption which may→
    - −Hypophosphatemia

SELECTIVE DIGESTIVE DECONTAMINATION	
Location	Dose
Oropharynx	A methylcellulose paste† containing •2% Amphotericin •2% Polymyxin E •2% Tobramycin ...applied to the buccal mucosa & tongue via a gloved finger q6hours
Distal gastrointestinal tract	A solution containing •500mg Amphotericin •100mg Polymyxin E •80mg Tobramycin ...administered via nasogastric tube q6hours

†The hospital pharmacy will make the paste

Mechanism:
- **Eradication of Pseudomonas aeruginosa, as well as most gastrointestinal fungi & enterobacteriaceae @ 1week**
- The normal gastrointestinal bacterial flora, composed mostly of anaerobes, is relatively unaffected
...→treatment & prevention of gastrointestinal colonization by the organisms typically responsible for hospital acquired:
  - •Pneumonia
  - •Urinary tract infections
  - •Bacteremia/ fungemia via mucocutaneous routes:
    - ∘Cutaneous lesion
    - ∘Gastrointestinal translocation
    - ∘Intravascular catheter

Side effects:
- •The antimicrobials used are nonabsorbable, & thus do not cause systemic toxicity

VENTILATOR ASSOCIATED PNEUMONIA–1%/ 24hours
Pathophysiology:
- •Due to pericuff microaspiration of:
  - ∘Esophagogastric mucus
  - ∘Saliva
  - ∘Tube feedings
Outcomes:
- •30% mortality
Additional prophylaxis:
- •Avoidance of gastric distention
- •Routine orotracheal suctioning w/ continuous subglottic suctioning
- •Semirecumbent positioning of the patient

DELIVERY MODE SPECIFIC COMPLICATIONS
- **Assist–control–AC ventilation** sets no maximum limit to the inhalations the patient can initiate, w/ tachypnea→
  - ∘**Respiratory alkalemia**
  - ∘↓Exhalation time→
    - –**Intrinsic peep**
- **Synchronized intermittent mandatory ventilation–SIMV** requires spontaneous, unassisted breathing to overcome a high resistance circuit (tracheal tube & ventilator tubing)→
  - ∘↑Work of breathing (being ↓ w/ concomitant pressure support ventilation)→
    - –**Respiratory muscle fatigue**↔↑ventilator dependence
- **Pressure control ventilation** causes tidal volume to be dependent on airways resistance & thoracic compliance→
  - ∘**Hypoventilation risk**
- **Positive end expiratory pressure–PEEP** is most useful w/ diffuse thoracic disease, as localized disease may lead to overdistention of unaffected alveoli→
  - ∘↑Perialveolar capillary pressure→↓flow→
    - –↑Dead space ventilation→ventilation/ perfusion mismatch→**hypoxemia**
    - –**Alveolar rupture**

182

- **Mask mediated ventilation**
  - ○Abnormal swallowing of air=aerophagia→
    - −Gastric distention
  - ○↑Aspiration risk
  - ○Difficult exhalation
  - ○Mucocutaneous effects
    - −Dry mucosa→epistaxis &/or rhinorrhea
    - −Dry conjunctiva→eye irritation
    - −Facial skin irritation ± necrosis

WEANING

- Place the patient on pressure support ventilation of 5−8cm H_2O in order to overcome the high resistance circuit (endotracheal tube & ventilator tubing), thus allowing for spontaneous respirations w/ concomitant monitoring of tidal volume & respiratory rate. If the patient tolerates pressure support ventilation for 2hours, the patient is extubated. If unsuccessful, the patient is returned to full ventilatory support for ≥24hours prior to another trial.

Weaning parameters:
- Hemodynamic stability
- PaO_2 >60% on an FiO_2 ≤40%, w/ a PEEP of ≤5cm H_2O
- Taper sedative medications
- Ensure adequate magnesium & phosphate levels, as depletion→
  - ○↓Respiratory muscle strength
- Ensure reversal of bronchospasm
- Minimize pulmonary edema via diuresis
- Optimize blood O_2 carrying capacity via a Hb ≥10g/ dL
- Consider the administration of anti−anginal medications
- Suppress fever w/ antipyretics
- Consider possible medication induced neuromuscular blockade:
  - ○Non−depolarizing neuromuscular blocking medications
    - −Residual paralytic medication (Atracurium, Cisatracurium, Pancuronium, Rocuronium, Tubocurarine, Vecuronium) w/ possible prolonged neuromuscular paralysis occurring after discontinuation
    - Mechanism:
      - •Bind to neuromuscular postsynaptic skeletal muscle nicotinic−Nm receptors→
        - ○↓Acetylcholine mediated activation→
          - −Flaccid skeletal muscle paralysis
  - ○Aminoglycosides
    - Mechanism:
      - •↓Presynaptic acetylcholine release
      - •↓Postsynaptic sensitivity to acetylcholine
    - Treatment:
      - •Calcium chloride

OTHER PARAMETERS		
Parameters	Normal	Weaning threshold
Max inspiratory pressure	< −100cm H_2O	< −25cm H_2O†
Resp. rate / tidal volume=RSBI‡	<50 breaths/min./L	<100 breaths/min./L†
Minute ventilation	5−7L/ min.	<10L/ min.
Respiratory rate	12/ min.	<25/ min.
Spontaneous tidal volume	5−7mL/ kg	≥5mL/ kg
Vital capacity°	~4L	≥10mL/ kg

†Failure to meet this weaning threshold indicates a >95% weaning failure rate
‡Rapid−shallow breathing index−RSBI
°Vital capacity: Maximum amount of air that can be exhaled

Indicators of weaning intolerance:
- •↑Autonomic sympathetic tone→
  - ○Anxiety†
  - ○Diaphoresis
  - ○Tachycardia
  - ○Tachypnea/ dyspnea†
- Deteriorating arterial blood gases
- Hemodynamic instability

183

†Dyspnea & anxiety can usually be alleviated by either:
- •Morphine
- •Haloperidol in chronic CO_2 retainers, as it does not cause respiratory depression

ENDOTRACHEAL INTUBATION

Procedure:
1. Ensure adequate equipment is within reach:
   - •100% non–rebreather mask & mask–reservoir bag
   - •A suction tube which is hooked up & works
   - •Laryngoscope w/ working light, & blades of various sizes
   - •Lubricated endotracheal tubes of various sizes, containing a tube stylet
     - ◦Endotracheal tube size can be estimated via the patients 5th digit=pinky finger, diameter in millimeters, usually being 7–8mm in adults
   - •Check for endotracheal tube cuff leak by inflating the cuff in fluid, checking for the presence of air bubbles. Deflate the cuff prior to proceeding
   - •Working intravenous access & appropriate medications
     - ◦Code cart
     - ◦Non–depolarizing neuromuscular blocking medications
     - ◦Sedative/ hypnotics (see below)
2. Anesthetize the oropharynx w/ anesthetic spray if the patient is awake
3. If possible, preoxygenate the patient via:
   - •100% non–rebreather mask, if the patient is spontaneously ventilating
   - •Bag–valve mask, if the patient is not spontaneously ventilating
   - …while monitoring the SaO_2 & the corresponding rise & fall of the chest & abdominal wall if ventilating the patient
   Bag–valve mask technique:
   A. Place the patients head in the sniffing position via tilting the head backwards (except if suspect cervical spine injury†) & thrust the mandible forward w/ your 3rd–5th digits under the bilateral mandibular rami→
      - •**Open airway**. This position must be maintained for adequate ventilation until the patient is intubated
   B. Insert a plastic oral airway (which serves to keep the tongue forward), & place a bag–valve mask on the patient
   C. Use your 3rd–5th digits to maintain the head position, while placing your thumbs & index fingers around the mask in a 'C' like shape, maintaining a strong skin–mask seal
      - •You may use both hands while another person ventilates or maintain position & seal w/ your dominant hand alone
4. View the airway
   - •During intubation attempts, ventilation should not be held for >20seconds, after which time the laryngoscope should be withdrawn & ventilation resumed until the next intubation attempt
   A. **Using your right hand**, open the mouth widely using the crossed finger technique, w/ your thumb on the lower incisors & index finger crossing under it on the upper incisors
   B. Have someone apply cricoid pressure throughout the procedure→
      - •Esophageal compression→
        - –↓Gastric aspiration risk
   C. **Using your left hand**, insert the laryngoscope in the right corner of the mouth, w/ subsequent advancement, sweeping the tongue to the left
   D. When the epiglottis is visualized, place the tip of the laryngoscope above (curved blade) or below (straight blade) the epiglottis
   E. Lift the handle of the laryngoscope upwards in order to visualize the vocal cords
5. Under direct vision, insert the tracheal tube through the vocal cords & inflate the cuff w/ the minimal amount of air that will both prevent leakage around the cuff during ventilation & reduce tracheal necrosis risk (<20mmHg). Remove the stylet, & assess for adequate placement via:
   - •End tidal CO_2 monitor
   - •Auscultation of the thorax for corresponding bilateral breath sounds‡
   - •Looking & feeling for the corresponding symmetric rise & fall of the chest & abdominal wall
   - •Monitoring the SaO_2
6. Once the patient is intubated, detach the bag device from the mask & attach it to the endotracheal tube
7. Secure the endotracheal tube w/ adhesive tape to prevent dislodgement
8. Check endotracheal tube position by chest x ray

Complications:
- **Endotracheal tube malposition**
  - ○Mainstem bronchus intubation, esp. the right mainstem bronchus as it runs a straighter course from the trachea→
  - −Obstruction of the contralateral mainstem bronchus
  - Prevention:
    - •Advancing the endotracheal tube no further than ♂: 23cm, ♀: 21cm from the teeth
- •Esophageal intubation

---

†Nasotracheal intubation is the method of choice in patients w/ possible cervical spine injury
‡The presence of bilateral breath sounds does not rule out either esophageal or mainstem bronchus intubation. Therefore, a **chest x ray is required to determine endotracheal tube position**, the tip of which should be midway between the vocal cords (C5 interspace) & the carina (T5 interspace) @ 3−5cm above the carina, w/ the head in the neutral position (inferior mandible over C5), as the tube is displaced 2cm up or down w/ extension & flexion respectively, following the movement of the chin

MEDICATIONS FOR INTUBATION & MECHANICAL VENTILATION				
SEDATIVE/ HYPNOTICS				
Generic (Trade)	M	♀	Dose	Max
ANESTHETICS				
Etomidate (Amidate)	L	?		
•Induction			0.5mg/ kg IV	
○Onset: <30seconds				
○Duration: <10min.				
Advantages:				
•Rapid onset & offset				
•Minimal hypotension or respiratory depression				
•↓Intracranial pressure				
Limitations:				
•No analgesic effect				
Propofol (Diprivan)	L	P		
•Induction			1mg/ kg IV	
○Onset: <1min.				
○Duration: <10min.				
•Maintenance			1mg/kg/hour	6mg/kg/hour
Dose adjustment:				
•As the medication is lipophilic, accumulation is prominent in obese patients, requiring dosage to be based on ideal, rather than actual body weight				
Adjusted weight= Ideal weight† + **0.4 (actual weight − ideal weight)**				
†Ideal weight:				
•♂: 50kg + 2.3kg per inch > 5'				
•♀: 45.5kg + 2.3kg per inch > 5'				
Advantages:				
•Rapid onset & offset				
•Anti−emetic action				
Limitations:				
•Expense				
•No analgesic effects				
Contraindications:				
•Egg or soy allergies				
BENZODIAZEPINES				
Midazolam (Versed)	LK	U		
•Induction			0.1mg/ kg IV over 30seconds	
○Onset: <5min.				
○Duration: Varies w/ infusion time				
•Maintenance			0.04mg/kg/hour	0.15mg/kg/hour
Dose adjustment:				
•As the medication is lipophilic, accumulation is prominent in obese patients, requiring dosage to be based on ideal, rather than actual body weight				
Adjusted weight= Ideal weight†† + **0.4 (actual weight − ideal weight)**				
†Ideal weight:				
•♂: 50kg + 2.3kg per inch > 5'				
•♀: 45.5kg + 2.3kg per inch > 5'				
Advantages:				
•Anti−seizure				

Limitations:
- **No analgesic effects**
- •Numerous medication interactions
Contraindications:
- •Narrow-angle glaucoma

BARBITURATES

Thiopental (Pentothal)   L   ?
- •Induction   5mg/ kg IV over 2min.
  ◦Onset: <30seconds
  ◦Duration: 5min.
Advantages:
- •Rapid onset & offset
- •Anti-seizure
Limitations:
- **No analgesic effects**

Anesthetic specific mechanism:
- •Bind to a receptor site on the neuronal inhibitory gamma aminobutyric acid–GABA$_A$ chloride ion channel→
  ◦↑Channel opening in the concomitant presence of GABA→
    –Neuronal inhibition

Benzodiazepine specific mechanism:
- •Bind to a benzodiazepine receptor site on the neuronal inhibitory gamma aminobutyric acid–GABA$_A$ chloride ion channel→
  ◦↑**Frequency** of channel opening in the concomitant presence of GABA→
    –Neuronal inhibition

Barbiturate specific mechanism:
- •Bind to a barbiturate receptor site on the neuronal inhibitory gamma aminobutyric acid–GABA$_A$ chloride ion channel→
  ◦↑**Duration** of channel opening in the concomitant presence of GABA→
    –Neuronal inhibition

Etomidate specific side effects:
General
- •Pain upon injection, due to its propylene glycol preparation
- •Sneezing
Endocrine
- •Adrenocortical suppression, rarely of clinical significance
Gastrointestinal
- •Nausea ± vomiting
Neurologic
- •Myoclonus

Propofol specific side effects:
General
- •Formulated as a milky white lipid emulsion (composed of egg lecithin, glycerol, & soybean oil) which supports microbial growth→
  ◦↑**Infection risk**
    –Strict aseptic technique should be used when withdrawing the medication
    –Once the vial is opened, infusion should commence promptly, w/ the tubing & any unused amount being discarded @ 12hours
Cardiovascular
- •**Bradycardia**
- •↓Myocardial contractility
- •Vasodilation→
  ◦**Hypotension**, which may be severe
Neurologic
- •Dystonic or choreoform movements
- •Intense dreams
Pulmonary
- •↑Caloric load (>1000 calories/ day as lipid)→
  ◦↑CO_2
- •Respiratory depression

186

Hematologic
- **Hypertriglyceridemia**→
  - ∘Pancreatitis

Midazolam specific side effects:
Cardiovascular
- **Hypotension**
Neurologic
- **Prolonged use**→
  - ∘Withdrawal syndrome upon discontinuation. Gradual withdrawal is recommended @ >1month of use
Pulmonary
- **Respiratory depression**

Thiopental specific side effects:
Cardiovascular
- **Hypotension**
Mucocutaneous
- **Tissue necrosis w/ extravasation**
Pulmonary
- **Respiratory depression**
- **Histamine release**→
  - ∘Laryngospasm

Propofol specific monitoring:
- **W/ prolonged use, check triglyceride levels periodically**

ANALGESIA

OPIOID RECEPTOR AGONISTS

Generic (Trade)	M ♀	Dose
Fentanyl (Sublimaze)	L ?	50–150μg IV bolus, then 30–100μg/ hour IV infusion

- **Onset: <2min.**
- **Duration: 1hour**

Advantages:
- In comparison w/ Morphine, Fentanyl:
  - ∘Has a more rapid onset, & shorter duration of action, as the medication is more lipophilic→
    - −↑Central nervous system infiltration & exit, allowing for more rapid titration
  - ∘Is less hypotensive, due to ↓histamine release
  - ∘Is more potent, due to its lipophilic nature, as wall as greater affinity for the mu opiate receptor

Side effects:
Cardiovascular
- **Vasodilation (venous >> arterial)**→
  - ∘↓Preload→
    - −↓Cardiac output→**hypotension**
- **Bradycardia**
Gastrointestinal
- Central nervous system chemoreceptor trigger zone activation→
  - ∘**Nausea ± vomiting**, exacerbated by ambulation
- Enteric nervous system opioid receptor activation→
  - ∘↓Gastrointestinal smooth muscle peristalsis→
    - −**Constipation**
- ↑Biliary tract smooth muscle contraction→
  - ∘Biliary colic
Genitourinary
- ↑Ureteral & urinary bladder smooth muscle peristalsis→
  - ∘Prostatic neoplastic syndrome exacerbation
- ↓Uterine muscle tone→
  - ∘Labor prolongation
Neurologic
- **Altered mental status**
- **Dysphoria**
- **Sedation**
- **Seizures**

Opthalmologic
- •Iris radial smooth muscle relaxation→
  - ◦↓Pupil size=**miosis**, being fixed

Pulmonary
- •Inhibition of medullary respiratory center response to CO_2 concentration→
  - ◦**Respiratory depression**→
    - −Hypercapnic respiratory failure→altered mental status
- •↓Cough reflex

Side effects of chronic use:
- •Development of **tolerance**† to its effects, as the dosage previously sufficient to produce effects progressively fails to do so, as both the central nervous system & liver adapt to its chronic presence by altering:
  - ◦Neuronal membrane constituents
  - ◦Neurotransmitter release & re−uptake
  - ◦Hepatic clearance
  - …which set the stage for the vicious cycle of **dependence** & craving for ever increasing amounts of the medication, regardless of the professional, social, or health risks

---

†Tolerance does not develop to:
- •Constipation
- •Miosis
- •Seizures

ANTIDOTE				
Generic (Trade)	**M**	♀	**Start**	**Max**
Naloxone (Narcan)	LK	P	2mg IV/ SC/ IM/ ET q2min. prn	10mg total

Mechanism:
- •μ receptor antagonist, which, in the absence of exogenous opioids, have no clinical effect

Duration:
- •1−2hours

Side effects:
- •**Acute opioid withdrawal/ reversal syndrome**
  - ◦Diaphoresis
  - ◦Goose flesh
  - ◦↑Lacrimation
  - ◦Nausea ± vomiting
  - ◦Rhinorrhea
  - ◦Tachypnea
  - …w/ rare:
    - •Hypo or hypertension
    - •Pulmonary edema
    - •Ventricular tachycardia &/or fibrillation

•Caused by **abnormal clot formation=thrombus** ± detachment & distal flow, termed thromboembolus→
  ◦Occlusion of distal vasculature
•Deep venous thrombosis–DVT occurs in 5million persons/ year, w/:
  ◦10% developing pulmonary embolism–PE (only 30% being detected pre–mortem)→
    –10% mortality

RISK FACTORS
•**Endothelial damage**
  ◦Trauma, including surgery (also causing immobility), esp. of the structures distal to the abdomen (pelvis & legs)
  ◦Previous stable deep venous thrombosis→
    –Incorporation into the venous endothelium→↓valve function→local venous stasis
  ◦Iatrogenic via intravascular devices
    –Cardiac valves
    –Peritoneovenous shunts
    –Venous catheters
    –Vessel grafts

•**Altered vascular flow**
  ◦**Immobilization**
    –Bed rest >4 days
    –Cerebrovascular accident
    –Morbid obesity
  ◦**Venous congestion**
    –Heart failure (also causing Immobility)
    –Varicose veins
    –Pregnancy

•**Acquired hypercoagulable states**
  ◦**Antiphospholipid antibodies** via antibody mediated interference of procoagulant glycoprotein function
    –Anticardiolipin antibody
    –Lupus anticoagulant
    –False positive syphilis serum VDRL or RPR test
  ◦**Antithrombin 3 deficiency**
    –Disseminated intravascular coagulation–DIC
    –Hepatic failure
    –Nephrotic syndrome
  ◦**Estrogen**
    –Medications (hormone replacement therapy–HRT, oral contraceptive pills–OCPs, mixed estrogen receptor agonists/ antagonists)→↓antithrombin 3
    –Pregnancy via ↓antithrombin 3, ↓protein S, ↓fibrinolytic acitivity, ↑platelet activation, activated protein C resistance, venous stasis, & ↑factors 1, 7, 8, 9, & 10
    –The puerperium (childbirth to 1.5months)
  ◦**Hyperlipidemia**
  ◦**Inflammatory bowel disease–IBD**
    –Crohn's disease
    –Ulcerative colitis
  ◦**Malignancy**
  ◦**Medications**
    –Heparin→Heparin induced thrombocytopenia ± thrombosis, esp. high molecular weight Heparin
  ◦**Nephrotic syndrome**
  ◦**Stem cell disease**
    –Myeloproliferative disease syndromes
    –Paroxysmal nocturnal hemoglobinuria
  ◦**Systemic thrombohemorrhagic syndromes**
    –Disseminated intravascular coagulation–DIC
    –Thrombotic thrombocytopenic purpura–TTP
    –Hemolytic uremic syndrome–HUS

- **Congenital hypercoagulable states†**
  - ∘↓&/or dysfunctional proteins
    - −Antithrombin 3
    - −Cystathionine β−synthase &/or the thermolabile variant of methylenetetrahydrofolate reductase→ homocystinemia
    - −Heparin cofactor 2
    - −Plasminogen
    - −Plasminogen activator
    - −Protein C
    - −Protein S
  - ∘Dysfunctional proteins
    - −Activated protein C resistance=factor 5 Leiden
    - −Fibrinogen
  - ∘↑Proteins
    - −Plasminogen activator inhibitor 1
    - −Prothrombin gene G20210A mutation
    - −Factor VIII
    - −Factor IX
    - −Factor XI

- **Virchow's triad** is the eponym describing the risk factors for thrombosis
  - ∘Endothelial damage
  - ∘Altered vascular flow
  - ∘Hypercoagulable states

†Indications for a congenital hypercoagulable state workup
  - •Any of the following, if it changes management:
    - ∘**Age <45 years**
    - ∘**Venous thrombosis above the pelvis**
    - ∘**Recurrent thrombosis**
    - ∘**Family history of thrombosis**
    - ∘**Thrombosis despite adequate anticoagulation**
    - ∘**Warfarin induced skin necrosis**, as may occur w/ either protein C or S deficiency or dysfunction

CLASSIFICATION

- **Deep venous thrombosis**
  - ∘Thrombus, formation in large diameter veins, being relatively deeper in location to small diameter veins

- **Superficial venous thrombosis**
  - ∘Thrombus formation in small diameter veins, being relatively superficial in location to large diameter veins
    - −Not associated w/ embolus formation unless distal growth occurs into a large diameter vein

- **Pulmonary thromboembolism**
  - ∘Thrombus detachment from the endothelium→
    - −Distal flow to the pulmonary arterial system
  - ∘**70% have a detectable deep venous thrombosis @ the time of diagnosis**
  - Sites of origination:
    - •**Lower extremity veins−95%**
      - ∘Occurring w/ 50% of untreated thrombi proximal to the calf
      - ∘Calf vein thromboses are not associated w/ embolus formation unless they encroach into the popliteal vein (occurring in 25% of untreated patients, usually within 1week)
    - •Upper extremity veins
    - •Inferior vena cava
    - •Renal veins
    - •Right atrium or ventricle
  - Severity based subclassification:
    - •**Massive pulmonary embolism**
      - ∘Occlusion of ≥2 lobar arteries
    - •**Saddle embolism**
      - ∘Occlusion of any vascular bifurcation
        - −May occlude the bifurcation of the left & right pulmonary arteries

•Non-thrombotic pulmonary embolism
　◦Flow of non-thrombotic material to the pulmonary arterial system, composed of either:
　　−Air
　　−Amniotic fluid
　　−Bacterial mass
　　−Bone marrow
　　−Fat
　　−Foreign body
　　−Neoplasm

DIAGNOSIS OF VENOUS THROMBOSIS
General
　•Inflammatory cytokines→
　　◦**Fever**, usually being low grade (<101°F=38.4°C)

Cardiovascular
　•Venous thrombosis→**unilateral:**
　　◦Venous inflammation=phlebtitis→
　　　−Palpable venous cord
　　◦Partial venous occlusion→
　　　−Proximal venous congestion
　　…→**edematous, erythematous,** & **painful** extremity

IMAGING
•Venous compression ultrasonography
　Findings:
　　•The force of compressing the ultrasound probe against the skin→
　　　◦Normal venous collapse vs. a non-collapsed thrombosed vein
　　•Doppler ultrasonography uses Doppler shift to detect vessel flow velocity, allowing differentiation of
　　veins from arteries
　　…both together are termed venous duplex compression ultrasonography=duplex ultrasonography
　Outcomes:
　　•Thigh deep venous thrombosis sensitivity: 95%, specificity: 95%
　Limitations:
　　•Calf veins are smaller & thus more difficult to visualize
　　•Differentiating acute from chronic thromboses may be difficult
　Follow-up:
　　•Being that 25% of untreated calf vein thrombi extend to the distal vasculature, perform a
　　follow-up ultrasonography @ 1week after a normal test result. If the test is negative at that time,
　　subsequent extension of a possible calf vein thrombus is unlikely

•Ascending venography
　Indications:
　　•A strong clinical suspicion of deep venous thrombosis, w/ a negative ultrasonography

COMPLICATIONS
•Post-thrombotic syndrome-25%
　Cardiovascular
　　•Thrombus organization & incorporation into the venous endothelium→
　　　◦Venous valve malfunction→**chronic venous insufficiency**→proximal venous congestion→
　　　stasis dermatitis characterized by:
　　　　−Erythema & scaling of the skin
　　　　−↓Lymphatic flow
　　　　−Ulceration
　　　　…→↑risk of:
　　　　　•Extremity infection, esp. cellulitis
　　　　　•Recurrent deep venous thrombosis

•Pulmonary embolism

General
- •Inflammatory cytokines→
  - ◦**Fever–50%**, usually being low grade (<101°F=38.4°C)

Cardiovascular
- •Pain, anxiety, &/or hypoxemia→
  - ◦Pulse ≥100/ min.=tachycardia
  - ◦Palpitations

Pulmonary
- •Pulmonary arterial occlusion, usually occurring in the lower lung fields to which there is relatively more blood flow→
  - ◦Local release of vascular & bronchial smooth muscle constrictors (bradykinin, prostaglandins, serotonin)→
    - –Further occlusion
    - …→distal ischemia ± infarction–10%→
      - •**Thoracic pain–90%**, which may be pleuritic, being exacerbated by either:
        - ◦Deep inhalation (including coughing & sneezing)
        - ◦Supine position
        - ◦Thoracic palpation
        - …& being relieved by leaning forward
      - •Cough ± **hemoptysis–30%**
      - •Pulmonary bronchospasm→
        - ◦Wheezing
  - ◦Difficulty breathing=**dyspnea**→
    - –Respiratory rate >16/ min.=**tachypnea**
    - –Accessory muscle usage (sternocleidomastoid muscles for inspiration & abdominal muscles for expiration)
    - –Speech frequently interrupted by inspiration=telegraphic speech
    - –Pursed lip breathing &/or grunting expirations→positive end-expiratory pressure–PEEP
    - –Paradoxical abdominal motion: Negative intrathoracic pressure→fatigued diaphragm being pulled into the thorax→inspiratory inward motion of the anterior abdominal wall, rather than expected outward motion due to diaphragmatic contraction
  - ◦Ventilation/ perfusion mismatch via:
    - –↑Alveolar dead space: Alveolar ventilation through relatively underperfused capillaries
    - –↑Vascular shunting†: Capillary blood flow through relatively underventilated alveoli. Usually occurring, or exacerbated via ↑venous return
    - …→↓diffusion of O_2 & CO_2→
      - •Hypoxemia (SaO_2 ≤ 91% or PaO_2 ≤ 60mmHg‡) on room air, w/ subsequent hypercapnia ($PaCO_2$ ≥45mmHg) due to either:
        - ◦Respiratory muscle fatigue
        - ◦Alveolar hypoventilation
        - …as CO_2 clearance is unimpaired (& may be ↑in the dyspneic patient) as long as adequate ventilation (including lack of diffuse severe ventilation/ perfusion mismatching) is maintained, as:
          - •CO_2 diffuses 20X as rapidly as O_2
          - •Hypercapnia→
            - ◦Immediate brain stem respiratory center mediated stimulation of pulmonary ventilation, which may correct the hypercapnia, but not necessarily the hypoxia
  - ◦↑Pulmonary artery pressure°→
    - –Right ventricular heave→a palpable lift over the left sternal border
    - –Tricuspid regurgitation murmur–25%
    - –↑Pulmonic component of the 2nd heart sound–55%
    - –Right sided heart failure
    - –Syncope–15%
    - –Pulseless electrical activity–PEA

---

†Being exacerbated by the supine position→
- •↑Systemic venous return→
  - ◦↑Vascular shunting→↑dyspnea, being termed:
    - –Orthopnea, if persistent
    - –Paroxysmal nocturnal dyspnea if intermittent
    - …causing the patient to either use multiple pillows or sleep in a chair

‡Age adjusted normal PaO_2 = 101 – (0.43 X age)

°Indicates limited cardiopulmonary reserve via either:
•Underlying heart failure
•Underlying chronic obstructive pulmonary disease–COPD
•Massive or recurrent pulmonary embolism→
  ◦Cor pulmonale

Hematologic
•↑**Fibrin d–dimers** (≥0.5µg/ mL)
  Mechanism:
  •Plasmin→
    ◦Thrombus fibrin degradation→
      −↑Fibrin degradation products, termed fibrin d–dimers
  Outcomes/ limitations:
  •Sensitivity: >90%, specificity: 30%
  …making this test **useful in helping to exclude a pulmonary embolus**, but unable to reliably
  confirm one, as the levels may be ↑ for any cause of thrombus formation, as occurs w/:
    •↑Age
    •Cancer
    •Heart failure
    •Myocardial infarction
    •Pneumonia
    •Pregnancy
    •Recent trauma, including surgery

•↑**Alveolar–arterial O_2 difference**†, termed the A–a gradient
  ◦The measured arterial partial pressure of O_2 (PaO_2) is subtracted from the calculated alveolar
  partial pressure of O_2 via the following formula, thus expressing the efficiency w/ which a lung
  exchanges oxygen:
    −**Room air:** $150 - (PaCO_2 \div 0.8) - PaO_2$
    −**Supplemental O_2:** $(713 \times FiO_2‡) - (PaCO_2 \div 0.8) - PaO_2$
  Physiology:
  •In a perfect lung, there should be no difference. However, the slight ventilation/ perfusion
  mismatch that occurs in a normal lung causes a mild difference to occur via the following
  formulas:
    ◦**Age adjusted normal:** A–a gradient = (age $\div$ 4) + 4
    ◦**Supplemental O_2:** Every 10%↑→
      −↑A–a gradient by 5mmHg

Additional features associated w/ a **fat embolism:**
•Bone fracture mediated fat marrow globulemia→
  ◦**Altered mental status**
  ◦**Petechiae**
  ◦Acute respiratory distress syndrome–ARDS
  ◦Disseminated intravascular coagulation–DIC

---

†W/ respiratory distress, an ↑alveolar–arterial O_2 gradient indicates ↑ventilation/ perfusion mismatch
from any cardiopulmonary disorder, whereas **a normal gradient indicates no disease vs. a sole
ventilatory defect**
‡Fraction of inspired air that is oxygen–FiO_2

ELECTRICAL STUDIES
•**Electrocardiogram–ECG**
  Findings:
  •**Sinus tachycardia–45%** (pulse ≥100bpm)
  •**Right ventricular strain** pattern via inverted T waves in leads V1–V4
  •**S1–Q3–T3:** S wave in lead I, Q wave & inverted T wave in lead III
  •↑Right atrial hydrostatic pressure†→
    ◦Premature atrial contractions–PACs
    ◦Atrial fibrillation
    ◦Right atrial dilation→p pulmonale, indicated by either:
      −P wave ≥0.11seconds
      −P wave ≥2.5mm in lead II
      −Initial portion of a biphasic p wave being ≥2mm in lead V1

- •↑Right ventricular hydrostatic pressure†→
  - ○Premature ventricular contractions–PVCs
  - ○Right bundle branch block (RR' in leads V1 &/or V2)→
    - –Right axis deviation
    - …w/ chronic effects→
      - •Right ventricular hypertrophy
- Limitations:
  - •Normal in 40% of patients
  - •Changes do not correlate w/ severity

---

†Right sided changes are present in only 5% of patients

IMAGING

•Venous thromboembolic mediated perfusion defects may persist unchanged for several years. Pulmonary angiography may help in determining whether a perfusion defect is acute or chronic via differing appearances.

- •**Chest x ray**
  - Findings:
    - •Pneumonitis→
      - ○Consolidation
      - ○Pleural effusion–35% (exudative–75% > transudative), w/ 60% being hemorrhagic
    - •Thromboembolism & local vasoconstriction→
      - ○↓Pulmonary vascularity–20%
      - ○**Radiolucent area due to abrupt vascular cutoff, termed Westermarks sign–7%**
    - •Pulmonary infarction→
      - ○**Wedge shaped, pleural based consolidation, termed Hampton's hump–35%**
        - –Occurs 12–36hours after symptoms begin
  - Limitations:
    - •Normal in 50% of patients

- •**Pulmonary ventilation/ perfusion mismatch**
  - Procedure:
    1. Intravenous injection of technetium–^{99}Tm labeled microaggregates of albumin→
       - •Images of the lung vasculature in 6 different planes
         - –If vascular cutoff seen, then→
    2. Inhalation of radioactive xenon–^{133}Xe gas→
       - •Images of lung aeration
    …w/ a **mismatch defect indicated by normal aeration in a region of vascular cutoff**
  - Interpretations:
    - •**Normal:** Pulmonary embolism–5%
    - •**Low or intermediate probability:** Pulmonary embolism 15–30%, w/ the diagnosis made via venous compression ultrasonography (@ days 0 & 7) or pulmonary angiography
    - •**High probability:** Pulmonary embolism–90%
  - Limitations:
    - •Nearby aeration may be affected by consolidation or atelectasis, so it is best performed in a patient w/ **no underlying lung disease**

- •**Thoracic computed tomographic–CT scan**
  - Findings:
    - •Vascular cutoff
  - Limitations:
    - •Unreliable in the subsegmental vessels

- •**Pulmonary angiography**
  - Findings:
    - •The **gold standard** in identifying vascular cutoff
  - Outcomes:
    - •0.3% mortality
  - Major nonfatal complications–0.8%:
    - •Hematoma requiring transfusion
    - •Renal failure
    - •Respiratory failure

TREATMENT OF THROMBOSIS

ANTICOAGULANTS: High molecular weight Heparin

Treatment duration:
- **Transient risk factor mediated:** 3months after risk factor has resolved
- **Idiopathic:** 6months
- **Persistent risk factor mediated:** Lifelong
- **Recurrent thrombosis:** Lifelong

- Anticoagulation treatment is not needed for asymptomatic, small (several millimeters) calf vein thrombosis (superficial or deep) not due to a hypercoagulable state

M	♀	Start
M	?	80units/ kg IV bolus (or 5000units empirically)
		18units/kg/hour infusion (or 1000units/ hour empirically)

- Titrated by 2.5units/kg/hour to achieve an activated partial thromboplastin time–aPTT of 1.5–2X control value or **50–70seconds**

aPTT (seconds)	Action	Obtain next aPTT
<40	Bolus 5000units & ↑infusion rate by 100units/ hour	6hours
40–49	↑Infusion rate by 50units/ hour	6hours
50–70 (or 1.5–2Xcontrol)	NO ACTION	24hours
71–85	↓Infusion rate by 50units/ hour	6hours
86–100	Hold infusion 30min., then ↓infusion rate by 100units/ hour	6hours
101–150	Hold infusion 60min., then ↓infusion rate by 150units/ hour	6hours
>150	Hold infusion 60min., then ↓infusion rate by 300units/ hour	6hours

Monitoring:
- Complete blood count q24hours to monitor for side effects

ANTICOAGULANTS: Low molecular weight Heparin

Generic (Trade)	M	♀	Start	Max
Enoxaparin (Lovenox)	KL	P	1.5mg/ kg SC q24hours or 1mg/ kg SC q12hours	180mg/ 24hours
Dalteparin (Fragmin)	KL	P	200 anti–factor Xa units/ kg SC q24hours or 100 anti–factor Xa units/ kg SC q12hours	18,000units q24h

Dose adjustment:
- Obesity
  - Most manufacturers recommend a maximum dose of that for a 90kg patient

Monitoring:
- Monitoring of anti–Xa levels is recommended in patients w/:
  - Abnormal coagulation/ hemorrhage
  - Obesity
  - Renal failure
  - Underweight
- Check 4h after 2nd SC dose. Further monitoring is not necessary once the correct dose is established in obese patients

Administration frequency	Therapeutic anti–Xa levels
Q12hours	0.6–1 units/ mL
Q24hours	1–2 units/ mL

Mechanism:
- Heparin combines w/ plasma antithrombin 3→
  - ↑Antithrombin 3 activity in removing thrombin & activated factors 9, 10, 11,& 12→
    - ↓Coagulation→↓vascular & mural thrombus formation &/or propagation
- Heparin is metabolized by the plasma enzyme heparinase

Outcomes:
- ↓Morbidity & mortality

Side effects:
Cardiovascular
- **Hemorrhage**
- **Heparin induced thrombocytopenia–HIT 10%**, esp. w/ high molecular weight Heparin
  Mechanism:
  - Heparin mediated platelet agglutination→
    - Monocyte/ macrophage mediated extravascular removal via the splenic trabecular network=red pulp, & hepatic sinusoids→
      - **Thrombocytopenia**
  Outcomes:
  - Benign, as it resolves spontaneously, even w/ continued exposure

195

- **Heparin induced thrombocytopenia ± thrombosis–HITT ≤3%**, esp. w/ high molecular weight Heparin
  - Mechanism:
    - •Heparin mediated platelet agglutination→
      - ∘Monocyte/ macrophage mediated extravascular removal via the splenic trabecular network=red pulp, & hepatic sinusoids→
        - **–Thrombocytopenia**
      - ∘Platelet release of Heparin neutralizing factor=platelet factor 4–PF4, which complexes w/ Heparin→
        - –Production of anti–complex antibodies→↑platelet activation↔↑platelet factor 4 release→ a vicious cycle of **platelet mediated arterial &/or venous thrombus formation, termed the "white clot syndrome,"** being as the clot is relatively devoid of erythrocytes
  - Outcomes:
    - •Must discontinue treatment as **20% develop thromboembolic complications**. Being that both Heparins may cross–react w/ the etiologic antibodies, their further use is contraindicated. Consider continued treatment w/ direct thrombin inhibitors
      - ∘Antibody cross–reactivity:
        - –Low molecular weight Heparins–85%
        - –Heparinoids–5%
- **Mucocutaneous**
  - •Skin necrosis–rarely occurring w/ high molecular weight Heparins, & not being associated w/ anticoagulant deficiency
- **Musculoskeletal**
  - •Osteoporosis, esp. w/ high molecular weight Heparin
    - ∘Usually @ use ≥1month
- **Hematologic**
  - •↓Aldosterone production→
    - ∘**Hyperkalemia–8%**

CHARACTERISTICS OF HEPARIN INDUCED THROMBOCYTOPENIC SYNDROMES

	HIT	HITT
Onset	<2days	4–10 days
Re-exposure	<2days	Earlier if re–exposed within 3 months
Platelet count	↓, being <150,000 or ≥50%	
Platelet median nadir	~90,000	~60,000

- •^{14}C–Serotonin release assay
  - Indications:
    - •Suspected HITT
  - Procedure:
    - •Normal donor platelets are radiolabeled w/ ^{14}C–serotonin. They are then washed & combined w/ patient serum & therapeutic Heparin concentrations (0.1 U/ mL). Induction of ^{14}C–serotonin release from platelets constitutes a positive test
  - Limitations:
    - •Expense, due to the use of radioactive material
  - Outcomes:
    - •Considered the gold standard in the detection of HITT
- •**Enzyme linked immunosorbent assay–ELISA**
  - Indications:
    - •Suspected HITT
  - Procedure:
    - •Heparin–PF4 complexes affixed to a plastic plate are incubated w/ the patient's serum. If the patient has produced antibodies, then the addition of enzymatically (horseradish peroxidase) labeled anti–human IgG allows for color visualization via spectrophotometer
  - Limitations:
    - •Many antibody positive patients do not develop clinical HITT
    - •30% false positive

Contraindications:
- •Active hemorrhage
- •Severe bleeding diathesis
- •Severe thrombocytopenia (platelet count ≤20,000/ µL)
- •Recent significant trauma
- •Neurosurgery, ocular surgery, or intracranial hemorrhage within 10days

ANTIDOTE				
Generic	M ♀	Amount IV over 10min.	Max	
Protamine	P ?	1mg/ 100units of HMWH	50mg	
		1mg/ 100units Dalteparin	"	
		1mg/ 1mg Enoxaparin	"	

Mechanism:
- •Protamine combines electrostatically w/ Heparin→
  - ◦Inability to bind to antithrombin 3

FOLLOWED BY

ANTICOAGULANTS		
Generic	M ♀	Start

Warfarin (Coumadin) L U   5mg PO q24hours
- •Because the anticoagulant proteins↓ relatively faster than the procoagulant proteins, an initial transient hypercoagulable state develops. Due to this, warfarin is started once the patient is therapeutic on Heparin, via either:
  - ◦Goal aPTT w/ high molecular weight Heparin
  - ◦Evening of initiation of low molecular weight Heparin
  - …requiring ~7days (corresponding to 2 half lives of factor 2, or a 75% reduction) to reach a true therapeutic level of an **international normalized ratio–INR of 2–3**

INR	Action	Obtain next INR
<1.5	↑Weekly dose by 15%	1 week
1.5–1.9	↑Weekly dose by 10%	2 weeks
2–3	NO ACTION	1 month if stable
3.1–3.9	↓Weekly dose by 10%	2 weeks
4–5	Skip 1 day, then ↓weekly dose by 15%	1 week
>5	DISCONTINUE WARFARIN	Q day until ≤3, then ↓weekly dose by 50%

Mechanism:
- •Competitively inhibits hepatocyte enzymatic vitamin K reactive sites→
  - ◦↓Formation of both:
    - −Procoagulant proteins 2, 7, 9, & 10
    - −Anticoagulant proteins C & S
    - …w/ the anticoagulant effect requiring several days, as it must await the metabolism of the pre–existing plasma procoagulant proteins, w/ normal coagulation returning within several days of discontinuation

Side effects:
  Cardiovascular
  - •**Hemorrhage**
    - ◦Fatal: 0.6%/ year
    - ◦Major: 3%/ year
    - ◦Minor: 7%/ year
  Cutaneous
  - •Tissue necrosis w/ protein C or S deficiency or dysfunction

Contraindications:
- •Active hemorrhage
- •Severe bleeding diathesis
- •Severe thrombocytopenia (platelet count ≤20,000/ μL)
- •Recent significant trauma
- •Neurosurgery, ocular surgery, or intracranial hemorrhage within 10days
- •Injury risk (including falls & sports) or compliance risk via:
  - ◦Alcoholism
  - ◦Altered mental status
  - ◦Illicit drug abuse
  - ◦Orthostatic hypotension
  - ◦Poor compliance
  - ◦Seizure disease
  - ◦Syncope
  - ◦Unstable gait

Special considerations:
- •**If undergoing elective surgery during treatment**
  - ◦Stop warfarin 5 days prior to surgery, & begin Heparin
- •**Anticoagulation during pregnancy**
  - ◦Substitute low molecular weight Heparin for warfarin, followed by warfarin treatment postpartum if necessary

197

ANTIDOTES
•**Gastric lavage & activated charcoal** if recently administered; forced emesis at home

VITAMIN K=Phytonadione
Indications:
•To correct the international normalized ration-INR or prothrombin time-PT
Dose
10mg SC/ IV slow push @ 1mg/ min. in order to ↓anaphylactoid reaction risk
Mechanism:
•Requires several hours to days for effect
Side effects:
•Avoid intramuscular administration which may→
∘Intramuscular hemorrhage

FRESH FROZEN PLASMA-FFP
Indications:
•To correct the international normalized ration-INR or prothrombin time-PT under the following conditions:
∘**INR >20**
∘**Severe hemorrhage**
∘**Other need for rapid reversal, such as an emergent procedure**
Dose†
15mL/ kg IV (w/ ~200mL FFP/ unit) q4hours prn ↑INR
Mechanism:
•Contains clotting factors 2, 7, 9-13, & heat labile 5 & 7→
∘Immediate onset of action
•Each unit→
∘8% ↑coagulation factors
∘4% ↑blood volume

•**Inferior vena cava-IVC filter**
  Indications:
    •Contraindication to anticoagulation
    •Thrombosis during appropriate anticoagulation
    •Massive pulmonary embolism→
      ∘↓↑Pulmonary reserve→
        -↑Fatal pulmonary embolism risk
    •Underlying severe cardiopulmonary disease→
      ∘↓Pulmonary reserve→
        -↑Fatal pulmonary embolism risk
    •Primary long term prophylaxis
      ∘Paraplegic patients
      ∘Those at high risk for thromboembolism
    •Patients who require urgent surgery which precludes the use of anticoagulants
  Procedure:
    •A mesh-like filter (usually the conical shaped Greenfield filter) is inserted percutaneously via a catheter, into the femoral or internal jugular vein→
      ∘Inferior vena cava placement, below the level of the renal veins†→
        -**Entrapment of thromboemboli**
  Outcomes:
    •Recurrent, symptomatic pulmonary thromboembolism risk is 3%, w/ fatal a embolism being rare
  Limitations:
    •Eventually, the filter becomes obstructed→
      ∘↓Blood flow→
        -Collateral venous formation→↓protective effect. Therefore, **concomitant anticoagulation→ prolonged filter patency**, & continued treatment during the presence of collateral vasculature

---

†Unless the thrombus extends to the renal veins without impairment of renal venous flow→
  •Placement above the renal veins

•**Thrombectomy**
  Indications:
    •Patients in whom ↓venous flow→
      ∘**Severe limb ischemia**

ADDITIONAL TREATMENT OF ACUTE PULMONARY EMBOLISM ▬▬▬▬▬▬

•**Oxygen** to maintain SaO_2 >92% or PaO_2 >60mmHg, usually accomplished via nasal cannula @ 2–4L/ min.

Indications:
•Hypoxemia (SaO_2 ≤ 91% or PaO_2 ≤ 60mmHg)

Duration:
•24–48hours or longer if needed for oxygenation

THROMBOLYTIC MEDICATIONS			
Indications: •Pulmonary embolism→ ∘Hemodynamic compromise •Deep venous thrombosis being limb threatening within 1 week			
Generic (trade)	M	♀	Dose
Alteplase (Tissue plasminogen activator–tPA)	L	?	PE: 100mg IV over 2hours

Streptokinase (Kabikinase, Streptase)	L	?	PE or DVT: 250,000 units IV over 30min. (loading dose), then 100,000 units/ hour IV
			  •X 24h for PE
			  •X 72h for DVT

Urokinase (Abbokinase)	L	P	PE: 4400units/ kg IV over 10min. (loading dose), then 4400units/kg/hour X 12hours

•IV Heparin therapy must be administered promptly upon thrombolytic therapy discontinuation→
  ∘↓Reocclusion rate

Mechanism:
•Fibrinolysis→
  ∘↑Pulmonary perfusion ± venous return

Outcomes:
•Effective if initiated within 1 week after symptom onset

Complications:
Cardiovascular
•**Hemorrhage**
  ∘Most important being **intracranial hemorrhage**
    –Streptokinase–0.5%
    –Alteplase–0.7%
    –Lanetoplase, Reteplase or Tenecteplase–1%
  …→**cerebrovascular accident syndrome** having a 65% overall mortality, being 95% @ age
      >75years
  Risk factors:
    •Elderly
    •Hypertension
    •History of cerebrovascular accident

Absolute contraindications:
•Lifetime history of hemorrhagic stroke
•Ischemic stroke within 1year
•Suspected aortic dissection
•Acute pericarditis
•Active internal hemorrhage, not including menses
•Intracranial or spinal:
  ∘Aneurysm
  ∘Arteriovenous malformation–AVM
  ∘Neoplasm

Relative contraindications:
•≥Severe hypertension refractory to medical treatment, via either:
  ∘Systolic blood pressure ≥180mmHg
  ∘Diastolic blood pressure ≥110mmHg
•History of ischemic stroke @ >1year
•Significant trauma or surgery within 1month
•Prolonged (>10min.) or traumatic CPR, or traumatic intubation
•Non–compressible vascular punctures
•Active peptic ulcer
•Internal hemorrhage within 1month

- •Known bleeding diathesis
- •Current anticoagulation treatment w/ INR ≥2
- •Pregnancy
- •Liver failure
- •Diabetic hemorrhagic retinopathy
- •Hypersensitivity reaction to Streptokinase or Anistreplase, which contains Streptokinase. Also, patients should not receive Streptokinase if it was administered within 2years

Monitoring:
- •Vital signs & neurologic examination q15min. during infusion, then:
  - ∘Q30min. X 6hours, then
    - –Q1hour X 16hours

Streptokinase specific:
- •Obtain the thrombin time (normal: 6–11seconds) several hours into therapy, which should be 2X the upper limit of normal, indicating adequate plasma proteolytic action. If inadequately prolonged, re-load w/ 500,000units IV over 30min. to overcome binding by anti–streptokinase antibodies, & re–measure the thrombin time in several hours. If the thrombin time remains inadequately prolonged, switch to a different thrombolytic medication

- •If severe headache, acute hypertension, altered mental status, nausea, or vomiting occur, discontinue the infusion, if still running, give cryoprecipitate, & obtain an emergent non–contrast computed tomography–CT scan to rule out intracranial hemorrhage

OTHER TREATMENT OPTIONS
- •Embolectomy
  Indications:
  - •Cardiac arrest due to pulmonary embolism is an indication for immediate thoracotomy
  - •Pulmonary embolism→
    - ∘Hemodynamic compromise despite thrombolytic therapy
  - •Thrombolytic therapy is contraindicated
  Procedure:
  - •Surgical, via either:
    - ∘Intravascular catheter
    - ∘Thoracotomy

PROGNOSIS
- •≤50% mortality if hemodynamically unstable
- •Of patients who die of pulmonary embolism:
  - ∘80% die during the first several hours
  - ∘20% die due to recurrent emboli, usually within 2weeks
- •Recurrent thromboembolism mediated pulmonary hypertension–0.5%

PROPHYLAXIS
- •Graduated elastic compression stockings=thromboembolic deterrent–TED stockings
  Mechanism:
  - •↑Venous flow by providing 18mmHg distal leg pressure @ the ankle, w/ graduated ↓proximal pressure to 8mmHg @ the thigh
- •Intermittent pneumatic compression stockings
  Mechanisms:
  - •↑Venous flow by providing 35mmHg distal leg pressure @ the ankle, w/ a proximal pressure of 20mmHg @ the thigh
  - •Vascular compression→
    - ∘↑Systemic fibrinolysis

200

ANTICOAGULATION MEDIATED PROPHYLAXIS

MEDICAL PROPHYLAXIS

Disease	Preferred prophylactic method
Limited mobility	•Enoxaparin 40mg SC q24hours •Low dose Heparin 5000units SC q12hours

SURGICAL PROPHYLAXIS

Surgery	Preferred prophylactic method
Hip or knee replacement	•Enoxaparin 30mg SC q12h, starting 12h post-op X 2weeks •Fondaparinux 2.5mg SC q24h, starting 6h post-op X 10days
Thoraco–abdomino–pelvic surgery	
•Without malignancy	•Enoxaparin 40mg SC q24h, starting 2h pre-op X 12days •Dalteparin 2,500units SC q24h, starting 2h pre-op X 10days •Low dose Heparin 5000units SC q12h, starting 2h pre-op X10days
•With malignancy	•Dalteparin 5,000units SC q24h, starting the evening prior to surgery X 10days •Low dose Heparin 5000units SC q8h, starting 2h pre-op X 10 days
Neurosurgery	•Pneumatic compression stockings
Prostate surgery	•Pneumatic compression stockings
Major trauma	•Enoxaparin 30mg SC q12hours, starting 12hours post-trauma, if hemodynamically stable

OTHER PROPHYLAXIS

Condition	Preferred prophylactic method
Paralysis	•Enoxaparin 30mg SC q12hours
Prophylaxis during pregnancy	•Enoxaparin 40mg SC q24hours •Dalteparin 5,000units SC q24hours •Low dose Heparin 5,000units SC q12hours
Long term central venous catheterization	•Warfarin 1mg q24hours
↑Risk patient on long airplane flight (>10hours)	•Enoxaparin 1mg/kg SC X 1dose 4hours prior to flight

201

CHRONIC OBSTRUCTIVE PULMONARY DISEASE–COPD

•Chronic, intermittently symptomatic airways inflammation→tissue damage→
  ◦**Chronic, incompletely reversible airflow obstruction**
Statistics:
  •Affects 15.5million persons in the U.S.→
    ◦**#4 cause of mortality in the U.S.**
    ◦#6 cause of mortality worldwide

RISK FACTORS

•**Cigarette smoking–90%** (active & passive="secondhand")
  ◦**Only 15% of smokers develop COPD,** esp. those w/:
    –Gender: ♂ > ♀, reflecting the greater prevalence of smoking
    –Family history of COPD
    –↓Socioeconomic status
    –↓Birth weight
    –Air pollution exposure
•**Asthma**
•**α1–antitrypsin deficiency–2%,** being an autosomal recessive disease→
  ◦↓Hepatocyte α1–antiprotease†, w/ plasma levels <10% of normal→
    –Relatively ↑protease activity→premature emphysema, esp. if the patient smokes

---

†An enzyme which normally protects organs (esp. the lungs & liver) from proteolytic digestion by inflammation mediated leukocyte cytokine release, esp. elastases & proteases

CLASSIFICATION

•Patients usually have a composite of chronic obstructive pulmonary diseases:
  ◦**Chronic bronchitis**
    –**Cough, being productive of mucus on most days for ≥3 months X ≥2 consecutive years,** not resulting from another identifiable cause
  ◦**Emphysema†**
    –Destruction of alveolar septa & pulmonary connective tissue→↑air spaces & bronchiole collapsibility
  ◦**Intrinsic asthma**
  ◦**Bronchiectasis**

---

†Not a clinical diagnosis, as is only diagnosed by pulmonary function testing or histology

DIAGNOSIS

Pulmonary
•Tracheobronchial inflammation→
  ◦**Cough**
  ◦**Edema**
  ◦**Mucus congestion** ± plugging of the small airways
  ◦**Loss of supporting connective tissue**
  …→chronic, incompletely reversible airways obstruction→
      •**Expiratory wheezing,** esp. on forced expiration
      •Bronchoalveolar air trapping→
        ◦Alveolar hypoventilation
        ◦Connective tissue loss→**enlarged, thin–walled air spaces, termed bullae**→
          –↑**Thoracic anteroposterior diameter**
          –Clavicle elevation
          –**Diaphragm flattening**
          …→↑breathing effort, as the patient must overcome progressive lung expansion to initiate a breath
              •Difficulty breathing=**dyspnea**→
                ◦Respiratory rate >16/ min.=**tachypnea**
                ◦Accessory muscle usage (sternocleidomastoid muscles for inspiration & abdominal muscles for expiration)
                ◦Speech frequently interrupted by inspiration=telegraphic speech
                ◦Pursed lip breathing &/or grunting expirations→positive end–expiratory pressure–PEEP
                ◦Paradoxical abdominal motion: Negative intrathoracic pressure→fatigued diaphragm being pulled into the thorax→inspiratory inward motion of the anterior abdominal wall, rather than expected outward motion due to diaphragmatic contraction

202

∘Ventilation/ perfusion mismatch via:
 −↑Alveolar dead space: Alveolar ventilation through relatively underperfused capillaries
 −↑Vascular shunting†: Capillary blood flow through relatively underventilated alveoli.
 Usually occurring, or exacerbated via ↑venous return
 …→↓diffusion of O_2 & CO_2→
  •Hypoxemia (SaO_2 ≤ 91% or PaO_2 ≤ 60mmHg‡) on room air, w/ subsequent
  hypercapnia ($PaCO_2$ ≥45mmHg) due to either:
   ∘Respiratory muscle fatigue
   ∘Alveolar hypoventilation
  …as CO_2 clearance is unimpaired (& may be ↑in the dyspneic patient) as long
  as adequate ventilation (including lack of diffuse severe ventilation/ perfusion
  mismatching) is maintained, as:
   •CO_2 diffuses 20X as rapidly as O_2
   •Hypercapnia→
    ∘Immediate brain stem respiratory center mediated stimulation of
    pulmonary ventilation, which may correct the hypercapnia, but not
    necessarily the hypoxia

---

†Being exacerbated by the supine position→
 •↑Systemic venous return→
  ∘↑Vascular shunting→↑dyspnea, being termed:
   −Orthopnea, if persistent
   −Paroxysmal nocturnal dyspnea if intermittent
  …causing the patient to either use multiple pillows or sleep in a chair
‡Age adjusted normal PaO_2 = 101 − (0.43 X age)

COMPARATIVE THORACIC EXAMINATION FINDINGS			
Physical examination	Consolidation/ empyema	Pleural effusion	Pneumothorax†
Chest expansion	⬇	⬇	⬇‡
Auscultation	⬇Breath sounds w/ crackles, rhonchi, wheezes, &/or egophony°		⬇Breath sounds
Percussion	⬇	⬇	⬆^
Tactile or auscultatory fremitus	⬆n	⬇	⬆⬇

Note: Outlining lung compression by all 3 etiologies→
     •Atelectasis→
       ∘Signs of consolidation
†If via bronchopleural fistula, may be accompanied by:
 •Hemothorax (a pleural effusion)
 •Pyothorax=empyema
‡Loss of intrapleural negative pressure→
 •Ipsilateral chest wall expansion→
  ∘↑Anteroposterior diameter→
   −↓Respiratory movement
°A patients verbalization of the sound 'E' is heard as 'A'
^Best detected over the midclavicle w/ the patient sitting or standing. The ipsilateral ↓breath sounds
should guide you, as otherwise, you may be fooled by the contralateral side being relatively dull to
percussion, assuming it to be the diseased lung
nUnless accompanied by a concomitant pleural effusion

Cardiovascular
 •↓Heart sounds, as the lungs envelop the heart
  ∘Usually heard best at the subxiphoid area, as diaphragmatic flattening→
   −Downward cardiac displacement
 •Hypoxemia (SaO_2 ≤ 91% or PaO_2 ≤ 60mmHg)→
  ∘**Dysrhythmias**
  ∘Reflex pulmonary arteriole vasoconstriction, in order to ↓ventilation/ perfusion mismatch, which,
   when chronic→**pulmonary hypertension**†→↑right ventricular pressure→**right ventricular
   hypertrophy**, being termed **cor pulmonale** when due to primary lung disease (COPD being the #1
   cause)→
    −Right ventricular heave→a palpable lift over the left sternal border
    −Tricuspid regurgitation murmur
    −↑**Pulmonic component of the 2nd heart sound**
    −**Right sided heart failure**

†Indicates limited cardiopulmonary reserve via either:
- •Underlying heart failure
- •Underlying chronic obstructive pulmonary disease–COPD
- •Massive or recurrent pulmonary embolism→
  - ◦Cor pulmonale

Hematologic
- •Chronic hypoxemia→
  - ◦Compensatory ↑renal erythropoietin production→
    - –↑Bone marrow erythrocyte production→secondary polycythemia (hematocrit ♂ ≥52%, ♀ ≥48%)
- •**Plasma electrophoresis**
  Indications:
  - •Suspected α1–antitrypsin deficiency in the following patients:
    - ◦Symptomatic non–smokers
    - ◦Symptomatic smokers @ age <50years

IMAGING

- •**Chest x ray**
  Findings:
  - •Lung hyperinflation→
    - ◦Flattened diaphragm (w/ the right dome being ≤7th rib)→
      - –Downwardly displaced & narrowed cardiac silhouette (w/ the cardiac diameter being <11.5cm)
      - –↑Costophrenic & sternophrenic angles (w/ the retrosternal space being >4.4cm)
      - –↓Vascular markings, also being due to alveolar capillary loss
  - •Connective tissue loss→
    - ◦Enlarged, thin walled airspaces=bullae
  - •**Cigarette smoke or pollution**→
    - ◦Pulmonary inflammation @ the **apex > base**, following the relative distribution of inhaled air
  - •**α1–antitrypsin deficiency**→
    - ◦Pulmonary inflammation @ the **base > apex**, following the relative distribution of blood flow

ELECTRICAL STUDIES

- •**Electrocardiogram–ECG**
  - •Air trapping→
    - ◦↑Thoracic antero–posterior diameter, causing the lungs to envelop the heart→
      - –↓Electrical current conduction→↓**voltage**†
  - •Right ventricular hypertension→
    - ◦Right ventricular strain pattern via inverted T waves in leads V1–V4

  Evidence of Cor pulmonale
  - •Right ventricular myocardial hypertrophy→
    - ◦↑Depolarization time→
      - –Axis deviation toward the hypertrophied right ventricle=**right axis deviation** (> +90°)
  - •Right sided heart failure→
    - ◦↑Right atrial pressure→
      - –Right atrial dilation→**p pulmonale**‡

---

†Low voltage criteria being either:
- •Peak to peak QRS complex <5mm in the limb leads (I, II, III, aVR, aVL, aVF)
- •Peak to peak QRS complex <10mm in the precordial leads (V1–V6)
‡P pulmonale criteria being either:
- •P wave ≥2.5mv in lead II
- •Initial portion of a biphasic p wave ≥2mv in lead V1

PULMONARY FUNCTION TESTING–PFT

- •The forced expiratory volume in the 1st second of forceful exhalation–**FEV1** is the most important variable in determining disease severity & prognosis, as it has been shown to predict long term mortality from all causes. It is normally 80% of the entire amount exhaled, termed the forced vital capacity–FVC
  - ◦Normal FVC values: ♂ 4.6L, ♀ 3.7L
  - ◦Normal FEV1 values: ♂ 3.7L, ♀ 3L
- •The diffusion capacity of carbon monoxide–**DLCO** is ↓w/ emphysema, being normal w/ other chronic obstructive pulmonary diseases

Monitoring disease progression:
- **FEV1** is used to monitor disease progression, w/:
  - ∘Normal aging→
    - −↓FEV1 of 30mL/ year, beginning @ age 30years
  - ∘**Smoking in a susceptible patient**→
    - −↓FEV1 of 60−90mL/ year, w/ smoking cessation→normal FEV1 loss from that point

Clinical correlations of FEV1:
- •≤60% predicted value ($\male$ ≤~2.2L, $\female$ ≤~1.8L)→
  - ∘**Exertional dyspnea**
- •≤30% predicted value ($\male$ ≤~1.1L, $\female$ ≤~0.9L)→
  - ∘**Dyspnea on activities of daily living**, leading many to finally stop smoking

CHRONIC TREATMENT

- •**Smoking cessation** via smoking cessation clinic
  - ∘Cigarette smoking contributes to 20% of deaths in the U.S., & is the #1 modifiable cause of premature death
- •**Exercise**
  - ∘An enjoyable form of aerobic exercise on a regular basis (≥3X/ week) for 20−30min., preceded by stretching
  - ∘Reassure both the patient & family that exertional dyspnea is not dangerous
- •**Pulmonary rehabilitation**
  - Outcomes in patients w/ severe COPD:
    - •↓Dyspnea
    - •↑Exercise capacity
    - •↑Quality of life
    - •↓Frequency & duration of hospitalization related to pulmonary disease
- •**Intravenous enzyme replacement if deficient in α1−antitrypsin**

- •Anticholinergic & β_2 selective receptor agonist medications relieve bronchospasm (w/ **combination treatment being more efficacious than either used alone**), but not the underlying bronchopulmonary inflammation→
  - ∘↑Parenchymal damage if not treated as well
- •The medications are available in several possible forms:
  - ∘Metered dose inhaler−MDI
  - ∘Dry powder inhaler−DPI
  - ∘Nebulizer

INHALED GLUCOCORTICOIDS				
Generic (Trade)	M ♀	Dose	Start	
Beclomethasone (Vanceril)	L ?	80µg	2 inhalations/ 24hours	
Budesonide (Pulmicort)	L ?	200µg	2 inhalations/ 24hours	
Flunisolide (Aerobid)	L ?	250µg	2 inhalations/ 24hours	
Fluticasone (Flovent)	L ?			
•MDI		220µg	1 inhalation/ 24hours	
•DPI		250µg	1 inhalation/ 24hours	

- •Chronic treatment w/ inhaled glucocorticoids has not been shown to ↑osteoporosis or bone fracture risk

β_2 SELECTIVE RECEPTOR AGONISTS: Long acting			
Generic (Trade)	M ♀	Dose	Start
Salmeterol (Serevent)	L ?		
•MDI		25µg	2 q12hours
•DPI		50µg	1 q12hours
Formoterol DPI (Foradil)	L ?	12µg	1 q12hours

Onset: 15min.

Additional mechanism:
- •↓Bacterial adhesion to airway epithelial cells→
  - ∘↓Infection risk

•**Oxygen** to maintain SaO_2 >92% or PaO_2 >60mmHg at rest & exertion, usually accomplished via nasal cannula @ 2–4L/ min.
  Indications:
    •Hypoxemia (SaO_2 ≤ 91% or PaO_2 ≤ 60mmHg)
  Dose adjustment:
    •As hypoxemia may worsen during air travel, a general recommendation is to ↑oxygen flow rate by 2L/ min. during flight
  Mechanism:
    •Continuous† (≥18h/ day) low flow oxygen treatment via nasal cannula→
      ∘↓Formation or progression of cor pulmonale
  Outcomes:
    •**The only medication shown to ↑survival**
  Side effects:
    •↓Brainstem respiratory center hypoxemic drive→
      ∘↓Ventilation→**hypercapnic respiratory failure**→$PaCO_2$ >55mmHg (normal 35–45mmHg)→ respiratory acidemia→
        −Altered mental status
        −Dysrhythmia
        −Seizures

---

†Patients must understand that the medication is not used to treat dyspnea, & thus is not to be reserved for symptomatic treatment

ALTERNATE/ ADDITIONAL TREATMENT

β₂ SELECTIVE RECEPTOR AGONISTS: Long acting

Generic	M ♀	Start	Max
Albuterol	L ?		
•XR form		4mg PO q12hours	16mg q12hours

METHYLXANTHINES

Generic	M ♀	Start	Max
Theophylline	L ?		
•XR form		300mg PO/ 24hours	900mg/ 24hours

Mechanism:
  •Both bronchodilatory & anti–inflammatory activity

Side effects: Dose related & may occur @ therapeutic levels
  General
    •Anorexia
    •Anxiety
    •Headache
    •Insomnia
    •Tremors
  Cardiovascular
    •Atrial dysrhythmias
    •Hypotension
    •Tachycardia
  Gastrointestinal
    •Diarrhea
    •Nausea ± vomiting
    •Gastroesophageal reflux disease–GERD
  Neurologic
    •Altered mental status
  Hematologic
    •Hypokalemia

Overdose @ plasma level >20µg/ L:
  •**Coma**
  •**Seizures**
  •**Ventricular dysrhythmias**

Monitoring:
  •Check plasma Theophylline concentration
    ∘8hours after am QD–XR dose
    ∘5hours after am BID–XR dose
    …which should be maintained at **10–15µg/ mL as overdose may be lethal, & without side effects**

ANTIDOTES			
Generic	M	♀	Dose
Charcoal	Ø	S	20g PO q2hours, w/ every other dose given concomitantly w/ 75mL of 70% Sorbitol in order to ↑gastrointestinal transit time

Charcoal or resin hemoperfusion
- Preferred to **hemodialysis** (peritoneal dialysis does not ↑Theophylline clearance)

Indications:
- Severe complication(s)
- Plasma level >60µg/ mL

Charcoal mechanism:
- Theophylline removal from the body by way of the gastrointestinal mucosa

THIRD LINE TREATMENT ▄▄▄▄▄▄▄▄▄▄▄▄▄▄▄▄▄▄▄▄▄▄▄▄▄▄▄▄▄▄
- **Lung volume reduction surgery**

Procedure:
- Removal of the most severely affected lung segment(s)→
  - ↓Hyperinflation

Outcomes:
- ↑FEV1
- ↑Exercise capacity
- ↑Respiratory muscle function
- ↑Quality of life
- ↓Total lung capacity .
- ↓Functional residual capacity
- Overall mortality unaffected
  - ↓Mortality in patients w/ predominantly upper lobe emphysema & ↓exercise tolerance
  - ↑Mortality in patients w/ either:
    - FEV1 ≤20% of the predicted normal value & homogenous emphysema
    - DLCO ≤20% of the predicted normal value

- **Lung transplantation**
  - Chronic obstructive pulmonary disease–COPD is the #1 cause of lung transplantation referrals

Procedure:
- Single or double lung transplantation

Indications: Any of the following:
- FEV_1 <25% of the predicted normal value after the administration of a bronchodilator
- $PaCO_2$ ≥55mmHg
- Pulmonary hypertension syndrome

Outcomes:
- 20–50% ↑FEV1
- The 1, 3, & 5 year post–transplantation survival rates are 80%, 60%, & 40% respectively

PROGNOSIS
- **50% of patients die within 10years after diagnosis due to cor pulmonale→**
  - **Cardiopulmonary failure**
- Patients w/ a FEV1 <1L have a median 5 year survival of 50%

Major causes of exacerbations:
- **Pulmonary infections**
- **Air pollution**
- **Atelectasis**
- **Left sided heart failure**
- **Pneumothorax**
  - ∘COPD→
    - −↑Risk of thoracentesis mediated pneumothorax
- **Pulmonary embolism**

PEAK EXPIRATORY FLOW RATES–PEFR FOR HEALTHY ADULTS

•If the patient is unsure of their best peak expiratory flow rate (in L/ min.), then use the following table to help classify exacerbation severity

Height (inches):	5'=60"		5' 5"=65"		5'10"=70"		6'=72"		6'5"=78"	
Age (years)	♂	♀	♂	♀	♂	♀	♂	♀	♂	♀
20	555	425	600	460	650	495	670	510	725	550
25	545	420	590	455	635	490	655	505	710	545
30	530	415	580	450	620	485	640	495	690	540
35	520	410	565	440	610	475	625	490	680	530
40	510	405	550	435	595	470	610	485	665	525
45	500	400	540	430	580	465	600	475	650	515
50	490	390	530	425	570	460	585	470	635	510
55	475	385	515	420	555	450	570	465	620	500
60	465	380	500	410	540	445	560	455	605	495
65	450	375	490	405	530	440	545	450	590	490
70	440	370	480	400	515	430	530	445	575	480

MILD EXACERBATION

Criteria: Both:
- **Symptoms only during physical activity**
- •Peak expiratory flow rate–PEFR >80% predicted or personal best

Outpatient action:
- •Patients should promptly take the following medications as either:
  - ∘**2–4 inhalations X 3**
  - ∘**Nebulizer treatment q20min. X 3**
  - …or until the exacerbation resolves, w/ subsequent treatment q4h for 24–48hours, & contact physician for follow up instructions
- •If taking inhaled glucocorticoid treatment, double the dose for 10days

ANTICHOLINERGIC MEDICATIONS			
Generic (Trade)	**M ♀**	**Duration**	
Ipratropium (Atrovent)	L	P	5hours

&

β₂ SELECTIVE RECEPTOR AGONISTS: Short acting			
Generic (Trade)	**M ♀**	**Duration**	
Albuterol (Ventolin)	L	?	5hours

Onset: ~5min.
•Patients must have access to this medication regardless of the use of chronic agents, as **anticholinergic medications are of slower onset**

MODERATE EXACERBATION

Criteria: Either:
- **Symptoms at rest**
- •Peak expiratory flow rate–PEFR 50–80% predicted or personal best

Outpatient action:
- •As for mild exacerbation, & **proceed to a nearby emergency department**

SEVERE EXACERBATION

Criteria: Either:
- Syndrome
  - Inspiratory wheezing
  - Accessory muscle use
  - Paradoxical abdominal motion
  - Pulse >120/ min.
  - Hypoxemia
  - Pulsus paradoxus
- Pulmonary function
  - Peak expiratory flow rate–PEFR <50% predicted or personal best

Outpatient action:
- As for mild exacerbation, & **call 911, as CO_2 retention usually occurs @ PEFR <25%**

Inpatient action:
- **Oxygen** to maintain SaO_2 >92% or PaO_2 >60mmHg
  - Side effects:
    - ↓Brainstem respiratory center hypoxemic drive→
      - ↓Ventilation→**hypercapnic respiratory failure**→$PaCO_2$ >55mmHg (normal 35–45mmHg)→ respiratory acidemia→
        - Altered mental status
        - Dysrhythmia
        - Seizures
  - Monitoring:
    - Draw an arterial blood gas panel 30min. after initiation of oxygen treatment
      - If adequate oxygenation cannot be maintained, then invasive mechanical ventilation is needed
- **Intravenous hydration**
  - As the patient is likely dehydrated due to poor intake &/or respiratory losses
  - ↓Pulmonary mucus viscosity→
    - Easier expectoration→↓mucus plugging
- **Empiric antibiotic treatment** X 5–10 days as per the pneumonia section
  - Gram stain & sputum culture are usually not necessary unless there is evidence of pneumonia or resistant infection
- **Do not use mucolytic agents** such as Acetylcysteine (Mucomyst), as they may→
  - Mucosal irritation→
    - ↑Bronchospasm

β$_2$ SELECTIVE RECEPTOR AGONISTS: Short acting		
Generic (Trade) M ♀	**Dose**	
Albuterol (Ventolin) L ?		
• Nebulizer	5mg q20min. X 3, then	
	5–10mg q1–4hours prn or 10–15mg/ hour **continuous**	
• MDI + spacer device†	4–8 inhalations q20min. X3, then	
	q1–6hours prn	

†Equivalent efficacy to noncontinuous nebulizer treatment

ANTICHOLINERGIC MEDICATIONS		
Generic (Trade) M ♀	**Dose**	
Ipratropium (Atrovent) L P		
• Nebulizer	0.5mg q20min. X 3, then	
	q1–4hours prn	
• MDI + spacer device†	4–8 inhalations q20min. X 3, then	
	q1–6hours prn	

†Equivalent efficacy to noncontinuous nebulizer treatment

SYSTEMIC GLUCOCORTICOID TREATMENT			
Generic	M ♀	Dose	
Methylprednisolone	L ?	60mg PO/ IV q6hours X 3days, then q24hours X 1week	
Prednisolone	L ?	60mg PO/ IV q6hours X 3days, then q24hours X 1week	
Prednisone	L ?	60mg PO q6hours X 3days, then q24hours X 1week	

•Once disease control is achieved, switch to inhaled therapy
•If the total duration of systemic glucocorticoid therapy is ≤2weeks, there is no need to taper
•Both the IV & PO routes have equal efficacy
•There is no advantage in administering very high or more frequent dosing of glucocorticoids

	Relative potencies			
Glucocorticoids	Anti-inflammatory	Mineralocorticoid	Duration	Dose equiv.
Cortisol (physiologic†)	1	1	10hours	20mg
Cortisone (PO)	0.7	2	10hours	25mg
Hydrocortisone (PO, IM, IV)	1	2	10hours	20mg
Methylprednisolone (PO, IM, IA, IV)	5	0.5	15-35hours	5mg
Prednisone (PO)	5	0.5	15-35hours	5mg
Prednisolone (PO, IM, IV)	5	0.8	15-35hours	5mg
Triamcinolone (PO, IM)	5	~0	15-35hours	5mg
Betamethasone (PO, IM, IA)	25	~0	35-70hours	0.75mg
Dexamethasone (PO)	25	~0	35-70hours	0.75mg
Fludrocortisone (PO)	10	125	10hours	

†The physiologic rate of adrenal cortical cortisol production is 20-30mg/ 24hours

Side effects of chronic use:
General
  •Anorexia→
    ∘Cachexia
  •↑Perspiration
Cardiovascular
  •Mineralocorticoid effects→
    ∘↑Renal tubular NaCl & water retention as well as potassium secretion→
      –**Hypertension**
      –**Edema**
      –**Hypokalemia**
  •Counter-regulatory=anti-insulin effects→
    ∘↑Plasma glucose→
      –**Secondary diabetes mellitus**, which may→ketoacidemia
    ∘Hyperlipidemia→↑atherosclerosis→
      –**Coronary artery disease**
      –Cerebrovascular disease
      –Peripheral vascular disease
Cutaneous/ subcutaneous
  •↓Fibroblast function→
    ∘↓Intercellular matrix production→
      –↑Bruisability→ecchymoses
      –Poor wound healing
      –Skin striae
  •Androgenic effects→
    ∘Acne
    ∘↑Facial hair
    ∘Thinning scalp hair
  •Fat redistribution from the extremities to the:
    ∘Abdomen→
      –Truncal obesity
    ∘Shoulders→
      –Supraclavicular fat pads
    ∘Upper back→
      –Buffalo hump
    ∘Face→
      –Moon facies
    …w/ concomitant thinning of the arms & legs
Endocrine
  •**Adrenal failure** upon abrupt discontinuation after 2weeks

210

Gastrointestinal
- Inhibition of phospholipase A_2 mediated conversion of cell membrane lipids to arachidonic acid, which is the precursor for both cyclooxygenase–COX enzymes, w/ the cyclooxygenase–COX1 enzyme found in most cells of the body, responsible for normal physiologic function. Inhibition of the cyclooxygenase–COX1 enzyme→↑peptic inflammatory disease risk→↑**upper gastrointestinal hemorrhage risk** via:
  - ∘↓Gastric mucosal prostaglandin synthesis→
    - –↓Epithelial cell proliferation
    - –↓Mucosal blood flow→↓bicarbonate delivery to the mucosa
    - –↓Mucus & bicarbonate secretion from gastric mucosal cells

Musculoskeletal
- **Avascular necrosis of bone**
- **Osteoporosis**
- Proximal muscle weakness

Neurologic
- Anxiety
- Insomnia
- Psychosis

Opthalmologic
- **Cataracts**

Immunologic
- Inhibition of phospholipase A_2 mediated conversion of cell membrane lipids to arachidonic acid, which is the precursor for both cyclooxygenase–COX enzymes (COX1 & COX2) being responsible for the production of neuronal & inflammatory cell prostaglandins respectively→
  - –↓Pain
  - –↓Temperature (antipyretic)
  - –↓**Inflammation**
- Stabilization of lisosomal & cell membranes→
  - ∘↓Cytokine & proteolytic enzyme release
- ↓Lymphocyte & eosinophil production
  ...all→
  - **Immunosuppression**→
    - –↑**Infection** &/or neoplasm risk

Hematologic
- ↑Erythrocyte production→
  - ∘Polycythemia
- ↑Neutrophil demargination→
  - ∘Neutrophilia→
    - –**Leukocytosis**

SECOND LINE TREATMENT

METHYLXANTHINES

Generic	M ♀	Start	Max
Theophylline	L ?		
•XR form		300mg PO/ 24hours	900mg/ 24hours

Indications for assisted ventilation:
- **Severe hypoxemic respiratory failure**
  - ∘PaO_2 <55mmHg (normal >60mmHg) on 100% O_2 via a non–rebreathing mask
- **Severe hypercapnic respiratory failure**
  - ∘$PaCO_2$ >55mmHg (normal 35–45mmHg)→
    - –Respiratory acidemia
- **Respiratory distress** (respiratory rate >35/ min., accessory muscle use, or paradoxical abdominal motion) or **shock**
  - ∘In order to ↓breathing work, which can account for 50% of total O_2 consumption
- **Airways protection**
  - ∘Patients w/ a condition that predisposes to aspiration via ↓cough reflex:
    - –Altered mental status
    - –Dysphagia
    - –Neurologic deficits
- **Pulmonary toilet**
  - ∘Prevention &/or reversal of atelectasis
- **Pulmonary procedure**
  - ∘Allows for sedation or neuromuscular blockade

- •↑Intracranial pressure
  - ○Hyperventilation→
    - −↓Cerebral blood flow
- •Thoracic stabilization
  - ○Massive flail chest

Outcomes of mask mediated ventilation during a COPD exacerbation†:
- •Successful in adequately ventilating 70% of patients→
  - ○↓In hospital mortality (30%→10%)
  - ○↓Need for intubation (75%→25%)
  - ○↓Length of hospital stay

Indications for switch to endotracheal intubation:
- •Worsening, or lack of improvement within 1 hour

Contraindications to mask mediated ventilation:
- •Apnea
- •Hemodynamic instability
  - ○Hypotension
- •Inability to tolerate the mask
- •↓Ability to protect the airway
  - ○Absent gag reflex
  - ○Altered mental status
  - ○Status epilepticus
  - ○Unconsciousness
  - ○Uncontrollable vomiting
- •↑Need for suctioning
  - ○Secretions >50mL/ hour
- •↓Skin−mask air seal
  - ○Abnormal facial anatomy
  - ○Beard (which should be shaved)

---

†Patient must be admitted to the intensive care unit to ensure close monitoring, w/ the ability for prompt endotracheal intubation if necessary

ADMISSION CRITERIA
- •Exacerbation which does not meet the criteria for mild exacerbation after 3hours of treatment
- •Any history of intensive care unit admission
- •Any history of intubation for exacerbation
- •Pneumothorax

ASTHMA

•A chronic, intermittently symptomatic, incompletely reversible airflow obstruction, being either:
  ○IgE–mediated, termed allergic or **extrinsic asthma**
  ○Non–IgE mediated, termed pseudoallergic or **intrinsic asthma**
  ...→histamine/ leukotriene based inflammation of the tracheobronchial tract→
    •**Bronchoconstriction** due to both:
      ○**Airways edema**
      ○**Smooth muscle contraction**
      ...→↓airflow & air trapping
Statistics:
  •Affects 5% of the U.S. population at some point in their lives, w/ acute exacerbations→
    ○>4000 deaths/ year
  •Is often present concomitantly w/ chronic bronchitis &/or emphysema

RISK FACTORS

•**Genetic**
  ○Family history of allergic disease

CLASSIFICATION

•Patients usually have both the extrinsic & intrinsic forms of asthma, & may not always experience a hypersensitivity reaction upon exposure to a known inciting agent

•**Extrinsic asthma–10%**
  ○Symptoms, **usually beginning in childhood**, are precipitated by **exposure to a specific allergen**, being an antigen which incites plasma cell IgE formation, w/ some binding to mast cell membrane IgE Fc receptors. Subsequent antigen exposure→
    –Cell membrane IgE mediated mast cell degranulation→an immediate phase hypersensitivity reaction, such as asthma, usually being accompanied by other hypersensitivity reactions, such as allergic rhinitis=hay fever, allergic dermatitis=eczema, &/or urticaria=hives
    –Cytokine mediated basophil & eosinophil degranulation→a late phase hypersensitivity reaction, occurring 4–6hours after exposure
Risk factors:
  •**Seasonal allergens**
    ○Grass, tree, &/or weed microspores, termed **pollens**, carried by the wind, insects, & animals
  •**Year long allergens, termed perennial**
    ○Warm blooded **animal dander**, being shedded skin &/or hair
    ○**Insect detritus**, being feces or decaying dead body parts, esp. of the:
      –Dust mite
      –Cockroach
    ○Mold spores
    ○Aspergillus sp. (esp. Aspergillus fumigatus) bronchial colonization→**allergic bronchopulmonary aspergillosis–ABPA** via:
      –Extrinsic allergic asthma
      –Pulmonary infiltrate w/ eosinophilia–PIE syndrome

•**Intrinsic asthma–90%**
  ○Symptoms, **usually beginning in adulthood**, are precipitated by exposure to various:
    –**Dusts**, esp. coffee, grain, soybeans, or wood
    –**Industrial chemicals**, esp. laundry detergents
    –**Irritants**, esp. cigarette &/or cigar smoke, perfumes, strong smells, air pollution, or gastroesophageal reflux disease–GERD
    –**Pulmonary infections**
    –**Exercise** via heat &/or water loss from the airways, esp. in cold &/or low humidity weather, occurring in asthmatics in general
    –**Nonsteroidal anti–inflammatory drugs–NSAIDs**, including Aspirin→inhibition of both cyclooxygenase enzymes (COX 1 & COX2)→↑lipoxygenase activity→↑leukotriene synthesis→ symptomatic asthma within 2hours of ingestion in 5% of asthmatics. Often being associated w/ an ↑incidence of sinusitis & nasal polyps, w/ the presence of all three being termed **Samter's triad** (♀ > ♂)
    –**Psychologic factors**
    ...all→unknown intrinsic factor mediated (non–IgE) hypersensitivity reaction, such as asthma, usually being accompanied by other hypersensitivity reactions, such as allergic rhinitis=hay fever, allergic dermatitis=eczema, &/or urticaria=hives

•Other
  ∘**β receptor blocker induced asthma** (esp. nonselective medications)
   Mechanism:
    •β_2 receptor blockade→
     ∘↑Vascular & organ smooth muscle contraction→
      −Bronchoconstriction, possibly being symptomatic in persons w/ chronic obstructive pulmonary
      diseases−COPD (asthma, emphysema, &/or chronic bronchitis)

DIAGNOSIS

Pulmonary
  •Mast cell degranulation→cytokine release, esp. histamine, leukotrienes, eosinophilic chemotactic
  factor, & bradykinin→tracheobronchial inflammation→
   ∘**Cough**
   ∘**Edema**
   ∘**Mucus congestion** ± plugging of the small airways
   ∘**Smooth muscle contraction**
   ...→chronic, incompletely reversible airways obstruction→
    •**Expiratory wheezing**, esp. on forced expiration
    •Bronchoalveolar air trapping→
     ∘Alveolar hypoventilation
     ∘↑Intra−alveolar pressure→
      −↑**Thoracic anteroposterior diameter**
      −Clavicle elevation
      −**Diaphragm flattening**
     ...→↑breathing effort, as the patient must overcome progressive lung expansion to initiate
     a breath
      •Difficulty breathing=**dyspnea**→
       ∘Respiratory rate >16/ min.=**tachypnea**
       ∘Accessory muscle usage (sternocleidomastoid muscles for inspiration &
       abdominal muscles for expiration)
       ∘Speech frequently interrupted by inspiration=telegraphic speech
       ∘Pursed lip breathing &/or grunting expirations→positive end−expiratory
       pressure−PEEP
       ∘Paradoxical abdominal motion: Negative intrathoracic pressure→fatigued
       diaphragm being pulled into the thorax→inspiratory inward motion of the anterior
       abdominal wall, rather than expected outward motion due to diaphragmatic
       contraction
     ∘Ventilation/ perfusion mismatch via:
      −↑Alveolar dead space: Alveolar ventilation through relatively underperfused capillaries
      −↑Vascular shunting†: Capillary blood flow through relatively underventilated alveoli.
      Usually occurring, or exacerbated via ↑venous return
      ...→↓diffusion of O_2 & CO_2→
       •Hypoxemia (SaO_2 ≤ 91% or PaO_2 ≤ 60mmHg‡) on room air, w/ subsequent
       hypercapnia ($PaCO_2$ ≥45mmHg) due to either:
        ∘Respiratory muscle fatigue
        ∘Alveolar hypoventilation
       ...as CO_2 clearance is unimpaired (& may be ↑in the dyspneic patient) as long
       as adequate ventilation (including lack of diffuse severe ventilation/ perfusion
       mismatching) is maintained, as:
        •CO_2 diffuses 20X as rapidly as O_2
        •Hypercapnia→
         ∘Immediate brain stem respiratory center mediated stimulation of
         pulmonary ventilation, which may correct the hypercapnia, but not
         necessarily the hypoxia

  Effects of chronic, inadequately controlled disease:
    •Asthmatics (even during the asymptomatic phase) have persistent airways inflammation→
     ∘Interstitial damage→
      −Fibrosis→emphysema

---

†Being exacerbated by the supine position→
  •↑Systemic venous return→
   ∘↑Vascular shunting→↑dyspnea, being termed:
    −Orthopnea, if persistent
    −Paroxysmal nocturnal dyspnea if intermittent
    ...causing the patient to either use multiple pillows or sleep in a chair

‡Age adjusted normal PaO_2 = 101 − (0.43 X age)

COMPARATIVE THORACIC EXAMINATION FINDINGS			
Physical examination	Consolidation/ empyema	Pleural effusion	Pneumothorax†
Chest expansion	⬇	⬇	⬇‡
Auscultation	⬇Breath sounds w/ crackles, rhonchi, wheezes, &/or egophony°		⬇Breath sounds
Percussion	⬇	⬇	⬆^
Tactile or auscultatory fremitus	⬆n	⬇	⬇

Note: Outlining lung compression by all 3 etiologies→
    •Atelectasis→
      ∘Signs of consolidation
†If via bronchopleural fistula, may be accompanied by:
    •Hemothorax (a pleural effusion)
    •Pyothorax=empyema
‡Loss of intrapleural negative pressure→
    •Ipsilateral chest wall expansion→
      ∘↑Anteroposterior diameter→
        −↓Respiratory movement
°A patients verbalization of the sound 'E' is heard as 'A'
^Best detected over the midclavicle w/ the patient sitting or standing. The ipsilateral ↓breath sounds
should guide you, as otherwise, you may be fooled by the contralateral side being relatively dull to
percussion, assuming it to be the diseased lung
nUnless accompanied by a concomitant pleural effusion

Hematologic
    •Intrinsic asthma component→
      ∘Eosinophilia (>500/ μL)

MICROSCOPY
•Sputum examination
Findings:
    •Charcot−Leyden crystals, composed of the crystallized enzyme, lisophospholipase, derived from
    eosinophil granules
    •Creola bodies, being aggregates of desquamated epithelial cells
    •Curschmann's spirals, being mucus casts of small airways

HYPERSENSITIVITY TESTING
Indications:
    •To test for extrinsic etiologies, via allergenic proteins available as commercial extracts. Be careful to
    keep anaphylaxis medications nearby in case of a severe reaction

•Skin testing
Procedure:
    •Intradermal injection of both the suspected allergen & saline control on the forearm or back
Interpretation:
    •Positive: Local allergen area urticaria within 30 min., w/ a nonreactive saline area

•Serologic testing
Procedure:
    1. Placement of the patients diluted serum over a solid phase carrier embedded w/ the suspected
    allergen
    2. Incubation, serum wash off, & subsequent addition of either radioactive or enzymatic (horseradish
    peroxidase) labeled anti−IgE antibody, allowing for Geiger counter detection or color visualization
    respectively, if the patients serum contains anti−allergen IgE

•**Avoidance of known precipitants**

•Anticholinergic & β_2 selective receptor agonist medications relieve bronchospasm (w/ **combination treatment being more efficacious than either used alone**), but not the underlying bronchopulmonary inflammation→

  ∘↑Parenchymal damage if not treated as well

•The medications are available in several possible forms:

  ∘Metered dose inhaler–MDI

  ∘Dry powder inhaler–DPI

  ∘Nebulizer

INHALED GLUCOCORTICOIDS				
Generic (Trade)	M	♀	Dose	Start
Beclomethasone (Vanceril)	L	?	80μg	2 inhalations/ 24hours
Budesonide (Pulmicort)	L	?	200μg	2 inhalations/ 24hours
Flunisolide (Aerobid)	L	?	250μg	2 inhalations/ 24hours
Fluticasone (Flovent)	L	?		
•MDI			220µg	1 inhalation/ 24hours
•DPI			250µg	1 inhalation/ 24hours

•Chronic treatment w/ inhaled glucocorticoids has not been shown to ↑osteoporosis or bone fracture risk

β_2 SELECTIVE RECEPTOR AGONISTS: Long acting				
Generic (Trade)	M	♀	Dose	Start
Salmeterol (Serevent)	L	?		
•MDI			25µg	2 q12hours
•DPI			50µg	1 q12hours
Formoterol DPI (Foradil)	L	?	12µg	1 q12hours

Onset: 15min.

Additional mechanism:
  •↓Bacterial adhesion to airway epithelial cells→
    ∘↓Infection risk

ALTERNATE/ ADDITIONAL ANTI–INFLAMMATORY TREATMENT

LEUKOTRIENE INHIBITORS			
Generic	M	♀	Dose
Montelukast (Singulair)	L	P	10mg PO qpm
Zafirlukast (Accolate)	L	P	20mg PO q12hours on an empty stomach

Side effects:
  Gastrointestinal
    •Nausea ± vomiting

MAST CELL STABILIZERS			
Generic (Trade)	M	♀	Dose
Cromolyn sodium (Gastrocrom)	LK	P	800μg @ 2–4 inhalations q6hours
Nedocromil (Tilade)	L	P	1.75mg @ 2 inhalations q6hours

Cromolyn sodium specific side effects:
  Mucocutaneous
    •Pharyngitis

Nedocromil specific side effects:
  Gastrointestinal
    •Altered taste=dysgeusia
  Pulmonary
    •Dysphonia

216

METHYLXANTHINES			
Generic M ♀	**Start**		**Max**
Theophylline L ?			
•XR form	300mg PO/ 24hours		900mg/ 24hours

Mechanism:
•Both bronchodilatory & anti-inflammatory activity

Side effects: Dose related & may occur @ therapeutic levels
General
  •Anorexia
  •Anxiety
  •Headache
  •Insomnia
  •Tremors
Cardiovascular
  •Atrial dysrhythmias
  •Hypotension
  •Tachycardia
Gastrointestinal
  •Diarrhea
  •Nausea ± vomiting
  •Gastroesophageal reflux disease–GERD
Neurologic
  •Altered mental status
Hematologic
  •Hypokalemia

Overdose @ plasma level >20µg/ L:
  •**Coma**
  •**Seizures**
  •**Ventricular dysrhythmias**

Monitoring:
•Check plasma Theophylline concentration
  ◦8hours after am QD–XR dose
  ◦5hours after am BID–XR dose
  …which should be maintained at **10–15µg/ mL** as **overdose may be lethal, & without side effects**

ANTIDOTES		
Generic M ♀		**Dose**
Charcoal Ø S		20g PO q2hours, w/ every other dose given concomitantly w/ 75mL of 70% Sorbitol in order to ↑gastrointestinal transit time

Charcoal or resin hemoperfusion
•Preferred to **hemodialysis** (peritoneal dialysis does not ↑Theophylline clearance)
Indications:
  •Severe complication(s)
  •Plasma level >60µg/ mL

Charcoal mechanism:
•Theophylline removal from the body by way of the gastrointestinal mucosa

SYSTEMIC GLUCOCORTICOID TREATMENT

Indications:
- •Severe disease, indicated by either of the following, if uncontrolled via inhaled glucocorticoid treatment
  - ◦Continuous symptoms
  - ◦Frequent exacerbations
  - ◦Frequent nocturnal symptoms
  - ◦Limited physical activity
  - ◦Hypoxemia ($SaO_2 \leq 91\%$ or $PaO_2 \leq 60mmHg$)
  - ◦$PaCO_2 > 42mmHg$
  - ◦FEV1 or PEFR ≤60% predicted

Generic	M ♀	Dose
Methylprednisolone	L ?	5–60mg PO q24–48hours
Prednisolone	L ?	5–60mg PO q24–48hours
Prednisone	L ?	5–60mg PO q24–48hours

•Once disease control is achieved, taper to the lowest effective maintenance dose in order to minimize serious side effects, w/ the goal of discontinuation if possible, w/ attention to relapse syndrome

	Relative potencies			
Glucocorticoids	Anti–inflammatory	Mineralocorticoid	Duration	Dose equiv.
Cortisol (physiologic†)	1	1	10hours	20mg
Cortisone (PO)	0.7	2	10hours	25mg
Hydrocortisone (PO, IM, IV)	1	2	10hours	20mg
Methylprednisolone (PO, IM, IA, IV)	5	0.5	15–35hours	5mg
Prednisone (PO)	5	0.5	15–35hours	5mg
Prednisolone (PO, IM, IV)	5	0.8	15–35hours	5mg
Triamcinolone (PO, IM)	5	~0	15–35hours	5mg
Betamethasone (PO, IM, IA)	25	~0	35–70hours	0.75mg
Dexamethasone (PO)	25	~0	35–70hours	0.75mg
Fludrocortisone (PO)	10	125	10hours	

†The physiologic rate of adrenal cortical cortisol production is 20–30mg/ 24hours

Side effects of chronic use:
General
- •Anorexia→
  - ◦Cachexia
- •↑Perspiration

Cardiovascular
- •Mineralocorticoid effects→
  - ◦↑Renal tubular NaCl & water retention as well as potassium secretion→
    - –**Hypertension**
    - –**Edema**
    - –**Hypokalemia**
- •Counter–regulatory=anti–insulin effects→
  - ◦↑Plasma glucose→
    - –**Secondary diabetes mellitus**, which may→ketoacidemia
  - ◦Hyperlipidemia→↑atherosclerosis→
    - –**Coronary artery disease**
    - –Cerebrovascular disease
    - –Peripheral vascular disease

Cutaneous/ subcutaneous
- •↓Fibroblast function→
  - ◦↓Intercellular matrix production→
    - –↑Bruisability→ecchymoses
    - –Poor wound healing
    - –Skin striae
- •Androgenic effects→
  - ◦Acne
  - ◦↑Facial hair
  - ◦Thinning scalp hair
- •Fat redistribution from the extremities to the:
  - ◦Abdomen→
    - –Truncal obesity
  - ◦Shoulders→
    - –Supraclavicular fat pads

218

  ∘Upper back→
   -Buffalo hump
  ∘Face→
   -Moon facies
  ...w/ concomitant thinning of the arms & legs
Endocrine
- **Adrenal failure** upon abrupt discontinuation after 2weeks

Gastrointestinal
- Inhibition of phospholipase A_2 mediated conversion of cell membrane lipids to arachidonic acid, which is the precursor for both cyclooxygenase–COX enzymes, w/ the cyclooxygenase–COX1 enzyme found in most cells of the body, responsible for normal physiologic function. Inhibition of the cyclooxygenase–COX1 enzyme→↑peptic inflammatory disease risk→↑**upper gastrointestinal hemorrhage risk** via:
  - ∘↓Gastric mucosal prostaglandin synthesis→
    - -↓Epithelial cell proliferation
    - -↓Mucosal blood flow→↓bicarbonate delivery to the mucosa
    - -↓Mucus & bicarbonate secretion from gastric mucosal cells

Musculoskeletal
- **Avascular necrosis of bone**
- **Osteoporosis**
- Proximal muscle weakness

Neurologic
- Anxiety
- Insomnia
- Psychosis

Opthalmologic
- **Cataracts**

Immunologic
- Inhibition of phospholipase A_2 mediated conversion of cell membrane lipids to arachidonic acid, which is the precursor for both cyclooxygenase–COX enzymes (COX1 & COX2) being responsible for the production of neuronal & inflammatory cell prostaglandins respectively→
  - -↓Pain
  - -↓Temperature (antipyretic)
  - -↓**Inflammation**
- Stabilization of lisosomal & cell membranes→
  - ∘↓Cytokine & proteolytic enzyme release
- ∘↓Lymphocyte & eosinophil production
  ...all→
  - **Immunosuppression**→
    - -↑**Infection** &/or neoplasm risk

Hematologic
- ↑Erythrocyte production→
  - ∘Polycythemia
- ↑Neutrophil demargination→
  - ∘Neutrophilia→
    - -**Leukocytosis**

Major causes of exacerbations:
- **Pulmonary infections**
- **Air pollution**
- **Atelectasis**
- **Left sided heart failure**
- **Pneumothorax**
- **Pulmonary embolism**

PEAK EXPIRATORY FLOW RATES-PEFR FOR HEALTHY ADULTS

- If the patient is unsure of their best peak expiratory flow rate (in L/ min.), then use the following table to help classify exacerbation severity

Height (inches):	5'=60"		5' 5"=65"		5'10"=70"		6'=72"		6'5"=78"	
Age (years)	♂	♀	♂	♀	♂	♀	♂	♀	♂	♀
20	555	425	600	460	650	495	670	510	725	550
25	545	420	590	455	635	490	655	505	710	545
30	530	415	580	450	620	485	640	495	690	540
35	520	410	565	440	610	475	625	490	680	530
40	510	405	550	435	595	470	610	485	665	525
45	500	400	540	430	580	465	600	475	650	515
50	490	390	530	425	570	460	585	470	635	510
55	475	385	515	420	555	450	570	465	620	500
60	465	380	500	410	540	445	560	455	605	495
65	450	375	490	405	530	440	545	450	590	490
70	440	370	480	400	515	430	530	445	575	480

MILD EXACERBATION ▬▬▬▬▬▬▬

Criteria: Both:
- **Symptoms only during physical activity**
- Peak expiratory flow rate-PEFR >80% predicted or personal best

Outpatient action:
- Patients should promptly take the following medications as either:
  - **2–4 inhalations X 3**
  - **Nebulizer treatment q20min. X 3**
  ...or until the exacerbation resolves, w/ subsequent treatment q4h for 24–48hours, & contact physician for follow up instructions
- If taking inhaled glucocorticoid treatment, double the dose for 10days

ANTICHOLINERGIC MEDICATIONS			
Generic (Trade)	M	♀	**Duration**
Ipratropium (Atrovent)	L	P	5hours

&

β₂ SELECTIVE RECEPTOR AGONISTS: Short acting			
Generic (Trade)	M	♀	**Duration**
Albuterol (Ventolin)	L	?	5hours

Onset: ~5min.
- Patients must have access to this medication regardless of the use of chronic agents, as **anticholinergic medications are of slower onset**

MODERATE EXACERBATION ▬▬▬▬▬▬▬

Criteria: Either:
- **Symptoms at rest**
- Peak expiratory flow rate-PEFR 50–80% predicted or personal best

Outpatient action:
- As for mild exacerbation, & **proceed to a nearby emergency department**

SEVERE EXACERBATION ▬▬▬▬▬

Criteria: Either:
- ∘Syndrome
  - –Inspiratory wheezing
  - –Accessory muscle use
  - –Paradoxical abdominal motion
  - –Pulse >120/ min.
  - –Hypoxemia
  - –Pulsus paradoxus
- ∘Pulmonary function
  - –Peak expiratory flow rate–PEFR <50% predicted or personal best

Outpatient action:
- •As for mild exacerbation, & **call 911, as CO$_2$ retention usually occurs @ PEFR <25%**

Inpatient action:
- •**Oxygen** to maintain SaO$_2$ >92% or PaO$_2$ >60mmHg
  - Side effects:
    - •↓Brainstem respiratory center hypoxemic drive→
      - ∘↓Ventilation→**hypercapnic respiratory failure**→PaCO$_2$ >55mmHg (normal 35–45mmHg)→ respiratory acidemia→
        - –Altered mental status
        - –Dysrhythmia
        - –Seizures
  - Monitoring:
    - •Draw an arterial blood gas panel 30min. after initiation of oxygen treatment
      - ∘If adequate oxygenation cannot be maintained, then invasive mechanical ventilation is needed
- •**Intravenous hydration**
  - ∘As the patient is likely dehydrated due to poor intake &/or respiratory losses
  - ∘↓Pulmonary mucus viscosity→
    - –Easier expectoration→↓mucus plugging
- •**Empiric antibiotic treatment** X 5–10 days as per the pneumonia section
  - ∘Gram stain & sputum culture are usually not necessary unless there is evidence of pneumonia or resistant infection
- •**Do not use mucolytic agents** such as Acetylcysteine (Mucomyst), as they may→
  - ∘Mucosal irritation→
    - –↑Bronchospasm

β$_2$ SELECTIVE RECEPTOR AGONISTS: Short acting			
Generic (Trade)	**M**	♀	**Dose**
Albuterol (Ventolin)	L	?	
•Nebulizer			5mg q20min. X 3, then
			5–10mg q1–4hours prn or 10–15mg/ hour **continuous**
•MDI + spacer device†			4–8 inhalations q20min. X3, then
			q1–6hours prn

†Equivalent efficacy to noncontinuous nebulizer treatment

ANTICHOLINERGIC MEDICATIONS			
Generic (Trade)	**M**	♀	**Dose**
Ipratropium (Atrovent)	L	P	
•Nebulizer			0.5mg q20min. X 3, then
			q1–4hours prn
•MDI + spacer device†			4–8 inhalations q20min. X 3, then
			q1–6h prn

†Equivalent efficacy to noncontinuous nebulizer treatment

SYSTEMIC GLUCOCORTICOID TREATMENT			
Generic	**M**	♀	**Dose**
Methylprednisolone	L	?	60mg PO/ IV q6hours X 3days, then q24hours X 1week
Prednisolone	L	?	60mg PO/ IV q6hours X 3days, then q24hours X 1week
Prednisone	L	?	60mg PO q6hours X 3days, then q24hours X 1week

- •Once disease control is achieved, switch to inhaled therapy
- •If the total duration of systemic glucocorticoid therapy is ≤2weeks, there is no need to taper

•Both the IV & PO routes have equal efficacy	
•There is no advantage in administering very high or more frequent dosing of glucocorticoids	

SECOND LINE TREATMENT
•**Heliox**, being a helium–oxygen mixture delivered via a non–rebreathing mask
  Mechanism:
    •Being that airways resistance in turbulent flow is directly related to the density of a gas, heliums low
    density (having the lowest density of any gas except hydrogen)→
      ∘↓Turbulent airflow→↓airways resistance→
      −↑Ventilation

†Helium is an inert element, being tasteless, odorless, & non–combustible

SYMPATHOMIMETIC MEDICATIONS			
Generic	M ♀	Dose	
Epinephrine	P ?	0.5mL of a 1/1000 solution=0.5mg SC/ IM q10min. prn or	
		5mL of a 1/10,000 solution=0.5mg IV slow push over 10min.	

Outcomes:
  •No advantage over inhaled β_2 selective receptor agonists

MAGNESIUM SULFATE		
M ♀	Dose	Max
K S	2g IV infusion over 20min. q1hour prn	8g total

Mechanism:
  •Vascular & organ smooth muscle relaxation→
    ∘Bronchodilation
    ∘Vasodilation
  •Anti–dysrhythmic
  •↓Platelet function

Side effects:
Pulmonary
  •Pulmonary edema
Neurologic
  •Magnesium sulfate→
    ∘Neuromuscular junction toxicity→
      −Plasma concentration dependent side effects as below

  Plasma $MgSO_4$ concentration effects (mg/ mL):
  •**8**→
    ∘Central nervous system depression
  •**10**→
    ∘Loss of deep tendon reflexes
  •**15**→
    ∘Respiratory depression (<10 breaths/ min.)
  •**17**→
    ∘Coma
  •**>20**→
    ∘Cardiac arrest

Monitoring:
  •Qhour for:
    ∘Altered mental status
    ∘↓Patellar reflexes
    ∘Respiratory depression
    ∘↓Urinary output, as ≤25mL/ hour requires ↓infusion dose

ANTIDOTE		
Generic	Dose	Max
10% Calcium chloride†	10mL (1 ampule) IV slow push over 3min. q5min. prn	
•Continuous infusion	0.3mEq/ hour	0.7mEq/ hour

Onset: 1–2 min., Duration: 30–60 min.

•Use cautiously in patients taking Digoxin, as hypercalcemia→
  ∘Digoxin cardiotoxicity
†Preferred to calcium gluconate, as it contains 3X more elemental calcium

Indications for assisted ventilation:
- **Severe hypoxemic respiratory failure**
  - PaO_2 <55mmHg (normal >60mmHg) on 100% O_2 via a non-rebreathing mask
- **Severe hypercapnic respiratory failure**
  - $PaCO_2$ >55mmHg (normal 35–45mmHg)→
    - −Respiratory acidemia
- **Respiratory distress** (respiratory rate >35/ min., accessory muscle use, or paradoxical abdominal motion) or **shock**
  - In order to ↓breathing work, which can account for 50% of total O_2 consumption
- **Airways protection**
  - Patients w/ a condition that predisposes to aspiration via ↓cough reflex:
    - −Altered mental status
    - −Dysphagia
    - −Neurologic deficits
- **Pulmonary toilet**
  - Prevention &/or reversal of atelectasis
- **Pulmonary procedure**
  - Allows for sedation or neuromuscular blockade
- **↑Intracranial pressure**
  - Hyperventilation→
    - −↓Cerebral blood flow
- **Thoracic stabilization**
  - Massive flail chest

Outcomes of mask mediated ventilation during a COPD exacerbation†:
- **Successful in adequately ventilating 70% of patients**→
  - ↓In hospital mortality (30%→10%)
  - ↓Need for intubation (75%→25%)
  - ↓Length of hospital stay

Indications for switch to endotracheal intubation:
- Worsening, or lack of improvement within 1 hour

Contraindications to mask mediated ventilation:
- **Apnea**
- **Hemodynamic instability**
  - Hypotension
- **Inability to tolerate the mask**
- **↓Ability to protect the airway**
  - Absent gag reflex
  - Altered mental status
  - Status epilepticus
  - Unconsciousness
  - Uncontrollable vomiting
- **↑Need for suctioning**
  - Secretions >50mL/ hour
- **↓Skin−mask air seal**
  - Abnormal facial anatomy
  - Beard (which should be shaved)

†Patient must be admitted to the intensive care unit to ensure close monitoring, w/ the ability for prompt endotracheal intubation if necessary

ADMISSION CRITERIA
- Exacerbation which does not meet the criteria for mild exacerbation after 3hours of treatment
- Any history of intensive care unit admission
- Any history of intubation for exacerbation
- Pneumothorax

ACUTE RESPIRATORY DISTRESS SYNDROME-ARDS

•Inflammation→
  ◦Cytokine mediated, **severe, diffuse pneumonitis**→
  -↑Permeability of the alveolar-capillary membranes→protein-rich pulmonary edema

RISK FACTORS

•**Direct lung injury**
  ◦**Aspiration of gastric contents**
  ◦**Pneumonia**
  ◦↑Altitude
  ◦Fat embolism
  ◦Inhalation injury
    -Irritant gas (ammonia, chloride, NO_2, SO_2)
    -Oxygen toxicity, occurring @ an FiO_2 >60%, being directly proportional to the degree & duration of treatment
    -Smoke
  ◦Near drowning
  ◦Pulmonary contusion
  ◦Radiation
  ◦Reperfusion pulmonary edema after either:
    -Lung transplantation
    -Pulmonary embolectomy
  ◦Venous air embolism

•**Indirect lung injury**
  ◦Systemic inflammatory response syndrome-SIRS
    -**Sepsis-40%**
  ◦**Severe non-thoracic trauma**
  ◦Blood product transfusion
  ◦Burns
  ◦Cardiopulmonary bypass
  ◦Disseminated intravascular coagulation-DIC
  ◦Drug overdose
  ◦↑Intracranial pressure
  ◦Pancreatitis
  ◦Shock

DIAGNOSIS

American-European Consensus Conference Criteria: All must be present:
1. **Acute onset of severe dyspnea**
2. **Bilateral infiltrative disease**
   •May be patchy or asymmetric
3. **Lack of left ventricular heart failure,** via either:
   •Lack of clinical syndrome
   •Pulmonary capillary wedge pressure (reflecting left atrial pressure) <18mmHg
4. **PaO_2 / FiO_2 < 200**

•Although not a criteria, the majority of patients have **hypoxemic respiratory failure refractory to** ↑**inspired O_2 concentration**

224

•**Treat the etiologic cause,** w/ considerable attention to possible infection

MECHANICAL VENTILATION ━━━━━━━━━━━━━━━━━━━━━━
•90% of patients who develop ARDS require mechanical ventilation within 3 days of the initiating insult
•**Lung protective ventilation** via:
  ◦**Inflation volume of 5–8mL/ kg** (which may need to be ↓to <5mL/ kg), a ventilatory strategy of intentional hypoventilation termed **permissive hypercapnia**†, in order to maintain a **plateau pressure‡ ≤35 cmH₂O**→
    –↓Barotrauma mediated inflammation
Goals
  •FiO₂ <60%→either:
    ◦SaO₂ >90%
    ◦PaO₂ >60%
Outcomes:
  •22%↓ mortality when compared to the previously used 12mL/ kg
  •↓Days requiring mechanical ventilation

Strategies to improve oxygenation:
  •The following strategies allow for the reduction of the inspired O₂ concentration→
    ◦↓O₂ toxicity
  •↑**Positive end–expiratory pressure–PEEP** of 5–10cm H₂O→
    ◦↓Compression atelectasis→
      –↑Oxygenation
    ◦↓Phasic bronchoalveolar collapse→
      –↓Pneumonitis
  •↑**Inspiratory time**
  •**Prone ventilation**
    ◦The prone position directs blood toward the ventral lung regions which are better aerated→
      –↓Right to left intrapulmonary shunt→↓ventilation perfusion mismatch→↑**oxygenation**
      –↑Cardiac output
      –↑Secretions clearance
Outcomes:
  •↑PaO₂ in 50–75% of patients
  •No mortality benefit
  •**Inhaled nitric oxide**→
    ◦Selective pulmonary vasodilation of ventilated alveoli→
      –↓Right to left intrapulmonary shunt→↓ventilation perfusion mismatch→↑**oxygenation**
Outcomes:
  •↓Pulmonary artery pressures
  •No mortality benefit
  •**Extracorporeal treatment**
    ◦Membrane oxygenation–ECMO
    ◦CO₂ removal–ECCO₂R

---

†In order to achieve a safe peak inspiratory pressure &/or plateau pressure. Tidal volume may need to be decreased to <5mL/ kg, a ventilatory strategy of intentional hypoventilation termed **permissive hypercapnia**, allowing for:
  •PaCO₂ <80mmHg
  •pH >7.2, w/ some infusing bicarbonate to minimize acidemia
Contraindications:
  •Cerebrovascular disease
  •Hemodynamic instability
  •Pulmonary hypertension
  •Renal failure
†Measurement of airways pressure at end–inspiration, prior to expiration, when there is no airflow, being determined by thoracic compliance alone (↓thoracic compliance→↑Pplat) as airways resistance is not a factor due to lack of airflow

PROGNOSIS

•**Mortality is 65%,** being mainly due to sepsis or multiple organ failure syndrome, rather than primary pulmonary disease
  ◦35% of deaths occur within 3 days, w/ most of the remaining deaths occurring within 2 weeks
  ◦↑Mortality risk†:
    −↑Age
    −Chronic liver disease
    −Extrapulmonary organ failure
    −Sepsis
•In most survivors, pulmonary function nearly normalizes within 1year, w/ any residual pulmonary abnormalities consisting of:
  ◦Obstruction
  ◦Restriction
  ◦↓Diffusing capacity for carbon monoxide
  …usually being asymptomatic, but possibly→
      •Pulmonary hypertension

---

†Surprisingly, initial indexes of oxygenation do not predict outcome

226

OBSTRUCTIVE SLEEP APNEA–OSA

•Sleep mediated oropharyngeal airways musculature relaxation→
◦Intermittent, recurrent, oropharyngeal obstruction, being terminated only by arousal (partial to complete)
Statistics:
•Affects 3% of persons age >40years in the U.S.

RISK FACTORS

•**Body habitus**
◦**Overweight/ obese** via ↑peri–oropharyngeal pressure, being the #1 cause
◦↑Neck circumference
•**Age:** 40–70years
•**Gender:** ♂ 2 X ♀, w/ ↑risk postmenopausally
•**Endocrine**
◦Acromegaly
◦Hypothyroidism
•**Sedative–hypnotic substances/ medications**
◦Ethanol
◦Barbiturates
◦Benzodiazepines
◦Histamine–1 receptor blockers
•**Altered oropharyngeal anatomy–8%**
◦Craniofacial abnormailities
◦Enlarged tonsils
◦Micrognathia, being an abnormally small maxillae &/or mandible
◦Retrognathia, in which the mandible is located posterior to its normal position relative to the maxillae

DIAGNOSIS

Pulmonary
•Partial obstruction→
◦**Snoring,** as reported by family &/or housemates
◦Markedly ↓tidal volume, termed hypopnea, defined as either:
  −↓Tidal volume w/ either a ≥4% ↓SaO$_2$ or arousal
  −≥50% ↓tidal volume
•Complete obstruction→
◦**Cessation of airflow despite continued respiratory effort, termed apnea**
...both→
  •Ventilation/ perfusion mismatch via ↑vascular shunting†→
  ◦↓Diffusion of O$_2$ & CO$_2$→
    −Hypoxemia (SaO$_2$ ≤ 91% &/or PaO$_2$ ≤ 60mmHg)→difficulty breathing=**dyspnea**→
    partial to complete arousal, gasping for air→fragmented & ↓ sleep time→**daytime sleepiness‡**→frequent napping, ↓cognitive function, personality change, &/or ↓libido

---

†Capillary blood flow through relatively underventilated alveoli. Usually occurring, or exacerbated via ↑venous return
‡The severity of daytime sleepiness is directly proportional to the frequency of sleep apnea/ hypopnea, ranging from daytime sleepiness during sedentary activities, such as watching television or reading, to pathologic hypersomnolence, such as occurs while driving a car, or even while talking or eating

Neurologic
•Obstruction mediated respiratory effort & hypoxemia→
◦Morning headaches
Genitourinary
•Partial to complete arousal→
◦Nocturia ± enuresis

Cardiovascular
- Hypoxemia (SaO_2 ≤ 91% or PaO_2 ≤ 60mmHg)→
  - ∘**Dysrhythmias**
  - ∘Reflex pulmonary arteriole vasoconstriction, in order to ↓ventilation/ perfusion mismatch, which, when chronic→**pulmonary hypertension†→↑**right ventricular pressure→**right ventricular hypertrophy**, being termed **cor pulmonale** when due to primary lung disease (COPD being the #1 cause)→
    - −Right ventricular heave→a palpable lift over the left sternal border
    - −Tricuspid regurgitation murmur
    - −↑**Pulmonic component of the 2nd heart sound**
    - −**Right sided heart failure**
- **Hypertension−50%**, correlating w/ apneic/ hypopneic events/ hour
  - ∘Also being due to obesity mediated essential hypertension

---

†Indicates limited cardiopulmonary reserve via either:
- Underlying heart failure
- Underlying chronic obstructive pulmonary disease−COPD
- Massive or recurrent pulmonary embolism→
  - ∘Cor pulmonale

Hematologic
- Chronic hypoxemia→
  - ∘Compensatory ↑renal erythropoietin production→
    - −↑Bone marrow erythrocyte production→secondary polycythemia (hematocrit ♂ ≥52%, ♀ ≥48%)

SLEEP STUDY=Polysomnography

Indications:
- To diagnose obstructive sleep apnea/ hypopnea syndrome
- To determine the optimal level of continuous positive airways pressure−CPAP needed during sleep in order to prevent upper airways collapse in patients who are diagnosed w/ the syndrome
  - ∘Determined via a ↓apnea/ hypopnea severity index

Procedure:
- The simultaneous overnight continuous monitoring of:
  - ∘Sleep stage via:
    - −Electroencephalography−EEG
    - −Electro−oculography−EOG to detect eye movements
    - −Electromyography−EMG to detect chin & leg movements
  - ∘Cardiac rhythm via electrocardiogram−ECG
  - ∘Oxygen saturation via pulse oximetry
  - ∘Airflow and respiratory effort via respiratory gauges

Classification via the apnea/ hypopnea index:
- Normal: <5 episodes/ hour
- Mild: 5−30 episodes/ hour
- Moderate: 31−60 episodes/ hour
- Severe: >60 episodes/ hour

TREATMENT

- **Weight loss via goal daily caloric requirement**
  - ∘The caloric total needed to reach & maintain a goal weight depends on physical activity level
  - ∘10 calories/ lb of goal weight +
    - −33% if sedentary
    - −50% if moderately physically active
    - −75% if very physically active
  - ∘3500 calories are roughly equivalent to 1 lb of body fat
    - −Consuming 500calories less/ day X 1week→1 lb weight loss
    - −Exercising 500calories/ day X 1week→1 lb weight loss
    - …w/ the average human body being able to lose 3.5 lbs/ week maximum, aside from a diuretic effect
- **Avoid sedative hypnotic substances/ medications**
  - ∘Ethanol
  - ∘Barbiturates
  - ∘Benzodiazepines
  - ∘Histamine−1 receptor blockers
- **Continuous positive airways pressure−CPAP**
  - Mechanism:
    - Provides a preset, continuous positive airways pressure in order to produce extrinsic PEEP during sleep, in order to prevent upper airways collapse

228

<u>Settings:</u>
- Start w/:
  - A positive airways pressure of 5cm H_2O (max 15cm H_2O)
  - 2L O_2/ min.
  - ...then titrate the pressure by 2cm H_2O q20min., & O_2 prn, as tolerated, to reach goal parameters. Most patients cannot tolerate an expiratory positive airways pressure–EPAP >10cm H_2O

<u>Goal:</u>
- To achieve an $SaO_2 \geq 91\%$ during sleep, while minimally ↓cardiac output

<u>Adverse consequences:</u>
- Abnormal swallowing of air=aerophagia→
  - Gastric distention
- ↑Aspiration risk
- Difficult exhalation
- Mucocutaneous effects
  - Dry mucosa→
    - Epistaxis
    - Rhinorrhea
  - Dry conjunctiva→
    - Eye irritation
  - Facial skin irritation ± necrosis
- ↓**Venous return/ cardiac output**
  - Positive end expiratory pressure–PEEP→↑mean intrathoracic pressure, being determined by:
    - Airways resistance
    - Thoracic compliance
    - Added PEEP
  - ...→↑atrial & vena caval pressure→
    - ↓Systemic & pulmonary venous return→
      - ↓Ventricular preload→
        - ↓Cardiac output→**heart failure**→hypotension→obstructive shock (hypotension + organ failure unresponsive to fluid resuscitation

<u>Advantages:</u>
- ↓**Venous return**→
  - ↓Pulmonary congestion→
    - ↓Dyspnea→↓autonomic sympathetic tone
  - ↓Myocardial contractile strength
    - ...→↓myocardial O_2 & nutrient demand
- ↓Transmural aortic pressure→
  - ↓**Afterload**
  - ...→**improved heart failure syndrome**

SECOND LINE TREATMENT ━━━━━━━━━━━━━━━━━━━━━━━━
- **Uvulopalatopharyngoplasty**
  <u>Procedure:</u>
  - Removal of the tonsils, uvula, rim of the soft palate, & redundant pharyngeal mucosa
  <u>Outcomes:</u>
  - 45% cure overall, being ↑in patients w/ altered oropharyngeal anatomy

- **Maxillofacial surgery**
  <u>Indications:</u>
  - Altered oropharyngeal anatomy

THIRD LINE TREATMENT ━━━━━━━━━━━━━━━━━━━━━━━━
- **Tracheostomy**
  <u>Indications:</u>
  - Severe disease failing to respond to the above treatments
  <u>Outcomes:</u>
  - 100% cure, as the area of pharyngeal collapse is bypassed

•Caused by any process→
  ∘Fluid accumulation in the pleural space

•**90% being due to either:**
  ∘**Heart failure**
  ∘**Malignancy**
  ∘**Pneumonia**
  ∘**Pulmonary embolism**

TRANSUDATIVE PLEURAL EFFUSION ▬▬▬▬▬▬▬

Fluid escaping through normal vasculature:
•↑**Pulmonary vascular hydrostatic pressure**†
  ∘Heart failure–40%, esp. w/ biventricular failure, as right ventricular failure→
    –↑Lymphatic hydrostatic pressure
•↑**Interstitial fluid oncotic pressure**
  ∘Hypothyroidism→
    –↑Interstitial fluid albumin
•↓**Vascular oncotic pressure**
  ∘Liver cirrhosis
    –Usually being right sided
    –May be massive without concomitant marked ascites
  ∘Malnutrition
  ∘Nephrotic syndrome
  ...→↓plasma albumin
•↑**Negative pleural pressure**
  ∘Atelectasis
•↑**Lymphatic hydrostatic pressure**
  ∘Right sided heart failure
  ∘Tumor→
    –Lymphatic obstruction

Other:
  •**Trauma**→
    ∘Lymphatic laceration
  •**Diaphragmatic defect mediated flow from the peritoneal cavity**
    ∘Transudative ascites
    ∘Peritoneal dialysis

---

†Occasionally being exudative

EXUDATIVE PLEURAL EFFUSION ▬▬▬▬▬▬▬

Fluid escaping through damaged vasculature:
•**Pneumonia–25%:** Infection mediated pulmonary inflammation→
  ∘**Parapneumonic effusion**, being termed **complicated** via either:
    –pH <7.2, indicating empyema
    –Glucose ≤40mg/ dL
    –Lactate dehydrogenase–LDH >1000 U/ L
    –Positive gram stain or culture
    Note: If bacterial, esp. anaerobic organisms (esp. Streptococcus sp. or Bacteroides sp.)→
        •Pus within the pleural space, indicating >30,000 leukocytes/ µL, being termed **empyema**
•**Pneumonitis:** Non-infection mediated pulmonary inflammation
  ∘**Asbestos**
  ∘**Autoimmune syndromes**
    –Dressler's syndrome
    –Rheumatoid arthritis
    –Systemic lupus erythematosus–SLE
    –Vasculitides
  ∘**Medications**
    –Amiodarone
    –Bromocriptine
    –Cancer chemotherapy
    –Methysergide
    –Minoxidil
    –Nitrofurantoin

230

  ◦Pulmonary embolism ± infarction–10%
    –Pleural effusion–35% (exudative–75% > transudative), w/ 60% being hemorrhagic
  ◦**Radiation treatment**
  ◦**Uremia**
•**Malignancy–20%**
  ◦Bronchogenic cancer, being the #1 malignancy
  ◦Extrapulmonary cancer w/ secondary metastasis to the lung
  ◦Lymphoma
  ◦Ovarian fibroma→
    –**Meigs'** syndrome, being a triad of ovarian fibroma, hydrothorax (right > left), & ascites
  ◦Pleural mesothelioma
•**Thoracic hemorrhage**
  ◦Aortic perforation
  ◦Esophageal perforation
  ◦Trauma
•**Coronary artery bypass–CABG**
  ◦Left sided
  ◦Initially being hemorrhagic, & clearing after several weeks

<u>Other:</u>
•**Inflammatory lymphatic drainage**
  <u>Mechanism:</u>
    •**Abdominal &/or pelvic inflammation→**
     ◦Inflammatory lymphatic flow through the thoracic duct, which ascends to ~T5 on the right side,
      then on the left thereafter→
       –Left > right sided pleural effusion
•**Diaphragmatic defect mediated flow from the peritoneal cavity**
  ◦Exudative ascites

DIAGNOSIS

Pulmonary
<u>Laterality of pleural effusions:</u>
•**Usually right sided**
  ◦Heart failure
  ◦Liver cirrhosis
•**Usually left sided**
  ◦Chylothorax
  ◦Pancreatitis
  ◦Pericarditis
  ◦Coronary artery bypass graft–CABG

COMPARATIVE THORACIC EXAMINATION FINDINGS			
Physical examination	Consolidation/ empyema	Pleural effusion	Pneumothorax†
Chest expansion	⬇	⬇	⬇‡
Auscultation	⬇Breath sounds w/ crackles, rhonchi, wheezes, &/or egophony°		⬇Breath sounds
Percussion	⬇	⬇	⬆^
Tactile or auscultatory fremitus	⬆n	⬇	⬇

Note: Outlining lung compression by all 3 etiologies→
    •Atelectasis→
     ◦Signs of consolidation
†If via bronchopleural fistula, may be accompanied by:
  •Hemothorax (a pleural effusion)
  •Pyothorax=empyema
‡Loss of intrapleural negative pressure→
  •Ipsilateral chest wall expansion→
   ◦↑Anteroposterior diameter→
    –↓Respiratory movement
°A patients verbalization of the sound 'E' is heard as 'A'
^Best detected over the midclavicle w/ the patient sitting or standing. The ipsilateral ↓breath sounds
should guide you, as otherwise, you may be fooled by the contralateral side being relatively dull to
percussion, assuming it to be the diseased lung
nUnless accompanied by a concomitant pleural effusion

•**Tension hydrothorax**–a medical emergency
Pathophysiology:
  •↑Pleural space hydrostatic pressure→
    ∘↑Atrial & vena caval hydrostatic pressure→↑intra–thoracic pressure→
    –↓Systemic & pulmonary venous return→**biventricular heart failure**
    ...w/ eventual:
      •**Hypotension**, being refractory to intravenous fluid infusion→
        ∘Cerebral failure→
          –Altered mental status
        ∘Pre–renal renal failure
        ∘Lactic acidemia
      ...termed **obstructive shock**

•**Chest x ray**
Findings:
  •Pleural effusion, which if present, should undergo diagnostic ± therapeutic thoracentesis
    ∘Requires ≥300mL of fluid to be visualized via posteroanterior chest x ray
      –Posteroanterior view: Blunting of the costophrenic angle
      –Lateral view: Blunting of the posterior diaphragm
      ...w/ fluid usually tapering slightly up the lateral pleural wall, forming a **meniscus**, unless the
        effusion is accompanied by either:
        •Fluid loculation
          Pathophysiology:
          •Current &/or previous pleural inflammation→
            ∘Outlining pleural layer fibrosis→**loculation of effusion** ± bulging into the lung
              –**Interpleural effusion:** Between the lung & chest wall
              –**Infrapulmonary effusion:** Between the lung & diaphragm
              –**Interlobular effusion:** Between 2 lung lobes, esp. the horizontal fissure
        •Pneumothorax, being almost always due to a bronchopleural fistula
          ...→loss of the meniscus
    ∘Requires ≥15mL of fluid to be visualized via decubitus CXR
      Indications:
      •Pleural effusion present on posteroanterior CXR, in order to check for loculation

•**Thoracic computed tomographic–CT scan**
Findings:
  •Shows decubitus findings, w/ increased visualization of:
    ∘A small pleural effusion
    ∘Parenchymal infiltration ± alveolar consolidation
    ∘Parenchymal nodule or mass
    ∘Lymphadenopathy
    ∘Separation of lung, mediastinal, pleural, & chest wall structures

•**Thoracentesis**
Indications:
  •**Any new pleural effusion >1cm on decubitus view**, except those clearly a result of heart failure
    (which should resolve w/ diuresis), allowing for:
    ∘Fluid analysis
    ∘Symptom relief
    ∘↑Visualization of the lung fields
    ...w/ ultrasound allowing for localization of:
      •Loculated fluid
      •The proximal border of free pleural fluid , esp. w/ a small pleural effusion
        ...both of which should be identified via a skin marker
  •Emergently w/ either a tension pneumo-, hemo-, or hydrothorax
Procedure:
  1. If possible, obtain patient informed consent for the procedure
  2. Have the patient remove all thoracic clothing & sit at the bedside w/ arms & head resting on a
     bedside adjustable table
  3. Identify & mark the proximal end of the effusion by percussion or ultrasound
  4. Place another small mark along the mid–axillary line at the superior margin of the rib below the
     previous marking, in order to avoid damaging the intercostal nerve which courses at the inferior
     margin of the upper rib

5. Use aseptic technique to clean the chosen area & a large surrounding margin, several times w/ progressively widening circular motions w/ a povidone–iodine solution, allowing several min. to dry
6. Anesthetize the overlying skin & subcutaneous tissue w/ 1–2% lidocaine solution. Always gently aspirate while advancing any needle in order to realize if you have entered a vessel or the pleural space
7. Using the previous puncture site, insert a 17–20 gauge needle & anesthetize the deeper structures (fascia, muscle, pleura) w/ 1–2% lidocaine, w/ advancing gentle aspiration until pleural fluid is noted. Use the hemostat to prevent inadvertent to & fro needle movement, & aspirate the pleural fluid:
   - **100mL for diagnostic**
   - **≤1.5L for therapeutic**
8. When finished, remove the needle & obtain the studies listed below, as well as a **post-thoracentesis chest x ray for possible iatrogenic pneumothorax**
   Note: A trauma induced pneumothorax may require 48hours to become radiographically evident. Therefore, serial chest x rays are needed only if the patient becomes symptomatic

Complications:
- •Attempts to completely drain the effusion→
   - ∘↑Risk of visceral pleural needle laceration→
      - –**Pneumothorax-7%**
      - –**Hemothorax-1%**
      - –Hemoptysis
   - ∘**Organ perforation**, esp. the liver or spleen depending on side
- •Removal of >1.5L of fluid→
   - ∘Hypotension
   - ∘**Re-expansion pulmonary edema-rare**, due to overly rapid lung re-expansion (esp. after prolonged collapse). Also occurring w/ rapid removal of pleural gas
      - Timing:
         - •Within 1hour post re-expansion-65%
         - •Within 24hours post re-expansion-100%

Contraindications:
- •Coagulopathy (INR >1.3 &/or PTT >35seconds) &/or thrombocytopenia (<150,000/ μL)→
   - ∘↑Hemothorax risk
- •Ventilator dependent patient, continuous cough &/or hiccups, &/or uncooperative patient→↑risk of:
   - ∘Air embolism
   - ∘Hemothorax
   - ∘Organ perforation, esp. the liver or spleen depending on side
   - ∘Pneumothorax
- •Overlying skin infection→
   - ∘↑Deep tissue infection risk

Lab studies:
- •**Tube 1:** Albumin, total protein, lactate dehydrogenase-LDH, & glucose
   - ∘Send plasma samples for comparative analysis
- •**Tube 2:** Cell count & differential
- •**Tube 3:** Gram stain & culture (bacterial, fungal, & mycobacterial)
- •**Tube 4:** Other studies as clinically indicated
- •**Arterial blood gas tube:** pH

PLEURAL FLUID STUDIES

Studies†	Transudate	Exudate
Gross appearance	Serous=clear straw colored	•**Serous**=clear straw colored •**Turbid:** Leukocytes, lipid, organisms •**Purulent:** Empyema •**Bloody:** Malignancy, pneumonia (esp. mycobacterial infection), pulmonary embolism, trauma (including traumatic tap), coagulopathy, aortic dissection, leaking aortic aneurysm, pulmonary arterio–venous malformation, post-coronary artery bypass •**Milky=chylothorax:** Lymphatic obstruction vs. perforation •**Anchovy paste:** Amebiasis •**Black:** Aspergillus sp. infection •**Green:** Rheumatoid arthritis
Smell	None	Foul odor=anaerobic infection
Protein level (1–1.5g/ dL)	<3g/ dL (CHF may ≥3g/ dL)	≥3g/ dL
Peritoneal/ plasma protein level	<0.50=50%	≥0.50=50%‡
LDH level	<200 IU	≥200 IU or ≥2/3rds upper normal plasma limit‡
Pleural/ plasma LDH level	<0.60=60%	≥0.60=60%‡
Plasma–effusion albumin	>1.1	≤1.1
Cholesterol	<45mg/ dL	>55mg/ dL
Glucose level	Same as serum	<60mg/ dL <20mg/ dL: Empyema or rheumatoid arthritis
Leukocytes	<1000/μL	>1000/ μL° >30,000/ μL: Empyema
Differential	Mononuclear predominant	•**Mononuclear^:** Malignancy, mycobacterial, fungal, or viral pneumonia; rheumatoid arthritis, vasculitides •**Eosinophils >10%:** Asbestos, Churg–Strauss syndrome, medication mediated, paragonomiasis •**Neutrophil predominant:** All others
Erythrocytes (0–5/μL)	<1,000/ μL	≥1000/ μL >50% plasma hematocrit: Hemothorax
Amylase	60–130 U/ L	>2X plasma level: Esophageal rupture, pancreatitis, malignancy
pH	7.38–7.44	**<7.2: Empyema** <6: Esophageal rupture
Adenosine deaminase–ADA		Positive in granulomatous disease >70: Possible mycobacterial infection <40: Excludes mycobacterial pneumonia
Fibrinogen	Negative	Positive
Specific gravity	<1.016	≥1.016
Triglyceride		>110mg/ dL: Chylothorax
Sudan III staining	Negative	Positive: Chylothorax
Microscopy	–	•AFB stain positive: Mycobacterial pneumonia •Cytology positive: Malignancy °Sensitivity: 60–90% •Gram stain positive: Bacterial
Culture (aerobic & anaerobic)	Negative	±

†Consider transudative values to be normal
‡The presence of any of these, termed **Light's criteria**, indicate an exudative effusion
°To correct for the neutrophil count in a traumatic tap, subtract 1 neutrophil for every 250 erythrocytes
^Lymphocyte & monocyte

•Chest tube insertion=thoracostomy
  Indications:
  •Symptomatic
  •Complicated parapneumonic effusion
  •Chylothorax
  •Hemothorax
  •Recurrent pleural effusion
  Procedure:
  •Usually, small caliber, termed pigtail chest tubes, are placed by interventional radiology, whereas larger chest tubes are placed by thoracic surgery at the 4th or 5th **intercostal space, along the mid-axillary line, at the superior margin of the lower rib†**
  Duration:
  •**Uncomplicated effusion:** Until drainage <50mL/ 24hours
  •**Complicated effusion:** Until drainage <20mL/ 24hours
  •**Pneumothorax:** The chest tube should be left in place for 2–4 days in order for the damaged pleura to heal. Prior to the removal of the chest tube, clamp the tube to simulate its absence, & perform a chest x ray @ 4hours to check for a pneumothorax, indicating a residual unhealed visceral tear
  Complications:
  •Hemorrhage
  •Infection
  •Lung infarction
  •Lung trauma
  •**Re-expansion pulmonary edema-rare,** due to overly rapid lung re-expansion (esp. after prolonged collapse)
  •Subcutaneous emphysema
  3 chamber collecting system:
  •Chamber 1, termed the **collecting chamber:**
    ◦Collects pleural fluid, allowing gas to travel to the next chamber, as the inlet is not in direct contact w/ fluid
  •Chamber 2, termed the **water seal chamber:**
    ◦Fluid contact w/ the inlet creates a water seal, w/ gas bubbling out to the next chamber, w/ no backflow. **Air bubbles are thus evidence of a continuing pleural air leak**
  •Chamber 3, termed the **suction control chamber:**
    ◦Sets limit to suction pressure drawing air into the wall

•Parietal pleural biopsy
  Indications:
  •Exudates suspected of being due to either:
    ◦Malignancy
    ◦Mycobacterial pneumonia
      –Sensitivity: 75%

<hr>

TREATMENT

•Transudative effusions
  ◦Treat the underlying cause
  ◦Do not require therapeutic thoracentesis or chest tube placement unless they are very large (>1/2 hemithorax)→
    –Unmanageable dyspnea

•Parapneumonic effusions
  ◦**Uncomplicated:** Usually resolve w/ antimicrobial treatment alone, & do not require chest tube placement
  ◦**Complicated:** Require **chest tube placement in order to prevent the formation of fibrin mediated loculations & subsequent restrictive fibrotic pleural "peels" that may trap lung→**
    –↓Lung function

•Loculated effusions
  ◦Requires the placement of ≥1 chest tube(s) w/ subsequent:
    –Administration of intrapleural tissue plasminogen activator–tPA or
    –Surgical decortication via video–assisted thoracoscopic surgery–VATS or thoracotomy

•Pleural peels
  ◦Surgical decortication via video–assisted thoracoscopic surgery–VATS or thoracotomy

•Malignant effusions
  ○Usually indicate unresectable cancer
  ○Recurrence after thoracentesis is an indication for chemical pleurodesis, which is 80% successful

SECOND LINE TREATMENT ━━━━━━━━━━━━━━━━━━━━━━━━━━━━━━
•Chemical pleurodesis
  Indications: Effusion being either:
    •Recurrent
    •Unresponsive to chest tube placement
  Procedure:
    •Instillation of sterile Bleomycin, Doxycycline, Mitoxantrone, or talc slurry into the pleural space→
      ○Pleuritis→
        −Fibrous adhesion of the visceral & parietal pleura→obliteration of the pleural space

236

•Caused by any process→
  ◦Perforation of the visceral pleura→
    −Bronchopleural fistula
  ◦Perforation of the parietal pleura
  ◦Introduction of bacteria within the pleural space
  ...→gas within the pleural cavity→
    •Lung collapse &/or compression

CLASSIFICATION/ RISK FACTORS

•**Primary Pneumothorax**
  Etiology:
    •**Spontaneous rupture of apical sub-pleural blebs**
  Risk factors:
    •Tall, thin ♂ age 20–40years
    •Cigarette smoking
    •Genetic
      ◦Family history of primary pneumothorax

•**Secondary pneumothorax**
  Etiology:
    •**Secondary to trauma or pulmonary disease**
  Risk factors:
    •**Chronic obstructive pulmonary disease–COPD**
      ◦**Emphysema, being the #1 cause**
      ◦Asthma
      ◦Cystic fibrosis
    •**Interstitial lung disease**
      ◦Eosinophilic granulomatosis
      ◦Idiopathic pulmonary fibrosis
      ◦Lymphangioleiomyomatosis
      ◦Sarcoidosis
      ◦Tuberous sclerosis
    •**Infection**
      ◦Pneumonia→
        −Bronchopleural fistula
        −Empyema→intra-pleural gas production
    •**Neoplasm**
    •**Connective tissue disease**
      ◦Ehlers−Danlos syndrome
      ◦Marfan's syndrome
    •**Catamenial Pneumothorax**
      ◦Endometriosis via ? pathogenesis
    •**Trauma:** Any form of chest trauma (penetrating or non−penetrating), including:
      ◦Iatrogenic
        −Central line insertion, esp. subclavian venous line placement
        −Lung biopsy: Transthoracic−15% > transbronchial−5%
        −Pleural biopsy
        −Mechanical ventilation mediated volutrauma or barotrauma
        −Thoracentesis

DIAGNOSIS

•Patients may be asymptomatic

Pulmonary
  •Bronchoalveolar collapse→
    ◦**Cough** ± sputum production ± blood=hemoptysis
    ◦Pleurisy−30%, being thoracic pain exacerbated by either:
      −Deep inhalation (including coughing & sneezing)
      −Supine position
      −Thoracic palpation
      ...& being relieved by leaning forward

∘Difficulty breathing=**dyspnea-60%**→
  –Respiratory rate >16/ min.=**tachypnea**
  –Accessory muscle usage (sternocleidomastoid muscles for inspiration & abdominal muscles for expiration)
  –Speech frequently interrupted by inspiration=telegraphic speech
  –Pursed lip breathing &/or grunting expirations→positive end–expiratory pressure–PEEP
  –Paradoxical abdominal motion: Negative intrathoracic pressure→fatigued diaphragm being pulled into the thorax→inspiratory inward motion of the anterior abdominal wall, rather than expected outward motion due to diaphragmatic contraction
∘Ventilation/ perfusion mismatch via:
  –↑Alveolar dead space: Alveolar ventilation through relatively underperfused capillaries
  –↑Vascular shunting†: Capillary blood flow through relatively underventilated alveoli. Usually occurring, or exacerbated via ↑venous return
  …→↓diffusion of O_2 & CO_2→
    •Hypoxemia (SaO_2 ≤ 91% or PaO_2 ≤ 60mmHg‡) on room air, w/ subsequent hypercapnia ($PaCO_2$ ≥45mmHg) due to either:
      ∘Respiratory muscle fatigue
      ∘Alveolar hypoventilation
    …as CO_2 clearance is unimpaired (& may be ↑in the dyspneic patient) as long as adequate ventilation (including lack of diffuse severe ventilation/ perfusion mismatching) is maintained, as:
      •CO_2 diffuses 20X as rapidly as O_2
      •Hypercapnia→
        ∘Immediate brain stem respiratory center mediated stimulation of pulmonary ventilation, which may correct the hypercapnia, but not necessarily the hypoxia

•Alveolar rupture or tracheal/ chest wall trauma→
  ∘Pneumothorax
  ∘Pneumomediastinum
  ∘Pneumoperitoneum, via passage through diaphragmatic rents
  ∘Subcutaneous emphysema, via gaseous dissection into the neck→skin distention→
    –"Puffy" appearance
    –Palpation of air bubbles ± crackling sound=crepitus

---

†Being exacerbated by the supine position→
  •↑Systemic venous return→
    ∘↑Vascular shunting→↑dyspnea, being termed:
      –Orthopnea, if persistent
      –Paroxysmal nocturnal dyspnea if intermittent
      …causing the patient to either use multiple pillows or sleep in a chair
‡Age adjusted normal PaO_2 = 101 – (0.43 X age)

COMPARATIVE THORACIC EXAMINATION FINDINGS			
Physical examination	Consolidation/ empyema	Pleural effusion	Pneumothorax†
Chest expansion	↓	↓	↓‡
Auscultation	↓Breath sounds w/ crackles, rhonchi, wheezes, &/or egophony°		↓Breath sounds
Percussion	↓	↓	↑^
Tactile or auscultatory fremitus	↑n	↓	↓

Note: Outlining lung compression by all 3 etiologies→
  •Atelectasis→
    ∘Signs of consolidation
†If via bronchopleural fistula, may be accompanied by:
  •Hemothorax (a pleural effusion)
  •Pyothorax=empyema
‡Loss of intrapleural negative pressure→
  •Ipsilateral chest wall expansion→
    ∘↑Anteroposterior diameter→
      –↓Respiratory movement
°A patients verbalization of the sound 'E' is heard as 'A'
^Best detected over the midclavicle w/ the patient sitting or standing. The ipsilateral ↓breath sounds should guide you, as otherwise, you may be fooled by the contralateral side being relatively dull to percussion, assuming it to be the diseased lung
nUnless accompanied by a concomitant pleural effusion

•**Tension pneumothorax**–a medical emergency
Pathophysiology:
  •Any cause of pneumothorax→
    ◦"Ball-valve" mechanism of air entering the pleural space (being drawn in via inhalation, or forced in via assisted ventilation), but prevented from escaping during exhalation→↑pleural space pressure→↑intra-thoracic pressure→
      ‑↑Atrial & vena caval pressure→↓systemic & pulmonary venous return→**biventricular heart failure**
      ...w/ eventual:
        •**Hypotension**, being refractory to intravenous fluid infusion→
          ◦Cerebral failure→
            ‑Altered mental status
          ◦Pre-renal renal failure
          ◦Lactic acidemia
          ...termed **obstructive shock**

•**Chest x ray**
Procedure:
  •**End-expiratory films**→
    ◦↓Lung air volume, having no effect on the pleural air volume→
      ‑Relative ↑pleural air→↑visualization
  •25% of patients have either a concomitant:
    ◦Pleural effusion
    ◦Hemorrhage, termed hemopneumothorax
Findings:
  •Pleural space air→
    ◦Lung compression→
      ‑A sharp **white line, outlining the compressed lung tissue & visceral pleura**
      ‑A hyperlucent area w/ ↓vascular markings at the most superior pleural space region (unless loculated), being apical in the sitting or standing position & basilar in the supine position
      ‑**Thoracic structure deviation to the contralateral hemithorax**→heart & lung compression ± tracheal deviation
Limitations
  •False Positive:
    ◦Portable chest x ray cartridges placed under the patient's back may→skin folding over on itself, termed a redundant skin fold→
      ‑Gradually ↑radiodensity, blending into a line. If this is suspected, ask the technician to repeat the chest x ray w/ the cartridge placed flat on the patients back→skin fold line disappearance
  •False negative:
    ◦A trauma induced pneumothorax may require 48hours to become radiographically evident (esp. post-central venous line placement)

•**Oxygen** via nasal cannula @ 2–4L/ min.
  Mechanisms:
    •↑Nitrogen gradient from the pleura to the lung parenchyma & vasculature→
      ◦Pleural nitrogen diffusion down its gradient→
        ‑↑Pleural gas absorption

•**Emergent thoracentesis**
Indications:
  •Tension pneumo-, hemo-, or hydrothorax
Procedure:
  1. Place a large bore needle through the **anterior 2nd or 3rd intercostal space, along the midclavicular line, at the superior margin of the lower rib**† on the affected side →
    •Urgent pleural decompression
  2. Chest tube insertion should follow

239

•Chest tube insertion=thoracostomy
　Indications:
　　•Symptomatic
　　•Complicated parapneumonic effusion
　　•Chylothorax
　　•Hemothorax
　　•Recurrent pleural effusion
　Procedure:
　　•Usually, small caliber, termed pigtail chest tubes, are placed by interventional radiology, whereas larger chest tubes are placed by thoracic surgery at the **4th or 5th intercostal space, along the mid-axillary line, at the superior margin of the lower rib†**
　Duration:
　　•The chest tube should be left in place for 2-4 days in order for the damaged pleura to heal. Prior to the removal of the chest tube, clamp the tube to simulate its absence, & perform a chest x ray @ 4hours to check for a pneumothorax, indicating a residual unhealed visceral tear
　Complications:
　　•Hemorrhage
　　•Infection
　　•Lung infarction
　　•Lung trauma
　　•**Re-expansion pulmonary edema-rare**, due to overly rapid lung re-expansion (esp. after prolonged collapse)
　　•Subcutaneous emphysema
　3 chamber collecting system:
　　•Chamber 1, termed the **collecting chamber**:
　　　◦Collects pleural fluid, allowing gas to travel to the next chamber, as the inlet is not in direct contact w/ fluid
　　•Chamber 2, termed the **water seal chamber**:
　　　◦Fluid contact w/ the inlet creates a water seal, w/ gas bubbling out to the next chamber, w/ no backflow. **Air bubbles are thus evidence of a continuing pleural air leak**
　　•Chamber 3, termed the **suction control chamber:**
　　　◦Sets limit to suction pressure drawing air into the wall

---

†In order to avoid damaging the intercostal nerve, which courses at the inferior margin of the upper rib

SECOND LINE TREATMENT ■■■■■■■■■■■■■■■■■■■■■■■■■■■■■■■■■■■■■
•Thoracoscopy
　Procedure:
　　•Stapling of the visceral tear

•Thoracotomy
　Procedure:
　　•Stapling &/or laser pleurodesis of the visceral tear

PREVENTION
•Due to ↑recurrence rates
　◦Primary pneumothorax: 30%
　◦Secondary pneumothorax: 50%
　...usually occurring within 2years, patients should avoid:
　　•High altitude exposure
　　•Flying in unpressurized aircraft
　　•Scuba diving

240

•A chronic, intermittently symptomatic, systemic disease of uncertain etiology→
∘**Noncaseating granulomatous inflammation**
<u>Statistics:</u>
•**#1 chronic interstitial lung disease**

RISK FACTORS

•**Age:** 20–40years
•**Gender:** ♀ 3X ♂
•**Skin color: Blacks** 12 X whites in the U.S.
•**Ethnicity**
∘Northern Europeans

DIAGNOSIS

•50% of patients are asymptomatic

General
•Inflammatory cytokines→
∘Anorexia→
–Cachexia
∘Chills
∘Fatigue
∘**Fever**
∘Headache
∘Malaise
∘Night sweats
∘Weakness

---

†Temperature may be normal in patients w/:
•Chronic kidney disease, esp. w/ uremia
•Cirrhosis
•Heart failure
•Severe debility
...or those who are:
•Intravenous drug users
•Taking certain medications:
∘Acetaminophen
∘Antibiotics
∘Glucocorticoids
∘Nonsteroidal anti–inflammatory drugs

Pulmonary–100%
•Bronchoalveolar inflammation→
∘**Cough** ± sputum production ± blood=hemoptysis
∘Pleurisy–30%, being thoracic pain exacerbated by either:
–Deep inhalation (including coughing & sneezing)
–Supine position
–Thoracic palpation
...& being relieved by leaning forward
∘Difficulty breathing=**dyspnea**→
–Respiratory rate >16/ min.=**tachypnea**
–Accessory muscle usage (sternocleidomastoid muscles for inspiration & abdominal muscles for expiration)
–Speech frequently interrupted by inspiration=telegraphic speech
–Pursed lip breathing &/or grunting expirations→positive end–expiratory pressure–PEEP
–Paradoxical abdominal motion: Negative intrathoracic pressure→fatigued diaphragm being pulled into the thorax→inspiratory inward motion of the anterior abdominal wall, rather than expected outward motion due to diaphragmatic contraction

∘Ventilation/ perfusion mismatch via:
−↑Alveolar dead space: Alveolar ventilation through relatively underperfused capillaries
−↑Vascular shunting†: Capillary blood flow through relatively underventilated alveoli. Usually occurring, or exacerbated via ↑venous return
...→↓diffusion of O_2 & CO_2→
    •Hypoxemia (SaO_2 ≤ 91% or PaO_2 ≤ 60mmHg‡) on room air, w/ subsequent hypercapnia ($PaCO_2$ ≥45mmHg) due to either:
    ∘Respiratory muscle fatigue
    ∘Alveolar hypoventilation
    ...as CO_2 clearance is unimpaired (& may be ↑in the dyspneic patient) as long as adequate ventilation (including lack of diffuse severe ventilation/ perfusion mismatching) is maintained, as:
      •CO_2 diffuses 20X as rapidly as O_2
      •Hypercapnia→
      ∘Immediate brain stem respiratory center mediated stimulation of pulmonary ventilation, which may correct the hypercapnia, but not necessarily the hypoxia

Effects of chronic, inadequately controlled disease:
•**Pulmonary fibrosis**→
∘Chronic restrictive pulmonary disease

---

†Being exacerbated by the supine position→
•↑Systemic venous return→
∘↑Vascular shunting→↑dyspnea, being termed:
−Orthopnea, if persistent
−Paroxysmal nocturnal dyspnea if intermittent
...causing the patient to either use multiple pillows or sleep in a chair
‡Age adjusted normal PaO_2 = 101 − (0.43 X age)

COMPARATIVE THORACIC EXAMINATION FINDINGS			
Physical examination	Consolidation/ empyema	Pleural effusion	Pneumothorax†
Chest expansion	↓	↓	↓‡
Auscultation	↓Breath sounds w/ crackles, rhonchi, wheezes, &/or egophony°		↓Breath sounds
Percussion	↓	↓	↑^
Tactile or auscultatory fremitus	↑ⁿ	↓	↓

Note: Outlining lung compression by all 3 etiologies→
•Atelectasis→
∘Signs of consolidation
†If via bronchopleural fistula, may be accompanied by:
•Hemothorax (a pleural effusion)
•Pyothorax=empyema
‡Loss of intrapleural negative pressure→
•Ipsilateral chest wall expansion→
∘↑Anteroposterior diameter→
−↓Respiratory movement
°A patients verbalization of the sound 'E' is heard as 'A'
^Best detected over the midclavicle w/ the patient sitting or standing. The ipsilateral ↓breath sounds should guide you, as otherwise, you may be fooled by the contralateral side being relatively dull to percussion, assuming it to be the diseased lung
ⁿUnless accompanied by a concomitant pleural effusion

Cardiovascular−5%
•Chronic granulomatous inflammation→
∘Dysrhythmias
∘Restrictive cardiomyopathy
Lymphatic
∘Inflammatory cytokines→extramedullary hematopoeisis→
−**Lymphadenopathy**, usually being **firm & non−tender**, which may remain stable, or wax & wane in size for many months ± spontaneous regression
−**Hepatomegally**
−**Splenomegally**, which may retain a relatively ↑proportion of circulating cells, termed hypersplenism→anemia, granulocytopenia, &/or thrombocytopenia
...w/ organ destruction

242

Mucocutaneous–20%
- Chronic granulomatous inflammation→
  - Alopecia
  - Cutaneous anergy–70%→
    - ↓Delayed type hypersensitivity to recall antigens, such as Mycobacterium tuberculosis, Candida albicans, & mumps virus
  - Flat violaceous skin plaques, esp. on the cheeks, nose, &/or digits
  - Painful nodes on the extensor surfaces of the lower extremities, termed erythema nodosum
  - Parotid gland inflammation & fibrosis→
    - Gland enlargement
    - ↓Saliva production→dry mouth

Musculoskeletal
- Usually occurring w/ concomitant cutaneous involvement
- Chronic granulomatous inflammation of:
  - Joints→
    - **Arthritis–25%**
      Affected joints:
      - Small joints > large weight bearing joints
        - Hands
          - Proximal interphalangeal joints–PIPs
          - Distal interphalangeal joints–DIPs
        - Wrist
          - Carpometacarpal joints
        - Shoulder
        - Knee
        - Ankle
  - Bursae (olecranon, popliteal, subacromial, retrocalcaneal)→
    - Bursitis
  - Tendon sheaths→
    - Tenosynovitis
  - Tendons→
    - Tendonitis
  - Skin→
    - Cellulitis
  - The site of the insertion of tendons, ligaments, & fascia into bones or joint capsules, termed **enthesopathy†**→
    - Sausage–like swelling of an entire finger or toe, termed **dactylitis**
    - Inflammation of the plantar fascia at its insertion into the calcaneous→heel pain
    - Swelling of the Achilles tendon
  - ...→edematous, erythematous, warm, & extremely painful joints, bursae, tendon sheaths, &/or periarticular tissue, usually **being worse in the morning, w/ joint stiffness after prolonged inactivity (even several hours), being termed the gel phenomenon**

Effects of chronic, inadequately controlled disease:
- Progressive inflammation→
  - Inflammatory, hypertrophied synovial mass, termed pannus, extending to overlie the articular cartilage→
    - **Osteo–cartilagenous erosions, termed "rat–bite" or "punched out" erosions, beginning at the joint margins,** where bone is not protected by cartilage
  - Knee synovitis→synovial cyst formation, esp. popliteal &/or sub-popliteal, termed Baker's cyst→
    - Venous &/or lymphatic compression→distal lower extremity pitting edema
    - Rupture→calf dissection→deep venous thrombosis–like=pseudothrombophlebitis syndrome
  - Periarticular osteopenia→
    - Osteoporosis→↑fracture risk
  - ↓Ligament attachment→
    - Damaged joint structure→bone malalignment=subluxation
  - Tenosynovitis→palpable tendon synovial sheath, w/ the inflamed, edematous synovium & surrounding tissue→
    - Median nerve compression→carpal tunnel syndrome→finger paresthesia, esp. numbness &/or tingling

∘Tendinitis→fibrosis→contracture→
  −**Boutonniere deformity:** Flexion of the proximal interphalangeal joint−PIP, & hyperextension of distal interphalangeal joint−DIP
  −**Swan neck deformity:** Extension of the proximal interphalangeal joint−PIP, & flexion of the distal interphalangeal joint−DIP
  −**Ulnar deviation of the phalanges**
  −Tendon rupture, esp. the 4th &/or 5th extensor tendons→tendon displacement & inability to extend the involved digits
  …w/ pain, stiffness, & malalignment→
      •↓Function
        ∘Hip or knee arthritis→
          −↓Ambulation
        ∘Finger arthritis→
          −Inability to use hands
      …→periarticular muscle atrophy↔
        •Muscle weakness

---

†Enthesopathy is limited to sarcoidosis & seronegative spondyloarthropathies

Neurologic
•Chronic granulomatous inflammation→
  ∘Aseptic meningitis, for which no microorganism can be isolated using conventional staining & cultures
  ∘Cranial nerve (esp. the facial nerve) &/or peripheral motor nerve palsies
  ∘Sensory neuropathy
  ∘Localized space occupying lesions or diffuse central nervous system disease→encephalopathy→
    −Altered mental status
    −Dementia
  ∘Seizures
  ∘Has a **predilection for midline structures at the base of the brain,** such as the:
    −Optic chiasm→↓vision
    −Hypothalamus→↓neuroendocrine function
    −Pituitary gland→↓neuroendocrine function &/or ↓vision
Opthalmologic−25%
•Chronic granulomatous inflammation→
  ∘Uveal tract† inflammation & fibrosis, termed uveitis, being either anterior or posterior→
    −↓Vision
  ∘Lacrimal gland inflammation & fibrosis→
    −Gland enlargement
    −↓Lacrimation→conjunctival inflammation=conjunctivitis→erythema, termed conjunctival injection

---

†The iris & ciliary body comprise the anterior portion, w/ the choroid comprising the posterior portion

Hematologic
•Granuloma macrophage mediated hydroxylation of 25−hydroxycholecalciferol→
  ∘↑1,25−dihydrocholecalciferol, being the active form of vitamin D→
    −**Hypercalcemia−10%**
•↑**Angiotensin converting enzyme−ACE levels** (>35 U/ L)−**80%**
  ∘>2 X the upper limit of normal is almost always due to Sarcoidosis
•Anemia
•Leukopenia
•Eosinophilia
•Polyclonal IgG gammopathy
•Inflammatory cytokines→
  ∘↑Acute phase proteins
    −↑Erythrocyte sedimentation rate−ESR (normal: 5mm/ decade aged + ♂ ≤10mm/h or ♀ ≤20mm/h)
    −↑C−reactive protein−CRP (normal: <2mg/ L), responding more acutely than ESR, as it rises within several hours & falls within 3days upon partial resolution
    −↑Fibrinogen
    −↑Platelets→thrombocytosis

Chest x ray
Findings:
- •**Hilar (usually being bilateral) & mediastinal lymphadenopathy**
- •Interstitial infiltrates
- •Pulmonary fibrosis→
  - ∘Honeycombing
- •Chronic airways inflammation→
  - ∘Interstitial damage→
    - −Bronchiectasis
    - −Fibrosis→restrictive pulmonary disease

•**Kveim test**
Procedure:
- •Intradermal injection of sarcoid spleen tissue→
  - ∘Noncaseating granuloma formation at the injections site @ 4−6weeks
Outcomes/ limitations:
- •↑Specificity w/ ↓sensitivity, making this test **useful in helping to reliably confirm sarcoidosis**, but unable to exclude the diagnosis

•**Transthoracic needle biopsy**
Indications:
- •**Small peripheral lesion**
Outcomes:
- •Sensitivity: 80%

•**Transtracheal vs. transbronchial needle biopsy**
Indications:
- •**Central lesion**
- •**Lymphadenopathy** (mediastinal or paratracheal)
Procedures:
- •Fiberoptic bronchoscopy performed w/ fluoroscopic guidance
Complications:
- •**Pneumothorax**
  - ∘Transthoracic approach: 15%
  - ∘Transtrachial/ bronchial approach: 5%
  - ...both being ↑in patients w/ chronic obstructive pulmonary disease−COPD
- •**Pulmonary hemorrhage**→
  - ∘Blood in the pleural space=hemothorax
  - ∘Coughing blood=hemoptysis
- •**Transient cardiac dysrhythmias** in 5% of elderly patients
- •**Bacteremia−2%**
- •**Laryngospasm &/or bronchospasm**
- •**Low grade fever−15%**
- •**Organ perforation**, esp. of the liver or spleen, depending on the side
Contraindications:
- •Coagulopathy (INR >1.3 &/or aPTT >35seconds) &/or thrombocytopenia (<150,000/ μL)→
  - ∘↑Hemothorax risk
- •Ventilator dependent patient, continuous cough &/or hiccups, &/or uncooperative patient→↑risk of:
  - ∘Air embolism
  - ∘Hemothorax
  - ∘Organ perforation
  - ∘Pneumothorax
- •Overlying skin infection→
  - ∘↑Deep tissue infection risk

•**Cervical mediastinoscopic biopsy**
Indications:
•To biopsy the anterior mediastinal area:
  ◦Above or at the carina
  ◦Right paratracheal lesions
  ◦Left paratracheal lesions above the aorta
  …when inaccessible via transthoracic or transbronchial biopsy
Procedure:
•Performed by inserting a rigid endoscope through a small suprasternal incision

•**Open lung biopsy via thoracotomy**
Indications:
•A lesion otherwise inaccessible or too small, w/ both:
  ◦The clinical suspicion of cancer
  ◦Resection being potentially curative

TREATMENT

Indications:
•Symptomatic patients
•Hypercalcemia
•Organ dysfunction
•Pulmonary infiltrates >2years→
  ◦↑Pulmonary fibrosis risk

SYSTEMIC GLUCOCORTICOID TREATMENT

Generic	M ♀	Dose
Prednisone	L ?	40mg PO q24hours X 2weeks or until disease control is achieved, then
		30mg PO q24hours X 2weeks, then
		25mg PO q24hours X 2weeks, then
		20mg PO q24hours X 2 weeks, then
		15mg PO q24hours X 6months, then
		Taper by 2.5mg qmonth

•Once disease control is achieved, taper to the lowest effective maintenance dose in order to minimize serious side effects, w/ the goal of discontinuation if possible, w/ attention to relapse syndrome
•Both the IV & PO routes have equal efficacy

	Relative potencies			
Glucocorticoids	Anti-inflammatory	Mineralocorticoid	Duration	Dose equiv.
Cortisol (physiologic†)	1	1	10hours	20mg
Cortisone (PO)	0.7	2	10hours	25mg
Hydrocortisone (PO, IM, IV)	1	2	10hours	20mg
Methylprednisolone (PO, IM, IA, IV)	5	0.5	15-35hours	5mg
Prednisone (PO)	5	0.5	15-35hours	5mg
Prednisolone (PO, IM, IV)	5	0.8	15-35hours	5mg
Triamcinolone (PO, IM)	5	~0	15-35hours	5mg
Betamethasone (PO, IM, IA)	25	~0	35-70hours	0.75mg
Dexamethasone (PO)	25	~0	35-70hours	0.75mg
Fludrocortisone (PO)	10	125	10hours	

†The physiologic rate of adrenal cortical cortisol production is 20-30mg/ 24hours

Side effects of chronic use:
General
  •Anorexia→
    ◦Cachexia
  •↑Perspiration
Cardiovascular
  •Mineralocorticoid effects→
    ◦↑Renal tubular NaCl & water retention as well as potassium secretion→
    −**Hypertension**
    −**Edema**
    −**Hypokalemia**
  •Counter−regulatory=anti−insulin effects→
    ◦↑Plasma glucose→
    −**Secondary diabetes mellitus**, which may→ketoacidemia

246

∘Hyperlipidemia→↑atherosclerosis→
-**Coronary artery disease**
-Cerebrovascular disease
-Peripheral vascular disease
Cutaneous/ subcutaneous
•↓Fibroblast function→
∘↓Intercellular matrix production→
-↑Bruisability→ecchymoses
-Poor wound healing
-Skin striae
•Androgenic effects→
∘Acne
∘↑Facial hair
∘Thinning scalp hair
•Fat redistribution from the extremities to the:
∘Abdomen→
-Truncal obesity
∘Shoulders→
-Supraclavicular fat pads
∘Upper back→
-Buffalo hump
∘Face→
-Moon facies
...w/ concomitant thinning of the arms & legs
Endocrine
•**Adrenal failure** upon abrupt discontinuation after 2weeks
Gastrointestinal
•Inhibition of phospholipase A_2 mediated conversion of cell membrane lipids to arachidonic acid,
which is the precursor for both cyclooxygenase–COX enzymes, w/ the cyclooxygenase–COX1
enzyme found in most cells of the body, responsible for normal physiologic function. Inhibition of
the cyclooxygenase–COX1 enzyme→↑peptic inflammatory disease risk→↑**upper
gastrointestinal hemorrhage risk** via:
∘↓Gastric mucosal prostaglandin synthesis→
-↓Epithelial cell proliferation
-↓Mucosal blood flow→↓bicarbonate delivery to the mucosa
-↓Mucus & bicarbonate secretion from gastric mucosal cells
Musculoskeletal
•**Avascular necrosis of bone**
•**Osteoporosis**
•Proximal muscle weakness
Neurologic
•Anxiety
•Insomnia
•Psychosis
Opthalmologic
•**Cataracts**
Immunologic
•Inhibition of phospholipase A_2 mediated conversion of cell membrane lipids to arachidonic acid,
which is the precursor for both cyclooxygenase–COX enzymes (COX1 & COX2) being
responsible for the production of neuronal & inflammatory cell prostaglandins respectively→
-↓Pain
-↓Temperature (antipyretic)
-↓**Inflammation**
•Stabilization of lisosomal & cell membranes→
∘↓Cytokine & proteolytic enzyme release
•↓Lymphocyte & eosinophil production
...all→
•**Immunosuppression**→
-↑**Infection** &/or neoplasm risk
Hematologic
•↑Erythrocyte production→
∘Polycythemia
•↑Neutrophil demargination→
∘Neutrophilia→
-**Leukocytosis**

247

•The following medications usually require 1–6 months for symptomatic improvement, making these medications not useful in the control of acute disease, but rather, useful when prolonged treatment is planned.

Generic (Trade)	M	♀	Dose
Hydroxychloroquine (Plaquenil)	K	?	200mg PO q48hours X alternating 6month periods prn

•Once disease control is achieved, taper to the lowest effective maintenance dose in order to minimize serious side effects

Mechanism: Unknown

Side effects:
Gastrointestinal
- •↓Mucosal cell proliferation→
  - ◦Mucosal inflammation=mucositis, including inflammation of the oral mucosa=stomatitis→
    - −Diarrhea
    - −Nausea ± vomiting

Opthalmologic
- •Accommodation defects
- •Blurred vision scotomas
- •Corneal deposits
- •Extraocular muscle weakness
- •Night blindness
- •**Retinopathy–rare**, being related to cumulative dose, which may→
  - ◦Irreversible visual loss

Mucocutaneous
- •↓Hair formation→
  - ◦Alopecia
- •↓Epithelial cell proliferation→
  - ◦Dermatitis
- •Skin pigmentation
- •Stevens–Johnson syndrome

Musculoskeletal
- •Myopathy

Neurologic
- •Headache
- •Insomnia
- •Neuropathy
- •Tinnitus
- •Vertigo

Hematologic
- •**Myelosuppression→**
  - ◦Macrocytic anemia→
    - −Fatigue
  - ◦Leukopenia→immunosuppression→
    - −↑Infection & neoplasm risk
  - ◦Thrombocytopenia→
    - −↑Hemorrhage risk, esp. petechiae

Monitoring:
•Baseline ophthalmologic examination, then
  ◦Q6months

•As spontaneous remissions are common (whites > blacks), asymptomatic patients without organ dysfunction or hypercalcemia can be observed for up to 2years, w/ monitoring to include:
  ◦Occasional chest x ray
  ◦Occasional pulmonary function testing

•Erythema nodosum indicates an excellent prognosis
•Spontaneous remission: 40%, w/ rare relapse
•Control/ remission w/ treatment: 40%
•Develop irreversible pulmonary fibrosis: 20%, w/ a 50% mortality

248

ACUTE RENAL FAILURE

- •Any disease→
  - ∘↓**Renal function over hours to days**→
    - –↓Excretion of nitrogenous waste products (ammonia, blood urea nitrogen–BUN, creatinine, uric acid, etc...) which are the end–products of protein catabolism→**uremia, w/ altered fluid & electrolyte regulation**
- •**Age** mediated nephron loss→
  - ∘↓Functional reserve to withstand acute insults

Statistics:
  - •Develops in 5% of hospitalized patients

PATHOPHYSIOLOGY OF NITROGENOUS WASTE PRODUCTS

- •Cellular amino acid metabolism→
  - ∘**Ammonia (NH₃)** formation, w/ subsequent extracellular diffusion→hepatocyte metabolism (via the cytoplasmic urea cycle enzymes) to **urea**, w/ subsequent extracellular diffusion→
    - –Urinary excretion, via both glomerular filtration & renal tubular secretion
    - –Gastrointestinal diffusion→bacterial urease mediated metabolism to CO_2 & ammonia, w/ subsequent extracellular reabsorption
- •Hepatocyte amino acid metabolism→
  - ∘Creatine formation, w/ subsequent myocyte creatine kinase mediated reversible phosphorylation→
    - –Creatine phosphate (being proportional to muscle mass), which provides a rapidly metabolizeable reserve of high energy phosphates, serving to maintain the intracellular ATP level during the first several min. of myocyte contraction. Creatine phosphate is slowly metabolized to **creatinine**, being excreted via both glomerular filtration & renal tubular secretion
- •**Uric acid** is a metabolic byproduct of purine metabolism, which are essential components of DNA synthesis

CLASSIFICATION

Urinary output based classification:
  - •**Non–oliguric renal failure, being most common:** Urine output ≥400mL/ 24hours
  - •**Oliguric renal failure:** Urine output <400mL/ 24hours
  - •**Anuric renal failure:** Urine output <100mL/ 24hours

PSEUDO–RENAL FAILURE

- •**Medications**
  - ∘Trimethoprim

    Mechanism:
    - •Competes w/ creatinine for tubular secretion→
      - ∘↑Plasma creatinine without concomitantly ↑blood urea nitrogen–BUN

249

- ↓Renal blood flow→
  - ↓Glomerular filtration rate, w/ intact tubular & glomerular function

RISK FACTORS

Hypovolemia:
- **Direct vascular loss**
  - Hemorrhage
- **Gastrointestinal loss**
  - Diarrhea
  - Nasogastric tube suctioning
  - Poor oral intake
  - Surgical drainage
  - Vomiting
- **Cutaneous loss**
  - Diaphoresis
  - Fever
  - Severe burn
- **Renal loss**
  - Diuretic use
  - Osmotic diuresis
    - Diabetes mellitus
    - Hypercalcemia
- **Hypoalbuminemia**
  - Cirrhosis
  - Malnutrition
  - Nephrotic syndrome
  - ...→systemic edema, termed anasarca, as well as transudative peritoneal, pleural, pericardial, & synovial effusions
- **Abdominal organ inflammation**→
  - Exudative effusion→
    - Ascites

Distributive disease:
- ↓**Cardiac output**
  - **Heart failure**
  - Cross clamping of the aorta during surgery
- **Systemic vasodilation**
  - Distributive shock
    - Anaphylactic shock
    - Septic shock
  - Medications
    - Anesthetics
    - Anti-hypertensives
- **Renal arteriole vasoconstriction**
  - Electrolytes
    - Hypercalcemia
  - Medications
    - Amphotericin B
    - Catecholamines (epinephrine, norepinephrine, or high dose dopamine)
    - Cyclosporine
    - FK506
  - **Radiocontrast dye**

Renal artery obstruction†:
- **Atherosclerosis**
- **Dissecting aneurysm**
- **Embolus**
- **Fibromuscular dysplasia**
- **Thrombosis**
- **Vasculitis**

---

†Being ≥95% occlusive bilaterally (or unilateral w/ 1 functional kidney), or less w/ concomitant risk factors

250

Altered renal arteriole autoregulation:
- Hepatorenal syndrome
- Medications
  - **Nonsteroidal anti-inflammatory drugs–NSAIDs**, including Aspirin
  - **Angiotensin converting enzyme inhibitors–ACEi** or **angiotensin 2 receptor blockers–ARB**

Mechanism:
- Patients w/ pre-existing bilateral ↓renal perfusion, not necessarily failure:
  - Heart failure
  - Bilateral renal artery stenosis
  - Hypovolemia
  - Renal failure
  …rely more on the compensatory production of:
  - Prostaglandin→
    - Afferent arteriole dilation→maintained glomerular filtration rate, whereas NSAIDs→
      - ↓Prostaglandin production→pre-renal renal failure
  - Angiotensin 2→
    - Efferent arteriole constriction→maintained glomerular filtration rate, whereas either:
      - Angiotensin converting enzyme inhibition
      - Angiotensin 2 receptor blockade
      …→↓angiotensin 2 production & action respectively→
        - Pre-renal renal failure

251

•Intrarenal disease→
  ◦↓Glomerular filtration rate, w/ ↓tubular &/or glomerular function

CLASSIFICATION/ RISK FACTORS
ACUTE TUBULAR NECROSIS-ATN 85% ▬▬▬▬▬▬▬▬▬▬▬▬▬▬▬
•**Disease of the tubulointerstitium** (sparing the glomeruli)→
  ◦Sloughed tubular epithelial cells
  ◦Clumped proteins
  ◦Interstitial edema
  ...→tubular stenosis→
    •Proximal tubular congestion→
      ◦↓Glomerular filtration rate

RISK FACTORS_____
•**Extra-renal renal failure**
  ◦**Prolonged or severe pre-renal renal failure-50%**→
    -Renal ischemia
  ◦Prolonged post-renal renal failure
•**Tubular toxins-35%**
  ◦Pigments
    -Hemolysis→hemoglobinuria
    -Rhabdomyolysis→myoglobinuria
  ◦Crystals
    -Calcium oxalate
    -Hyperuricemia via gout, hematologic malignancy (or its treatment)
  ◦Antibodies
    -Multiple myeloma immunoglubulin light chain proteins or altered heavy chain proteins
    ...also→obstructive tubular casts
  ◦**Radiocontrast dye**
    Risk factors:
      •Age >60years
      •Gender: ♀ > ♂
      •Concurrent administration of nephrotoxic medications
      •↑Volume administration
        ◦Coronary angiography w/ left ventriculogram
      •**Underlying renal disease**, esp. w/ a creatinine >1.5mg/ dL (30% of whom experience renal failure, as opposed to 2% w/ lower values)
      •**Diabetes mellitus**
      •Hypertension
      •Hypovolemia
      •Multiple myeloma
    Timing:
      •Renal failure @ 1-2days after administration, w/ peak uremia @ 3-5days, & resolution usually within 10days
  ◦Medications
    -Acyclovir
    -**Aminoglycosides** (Gentamicin > Tobramycin > Amikacin > Neomycin)
      Timing:
        •Renal failure @ ≥1week
      Risk factors:
        •↑Age
        •Cirrhosis
        •Hypovolemia
        •Hypokalemia
        •Hypomagnesemia
        •Pre-existing renal failure
    -Amphotericin B
    -Cisplatin
    -Cyclosporine
    -Foscarnet
    -Intravenous immune globulin-IVIG
    -Intravenous anti-Rhd immunoglobulin
    -Methotrexate
    -Pentamidine
    -Sulfonamide

252

-Tacrolimus
∘Heavy metals
  -Cadmium
  -Lead
  -Mercury
∘Propylene glycol, being a nonpolar solvent used for intravenous medications that do not readily dissolve in aqueous solutions, such as:
  -Diazepam
  -Digoxin
  -Etomidate
  -Lorazepam
  -Nitroglycerin
  -Phenobarbital
  -Phenytoin
  -Trimethoprim-Sulfamethoxazole
∘Toxins
  -Carbon tetrachloride
  -Ethylene glycol, being a major component of antifreeze
  -Insecticides
  -Poison mushrooms
•**Renal vein obstruction**
∘Nephrotic syndrome
∘↑Plasma viscosity
  -Acute leukemia
  -Myeloma
  -Polycythemia
•**Small vessel obstruction**
∘Atheroembolism, usually being due to extensive angiographic exploration or vascular surgery→
  -Hollenhorst plaques
  -Petechiae
  -↓Complement levels
  -Eosinophilia
∘Autoimmune disease
∘Gestational hypertensive syndromes (pre-eclampsia/ eclampsia)
∘Scleroderma renal crisis
∘Severe hypertension
∘Systemic thrombohemorrhagic syndromes
  -Disseminated intravascular coagulation-DIC
  -Hemolytic uremic syndrome-HUS/ thrombotic thrombocytopenic purpura-TTP
∘Sickle cell anemia
∘Transplant rejection

ACUTE INTERSTITIAL NEPHRITIS–AIN 10% ━━━━━━━━
•**Inflammation of the tubulointerstitium** (sparing the glomeruli)→
∘Sloughed tubular epithelial cells
∘Interstitial edema
...→tubular stenosis→
    •Proximal tubular congestion→
      ∘↓Glomerular filtration rate

RISK FACTORS
•**Hypersensitivity reaction**
∘Medications, esp.:
  -Allopurinol
  -Captopril
  -Cimetidine
  -β lactam medications (carbapenems, cephalosporins, penicillins)
  -Loop diuretics
  -Nonsteroidal anti-inflammatory drugs-NSAIDs
  -Oral hypoglycemic medications
  -Phenacetin
  -Phenytoin
  -Rifampin
  -Sulfonamides
  -Thiazide diuretics
  -Trimethoprim

<u>Clinical features:</u>
  •May be accompanied by arthralgia, dermatitis, &/or fever

•**Infection**
  ∘Bacterial
    −Fulminant bacterial pyelonephritis
    −Legionella sp.
    −Leptospira interrogans
    −Rickettsia Rickettsiae
  ∘Viral
    −Cytomegalovirus−CMV
    −Hantavirus
  ∘Fungal
    −Candida sp.
    −Histoplasma capsulatum
•**Infiltrative disease**
  ∘Leukemia
  ∘Lymphoma
  ∘Sarcoidosis

ACUTE GLOMERULONEPHRITIS−AGN 5% ▬▬▬▬▬▬▬▬▬▬▬▬▬▬
•Immune complex deposition→**inflammation of the glomeruli** (sparing the tubulointerstitium)→
  ∘↓Glomerular filtration rate

RISK FACTORS_____
•**Infection**
  ∘Streptococcus pyogenes
  ∘Viral infections
•**Autoimmune disease**
  ∘Goodpasture's syndrome
  ∘Systemic lupus erythematosus−SLE
  ∘Wegener's granulomatosis

254

•**Urinary outflow tract obstruction**→
　◦↓Glomerular filtration rate

RISK FACTORS_____
•**Ureteral obstruction**, being either bilateral or unilateral w/ 1 functional kidney
　◦Blood clot
　◦Lymphadenopathy
　◦Malignancy, esp. cervical & colorectal cancer
　◦Nephrolithiasis
　◦Pelvic adhesions
　◦Retroperitoneal fibrosis
　◦Sloughed papillae
•**Urinary bladder outlet obstruction**
　◦Bladder cancer
　◦Blood clot
　◦Nephrolithiasis
　◦Obstructed bladder catheter
　◦Neurologic
　　−Anticholinergic medications
　　−Neuropathy
•**Urethral obstruction**
　◦**Benign prostatic hyperplasia−BPH**
　◦Congenital urethral valve
　◦Phimosis
　◦**Prostate cancer**
　◦Sricture

Diagnostic criteria for acute renal failure:
- Creatinine ↑≥0.5mg/ dL or >50% above baseline
- Glomerular filtration rate ↓≥50%
- Requiring dialysis

General
- Uremia→
  - Anorexia→
    - ↓Cachexia
  - Malaise
- Hypovolemia→
  - ↓Weight (1L fluid=1kg=2.2 lbs)
- ↓Fluid excretion→
  - Hypervolemia→
    - ↑Weight (1L fluid=1kg=2.2 lbs)
    - Pitting edema, requiring ≥3L of fluid

Cardiovascular
- Uremia→
  - Pericardial inflammation=pericarditis, esp. @ >100mg/ dL
- ↓Intravascular volume→
  - ≥10% blood volume loss→
    - ↑Autonomic sympathetic tone→↑pulse
  - ≥20% blood volume loss→
    - Orthostatic hypotension (supine to standing→↑20 pulse, ↓20 SBP, &/or ↓10 DBP)→ lightheadedness upon standing
    - Urine output 20–30mL/ hour (normal being >30mL/ hour)
  - ≥30% blood volume loss→
    - Recumbent hypotension &/or tachycardia
  - ≥40% blood volume loss→
    - Altered mental status &/or urine output <20mL/ hour
    - Hypovolemic shock, being hypotension + organ failure, unresponsive to fluid resuscitation
- ↓Fluid excretion→
  - Heart failure
  - Hypertension

Endocrine
- Uremia→
  - Hyperglycemia, termed **secondary diabetes mellitus**
- ↓Phosphate excretion→
  - Hyperphosphatemia→hypocalcemia→
    - ↑Parathyroid hormone–PTH secretion, termed **secondary hyperparathyroidism**

Gastrointestinal
- Uremia→
  - Metabolism to ammonia in saliva→
    - Metallic taste sensation
    - Urine-like odored breath, termed uremic fetor
  - Inflammation anywhere along the gastrointestinal tract, from the oropharnyx to the anus
- Prostate enlargement→
  - Urinary retention†→
    - Urinary bladder distention→pelvic, back, &/or flank pain

---

†Perform bladder catheterization to determine the post–void residual, w/ >100mL indicating incomplete voiding via either:
- Obstruction
- Autonomic neuropathy

Immunologic
- Uremia→
  - ↓Lymphocyte function→
    - Immunosuppression→**infection, being the #1 cause of mortality**

Neurologic
- ↓Excretion of nitrogenous waste products→central nervous system dysfunction, termed **renal encephalopathy**→
  - ○**Altered mental status**
  - ○Cerebral edema
  - ○Headache
  - ○Nausea ± vomiting
  - ○Altered neuromuscular function→
    - −**Asterixis**, being an inability to maintain a posture
      Examination:
      - •Usually assessed using the upper extremities, but may viewed via any attempt at voluntary posture maintenance. Best viewed by asking the patient to hold out extended arms & dorsiflexed hands, w/ fingers spread as though signaling traffic to stop→
        - ○An intermittent, nonrhythmic flapping tremor of the wrist & metacarpophalangeal joints due to **intermittent inhibition of wrist extensors**→
          - −Brief lapses of posture. If the patient cannot comply, simply ask them to squeeze your extended fingers→intermittently ↓grip strength
      Limitations: Also found w/:
      - •Hepatic failure→
        - ○Hyperammonemia
      - •Chronic heart failure
      - •Chronic lung disease→
        - ○Respiratory failure

Precipitants of renal encephalopathy:
- •↑**Protein metabolism**
  - ○Blood transfusion
  - ○↑Dietary protein
  - ○Gastrointestinal hemorrhage
  - ○Inflammation
  - …→↑ammonia production
- •**Hypovolemia**→
  - ○↑Plasma concentration of the various possible causative substances
  - ○↓Hepatic & renal perfusion→
    - −↓Filtration
- •Certain medications, esp.
  - ○Analgesics (opiates)
  - ○Sedatives (benzodiazepines, barbiturates)
- •↑Bacterial contact w/ colonic substrates via:
  - ○Constipation
  - ○Ileus (obstructive or paralytic)
  - …→↑ammonia production
- •Hepatic failure→
  - ○↓Conversion of ammonia to urea
- •↑Renal production of ammonia
  - ○Hypokalemia
- •↑Diffusion of ammonia across the blood brain barrier
  - ○Alkalemia
- •Iatrogenic
  - ○Peritoneojugular shunt
  - ○Portosystemic shunting
    - −Transjugular intrahepatic portosystemic shunt−TIPS

Pulmonary
- •Hiccoughs

Hematologic
- •↓Excretion of nitrogenous waste products→
  - ○↑Ammonia
  - ○↑**Blood urea nitrogen−BUN**
    - −↓Platelet & factor 8 function→↑hemorrhage risk, termed coagulopathy, w/ ↑bleeding time being the best predictor of hemorrhage risk
  - ○↑**Creatinine**
    - −Being that the plasma creatinine does not become abnormal until the glomerular filtration rate ↓ by 50%↑, creatinine clearance allows for a more accurate assessment of renal function
  - ○↑Uric acid

257

•**Hyperkalemia** via:
  ○↓Tubular secretion, occurring @ a:
    –Glomerular filtration rate <10mL/ min.
    –Urine output <1L/ 24h
    ...→potassium homeostasis adaptive mechanism failure
  ○Acidemia, as every 0.1↓ in pH→0.5mEq/ L↑ in potassium via the H^+/K^+ cell membrane exchange protein→
    –Potassium extracellular shift
  ○Coagulopathy→
    –Gastrointestinal hemorrhage→intestinal absorption
    –Hematoma→absorption
  ○Low grade, chronic hemolysis
•**Hypermagnesemia** via ↓excretion
•**Hypervolemic hyponatremia** via total body water > NaCl, which may be due to either:
  ○↑Intake, due to thirst
  ○Relatively ↑renal tubular water absorption, due to antidiuretic hormone–ADH
•**Hyperphosphatemia @ a glomerular filtration rate <50mL/ min.**, via ↓excretion
•**Hypocalcemia @ a glomerular filtration rate <50mL/ min.**, via hyperphosphatemia→
  ○↑Calcium binding
  ○↓Renal mediated 1,25–dihydroxycholecalciferol production (also due to primary renal disease)→↓intestinal calcium absorption
•**Metabolic acidemia @ a glomerular filtration rate <25mL/ min.**, via ↓excretion of sulfuric & phosphoric acids→
  ○Widened, anion gap, metabolic acidemia‡

Additional serologic testing for Intrarenal renal failure:
•**Cryoglobulinemic glomerulonephritis**
  ○Cryoglobulins
  ○Hepatitis C virus antibodies
•**Goodpasture's syndrome**
  ○Antiglomerular basement membrane–GBM antibodies, w/ hemoptysis
•**Myeloma**
  ○Plasma & urine protein electrophoresis
•**Polyarteritis nodosa**
  ○Perinuclear antineutrophil cytoplasmic antibodies P–ANCA
•**Post–infectious glomerulonephritis**
  ○↓Complement 3
•**Post–streptococcal glomerulonephritis**
  ○Anti–deoxyribonuclease–DNase B
  ○Anti–streptolysin O–ASO
  ○↓Complement 3
•**Systemic lupus erythematosus–SLE**
  ○Antinuclear antibodies–ANA
    –Anti–dsDNA
    –Anti–Sm (Smith)
  ○↓Complement 3 & 4
•**Wegener's granulomatosis**
  ○Circulating antineutrophil cytoplasmic antibodies C–ANCA, w/ hemoptysis

---

†Correlation of creatinine w/ glomerular filtration rate:
  •Creatinine 1→2mg/ dL, indicates a 50%↓GFR
  •Creatinine 3→4mg/ dL, indicates a 5%↓GFR
‡Plasma anion gap= $[Na^+] - ([Cl^-] + [HCO_3])$
  •**Normal value: 8–12 mEq/ L**
  •Equation value: 12 mEq/ L
Correction:
  •**Hypoalbuminemia:** For each 1g/ dL ↓in albumin below 4, add 2.5 to the calculated anion gap
  •**Acidemia:** Add 2 to the calculated anion gap
  •**Alkalemia:** Add 4 to the calculated anion gap
Interpretation:
  •A widened gap indicates the **presence of excess unmeasured anions**, via either:
    ○Organic acids
    ○Phosphates
    ○Sulfates

CREATININE CLEARANCE MEDIATED GFR ESTIMATION

Gender	Cockcroft–Gault formula (mL/ min.)	Normal	Age adjusted norm
♂	$\dfrac{(140 - age) \times weight\ (kg)}{72 \times plasma\ creatinine\ (mg/ dL)}$†	100–140	133 – (0.64 X age)
♀	♂ X 0.85	85–115	[133 – (0.64 X age)] X 0.85

†Does not require a 24hour urine collection
•**Creatinine clearance becomes an unreliable indicator of glomerular filtration rate @ <30mL/ min.**, as renal tubular creatinine secretion makes up an increasing fraction of the total creatinine eliminated→
  •Falsely ↑amount

URINE EVALUATION

	EXTRARENAL Pre-renal	Post-renal	INTRARENAL ATN	AIN	AGN
Dipstick proteinuria	≤T r a c e		Mild–mod (1–2+)		Severe (3–4+)
Quantitative proteinuria†	0–20mg/ dL		25–100mg/ dL 1–2g/ 24hours		≥200mg/ dL >3g/ 24hours
Casts	Hyaline		Granular, Tubular	Leukocyte, Tubular	Erythrocyte, Leukocyte
Erythrocytes		+	+	+	+‡
Leukocytes		+	+	+°	
Tubular epithelial cells			+		
Crystals^		+			
↑Plasma IgE				+	+

	EXTRARENAL Pre-renal	Post-renal	INTRARENAL ATN	AIN	AGN
RENAL TUBULAR CONCENTRATING ABILITY	Preserved		I m p a i r e d		Preserved
Serum BUN:Cr	>20:1	>20:1	<20:1	<20:1	>20:1
Urine/ serum urea	>8	<3	<3	>8	
Urine/ serum creatinine	>40	<20	<20	>40	
Urine/ serum osmolarity	>1.2	<1	<1	>1.2	
Osmolarity (mosm/ kg)	>500	<350	<350	<350	>500
Urine sodium (meq/ L)	<20	Variable	>40	Variable	<20
Urine specific gravity	>1.025	<1.015	<1.015	<1.015	>1.025
FENa (%)^n	<1	>1	>1‡	>1	<1
FE$_{UN}$^{n}	<35%				
Urine volume (mL/ 24h)	<400	<400	V a r i a b l e (usually >400)		

•ATN, AIN, & AGN may have aspects of each other, as inflammation has no borders
•In the absence of sediment erythrocytes, heme–positive urine suggests the presence of either hemoglobin or myoglobin. Check the plasma creatine kinase for possible rhabdomyolysis
†Grams of protein/ 24hours ≈ $\dfrac{\text{Spot urine protein}}{\text{Spot urine creatinine}}$
‡May be dysmorphic
°Acute interstitial nephritis etiology differentiation:
  •Lymphocytes indicate nonsteroidal anti–inflammatory drug–NSAID mediated disease
  •**Eosinophils** >1% (per 100 cells, via Wright's stain or Hansel's stain) indicate antibiotic mediated disease
    Limitations: Also present w/:
      •Atheroembolism
      •Pyelonephritis
^Oxalate crystals are seen w/ ethylene glycol ingestion, being a major component of antifreeze
^{n}**Fractional excretion of Na–FENa**= $\dfrac{\text{Urine Na X plasma creatinine}}{\text{Plasma Na X urine creatinine}}$ X 100

Interpretation:
  •Indicates the percent of filtered sodium excreted in the urine
    °<1% indicates either:
      –**Pre–renal renal failure**
      –Acute glomerulonephritis
      –Contrast nephropathy→acute tubular necrosis
      –Pigment nephropathy (hemoglobin or myoglobin)→acute tubular necrosis

259

○>1% indicates either:
    −Acute interstitial nephritis
    −Acute tubular necrosis other than contrast or pigment nephropathy
    −Post−renal renal failure
Limitations:
•Only useful in oliguric renal failure (<400mL urine/ hour)
•Both the FENa & urine sodium may be falsely ↑ in:
    ○Elderly
    ○Underlying chronic renal failure
    ○Diuretic use, in which case, calculate the fractional excretion of urea nitrogen−FE$_{UN}$
        Urine BUN X plasma creatinine   X 100
        Plasma BUN X urine creatinine
        ...→↑urine sodium excretion

ELECTRICAL STUDIES

•Electrocardiography−ECG
Findings:
•>5 mEq/ L→
    ○Atrial &/or ventricular dysrhythmia, not correlating w/ plasma potassium
•≥5.5 mEq/ L→
    ○↑T wave height & duration, termed "peaked" T waves
•≥6 mEq/ L→
    ○Atrioventricular conduction delay→
        −Bradycardia
    ○↑PR interval
    ○↑QRS duration
    ○↓QT interval
•≥7 mEq/ L→
    ○P wave flattening, indicating atrial arrest
    ○Progressive QRS widening→
        −Merging w/ T wave→sine−wave pattern
    ○↓ST segment

IMAGING

•Renal & pelvic ultrasound
Indications/ findings:
•To look for obstruction
    ○Dilated pyelocalceal outflow tract, indicating hydronephrosis. A non−dilated tract does not exclude
      obstruction, esp. in the acute setting
    ○Distended bladder or residual urine if recent urination
    ○Nephrolithiasis
•To look for possible chronic renal disease
    ○Small kidneys, being <8cm
        −Consider renal artery stenosis if unilateral
    ○Large kidneys indicate either:
        −Diabetes mellitus
        −HIV nephropathy
        −Infiltrative disease (amyloidosis, multiple myeloma)
        −Polycystic kidney disease

•Pyelography
Mechanism:
    ○Retrograde or percutaneous antegrade
Indications:
•Suspected partial outflow obstruction & a relatively normal plasma creatinine

•Renal magnetic resonance imaging−MRI or angiography−MRA
Indications:
•Suspected vascular stenosis

260

Percutaneous renal biopsy
Indications:
- •Suspected systemic disease→
  - ∘Intra-renal renal failure
- •Unexplained, persistent renal failure
- •Suspected renal transplant rejection

Outcomes:
- •Renal histology will affect treatment in 70% of patients undergoing biopsy

Complications–<1% overall:
- •Hematoma
- •Infection
- •Death

TREATMENT OF ACUTE RENAL FAILURE

- •**Treat the etiologic disease**
- •**Discontinue nephrotoxic, dysautoregulatory, & potassium retaining medications**
- •**Adjust medications** according to renal failure severity, & use caution w/ the following:
  - ∘Allopurinol
  - ∘Aminoglycosides→
    - −Acute tubular necrosis
  - ∘Atenolol→
    - −Bradycardia (Atenolol > Metoprolol)
  - ∘Digoxin
  - ∘Histamine 2 selective receptor blockers
  - ∘Lithium
  - ∘Magnesium containing medications
    - −Antacids
    - −Laxatives
  - ∘Meperidine†→
    - −Seizure
  - ∘Metformin†→
    - −Lactic acidemia
  - ∘NSAIDs & COX−2 inhibitors→
    - −Pre-renal renal failure
  - ∘Sucralfate→
    - −Aluminum toxicity via aluminum content
  - ∘Sulfonylureas→
    - −Hypoglycemia (Glyburide > Glipizide)
- •**Potassium restriction:** 40mEq/ 24hours
  Foods w/ ↑potassium content:
  - •Bananas
  - •Melons
  - •Oranges
  - •Potatoes
  - •Tomatoes
- •**Protein restriction:** 0.7g/kg/24hours, w/ a total caloric intake of 40kcal/kg/24hours to avoid catabolism
  Dose adjustment:
  - •Patients w/ ↑catabolic states require ↑amounts

---

†Should be avoided in all patients w/ renal failure

HYPERVOLEMIA ━━━━━━━━━━━━━━━━
- •**Fluid restriction** to ≤1.5L/ 24h (~6 cups)
  Guide:
  - •1oz = 30mL
  - •1cup = 8oz = 240mL
  - •4cups = 32oz = ~1L
- •↓**Sodium intake**
  - ∘≤100mmol sodium/ 24h=2g elemental sodium or 6g salt/ 24h, which can usually be achieved w/ a no–added salt diet. Patients w/ poorly compensated renal failure should only consume 0.5–1g elemental sodium or 1.5–3g salt/ 24h
  - ∘→↓Renal potassium loss if taking a diuretic

LOOP DIURETICS

Indications:
- Pulmonary edema
- To convert oliguric to non-oliguric renal failure, which has a better prognosis

Generic (Trade)	M	♀	Start	Max
Furosemide (Lasix)	K	?	20mg q24–q12hours PO/ IM/ IV	600mg/ 24hours
• IV infusion†:			0.05mg/kg/hour	160mg/ hour

Onset: 1hour, Duration: 6hours (La**six** lasts **six** hours)

- There is synergistic efficacy of combination treatment w/ a thiazide diuretic
- Intravenous administration may be preferred, as intestinal edema→
  - ↓Absorption
- Administer 2nd dose in the mid-afternoon to avoid nocturia
- †Furosemide→
  - ↑Juxtaglomerular cell renin secretion→
    - −↑Angiotensin 2 & aldosterone levels→vasoconstriction→↑afterload→↓cardiac output, which may→clinical deterioration during acute decompensated heart failure. Being that the diuretic effect is related predominantly to its renal tubular secretion rate (as it is not filtered by the glomerulus), while its vasoconstricting effects are related to its plasma concentration, some advocate the **administration of continuous intravenous Furosemide** when >80mg IV is needed for adequate diuresis, thus providing a means for ↑diuretic effectiveness

Dose adjustment:
- For patients currently on chronic loop diuretic treatment, starting dose=current dose + above starting dose
- Once organ edema has resolved, consider maintenance dosing @ same dose q24h w/ titration

Conversion equivalents
40mg PO = 20mg IV

Limitations:
- ↓Efficacy in patients w/ a glomerular filtration rate <10mL/ min.

Side effects:
- **Genitourinary**
  - Acute interstitial nephritis
- **Neurologic**
  - **Ototoxicity**
- **Hematologic**
  - Acid base disturbances
    - Hypochloremic metabolic alkalemia
  - Dyslipidemia
    - ↑Cholesterol & triglycerides
  - Electrolyte disturbances
    - **Hypokalemia**
    - Hypomagnesemia
    - Hyponatremia
    - Hypercalcemia
  - Hyperglycemia
  - Hyperuricemia

Contraindications:
- **Sulfa allergy**, as all thiazide & loop diuretics (except Ethacrynic acid) contain a sulfa component

262

HYPERPHOSPHATEMIA/ HYPOCALCEMIA

•**Phosphate restriction** to ≤10g/kg/24hours
  Indications:
    •Hyperphosphatemia
  Goal levels:
    •Plasma phosphorus 4–6mg/ dL (normal 3–4.5mg/ dL)
    •Normalized plasma calcium

INTESTINAL PHOSPHATE BINDERS			
Generic (Trade)	M ♀		Dose
Aluminum hydroxide† (Alternagel)	K ?		30–60ml PO tid, w/ meals
Calcium carbonate (Mylanta, Rolaids, Tums)	K ?		500mg elemental calcium PO tid, w/ meals
Calcium acetate (PhosLo)	K P		2tabs (169mg elemental Ca^{+2}/ tab) PO, tid w/ meals
Sevelamer (Renagel)‡	Ø ?		800–1600mg PO q8hours, w/ meals

†Initially, consider the use of aluminum hydroxide, as it is more effective than calcium containing phosphate binders, & avoids the risk of precipitating **metastatic tissue calcification** (occurring w/ a calcium–phosphate product ≥60)→
  •Finger &/or toe small vessel calcification→
    ◦Painful ischemic gangrene, termed calciphylaxis
However, once the phosphate is normalized, switch to calcium carbonate or acetate to both treat possible concomitant hypocalcemia & avoid the risk of renal failure mediated aluminum accumulation
‡May be used w/ concomitant hypercalcemia

SECOND LINE TREATMENT

ACTIVATED VITAMIN D			
Generic	M ♀	Start	Titrate
•1,25–dihydroxycholecalciferol (Rocaltrol)	L ?	0.25µg PO q24hours	qmonth by 0.25µg prn

METABOLIC ACIDEMIA

BICARBONATE		
Generic	M ♀	Dose
Sodium bicarbonate	K ?	
•**Moderate disease** (HCO^{-3} <16mEq/ L)		650–1300mg PO q8hours
•**Severe disease** (HCO^{-3} <12mEq/ L or pH<7.2)		2–5mEq/kg/dose IV infusion over 4–8hours prn

Goal plasma bicarbonate:
  •>20mEq/ L (normal 23–28mEq/ L)
Side effects:
  •May exacerbate volume overload due to sodium content

HEMORRHAGE ▬▬▬▬▬
•**Fluid resuscitation**

ANTI–DIURETIC HORMONE ANALOGUE: Long acting					
Generic (Trade)	M ♀	Dose		Onset	Duration
Desmopressin (DDAVP)	LK P	0.3µg/ kg IV q12h prn		1–2hours	7hours

FACTOR 8	
Generic	Dose
Cryoprecipitate	10–15 units typically transfused at a time (25mL cryoprecipitate/ unit)
Mechanism:	
•Contains factors 8, 13, von Willebrand factor, & fibrinogen	

ALLERGIC ACUTE INTERSTITIAL NEPHRITIS ▬▬▬

SYSTEMIC GLUCOCORTICOID TREATMENT

Generic	M ♀	Dose
Methylprednisolone	L ?	60mg PO/ IV q6hours X 1week
Prednisolone	L ?	60mg PO/ IV q6hours X 1week
Prednisone	L ?	60mg PO q6hours X 1week

•Both the IV & PO routes have equal efficacy

Glucocorticoids	Relative potencies Anti-inflammatory	Mineralocorticoid	Duration	Dose equiv.
Cortisol (physiologic†)	1	1	10hours	20mg
Cortisone (PO)	0.7	2	10hours	25mg
Hydrocortisone (PO, IM, IV)	1	2	10hours	20mg
Methylprednisolone (PO, IM, IA, IV)	5	0.5	15–35hours	5mg
Prednisone (PO)	5	0.5	15–35hours	5mg
Prednisolone (PO, IM, IV)	5	0.8	15–35hours	5mg
Triamcinolone (PO, IM)	5	~0	15–35hours	5mg
Betamethasone (PO, IM, IA)	25	~0	35–70hours	0.75mg
Dexamethasone (PO)	25	~0	35–70hours	0.75mg
Fludrocortisone (PO)	10	125	10hours	

†The physiologic rate of adrenal cortical cortisol production is 20–30mg/ 24hours

OTHER COMPLICATIONS ▬▬▬
•Careful w/ urethral catheterization, which may→
 •Decompression hemorrhagic cystitis, due to overly rapid urinary bladder decompression (esp. after prolonged expansion) via the rapid removal of >1L of urine
•Treatment of severe acute obstruction may→
 ∘Post–obstructive diuresis→
  −Fluid & electrolyte loss, which should be replenished

PROGNOSIS
•30% of patients w/ acute renal failure require dialysis
Mortality:
 •Infection–75% >> cardiopulmonary complications > others

RENAL REPLACEMENT THERAPY
Indications:
 •Hyperkalemia refractory to medical treatment
 •Metabolic acidemia refractory to bicarbonate treatment, or if unable to administer bicarbonate due to hypervolemia
 •Intoxication
  ∘Acetylsalicylic acid
  ∘Ethylene glycol
  ∘Lithium
  ∘Methanol
 •Volume overload→
  ∘Pulmonary edema refractory to diuretic treatment
 •Uremia mediated:
  ∘Encephalopathy
  ∘Hemorrhage
  ∘Intractable nausea ± vomiting
  ∘Pericarditis
  ∘Progressive neuropathy
 •Severe malnutrition, as required replenishment would→
  ∘↑Uremia
  Malnutrition indices: Either:
   •Albumin <3.8g/ dL
   •Pre–albumin <18mg/ dL
   •Transferrin <180μg/ dL
 •Creatinine clearance
  ∘<10mL/ min. for non–diabetics
  ∘<15mL/ min. for diabetics
Frequency:
 •Usually q48hours, w/ attention to medications affected by dialysis

<u>Outcomes:</u>
- •Hemodialysis does not ↓mortality in acute renal failure

PROPHYLAXIS

- •**Radiocontrast dye**
  - ◦Administration of the smallest amount necessary
  - ◦Use of a nonionic & iso−osmolar dye
  - ◦Hydration 12−24hours before & after the imaging study, via either:
    - −Intravenous fluid administration
    - −Holding the administration of diuretic medications & dysautoregulatory medications (ACEi, ARB, NSAIDs)

&

N−ACETYLCYSTEINE		
M ♀	Dose	
L P	600mg PO q12hours, on the day before & of imaging	

- •**Aminoglycosides**
  - ◦Use the lowest dose necessary
  - ◦Extended interval dosing
  - ◦Treatment limitation to ≤10days
  - <u>Note:</u> Upon discontinuation, renal failure may persist or worsen over the following week due to accumulation in the renal cortex

CHRONIC RENAL FAILURE

•Any disease→
  ◦**Intra-renal disease**→**chronic** ↓**renal function**→
    −↓Excretion of nitrogenous waste products (ammonia, blood urea nitrogen–BUN, creatinine, uric acid, etc...) which are the end-products of protein catabolism→**uremia, w/ altered fluid & electrolyte regulation**
Statistics:
  •Affects 11% of the U.S. population

PATHOPHYSIOLOGY OF NITROGENOUS WASTE PRODUCTS

•Cellular amino acid metabolism→
  ◦**Ammonia (NH₃)** formation, w/ subsequent extracellular diffusion→hepatocyte metabolism (via the cytoplasmic urea cycle enzymes) to **urea**, w/ subsequent extracellular diffusion→
    −Urinary excretion, via both glomerular filtration & renal tubular secretion
    −Gastrointestinal diffusion→bacterial urease mediated metabolism to CO_2 & ammonia, w/ subsequent extracellular reabsorption
•Hepatocyte amino acid metabolism→
  ◦Creatine formation, w/ subsequent myocyte creatine kinase mediated reversible phosphorylation→
    −Creatine phosphate (being proportional to muscle mass), which provides a rapidly metabolizeable reserve of high energy phosphates, serving to maintain the intracellular ATP level during the first several min. of myocyte contraction. Creatine phosphate is slowly metabolized to **creatinine**, being excreted via both glomerular filtration & renal tubular secretion
•**Uric acid** is a metabolic byproduct of purine metabolism, which are essential components of DNA synthesis

RISK FACTORS

•**Diabetes mellitus–35%**
•**Hypertension–25%**
•**Glomerulonephritis–15%**
•**Interstitial nephritis–5%**
•**Polycystic kidney disease–5%**
•**Other–15%**, which may be due to prolonged pre-renal or post-renal disease

CLASSIFICATION

SEVERITY CLASSIFICATION		
Stage	Severity	GFR (mL/min./1.73m^2)
1	Renal dysfunction†	>90
2	Mild failure†	60–89
3	Moderate failure	30–59 or biochemical evidence of renal failure
4	Severe failure	15–29 or symptomatic renal failure
5	ESRD	Permanently <15 or dependence on renal replacement therapy (dialysis or transplantation) in order to avoid lethal uremia‡

†May be normal for age &/or gender, w/ absolute chronic renal failure @ a glomerular filtration rate <60mL/ min.
‡Usually @ a glomerular filtration rate of:
  •<10mL/ min. for non-diabetics
  •<15mL/ min. for diabetics

DIAGNOSIS

General
•Uremia→
  ◦Anorexia→
    −↓Cachexia
  ◦Malaise
•Hypovolemia→
  ◦↓Weight (1L fluid=1kg=2.2 lbs)
•↓Fluid excretion→
  ◦Hypervolemia→
    −↑Weight (1L fluid=1kg=2.2 lbs)
    −Pitting edema, requiring ≥3L of fluid

266

Cardiovascular
- Uremia→
  - Pericardial inflammation=pericarditis, esp. @ >100mg/ dL
  - ↓Lipoprotein lipase & hepatic lipase function→
    - **Hypertriglyceridemia→↑atherosclerosis**
- ↓Intravascular volume→
  - ≥10% blood volume loss→
    - ↑Autonomic sympathetic tone→↑pulse
  - ≥20% blood volume loss→
    - Orthostatic hypotension (supine to standing→↑20 pulse, ↓20 SBP, &/or ↓10 DBP)→ lightheadedness upon standing
    - Urine output 20–30mL/ hour (normal being >30mL/ hour)
  - ≥30% blood volume loss→
    - Recumbent hypotension &/or tachycardia
  - ≥40% blood volume loss→
    - Altered mental status &/or urine output <20mL/ hour
    - Hypovolemic shock, being hypotension + organ failure, unresponsive to fluid resuscitation
- ↓Fluid excretion→
  - Heart failure
  - Hypertension

Endocrine
- Uremia→
  - Hyperglycemia, termed **secondary diabetes mellitus**
  - ↑Anterior pituitary prolactin secretion→hyperprolactinemia, w/ concomitant ↓renal clearance→
    - ♂: Gynecomastia, galactorrhea, &/or hypogonadism
    - ♀: Amenorrhea
- ↓Phosphate excretion→
  - Hyperphosphatemia→hypocalcemia→
    - ↑Parathyroid hormone–PTH secretion, termed **secondary hyperparathyroidism**

Gastrointestinal
- Uremia→
  - Metabolism to ammonia in saliva→
    - Metallic taste sensation
    - Urine-like odored breath, termed uremic fetor
  - Inflammation anywhere along the gastrointestinal tract, from the oropharnyx to the anus
- Prostate enlargement→
  - Urinary retention†→
    - Urinary bladder distention→pelvic, back, &/or flank pain

---

†Perform bladder catheterization to determine the post–void residual, w/ >100mL indicating incomplete voiding via either:
- Obstruction
- Autonomic neuropathy

Immunologic
- Uremia→
  - ↓Lymphocyte function→
    - Immunosuppression→**infection, being the #1 cause of mortality**

Mucocutaneous
- Uremia→
  - Acne
  - Dryness→
    - Pruritus
  - White urea crystal deposition on the skin via sweat→
    - Uremic frost
- Hyperpigmentation

Musculoskeletal
- Aluminum containing medications or dialysate→
  - Bone aluminum deposits→
    - Bone demineralization (calcium & phosphate)

- •Secondary hyperparathyroidism→
  - ○Subperiosteal bone resorption
  - ○**Osteitis fibrosa cystica**
  - ○↓Osteoblast activity→relatively ↑osteoclast activity→
    - −↓Bone demineralization (calcium & phosphate)
    - −↓Bone matrix formation
    - ...→↓**bone density**, being greater than the age expected norm→
      - •Diffuse osteopenia→
        - ○Secondary osteoporosis
  - ...all→bone weakening→
    - •↑**Fracture risk**

Neurologic
- •↓Excretion of nitrogenous waste products→central nervous system dysfunction, termed **renal encephalopathy**→
  - ○**Altered mental status**
  - ○Cerebral edema
  - ○Headache
  - ○Nausea ± vomiting
  - ○Altered neuromuscular function→
    - −**Asterixis**, being an inability to maintain a posture
      - Examination:
        - •Usually assessed using the upper extremities, but may viewed via any attempt at voluntary posture maintenance. Best viewed by asking the patient to hold out extended arms & dorsiflexed hands, w/ fingers spread as though signaling traffic to stop→
          - ○An intermittent, non−rhythmic flapping tremor of the wrist & metacarpophalangeal joints due to **intermittent inhibition of wrist extensors**→
            - −Brief lapses of posture. If the patient cannot comply, simply ask them to squeeze your extended fingers→intermittently ↓grip strength
      - Limitations: Also found w/:
        - •Hepatic failure→
          - ○Hyperammonemia
        - •Chronic heart failure
        - •Chronic lung disease→
          - ○Respiratory failure
  - ○Segmental axonal demyelination→
    - −Nerve disease=**neuropathy**, over years

  - Peripheral symmetric polyneuropathy (sensory >> motor)
    - •**Abnormal sensations, termed paresthesias** (numbness, pain, &/or tingling) beginning in the hands & feet (as longer neurons have ↑myelination, & so are affected sooner), w/ proximal progression
      - ○Numbness→
        - −**Unrecognized foot trauma** (cut, blister)→↑infection risk
    - Diagnosis:
      - •**A nylon monofilament** designated 5.07 is pressed against the skin to the point of buckling. A patients inability to feel the buckled monofilament indicates neuropathy
    - Additional exacerbatory factors:
      - •Atherosclerosis mediated ↓blood supply, & hyperglycemia mediated immunosuppression→
        - ○↓**Wound healing**, w/ ↑ulcer formation

  - Autonomic neuropathy
    - •↓**Sympathetic tone:**
      - ○Orthostatic hypotension→
        - −Falls
      - ○↑Gastrointestinal tone→
        - −Diarrhea
      - ○↓Hypoglycemic response, termed hypoglycemic unawareness
    - •↓**Parasympathetic tone:**
      - ○Fixed, resting tachycardia
      - ○Impotence
      - ○↓Gastrointestinal tone→
        - −Abdominal distention
        - −Constipation
        - −Nausea ± vomiting
      - ○Incomplete urinary bladder emptying, termed neurogenic bladder→
        - −Overflow incontinence
        - −↑Urinary tract infection risk

Precipitants of renal encephalopathy:
- •↑**Protein metabolism**
  - ◦Blood transfusion
  - ◦↑Dietary protein
  - ◦Gastrointestinal hemorrhage
  - ◦Inflammation
  - …→↑ammonia production
- •**Hypovolemia→**
  - ◦↑Plasma concentration of the various possible causative substances
  - ◦↓Hepatic & renal perfusion→
    - –↓Filtration
- •Certain medications, esp.
  - ◦Analgesics (opiates)
  - ◦Sedatives (benzodiazepines, barbiturates)
- •↑Bacterial contact w/ colonic substrates via:
  - ◦Constipation
  - ◦Ileus (obstructive or paralytic)
  - …→↑ammonia production
- •Hepatic failure→
  - ◦↓Conversion of ammonia to urea
- •↑Renal production of ammonia
  - ◦Hypokalemia
- •↑Diffusion of ammonia across the blood brain barrier
  - ◦Alkalemia
- •Iatrogenic
  - ◦Peritoneojugular shunt
  - ◦Portosystemic shunting
    - –Transjugular intrahepatic portosystemic shunt–TIPS

Pulmonary
- •Hiccoughs

Hematologic
- •↓Excretion of nitrogenous waste products→
  - ◦↑Ammonia
  - ◦↑**Blood urea nitrogen–BUN**
    - –↓Platelet & factor 8 function→↑hemorrhage risk, termed coagulopathy, w/ ↑bleeding time being the best predictor of hemorrhage risk
  - ◦↑**Creatinine**
    - –Being that the plasma creatinine does not become abnormal until the glomerular filtration rate ↓ by 50%↑, creatinine clearance allows for a more accurate assessment of renal function
  - ◦↑Uric acid
- •**Hyperkalemia** via:
  - ◦↓Tubular secretion, occurring @ a:
    - –Glomerular filtration rate <10mL/ min.
    - –Urine output <1L/ 24h
    - …→potassium homeostasis adaptive mechanism failure
  - ◦Acidemia, as every **0.1↓ in pH→0.5mEq/ L↑ in potassium** via the H^+/K^+ cell membrane exchange protein→
    - –Potassium extracellular shift
  - ◦Coagulopathy→
    - –Gastrointestinal hemorrhage→intestinal absorption
    - –Hematoma→absorption
  - ◦Low grade, chronic hemolysis
- •**Anemia @ a glomerular filtration rate <30mL/ min.**, via:
  - ◦↓Erythropoietin production
  - ◦Low grade chronic hemolysis
  - ◦Uremia mediated ↓erythropoiesis
    - …→**normocytic, normochromic anemia**, w/ a ↓reticulocyte count
- •**Hypermagnesemia** via ↓excretion
- •**Hypervolemic hyponatremia** via total body water > NaCl, which may be due to either:
  - ◦↑Intake, due to thirst
  - ◦Relatively ↑renal tubular water absorption, due to antidiuretic hormone–ADH
- •**Hyperphosphatemia @ a glomerular filtration rate <50mL/ min.**, via ↓excretion
- •**Hypocalcemia @ a glomerular filtration rate <50mL/ min.**, via hyperphosphatemia→
  - ◦↑Calcium binding
  - ◦↓Renal mediated 1,25–dihydroxycholecalciferol production (also due to primary renal disease)→↓intestinal calcium absorption

269

- **Metabolic acidemia @ a glomerular filtration rate <25mL/ min.**, via ↓excretion of sulfuric & phosphoric acids→
  - ○Widened, anion gap, metabolic acidemia‡

Additional serologic testing for Intrarenal renal failure:
- **Cryoglobulinemic glomerulonephritis**
  - ○Cryoglobulins
  - ○Hepatitis C virus antibodies
- **Goodpasture's syndrome**
  - ○Antiglomerular basement membrane–GBM antibodies, w/ hemoptysis
- **Myeloma**
  - ○Plasma & urine protein electrophoresis
- **Polyarteritis nodosa**
  - ○Perinuclear antineutrophil cytoplasmic antibodies P–ANCA
- **Post-infectious glomerulonephritis**
  - ○↓Complement 3
- **Post–streptococcal glomerulonephritis**
  - ○Anti–deoxyribonuclease–DNase B
  - ○Anti–streptolysin O–ASO
  - ○↓Complement 3
- **Systemic lupus erythematosus–SLE**
  - ○Antinuclear antibodies–ANA
    - –Anti–dsDNA
    - –Anti–Sm (Smith)
  - ○↓Complement 3 & 4
- **Wegener's granulomatosis**
  - ○Circulating antineutrophil cytoplasmic antibodies C–ANCA, w/ hemoptysis

---

†Correlation of creatinine w/ glomerular filtration rate:
- Creatinine 1→2mg/ dL, indicates a 50%↓GFR
- Creatinine 3→4mg/ dL, indicates a 5%↓GFR

‡Plasma anion gap= $[Na^+] - ([Cl^-] + [HCO_3])$
- **Normal value: 8–12 mEq/ L**
- Equation value: 12 mEq/ L

Correction:
- **Hypoalbuminemia:** For each 1g/ dL ↓in albumin below 4, add 2.5 to the calculated anion gap
- **Acidemia:** Add 2 to the calculated anion gap
- **Alkalemia:** Add 4 to the calculated anion gap

Interpretation:
- A widened gap indicates the **presence of excess unmeasured anions**, via either:
  - ○Organic acids
  - ○Phosphates
  - ○Sulfates

CREATININE CLEARANCE MEDIATED GFR ESTIMATION			
Gender	Cockcroft–Gault formula (mL/ min.)	Normal	Age adjusted norm
♂	(140 − age) X weight (kg) / 72 X plasma creatinine (mg/ dL)†	100–140	133 − (0.64 X age)
♀	♂ X 0.85	85–115	[133 − (0.64 X age)] X 0.85

†Does not require a 24hour urine collection
- **Creatinine clearance becomes an unreliable indicator of glomerular filtration rate @ <30mL/ min.**, as renal tubular creatinine secretion makes up an increasing fraction of the total creatinine eliminated→
  - Falsely ↑amount

URINE EVALUATION
- Inactive sediment (lacking cells, organisms, & crystals) w/ broad casts indicate **chronic** tubulointerstitial scarring & tubular atrophy→
  - ○Widened tubular diameter

270

•Renal & pelvic ultrasound
Indications/ findings:
- •To look for obstruction
  - ∘Dilated pyelocalceal outflow tract, indicating hydronephrosis. A non–dilated tract does not exclude obstruction, esp. in the acute setting
  - ∘Distended bladder or residual urine if recent urination
  - ∘Nephrolithiasis
- •To look for possible chronic renal disease
  - ∘Small kidneys, being <8cm
    - –Consider renal artery stenosis if unilateral
  - ∘Large kidneys indicate either:
    - –Diabetes mellitus
    - –HIV nephropathy
    - –Infiltrative disease (amyloidosis, multiple myeloma)
    - –Polycystic kidney disease

•Renal magnetic resonance imaging–MRI or angiography–MRA
Indications:
- •Suspected vascular stenosis

Percutaneous renal biopsy
Indications:
- •Suspected systemic disease→
  - ∘Intra–renal renal failure
- •Unexplained, persistent renal failure
- •Suspected renal transplant rejection
Outcomes:
- •Renal histology will affect treatment in 70% of patients undergoing biopsy
Complications–<1% overall:
- •Hematoma
- •Infection
- •Death

•Treat the etiologic disease
•Hypertension control
- ∘Systolic blood pressure <120mmHg & diastolic blood pressure <80 mmHg
•Discontinue nephrotoxic, dysautoregulatory, & potassium retaining medications
•Adjust medications according to renal failure severity, & use caution w/ the following:
- ∘Allopurinol
- ∘Aminoglycosides→
  - –Acute tubular necrosis
- ∘Atenolol→
  - –Bradycardia (Atenolol > Metoprolol)
- ∘Digoxin
- ∘Histamine 2 selective receptor blockers
- ∘Lithium
- ∘Magnesium containing medications
  - –Antacids
  - –Laxatives
- ∘Meperidine†→
  - –Seizure
- ∘Metformin†→
  - –Lactic acidemia
- ∘NSAIDs & COX–2 inhibitors→
  - –Pre–renal renal failure
- ∘Sucralfate→
  - –Aluminum toxicity via aluminum content
- ∘Sulfonylureas→
  - –Hypoglycemia (Glyburide > Glipizide)

- **Potassium restriction:** 40mEq/ 24hours
  Foods w/ ↑potassium content:
  - Bananas
  - Melons
  - Oranges
  - Potatoes
  - Tomatoes
- **Protein restriction:** 0.7–1g/kg/24hours, w/ a total caloric intake of 40kcal/kg/24hours, to avoid catabolism
  Dose adjustment:
  - Patients w/ ↑catabolic states require ↑amounts
  - If concurrent nephrotic syndrome: 0.8g/kg/24hours + 1g protein/ g proteinuria
  Outcomes:
  - ↓Uremia
  - **↓Progression of renal disease**

†Should be avoided in all patients w/ renal failure

RENAL PROTECTION

ANGIOTENSIN CONVERTING ENZYME INHIBITORS–ACEi				
Generic (Trade)	M	♀	Start	Max
Benazepril (Lotensin)	LK	U	10mg PO q24hours	40mg/ 24hours
Captopril (Capoten)	LK	U	12.5mg PO q12hours	450mg/ 24hours
Enalapril (Vasotec)	LK	U	5mg PO q24hours	40mg/ 24hours
Fosinopril (Monopril)	LK	U	10mg PO q24hours	40mg/ 24hours
Lisinopril (Prinivil, Zestril)	K	U	10mg PO q24hours	40mg q24hours

Dose adjustment:
- ↓Initial dose by 50% if:
  ○ Elderly
  ○ Concomitant diuretic use
  ○ Renal disease

Mechanism:
- Reversibly inhibits angiotensin converting enzyme–ACE→
  ○ ↓Bradykinin degradation→
    – Vasodilation
  ○ ↓Angiotensin 2 formation→
    – Vasodilation (**arterial** > venous)
    – ↓Renal NaCl & water retention
    – ↓Adrenal cortex aldosterone release→↓renal NaCl & water retention
    – ↓Facilitation of adrenal medullary & presynaptic norepinephrine release→vasodilation
    – Glomerular efferent arteriole vasodilation→↓intraglomerular hydrostatic pressure→↓filtration→ ↓proteinuria in patients w/ nephropathy
  ○ ↓Cardiovascular remodeling

Side effects:
  Cardiovascular
  - Hypotension
  Gastrointestinal
  - Altered gustatory sense=dysguesia–3%
  Genitourinary
  - Acute interstitial nephritis
  - Patients w/ pre–existing bilateral ↓renal perfusion, not necessarily failure:
    ○ Heart failure
    ○ Bilateral renal artery stenosis
    ○ Hypovolemia
    ○ Renal failure
    …rely more on the compensatory production of angiotensin 2→
      - Efferent arteriole constriction→
        ○ Maintained glomerular filtration rate–GFR, whereas either:
          – Angiotensin converting enzyme inhibition
          – Angiotensin 2 receptor blockade
          …→↓angiotensin 2 production & action respectively, which may→
            - **Pre–renal renal failure**

Mucocutaneous
- •↓Bradykinin & substance P degradation→↑levels→hypersensitivity–like syndrome→
  - ∘**Angioedema–0.4%**, usually within 2weeks of treatment, but may manifest @ months to years→
    - −Soft tissue edema of the epiglottis, face, lips, oropharynx, &/or tongue
  - ∘**Dermatitis–10%**

Pulmonary
- •↑Bradykinin levels→
  - ∘**Chronic cough–20%**, usually being dry & involuntary

Materno–fetal
- •**Fetal & neonatal morbidity & mortality**

Hematologic
- •↓Aldosterone production ± renal failure→
  - ∘**Hyperkalemia**
- •Neutropenia

Monitoring:
- •Check creatinine & potassium @ 3–10days after initiation or dose↑, then
  - ∘Q3–6months

Contraindications:
Genitourinary
- •Acute renal failure
- •Bilateral renal artery stenosis
- •Unilateral renal artery stenosis of a solitary functioning kidney

Mucocutaneous
- •Angiotensin converting enzyme inhibitor induced angioedema or dermatitis

Materno–fetal
- •Breast feeding
- •**Pregnancy**

Hematologic
- •**Potassium >5mEq/ L**

ANGIOTENSIN 2 RECEPTOR BLOCKERS–ARBs

Generic (Trade)	M	♀	Start	Max
Candesartan (Atacand)	K	?	16mg PO q24hours	32mg q24hours
Eprosartan (Teveten)	F	U	600mg PO q24hours	800mg/ 24hours
Irbesartan (Avapro)	L	U	150mg PO q24hours	300mg q24hours
Olmisartan (Benicar)	K	U	20mg PO q24hours	40mg q24hours
Losartan (Cozaar)	L	U	50mg PO q24hours	100mg/ 24hours
Telmisartan (Micardis)	L	U	40mg PO q24hours	80mg q24hours
Valsartan (Diovan)	L	U	80mg PO q24hours	320mg q24hours

Dose adjustment:
- •↓Initial dose by 50% if:
  - ∘Elderly
  - ∘Concomitant diuretic use
  - ∘Renal disease

Losartan specific dose adjustment:
- •Starting dose is halved if concomitant hepatic disease

Mechanism:
- •Angiotensin 2 receptor blockade→
  - ∘↓Angiotensin 2 action→
    - −Vasodilation (**arterial** > venous)
    - −↓Renal NaCl & water retention
    - −↓Adrenal cortex aldosterone release→↓renal NaCl & water retention
    - −↓Facilitation of adrenal medullary & presynaptic norepinephrine release→vasodilation
    - −Glomerular efferent arteriole vasodilation→↓intraglomerular hydrostatic pressure→↓filtration→ ↓proteinuria in patients w/ nephropathy
  - ∘↓Cardiovascular remodeling

Side effects†:
Cardiovascular
- •Hypotension

Gastrointestinal
- •Altered gustatory sense=dysguesia–3%

273

Genitourinary
- Acute interstitial nephritis
- Patients w/ preexisting bilateral ↓renal perfusion, not necessarily failure:
  - Heart failure
  - Bilateral renal artery stenosis
  - Hypovolemia
  - Renal failure
  - …rely more on the compensatory production of angiotensin 2→
    - Efferent arteriole constriction→
      - Maintained glomerular filtration rate–GFR, whereas either:
        - –Angiotensin converting enzyme inhibition
        - –Angiotensin 2 receptor blockade
        - …→↓angiotensin 2 production & action respectively, which may→
          - **Pre–renal renal failure**

Materno–fetal
- **Fetal & neonatal morbidity & mortality**

Hematologic
- ↓Aldosterone production ± renal failure→
  - **Hyperkalemia**
- Neutropenia

---

†Do not cause the hypersensitivity–like syndrome associated w/ ACE inhibitors, due to lack of bradykinin & substance P elevation

Monitoring:
- Check creatinine & potassium @ 3–10days after initiation or dose↑, then
  - Q3–6months

Contraindications:
Genitourinary
- Acute renal failure
- Bilateral renal artery stenosis
- Unilateral renal artery stenosis of a solitary functioning kidney

Materno–fetal
- Breast feeding
- **Pregnancy**

Hematologic
- **Potassium >5mEq/ L**

HYPERVOLEMIA
- **Fluid restriction** to ≤1.5L/ 24h (~6 cups)
  - Guide:
    - 1oz = 30mL
    - 1cup = 8oz = 240mL
    - 4cups = 32oz = ~1L
- **↓Sodium intake**
  - ≤100mmol sodium/ 24h=2g elemental sodium or 6g salt/ 24h, which can usually be achieved w/ a no-added salt diet. Patients w/ poorly compensated renal failure should only consume 0.5–1g elemental sodium or 1.5–3g salt/ 24h
  - →↓Renal potassium loss if taking a diuretic

THIAZIDE DIURETICS

Generic (Trade)	M ♀		Start	Max
Hydrochlorothiazide	L	U	12.5mg PO q24hours	50mg q24hours
Metolazone (Zaroxolyn)	L	U	5mg PO q24hours	10mg q24hours

Duration: 6–12hours

- There is synergistic efficacy of combination treatment w/ a loop diuretic

Mechanism:
- Inhibits NaCl reabsorption in the early distal convoluted tubule→
  - ↑Urination→
    - –↓Intravascular volume→↓cardiac preload→↓cardiac output→eventual compensatory intravascular volume repletion to near pre–treatment levels, but w/ peripheral vascular resistance falling below pre–treatment baseline being responsible for the chronic hypotensive effect

Limitations:
- ↓Efficacy in patients w/ a glomerular filtration rate <30mL/ min.

274

Side effects:
Genitourinary
•Acute interstitial nephritis
Neurologic
•**Ototoxicity**
Hematologic
•Acid base disturbances
  ∘Hypochloremic metabolic alkalemia
•Dyslipidemia
  ∘↑Cholesterol & triglycerides
•Electrolyte disturbances
  ∘**Hypokalemia**
  ∘Hypomagnesemia
  ∘Hyponatremia
  ∘Hypercalcemia
•Hyperglycemia
•Hyperuricemia

Contraindications:
•**Sulfa allergy**, as all thiazide & loop diuretics (except Ethacrynic acid) contain a sulfa component

LOOP DIURETICS			
Generic (Trade)	M ♀	**Start**	**Max**
Furosemide (Lasix)	K ?	20mg q24-12hours PO	600mg/ 24hours
Onset: 1hour, Duration: 6hours (La**six** lasts **six** hours)			

•There is synergistic efficacy of combination treatment w/ a thiazide diuretic
•Administer 2nd dose in the mid-afternoon to avoid nocturia

Mechanism:
•Inhibits $Na^+/K^+/2Cl^-$ reabsorption in the thick ascending limb of the loop of Henle→
  ∘↑Urination→
    −↓Intravascular volume→↓cardiac preload→↓cardiac output→eventual compensatory intravascular volume repletion to near pre-treatment levels, but w/ peripheral vascular resistance falling below pre-treatment baseline being responsible for the chronic hypotensive effect

Limitations:
•↓Efficacy in patients w/ a glomerular filtration rate <10mL/ min.

Side effects:
Genitourinary
•Acute interstitial nephritis
Neurologic
•**Ototoxicity**
Hematologic
•Acid base disturbances
  ∘Hypochloremic metabolic alkalemia
•Dyslipidemia
  ∘↑Cholesterol & triglycerides
•Electrolyte disturbances
  ∘**Hypokalemia**
  ∘Hypomagnesemia
  ∘Hyponatremia
  ∘Hypercalcemia
•Hyperglycemia
•Hyperuricemia

Contraindications:
•**Sulfa allergy**, as all thiazide & loop diuretics (except Ethacrynic acid) contain a sulfa component

275

HYPERPHOSPHATEMIA/ HYPOCALCEMIA ━━━━━
•**Phosphate restriction** to ≤10g/kg/24hours
Indications:
 •Hyperphosphatemia
 Goal levels:
 •Plasma phosphorus 4–6mg/ dL (normal 3–4.5mg/ dL)
 •Normalized plasma calcium

INTESTINAL PHOSPHATE BINDERS			
Generic (Trade)	M ♀		Dose
Aluminum hydroxide† (Alternagel)	K	?	30–60ml PO tid, w/ meals
Calcium carbonate (Mylanta, Rolaids, Tums)	K	?	500mg elemental calcium PO tid, w/ meals
Calcium acetate (PhosLo)	K	P	2tabs (169mg elemental Ca^{+2}/ tab) PO, tid w/ meals
Sevelamer (Renagel)‡	Ø	?	800–1600mg PO q8hours, w/ meals

†Initially, consider the use of aluminum hydroxide, as it is more effective than calcium containing phosphate binders, & avoids the risk of precipitating **metastatic tissue calcification** (occurring w/ a calcium–phosphate product ≥60)→
 •Finger &/or toe small vessel calcification→
  ∘Painful ischemic gangrene, termed calciphylaxis
However, once the phosphate is normalized, switch to calcium carbonate or acetate to both treat possible concomitant hypocalcemia & avoid the risk of renal failure mediated aluminum accumulation
‡May be used w/ concomitant hypercalcemia

SECOND LINE TREATMENT

ACTIVATED VITAMIN D			
Generic	M ♀	Start	Titrate
•1,25–dihydroxycholecalciferol (Rocaltrol) L ?		0.25µg PO q24hours	qmonth by 0.25µg prn

METABOLIC ACIDEMIA ━━━━━━━━━

BICARBONATE	
Generic M ♀	Dose
Sodium bicarbonate K ?	
•**Moderate disease** (HCO^{-3} <16mEq/ L)	650–1300mg PO q8hours
•**Severe disease** (HCO^{-3} <12mEq/ L or pH<7.2)	2–5mEq/kg/dose IV infusion over 4–8hours prn
Goal plasma bicarbonate:	
•>20mEq/ L (normal 23–28mEq/ L)	
Side effects:	
•May exacerbate volume overload due to sodium content	

HEMORRHAGE ━━━━━━
•**Fluid resuscitation**

ANTI-DIURETIC HORMONE ANALOGUE: Long acting				
Generic (Trade)	M ♀	Dose	Onset	Duration
Desmopressin (DDAVP)	LK P	0.3µg/ kg IV q12hours prn	1–2hours	7hours

FACTOR 8	
Generic	Dose
Cryoprecipitate	10–15 units typically transfused at a time (25mL cryoprecipitate/ unit)
Mechanism:	
•Contains factors 8, 13, von Willebrand factor, & fibrinogen	

276

ANEMIA

RECOMBINANT HUMAN ERYTHROPOIETIN

Generic (Trade)	M	♀	Start
Darbopoetin (Aranesp)	†	?	0.45µg/ kg SC/ IV qweek
Erythropoietin (Epogen, Procrit)	L	?	50–100 units/ kg SC/ IV 3 times/ week

&

Generic	M	♀	Dose
Ferrous sulfate	K	P	325mg PO q8hours
Folic acid	K	S	1mg PO q24hours
Multivitamin			1q24hours

CONVERSION SCALE

Erythropoietin/ week (units)	Darbopoetin qweek† (µg)
<2,500	6.25
2,500–4,999	12.5
5,000–10,999	25
11,000–17,999	40
18,000–33,999	60
34,000–89,999	100
≥90,000	200

•Administer Darbopoetin q 2weeks in patients receiving erythropoietin once weekly
†Darbopoetin is metabolized by cellular enzymes termed sialidases

Goal parameters:
•Goal hematocrit/ hemoglobin of 33–36%/ 11–12g/dL
  ◦The ideal hemoglobin level remains a topic of debate, as the current goal parameters were set by
  the U.S. government to meet Medicare reimbursement goals, rather than to reflect scientific
  consensus

Dose adjustment:
•↑Dose by 25% if hemoglobin rises <1g/ dL over 1month
•↓Dose by 25% if hemoglobin 12–13g/ dL
  ◦Hold & ↓reinstated dose if hemoglobin >13g/ dL

Mechanism:
•↑Bone marrow erythrocyte production
•↑Erythrocyte intravascular survival

Outcomes:
•↑Hematocrit/ hemoglobin by 6%/ 2g/dL over 1 month

Side effects:
Cardiovascular
  •↑Blood viscosity
  •Hypertension

Contraindications:
•Uncontrolled hypertension

Monitoring:
•Blood pressure
•Hemoglobin qweek until stable, then
  ◦Qmonth

RENAL REPLACEMENT THERAPY

Indications:
•**Hyperkalemia** refractory to medical treatment
•**Metabolic acidemia** refractory to bicarbonate treatment, or if unable to administer bicarbonate due to
hypervolemia
•**Intoxication**
  ◦Acetylsalicylic acid
  ◦Ethylene glycol
  ◦Lithium
  ◦Methanol
•**Volume** overload→
  ◦**Pulmonary edema** refractory to diuretic treatment

- •Uremia mediated:
  - ∘Encephalopathy
  - ∘Hemorrhage
  - ∘Intractable nausea ± vomiting
  - ∘Pericarditis
  - ∘Progressive neuropathy
- •Severe malnutrition, as required replenishment would→
  - ∘↑Uremia
  <u>Malnutrition indices:</u> Either:
    - •Albumin <3.8g/ dL
    - •Pre−albumin <18mg/ dL
    - •Transferrin <180µg/ dL
- •Creatinine clearance
  - ∘<10mL/ min. for non−diabetics
  - ∘<15mL/ min. for diabetics

<u>Frequency:</u>
- •Usually q48hours, w/ attention to medications affected by dialysis

<u>Outcomes:</u>
- •Hemodialysis does not ↓mortality in acute renal failure

•Mucosal inflammation→
 ◦Erosion ± ulceration, along the stomach, termed gastritis, &/or duodenum, termed duodenitis

•**Gender:** ♂ 3X ♀ for duodenal ulcers
•**Genetic:**
 ◦First degree relative w/ a history of a gastric ulcer
•↑**Gastric acid secretion**, w/ basal output being >10mEq/ hour
 ◦Electrolyte abnormality
  –Hypercalcemia
 ◦Neoplasm
  –Gastrinoma→↑gastrin secretion→↑gastric acid secretion, termed the Zollinger–Ellison syndrome
•**Ectopic acid secretion**
 ◦Anatomic defect
  –Meckel's diverticulum containing ectopic gastric mucosa
•**Infection**
 ◦**Helicobacter pylori colonization/ infection**†→↑risk of:
  –Gastric &/or duodenal ulcers
  –Gastric adenocarcinoma
  –Gastric non–Hodgkin's lymphoma
  …via:
   ◦Release of cytotoxic enzymes (ex. proteases, urease)
   ◦↑Gastrin secretion→
    –↑Gastric acid secretion
•**Lifestyle:**
 ◦**Alcohol**→
  –Direct gastroduodenal mucosal toxicity
  –↑Gastric mucosal HCl & pepsin secretion
 ◦**Cigarette smoking** via unknown mechanisms
•↓**Mucosal defenses**
 ◦Medications
  –**Aspirin** & other **nonsteroidal anti–inflammatory drugs–NSAIDs**→respectively to
  irreversible & reversible inhibition of both cyclooxygenase enzymes (COX–1 & COX–2), w/ COX–1
  being responsible for the maintenance of gastroduodenal mucosal integrity. These medications
  also→local toxic effects on the gastroduodenal mucosa (less so w/ enteric coated preparations)
  –**Glucocorticoids**→Inhibition of phospholipase A_2 mediated conversion of cell membrane lipids to
  arachidonic acid, which is the precursor for both cyclooxygenase–COX enzymes
  Mechanism:
   •Inhibition of the cyclooxygenase COX–1 enzyme→
    ◦↓Gastric mucosal prostaglandin synthesis→
     –↓Epithelial proliferation
     –↓Mucosal blood flow→↓bicarbonate delivery to the mucosa
     –↓Mucus & bicarbonate secretion from gastric mucosal cells
     …→↑peptic inflammatory disease risk
•**Other**
 ◦**Chronic obstructive pulmonary disease–COPD**

---

†In industrialized countries, 50% of persons age >50years are infected

•**Duodenitis ± ulcer–75%**
•**Gastritis ± ulcer–25%**

Gastrointestinal
- Mucosal irritation→↑gastrointestinal smooth muscle contraction→↑peristalsis→
  - **Abdominal pain** (burning, gnawing, &/or tightness), gradually worsening for 1–2hours, w/ subsequent gradual relief. The pain may be precipitated or relieved by eating, termed **dyspepsia**
    - Gastric inflammation is usually worsened by meals→avoidance of food→cachexia
    - Duodenal inflammation is usually relieved by meals
      <u>Areas of pain reference:</u>
      - Stomach &/or duodenum: Epigastrium
      - Small intestine: Periumbilical area
      - Large intestine: Hypogastrium &/or suprapubic area
      - Rectum: Suprapubic, sacral, &/or perineal areas
  - Anorexia
  - ↑Bowel sounds→audible gastrointestinal gurgling, termed borborygmi
  - Diarrhea
  - Retrograde peristalsis→
    - Nausea ± vomiting

<u>Other causes of dyspepsia:</u>
- Myocardial ischemia
- Cholecystitis
- Colorectal cancer
- Delayed gastric emptying
- Ovarian cancer
- Pancreatitis
- Pancreatic cancer
- Renal cell cancer

- **Stool antigen assay†**
  <u>Mechanism:</u>
  - Helicobacter pylori antigen detected in feces via immunoassay
  <u>Limitations:</u>
  - False positive:
    - Gastrointestinal hemorrhage, via possible cross reactivity w/ blood constituents
  <u>Outcomes:</u>
  - Sensitivity–95%
  - Specificity–90%

- **Urease breath test†**
  <u>Mechanism:</u>
  - Helicobacter pylori releases the enzyme urease‡→
    - Metabolism of radiolabeled urea ingested by the patient→
      - Radiolabeled CO_2 detected in the breath, which if positive, indicates current infection
  <u>Outcomes:</u>
  - Sensitivity–93%
  - Specificity–98%

- **Helicobacter pylori serology**
  <u>Findings:</u>
  - Anti–Helicobacter pylori IgG antibodies
  <u>Limitations:</u>
  - Indicate exposure at some point in lifetime, not necessarily current infection

---

†These tests can also be used to monitor for eradication after treatment
‡Urease is an enzyme that catalyzes the conversion of urea & water to carbon dioxide & ammonia:
H_2O + urea —— urease ——> $2NH_3$ (ammonia) + CO_2

•Esophagogastroduodenoscopy–EGD

Indications†:

- •Gastrointestinal hemorrhage, for diagnosis (including biopsy), risk stratification, & appropriate treatment
- •Diagnosis of abdominal pain of uncertain etiology
- •Possible gastric cancer, via:
  - ∘**Biopsy of gastric ulcer (duodenal ulcers are not associated w/ malignancy).** Gastric ulcers↔gastric cancer, w/ both leading to similar syndromes, which may be relieved by the same medications. The following findings are indications for visualization & biopsy:
    - –Age >40 years
    - –Anorexia→cachexia
    - –Anemia
    - –Hemorrhage, being either occult (via fecal occult blood testing) or gross (hematemesis, melena)
    - –Lack of response to medical treatment X 6weeks

Findings:

- •90% of gastric ulcers are on the lesser curvature
- •95% of duodenal ulcers are in the duodenal bulb

Ulceration features suggesting malignancy:

- •Diameter >1cm
- •Mucosal folds not radiating toward the center of the crater
- •Shallow mucosal edges

---

†Esophagogastroduodenoscopy should be accompanied by a search for possible helicobacter pylori infection if a lesion is visualized, via:

- •Biopsy for histology
- •Rapid urease testing, which if positive, allows for diagnosis without the need for histologic confirmation
- •Culture, which may be obtained to perform antibiotic sensitivity testing to detect possible resistant organisms

Limitations:

- •False negative: Recent antibiotic use

•Gastrointestinal hemorrhage 5–20%

- ∘Thrombolytic or anticoagulant medications may initiate or exacerbate hemorrhage via underlying gastrointestinal lesions, but are unlikely to cause normal mucosal hemorrhage

•Gastroduodenal perforation 5–10%→

- ∘Hemorrhage
- ∘Release of contents (air, mucus, digestive enzymes, ± food)→generalized peritonitis

•Gastric outlet obstruction <5%

- ∘Gastric &/or duodenal inflammation near the pylorus→
  - –**Pyloric stenosis**→nausea ± vomiting, w/ chronic pyloric inflammation→fibrotic pyloric stenosis

Physical findings:

- •Succussion splash, indicating excess fluid in the stomach due to outlet obstruction
- •**Saline load test**
  - Procedure:
    1. Place a nasogastric tube (check placement w/ chest x ray) for infusion of 750mL of saline into the stomach
    2. Aspirate the stomach contents 30 min. later, w/ a residual ≥400mL indicating gastric outlet obstruction, in which case, the nasogastric tube then may be used for intermittent suctioning→
       - •↓Mucus & sputum accumulation→
         - ∘↓Risk of gastric content aspiration

281

•**Smoking cessation** via smoking cessation clinic
   ∘Cigarette smoking contributes to 20% of deaths in the U.S., & is the #1 modifiable cause of premature death
•↓**Alcohol consumption**
   ∘If symptoms occur in moderation, then cessation is necessary
•**Avoidance of certain medications**
   ∘Glucocorticoids
   ∘Nonsteroidal anti–inflammatory medications, including Aspirin
   Note: If for some reason, these substances cannot be discontinued, either:
      •↓Dosage
      •Co–administer w/ meals &/or an acid suppressing medication
•**Avoidance of other exacerbatory substances** (ex. caffeine, spicy foods) if they cause symptoms in that individual patient, as there is no evidence that a bland diet or other diet modification improves symptoms, or affects ulcer healing
•**Emotional stress management**
   ∘Psychological therapy
   ∘Regular exercise
   ∘Biofeedback
   ∘Yoga
   ∘Listening to music
   ∘Gardening

Medical treatment duration:
•3months, w/ indications for continued maintenance treatment being:
   ∘**Severe gastrointestinal hemorrhage**
   ∘**If the patient must continue on causative medications**
   Maintenance treatment:
      •Simply continue the acid suppressive medication which was used to treat the acute disease
      ∘Histamine 2 selective receptor blockers: Half treatment dose qhs
      ∘Proton pump inhibitors–PPIs: Same as treatment dose
      ∘Sucralfate: Same as treatment dose

MUCOSAL COATING MEDICATIONS			
Generic (Trade)	M ♀	Dose	
Sucralfate (Carafate) Ø P		2g PO q12hours (1h prior to meals &/or qhs)	
•Do not administer concomitantly w/ other acid suppressing medications, as ↑gastric pH→ ∘↓Efficacy, as this medication requires an acidic environment			

Mechanism:
•An aluminum hydroxide complex of sucrose that:
  ∘Forms a protective coating over the inflammatory/ ulcerated area
  ∘↑Prostaglandin synthesis
  ∘Binds to bile salts
  ...and does not ↑gastric pH			

Side effects:
Gastrointestinal
•Constipation
Genitourinary
•Aluminum toxicity, in the presence of renal failure
Hematologic
•Aluminum binding to intestinal phosphate→
  ∘↓Intestinal phosphate absorption which may→
    –Hypophosphatemia			

HISTAMINE 2 SELECTIVE RECEPTOR BLOCKERS			
Generic (Trade)	M	♀	Dose
Cimetidine (Tagamet)	LK	P	800mg PO qhs
Famotidine (Pepcid)	LK	P	40mg PO qhs
Nizatadine (Axid)	K	?	300mg PO qhs
Ranitidine (Zantac)	K	P	300mg PO qhs

Mechanism:
- •Block parietal cell histamine 2 receptors→
  - ∘50–80%↓gastric acid production

Side effects:
General
- •Headache

Gastrointestinal
- •Constipation
- •Diarrhea

Neurologic
- •Altered mental status
- •Depression
- •Dizziness
- •Hallucinations

Hematologic/ neurologic
- •Chronic use→
  - ∘Vitamin B_{12} deficiency

Cimetidine specific:
Endocrine
- •Anti–androgen effect→
  - ∘Gynecomastia, being the ↑development of male mammary glands
  - ∘Impotence, being the inability to achieve &/or maintain an erection
  - ...being reversible upon discontinuation

PROTON PUMP INHIBITORS			
Generic (Trade)	M	♀	Dose
Esomeprazole (Nexium)	L	P	40mg PO q24hours
Lansoprazole (Prevacid)	L	P	30mg PO q24hours
Omeprazole (Prilosec)	L	?	40mg PO q24hours
Pantoprazole (Protonix)	L	P	40mg PO/ IV q24hours
Rabeprazole (Aciphex)	L	P	40mg PO q24hours

Mechanism:
- •Inhibit parietal cell hydrogen/ potassium ATPase, located on the luminal border→
  - ∘90%↓gastric acid secretion

Side effects:
Gastrointestinal
- •Abdominal pain
- •Constipation
- •Diarrhea
- •Flatulence
- •Hepatitis–rare
- •Nausea ± vomiting

Mucocutaneous
- •Gynecomastia–rare

Neurologic
- •Headaches

Hematologic/ neurologic
- •Chronic use→
  - ∘Vitamin B_{12} deficiency

Interactions
- •↓Absorption of Ampicillin, Digoxin, iron, Itraconazole, & Ketoconazole

ANTACIDS

Indications:
- •Supplemental therapy for acute breakthrough pain relief, rather than chronic treatment, due to their short duration of action

Generic (Trade)	M ♀	Dose
Aluminum hydroxide (Amphogel, Alternagel)	K S–? 1st trimester	45mL or 3tabs PO
Calcium carbonate (Tums)	K S–? 1st trimester	3g PO
Aluminum & magnesium hydroxide (Maalox)	K S–? 1st trimester	45mL PO

- •Liquid formulations are typically more effective

Side effects:
Gastrointestinal
- •Constipation (aluminum, calcium)
- •Diarrhea (magnesium)

HELICOBACTER PYLORI ERADICATION TREATMENT
- •Combination therapy via the following, as the organism rapidly attains resistance
  - ◦Acid suppression treatment via either:
    - −Histamine 2 selective receptor blocker
    - −Proton pump inhibitor−PPI
    - ...as above
  - ◦Antibiotic treatment:
    - −Clarithromycin & either amoxicillin or metronidazole
    - −Bismuth subsalicylate, metronidazole, & tetracycline

Treatment duration:
- •2weeks

Indications to confirm eradication:
- •A complicated ulcer
- •Gastric malignancy
- •Lack of symptomatic improvement by 2weeks
- •Symptom recurrence after treatment

MACROLIDES

Generic (Trade)	M ♀	Dose
Clarithromycin (Biaxin)	KL ?	500mg PO q12hours

Mechanism:
- •Affects the ribosomal 50S subunit→
  - ◦↓Transfer RNA translocation

Side effects:
Hematologic
- •Eosinophilia
Gastrointestinal
- •Gastroenteritis→
  - ◦Diarrhea
  - ◦Nausea ± vomiting
- •Hepatitis
Neurologic
- •Transient deafness

284

PENICILLINS

Generic (Trade)	M	♀	Dose
Amoxicillin (Amoxil)	K	P	1g PO q12hours

Mechanism:
- A β-lactam ring structure which binds to bacterial transpeptidase→
  - ↓Transpeptidase function→
    - ↓Bacterial cell wall peptidoglycan cross-linking→↓cell wall synthesis→osmotic influx of extracellular fluid→↑intracellular hydrostatic pressure→cell rupture→cell death=bactericidal
- ↑Bacterial autolytic enzymes→
  - Peptidoglycan degradation

- Certain bacteria produce β-lactamase→
  - Cleavage of this essential structural component of cephalosporins & certain penicillins (as the other β-lactam medications differ sufficiently to prevent ring cleavage)→
    - Antibiotic inactivation. This process may be antagonized by the concomitant administration of **β-lactamase inhibitors** (Clavulanic acid=clavulanate, Sulbactam, or Tazobactam)→renewed susceptibility

Side effects:
General
- **Hypersensitivity reactions ≤10%**
  - Anaphylaxis−0.5%→
    - Death−0.002% (1:50,000)
  - Acute interstitial nephritis
  - Dermatitis
  - Drug fever
  - Hemolytic anemia
  …having cross−hypersensitivity to other β lactam medications (cephalosporins, carbapenems), except monobactams (ex. Aztreonam)

METRONIDAZOLE (Flagyl)

M	♀	Dose
KL	P−U in 1st trimester	500mg PO q12hours

Mechanism:
- DNA binding→
  - DNA strand breakage

Side effects:
General
- **Disulfuram−like reaction to alcohol**
  - Avoid alcoholic beverages during, & for 48hours after completion of treatment
Gastrointestinal
- Nausea ± vomiting−10%
- Taste changes=dysgeusia (esp. metallic taste)
Genitourinary
- Dark urine, being common, but harmless
Neurological
- Peripheral neuropathy
- Seizures
Hematologic
- Transient neutropenia−8%

TETRACYCLINES

Generic (Trade)	M	♀	Dose
Tetracycline (Sumycin)	LK	U	500mg PO q6hours

Mechanism:
- Affects the ribosomal 30S subunit→
  - ↓Ribosomal binding to transfer RNA

Side effects:
Gastrointestinal
- Acute hepatic fatty necrosis
- Gastroenteritis→
  - Abdominal pain
Genitourinary
- Acute tubular necrosis

285

```
Mucocutaneous
 •Photosensitivity
Neurologic
 •Pseudotumor cerebri
Materno-fetal
 •Fetus to age 10 years→
  ∘Tooth staining
  ∘↓Bone growth
```

ANTIPERISTALSIS MEDICATIONS			
Generic	M	♀	Start
Bismuth subsalicylate (Pepto-Bismol)	K	U	524mg PO q6hours

Side effects:
 Gastrointestinal
 •Blackening of the tongue &/or stool

INVASIVE PROCEDURES
•Endoscopic balloon dilation
Indications:
 •Fibrotic pyloric stricture

•Gastric surgery
Indications/ procedures:
 •Nonhealing gastric ulcers via:
  ∘Wedge resection &
  ∘Nonselective vagotomy, termed truncal vagotomy→
   −↓Gastric emptying, necessitating a drainage procedure, via either antrectomy, pyloroplasty, or
    gastroenterostomy
 •Nonhealing duodenal ulcers via:
  ∘Selective vagotomy, termed proximal gastric vagotomy, which does not affect gastric emptying
 •Fibrotic pyloric stricture refractory to endoscopic balloon dilation

PREVENTION
Indications for peptic inflammatory disease prophylaxis in patients taking NSAIDs:
 •Prophylax w/ either:
  ∘Histamine 2 selective receptor blockers: Half treatment dose qhs
  ∘Proton pump inhibitors−PPIs: Same as treatment dose
  ∘Sucralfate: Same as treatment dose
 ...in patients w/ any of the following:
  •Age >60 years w/ a history of peptic inflammatory disease
  •Anticipated therapy >3 months
  •Concurrent glucocorticoid use
  •Moderate to high dose NSAID use
Note: Newer NSAIDs (Etodolac, Nabumetone, Salsalate) & cyclooxygenase COX-2 selective
  inhibitors→
  •↓Risk of NSAID induced peptic inflammation

SEVERE ILLNESS INDUCED GASTRIC INFLAMMATION/ ULCERATION PROPHYLAXIS
Mechanism:
 •↓Mucosal blood flow→
  ∘↓Bicarbonate delivery to the mucosa
  ∘↓Mucus & bicarbonate secretion from gastric mucosal cells
  ∘↓Epithelial proliferation
Indications:
 •Emergent or major surgery
 •Severe illness
 •Severe trauma, esp. head injury
Prophylaxis:
 •Proton pump inhibitors, histamine 2 selective receptor blockers, antacids, or pernicious anemia→
  ∘Loss of the protective gastic acid coating→gastroesophageal colonization by oropharyngeal
   organisms→
   −↑**Hospital acquired pneumonia risk via aspiration**
   −↑**Stress erosion/ ulceration mediated organism translocation risk**→bacteremia
   ...all being ↓risk w/ the use of **sucralfate**, which typically does not ↑gastric pH

286

MUCOSAL COATING MEDICATIONS			
Generic (Trade)	**M**	**♀**	**Dose**
Sucralfate (Carafate)	Ø	P	2g PO q12hours (1hour prior to meals &/or qhs)

•Do not administer concomitantly w/ other acid suppressing medications, as ↑gastric pH→
  ○↓Efficacy, as this medication requires an acidic environment

•Esophageal mucosal inflammation=esophagitis→
  ◦Erosion ± ulceration

•**Gastroesophageal reflux disease–GERD, being the #1cause**
  ◦↓**Lower esophageal sphincter–LES tone**
    –**Alcohol**
    –**Caffeine**
    –Chocolate
    –Mints
    –Smoking
    –Scleroderma
    –Medications (anticholinergics, benzodiazepines, β receptor agonists, calcium channel blockers, nitrates, & Theophylline)→↓esophageal motility→↓lower esophageal sphincter–LES tone
  ◦↑**Intra–abdominal pressure**
    –Abdominal or pelvic tumor, including pregnancy
    –**Obesity**
    –Tight belt
•**Medications**
  ◦Nonsteroidal anti–inflammatory drugs–NSAIDs, including Aspirin, esp. enteric coated versions due to ↑size→
    –↑Risk of lodging in the esophagus
  ◦Bisphosphonates
  ◦Iron
  ◦Potassium
  ◦Quinidine
  ◦Tetracycline
    ...→local toxic effects on the esophageal mucosa
•**Esophageal infections in immunosuppressed patients**
  ◦Candida sp., esp. Candida albicans
  ◦Cytomegalovirus–CMV
  ◦Herpes simplex virus–HSV 1 or 2

Gastrointestinal
•**Substernal chest discomfort &/or pain** (burning, gnawing, &/or tightness) ± radiation to the neck
•Pain on swallowing=odynophagia, esp. w/ medication & infectious etiologies
•Acid reflux→
  ◦**Sour or bitter taste, termed waterbrash**
  ◦Vocal cord inflammation→
    –**Asthma exacerbation**
    –**Cough**
    –Hoarseness
  ◦↑Aspiration pneumonia risk

Effects of chronic, inadequately controlled disease:
•Chronic esophagitis→
  ◦Fibrosis→
    –Esophageal stricture ± webs &/or rings→difficulty swallowing=dysphagia
  ◦Esophageal metaplasia→
    –**Barrett's esophagus–7%** via replacement of the normal squamous epithelium w/ more acid resistant columnar epithelium (as in the stomach), being salmon colored→**esophageal adenocarcinoma–10%**, esp. those w/ dysplasia

•**Esophagogastroduodenoscopy–EGD**
  Indications:
  •Suspected:
    ◦Esophagitis (any cause)
    ◦Esophageal ulceration
    ◦Esophageal stricture
  •Severe symptoms unresponsive to medical therapy
  •pH monitoring showing severe reflux

•**24 hour pH monitoring**
  Indications:
  •Lack of response to diet & lifestyle
  Mechanism:
  •An intra-esophageal pH electrode records esophageal pH to test for the occurrence, frequency, severity, & relation to the symptoms of gastroesophageal reflux-GERD

TREATMENT OF GASTROESOPHAGEAL REFLUX DISEASE

•**Smoking cessation** via smoking cessation clinic
  ◦Cigarette smoking contributes to 20% of deaths in the U.S., & is the #1 modifiable cause of premature death
•**Eat more frequent, smaller meals**, & avoid eating within 3hours of bedtime
•**Avoid substances known to irritate the esophagus**
  ◦Caffeine
  ◦Citrus juice
  ◦Spices
•**Avoid substances which ↓lower esophageal sphincter-LES tone**
•**Elevate head of bed** w/ either:
  ◦6-8" blocks
  ◦Wedge under the mattress
  ...→upper body elevation→
    •Gravity mediated ↓GERD risk
  Note: Avoid simply using pillows to prop the head up, as this may→
    •↑Intra-abdominal pressure→
      ◦↑Reflux

ANTACIDS
Indications:
•Supplemental therapy for acute breakthrough pain relief, rather than chronic treatment, due to their short duration of action

Generic (Trade)	M ♀		Dose
Aluminum hydroxide (Amphogel, Alternagel)	K	S-? 1st trimester	45mL or 3tabs PO
Calcium carbonate (Tums)	K	S-? 1st trimester	3g PO
Aluminum & magnesium hydroxide (Maalox)	K	S-? 1st trimester	45mL PO

•Liquid formulations are typically more effective

Side effects:
  Gastrointestinal
    •Constipation (aluminum, calcium)
    •Diarrhea (magnesium)

ADJUNCTIVE MEDICAL TREATMENT ▬▬▬▬▬▬▬▬▬▬▬▬▬▬▬▬
Indications:
•Severe GERD
•Mild to moderate GERD, refractory to lifestyle modification X 3 weeks
•Documented:
  ◦Esophagitis
  ◦Esophageal ulcer
  ◦Esophageal stricture
  ◦Barrett's esophagus

Medical treatment duration:
•1.5 months. However, being that gastroesophageal reflux is a chronic disease, w/ endoscopic recurrence of esophagitis occurring in the majority of patients who were initially successfully treated, most patients benefit from maintenance treatment
  Maintenance treatment:
    •Simply continue the acid suppressive medication which was used to treat the acute disease
      ◦Histamine 2 selective receptor blockers: Half treatment dose qhs
      ◦Proton pump inhibitors-PPIs: Same as treatment dose
      ◦Sucralfate: Same as treatment dose

289

HISTAMINE 2 SELECTIVE RECEPTOR BLOCKERS

Generic (Trade)	M	♀	Dose
Cimetidine (Tagamet)	LK	P	800mg PO qhs
Famotidine (Pepcid)	LK	P	40mg PO qhs
Nizatadine (Axid)	K	?	300mg PO qhs
Ranitidine (Zantac)	K	P	300mg PO qhs

Mechanism:
- •Block parietal cell histamine 2 receptors→
  - ◦50–80%↓gastric acid production

Side effects:
General
- •Headache

Gastrointestinal
- •Constipation
- •Diarrhea

Neurologic
- •Altered mental status
- •Depression
- •Dizziness
- •Hallucinations

Hematologic/ neurologic
- •Chronic use→
  - ◦Vitamin B$_{12}$ deficiency

Cimetidine specific:
Endocrine
- •Anti–androgen effect→
  - ◦Gynecomastia, being the ↑development of male mammary glands
  - ◦Impotence, being the inability to achieve &/or maintain an erection
    ...being reversible upon discontinuation

PROTON PUMP INHIBITORS

Generic (Trade)	M	♀	Dose
Esomeprazole (Nexium)	L	P	40mg PO q24hours
Lansoprazole (Prevacid)	L	P	30mg PO q24hours
Omeprazole (Prilosec)	L	?	40mg PO q24hours
Pantoprazole (Protonix)	L	P	40mg PO/ IV q24hours
Rabeprazole (Aciphex)	L	P	40mg PO q24hours

Mechanism:
- •Inhibit parietal cell hydrogen/ potassium ATPase, located on the luminal border→
  - ◦90%↓gastric acid secretion

Side effects:
Gastrointestinal
- •Abdominal pain
- •Constipation
- •Diarrhea
- •Flatulence
- •Hepatitis–rare
- •Nausea ± vomiting

Mucocutaneous
- •Gynecomastia–rare

Neurologic
- •Headaches

Hematologic/ neurologic
- •Chronic use→
  - ◦Vitamin B$_{12}$ deficiency

Interactions
- •↓Absorption of Ampicillin, Digoxin, iron, Itraconazole, & Ketoconazole

PROKINETIC MEDICATIONS				
Generic (Trade)	M	♀	Dose	Max
Cisapride (Propulsid)	LK	?	10mg PO q6hours, 30min. prior to meals & qhs	20mg q6hours
Metoclopramide (Reglan)	K	P	5mg PO q6hours, 30min. prior to meals & qhs	15mg q6hours

Mechanism:
- ↑Esophageal motility→
  - ∘↑Lower esophageal sphincter–LES tone

Cisapride specific side effects:
General
  - Headache
Cardiovascular
  - Dysrhythmias
Gastrointestinal
  - Diarrhea
  - Nausea ± vomiting
Mucocutaneous
  - Rhinitis

Metoclopramide specific side effects:
Neurologic
  - Dopamine receptor blockade→
    - ∘**Extrapyramidal dysfunction** (treat w/ Diphenhydramine)

Metoclopramide specific contraindications:
  - Parkinson's disease/ syndrome

INVASIVE PROCEDURES
•Endoscopic balloon dilation
Indications:
  - Esophageal stenosis via fibrotic webs or rings

•Nissen fundoplication
Indications:
  - Patients unresponsive to dietary, lifestyle, & medical therapy

GASTROINTESTINAL HEMORRHAGE

- Caused by hemorrhage from anywhere along the gastrointestinal tract, from the oropharynx to the anus
- Most acute gastrointestinal hemorrhages are episodic, lasting ≤30 min.

CLASSIFICATION/ RISK FACTORS

- **Age ≥60years**
- **Medications**
  - Thrombolytic or anticoagulant medications may initiate or exacerbate hemorrhage via underlying gastrointestinal lesions, but are unlikely to cause normal mucosal hemorrhage

UPPER GASTROINTESTINAL HEMORRHAGE–80%
- Hemorrhage proximal to the ligament of Treitz=suspensory muscle of the duodenum, being a fibromuscular attachment from the right crus of the diaphragm to the duodenal/ jejunal junction

- **Capillary/ arterial hemorrhage**
  - **Peptic inflammatory disease–80%**
    - Ulceration–45%→arterial hemorrhage
    - Erosion–35% (gastritis–25% >> esophagitis–5%, duodenitis–5%)→capillary hemorrhage
  - **Neoplasm–3%**
    - Polyps
    - Cancer

- **Venous hemorrhage–10%**
  - **Gastroesophageal varices**, being the #1 cause of mortality in patients w/ cirrhosis

- **Arterial hemorrhage**
  - **Mallory–Weiss Tear–7%**
    - Persistent lifting, vomiting, &/or retching†→↑intra–abdominal pressure→↑intra–gastric pressure→ **gastroesophageal junction mucosal horizontal tear**
  - **Angiodysplasia**
    - Arterio–venous malformations–AVMs
  - **Aorto–enteric fistula** s/p aortic graft
  - **Dielafoy's anomaly**
    - An arteriole penetrating the gastric mucosal surface, usually in the fundus
  - **Vasculitis**

---

†Gastroesophageal reverse peristaltic contractions without expulsion of vomitus, esp. after an alcoholic binge

LOWER GASTROINTESTINAL HEMORRHAGE–20%
- Hemorrhage distal to the ligament of Treitz

- **Arterial hemorrhage**
  - **Diverticulosis ± diverticulitis→diverticular hemorrhage–40%,** being the #1 cause of massive lower gastrointestinal hemorrhage
  - **Angiodysplasia–3%**
    - Arterio–venous malformations–AVMs
  - **Vasculitis**

- **Venous hemorrhage**
  - **Hemorrhoids–5%**

- **Capillary/ arterial hemorrhage**
  - **Anal & rectal lesions**
    - Anal fissure
  - **Neoplasm–10%**
    - Polyps
    - Cancer
  - **Colitis**
    - Inflammatory bowel disease–IBD (Ulcerative colitis >> Crohn's disease)
    - Infection–5%
    - Ischemic colitis–10%
    - Radiation mediated, which may occur months to years after initial exposure
  - **Meckel's diverticulum**

Cardiovascular
- Acute hemorrhage→↓intravascular volume→
  - ≥10% blood volume loss→
    - ↑Autonomic sympathetic tone→↑pulse
  - ≥20% blood volume loss→
    - Orthostatic hypotension (supine to standing→↑20 pulse, ↓20 SBP, &/or ↓10 DBP)→ lightheadedness upon standing
    - Urine output 20–30mL/ hour (normal being >30mL/ hour)
  - ≥30% blood volume loss→
    - Recumbent hypotension &/or tachycardia
  - ≥40% blood volume loss→
    - Altered mental status &/or urine output <20mL/ hour
    - Hypovolemic shock, being hypotension + organ failure, unresponsive to fluid resuscitation
  - …w/ arterial hemorrhage→
    - Reflex autonomic sympathetic splanchnic vasoconstriction→
      - Clot formation. However, intravascular volume is partially repleted via:
        - Interstitial fluid drawn in from the extravascular space
        - Large intestinal absorption
      - …→↑intravascular volume→
        - ↓Splanchnic vasoconstriction→
          - Possible rebleeding in as early as 1 hour

Gastrointestinal
- **Hemorrhage**, which may occur intermittently→
  - Mucosal irritation→↑gastrointestinal smooth muscle contraction→↑peristalsis→
    - **Abdominal pain**, being referred & episodic or "wave like", termed colic
      Areas of reference:
      - Stomach &/or duodenum: Epigastrium
      - Small intestine: Periumbilical area
      - Large intestine: Hypogastrium &/or suprapubic area
      - Rectum: Suprapubic, sacral, &/or perineal areas
    - Anorexia
    - ↑Bowel sounds→audible gastrointestinal gurgling, termed borborygmi
    - Diarrhea
    - Retrograde peristalsis→nausea ± vomiting
  - **Hematemesis:** Vomiting of blood, including very dark, tarry looking blood termed 'coffee ground' emesis
    Lesion localization:
    - Upper gastrointestinal hemorrhage
  - **Hematochezia:** Passage of bright red blood per rectum
    Lesion localization:
    - Lower gastrointestinal hemorrhage >> upper gastrointestinal hemorrhage via massive hemorrhage (≥1L) &/or ↑↑peristalsis
  - **Melena†‡:** Passage of sticky, very dark, tarry looking stool, w/ a characteristic odor, requiring ≥50mL of blood, indicating gastrointestinal hemorrhage proximal to ileocecal sphincter >> colonic gastrointestinal hemorrhage via slow hemorrhage &/or ↓peristalsis
  - **Fecal occult blood:** Passage of blood detectable only by laboratory testing, requiring ≥20mL of blood. Not helpful in the anatomic determination of the lesion

- **Digital rectal exam–DRE**
  Indications:
  - To palpate a possible distal rectal tumor
  - Visualization of fecal streaks on glove, in order to identify possible melena &/or hematochezia

- **Fecal occult blood test–FOBT**
  Procedure:
  - 2 samples are taken from 1 bowel movement/ day X 3 days=6 total samples, which may be stored for <1 week
  Mechanism:
  - Uses the peroxidase activity of hemoglobin to cause a change in the reagent, w/ the patient to avoid the following for ≥3 days prior to, & during testing:

Limitations:
- •False positive:
  - ◦Hemoglobin rich foods:
    - −Raw red meat
  - ◦Peroxidase rich foods:
    - −Uncooked vegetables, esp. broccoli, cauliflower, or turnips
  - ◦Gastrointestinal mucosal irritants:
    - −Laxatives
    - −Nonsteroidal anti−inflammatory drugs−NSAIDs, including Aspirin
- •False negative:
  - ◦↑Dose vitamin C

---

†Iron→
- •Melanotic looking stools ± constipation &/or diarrhea

‡Bismuth subsalicylate (Pepto−Bismol)→
- •Melanotic looking stools &/or dark tongue

Mucocutaneous
- •Hypovolemia→
  - ◦Dry mucous membranes
  - ◦Dry skin→
    - −↓Skin turgor→skin tenting
- •↓Hemoglobin→
  - ◦Skin & mucus membrane pallor
    - −Extended palmar crease pallor @ a hemoglobin ≤7g/ dL
- •Coagulopathy &/or thrombocytopenia→
  - ◦Ecchymoses or petechiae respectively
  - ◦Mucosal hemorrhage→
    - −Bleeding gums, esp. w/ brushing
    - −Nasal hemorrhage=epistaxis
- •Cirrhosis or hemolysis→↑plasma bilirubin→subcutaneous deposition→
  - ◦Yellow staining of tissues @ >3mg/ dL
    - −Skin→jaundice
    - −Sclera→scleral icterus
    - −Mucus membranes
  - ◦Pruritus

Pulmonary
- •Nasal hemorrhage=epistaxis (not a gastrointestinal hemorrhage)→
  - ◦Swallowed blood→
    - −Vomiting of blood=hematemesis
    - −Fecal occult blood
    - −Melena
  - ◦Aspirated blood→
    - −Coughing of blood=hemoptysis

Hematologic
- •↓Hemoglobin & hematocrit, **requiring ≥8hours to be evident & ≥24hours to be complete**, are not useful indices of the amount of blood loss. Within the 1st several hours after blood loss, hypovolemia is indicated via intravenous fluid resuscitation→↑plasma→↓hemoglobin/ hematocrit via a dilutional effect
- •Search for coagulopathy via:
  - ◦↑Prothrombin time−PT (normal 11−13seconds) or ↑international normalized ratio−INR (normal <1.3)
  - ◦↑Partial thromboplastin time−PTT (normal 25−35seconds)
- •Search for thrombocytopenia via:
  - ◦↓Platelet count (normal 150,000−350,000/ µL)
- •Intravascular volume loss→
  - ◦↑Creatinine & blood urea nitrogen−BUN†, indicating pre−renal renal failure
- •Search for hepatitis via:
  - ◦↑Liver function tests
- •Search for chronic gastrointestinal hemorrhage via:
  - ◦Iron deficiency anemia

---

†Upper gastrointestinal hemorrhage→
- •↑Blood urea nitrogen−BUN via gastrointestinal mucosa mediated erythrocyte protein absorption→
  - ◦↑Ammonia, which diffuses into the intestinal blood, being filtered via hepatocytes→
    - −Urea cycle→↑urea

294

•Nasogastric–NG lavage
Indications:
  •Suspected upper gastrointestinal hemorrhage
  •Differentiation of active vs. inactive upper gastrointestinal hemorrhage
  •Clearing of gastric contents in order to:
    ○↓Aspiration risk
    ○Enable better visualization for possible forthcoming esophagogastroduodenoscopy–EGD
Mechanism:
  •Lavage the stomach w/ 500mL of tap water. If positive for blood, continue lavage until fluid clears.
    ○Active hemorrhage→
      −Bright red blood ± coffee ground blood
    ○Inactive hemorrhage→
      −Coffee ground blood which clears
Limitations:
  •In the setting of a known gastrointestinal hemorrhage, a clear nasogastric lavage, defined as bilious
    aspirate without blood, indicates 1 of the following:
    ○Lower gastrointestinal hemorrhage
    ○Upper gastrointestinal hemorrhage which has stopped w/ sufficient time for blood to flow out of the
      proximal duodenum
Caution:
  •The placement of a nasogastric tube in a patient w/ known gastroesophageal varices is considered
    safe, unless they have undergone recent banding, in which case the procedure should be avoided
Note: Occult blood may be detected in clear lavaged fluid via urine dipstick

•Endoscopy
Indications:
  •Diagnosis, risk stratification, & appropriate treatment
  •Acute hemorrhage
    ○If the nasogastric fluid is clear, or subsequently clears, & the patient is fluid resuscitated, perform
      an esophagogastroduodenoscopy–EGD ± push enteroscopy†. If no lesion is noted, & a lower
      gastrointestinal hemorrhage is suspected, perform an anoscopy & colonoscopy
  •Chronic hemorrhage
    ○Esophagogastroduodenoscopy–EGD ± colonoscopy
Preparation:
  •Golytely™ lavage administered PO/ nasogastric tube
Injection treatment methods:
  •Epinephrine
  •Sclerotherapy via:
    ○Alcohol
    ○Ethanolamine
Thermal treatment methods:
  •Heat probe
  •Multipolar electrocoagulation
  •Argon plasma coagulator
Other:
  •Metallic clip placement
  •Variceal banding
Outcomes:
  •Esophagogastroduodenoscopy–EGD→
    ○Identification of 90% of upper gastrointestinal hemorrhage sites
    ○↓Rebleeding rates
    ○↓Surgeries performed
    ○↓Packed red blood cell transfusion requirements

---

†Involves passing an enteroscope or pediatric colonoscope, as distal into the jejunum as possible

•Barium swallow study
Indications:
  •Endoscopy does not localize the lesion
  •Age <30years, for possible Meckel's diverticulum
Procedure:
  •Barium mediated small intestinal follow through via sequential radiographs
Limitations:
  •The procedure is not therapeutic

•Radionuclide scintigraphy=tagged red blood cell scan
Indications:
- **•Active gastrointestinal hemorrhage in a stable patient, while being prepared for colonoscopy**
- **•Endoscopy does not localize the lesion†**
- **•Age <30years, for possible Meckel's diverticulum**

Procedure:
- •Intravenous infusion of the patients previously labeled (technetium Tc 99m pertechnetate) erythrocytes→
  - ◦Abdominal & pelvic scintiscans, obtained at regular intervals over the following 24–48hours, to localize active hemorrhage

Limitations:
- •Requires active hemorrhage @ a rate of **≥0.1mL/ min.**
- •The procedure is not therapeutic
- •Useful only to determine the general region of hemorrhage

---

†If radionuclide scintigraphy is unhelpful, upper and lower endoscopy should be repeated→
- •Detection of 35% of lesions missed on initial examination

•Arteriography
Indications:
- **•Active gastrointestinal hemorrhage**
- **•Unstable patient**
- **•Endoscopy does not localize the lesion**

Procedure:
- •Imaging of the celiac artery (for upper gastrointestinal hemorrhage) ± superior & inferior mesenteric arteries (for lower gastrointestinal hemorrhage), in order to:
  - ◦Localize active hemorrhage, via visualization of the extravasation of contrast into the intestinal lumen
  - ◦Identify suspect lesions not actively hemorrhaging by demonstrating typical vascular patterns seen w/ angiodysplasia or neoplasia
- •If the lesion is found, the following may be performed:
  - ◦**Infusion of a vasoconstricting medication**
    - –Vasopressin
  - ◦**Embolization of the vessel**, via:
    - –Gelatin sponge pledgets
    - –Microcoils
    - –Polyvinyl alcohol particles

Complications:
- •Myocardial &/or intestinal ischemia ± infarction

Limitations:
- •Requires active hemorrhage @ a rate of **≥0.5mL/ min.** in order to identify the causative lesion

•Exploratory laparotomy ± intraoperative enteroscopy
Indications:
- **•Active hemorrhage**
- **•Unstable patient**

OTHER STUDIES ▬▬▬▬▬▬▬▬▬▬▬▬▬▬▬▬▬▬▬▬▬▬▬
•3–dimensional computed tomographic–CT colography=virtual colonoscopy
Procedure:
- •A noninvasive procedure combining the use of computed tomography–CT w/ computer software capable of rendering images of the entire colon, meant to simulate an endoscopic view

Advantages:
- •No sedation required
- •Less time consuming
- •Ability to view both sides of the bowel folds
- •Precise lesion localization
- •Ability to re–examine the images

Limitations:
- •? Sensitivity/ specificity
- •Requires prior colonic cleansing
- •Requires colonic insufflation
- •Requires subsequent colonoscopy if a lesion is detected, as it does not allow for biopsy

•Pill camera
  Mechanism:
  •An 11mm X 26mm pill, functioning as a camera, allows visualization of the gastrointestinal tract
  distal to the esophagus (stomach, small intestine, & large intestine), taking 2 images/ second, w/ the
  images being transmitted to, & stored on, a recording device worn on a belt around the patients
  abdomen. The study usually lasts ~8hours, after which the recording device is removed, w/ its
  images loaded into a computer
  Preparation:
  •12 hour fast prior to capsule ingestion
  •4 hour fast following capsule ingestion
  Contraindications:
  •History of intestinal obstruction or major abdominal surgery→
    ∘↑Capsule enlodgement risk, which may require surgical removal
  •Automated internal cardioverter–defibrillator–AICD
  •Pacemaker

TREATMENT OF ACUTE GASTROINTESTINAL HEMORRHAGE

•All patients should be admitted to the hospital for treatment & monitoring, w/ gastroenterology consult
for possible urgent endoscopy
•Endotracheal intubation
  Indications:
  •Altered mental status, in order to ↓aspiration risk
•Intravenous access via 2 large bore (≤ #18 gauge) peripheral lines
•Nil per os–NPO, w/ duration dependant on severity
  ∘Eating >> drinking→
    −↑Peristalsis
    −↑Gastric acid & digestive enzyme release
    ...→↑pain & organ destruction→
        •↑Rebleeding risk
  ∘Possible endoscopy
•Intravenous fluid, w/ attention to both:
  ∘**Intravascular volume repletion via Normal saline** (0.9% NaCl) or **lactated Ringer's solution**, as
  per:
    −Vital signs
    −Physical examination
    −Urine output (normal being ≥0.5mL/kg/h)
    −Blood urea nitrogen–BUN & creatinine
  ∘**Intravascular volume maintenance via Normal saline** (0.9% NaCl) or **lactated Ringer's solution**
  Adult maintenance fluid:
    •Weight (kg) + 40= #mL/ hour
  Additional febrile requirements:
    •1L/ 24hours for every 1°F >100°F
  Additional:
    •Estimate loss for:
      ∘Diaphoresis
      ∘Diarrhea
      ∘Polyuria
      ∘Tachypnea
  ...followed by oral rehydration w/ a glucose based electrolyte solution upon both clinical stability &
  ability to tolerate PO
•Type & cross match the patients blood for possible transfusion of 2−8units of packed red blood cells,
depending on the clinical severity. O−negative blood may be used if needed emergently

297

PACKED RED BLOOD CELLS

Dose

1unit is composed of 450mL of blood & 50mL of plasma=500mL total

Indications:
- **Hemoglobin <10g/ dL** w/:
  - ∘Active hemorrhage
  - ∘Cardiovascular disease
  - ∘Cerebrovascular disease
  - ∘Peripheral vascular disease
  - ∘Pulmonary disease
  - ∘Sepsis
  - ∘Hemoglobinopathy
  - ∘Otherwise critically ill
- **Hemoglobin <7–8g/ dL** otherwise

Mechanism:
- •1unit→
  - ∘1g/ dL ↑hemoglobin
  - ∘3% ↑hematocrit
  - ∘~10% ↑blood volume

PLATELETS

Indications:
- •Platelet count <50,000/ µL w/ either hemorrhage or pre–procedure
- •Prophylactically w/ a platelet count <20,000/ µL

Thrombocytopenia mediated hemorrhage risk:
- •Platelet count
  - ∘20,000–50,000/ µL w/ minimal trauma
  - ∘10,000–20,000/ µL, possibly spontaneous
  - ∘<10,000/ µL, commonly spontaneous

Dose

6–10 units typically being transfused at a time (50mL/ unit)

Mechanism:
- •↑Platelet count by 5,000–10,000/ µL per unit

VITAMIN K=Phytonadione

Indications:
- •To correct the international normalized ration–INR or prothrombin time–PT

Dose

10mg SC/ IV slow push @ 1mg/ min. in order to ↓anaphylactoid reaction risk

Mechanism:
- •Requires several hours to days for effect

Side effects:
- •Avoid intramuscular administration, which may→
  - ∘Intramuscular hemorrhage

FRESH FROZEN PLASMA–FFP

Indications:
- •To correct the international normalized ration–INR or prothrombin time–PT under the following conditions:
  - ∘**INR >20**
  - ∘**Severe hemorrhage**
  - ∘**Other need for rapid reversal, such as an emergent procedure**

Dose†

15mL/ kg IV (w/ ~200mL FFP/ unit) q4hours prn ↑INR

Mechanism:
- •Contains clotting factors 2, 7, 9–13, & heat labile 5 & 7→
  - ∘Immediate onset of action
- •Each unit→
  - ∘8% ↑coagulation factors
  - ∘4% ↑blood volume

FIBRINOGEN	
Indications:	
•Fibrinogen level <100mg/ dL w/ either hemorrhage or pre-procedure	
Generic	**Dose**
Cryoprecipitate	10-15 units being transfused at a time (25mL cryoprecipitate/ unit)
Mechanism:	
•Contains factors 8, 13, von Willebrand factor, & fibrinogen •Each unit→ ◦7mg/ dL ↑plasma fibrinogen	

ADDITIONAL TREATMENT FOR UPPER GASTROINTESTINAL HEMORRHAGE ████████
•No medical treatments have proven to prevent upper gastrointestinal rebleeding episodes within 72hours, which is the highest risk period

ANTACIDS			
Indications:			
•Supplemental therapy for acute acid suppression until the effects of a proton pump inhibitor–PPI occur			
Generic (Trade)	**M** ♀		**Dose**
Aluminum hydroxide (Amphogel, Alternagel)	K S-? 1st trimester		45mL or 3tabs PO
Calcium carbonate (Tums)	K S-? 1st trimester		3g PO
Aluminum & magnesium hydroxide (Maalox)	K S-? 1st trimester		45mL PO
•Liquid formulations are typically more effective			
Side effects:			

Gastrointestinal
  •Constipation (aluminum, calcium)
  •Diarrhea (magnesium)			

PROTON PUMP INHIBITORS		
Generic (Trade)	**M** ♀	**Dose**
Esomeprazole (Nexium)	L P	40mg PO q12hours
Lansoprazole (Prevacid)	L P	30mg PO q12hours
Omeprazole (Prilosec)	L ?	40mg PO q12hours
Pantoprazole (Protonix)	L P	40mg PO/ IV q12hours
Rabeprazole (Aciphex)	L P	40mg PO q12hours
Mechanism:		
•Inhibit parietal cell hydrogen/ potassium ATPase, located on the luminal border→ ◦90%↓gastric acid secretion		
Side effects:		

Gastrointestinal
  •Abdominal pain
  •Constipation
  •Diarrhea
  •Flatulence
  •Hepatitis-rare
  •Nausea ± vomiting
Mucocutaneous
  •Gynecomastia-rare
Neurologic
  •Headaches
Hematologic/ neurologic
  •Chronic use→
    ◦Vitamin B_{12} deficiency
Interactions
  •↓Absorption of Ampicillin, Digoxin, iron, Itraconazole, & Ketoconazole		

ANTIBACTERIAL PROPHYLAXIS

•50% of patients w/ advanced liver disease (Childs–Pugh class C) develop an infection (usually due to enterobacteriaceae) such as:
　◦Spontaneous bacterial peritonitis–SBP
　◦Sepsis
　…within 48hours after an acute gastrointestinal hemorrhage, X 1week

FLUOROQUINOLONES			
Generic (Trade)	M	♀	Dose
Gatifloxacin (Tequin)	K	?	400mg PO/ IV q24hours
Levofloxacin (Levaquin)	KL	?	500mg PO/ IV q24hours
Moxifloxacin (Avelox)	LK	?	400mg PO/ IV q24hours

Mechanism:
•↓DNA gyrase=topoisomerase action→
　◦↓Bacterial DNA synthesis

Side effects:
General
•Hypersensitivity reactions
Gastrointestinal
•Gastroenteritis→
　◦Diarrhea
　◦Nausea ± vomiting
Mucocutaneous
•Phototoxicity
Neurologic
•Dizziness
•Drowsiness
•Headache
•Restlessness
Materno–fetal
•Fetal & child tendon malformation (including breast fed)→
　◦↑Tendon rupture risk

PROGNOSIS

•80% of all gastrointestinal hemorrhages resolve w/ supportive care alone
•The overall mortality rate for acute upper gastrointestinal hemorrhage is 10%
•The overall mortality rate for acute lower gastrointestinal hemorrhage is 5%

•**Variceal hemorrhage**
　◦50% of patients w/ cirrhosis develop gastroesophageal varices, 30% of which experience hemorrhage, comprising 85% of hemorrhagic episodes in these patients→
　　–20% mortality @ 1st hemorrhage
　　–50% of survivors rebleeding within 6months (usually within 6weeks)
　　–Overall 35% mortality, being the **#1 cause of death in patients w/ cirrhosis**

Poor prognostic indicators of an acute upper GI hemorrhage necessitating ICU admission:
•**Clinical**
　◦Age >75 years
　◦Coagulopathy
　◦Major comorbid illness
　◦Active hemorrhage during hospitalization
　◦Hypotension ± shock
•**Endoscopic**
　◦Active hemorrhage
　◦Non–bleeding visible vessel
　◦Adherent clot
　◦Gastroesophageal variceal etiology
　◦Neoplasm

•Any process→
  ◦Infiltration of the pancreas by its own enzymatic secretions→
    –Inflammation=pancreatitis

RISK FACTORS
•**Obstructive**
  ◦**Gallstone enlodgement in the ampulla of vater–45%**
  ◦Ampullary or pancreatic tumor
  ◦Lymphoma
  ◦Pancreas divisum, being the #1 congenital anomaly of the pancreas, occurring in 10% of the
    population, in which the embryonic dorsal & ventral buds of the pancreas fail to fuse during
    embryologic development→
    –Drainage of the main pancreatic duct of Wirsung through the accessory pancreatic duct of
      Santorini, w/ pancreatitis being due to stenosis of the minor papillae through which the accessory
      duct drains into the duodenum
•**Alcohol abuse–35%**
  ◦5% of alcoholics, rarely occurring in casual drinkers
•**Idiopathic–10%**
  ◦Microcholelithiasis, termed biliary sludge
  ◦Hypertensive sphincter of Oddi
    –Basal sphincter >40mmHg as measured endoscopically via manometry
•**Trauma**
  ◦Blunt abdominal trauma
  ◦Endoscopic retrograde cholangiopancreatography–ERCP (2–5%)
  ◦Endoscopic sphincterectomy
  ◦Manometry of the sphincter of Oddi
  ◦Postoperative, esp. involving cardiopulmonary bypass
•**Infectious**
  ◦**Viruses:** Adenovirus, Coxsackievirus, Cytomegalovirus–CMV, echovirus, Epstein–Barr virus–EBV,
    hepatitis A or B virus, Human immune deficiency virus–HIV, Mumps virus, Rubella virus,
    Varicella–zoster virus–VZV
  ◦**Protozoa:** Ascaris lumbricoides, Clonorchis sinensis
  ◦**Bacteria:** Campylobacter jejuni, Legionella sp., Leptospira interrogans, Mycobacterium
    avium–intracellulare complex–MAC, Mycobacterium tuberculosis, Mycoplasma pneumoneae
•**Medications**
  ◦**Diuretics:** Loop diuretics, thiazide diuretics
  ◦**Estrogen:** Oral contraceptive pills–OCPs, hormone replacement therapy–HRT
  ◦**Antimicrobials:** Erythromycin, Isoniazid–INH, Metronidazole, Nitrofurantoin, certain nucleoside
    reverse transcriptase inhibitors–NRTIs (Didanosine–ddI, Stavudine–d4T, Zalcitabine–ddC),
    Pentamidine, protease inhibitors, sulfonamides, Tetracycline
  ◦**Angiotensin converting enzyme inhibitors–ACEi**
  ◦**Acetaminophen**
  ◦**Glucocorticoids**
  ◦**Histamine 2 selective receptor blockers**
  ◦**Nonsteroidal anti–inflammatory drugs–NSAIDs, including Aspirin**
  ◦**Other:** Azathioprine (& its active metabolite 6–mercaptopurine), Cisplatin, Danazol, Diphenoxylate,
    Gold, L–asparaginase, Methyldopa, Procainamide, Valproic acid
•**Hypercalcemia**
•**Hypertriglyceridemia** >1000mg/ dL
•**Perforated peptic ulcer**
•**Vascular injury**
  ◦Cholesterol embolism
  ◦Vasculitis
•**Genetic**
  ◦Crohn's disease of the duodenum→
    –Pancreatic duct obstruction
  ◦Cystic fibrosis
•**Insecticides**
  ◦Organophosphorous
•**Scorpion venom**, being the #1 cause in Trinidad

301

•**Chronicity based classification:**
  ◦**Acute pancreatitis**
  ◦**Chronic relapsing pancreatitis**, being caused esp. by **alcoholism-90%**
    –Repeated episodes of acute pancreatitiis→parenchymal destruction→fibrosis→duct distortion & obstruction by proteinaceous plugs (which eventually calcify)→↓exocrine secretory flow→enzyme parenchymal extravasation→**eventual pancreatitis autonomous of the original stimulus**

•**Severity based classification**
  ◦**Mild pancreatitis-75%:** Lack signs &/or symptoms of severe pancreatitis, w/ an uneventful recovery
  ◦**Severe pancreatitis-25%**, via the presence of either:
    –Abscess formation
    –Compromised organ vascularity→necrosis & hemorrhage
    –Pseudocyst formation
    –Organ failure, including pancreatic failure→steatorrhea &/or secondary diabetes mellitus
    –Ranson's prognostic criteria score ≥3

General
•Inflammatory cytokines→
  ◦Anorexia (also being due to nausea &/or ↑pain upon eating)→
    –Cachexia (also being due to ↓intestinal absorption)
  ◦Chills
  ◦Fatigue
  ◦**Fever-75%**
  ◦Headache
  ◦Malaise
  ◦Night sweats
  ◦Weakness

---

†Temperature may be normal in patients w/:
  •Chronic kidney disease, esp. w/ uremia
  •Cirrhosis
  •Heart failure
  •Severe debility
  …or those who are:
    •Intravenous drug users
    •Taking certain medications:
      ◦Acetaminophen
      ◦Antibiotics
      ◦Glucocorticoids
      ◦Nonsteroidal anti-inflammatory drugs-NSAIDs

Gastrointestinal
•Viscous obstruction & inflammation (biliary tract or pancreatic ductal)→↑viscous peristalsis→
  ◦↑Generalized viscous peristalsis (gastrointestinal, biliary, & genitourinary)→
    –**Abdominal pain**, being referred & episodic or "wave like", termed colic
      Areas of reference:
        •Stomach &/or duodenum: Epigastrium
        •Small intestine: Periumbilical area
        •Large intestine: Hypogastrium &/or suprapubic area
        •Rectum: Suprapubic, sacral, &/or perineal areas
    –Anorexia
    –↑Bowel sounds→audible gastrointestinal gurgling, termed borborygmi
    –Diarrhea
    –Retrograde peristalsis→**nausea ± vomiting-80%**
•Biliary tract obstruction (either primary, or secondarily due to pancreatic edema)→
  ◦↓Intestinal bile flow→
    –↓Stool bile→↓stool bilirubin→**light colored/ pale stool, termed acholic stool**
•↓Intestinal bile &/or pancreatic lipase flow→
  ◦↓Fat absorption→
    –↑Stool fat→**foul smelling, floating stools**, leaving an oily residue on the toilet
    –Cachexia
    –Vitamin A, D, E, & K malabsorption

302

•Pancreatitis→
  ◦**Continuous abdominal pain**, being epigastric &/or periumbilical ± **radiation to the back–50%**, usually described as "knifelike" or "boring", being relieved by ↓peritoneal stretching, accomplished by sitting, leaning forward, & or hip flexion
  ◦Phlegmon formation, being viable & dead bacteria, leukocytes (predominantly neutrophils), & necrotic tissue, w/ eventual encapsulation by connective tissue, thus termed **abscess**, usually along the:
    –Inflammed organ
    –Pelvis, due to gravitational flow
    –Subphrenic area, due to diaphragmatic mediated negative pressure
  ◦Eventual spread to the parietal peritoneum→**parietal peritonitis**→
    –↑**Localized abdominal pain**, esp. to movement of the inflammed parietal peritoneum→patient lying "stone" still, w/ exacerbation upon any bodily movement, even diaphragmatic movement upon deep inspiration, cough, sneezing, or the Valsalva maneuver
    –**Referred rebound tenderness**, being the sudden release of gentle pressure remote from the painful area→parietal peritoneal movement→pain over the inflammed area
    –**Involuntary guarding**, being reflex contraction of the overlying abdominal muscles (in order to ↓pain), which persists despite attempts to relax
    –**Paralytic ileus**, being reflex relaxation of the regional intestinal smooth muscle (in order to ↓pain)→↓regional bowel sounds & constipation
    –Peritoneal effusion=**ascites** (being exudative)→localized rub to auscultation, shifting dullness to percussion, weight gain (1L fluid=1kg=2.2 lbs), & ↑**abdominal girth–75%** (also due to intestinal paralytic ileus)
    –Fibrous adhesions connecting the visceral & parietal peritoneum→intra-abdominal hernias

Cardiovascular
•Peritoneal effusion=ascites, which, along w/ diarrhea, vomiting, & anorexia→↓intravascular volume→
  ◦≥10% blood volume loss→
    –↑Autonomic sympathetic tone→↑pulse
  ◦≥20% blood volume loss→
    –Orthostatic hypotension (supine to standing→↑20 pulse, ↓20 SBP, &/or ↓10 DBP)→ lightheadedness upon standing
    –Urine output 20–30mL/ hour (normal being >30mL/ hour)
  ◦≥30% blood volume loss→
    –Recumbent hypotension &/or tachycardia
  ◦≥40% blood volume loss→
    –Altered mental status &/or urine output <20mL/ hour
    –Hypovolemic shock, being hypotension + organ failure, unresponsive to fluid resuscitation
Endocrine
•Chronic relapsing pancreatitis→
  ◦β–islet cell destruction→
    –↓Insulin secretion→secondary diabetes mellitus
Genitourinary
•Biliary tract obstruction→congestive hepatitis→
  ◦↑Plasma conjugated bilirubin→
    –↑Urine bilirubin→dark "coca-cola" colored urine
•↑Urine amylase
  ◦A 2hour urine collection for amylase may show elevation for ≤10days after the plasma value has normalized
Mucocutaneous
•Biliary tract obstruction→congestive hepatitis→↑plasma bilirubin→subcutaneous deposition→
  ◦Yellow staining of tissues @ >3mg/ dL
    –Skin→**jaundice–20%**
    –Sclera→**scleral icterus**
    –Mucus membranes
  ◦Pruritis
•Hemorrhagic pancreatitis→
  ◦Hemorrhagic retroperitoneal dissection→
    –**Abdominal flank ecchymoses, termed Grey-Turner's sign**
    –**Periumbilical ecchymosis, termed Cullen's sign**

Pulmonary
- •Liberation of phospholipase A→disruption of the alveolar surfactant layer→microatelectasis→
  - ○Ventilation/ perfusion mismatch via:
    - –↑Alveolar dead space: Alveolar ventilation through relatively underperfused capillaries
    - –↑Vascular shunting†: Capillary blood flow through relatively underventilated alveoli.
      Usually occurring, or exacerbated via ↑venous return
    - ...→↓diffusion of O_2 & CO_2→
      - •Hypoxemia (SaO_2 ≤ 91% or PaO_2 ≤ 60mmHg‡) on room air, w/ subsequent
        hypercapnia ($PaCO_2$ ≥45mmHg) due to either:
        - ○Respiratory muscle fatigue
        - ○Alveolar hypoventilation
        ...as CO_2 clearance is unimpaired (& may be ↑in the dyspneic patient) as long as
        adequate ventilation (including lack of diffuse severe ventilation/ perfusion mismatching)
        is maintained, as:
          - •CO_2 diffuses 20X as rapidly as O_2
          - •Hypercapnia→
            - ○Immediate brain stem respiratory center mediated stimulation of pulmonary
              ventilation, which may correct the hypercapnia, but not necessarily the hypoxia
- •Ascitic fluid movement from the abdomen to the pleural space through diaphragmatic defects→
  - ○Exudative pleural effusion (left > right) w/ an amylase level >2X plasma level

---

†Being exacerbated by the supine position→
- •↑Systemic venous return→
  - ○↑Vascular shunting→↑dyspnea, being termed:
    - –Orthopnea, if persistent
    - –Paroxysmal nocturnal dyspnea if intermittent
    ...causing the patient to either use multiple pillows or sleep in a chair
‡Age adjusted normal PaO_2 = 101 – (0.43 X age)

Hematologic
- •Inflammatory cytokines→
  - ○Leukocytosis
  - ○↑Acute phase proteins
    - –↑Erythrocyte sedimentation rate–ESR (normal: 5mm/ decade aged + ♂ ≤10mm/h or ♀ ≤20mm/h)
    - –↑C–reactive protein–CRP (normal: <2mg/ L), responding more acutely than ESR, as it rises
      within several hours & falls within 3days upon partial resolution
    - –↑Fibrinogen
    - –↑Platelets→thrombocytosis
- •Intravascular volume loss→
  - ○↑Creatinine & blood urea nitrogen–BUN indicating pre–renal renal failure
  - ○↑Hemoglobin/ hematocrit
- •Gallstone mediated pancreatitis→
  - ○**Alanine aminotransferase–ALT 2.5 X upper limit of normal**
- •Pancreatic inflammation→
  - ○Liberation of lipase→
    - –Lipid metabolism→calcium saponification→**hypocalcemia**
- •Hemorrhagic pancreatitis→
  - ○↓Hemoglobin & hematocrit, **requiring ≥8hours to be evident & ≥24hours to be complete**, are
    not useful indices of the amount of blood loss. Within the 1st several hours after blood loss,
    hypovolemia is indicated via intravenous fluid resuscitation→↑plasma→↓hemoglobin/ hematocrit via
    a dilutional effect

Pancreatic enzyme analysis:
- •↑**Plasma amylase–80%**, w/ peak @ ~24hours, being >300 U/ L (usually >1,000 U/ L)
- •↑**Plasma lipase**, w/ peak @ ~24hours, being >500 U/ L, **remaining ↑for several days longer than
  amylase**
Outcomes:
- •Sensitivity–95%, specificity–80%
Limitations:
- •Levels do not correlate w/ disease severity, which is why they are not incorporated into Ranson's
  prognostic criteria
- •Plasma amylase may normalize @ 48–72hours, despite persistent syndrome
- •Renal failure→
  - ○Falsely ↑levels
Etiologic differences:
- •A lipase/ amylase ratio >2 suggests alcoholic pancreatitis

•**Abdomino-pelvic ultrasound or computed tomographic-CT scan**
Findings:
  •Inflammation→
    ○**Enlarged edematous pancreas**
      –May appear normal in 30% of mild cases
    ○**Peri-organ stranding** seen on CT
    ○Lymphadenopathy
  •Biliary obstruction→
    ○Proximal biliary tract dilation
  •Ultrasound allows for the visualization of most gallstones, as only 15% are radiopaque
  •Peritonitis→
    ○Ascites
  •Paralytic ileus, being either:
    ○Generalized
    ○Localized to nearby intestine→
      –Air filled segment, termed the sentinel loop sign
      …→intestinal air fluid levels
  •Phlegmon, abscess, &/or peri-organ fluid, which may be subdiaphragmatic→
    –Diaphragm elevation
  •Perforation→
    ○Subdiaphragmatic air

Findings consistent w/ chronic pancreatitis:
  •**Calcification of ductal proteinaceous plugs-20%**
  •**Dilated pancreatic duct**

•**Endoscopic retrograde cholangiopancreatography-ERCP**
  Findings consistent w/ chronic pancreatitis:
    •**Beaded/ dilated main pancreatic duct, termed "chain of lakes" appearance**

PROGNOSIS

RANSON'S PROGNOSTIC CRITERIA

On admission	@48hours after admission
Age >55years (elderly)	Hematocrit ↓>10%
Glucose >200mg/ dL (diabetes mellitus)	**Blood urea nitrogen-BUN** ↑>5mg/ dL(dehydration)
Aspartate aminotransferase-AST >250 U/ L	Calcium <8mg/ dL (hypocalcemia)
Lactate dehydrogenase-LDH >350 U/ L	PaO₂ <60mmHg (hypoxemia)
Leukocytosis >16,000/ µL	Base deficit >4mEq/ L
	Fluid sequestration >6L (1L fluid=1kg=2.2 lbs)

Mortality based on number of criteria met @48hours†:
  •**≤2**: 1%
  •**3-4**: 15%
  •**5-6**: 40%
  •**≥7**: 100%
  …w/ an overall mortality of 10%, w/ **sepsis being the #1 cause of death**

†Hemorrhagic pancreatitis indicates a ≥50% mortality

COMPLICATIONS
•**Pancreatic necrosis**
Diagnosis:
  •Abdominal computed tomographic-CT scanning w/ rapid administration of intravenous contrast dye
  via a pressure injector, allowing for the assessment of the organ's vascular integrity, w/ **areas of
  hypoperfusion**→
    ○Non-enhancement, signifying necrosis
Treatment:
  •**Prophylactic antibiotic treatment** (Imipenem being preferred) as long as reasonably possible prior
  to surgical debridement via pancreatectomy or necrosectomy

Indications to proceed immediately w/ surgical treatment:
•Clinical instability
•**Infected pancreatic necrosis–70%,** diagnosed via percutaneous drainage for gram stain & culture, being treated w/ the administration of antibiotics (Imipenem being preferred), w/ surgical debridement of necrotic tissue via pancreatectomy or necrosectomy
  ◦**100% mortality if not adequately treated**
•Refractory to conservative treatment

•**Pancreatic abscess**
  ◦Usually occurring @ ≥6weeks after presentation, & suggested by **persistent fever & leukocytosis**
  Diagnosis:
    •Abdominal computed tomographic–CT scan guided percutaneous needle aspiration for gram stain & culture. Infected aspirate fluid is diagnostic
  Treatment:
    •Administration of antibiotics, w/ surgical removal

•**Pseudocyst formation–15%**
  ◦Pancreatitis→peripancreatic fluid collections, which may persist→
    –Fibrotic encapsulation over **6weeks,** at which time they are referred to as pancreatic pseudocysts, as they lack the epithelial lining of a true cyst
  ◦Formation is suggested by either:
    –**A palpable abdominal mass**
    –**Persistent pain**
    –**Persistently ↑amylase or lipase**
  Diagnosis:
    •Abdominal computed tomographic–CT scan
  Complications:
    •Mass effect→
      ◦Nearby organ compression (bile duct, duodenum, stomach, &/or colon)
    •**Hemorrhage** (acute or chronic), being diagnosed via angiography, & treated via embolization
    •**Superinfection:** Diagnosed via percutaneous drainage for gram stain & culture, being treated w/ the administration of antibiotics, Imipenem being preferred
    •**Rupture→**
      ◦15% mortality
  Treatment:
    •Most resolve spontaneously within 6weeks, esp. if ≤5cm diameter
  Indications for surgical treatment:
    •Surgical drainage of the pseudocyst, either percutaneously, or internally via the gastrointestinal tract, for the following indications:
      ◦Organ compression
      ◦Symptomatic @ >6weeks

OTHER ▬▬▬▬▬▬▬▬▬▬▬▬▬▬▬▬▬▬▬▬▬▬▬▬▬▬▬▬▬▬▬▬▬▬▬▬▬▬
•**Acute respiratory distress syndrome–ARDS**
•**Splenic vein thrombosis→**
  ◦Gastroesophageal varices. Being that the veins are thin walled, & poorly supported by the connective tissue of the submucosa, they commonly rupture→
    –Upper gastrointestinal hemorrhage
•**Arterial thrombosis,** esp. of the:
    –Gastroduodenal arteries
    –Splenic arteries
    –Colic branches of the superior mesenteric artery
    …→intestinal ischemia ± infarction
•**Purtscher's angiopathic retinopathy**
  ◦Visualized as discrete, flame shaped hemorrhages w/ soft exudates, termed cotton wool exudates, indicating ischemic or infarcted nerve fiber layers→
    –Acute blindness

306

•**Nil per os–NPO**, w/ duration dependant on severity
◦Eating >> drinking→
  −↑Peristalsis
  −↑Digestive enzyme release
  ...→↑pain & organ destruction
•**Parenteral hyperalimentation** via a central venous line
Indications:
  •Severe, prolonged acute pancreatitis, as ↓caloric intake→
  ◦Striking protein loss & catabolism
•**Alcohol cessation** via alcoholics anonymous
•**Intermittent nasogastric–NG suctioning**
◦Gastric acid delivery to the duodenum→
  −↑Pancreatic exocrine secretion
Indications:
  •As placement has not been shown to affect clinical outcome, it is reserved for patients w/ either:
  ◦Intractable vomiting
  ◦Paralytic ileus
  ◦Profound pain
  ◦Severe disease
•**Plasma monitoring q24h**, in order to follow the clinical course via Ranson's criteria
◦Arterial blood gas
◦Calcium
◦Chemistry
◦Complete blood count
•**Electrolyte repletion** as needed
◦Calcium
◦Potassium
◦Magnesium
•**Follow urine output & daily weights**
•**Intravenous fluid**, w/ attention to both:
◦**Intravascular volume repletion via Normal saline** (0.9% NaCl) or **lactated Ringer's solution**, as per:
  −Vital signs
  −Physical examination
  −Urine output (normal being ≥0.5mL/kg/h)
  −Blood urea nitrogen–BUN & creatinine
◦**Intravascular volume maintenance via Normal saline** (0.9% NaCl) or **lactated Ringer's solution**
  Adult maintenance fluid:
    •Weight (kg) + 40= #mL/ hour
  Additional febrile requirements:
    •1L/ 24hours for every 1°F >100°F
  Additional:
    •Estimate loss for:
    ◦Diaphoresis
    ◦Diarrhea
    ◦Polyuria
    ◦Tachypnea
  ...followed by oral rehydration w/ a glucose based electrolyte solution upon both clinical stability & ability to tolerate PO

OPIOID RECEPTOR AGONISTS			
Indications:			
•Acute pain			
Generic (Trade)	**M**	♀	**Start**
Hydromorphone (Dilaudid)	L	?	
•PO form			2mg q4hours
•SC/ IM/ IV forms			0.5mg q4hours
•PR form			3mg q6hours
Morphine sulfate	LK	?	10mg PO/ SC/ IM/ IV q4hours

•Titrate as high as necessary to relieve pain, w/ tolerable concomitant side effects

Side effects:
  Cardiovascular
  •Vasodilation (venous >> arterial)→
    ◦↓Preload→
      −↓Cardiac output→**hypotension**
  •**Bradycardia**
  Gastrointestinal
  •Central nervous system chemoreceptor trigger zone activation→
    ◦**Nausea ± vomiting**, exacerbated by ambulation
  •Enteric nervous system opioid receptor activation→
    ◦↓Gastrointestinal smooth muscle peristalsis→
      −**Constipation**
  •↑Biliary tract smooth muscle contraction→
    ◦Biliary colic
  Genitourinary
  •↑Ureteral & urinary bladder smooth muscle peristalsis→
    ◦Prostatic neoplastic syndrome exacerbation
  •↓Uterine muscle tone→
    ◦Labor prolongation
  Neurologic
  •**Altered mental status**
  •Dysphoria
  •Sedation
  •Seizures
  Opthalmologic
  •Iris radial smooth muscle relaxation→
    ◦↓Pupil size=**miosis**, being fixed
  Pulmonary
  •Inhibition of medullary respiratory center response to CO_2 concentration→
    ◦**Respiratory depression**→
      −Hypercapnic respiratory failure→altered mental status
  •↓Cough reflex

Side effects of chronic use:
  •Development of **tolerance**† to its effects, as the dosage previously sufficient to produce effects progressively fails to do so, as both the central nervous system & liver adapt to its chronic presence by altering:
    ◦Neuronal membrane constituents
    ◦Neurotransmitter release & re–uptake
    ◦Hepatic clearance
    …which set the stage for the vicious cycle of **dependence** & craving for ever increasing amounts of the medication, regardless of the professional, social, or health risks

---

†Tolerance does not develop to:
  •Constipation
  •Miosis
  •Seizures

ANTIDOTE

Generic (Trade)	M	♀	Start	Max
Naloxone (Narcan)	LK	P	2mg IV/ SC/ IM/ ET q2min. prn	10mg total

Mechanism:
  •μ receptor antagonist, which, in the absence of exogenous opioids, have no clinical effect
Duration:
  •1–2hours
Side effects:
  •**Acute opioid withdrawal/ reversal syndrome**
    ◦Diaphoresis
    ◦Goose flesh
    ◦↑Lacrimation
    ◦Nausea ± vomiting
    ◦Rhinorrhea
    ◦Tachypnea

...w/ rare:
- •Hypo or hypertension
- •Pulmonary edema
- •Ventricular tachycardia &/or fibrillation

ANTIEMETIC MEDICATIONS

Generic	M	♀	Start	Max
Prochlorperazine (Compazine)	LK	?	5mg PO/ IM/ IV q8hours	10mg q6hours
•PR form			25mg PR q12hpurs	
•XR form			15mg PO q24hours	30mg q24hours
Promethazine (Phenergan)	LK	?	12.5mg PO/ IM/ PR/ IV q6hours	25mg q4hours
Thiethylperazine (Torecan)	L	?	10mg PO/ IM q24hours	10mg q8hours
Trimethobenzamide (Tigan)	LK	?	200mg PO/ IM/ PR q6hours	

Prochlorperazine specific side effects:
- **Cardiovascular**
  - •Dysrhythmias
  - •Hypotension w/ IV administration
- **Mucocutaneous**
  - •Gynecomastia, being the ↑development of male mammary glands
- **Neurologic**
  - •Anticholinergic effects
  - •Extrapyramidal dysfunction
  - •Sedation
  - •Seizures
- **Hematologic**
  - •Leukopenia
  - •Thrombocytopenia

Promethazine specific side effects:
- **Cardiovascular**
  - •Hypotension w/ IV administration
- **Neurologic**
  - •Anticholinergic effects
  - •Extrapyramidal dysfunction
  - •Sedation

Trimethobenzamde specific side effects:
- **Neurologic**
  - •Sedation

INVASIVE PROCEDURES
- •**Endoscopic retrograde cholangiopancreatography–ERCP**
  - ◦Most cases of gallstone mediated pancreatitis do not require intervention via ERCP, as the majority of gallstones pass spontaneously into the duodenum
  - Indications:
    - •Within 24 to 48hours in patients w/ evidence of biliary tract obstruction, in order to either:
      - ◦Remove gallstones
      - ◦Place a biliary stent
  - Side effects:
    - •Cholangitis <1%
    - •Hemorrhage if sphincterectomy is performed
    - •Pancreatitis–1%
    - •Peritonitis
    - •Death–rare
  - Contraindications:
    - •Pregnancy, due to ionizing radiation

CHRONIC RELAPSING PANCREATITIS
- •Oral replacement of pancreatic enzymes for steatorrhea
- •Insulin to manage diabetes mellitus

SURGERY FOR PAIN CONTROL
- •↑**Pancreatic exocrine drainage**
  - Procedures:
    - •Sphincteroplasty
    - •Longitudinal pancreaticojejunostomy, termed the Puestow procedure

- ↓**Pancreatic tissue**
  Procedures:
    - Distal pancreatectomy
    - 95% pancreatectomy
    - Pancreaticoduodenectomy
    - Total pancreatectomy

- **Celiac plexus destruction**

•Obstruction of a hollow viscus→
∘Organ inflammation

CLASSIFICATION/ RISK FACTORS
•Appendicitis
Pathophysiology/ risk factors:
•Appendiceal obstruction via either:
∘Dehydrated feces, termed fecalith, being the #1 cause
∘Neoplasm
∘Parasitic infection
Additional risk factors:
•Age: 5–30 years
•Gender: ♂ 1.5 X ♀

•Diverticulitis
Pathophysiology/ risk factors:
•Diverticular obstruction, occurring in 25% of patients w/ diverticulosis, being:
∘8% of patients age >45years
∘80% of patients age >85years
Pathophysiology of diverticulosis:
•Diminished stool bulk due to **insufficient dietary fiber**→
∘Altered gastrointestinal transit time
∘↑Colonic intramural pressure→
  –Mucosal outpouchings through muscular defects in the intestinal wall, termed diverticula

•Ascending cholangitis
Pathophysiology/ risk factors:
•Common bile duct obstruction via either:
∘Gallstone, termed choledocholithiasis
∘Neoplasm, being either biliary or pancreatic in origin
∘Stricture

CHOLECYSTITIS
•Calculous–90%
Pathophysiology/ risk factors:
•Cystic duct obstruction via either:
∘**Gallstone, termed cholelithiasis–95%**
∘Microcholelithiasis, termed biliary sludge

•Acalculous
Pathophysiology/ risk factors:
•Non–obstructive disease† via either:
∘Fasting
∘Parenteral feeding
∘Prolonged illness
Additional risk factors:
•Age: ≥50 years
•Gender: ♂ X ♀

•Infectious–rare
Organisms:
•Salmonella sp.
•Cytomegalovirus–CMV or Cryptosporidia infection in severely immunocompromised patients

---

†Undetected biliary sludge formation may be the etiology

Gallstone types based on major constituent:
- **Cholesterol gallstone–90%**
  - ○Consider the **5 Fs**:
    - –Age: ≥Forty years
    - –Gender: Female (esp. Fertile) 4X ♂
    - –Obesity (Fat)
    - –Flatulent
  - ○**Endocrine**
    - –Diabetes mellitus
  - ○↑**Estrogen exposure**
    - –Nulliparity
    - –Early menarche (age <12years)
    - –Late menopause (age >50years)
    - –Late first pregnancy (age >35years)
    - –Absence of breast feeding
    - –Obesity
    - –Chronic anovulation
    - –Medications (hormone replacement treatment–HRT, oral contraception pills–OCP)
  - ○**Ethnicity**
    - –Pima Indians
    - –Scandanavians
  - ○**Genetic**
    - –Maternal family history of gallstones
  - ○**Ileal disease**
    - –Crohn's disease
    - –Ileal resection
    - –Gastrectomy
    - ...→↓enterohepatic circulation of bile salts→
      - •↑Bile lithogenicity→
        - ○Cholelithiasis
  - ○**Medications**
    - –Ceftriaxone
    - –Fibric acid derivatives
    - –Octreotide
  - ○**Other**
    - –Hyperlipidemia
- **Pigmented gallstone–10%**
  - ○Chronic hemolytic anemia→
    - –Black pigmented gallstones
  - ○Biliary tract infections→
    - –Brown pigmented gallstones
- **Mixed gallstone**

Mechanism:
- •Viscous obstruction→
  - ○↑Smooth muscle metabolic demand, w/ concomitant ↓vascular flow→
    - –Relative ischemia→inflammation
  - ○Inadequate mucous clearance→stagnant mucous proximal to the obstruction→
    - –↑Bacterial growth
    - ...→↑infection risk, usually being caused by >1 organism=**polymicrobial**

Organisms:
- •**Enterobacteriaceae**
  - ○**Escherichia coli**
  - ○Enterobacter cloacae
  - ○Enterococcus faecalis
  - ○Klebsiella pneumoniae
  - ○Proteus mirabilis & vulgaris
  - ○Providencia rettgeri
  - ○Pseudomonas aeruginosa
  - ○Serratia marcescens
- •**Anaerobes**
  - ○**Bacteroides sp., esp. fragilis**
  - ○Clostridium sp.
  - ○Peptococcus sp.
  - ○Streptococcus sp.
  - ○Peptostreptococcus sp.

312

General
- •Inflammatory cytokines→
  - ∘Anorexia (also being due to nausea &/or ↑pain upon eating)→
    - −Cachexia (also being due to ↓intestinal absorption)
  - ∘Chills
  - ∘Fatigue
  - ∘**Fever**
  - ∘Headache
  - ∘Malaise
  - ∘Night sweats
  - ∘Weakness

---

†Temperature may be normal in patients w/:
- •Chronic kidney disease, esp. w/ uremia
- •Cirrhosis
- •Heart failure
- •Severe debility
- …or those who are:
  - •Intravenous drug users
  - •Taking certain medications:
    - ∘Acetaminophen
    - ∘Antibiotics
    - ∘Glucocorticoids
    - ∘Nonsteroidal anti−inflammatory drugs−NSAIDs

Gastrointestinal
- •Viscous obstruction & inflammation (biliary tract or pancreatic ductal)→↑viscous peristalsis→
  - ∘↑Generalized viscous peristalsis (gastrointestinal, biliary, & genitourinary)→
    - −**Abdominal pain**, being referred & episodic or "wave like", termed colic
      - Areas of reference:
        - •Stomach &/or duodenum: Epigastrium
        - •Small intestine: Periumbilical area
        - •Large intestine: Hypogastrium &/or suprapubic area
        - •Rectum: Suprapubic, sacral, &/or perineal areas
    - −Anorexia
    - −↑Bowel sounds→audible gastrointestinal gurgling, termed borborygmi
    - −Diarrhea
    - −Retrograde peristalsis→**nausea ± vomiting−80%**
- •Biliary tract obstruction (either primary, or secondarily due to pancreatic edema)→
  - ∘↓Intestinal bile flow→
    - −↓Stool bile→↓stool bilirubin→**light colored/ pale stool, termed acholic stool**
- •↓Intestinal bile &/or pancreatic lipase flow→
  - ∘↓Fat absorption→
    - −↑Stool fat→**foul smelling, floating stools,** leaving an oily residue on the toilet
    - −Cachexia
    - −Vitamin A, D, E, & K malabsorption
- •Organ inflammation→
  - ∘**Continuous abdominal pain,** being epigastric &/or periumbilical ± **radiation to the back−50%,** usually described as "knifelike" or "boring", being relieved by ↓peritoneal stretching, accomplished by sitting, leaning forward, & or hip flexion
  - ∘Phlegmon formation, being viable & dead bacteria, leukocytes (predominantly neutrophils), & necrotic tissue, w/ eventual encapsulation by connective tissue, thus termed **abscess,** usually along the:
    - −Inflamed organ
    - −Pelvis, due to gravitational flow
    - −Subphrenic area, due to diaphragmatic mediated negative pressure
  - ∘Eventual spread to the parietal peritoneum→**parietal peritonitis**→
    - −↑**Localized abdominal pain,** esp. to movement of the inflamed parietal peritoneum→patient lying "stone" still, w/ exacerbation upon any bodily movement, even diaphragmatic movement upon deep inspiration, cough, sneezing, or the Valsalva maneuver
    - −**Referred rebound tenderness,** being the sudden release of gentle pressure remote from the painful area→parietal peritoneal movement→pain over the inflamed area
    - −**Involuntary guarding,** being reflex contraction of the overlying abdominal muscles (in order to ↓pain), which persists despite attempts to relax
    - −**Paralytic ileus,** being reflex relaxation of the regional intestinal smooth muscle (in order to ↓pain)→↓regional bowel sounds & constipation

313

-Peritoneal effusion=**ascites** (being exudative)→localized rub to auscultation, shifting dullness to percussion, weight gain (1L fluid=1kg=2.2 lbs), & ↑**abdominal girth-75%** (also due to intestinal paralytic ileus)
-Fibrous adhesions connecting the visceral & parietal peritoneum→intra-abdominal hernias
-Luminal connection w/ nearby epithelial surfaces, termed **fistula**, being **enterocutaneous, enteroenteric, enterovaginal,** &/or **enterovesical**
°**Perforation**→
-Release of contents (bacteria & digestive enzymes ± air, mucus, &/or feces)→generalized peritonitis

Appendicitis specific physical findings:
•Visceral peritonitis→
°Epigastric &/or periumbilical pain, w/ subsequent parietal peritonitis→
-**Right lower quadrant abdominal pain**
Note: Appendicitis occurs in 1/ 2000 pregnancies, w/ appendiceal displacement due to the enlarged uterus→
•Atypical presentations
•**Mcburney's point tenderness**
°Mcburney's point is located 1.5-2" medial to the anterior spinous process of the ileum, being tender to deep finger palpation
•**Obturator test**
°Flex the thigh of the supine patient, w/ subsequent internal rotation via pulling the ankle laterally & pushing the knee medially→
-Stretching of obturator muscle, & movement of surrounding tissues→pain if either the obturator muscle or nearby tissue is inflamed, indicating possible appendicitis if elicited solely w/ the right leg
Note: External rotation should not be associated w/ pain
•**Reverse psoas maneuver**
°Hyperextend the hip of the patient in the lateral decubitus position→
-Stretching of iliopsoas muscle, & movement of surrounding tissues→pain if either the iliopsoas muscle or nearby tissue is inflamed, indicating possible appendicitis if elicited solely w/ the right leg
Note: Hip flexion should not be associated w/ pain
•**Rovsing's sign**
°Deep palpation over the left iliac fossa→
-Pain over the right iliac fossa

Diverticulitis specific physical findings:
•85% occur in the descending or sigmoid colon, w/ visceral peritonitis→
°Right lower quadrant, epigastric, &/or periumbilical pain, w/ subsequent parietal peritonitis→
-**Left lower quadrant pain**, referred to as "left sided appendicitis"

Ascending cholangitis diagnostic findings:
•**Charcot's triad**
°Right upper quadrant abdominal pain
°Fever ± chills
°Jaundice

Cholecystitis specific physical findings:
•Visceral peritonitis→
°Right shoulder &/or scapular pain, w/ subsequent parietal peritonitis→
-**Right upper quadrant abdominal pain**
•**Murphy's sign**
°Place your left hand just beneath the supine right anterior rib cage (fingers pointed medially). Then, rotate the thumb into patients abdomen, & instruct the patient to inhale deeply→
-Diaphragm flattening, pushing the inflamed gallbladder at or near the thumb indentation→ pain→abrupt cessation of inspiration, whereas without thumb indentation, the patient experiences no pain
•**Boas' sign**
°↑Sensory sensitivity=hyperesthesia, beneath the right scapula→
-Pain to light touch
•**Mirizzi's syndrome**
°Cholecystitis→
-Gallbladder edema→compression of the common bile duct &/or hepatic ducts→jaundice

314

- **Gallstone ileus**
  - ∘Gallbladder inflammation↔
    - −Cholecyst−enteric (duodenal or gastric) fistula→gallstone passage through to the small intestine→ileocecal valve obstruction→mechanical ileus

Cardiovascular
- •Peritoneal effusion=ascites, which, along w/ diarrhea, vomiting, & anorexia→↓intravascular volume→
  - ∘≥10% blood volume loss→
    - −↑Autonomic sympathetic tone→↑pulse
  - ∘≥20% blood volume loss→
    - −Orthostatic hypotension (supine to standing→↑20 pulse, ↓20 SBP, &/or ↓10 DBP)→ lightheadedness upon standing
    - −Urine output 20−30mL/ hour (normal being >30mL/ hour)
  - ∘≥30% blood volume loss→
    - −Recumbent hypotension &/or tachycardia
  - ∘≥40% blood volume loss→
    - −Altered mental status &/or urine output <20mL/ hour
    - −Hypovolemic shock, being hypotension + organ failure, unresponsive to fluid resuscitation

Genitourinary
- •Biliary tract obstruction→congestive hepatitis→
  - ∘↑Plasma conjugated bilirubin→
    - −↑Urine bilirubin→dark "coca−cola" colored urine
- •Inflammation near the urinary tract→
  - ∘Urinary tract inflammation syndrome, w/ sterile pyuria, which occurs in 40% of cases of appendicitis

Mucocutaneous
- •Biliary tract obstruction→congestive hepatitis→↑plasma bilirubin→subcutaneous deposition→
  - ∘Yellow staining of tissues @ >3mg/ dL
    - −Skin→**jaundice−20%**
    - −Sclera→**scleral icterus**
    - −Mucus membranes
  - ∘Pruritis

Hematologic
- •Inflammatory cytokines→
  - ∘Leukocytosis
  - ∘↑Acute phase proteins
    - −↑Erythrocyte sedimentation rate−ESR (normal: 5mm/ decade aged + ♂ ≤10mm/h or ♀ ≤20mm/h)
    - −↑C−reactive protein−CRP (normal: <2mg/ L), responding more acutely than ESR, as it rises within several hours & falls within 3days upon partial resolution
    - −↑Fibrinogen
    - −↑Platelets→thrombocytosis
- •Intravascular volume loss→
  - ∘↑Creatinine & blood urea nitrogen−BUN indicating pre−renal renal failure
  - ∘↑Hemoglobin/ hematocrit

IMAGING
- •**Abdomino−pelvic ultrasound or computed tomographic−CT scan**
  - Findings:
    - •Inflammation→
      - ∘**Enlarged edematous organ**
      - ∘**Peri−organ stranding** seen on CT
      - ∘Lymphadenopathy
    - •Biliary obstruction→
      - ∘Proximal biliary tract dilation
    - •Ultrasound allows for the visualization of most gallstones, as only 15% are radiopaque
    - •Peritonitis→
      - ∘Ascites
    - •Paralytic ileus, being either:
      - ∘Generalized
      - ∘Localized to nearby intestine→
        - −Air filled segment, termed the sentinel loop sign
      - …→intestinal air fluid levels
    - •Phlegmon, abscess, &/or peri−organ fluid, which may be subdiaphragmatic→
      - −Diaphragm elevation
    - •Perforation→
      - ∘Subdiaphragmatic air

315

- **Hepatobiliary iminodiacetic acid—HIDA scan**
  Indications:
  - Suspected extrahepatic biliary tract obstruction, specifically, cystic duct obstruction
  Procedure:
  - Intravenous radiolabeled technetium Tc99m iminodiacetic acid→
    - Hepatocyte uptake→
      - Biliary excretion→extrahepatic biliary tract visualization, w/ cystic duct obstruction indicated by the inability to visualize the gallbladder
  Limitations:
  - False positive:
    - Chronic alcoholism
    - Chronic cholecystitis
    - Prolonged fasting states
    ...→gallbladder stasis w/ ↓filling
  - False negative:
    - Acalculous cholecystitis

- **Exploratory laparotomy**
  Indications:
  - Strongly suspected intra-abdominal inflammation requiring surgical treatment, not confirmed via imaging
  Outcomes:
  - 20% of patients who undergo an exploratory laparotomy due to suspected appendicitis prove to have a normal appendix

TREATMENT

- **Nil per os—NPO**, w/ duration dependant on severity
  - Eating >> drinking→
    - ↑Peristalsis
    - ↑Digestive enzyme release
    ...→↑pain & organ destruction
- **Parenteral hyperalimentation** via a central venous line
  Indications:
  - Severe, prolonged acute pancreatitis, as ↓caloric intake→
    - Striking protein loss & catabolism
- **Intermittent nasogastric—NG suctioning**
  - Gastric acid delivery to the duodenum→
    - ↑Pancreatic exocrine secretion
  Indications:
  - As placement has not been shown to affect clinical outcome, it is reserved for patients w/ either:
    - Intractable vomiting
    - Paralytic ileus
    - Profound pain
    - Severe disease
- **Follow urine output & daily weights**
- **Intravenous fluid**, w/ attention to both:
  - Intravascular volume repletion via Normal saline (0.9% NaCl) or **lactated Ringer's solution**, as per:
    - Vital signs
    - Physical examination
    - Urine output (normal being ≥0.5mL/kg/h)
    - Blood urea nitrogen—BUN & creatinine
  - Intravascular volume maintenance via Normal saline (0.9% NaCl) or **lactated Ringer's solution**
    Adult maintenance fluid:
    - Weight (kg) + 40= #mL/ hour
    Additional febrile requirements:
    - 1L/ 24hours for every 1°F >100°F
    Additional:
    - Estimate loss for:
      - Diaphoresis
      - Diarrhea
      - Polyuria
      - Tachypnea
    ...followed by oral rehydration w/ a glucose based electrolyte solution upon both clinical stability & ability to tolerate PO

316

•**Empiric antibiotic coverage** against:
  ◦Enterobacteriaceae, esp. Escherichia coli
  ◦Anaerobes, esp. Bacteroides fragilis
  Treatment duration:
    •**Non-perforated viscous:** 3 doses
    •**Perforated viscous:** Per clinical response

CEPHALOSPORINS: 3rd-4th generation			
Generic (Trade)	M	♀	Dose
Cefotetan (Cefotan)	KB	P	2g IV q12hours
Cefoxitin (Mefoxin)	K	P	2g IV q6hours

Mechanism:
•A β-lactam ring structure which binds to bacterial transpeptidase→
  ◦↓Transpeptidase function→
    −↓Bacterial cell wall peptidoglycan cross-linking→↓cell wall synthesis→osmotic influx of extracellular fluid→↑intracellular hydrostatic pressure→cell rupture→cell death=bactericidal
•↑Bacterial autolytic enzymes→
  ◦Peptidoglycan degradation

•Certain bacteria produce β-lactamase→
  ◦Cleavage of this essential structural component of cephalosporins & certain penicillins (as the other β-lactam medications differ sufficiently to prevent ring cleavage)→
    −Antibiotic inactivation. This process may be antagonized by the concomitant administration of **β-lactamase inhibitors** (Clavulanic acid=clavulanate, Sulbactam, or Tazobactam)→renewed susceptibility

Side effects:
General
  •**Hypersensitivity reactions ≤10%**
    ◦Anaphylaxis−0.5%→
      −Death−0.002% (1:50,000)
    ◦Acute interstitial nephritis
    ◦Dermatitis
    ◦Drug fever
    ◦Hemolytic anemia
    …having cross−hypersensitivity to other β lactam medications (penicillins, carbapenems), except monobactams (ex. Aztreonam)
  Gastrointestinal
  •Clostridium dificile pseudomembraneous colitis (3rd generation > others)

&

METRONIDAZOLE (Flagyl)		
M	♀	Dose
KL	P−U in 1st trimester	500mg IV q8hours

Mechanism:
•DNA binding→
  ◦DNA strand breakage

Side effects:
General
  •**Disulfuram−like reaction to alcohol**
    ◦Avoid alcoholic beverages during, & for 48hours after completion of treatment
Gastrointestinal
  •Nausea ± vomiting−10%
  •Taste changes=dysgeusia (esp. metallic taste)
Genitourinary
  •Dark urine, being common, but harmless
Neurological
  •Peripheral neuropathy
  •Seizures
Hematologic
  •Transient neutropenia−8%

OPIOID RECEPTOR AGONISTS

Indications:
- Acute pain

Generic (Trade)	M	♀	Start
Hydromorphone (Dilaudid)	L	?	
•PO form			2mg q4hours
•SC/ IM/ IV forms			0.5mg q4hours
•PR form			3mg q6hours
Morphine sulfate	LK	?	10mg PO/ SC/ IM/ IV q4hours

- Titrate as high as necessary to relieve pain, w/ tolerable concomitant side effects

Side effects:
- **Cardiovascular**
  - Vasodilation (venous >> arterial)→
    - ↓Preload→
      - –↓Cardiac output→**hypotension**
  - **Bradycardia**
- **Gastrointestinal**
  - Central nervous system chemoreceptor trigger zone activation→
    - **Nausea ± vomiting**, exacerbated by ambulation
  - Enteric nervous system opioid receptor activation→
    - ↓Gastrointestinal smooth muscle peristalsis→
      - –**Constipation**
  - ↑Biliary tract smooth muscle contraction→
    - ∘Biliary colic
- **Genitourinary**
  - ↑Ureteral & urinary bladder smooth muscle peristalsis→
    - ∘Prostatic neoplastic syndrome exacerbation
  - ↓Uterine muscle tone→
    - ∘Labor prolongation
- **Neurologic**
  - **Altered mental status**
  - Dysphoria
  - Sedation
  - Seizures
- **Opthalmologic**
  - Iris radial smooth muscle relaxation→
    - ∘↓Pupil size=**miosis**, being fixed
- **Pulmonary**
  - Inhibition of medullary respiratory center response to CO_2 concentration→
    - **Respiratory depression**→
      - –Hypercapnic respiratory failure→altered mental status
  - ↓Cough reflex

Side effects of chronic use:
- Development of **tolerance**† to its effects, as the dosage previously sufficient to produce effects progressively fails to do so, as both the central nervous system & liver adapt to its chronic presence by altering:
  - ∘Neuronal membrane constituents
  - ∘Neurotransmitter release & re-uptake
  - ∘Hepatic clearance
  - …which set the stage for the vicious cycle of **dependence** & craving for ever increasing amounts of the medication, regardless of the professional, social, or health risks

†Tolerance does not develop to:
- Constipation
- Miosis
- Seizures

318

ANTIDOTE

Generic (Trade)	M	♀	Start	Max
Naloxone (Narcan)	LK	P	2mg IV/ SC/ IM/ ET q2min. prn	10mg total

Mechanism:
- •µ receptor antagonist, which, in the absence of exogenous opioids, have no clinical effect

Duration:
- •1−2hours

Side effects:
- •**Acute opioid withdrawal/ reversal syndrome**
  - ∘Diaphoresis
  - ∘Goose flesh
  - ∘↑Lacrimation
  - ∘Nausea ± vomiting
  - ∘Rhinorrhea
  - ∘Tachypnea
  - …w/ rare:
    - •Hypo or hypertension
    - •Pulmonary edema
    - •Ventricular tachycardia &/or fibrillation

ANTIEMETIC MEDICATIONS

Generic	M	♀	Start	Max
Prochlorperazine (Compazine)	LK	?	5mg PO/ IM/ IV q8hours	10mg q6hours
•PR form			25mg PR q12hours	
•XR form			15mg PO q24hours	30mg q24hours
Promethazine (Phenergan)	LK	?	12.5mg PO/ IM/ PR/ IV q6hours	25mg q4hours
Thiethylperazine (Torecan)	L	?	10mg PO/ IM q24hours	10mg q8hours
Trimethobenzamide (Tigan)	LK	?	200mg PO/ IM/ PR q6hours	

Prochlorperazine specific side effects:
- **Cardiovascular**
  - •Dysrhythmias
  - •Hypotension w/ IV administration
- **Mucocutaneous**
  - •Gynecomastia, being the ↑development of male mammary glands
- **Neurologic**
  - •Anticholinergic effects
  - •Extrapyramidal dysfunction
  - •Sedation
  - •Seizures
- **Hematologic**
  - •Leukopenia
  - •Thrombocytopenia

Promethazine specific side effects:
- **Cardiovascular**
  - •Hypotension w/ IV administration
- **Neurologic**
  - •Anticholinergic effects
  - •Extrapyramidal dysfunction
  - •Sedation

Trimethobenzamde specific side effects:
- **Neurologic**
  - •Sedation

319

•Appendicitis
- ∘0.2–2% mortality, esp. if:
  - −Age >60years
  - −During pregnancy, having a fetal mortality of 8% w/ uncomplicated appendicitis, & 25% w/ perforation
- Indications for surgical resection:
  - **•All cases of acute appendicitis, on an emergent basis**
- Statistics:
  - •>250,000 appendectomies are performed in the U.S. each year, making it the #1 abdominal operation performed on an emergent basis

•Diverticulitis
- ∘85% resolve spontaneously, w/ surgical resection being ultimately indicated in 15% of patients
- Indications for hemicolectomy:
  - **•Elective:**
    - ∘Recurrent attacks
    - ∘Fistula formation
    - ∘Pericolic abscess formation
    - ...preferably after any inflammation resolves (usually @ 6weeks), as it obscures the anatomic landmarks, thereby ↑the risk of surgical injury
  - **•Emergent:**
    - ∘Acute clinical deterioration
    - ∘Generalized peritonitis
    - ∘Uncontrolled sepsis
    - ∘Visceral perforation

•Cholelithiasis
- ∘**Asymptomatic:** 70% of patients w/ gallstones ultimately become symptomatic via either:
  - −Biliary colic
  - −Cholecystitis−35% of patients w/ cholelithiasis
  - −Hepatitis
  - −Pancreatitis
  - −Ascending cholangitis
  - Indications for prophylactic cholecystectomy:
    - •Choledocholithiasis, after ERCP mediated gallstone extraction
    - •Patients thought to be at ↑risk for the development of gallbladder cancer:
      - ∘Calcified gallbladder
      - ∘Gallstone > 2.5cm diameter
      - ∘Gallbladder polyp >10mm diameter
      - ∘Pima Indians
- ∘**Symptomatic:**
  - −Biliary colic, having a 45%/ year recurrence rate, w/ a 1.5%/ year risk of an inflammatory complication (cholecystitis, hepatitis, pancreatitis, or ascending cholangitis)
  - Indications for cholecystectomy:
    - •**All cases of symptomatic cholelithiasis**, preferably after any inflammation resolves (usually @ 6weeks), as it obscures the anatomic landmarks, thereby ↑the risk of surgical injury to the:
      - ∘Extrahepatic biliary system (hepatic & common bile ducts)
      - ∘Hepatobiliary vasculature
    - •**Emergent:**
      - ∘Choledocholithiasis, after ERCP mediated gallstone extraction

•Cholecystitis
- ∘85% resolve spontaneously
- Indications for cholecystectomy:
  - •**All cases of symptomatic cholelithiasis**, preferably after any inflammation resolves (usually @ 6weeks), as it obscures the anatomic landmarks, thereby ↑the risk of surgical injury to the:
    - ∘Extrahepatic biliary system (hepatic & common bile ducts)
    - ∘Hepatobiliary vasculature
  - •**Emergent:**
    - ∘Choledocholithiasis, after ERCP mediated gallstone extraction
    - ∘Acute clinical deterioration
    - ∘Generalized peritonitis
    - ∘Uncontrolled sepsis
    - ∘Visceral perforation

320

•Any disease→
 ○↑Portal venous system intravascular pressure (normal: 5–10mmHg)

CLASSIFICATION/ RISK FACTORS
•Pre–hepatic etiology
 ○Portal vein obstruction
  –Thrombosis
  –Tumor mediated compression
 ○↑Portal blood flow
  –Arteriovenous fistula
  –Massive splenomegally

•Intra–hepatic etiology
 ○Hepatic fibrosis, termed **cirrhosis, being the #1 cause of portal hypertension**
  –Ethanol
  –Infection: Hepatitis B ± D virus(es), Hepatitis C virus, Schistosoma mansoni
  –Autoimmune: Autoimmune hepatitis, Primary biliary cirrhosis, Sclerosing cholangitis
  –Genetic: α1–antitrypsin deficiency, Hemochromatosis, Wilson's disease
  –Sarcoidosis
  –Idiopathic

•Post–hepatic etiology
 ○Hepatic vein obstruction–rare
  –Thrombosis
  –Tumor mediated compression
  ...→Budd–Chiari syndrome, being hepatomegally, ascites, & abdominal pain
 ○Heart failure
  –Hepatic congestion→hepatitis, which, if chronic→cirrhosis, termed cardiac cirrhosis

---

•Unlike pre–hepatic & intra–hepatic, **post–hepatic etiologies usually do not cause splenomegaly**

DIAGNOSIS
Cardiovascular
•Congestive portal venous pressure→
 ○Blood flow redirected through portal–systemic anastomoses→
  –Gastroesophageal varices, occurring in 50% of persons w/ cirrhosis
   Pathophysiology:
    •Left & right gastric venous congestion→esophageal venous congestion (which drain into the
     systemic azygous veins)→
     ○Gastroesophageal venous distention. Being that the veins are thin walled & poorly
      supported by the connective tissue of the submucosa, they commonly rupture→
      –Upper gastrointestinal hemorrhage
  –Rectal varices=hemorrhoids
   Pathophysiology:
    •Superior rectal venous congestion→
     ○Middle & inferior rectal venous congestion→
      –Internal & external hemorrhoids respectively
  –Abdominal subcutaneous varices
   Pathophysiology:
    •Paraumbilical venous congestion→
     ○Superficial & inferior radical epigastric venous congestion→
      –Periumbilical venous distention, w/ **blood flowing radially from the umbilicus** like the
       spokes of a wheel, being termed **caput Medusae†**, which when large→a vascular bruit,
       termed the Cruveilhier–Baumgarten syndrome
  –Retroperitoneal varices
   Pathophysiology:
    •Colon, renal, adrenal, & gonadal venous twig congestion→
     ○Retroperitoneal venous congestion
 ○Splenic venous congestion→enlarged, engorged spleen=**splenomegally‡**→cellular
  sequestration→pancytopenia, w/ the process termed hypersplenism→
   –Normocytic, normochromic anemia→fatigue
   –Leukopenia→immunosuppression→↑infection & neoplasm risk
   –Thrombocytopenia→↑hemorrhage risk, esp. petechiae

---

†Symbolizing the resemblance to the winding snakes comprising the hair of the Greek goddess Medusa

‡Degree not correlating w/ portal hypertension severity

CURATIVE INTENT TREATMENT

•**Liver transplantation**
  Indications:
    •Liver failure via either:
      ∘Fulminant hepatitis
      ∘Chronic disease→cirrhosis→portal hypertension syndrome→
        −Recurrent gastroesophageal variceal hemorrhage
        −Refractory ascites
        −Recurrent &/or severe encephalopathy
        −Spontaneous bacterial peritonitis−SBP
        −Hepatorenal syndrome
        −Total bilirubin >10mg/ dL
        −Plasma albumin <3g/ dL
        −Prothrombin time−PT prolonged >3seconds
    •Early stage hepatocellular cancer−HCC
  Outcomes:
    •Max 1 year survival: 90%
    •Max 5 year survival: 80%
  Contraindications:
    •Active substance abuse
    •Extrahepatic malignancy
    •HIV infection
    •Sepsis
    •Severe comorbidity

322

•As for gastroesophageal hemorrhage (see section) as well as:
•Stat gastrointestinal consult for **urgent esophagogastroduodenoscopy–EGD**

SOMATOSTATIN ANALOGUE			
Generic (Trade)	M ♀	Dose	
Octreotide (Sandostatin)	LK P	50µg IV push, then 50µg/ hour IV infusion X 5days	

Mechanism:
•↓Secretion of vasodilatory hormones (ex. glucagon)→splanchnic vasoconstriction→↓splanchnic blood flow→
  ∘↓Portal venous pressure→
    –↓Intravariceal pressure→↓hemorrhage risk

Outcomes:
•↓Rebleeding rate, but no mortality benefit

Side effects:
Cardiovascular
  •Dysrhythmias, esp. bradycardia
Endocrine
  •Hypothyroidism
Gastrointestinal
  •Abdominal cramping
Hematologic
  •Hypo or hyperglycemia

OR THE COMBINATION OF

VASOCONSTRICTING MEDICATIONS				
Generic	M ♀	Start	Titrate	Max
Vasopressin†	LK ?	0.4 units/ min. IV infusion	q30min. until hemorrhage stops	0.9 units/ min.

†Also known as Antidiuretic hormone–ADH

Mechanism:
•Splanchnic arteriole vasoconstriction→
  ∘↓Splanchnic blood flow→
    –↓Portal venous pressure→↓intravariceal pressure→↓hemorrhage risk

Outcomes:
•↓Rebleeding rate, but no mortality benefit

Side effects:
Cardiovascular
•Myocardial & intestinal ischemia ± infarction

&

NITROVASODILATORS: Long acting			
Generic	M ♀	Start	Max
Isosorbide dinitrate (Isordil, Sorbitrate)	L ?	5–20mg PO q8hours	40mg PO q8hours
•XR form (Isordil Tembids, Dilatrate SR)		40mg PO q12hours	80mg PO q12hours
Isosorbide mononitrate (ISMO, Monoket)	L ?	20mg PO q12hours	40mg PO bid
•XR form (Imdur)		30mg PO q24hours	240mg q24hours
Nitroglycerin–transdermal	L ?	Lowest dose, applied to non–hairy skin for 14hours/ day	

Trade	Available doses (mg/ hour)
Deponit	0.2, 0.4
Minitran	0.1, 0.2, 0.4, 0.6
Nitrodisc	0.2, 0.3, 0.4
Nitro–Dur	0.1, 0.2, 0.3, 0.4, 0.6, 0.8
Transderm–Nitro	0.1, 0.2, 0.4, 0.6, 0.8

Mechanism:
•Vasodilation (**venous** > arterial)→
  ∘↓Vasopressin mediated myocardial & intestinal ischemia ± infarction risk
  ∘↓Preload→
    –↓Myocardial contractile strength→↓O_2 & nutrient demand
  ∘↑Coronary artery dilation→↑perfusion
  ∘↓Intrahepatic vascular resistance

INVASIVE PROCEDURES_____
•**Esophagogastroduodenoscopy–EGD**
  Indications:
  •Therapeutic/ prophylactic, as it allows for:
    ∘**Sclerotherapy,** via a sclerosing agent (ethanol, morrhuate sodium, polidocanol, or sodium tetradecyl sulfate) being injected into varices
    ∘**Band ligation,** via small rubber bands being placed around varices
  Findings:
  •Varices ↑in size during inspiration
  Limitations:
  •Gastric varices are located deeper in the submucosa than esophageal varices→
    ∘↓Sclerotherapy & bind ligation efficacy. However, tissue glue (being composed of N−butyl−2−cyanocrylate) injection has been shown to be effective treatment & prophylaxis
  Outcomes:
  •When compared w/ sclerotherapy, bind ligation→
    ∘↓Complications:
    −Perforation
    −Ulceration
    −Stricture formation
    ∘↓Recurrent hemorrhage risk
    ∘↑Survival rate
    ∘↓Cost

324

ANTIBACTERIAL PROPHYLAXIS

- •50% of patients w/ advanced liver disease (Childs–Pugh class C) develop an infection (usually due to enterobacteriaceae) such as:
  - ∘Spontaneous bacterial peritonitis–SBP
  - ∘Sepsis
  - …within 48hours after an acute gastrointestinal hemorrhage, X 1week

FLUOROQUINOLONES			
Generic (Trade)	M	♀	Dose
Gatifloxacin (Tequin)	K	?	400mg PO/ IV q24hours
Levofloxacin (Levaquin)	KL	?	500mg PO/ IV q24hours
Moxifloxacin (Avelox)	LK	?	400mg PO/ IV q24hours

Mechanism:
- •↓DNA gyrase=topoisomerase action→
  - ∘↓Bacterial DNA synthesis

Side effects:
General
- •Hypersensitivity reactions

Gastrointestinal
- •Gastroenteritis→
  - ∘Diarrhea
  - ∘Nausea ± vomiting

Mucocutaneous
- •Phototoxicity

Neurologic
- •Dizziness
- •Drowsiness
- •Headache
- •Restlessness

Materno–fetal
- •Fetal & child tendon malformation (including breast fed)→
  - ∘↑Tendon rupture risk

REFRACTORY HEMORRHAGE–10%
- •**Gastroesophageal tamponade**
  Procedure:
  - •Placement of a specialized nasogastric tube (Sengstaken–Blakemore or Minnesota tube) containing both a gastric & esophageal balloon. The gastric balloon is inflated first to ~1kg of tension w/ 1L of water or normal saline. If hemorrhage continues, the esophageal balloon is inflated to a maximal pressure of 40mmHg for ≤36hours, being used as a temporizing measure, as hemorrhage often recurs after balloon decompression

  Complications:
  - •Airway obstruction due to misplaced tube, which is why endotracheal intubation is recommended prior to tube insertion
  - •Aspiration
  - •Esophageal tamponade→
    - ∘Ischemia, which if severe or prolonged→
      - –**Esophageal necrosis &/or perforation**

  …being followed by either:
  - •**Transjugular intra–hepatic portosystemic shunt–TIPS**
    Procedure:
    - •An expandable metal stent is placed between a hepatic vein & a major intra–hepatic branch of a portal vein, via angiographic catheterization

    Outcomes:
    - •Mortality in patients w/ advanced liver disease (Childs–Pugh class C) is ~100% within 1month

    Side effects:
    - •**Hepatic encephalopathy–25%**
    - •Infection
    - •Shunt stenosis
      - ∘30% @ 1year
      - ∘50% @ 2years
      - …requiring either balloon dilation or stent replacement

- **Other portal-systemic shunt**
  Indications:
  - If TIPS is either not available or technically feasible
  Types:
  - Distal splenorenal shunt
  - Mesocaval shunt
  - Portocaval shunt
- **Esophageal staple transection ± esophagogastric devascularization**
  Indications:
  - If TIPS is either not available or technically feasible
  Outcomes:
  - Mortality in patients w/ advanced liver disease (Childs-Pugh class C) is 80% within 1month

PROGNOSIS
- 50% of patients w/ cirrhosis develop gastroesophageal varices, 30% of which experience hemorrhage, comprising 85% of hemorrhagic episodes in these patients→
  - 20% mortality @ 1st hemorrhage
  - 50% of survivors rebleeding within 6months (usually within 6weeks)
  - Overall 35% mortality, being the **#1 cause of death in patients w/ cirrhosis**

PROPHYLAXIS
- **Esophagogastroduodenoscopy-EGD**
  Indications:
  - To screen for the presence of gastroesophageal varices in patients w/ cirrhosis, as it allows for:
    - **Sclerotherapy**, via a sclerosing agent (ethanol, morrhuate sodium, polidocanol, or sodium tetradecyl sulfate) being injected into varices
    - **Band ligation**, via small rubber bands being placed around varices
  Findings:
  - Varices ↑in size during inspiration
  Limitations:
  - Gastric varices are located deeper in the submucosa than esophageal varices→
    - ↓Sclerotherapy & bind ligation efficacy. However, tissue glue (being composed of N-butyl-2-cyanocrylate) injection has been shown to be effective prophylaxis
  Outcomes:
  - When compared w/ sclerotherapy, bind ligation→
    - ↓Complications:
      - -Perforation
      - -Ulceration
      - -Stricture formation
    - ↓Recurrent hemorrhage risk
    - ↑Survival rate
    - ↓Cost

- ↓Hepatic portal venous flow→
  - Compensatory ↑hepatic arterial flow, in order to maintain total hepatic flow near normal, thereby causing the liver to become more dependent upon arterial flow. Patients w/ advanced cirrhosis (Child-Pugh class C) will often not be able to compensate for the pharmacologic prophylaxis induced ↓arterial flow, making optimal treatment unclear

NONSELECTIVE β RECEPTOR BLOCKERS				
Generic (Trade)	M	♀	**Start**	**Max**
Nadolol (Corgard)	K	?	40mg PO q24hours	160mg q24hours
Propranolol (Inderal)	L	?	20mg PO q12hours	180 q12hours
α1 & NONSELECTIVE β RECEPTOR BLOCKERS				
Generic (Trade)	M	♀	**Start**	**Max**
Carvedilol (Coreg)	L	?	6.25mg PO q12hours	25mg q12hours
Labetalol (Normodyne)	LK	?	100mg PO q12hours	1200mg q12hours

Goal titration:
- To a pulse of 55bpm or 25% below baseline

Mechanism:
- Competitive antagonist of the β1 ± β2 receptor→
  - ↓Sinoatrial & atrioventricular node conduction (β1)→
    - -↓Pulse
  - Anti-dysrhythmic via nodal effects (β1)
  - ↓Cardiac muscle contractile strength (β1)

326

- ∘↓Juxtaglomerular cell renin release (β1)→
  - −↓Angiotensin 1, angiotensin 2, & aldosterone formation
- ∘↓Cardiovascular remodeling
- ∘↑Vascular/ organ smooth muscle contraction (β2)→
  - −Vasoconstriction→↓splanchnic blood flow→↓portal venous pressure→↓intravariceal pressure→ ↓hemorrhage risk
  - −Bronchoconstriction
  - −Uterine contraction
- ∘↓Tremor (β2)
- ∘↓Hepatocyte glycogenolysis (β2)
- •↓Extrathyroidal tetraiodothyronine−T4 (also termed thyroxine) conversion to the more metabolically active triiodothyronine−T3 form

Outcomes:
- •45%↓in primary variceal hemorrhage risk

Side effects:
General
- •Fatigue
- •Malaise

Cardiovascular
- •Bradycardia ± heart block
- •Hypotension
  - ∘Orthostatic hypotension
  - ∘Pelvic hypotension→
    - −Impotence, being the inability to achieve &/or maintain an erection
- •Initial worsening of systolic heart failure
- •Worsening symptoms of peripheral vascular disease
  - ∘Intermittent claudication
  - ∘Raynaud's phenomenon

Pulmonary
- •Bronchoconstriction

Endocrine
- •↑Risk of developing diabetes mellitus
- •May block catecholamine mediated:
  - ∘Physiologic reversal of hypoglycemia via:
    - −↓Hepatocyte gluconeogenesis
  - ∘↓Hypoglycemic symptoms, termed hypoglycemic unawareness→
    - −↓Tachycardia as a warning sign

Gastrointestinal
- •Diarrhea
- •Nausea ± vomiting
- •Gastroesophageal reflux

Mucocutaneous
- •Hair thinning

Neurologic
- •Sedation
- •Sleep alterations
- •↓Libido→
  - ∘Impotence

Psychiatric
- •Depression

Hematologic
- •↓High density lipoprotein−HDL levels

•Most patients w/ chronic obstructive pulmonary disease−COPD (including asthma), diabetes, &/or peripheral vascular disease can be safely treated w/ **cardioselective β1 receptor blockers**, as they have ↓peripheral effects

Contraindications:
Cardiovascular
- •**Acutely decompensated heart failure**
- •Hypotension
- •Pulse <50bpm
- •Atrioventricular heart block of any degree

Pulmonary
- •Moderate to severe chronic obstructive pulmonary disease−COPD, including asthma

Hyper-catacholamine state
- •Amphetamine use
- •**Cocaine use†**
- •Clonidine withdrawal
- •Monoamine oxidase inhibitor-MAOi mediated tyramine effect
- •Pheochromocytoma
- ...→relatively ↑vascular α1 receptor stimulation="unopposed α effect"→
  - •Vasoconstriction→
    - ∘Myocardial ischemic syndrome
    - ∘Cerebrovascular accident syndrome
    - ∘Peripheral vascular ischemic syndrome
- <u>Note</u>: **Carvedilol** & **Labetalol** may be used due to their α1 blocking property

---

†Cocaine use→
- •Varying ischemic syndrome onset per administration route, & may occur @ min. to days (usually within 3hours)

NITROVASODILATORS: Long acting

Generic	M ♀	Start	Max
Isosorbide dinitrate (Isordil, Sorbitrate)	L ?	5-20mg PO q8hours	40mg PO q8hours
•XR form (Isordil Tembids, Dilatrate SR)		40mg PO q12hours	80mg PO q12hours
Isosorbide mononitrate (ISMO, Monoket)	L ?	20mg PO q12hours	40mg PO bid
•XR form (Imdur)		30mg PO q24hours	240mg q24hours
Nitroglycerin-transdermal	L ?	Lowest dose, applied to non-hairy skin for 14hours/ day	

Trade	Available doses (mg/ hour)
Deponit	0.2, 0.4
Minitran	0.1, 0.2, 0.4, 0.6
Nitrodisc	0.2, 0.3, 0.4
Nitro-Dur	0.1, 0.2, 0.3, 0.4, 0.6, 0.8
Transderm-Nitro	0.1, 0.2, 0.4, 0.6, 0.8

SECOND LINE PROPHYLAXIS ▬▬▬▬▬
•**Transjugular intra-hepatic portosystemic shunt-TIPS**
  <u>Procedure:</u>
  - •An expandable metal stent is placed between a hepatic vein & a major intra-hepatic branch of a portal vein, via angiographic catheterization
  <u>Outcomes:</u>
  - •Mortality in patients w/ advanced liver disease (Childs-Pugh class C) is ~100% within 1month
  <u>Side effects:</u>
  - •**Hepatic encephalopathy-25%**
  - •Infection
  - •Shunt stenosis
    - ∘30% @ 1year
    - ∘50% @ 2years
    - ...requiring either balloon dilation or stent replacement

•**Other portal-systemic shunt**
  <u>Indications:</u>
  - •If TIPS is either not available or technically feasible
  <u>Types:</u>
  - •Distal splenorenal shunt
  - •Mesocaval shunt
  - •Portocaval shunt

THIRD LINE PROPHYLAXIS ▬▬▬▬▬
•**Esophageal staple transection ± esophagogastric devascularization**
  <u>Indications:</u>
  - •If TIPS is either not available or technically feasible
  <u>Outcomes:</u>
  - •Mortality in patients w/ advanced liver disease (Childs-Pugh class C) is 80% within 1month

ASCITES
•50% of patients w/ cirrhosis develop a peritoneal effusion=ascites within 10years→
  ○50% mortality within 2years

PATHOPHYSIOLOGY
•**Intra-hepatic or post-hepatic etiologies of portal hypertension†**
Mechanism:
  •↑Hepatic sinusoid intravascular pressure→
  ○↑Hepatic interstitial fluid→
    −Transudative effusion into the peritoneal cavity=**ascites**

•↓**Systemic intravascular osmotic pressure**
  ○Liver cirrhosis
  ○Malnutrition
  ○Nephrotic syndrome
  ...→↓plasma albumin→
    •↓Intravascular osmotic pressure→systemic fluid transudation→
      ○Interstitial edema→
        −↑Weight (1L fluid=1kg=2.2 lbs)
        −**Pitting edema**, requiring ≥3L of fluid, usually beginning in the most dependent body part
        (feet & ankles=pedal edema &/or sacral edema in bed−bound patients)→eventual
        generalized edema=**anasarca**
      ○Transudative peritoneal, pleural, pericardial, & synovial effusions

---

†Being that most ascitic fluid originates from the hepatic sinusoids, rarely are pre−hepatic etiologies of
portal hypertension responsible for its onset

DIAGNOSIS
Gastrointestinal
  •Congested gastrointestinal vasculature→
    ○↓Nutrient absorption→
      −↓Dry weight (careful, as weight loss may be offset by fluid gain)
  •Ascites→
    ○**Abdominal distention**
    ○**Bulging of the flanks**
    ○**Fluid wave**
    Examination:
      •W/ the patient lying supine, have the patient or an assistant, wedge the ulnar surface of their
      hand (being parallel to the axis of the patient) over the umbilicus, & into the abdomen. Then
      place your hands on the bilateral flank areas, using 1 hand to thump the flesh, & the other to
      palpate for a possible fluid wave crashing against the contralateral peritoneal wall→
        ○Light thump. Then repeat w/ subsequent reversal of roles
    Outcomes:
      •Sensitivity: 55%, specificity: 90%

    ○**Shifting dullness**
    Examination:
      •W/ the patient lying supine, percuss the abdomen circumferentially, from the periumbilical area,
      down the flanks, & mark the point @ which the note becomes dull, if found. If the dullness is due
      to fluid, you should be able to percuss a line of dullness parallel to the floor, being equal in
      height on both flanks. Then have the patient roll towards either side & repeat the percussion
      maneuver. If dullness is percussed above the previously drawn line, then fluid has accumulated
      toward the dependent side, thus proving the presence of ascites
    Outcomes:
      •Sensitivity: 90%, specificity: 55%

Genitourinary
- ↓Intravascular volume→↓arterial perfusion→
  - **Pre-renal renal failure**
  - Reflex ↑autonomic sympathetic tone
  - ...→↑juxtaglomerular cell renin release→
    - ↑Angiotensin 2 formation→
      - Efferent glomerular arteriole constriction→
        - ↑Glomerular filtrate→↓distal peritubular capillary hydrostatic pressure & osmolarity→
          ↑NaCl & water reabsorption
      - ↑Adrenal cortical aldosterone release→
        - Distal convoluted tubule NaCl & water reabsorption
      - ↑Posterior pituitary antidiuretic hormone–ADH release→
        - ↑Late distal convoluted tubule & collecting duct H_2O reabsorption→**hypervolemic hyponatremia**
      - ...→circulatory congestion (extracellular volume may ↑>200%) & ↑peripheral vascular resistance→
        - ↑Afterload
- Supine position→
  - ↓Systemic venous hydrostatic pressure→
    - ↑Venous return
    - Osmosis of interstitial edematous fluid to the intravascular space→↑venous return
    - ...→↑intravascular volume→
      - ↑Renal perfusion→
        - Nocturnal diuresis=**nocturia**

IMAGING

•Abdomino-pelvic ultrasound w/ doppler
Indications:
- Used to visualize:
  - Ascitic fluid, requiring ≥100mL of peritoneal fluid
  - Possible loculations
  - The peritoneum
  - The hepatic & splenic parenchyma
  - Biliary ductal size
- Doppler ultrasonography uses Doppler shift to detect vessel flow velocity→
  - Visualization of vasculature (portal, hepatic, & splenic veins) patency & flow

---

INVASIVE PROCEDURES

•Diagnostic paracentesis
- May require ultrasound guidance if mild
- Procedure is safe in coagulopathic patients
Complications–1%:
- Hematoma
- Hemoperitoneum
- Infection
- Intestinal perforation
Lab studies:
- **Tube 1:** Albumin, total protein, lactate dehydrogenase–LDH, & glucose
  - Send plasma samples for comparative analysis
- **Tube 2:** Cell count & differential
- **Tube 3:** Gram stain & culture (bacterial, fungal, & mycobacterial)
- **Tube 4:** Other studies as clinically indicated
- **Arterial blood gas tube:** pH

330

ASCITIC FLUID STUDIES

Studies	Transudate†	Exudate
Gross appearance	Serous=clear straw colored	•**Serous**=clear straw colored •**Turbid:** Leukocytes, lipid, organisms •**Purulent:** Empyema •**Bloody:** Malignancy, endometriosis, pancreatitis, mycobacterial infection, trauma (including traumatic tap), coagulopathy, perforated viscous, hepatic/ mesenteric thrombosis, mesenteric cyst, aortic dissection, leaking aortic aneurysm •**Milky=chylothorax:** Lymphatic obstruction vs. perforation
Smell	None	Foul odor=anaerobic infection
Protein level (1–1.5g/dL)	<3g/ dL (CHF may ≥3g/ dL)	≥3g/ dL
Peritoneal/ plasma protein level	<0.50=50%	≥0.50=50%‡
LDH level	<200 IU	**≥200 IU or ≥2/3rds upper normal plasma limit‡**
Pleural/ plasma LDH level	<0.60=60%	≥0.60=60%‡
Plasma–effusion albumin	>1.1	≤1.1
Cholesterol	<45mg/ dL	>55mg/ dL
Glucose level	Same as serum	<60mg/ dL <20mg/ dL: Empyema or rheumatoid arthritis
Leukocytes	<250/ µL	**>300/ µL°** >30,000/ µL: Empyema
Differential	Mononuclear predominant	•**Mononuclear^:** Malignancy, mycobacterial or fungal infections, rheumatoid arthritis, vasculitides •**Eosinophils >10%:** Eosinophilic enteritis •**Neutrophil predominant:** All others
Erythrocytes (0–5/µL)	<1,000/ µL	≥1000/ µL >50% plasma hematocrit: hemoperitoneum
Amylase	60–130 U/ L	>2X plasma level: Pancreatitis, malignancy
pH	7.38–7.44	<7.35 **<7.2: Empyema**
Adenosine deaminase–ADA		Positive in granulomatous disease >70: Possible mycobacterial infection <40: Excludes mycobacterial infection
Fibrinogen	Negative	Positive
Specific gravity	<1.016	≥1.016
Triglyceride		>110mg/ dL: Chylous ascites
Sudan III staining	Negative	Positive: Chylous ascites
Microscopy	–	•AFB stain positive: Mycobacterial infection •Cytology positive: Malignancy 　○Sensitivity: 60–90% •Gram stain positive: Bacterial
Culture (aerobic & anaerobic)	Negative	±
CEA		•>10mg/ mL: Malignant effusion 　○Sensitivity: 50%
Ascites/ plasma CEA		•>2: Malignant effusion 　○Sensitivity: 50%

†Consider transudative values to be normal
‡The presence of any of these, termed **Light's criteria**, indicate an exudative effusion
°To correct for the neutrophil count in a traumatic tap, subtract 1 neutrophil for every 250 erythrocytes
^Lymphocyte & monocyte

•Treat the underlying liver disease if possible
•**Daily weights** to monitor for fluid retention (edema &/or effusion)→
  ◦↑Weight (1L fluid=1kg=2.2 lbs)
•↓**Sodium intake**
  ◦≤100mmol sodium/ 24h=2g elemental sodium or 6g salt/ 24h, which can usually be achieved w/ a
  no–added salt diet. Patients w/ poorly compensated portal failure should only consume 0.5–1g
  elemental sodium or 1.5–3g salt/ 24h
  ◦→↓Renal potassium loss if taking a diuretic
•**Fluid restriction**
  ◦Patients w/ poorly compensated portal failure should restrict fluid intake to ≤1.5L/ 24h (~6 cups)
  Guide:
    •1oz = 30mL
    •1cup = 8oz = 240mL
    •4cups = 32oz = ~1L
•**Medication caution**
  ◦**Nonsteroidal anti–inflamatory drugs–NSAIDs,** including Aspirin
  ◦**Angiotensin converting enzyme inhibitors** or **angiotensin 2 receptor blockers**
  Mechanism:
    •Patients w/ pre–existing bilateral ↓renal perfusion, not necessarily failure:
    ◦Heart failure
    ◦Bilateral renal artery stenosis
    ◦Hypovolemia
    ◦Renal failure
    ...rely more on the compensatory production of:
      •Prostaglandin→
        ◦Afferent arteriole dilation→maintained glomerular filtration rate, whereas NSAIDs→
        –↓Prostaglandin production→pre–renal renal failure
      •Angiotensin 2→
        ◦Efferent arteriole constriction→maintained glomerular filtration rate, whereas either:
        –Angiotensin converting enzyme inhibition
        –Angiotensin 2 receptor blockade
        ...→↓angiotensin 2 production & action respectively→
          •Pre–renal renal failure
•**Diuretic treatment**
  Titration:
    •Diurese 1L/ day (1L fluid=1kg=2.2 lbs) during decompensated portal failure, as this is the usual
    maximum that the body can reabsorb from the interstitial tissue
  Outcomes:
    •Diuretic treatment is effective in 80% of patients
  Contraindications:
    •Pre–renal renal failure
    •Hepatic encephalopathy
    •Lack of weight loss despite maximal combination diuretic treatment

POTASSIUM SPARING DIURETICS: ↓Potassium & magnesium loss when used in combination w/ other diuretic types				
Generic (Trade)	M	♀	Start	Max
Spironolactone (Aldactone)	LK	U	100mg PO q24hours	400mg q24hours
Duration: 24–72hours				

Titration:
•Based on plasma potassium •A urinary sodium/ potassium ratio >1 indicates effective aldosterone antagonism

Mechanism:
•Structurally similar to aldosterone→
  ◦Competitive inhibition of the intracellular aldosterone receptor in the distal convoluted
  tubule & collecting duct→
    –↑Urination→↓intravascular volume→↓cardiac preload→↓cardiac output→↓blood pressure, w/
    eventual compensatory intravascular volume repletion to near pre–treatment levels, but w/
    peripheral vascular resistance falling below pre–treatment baseline being responsible for the
    chronic hypotensive effect

Side effects:
  Endocrine
    •Anti–androgenic effects→
      ◦**Gynecomastia**, being the ↑development of male mammary glands

Hematologic
- Acid base disturbances
  - Non–anion gap hypochloremic metabolic acidemia
- Electrolyte disturbances
  - **Hyperkalemia**
  - Hyponatremia
- **Hyperuricemia**

Monitoring:
- Monitor creatinine & potassium @ baseline, then
  - @ 1week, then
  - @ 1, 2, & 3months, then
  - Q3months for the remainder of the 1st year, then
  - Q6months thereafter

Contraindications:
- Potassium >5 mEq/ L

LOOP DIURETICS

Generic (Trade)	M	♀	Start	Max
Furosemide (Lasix)	K	?	20mg q24–12hours PO	600mg/ 24hours

Onset: 1hour, Duration: 6hours (Lasix lasts **six** hours)

- There is synergistic efficacy of combination treatment w/ a thiazide diuretic
- Administer 2nd dose in the mid–afternoon to avoid nocturia

Mechanism:
- Inhibits $Na^+/K^+/2Cl^-$ reabsorption in the thick ascending limb of the loop of Henle→
  - ↑Urination→
    - –↓Intravascular volume→↓cardiac preload→↓cardiac output→eventual compensatory intravascular volume repletion to near pre–treatment levels, but w/ peripheral vascular resistance falling below pre–treatment baseline being responsible for the chronic hypotensive effect

Limitations:
- ↓Efficacy in patients w/ a glomerular filtration rate <10mL/ min.

Side effects:
Genitourinary
- Acute interstitial nephritis

Neurologic
- **Ototoxicity**

Hematologic
- Acid base disturbances
  - Hypochloremic metabolic alkalemia
- Dyslipidemia
  - ↑Cholesterol & triglycerides
- Electrolyte disturbances
  - **Hypokalemia**
  - Hypomagnesemia
  - Hyponatremia
  - Hypercalcemia
- Hyperglycemia
- Hyperuricemia

Contraindications:
- **Sulfa allergy**, as all thiazide & loop diuretics (except Ethacrynic acid) contain a sulfa component

REFRACTORY ASCITES

•Being defined as urinary 24hour sodium excretion ≤10meq despite both:
  ∘Maximal combination diuretic treatment
  ∘Fluid & sodium restriction
  ...indicating ascites so severe, that the treatment required to produce adequate diuresis→
    ∘Hypovolemia→
      –Pre-renal renal failure

•**Therapeutic paracentesis**
  Indications:
    •Abdominal discomfort
    •Dyspnea
    •Early satiety
    •Refractory ascites
    •Tense ascites
  Procedure:
    •Remove 4–6L of fluid (over 30–90min.) ± albumin replacement IV
  Outcomes of albumin addition:
    •↓Asymptomatic chemical abnormalities. No mortality effect

•**Transjugular intra-hepatic portosystemic shunt–TIPS**
  Procedure:
    •An expandable metal stent is placed between a hepatic vein & a major intra-hepatic branch of
     a portal vein, via angiographic catheterization
  Outcomes:
    •Mortality in patients w/ advanced liver disease (Childs–Pugh class C) is ~100% within 1month
  Side effects:
    •**Hepatic encephalopathy–25%**
    •Infection
    •Shunt stenosis
      ∘30% @ 1year
      ∘50% @ 2years
      ...requiring either balloon dilation or stent replacement

•**Peritoneojugular shunt, termed the Le Veen shunt**
  Mechanism:
    •A subcutaneous tube, equipped w/ a one-way pressure valve, redirects ascites from the peritoneal
     cavity to the jugular vein or right atrium when the intra-abdominal pressure exceeds venous
     pressure
  Side effects:
    •Heart failure–3%
    •Disseminated intravascular coagulation–65%
      ∘Symptomatic–25%
      ∘Severe–5%
    •Infection–6%
    •Shunt stenosis w/ blood &/or debris
    •Variceal hemorrhage from acute intravascular volume expansion

334

SPONTANEOUS BACTERIAL PERITONITIS–SBP

•Any disease→↑peri–intestinal interstitial fluid→↓immune mediated defense→
∘↑**Bacterial transcolonic migration**→
  –Bacterial peritonitis not due to existing intra–abdominal inflammation (ex. appendicitis, cholecystitis, diverticulitis)
Statistics:
  •Occurs in 20% of cirrhotic patients

ORGANISMS

•**Enterobacteriaceae–70%**
  ∘Escherichia coli
  ∘Enterobacter cloacae
  ∘**Enterococcus faecalis**
  ∘Klebsiella pneumoniae
  ∘Proteus mirabilis & vulgaris
  ∘Providencia rettgeri
  ∘Pseudomonas aeruginosa
  ∘Serratia marcescens
•**Anaerobes**
  ∘Bacteroides sp.
  ∘Clostridium sp.
  ∘Peptococcus sp.
  ∘**Streptococcus sp., esp. pneumoniae**
  ∘Peptostreptococcus sp.

DIAGNOSIS

•The syndrome is unpredictable, so consider the diagnosis in anyone w/ cirrhosis who is ill

General
  •Inflammatory cytokines→
    ∘Anorexia→
      –Cachexia
    ∘Chills
    ∘Fatigue
    ∘**Fever–70%**
    ∘Headache
    ∘Malaise
    ∘Night sweats
    ∘Weakness

---

†Temperature may be normal in patients w/:
  •Chronic kidney disease, esp. w/ uremia
  •Cirrhosis
  •Heart failure
  •Severe debility
  …or those who are:
    •Intravenous drug users
    •Taking certain medications:
      ∘Acetaminophen
      ∘Antibiotics
      ∘Glucocorticoids
      ∘Nonsteroidal anti–inflammatory drugs–NSAIDs

Gastrointestinal
  •**Parietal peritonitis**→
    ∘Phlegmon formation, being viable & dead bacteria, leukocytes (predominantly neutrophils), & necrotic tissue w/ eventual encapsulation by connective tissue, thus termed **abscess**, usually along the:
      –Inflamed organ
      –Pelvis, due to gravitational flow
      –Subphrenic area, due to diaphragmatic mediated negative pressure
    ∘**Continuous abdominal pain–60%**, esp. to movement of the inflamed parietal peritoneum→
      –Patient lying "stone" still, w/ exacerbation upon any bodily movement, even diaphragmatic movement upon deep inspiration, cough, sneezing, or the Valsalva maneuver

o**Referred rebound tenderness**, being the sudden release of gentle pressure remote from the painful area→
  −Parietal peritoneal movement→pain over the inflammed area
o**Involuntary guarding**, being reflex contraction of the overlying abdominal muscles (in order to ↓pain), which persists despite attempts to relax
o**Paralytic ileus**, being reflex relaxation of the regional intestinal smooth muscle (in order to ↓pain)→
  −↓Regional bowel sounds & constipation

o Peritoneal effusion=**ascites** (being exudative)→
  −Localized rub to auscultation, shifting dullness to percussion, weight gain (1L fluid=1kg=2.2 lbs), & ↑**abdominal girth−75%** (also due to intestinal paralytic ileus)
o Fibrous adhesions connecting the visceral & parietal peritoneum→intra−abdominal hernias

Neurologic
•Inflammation→
  o↑Cell turnover→
    −↑Protein metabolsim→↑ammonia production→**hepatic encephalopathy−55%**

INVASIVE PROCEDURES

•**Diagnostic paracentesis**
  o May require ultrasound guidance if mild
  o Procedure is safe in coagulopathic patients
  Complications−1%:
    •Hematoma
    •Hemoperitoneum
    •Infection
    •Intestinal perforation
  Lab studies:
    •**Tube 1:** Albumin, total protein, lactate dehydrogenase−LDH, & glucose
      o Send plasma samples for comparative analysis
    •**Tube 2:** Cell count & differential
    •**Tube 3:** Gram stain & culture (bacterial, fungal, & mycobacterial), w/ organisms seen via gram stain in 25% of patients
    •**Tube 4:** Other studies as clinically indicated
    •**Arterial blood gas tube:** pH

BLOOD & EFFUSION STUDIES

•**Cultures**
  Procedure:
    •2 sets of aerobic & anaerobic culture mediums, w/ each bottle inoculated w/ ≥10mL of fluid
  Outcomes:
    •Bacteremia occurs in 75% of patients infected w/ aerobic organisms, being rare w/ anaerobic organisms
  Limitations:
    •Careful, as source may be contaminated via:
      o Concomitant infection
      o Lack of aseptic technique or intravascular line/ catheter→
        −Skin organism contamination

TREATMENT

•**Empiric intravenous antibiotics**
  o If treatment is initially begun w/ intravenous medication, the switch to PO medication should be attempted upon clinical improvement (fever resolution & clinical stabilization, usually by day 3) X 24 hours, if an acceptable PO medication is available, & the patient is able to take PO medication
  o**Organism−narrowed therapy** should be initiated promptly upon stain, culture, & sensitivities results
  o The following antibiotics achieve equivalent plasma levels via PO or intravenous administration in persons w/ a functioning gastrointestinal tract:
    −Chloramphenicol
    −Doxycycline
    −Minocycline
    −Most fluoroquinolones
    −Trimethoprim/ Sulfamethoxazole

<u>Bactericidal antibiotics</u>
- **Cell wall synthesis inhibitors**
  - ∘β lactam medications:
    - −Carbapenems
    - −Cephalosporins
    - −Monobactams
    - −Penicillins
  - ∘Vancomycin
- **DNA synthesis inhibitors**
  - ∘Fluoroquinolones
  - ∘Linezolid
  - ∘Metronidazole
  - ∘Rifampin
  - ∘Quinupristin & Dalfopristin
- **Aminoglycosides**

- **Albumin:** 1.5g/ kg @ diagnosis, & 1g/ kg on day 3
  <u>Outcomes:</u>
  - •↓Mortality
  - •↓Renal failure risk

<u>Treatment duration:</u>
- •5 days if culture negative
- •2 weeks if culture positive

CEPHALOSPORINS: 3rd generation			
Generic (Trade)	**M**	**♀**	**Dose**
Cefotaxime (Claforan)	KL	P	2g IV/ IM q8hours
Ceftriaxone (Rocephin)	KB	P	2g IV/ IM q24hours

Mechanism:
- •A β−lactam ring structure which binds to bacterial transpeptidase→
  - ∘↓Transpeptidase function→
    - −↓Bacterial cell wall peptidoglycan cross−linking→↓cell wall synthesis→osmotic influx of extracellular fluid→↑intracellular hydrostatic pressure→cell rupture→cell death=bactericidal
- •↑Bacterial autolytic enzymes→
  - ∘Peptidoglycan degradation

- •Certain bacteria produce β−lactamase→
  - ∘Cleavage of this essential structural component of cephalosporins & certain penicillins (as the other β−lactam medications differ sufficiently to prevent ring cleavage)→
    - −Antibiotic inactivation. This process may be antagonized by the concomitant administration of **β−lactamase inhibitors** (Clavulanic acid=clavulanate, Sulbactam, or Tazobactam)→renewed susceptibility

Side effects:
General
- •**Hypersensitivity reactions ≤10%**
  - ∘Anaphylaxis−0.5%→
    - −Death−0.002% (1:50,000)
  - ∘Acute interstitial nephritis
  - ∘Dermatitis
  - ∘Drug fever
  - ∘Hemolytic anemia
  ...having cross−hypersensitivity to other β lactam medications (penicillins, carbapenems), except monobactams (ex. Aztreonam)
Gastrointestinal
- •Clostridium dificile pseudomembraneous colitis (3rd generation > others)

OR

FLUOROQUINOLONES			
Generic (Trade)	**M**	**♀**	**Dose**
Gatifloxacin (Tequin)	K	?	400mg PO/ IV q24hours
Levofloxacin (Levaquin)	KL	?	750mg PO/ IV q24hours
Moxifloxacin (Avelox)	LK	?	400mg PO/ IV q24hours

Mechanism:
- •↓DNA gyrase=topoisomerase action→
  - ∘↓Bacterial DNA synthesis

Side effects:
  General
  •Hypersensitivity reactions
  Gastrointestinal
  •Gastroenteritis→
  ◦Diarrhea
  ◦Nausea ± vomiting
  Mucocutaneous
  •Phototoxicity
  Neurologic
  •Dizziness
  •Drowsiness
  •Headache
  •Restlessness
  Materno−fetal
  •Fetal & child tendon malformation (including breast fed)→
  ◦↑Tendon rupture risk

PROGNOSIS
•40% 1year survival, & 25% 2year survival in cirrhotic patients

PROPHYLAXIS
Indications:
  •A previous episode of spontaneous bacterial peritonitis−SBP
  •Ascetic albumin <1g/ dL
  •Current gastrointestinal hemorrhage†
Outcomes:
  •↓Spontaneous bacterial peritonitis−SBP risk
  ◦Primary prophylaxis: From 27% to 3%
  ◦Secondary prophylaxis: From 70% to 20% @ 1year
  •↓Spontaneous bacteremia risk

---

†50% of patients w/ advanced liver disease (Childs−Pugh class C) develop an infection (usually due to enterobacteriaceae) such as:
  ◦Spontaneous bacterial peritonitis−SBP
  ◦Sepsis
  …within 48hours after an acute gastrointestinal hemorrhage, X 1week

TRIMETHOPRIM−SULFAMETHOXAZOLE TMP−SMX (Bactrim, Septra)

M	♀	Dose
K	U	1 double strength−DS tab (160mg TMP/ 800mg SMX) PO q24hours

Trimethoprim specific mechanism:
  •↓Dihydrofolate reductase action→
  ◦↓Tetrahydrofolate, being required as a methyl donor for the synthesis of purines & pyrimidines→
  −↓Nucleotide synthesis

Sulfonamide specific mechanism:
  •A P−aminobenzoic acid−PABA analogue→
  ◦Competitive inhibition of dihydropteroate synthetase mediated PABA conversion to dihydrofolate→
  −↓Tetrahydrofolate, being required as a methyl donor for the synthesis of purines &
  pyrimidines→ ↓nucleotide synthesis

Side effects:
  Mucocutaneous
  •**Dermatitis** via maculopapular rash, urticaria >> exfoliative dermatitis, photosensitivity, Stevens−Johnson syndrome, or toxic epidermal necrolysis
  Genitourinary
  •Acute interstitial nephritis
  Neurologic
  •Aseptic meningitis
  Pulmonary
  •The sulfite component of the combination medication→
  ◦Asthma exacerbation in sensitive patients

338

Hematologic
- **Myelosuppression**→
  - ∘Anemia→
    - −Fatigue
  - ∘Leukopenia→immunosuppression→
    - −↑Infection & neoplasm risk
  - ∘Thrombocytopenia→
    - −↑Hemorrhage risk

Trimethoprim specific:
Genitourinary
- •Blocks distal renal tubule Na$^+$/K$^+$ exchange→
  - ∘**Hyperkalemia**
- •Competes w/ creatinine for tubular secretion→
  - ∘↑Creatinine, without concomitantly ↑blood urea nitrogen−BUN
Hematologic
- •↑Homocysteine levels

Sulfamethoxazole specific:
General
- •Anorexia
- •Drug fever via hypersensitivity syndrome
Gastrointestinal
- •Nausea ± vomiting
Genitourinary
- •Crystalluria→
  - ∘Acute tubular necrosis
- •Hepatitis
Hematologic
- •**G6PD deficiency mediated hemolytic anemia**

Contraindications:
- •Neonates or near term ♀s, as sulfamethoxazole competitively binds to albumin, thus displacing bilirubin→
  - ∘↑Kernicterus risk

OR

FLUOROQUINOLONES			
Generic (Trade)	**M**	**♀**	**Dose**
Ciprofloxacin (Cipro)	LK	?	750mg PO qweek
Norfloxacin (Noroxin)	LK	?	400mg PO q24hours

OR

FLUOROQUINOLONES			
Indications:			
•Gastrointestinal hemorrhage			
Generic (Trade)	**M**	**♀**	**Dose**
Gatifloxacin (Tequin)	K	?	400mg PO/ IV q24hours
Levofloxacin (Levaquin)	KL	?	500mg PO/ IV q24hours
Moxifloxacin (Avelox)	LK	?	400mg PO/ IV q24hours

•Liver failure→
  ∘↓Metabolism of:
    −Nitrogenous waste products (**ammonia**, uric acid), which are the end−products of protein catabolism
    −Biogenic amines (ex. gamma aminobutyric acid−GABA)
    −Endogenous benzodiazepine−like substances via GABA−ergic neurotransmission
    −Medications
    −Mercaptans derived from methionine metabolism
    −Toxic intestinal products
    ...as blood bypasses hepatic filtration via portal−systemic anastomoses→
      •Direct flow into the systemic circulation→
        ∘**Central nervous system dysfunction, termed hepatic encephalopathy**→
          −**Altered mental status**
          −Altered neuromuscular function

•↑**Protein metabolism**
  ∘Blood transfusion
  ∘↑Dietary protein
  ∘Gastrointestinal hemorrhage
  ∘Inflammation
  ...→↑ammonia production
•**Hypovolemia**→
  ∘↑Plasma concentration of the various possible causative substances
  ∘↓Hepatic & renal perfusion→
    −↓Filtration
•**Renal failure**→
  ∘↓Excretion of nitrogenous waste products
    −↓Ammonia filtration
    −↓Creatinine filtration & secretion
    −↓Urea nitrogen filtration→↑interstitial urea→↑gastrointestinal interstitial osmolarity→↑ammonia reabsorption
•Certain medications, esp.
  ∘Analgesics (opiates)
  ∘Sedatives (benzodiazepines, barbiturates)
•Superimposed hepatic damage
  ∘Hepatitis
  ∘Tumor
    −Hepatoma
    −Hepatocellular cancer
  ...→↓hepatic functional reserve
•↑Bacterial contact w/ colonic substrates via:
  ∘Constipation
  ∘Ileus (obstructive or paralytic)
  ...→↑ammonia production
•↑Renal production of ammonia
  ∘Hypokalemia
•↑Diffusion of ammonia across the blood brain barrier
  ∘Alkalemia
•Iatrogenic
  ∘Peritoneojugular shunt
  ∘Portosystemic shunting
    −Transjugular intrahepatic portosystemic shunt−TIPS

Neurologic
  •Central nervous system dysfunction→
    ∘**Altered mental status**
    ∘Cerebral edema
    ∘Headache
    ∘Nausea ± vomiting

○Altered neuromuscular function→
  −**Asterixis**, being an inability to maintain a posture
    Examination:
      •Usually assessed using the upper extremities, but may viewed via any attempt at voluntary posture maintenance. Best viewed by asking the patient to hold out extended arms & dorsiflexed hands, w/ fingers spread as though signaling traffic to stop→
        ○An intermittent, non−rhythmic flapping tremor of the wrist & metacarpophalangeal joints due to **intermittent inhibition of wrist extensors**→
          −Brief lapses of posture. If the patient cannot comply, simply ask them to squeeze your extended fingers→intermittently ↓grip strength
    Limitations: Also found w/:
      •Renal failure→
        ○Uremia
      •Chronic heart failure
      •Chronic lung disease→
        ○Respiratory failure

Encephalopathy severity scale:
  •**Grade 0**
    ○Consciousness:
      −Normal
    ○Cognitive:
      −Subclinical
    ○Motor:
      −Abnormalities only on psychometric analysis
  •**Grade 1**
    ○Consciousness:
      −Inverted sleep pattern
      −Restlessness
    ○Cognitive:
      −Anxiety
      −Irritability
      −Mild confusion→forgetfulness
    ○Motor:
      −Tremor
      −↓Coordination→impaired handwriting
  •**Grade 2**
    ○Consciousness:
      −Lethargy
    ○Cognitive:
      −Amnesia
      −↓Inhibitions→inappropriate behavior
      −Confusion→disorientation to time
    ○Motor:
      −Asterixis
      −↓↓Coordination→impaired movement
      −Difficulty speaking=dysarthria
      −Hypoactive reflexes
  •**Grade 3**
    ○Consciousness:
      −Somnolence
    ○Cognitive:
      −Aggressive behavior
      −Confusion→disorientation to place
    ○Motor:
      −Hyperactive reflexes
      −Muscle twitching &/or rigidity
      −Babinski's sign
      −Seizures−rare
  •**Grade 4**
    ○Motor
      −Decerebrate posturing

Hematologic
  •↑Ammonia in most patients, w/ the degree poorly correlating w/ the severity of encephalopathy→
    ○Little clinical value in diagnosis or treatment progression

•**Protein restriction**
  ◦**Grades 0-1:** Dietary restriction of 20g/ 24hours
  ◦**Grades ≥2:** Exclusion
  Titration:
    •Once the encephalopathy has resolved, titrate via 10g increments q5days, guided by clinical response

ZINC
Dose
600mg PO q24hours

Mechanism:
•Two of the five hepatocyte urea cycle enzymes responsible for the metabolism of ammonia to urea are zinc dependent
•Cirrhosis→
  ◦↑Renal zinc loss→
    −↓Ammonia metabolism

LAXATIVE MEDICATIONS			
Generic	**M**	**♀**	**Dose**
Lactulose	Ø	P	
•PO form			30-60mL liquid PO† q1h until the laxative effect is apparent, then titrate dose to produce 2-4 soft stools/ 24hours, then continue treatment until the patient can tolerate 50g protein/ 24h
•PR form			300mL in 700mL of water or normal saline as a retention enema for 30min. q4h

†May mix w/ juice to improve taste

Mechanism:
•A synthetic disaccharide (β−galactosidofructose) metabolized by intestinal bacteria→
  ◦Colonic acidification→ammonia (NH_3) conversion to ammonium (NH_4^+)→
    −Inability to be absorbed
    −↓Survival of urease† producing intestinal bacteria, w/ ↑growth of non−urease producing lactobacilli→↓ammonia production
  ◦Fermentative osmotic diarrhea→
    −↑Toxin elimination

†Urease is an enzyme that catalyzes the conversion of urea & water, to carbon dioxide & ammonia:
H_2O + urea —— urease ——> $2NH_3$ (ammonia) + CO_2

Side effects:
Gastrointestinal
  •Diarrhea→
    ◦Dehydration→
      −Paradoxically worsened encephalopathy
  •Flatulence

AMINOGLYCOSIDES				
Generic	**M**	**♀**	**Start**	**Max**
Neomycin	Small % absorbed	Ø	1g PO q6hours	2g q6hours

Mechanism:
•Affects the ribosomal 30S subunit→
  ◦↓Initiation complex function
  ◦Misreading of messenger RNA
  ...→colonic bacteriostasis→
    •↓Bacteria mediated urea metabolism→
      ◦↓Ammonia formation

Side effects:
•A small amount of the medication is absorbed which may→
Genitourinary
  •Nephrotoxicity† (Gentamicin > Tobramycin > Amikacin > Neomycin), w/ renal failure usually @ ≥1week via acute tubular necrosis
    Risk factors:
      •↑Age
      •Cirrhosis
      •Hypovolemia

- •Hypokalemia
- •Hypomagnesemia
- •Renal failure

Neurologic
- •**Ototoxicity‡,** being dose related & irreversible→
  - ∘High frequency sound loss
  - <u>Risk factors:</u>
    - •Concomitant use w/ other ototoxic medications such as loop diuretics
    - •Renal failure
    - •Use >2weeks
- •Neuromuscular blockade via:
  - ∘↓Presynaptic acetylcholine release
  - ∘↓Postsynaptic sensitivity to acetylcholine

---

†Early signs of nephrotoxicity include:
- •↓Ability to concentrate the urine (noted via ↓specific gravity)
- •Cylindrical urinary casts
- •Proteinuria

‡Audiometry is required to document ototoxicity, as the hearing loss occurs above the frequency range of normal human conversation

<u>Monitoring:</u>
- •Obtain baseline & serial audiometry w/ treatment >2weeks

METRONIDAZOLE (Flagyl)

M ♀	Dose
KL P–U in 1st trimester	800mg PO q24hours

<u>Mechanism:</u>
- •DNA binding→
  - ∘DNA strand breakage→
    - −Colonic bactericidal action→↓bacteria mediated urea metabolism→↓ammonia formation

<u>Side effects:</u>
General
- •**Disulfuram–like reaction to alcohol**
  - ∘Avoid alcoholic beverages during, & for 48hours after completion of treatment

Gastrointestinal
- •Nausea ± vomiting−10%
- •Taste changes=dysgeusia (esp. metallic taste)

Genitourinary
- •Dark urine, being common, but harmless

Neurological
- •Peripheral neuropathy
- •Seizures

Hematologic
- •Transient neutropenia−8%

BENZODIAZEPINE RECEPTOR ANTAGONIST

Generic (Trade)	M ♀	Dose	Max
Flumazenil (Romazicon)	LK ?	2mg IV over 15seconds, then 0.2mg q1min. prn	1mg total

<u>Contraindications due to seizure risk:</u>
- •Chronic benzodiazepine use
- •Acute tricyclic antidepressant overdose

HELICOBACTER PYLORI DIAGNOSIS & ERADICATION TREATMENT ▬▬▬

•Gastric ammonia production via **urease producing Helicobacter Pylori,** may contribute substantially to blood ammonia levels. For treatment protocol, see peptic inflammatory disease chapter

•Liver failure→
  ∘**Altered renal vascular autoregulation**→
    −Intra−renal vasoconstriction→progressive **pre−renal renal failure,** w/ the kidneys being histologically normal, having been used successfully as donor organs

RISK FACTORS

PRE−RENAL RENAL FAILURE
Hypovolemia:
  •**Direct vascular loss**
    ∘Hemorrhage
  •**Gastrointestinal loss**
    ∘Diarrhea
    ∘Nasogastric tube suctioning
    ∘Poor oral intake
    ∘Surgical drainage
    ∘Vomiting
  •**Cutaneous loss**
    ∘Diaphoresis
    ∘Fever
    ∘Severe burn
  •**Renal loss**
    ∘Diuretic use
    ∘Osmotic diuresis
      −Diabetes mellitus
      −Hypercalcemia
  •**Hypoalbuminemia**
    ∘Cirrhosis
    ∘Malnutrition
    ∘Nephrotic syndrome
    ...→systemic edema, termed anasarca, as well as transudative peritoneal, pleural, pericardial, & synovial effusions
  •**Abdominal organ inflammation**→
    ∘Exudative effusion→
      −Ascites

Distributive disease:
  •↓**Cardiac output**
    ∘**Heart failure**
    ∘Cross clamping of the aorta during surgery
  •**Systemic vasodilation**
    ∘Distributive shock
      −Anaphylactic shock
      −Septic shock
    ∘Medications
      −Anesthetics
      −Anti−hypertensives
  •**Renal arteriole vasoconstriction**
    ∘Electrolytes
      −Hypercalcemia
    ∘Medications
      −Amphotericin B
      −Catecholamines (epinephrine, norepinephrine, or high dose dopamine)
      −Cyclosporine
      −FK506
    ∘**Radiocontrast dye**

Renal artery obstruction†:
  •Atherosclerosis
  •Dissecting aneurysm
  •Embolus
  •Fibromuscular dysplasia
  •Thrombosis
  •Vasculitis

†Being ≥95% occlusive bilaterally (or unilateral w/ 1 functional kidney), or less w/ concomitant risk factors

Altered renal arteriole autoregulation:
- •Medications
  - ∘**Nonsteroidal anti-inflammatory drugs–NSAIDs,** including Aspirin
  - ∘**Angiotensin converting enzyme inhibitors–ACEi** or **angiotensin 2 receptor blockers–ARB**
- Mechanism:
  - •Patients w/ pre-existing bilateral ↓renal perfusion, not necessarily failure:
    - ∘Heart failure
    - ∘Bilateral renal artery stenosis
    - ∘Hypovolemia
    - ∘Renal failure
  - ...rely more on the compensatory production of:
    - •Prostaglandin→
      - ∘Afferent arteriole dilation→maintained glomerular filtration rate, whereas NSAIDs→
        - −↓Prostaglandin production→pre-renal renal failure
    - •Angiotensin 2→
      - ∘Efferent arteriole constriction→maintained glomerular filtration rate, whereas either:
        - −Angiotensin converting enzyme inhibition
        - −Angiotensin 2 receptor blockade
        - ...→↓angiotensin 2 production & action respectively→
          - •Pre-renal renal failure

OTHER
•**Aminoglycosides** via ?acute tubular necrosis

DIAGNOSIS
Genitourinary
- •**Altered renal vascular autoregulation→**
  - ∘Intra-renal vasoconstriction→
    - −**Pre-renal renal failure,** w/ a glomerular filtration rate <40mL/ min., in the **absence of intravascular volume depletion**
- Additional diagnostic criteria:
  - •**Oliguria,** being urine output <400mL/ 24h
  - •Absence of sustained improvement after volume expansion
  - •Absence of nephrotoxic medications
  - •**Urine sodium <10mEq/ L,** occurring in most patients
  - •Urine protein <500mg/ 24h
  - •Urine erythrocytes <50/ hpf

TREATMENT
•**Liver transplantation**
- Outcomes:
  - •Max 1 year survival: 90%
  - •Max 5 year survival: 80%
- Contraindications:
  - •Active substance abuse
  - •Extrahepatic malignancy
  - •HIV infection
  - •Sepsis
  - •Severe comorbidity

PROPHYLAXIS
•**Alcoholic hepatitis**
- ∘Alcoholic hepatitis severity is best predicted by the following formula, termed the discriminate function
  - −Discriminant function= 4.6 (prothrombin time–PT − control) + total bilirubin (mg/ dL)
- Outcomes:
  - •Either of the following indicate a 35% mortality within 6months
    - ∘**Score >32**
    - ∘**Encephalopathy** without a concomitant gastrointestinal hemorrhage or infection

NONSELECTIVE PHOSPHODIESTERASE INHIBITOR

Indications:
- Alcoholic hepatitis, w/ either:
  - Discriminate function score >32
  - Encephalopathy without a concomitant gastrointestinal hemorrhage or infection

Generic (Trade)	M	♀	Dose
Pentoxifylline (Trental)	L	?	400mg PO q8hours X 1month

Mechanism:
- ↑Intracellular cAMP & cGMP→
  - ↓Inflammatory cytokine production
  - ↓Endothelial adhesion molecule display
  - ↓Fibroblast mediated interstitial tissue formation

Outcomes:
- 40%↓ mortality
- 65%↓ new onset hepatorenal syndrome
  - 70%↓ mortality from hepatorenal syndrome

346

•A chronic, intermittently symptomatic autoimmune disease of unknown etiology→
  ◦Gastrointestinal inflammation=gastroenteritis

RISK FACTORS

•**Age:** ≤40years & 60–70years
•**Skin color:** Whites > blacks
•**Gender**
  ◦Crohn's disease ♂ > ♀
  ◦Ulcerative colitis ♀ > ♂
•**Genetic**
  ◦**Ashkenazic jewish ancestry**
  ◦Family history of either disease–20%
•**Lifestyle**
  ◦Smoking→
    –↑Crohn's disease risk, but ↓ulcerative colitis risk
•**Medications**
  ◦Nonsteroidal anti–inflammatory drugs–NSAIDs

CLASSIFICATION

•Distinction cannot be made in 10% of patients w/ colitis, necessitating a diagnosis of indeterminate colitis, at least initially

•**Crohn's disease**
  ◦Inflammation **anywhere along the gastrointestinal tract,** from the oropharnyx to the anus
  <u>Subsyndromes:</u>
    •**Gastritis &/or duodenitis–35%,** usually being asymptomatic
    •**Ileocolitis–40%:** Inflammation of the ileum (usually distal) & colorectum (usually proximal)
    •**Ileitis–30%:** Inflammation confined to the ileum
    •**Colitis &/or proctitis†–30%:** Inflammation confined to the colorectum

•**Ulcerative colitis**
  ◦Inflammation **confined to the colorectum,** being either:
    –Intermittently symptomatic–70%
    –Continuously symptomatic–20%
    –Rapidly progressive, termed fulminant–5%
    …w/ 5% achieving complete remission
  <u>Subsyndromes:</u>
    •**Distal ulcerative colitis–50%:** Inflammation distal to the splenic flexure
    •**Left sided ulcerative colitis–25%:** Inflammation extending to the splenic flexure
    •**Pancolitis–25%:** Inflammation extending beyond the splenic flexure

---

†50% of patients have inflammation of the rectum, termed proctitis, as either ileocolitis or proctitis

DIAGNOSIS

General
  •Inflammatory cytokines→
    ◦Anorexia (also being due to nausea &/or ↑pain upon eating)→
      –Cachexia (also being due to ↓intestinal absorption)
    ◦Chills
    ◦Fatigue
    ◦**Fever**
    ◦Headache
    ◦Malaise
    ◦Night sweats
    ◦Weakness

---

†Temperature may be normal in patients w/:
  •Chronic kidney disease, esp. w/ uremia
  •Cirrhosis
  •Heart failure
  •Severe debility

...or those who are:
- •Intravenous drug users
- •Taking certain medications:
  - ◦Acetaminophen
  - ◦Antibiotics
  - ◦Glucocorticoids
  - ◦Nonsteroidal anti–inflammatory drugs–NSAIDs

Gastrointestinal

- •Gastroenteritis→
  - ◦**Continuous abdominal pain**, usually described as "knifelike" or "boring", being relieved by ↓peritoneal stretching, accomplished by sitting, leaning forward, & or hip flexion
  - ◦↑Viscous peristalsis→↑generalized viscous peristalsis (gastrointestinal, biliary, & genitourinary)→
    - –↑**Abdominal pain**, being referred & episodic or "wave like", termed colic
      <u>Areas of reference:</u>
      - •Stomach &/or duodenum: Epigastrium
      - •Small intestine: Periumbilical area
      - •Large intestine: Hypogastrium &/or suprapubic area
      - •Rectum: Suprapubic, sacral, &/or perineal areas
    - –Anorexia
    - –↑Bowel sounds→audible gastrointestinal gurgling, termed borborygmi
    - –**Diarrhea**, esp. w/ Crohn's disease
    - –Retrograde peristalsis→**nausea ± vomiting**
  - ◦Hemorrhage, esp. w/ Ulcerative colitis
    - –**Hematemesis:** Vomiting of blood, including very dark, tarry looking blood termed 'coffee ground' emesis
      <u>Lesion localization:</u>
      - •Upper gastrointestinal hemorrhage
    - –**Hematochezia:** Passage of bright red blood per rectum
      <u>Lesion localization:</u>
      - •Lower gastrointestinal hemorrhage >> upper gastrointestinal hemorrhage via massive hemorrhage (≥1L) &/or ↑↑peristalsis
    - –**Melena:** Passage of sticky, very dark, tarry looking stool, w/ a characteristic odor, requiring ≥50mL of blood, indicating gastrointestinal hemorrhage proximal to ileocecal sphincter >> colonic gastrointestinal hemorrhage via slow hemorrhage &/or ↓peristalsis
    - –**Fecal occult blood:** Passage of blood detectable only by laboratory testing, requiring ≥20mL of blood. Not helpful in the anatomic determination of the lesion
  - ◦↑**Mucus production & pus formation** (being composed of viable & dead bacteria, leukocytes, & necrotic tissue), especially w/ ulcerative colitis
  - ◦Tissue edema→
    - –Luminal obstruction, esp. of the small intestine, occurring only w/ Crohn's disease
  - ◦Rectal inflammation=proctitis→
    - –Painful anal sphincter contraction, termed tenesmus→urgent desire to evacuate the bowel &/or bladder→urinary & bowel frequency
  - ◦Phlegmon formation, being viable & dead bacteria, leukocytes (predominantly neutrophils), & necrotic tissue, w/ eventual encapsulation by connective tissue, thus termed **abscess**, usually along the:
    - –Inflamed organ
    - –Pelvis, due to gravitational flow
    - –Subphrenic area, due to diaphragmatic mediated negative pressure
  - ◦Eventual spread to the parietal peritoneum→**parietal peritonitis**→
    - –↑**Localized abdominal pain**, esp. to movement of the inflamed parietal peritoneum→patient lying "stone" still, w/ exacerbation upon any bodily movement, even diaphragmatic movement upon deep inspiration, cough, sneezing, or the Valsalva maneuver
    - –**Referred rebound tenderness**, being the sudden release of gentle pressure remote from the painful area→parietal peritoneal movement→pain over the inflamed area
    - –**Involuntary guarding**, being reflex contraction of the overlying abdominal muscles (in order to ↓pain), which persists despite attempts to relax
    - –**Paralytic ileus**, being reflex relaxation of the regional intestinal smooth muscle (in order to ↓pain)→↓regional bowel sounds & constipation
    - –Peritoneal effusion=**ascites** (being exudative)→localized rub to auscultation, shifting dullness to percussion, weight gain (1L fluid=1kg=2.2 lbs), & ↑**abdominal girth** (also due to intestinal paralytic ileus)
    - –Fibrous adhesions connecting the visceral & parietal peritoneum→intra–abdominal hernias
    - –Luminal connection w/ nearby epithelial surfaces, termed **fistula**, being **enterocutaneous, enteroenteric, enterovaginal,** &/or **enterovesical**

348

○**Complete loss of intestinal smooth muscle tone**→
–Abdominal pain, tenderness, & **massive dilation, termed toxic megacolon**→intraluminal air
accumulation→↑intraluminal pressure→↓colonic vascular flow (venous > arterial)→congestive
ischemia→necrosis→**perforation & hemorrhage**→generalized peritonitis
Iatrogenic precipitants: Induced in patients w/ severe colitis by:
•**Anticholinergic medications**→
  ○↓Gastrointestinal tone
•**Opiates**→
  ○↓Gastrointestinal tone
•Barium enema preparation
•Lower endoscopy preparation
○**Perforation**→
–Release of contents (bacteria, digestive enzymes, air, mucus, & feces)→generalized peritonitis

Effects of chronic, inadequately controlled disease:
•Chronic gastroenteritis→
  ○↑**Intestinal fibrous tissue deposition**→
    –Luminal adhesions
    –Intestinal thickening
    ...→**luminal stenosis**
•Crohn's disease mediated chronic ileitis→
  ○Bacterial overgrowth
  ○↓Small intestinal absorption, occurring in the proximal 1/3rd portion→
    –↓Vitamin B12 & folic acid absorption→macrocytic anemia
    –↓Vitamin D absorption→osteoporosis
    –↓Enterohepatic circulation of bile salts→↑bile lithogenicity→cholelithiasis–12%
  ○↑Oxalate absorption→
    –Hyperoxaluria→oxalate nephrolithiasis

Musculoskeletal
•Inflammatory cytokines→
  ○↓Bone production in prepubertal children→
    –↓Growth
Hematologic
•Inflammatory cytokines→
  ○Leukocytosis
  ○↑Acute phase proteins
    –↑Erythrocyte sedimentation rate–ESR (normal: 5mm/ decade aged + ♂ ≤10mm/h or ♀ ≤20mm/h)
    –↑C-reactive protein–CRP (normal: <2mg/ L), responding more acutely than ESR, as it rises
      within several hours & falls within 3days upon partial resolution
    –↑Fibrinogen
    –↑Platelets→thrombocytosis
•Intravascular volume loss→
  ○↑Creatinine & blood urea nitrogen–BUN†, indicating pre-renal renal failure
•Crohn's disease mediated chronic ileitis→
  ○↓Small intestinal absorption, occurring in the proximal 1/3rd portion→
    –↓Vitamin B12 & folic acid absorption→macrocytic anemia
•Malnutrition→
  ○↓Albumin & blood urea nitrogen–BUN
•Search for chronic gastrointestinal hemorrhage via:
  ○Iron deficiency anemia
•Serology, being indicated w/ indeterminate colitis
  ○Perinuclear staining, anti-neutrophil cytoplasmic antibodies P-ANCA w/ Ulcerative Colitis–70%
  ○Anti-saccharomyces cerevisiae antibodies w/ Crohn's disease ≥50%

---

†Upper gastrointestinal hemorrhage→
  •↑Blood urea nitrogen–BUN via gastrointestinal mucosa mediated erythrocyte protein absorption→
    ○↑Ammonia, which diffuses into the intestinal blood, being filtered via hepatocytes→
      –Urea cycle→↑urea

•May accompany > precede gastrointestinal symptoms

Disease	Crohn's disease	Ulcerative colitis
Cirrhosis	<1%	Rare
Erythema nodosum	15%	5%
Pericholangitis	20%	30%
Peripheral arthritis	20%	10%
Pyoderma gangrenosum	1%	<5%
Sclerosing cholangitis	25%	30%
Spondylitis	17%	<5%
Stomatitis	10%	10%
Uveitis	7%	45%

IMAGING
•**Abdomino–pelvic ultrasound or computed tomographic–CT scan**
  Findings:
    •Inflammation→
      ◦**Enlarged edematous organ**
      ◦**Peri–organ stranding** seen on CT
      ◦Lymphadenopathy
    •Biliary obstruction→
      ◦Proximal biliary tract dilation
    •Ultrasound allows for the visualization of most gallstones, as only 15% are radiopaque
    •Peritonitis→
      ◦Ascites
    •Paralytic ileus, being either:
      ◦Generalized
      ◦Localized to nearby intestine→
        –Air filled segment, termed the sentinel loop sign
      …→intestinal air fluid levels
    •Phlegmon, abscess, &/or peri–organ fluid, which may be subdiaphragmatic→
        –Diaphragm elevation
    •Perforation→
      ◦Subdiaphragmatic air
  Differentiating radiographic features:
    •**Crohn's disease:**
      ◦Proliferation of the mesenteric fat, termed "**creeping fat**"

•**Abdominal, double contrast barium enema w/ computed tomographic–CT scanning**
  Differentiating radiographic features:
    •**Crohn's disease:**
      ◦Ulcerations→
        –Filling defects
      ◦Fistula formation
      ◦Intestinal stenosis→
        –Proximal dilation & distal 'string sign'
    •**Ulcerative colitis:**
      ◦Pseudopolyps→
        –Filling defects
      ◦'Lead pipe' sign
  Contraindications:
    •Acute exacerbation, as barium enema preparation→
      ◦↑Toxic megacolon risk. Rather, a flexible sigmoidoscopy & barium swallow study can be
      performed

INVASIVE PROCEDURES
•**Endoscopy**
  Differentiating endoscopic features:
    •**Crohn's disease:**
      ◦**Intermittent** lesions, w/ possible rectal involvement→
        –Friable mucosa, w/ longitudinal ulcerations, having a **cobblestone appearance**
        –Small mucosal ulcerations, termed **apthous ulcers**
    •**Ulcerative colitis:**
      ◦**Continuous** lesions **beginning at the rectum**, w/ proximal progression→
        –Friable mucosa, w/ regenerating areas having a polypoid appearance, termed **pseudopolyp**

350

Differentiating histologic features:
- **Crohn's disease:**
  - ○Usually being **transmural**, w/ **noncaseating granulomas**
- **Ulcerative colitis:**
  - ○Limited to the **mucosa & submucosa**, w/:
    - –Epithelial crypt necrosis & purulence, termed **crypt abscess**
    - –Lamina propria neutrophil infiltration

Contraindications:
- •Acute exacerbation, as lower endoscopy preparation→
  - ○↑Toxic megacolon risk. Rather, a flexible sigmoidoscopy & barium swallow study can be performed

TREATMENT				

MILD DISEASE

5-ACETYLSALICYLIC ACID–ASA COMPOUNDS

Generic (Trade)	M ♀	Dose	Max	Site of action
Balsalazide (Colazal)	† P	2.25g PO q8hours		Large intestine
Olsalazine (Dipentum)	L ?	500mg PO q12hours	3g/ 24h	Large intestine
Sulfasalazine (Azulfidine)	K U	500mg PO q6hours	6g/ 24h	Large intestine
Mesalamine	Gut P			
Trade name				
•**Asacol**		800mg PO q8hours	4.8g/ 24h	Distal ileum & large intestine
•**Pentasa**		800mg PO q8hours	4g/ 24h	Small & large intestine
•**Canasa supp**		500mg PR q12–q8h		Rectum
•**Rowasa supp**		500mg PR q12hours		Rectum
enema		4g (60mL) qhs		Distal colon & rectum

- •Available in various pH or time–dependent release capsules
- †Minimal absorption

Mechanism:
- •Inflammatory cell mediated prostaglandins are released at sites of inflammation (in addition to other inflammatory cytokines)→
  - ○Leukocyte migration→↑inflammation, via:
    - –Vasodilation→↑blood flow→erythema, edema, warmth, &/or tenderness/ pain via enhanced neuronal sensitivity
- •Interleukin–IL1→
  - ○↑Hypothalamic prostaglandin production→
    - –Fever
- •Topical, mucosal, nonsteroidal anti–inflammatory action→
  - ○Reversible inhibition of both cyclooxygenase enzymes (COX–1 & COX–2), being responsible for the production of neural & inflammatory cell prostaglandins respectively→
    - –↓Pain
    - –↓Temperature (antipyretic)
    - –↓Inflammation

In Brief:
- •**Cyclooxygenase–COX1 enzymes** are found in most cells of the body, being responsible for normal physiologic processes
- •**Cyclooxygenase–COX 2 enzymes** are responsible for the production of inflammatory cell prostaglandins

Side effects:
Gastrointestinal
- •Inhibition of the cyclooxygenase–COX1 enzyme→↑peptic inflammatory disease risk→↑**upper gastrointestinal hemorrhage risk** via:
  - ○↓Gastric mucosal prostaglandin synthesis→
    - –↓Epithelial cell proliferation
    - –↓Mucosal blood flow→↓bicarbonate delivery to the mucosa
    - –↓Mucus & bicarbonate secretion from gastric mucosal cells

Indications for peptic inflammatory disease prophylaxis:
- •Prophylax w/ proton pump inhibitors–PPI's, histamine 2 selective receptor blockers, or Misoprostol in patients w/ any of the following:
  - ○Age >60 years w/ a history of peptic inflammatory disease
  - ○Anticipated therapy >3 months
  - ○Concurrent glucocorticoid use
  - ○Moderate to high dose NSAID use

Genitourinary
- Patients w/ pre−existing bilateral ↓renal perfusion, not necessarily failure:
  - Heart failure
  - Bilateral renal artery stenosis
  - Hypovolemia
  - Renal failure
  ...rely more on the compensatory production of vasodilatory prostaglandins→
  - Afferent arteriole dilation→
    - Maintained glomerular filtration rate–GFR, whereas NSAIDs→
      - −↓Prostaglandin production, which may→renal failure

Pulmonary
- Inhibition of both cyclooxygenase enzymes (COX 1 & COX2)→
  - ↑Lipoxygenase activity→
    - −↑Leukotriene synthesis→symptomatic asthma within 2hours of ingestion in 5% of asthmatics

Rheumatologic
- Acetylsalicylic acid competes w/ uric acid secretion in the renal tubules→
  - ↑Uric acid levels→
    - −↑Risk of uric acid precipitation in the tissues=gout

Pediatric
- **Reye's syndrome**
  - A life threatening fulminant hepatitis→
    - −Hepatic encephalopathy in children age ≤16 years w/ a viral infection (esp. influenza or Varicella−zoster virus−VZV)

Olsalazine specific:
Gastrointestinal
- Diarrhea

Sulfasalazine specific:
General
- Orange/ yellow discoloration of body fluids, including sweat, tears, & urine, which stain clothing & contact lenses

Gastrointestinal
- **Hepatitis**

Genitourinary
- Infertility

Mucocutaneous
- Photosensitivity

Neurologic
- Neuropathy

Pulmonary
- Fibrosing alveolitis

Hematologic
- **Myelosuppression**→
  - Anemia→
    - −Fatigue
  - Leukopenia→immunosuppression→
    - −↑Infection & neoplasm risk
  - Thrombocytopenia→
    - −↑Hemorrhage risk, esp. petechiae

Mesalamine specific:
General
- Fever
- Headache
- Yellow/ brown discoloration of body fluids, including sweat, tears, & urine, which stain clothing & contact lenses

Mucocutaneous
- Dermatitis

Sulfasalazine specific monitoring:
- Complete blood count
- Liver function tests

SYSTEMIC GLUCOCORTICOID TREATMENT

Indications:
•↓Inflammation while an immunomodulating medication is taking effect

Generic	M ♀	Dose
Methylprednisolone	L ?	60mg PO/ IV q24hours
Prednisolone	L ?	60mg PO/ IV q24hours
Prednisone	L ?	60mg PO q24hours

•Once disease control is achieved (usually 7–10days), taper to the lowest effective maintenance dose X 2months, in order to minimize serious side effects, w/ the goal of discontinuation if possible, w/ attention to relapse syndrome
•Both the IV & PO routes have equal efficacy

	Relative potencies			
Glucocorticoids	Anti–inflammatory	Mineralocorticoid	Duration	Dose equiv.
Cortisol (physiologic†)	1	1	10hours	20mg
Cortisone (PO)	0.7	2	10hours	25mg
Hydrocortisone (PO, IM, IV)	1	2	10hours	20mg
Methylprednisolone (PO, IM, IA, IV)	5	0.5	15–35hours	5mg
Prednisone (PO)	5	0.5	15–35hours	5mg
Prednisolone (PO, IM, IV)	5	0.8	15–35hours	5mg
Triamcinolone (PO, IM)	5	~0	15–35hours	5mg
Betamethasone (PO, IM, IA)	25	~0	35–70hours	0.75mg
Dexamethasone (PO)	25	~0	35–70hours	0.75mg
Fludrocortisone (PO)	10	125	10hours	

†The physiologic rate of adrenal cortical cortisol production is 20–30mg/ 24hours

Side effects of chronic use:
General
  •Anorexia→
    ○Cachexia
  •↑Perspiration
Cardiovascular
  •Mineralocorticoid effects→
    ○↑Renal tubular NaCl & water retention as well as potassium secretion→
      –**Hypertension**
      –**Edema**
      –**Hypokalemia**
  •Counter–regulatory=anti–insulin effects→
    ○↑Plasma glucose→
      –**Secondary diabetes mellitus,** which may→ketoacidemia
    ○Hyperlipidemia→↑atherosclerosis→
      –**Coronary artery disease**
      –Cerebrovascular disease
      –Peripheral vascular disease
Cutaneous/ subcutaneous
  •↓Fibroblast function→
    ○↓Intercellular matrix production→
      –↑Bruisability→ecchymoses
      –Poor wound healing
      –Skin striae
  •Androgenic effects→
    ○Acne
    ○↑Facial hair
    ○Thinning scalp hair
  •Fat redistribution from the extremities to the:
    ○Abdomen→
      –Truncal obesity
    ○Shoulders→
      –Supraclavicular fat pads
    ○Upper back→
      –Buffalo hump
    ○Face→
      –Moon facies
      …w/ concomitant thinning of the arms & legs

Endocrine
•**Adrenal failure** upon abrupt discontinuation after 2weeks
Gastrointestinal
•Inhibition of phospholipase A_2 mediated conversion of cell membrane lipids to arachidonic acid, which is the precursor for both cyclooxygenase–COX enzymes, w/ the cyclooxygenase–COX1 enzyme found in most cells of the body, responsible for normal physiologic function. Inhibition of the cyclooxygenase–COX1 enzyme→↑peptic inflammatory disease risk→↑**upper gastrointestinal hemorrhage risk** via:
  ◦↓Gastric mucosal prostaglandin synthesis→
    –↓Epithelial cell proliferation
    –↓Mucosal blood flow→↓bicarbonate delivery to the mucosa
    –↓Mucus & bicarbonate secretion from gastric mucosal cells
Musculoskeletal
•**Avascular necrosis of bone**
•**Osteoporosis**
•Proximal muscle weakness
Neurologic
•Anxiety
•Insomnia
•Psychosis
Opthalmologic
•**Cataracts**
Immunologic
•Inhibition of phospholipase A_2 mediated conversion of cell membrane lipids to arachidonic acid, which is the precursor for both cyclooxygenase–COX enzymes (COX1 & COX2) being responsible for the production of neuronal & inflammatory cell prostaglandins respectively→
  –↓Pain
  –↓Temperature (antipyretic)
  –↓**Inflammation**
•Stabilization of lisosomal & cell membranes→
  ◦↓Cytokine & proteolytic enzyme release
•↓Lymphocyte & eosinophil production
  ...all→
        •**Immunosuppression**→
          –↑**Infection** &/or neoplasm risk
Hematologic
•↑Erythrocyte production→
  ◦Polycythemia
•↑Neutrophil demargination→
  ◦Neutrophilia→
    –**Leukocytosis**

IMMUNOMODULATING MEDICATIONS
•The following medications usually require 1–6 months for symptomatic improvement, making these medications not useful in the control of acute disease, but rather, useful when prolonged treatment is planned

Generic (Trade)	M	♀	Start	Max
6–mercaptopurine	L	U	50mg PO q24hours	
Azathioprine†(Imuran)	LK	U	1mg/ kg PO q24hours	2.5mg/kg/24hours

†Azathioprine's active metabolite is 6–mercaptopurine

Mechanism:
•Inhibition of enzymes involved in purine metabolism→
  ◦Cytotoxicity of differentiating lymphocytes (T cell >> B cell)

Side effects:
Gastrointestinal
•↓Mucosal cell proliferation→
  ◦Mucosal inflammation=mucositis, including inflammation of the oral mucosa=stomatitis→
    –Diarrhea
    –Nausea ± vomiting
•Hepatitis→
  ◦Cirrhosis–rare
Mucocutaneous
•↓Epithelial cell proliferation→
  ◦Dermatitis

354

Hematologic
•**Myelosuppression†→**
  ∘Macrocytic anemia→
   −Fatigue
  ∘Leukopenia→immunosuppression→
   −↑Infection & neoplasm risk
  ∘Thrombocytopenia→
   −↑Hemorrhage risk, esp. petechiae

---

†Esp. w/ concomitant:
•Renal failure
•Medications:
  ∘Allopurinol
  ∘Angiotensin converting enzyme inhibitor−ACEi

Monitoring:
•Baseline:
  ∘Complete blood count
  ∘Liver function tests, w/ treatment to be withdrawn @ plasma values >3 X the upper limit of normal
  …then q2weeks X 2months, then
    •Q2months

•**Prophylactic antibiotic coverage for perianal or fistulous Crohn's disease**, to cover:
  ∘Enterobacteriaceae, esp. Escherichia coli
  ∘Anaerobes, esp. Bacteroides fragilis

FLUOROQUINOLONES			
Generic (Trade)	M	♀	Dose
Gatifloxacin (Tequin)	K	?	400mg PO/ IV q24hours
Levofloxacin (Levaquin)	KL	?	750mg PO/ IV q24hours
Moxifloxacin (Avelox)	LK	?	400mg PO/ IV q24hours

Mechanism:
•↓DNA gyrase=topoisomerase action→
  ∘↓Bacterial DNA synthesis

Side effects:
General
  •Hypersensitivity reactions
Gastrointestinal
  •Gastroenteritis→
    ∘Diarrhea
    ∘Nausea ± vomiting
Mucocutaneous
  •Phototoxicity
Neurologic
  •Dizziness
  •Drowsiness
  •Headache
  •Restlessness
Materno−fetal
  •Fetal & child tendon malformation (including breast fed)→
    ∘↑Tendon rupture risk

&

METRONIDAZOLE (Flagyl)		
M	♀	Dose
KL	P−U in 1st trimester	500mg PO/ IV q8hours

Mechanism:
•DNA binding→
  ∘DNA strand breakage→
   −Colonic bactericidal action→↓bacteria mediated urea metabolism→↓ammonia formation

Side effects:
General
  •**Disulfuram−like reaction to alcohol**
    ∘Avoid alcoholic beverages during, & for 48hours after completion of treatment

355

Gastrointestinal
- Nausea ± vomiting–10%
- Taste changes=dysgeusia (esp. metallic taste)

Genitourinary
- Dark urine, being common, but harmless

Neurological
- Peripheral neuropathy
- Seizures

Hematologic
- Transient neutropenia–8%

SEVERE DISEASE ▬▬▬▬▬▬▬▬▬▬▬▬▬▬▬▬▬

- **Nil per os–NPO**, w/ duration dependant on severity
  - Eating >> drinking→
    - –↑Peristalsis
    - –↑Digestive enzyme release
    - …→↑pain & organ destruction
- **Parenteral hyperalimentation** via a central venous line
  Indications:
  - Severe, prolonged disease flare, as ↓caloric intake→
    - Striking protein loss & catabolism
- **Intermittent nasogastric–NG suctioning**
  - Gastric acid delivery to the duodenum→
    - –↑Pancreatic exocrine secretion
  Indications:
  - As placement has not been shown to affect clinical outcome, it is reserved for patients w/ either:
    - Intractable vomiting
    - Paralytic ileus
    - Profound pain
    - Severe disease
- **Follow urine output & daily weights**
- **Intravenous fluid**, w/ attention to both:
  - **Intravascular volume repletion via Normal saline** (0.9% NaCl) or **lactated Ringer's solution**, as per:
    - –Vital signs
    - –Physical examination
    - –Urine output (normal being ≥0.5mL/kg/h)
    - –Blood urea nitrogen–BUN & creatinine
  - **Intravascular volume maintenance via Normal saline** (0.9% NaCl) or **lactated Ringer's solution**
    Adult maintenance fluid:
    - Weight (kg) + 40= #mL/ hour
    Additional febrile requirements:
    - 1L/ 24hours for every 1°F >100°F
    Additional:
    - Estimate loss for:
      - Diaphoresis
      - Diarrhea
      - Polyuria
      - Tachypnea
    …followed by oral rehydration w/ a glucose based electrolyte solution upon both clinical stability & ability to tolerate PO
- **Prophylactic antibiotic coverage** (as for perianal or fistulous Crohn's disease) against:
  - Enterobacteriaceae, esp. Escherichia coli
  - Anaerobes, esp. Bacteroides fragilis
- **Serial abdominal physical & radiographic examinations** for possible:
  - Abscess formation
  - Dilation
  - Perforation

CROHN'S DISEASE

IMMUNOMODULATING MEDICATIONS
•The following medications usually require 1–6 months for symptomatic improvement, making these medications not useful in the control of acute disease, but rather, useful when prolonged treatment is planned. Consider combination therapy in patients who have failed 1medication

Generic (Trade)	M	♀	Dose
Methotrexate (Rheumatrex, Trexall)	LK	U	25mg PO qweek

•Once disease control is achieved, taper to the lowest effective maintenance dose in order to minimize serious side effects

Mechanism:
•Folate analog→
  ◦Dihydrofolate reductase inhibition→
    −↓DNA synthesis→cytotoxicity to all proliferating cells

Side effects:
•Concomitant use of **folic acid** 1mg PO q24h may ↓side effects without ↓efficacy
  Gastrointestinal
  •↓Mucosal cell proliferation→
    ◦Mucosal inflammation=mucositis, including inflammation of the oral mucosa=stomatitis→
      −Diarrhea
      −Nausea ± vomiting
  •Dyspepsia
  •Hepatitis→
    ◦Cirrhosis−rare
  Genitourinary
  •Bladder cancer
  •Hemorrhagic cystitis
  •Infertility
  •Miscarriage
  Lymphatic
  •Lymphadenopathy
  Mucocutaneous
  •↓Hair formation→
    ◦Alopecia
  Pulmonary
  •Interstitial fibrosis→
    ◦Pulmonary hypertension
  •**Interstitial pneumonitis−2%** (noninfectious lung inflammation), not being dose related→
    ◦Dyspnea
    ◦Nonproductive cough
    ◦Pulmonary hemorrhage→
      −Coughing blood=hemoptysis
  •Pleuritis→
    ◦Pleuritic thoracic pain
    ◦Pleural effusions
  Hematologic
  •**Myelosuppression→**
    ◦Macrocytic anemia→
      −Fatigue
    ◦Leukopenia→immunosuppression→
      −↑Infection & neoplasm risk
    ◦Thrombocytopenia→
      −↑Hemorrhage risk, esp. petechiae

Monitoring:
•Baseline:
  ◦Complete blood count
  ◦Liver function tests
  ◦Albumin
  ◦Renal function
  ◦Hepatitis B & C serologies
  ◦Chest x ray

357

...then q2month:
- •Complete blood count
- •Liver function tests, w/ treatment to be withdrawn @ plasma values >3 X the upper limit of normal
- •Albumin
- •Renal function

ANTICYTOKINE MEDICATIONS

Generic (Trade)	M	♀	Dose	Max
Adalimumab (Humira)	P	P	40mg SC qoweek	40mg qweek
Etanercept (Enbrel)	P	P	25mg SC 2X/ week	
Infliximab† (Remicade)	P	P	3mg/ kg IV over 2hours @ 0, 2, & 6weeks, then q2months	10mg/ kg
Anakinra (Kineret)	K	P	100mg SC q24hours	

†Ensure concomitant use w/ Methotrexate due to the frequent development of anti–infliximab antibodies

Adalimumab mechanism:
- •A human monoclonal antibody which binds to:
  - ◦Plasma tumor necrosis factor–TNF α, thus:
    - –Preventing its interaction w/ cell membrane TNF–α receptors
    - –↑Plasma clearance
  - ◦Cell membrane receptor bound TNF α→
    - –Antibody & cytokine dependent cytotoxicity

Etanercept mechanism:
- •A recombinant tumor necrosis factor–TNF receptor/ human IgG1 Fc domain† fusion protein, which binds to plasma TNF α & β, thus:
  - ◦Preventing their interaction w/ cell membrane TNF receptors
  - ◦↑Plasma clearance

Infliximab mechanism:
- •A chimeric IgG1 monoclonal antibody, which binds to:
  - ◦Plasma tumor necrosis factor–TNF α, thus:
    - –Preventing its interaction w/ cell membrane TNF–α receptors
    - –↑Plasma clearance
  - ◦Cell membrane receptor bound TNF–α→
    - –Antibody & cytokine dependent cytotoxicity

Anakinra mechanism:
- •Recombinant human interleukin–1 receptor antagonist–ILra

†Used to extend the in vivo half life of the receptor

Side effects:
General
- •Hypersensitivity syndrome

Gastrointestinal
- •Hepatitis–rare

Immunologic
- •Tumor necrosis factors & interleukins are required for appropriate granuloma formation & maintenance, in order to prevent progressive primary & **reactivation fungal & mycobacterial disease**, w/ suppression→
  - ◦**Severe infections (primary & reactivation)**
    - –Tuberculosis (reactivation >> primary), usually occurring within 5months of treatment, w/ extrapulmonary & widespread systemic disease, termed miliary tuberculosis, being common

Mucocutaneous
- •Mild injection site reactions

Neurologic–rare
- •Aseptic meningitis
- •Multiple sclerosis
- •Myelitis
- •Optic neuritis
- •Peripheral neuropathy

Hematologic
- •Aplastic anemia—rare
- •**Lymphoma**
- •Systemic lupus erythematosus—rare
- •Vasculitis
- •**Development of anti-medication antibodies**→
  - ∘↑Plasma clearance→
    - −↓Efficacy
  - ∘↑Infusion reactions

Adalimumab specific:
Interactions
- •Concomitant administration of Methotrexate→
  - ∘45% ↓plasma clearance

Infliximab specific:
General
- •**"Cytokine release syndrome"**→
  - ∘Fevers ± chills
  - ∘Headache
  - ∘Nausea ± vomiting
  - …associated w/ infusion
  - Risk reduction:
    - •Slower infusion rates
    - •Anti-histamine administration
    - •Antibodies containing less mouse sequence
Cardiovascular
- •**Heart failure**

Anakinra specific:
Hematologic
- •↓Neutrophil count→
  - ∘Severe neutropenia—0.3%
- •Thrombocytopenia→
  - ∘↑Hemorrhage risk, esp. petechiae

Monitoring:
- •Obtain a **purified protein derivative—PPD test** @ baseline
  - ∘Positive responders who have not previously been treated should receive appropriate treatment prior to the initiation of anti-cytokine treatment

Infliximab specific:
- •For heart failure syndrome

Anakinra specific:
- •Complete blood count @ baseline, then
  - ∘Qmonth X 3, then
  - ∘Q3months

Contraindications:
- •**Active infection**

Anakinra specific:
- •Do not use concomitantly w/ anti-TNFα medications, due to the possibility of marked immunosuppression

TOXIC MEGACOLON
- •**Decompression**, via patient rolling from side to side, & onto their abdomen

INDICATIONS FOR SURGICAL TREATMENT
- •75% of patients w/ Crohn's disease, & 25% of patients w/ Ulcerative colitis will eventually undergo a surgical procedure due to complications:
  - ∘Syndrome refractory to medical treatment
  - ∘Abscess formation
  - ∘Cancer
  - ∘Fistula formation
  - ∘Hemorrhage
  - ∘Perforation

359

∘Stricture formation
∘Toxic megacolon refractory to treatment X 48-72hours

COLORECTAL CANCER SCREENING

•**Ulcerative colitis or pancolonic Crohn's disease**
  ∘Colonoscopy, w/ multiple biopsies q1-2 years, starting @ 10years of disease, when risk ↑ 1%/ year
•**Non-pancolonic Crohn's disease**
  ∘Individualize screening

•A degenerative disease caused by any process→
 ◦**Hyperglycemia**
Statistics:
•Affects 8% of adults

 ◦Affecting 20% @ age ≥65years in the U.S. **(type 2–90% >> type 1–10%),** 50% of which are
  undiagnosed, w/ diabetes mellitus type 2 having an average diagnosis delay of 5 years
 •In the U.S., diabetes mellitus is **the #1 cause of adult:**
 ◦**Amputation**
 ◦**Renal failure**
 ◦**Vision loss**

•**Type 1 diabetes mellitus**
Mechanism:
 •**Autoimmune mediated** (anti–insulin antibodies, anti–islet cell antibodies, &/or anti–glutamic acid
  decarboxylase antibodies) **destruction of pancreatic β islet cells→**
  ◦↓Insulin secretion→
   –Hyperglycemia within several years
Risk factors:
 •**Age <40years**
 •**Body Habitus:** Normal to thin persons
 •**Genetic**
  ◦Family history
  ◦HLA haplotypes DR1, DR3, or DR4 (DR2 & DR5 being protective)

•**Type 2 diabetes mellitus**
Mechanism:
 •**Peripheral cellular insulin resistance** of unknown etiology (likely involving a post–receptor
  defect), & delayed pancreatic insulin secretion
Risk factors:
 •**Age >40years,** except gestational diabetes mellitus & MODY
 •**Body habitus: Overweight/ obese**
 •**Genetic**
  ◦Family history, having a strong genetic component
 •**Ethnicity**
  ◦Asians
  ◦Blacks
  ◦Hispanics
  ◦Native Americans
  ◦Pacific islanders
Outcomes:
 •35% require insulin at some point
Subtypes:
 •**Impaired fasting glucose** (pre–type 2)
  ◦Abnormal fasting glucose test not meeting the criteria for diabetes mellitus
  Outcomes:
   •35% progress to diabetes mellitus type 2
 •**Gestational diabetes mellitus** (type 2 of pregnancy)
  ◦Diabetes mellitus first diagnosed during pregnancy
  Outcomes:
   •75% become normoglycemic postpartum, but remain at risk for the future development of type 2
    diabetes mellitus
 •**Maturity onset diabetes mellitus of the young–MODY** (type 2 of children & adolescents)

•**Secondary diabetes mellitus**
 ◦**Medication induced**
  –Dextrose containing intravenous fluids
  –Diuretics (thiazide & loop)
  –Glucocorticoids
  –Protease inhibitors
 ◦**Stress induced,** via catecholamine & glucocorticoid release
 ◦**Pancreatic disease**
  –Chronic, relapsing pancreatitis
  –Infiltrative diseases, esp. hemochromatosis
  –Total pancreatectomy

361

- ∘**Neoplasms**, via endocrine mediated insulin antagonism
  - –↑Catecholamines: Pheochromocytoma
  - –↑Glucagon: Glucagonoma
  - –↑Glucocorticoids: Cushing's syndrome or disease
  - –↑Growth hormone: Acromegaly
  - –↑Thyroid hormones: Hyperthyroidism
- ∘**Renal failure**, via uremia

Cardiovascular
- •Hyperglycemia→
  - ∘Osmotic movement of water from the intracellular to the extracellular compartment→
    - –Cellular dehydration
    - –Plasma electrolyte dilution
  - ∘Glucosuria→
    - –↓Renal tubular fluid reabsorption
    - –↑Hunger→↑eating=polyphagia, w/ paradoxical **weight loss**
  - ...→↑**urination=polyuria**→extracellular dehydration→
    - •↑Thirst→
      - ∘↑**Drinking=polydipsia**
    - •↓intravascular volume→
      - ∘≥10% blood volume loss→
        - –↑Autonomic sympathetic tone→↑pulse
      - ∘≥20% blood volume loss→
        - –Orthostatic hypotension (supine to standing→↑20 pulse, ↓20 SBP, &/or ↓10 DBP)→ lightheadedness upon standing
        - –Urine output 20–30mL/ hour (normal being >30mL/ hour)
      - ∘≥30% blood volume loss→
        - –Recumbent hypotension &/or tachycardia
      - ∘≥40% blood volume loss→
        - –Altered mental status &/or urine output <20mL/ hour
        - –Hypovolemic shock, being hypotension + organ failure, unresponsive to fluid resuscitation
- •↓Insulin action→
  - ∘↑Activation of adipose cell lipase→triglyceride breakdown→↑plasma free fatty acids & glycerol, some of which are converted in hepatocytes to triglycerides, cholesterol, & phospholipids→ ↑lipoprotein formation→↑**atherosclerosis**†→
    - –**Coronary artery disease**→myocardial ischemic syndromes
    - –**Cerebrovascular disease**→cerebrovascular accident syndromes
    - –**Peripheral vascular disease**→renal artery stenosis, intermittent claudication, & thromboembolic disease, responsible for >50% of nontraumatic lower extremity amputations
  - ∘↑Fatty acid oxidation→
    - –**Hepatocyte ketone formation** (acetoacetic acid, β hydroxybutyric acid, & acetone) w/ acetoacetic acid being used by peripheral cells for energy (except neurons & neuroglia)
    - Note: Plasma & urine ketone measurements are based on acetoacetic acid level. The predominant ketone is β–hydroxybutyric acid, which is converted w/ treatment to acetoacetic acid→
      - •Continued ketonemia & ketonuria
  - ∘↓Protein synthesis & ↑protein catabolism (esp. within myocytes)→
    - –↑Plasma amino acids, used by peripheral cells for energy (except neurons & neuroglia)→protein wasting→weakness & other impaired organ function

---

†All patients w/ diabetes mellitus should be assumed to have underlying coronary, cerebral, & peripheral vascular disease. If the patient is found to have vascular disease, consider it as diffuse in nature

Genitourinary
- •Neuropathy, as well as hyperglycemia induced microvascular & hyperlipidemia induced macrovascular disease→
  - ∘Impotence, being the inability to achieve &/or maintain an erection–>50%, via:
    - –↓Parasympathetic tone
    - –↓Vascular blood filling of the bulbus cavernosi
- •Hyperglycemia→
  - ∘Glucosuria @ a plasma level >200mg/ dL, reflecting mean glycemia over the previous several hours
  - ∘Microvascular disease, including the glomerulus→renal disease=nephropathy, via:
    - –**Albuminuria↔renal failure**, usually @ >8years, being unlikely to occur if not evident @ ≥20 years

Categorization of albuminuria via urinary albumin (μg) ÷ urinary creatinine (mg)†:
•**<30:** Normal
•**30-299:** Microalbuminuria
•**≥300:** Macroalbuminuria
Limitations:
•The following ↑urinary albumin excretion:
  ◦Heart failure
  ◦Exercise within 24hours
  ◦Fever
  ◦Infection
  ◦Severe hyperglycemia
  ◦Severe hypertension

---

†Via a spot or 24hour urine collection. The measurement of urinary albumin without the concomitant measurement of urinary creatinine→
•Falsely ↑ or ↓determinations, as a result of variation of urine concentration

Immunologic
•Hyperglycemia→
  ◦↓Neutrophil function→
    –**Immunosuppression**→↑infection & neoplasm risk
Mucocutaneous
•Hypovolemia→
  ◦Dry mucous membranes
  ◦Dry skin→
    –↓Skin turgor→skin tenting
•**Necrobiosis lipoidoca diabeticorum**, being violet colored, thinned skin lesions ≥2cm in diameter (usually being pretibial), w/ fine superficial veins ± ulceration
•**Shin spots**, being hyperpigmented round lesions ~1cm in diameter, due to skin hypertrophy or atrophy
Neurologic
•Hyperglycemia→
  ◦Segmental axonal demyelination
  ◦Microvascular disease, including the vasa nervorum, being the vasculature supplying nerves
  …→nerve disease=**neuropathy**, over years

Peripheral symmetric polyneuropathy (sensory >> motor)
  •**Abnormal sensations, termed paresthesias** (numbness, pain, &/or tingling) beginning in the hands & feet (as longer neurons have ↑myelination, & so are affected sooner), w/ proximal progression
    ◦Numbness→
      –**Unrecognized foot trauma** (cut, blister)→↑infection risk
  Diagnosis:
    •**A nylon monofilament** designated 5.07 is pressed against the skin to the point of buckling. A patients inability to feel the buckled monofilament indicates neuropathy
  Additional exacerbatory factors:
    •Atherosclerosis mediated ↓blood supply, & hyperglycemia mediated immunosuppression→
      ◦↓**Wound healing**, w/ ↑ulcer formation

Autonomic neuropathy
    •↓**Sympathetic tone:**
      ◦Orthostatic hypotension→
        –Falls
      ◦↑Gastrointestinal tone→
        –Diarrhea
      ◦↓Hypoglycemic response, termed hypoglycemic unawareness
    •↓**Parasympathetic tone:**
      ◦Fixed, resting tachycardia
      ◦Impotence
      ◦↓Gastrointestinal tone→
        –Abdominal distention
        –Constipation
        –Nausea ± vomiting
      ◦Incomplete urinary bladder emptying, termed neurogenic bladder→
        –Overflow incontinence
        –↑Urinary tract infection risk

Ischemic neuropathy, via occlusion of the vasa nervorum, w/ sudden onset, & gradual improvement over 2–6months
- •**Mononeuropathy**, termed mononeuropathy multiplex when multiple single nerves are involved→
  - ◦Dermatomal paresthesias
  - ◦Weakness
- •**Cranial nerve palsy**, listed in order of occurrence:
  - ◦Oculomotor nerve palsy→
    - –↓Extraocular muscle contraction, except the superior oblique & lateral rectus→ptosis w/ lateral & downward eye deviation
    - –↓Iris circular smooth muscle contraction→pupil dilation=mydriasis
  - ◦Abducens nerve palsy→
    - –↓Lateral rectus muscle contraction→horizontal strabismus (lack of parallelism of the eyes, termed crossed eyes) ± diplopia
  - ◦Trochlear nerve palsy→
    - –↓Superior oblique muscle contraction→weakening of downward eye movement when looking medial ± diplopia
  - ◦Facial nerve palsy, w/ lesion of, or distal to, the facial nucleus→
    - –Ipsilateral facial muscle weakness→drooping of the lateral aspect of the lips, loss of the nasolabial fold, & inability to close the eye, raise the eyebrow, & crease the forehead†
    - –Chorda tympani nerve dysfunction→dry mouth & ↓taste of the ipsilateral soft palate & anterior 2/3rd of tongue
    - –Stapedius nerve dysfunction→stapedius muscle paralysis→hyperacusis
- •**Lumbar plexopathy**→
  - ◦Proximal pelvic &/or lower extremity paresthesias, weakness, & atrophy

---

†The ability to close the eye, raise the eyebrow, or crease the forehead indicates a lesion proximal to facial nucleus (not considered facial palsy), as the upper facial muscles receive bilateral motor cortex innervation

Opthalmologic
- •Hyperglycemia→
  - ◦Cataracts
  - ◦Glaucoma
  - ◦Microvascular disease, including the retinal vasculature→
    - –**Retinal disease=retinopathy** (visible in the macula via opthalmoscopic examination), which may be asymptomatic despite the presence of severe disease, w/ **vision loss associated w/ either macular edema &/or proliferative retinopathy**

Additional risk factors:
- •Pregnancy in diabetics may→
  - ◦Development, or transient worsening of retinopathy for up to 1year postpartum

Pre–proliferative retinopathy:
- •Initial findings, rarely impairing vision:
  - ◦**Hard exudates**, being white/ yellow lipid deposits in the outer retinal layers
  - ◦**Microaneurysms**
  - ◦**Punctate retinal hemorrhages**
  - ◦**Larger blot hemorrhages**
- •Subsequent findings, which may impair vision:
  - ◦**Soft exudates=cotton wool spots**, being superficial white lesions w/ feathery edges, indicating infarcted retinal nerve fiber layers
  - ◦**Macular edema** via damaged vasculature leaking plasma into the macula→
    - –Blurred vision
  - ◦**Intra–retinal microvascular abnormalities**
  - ◦**Venous hemorrhage**

Proliferative retinopathy:
- •**Retinal angiogenesis**→
  - ◦Growth of new blood vessels within, or on the surface of the retina &/or optic disc, which can extend into the vitreous body→
    - –**Pre–retinal, retinal, &/or vitreous hemorrhages**→unilateral blindness over hours, which may resolve, w/ the subsequent development of fibrous bands→contraction→retinal detachment→**blindness**

Hematologic
- Hyperglycemia→
  - Dehydration→
    - Pre−renal renal failure
  - Nephropathy→
    - Intra−renal renal failure
  ...→↑blood urea nitrogen−BUN & creatinine
  - A condensation reaction between glucose & hemoglobin→glycated hemoglobin, termed **hemoglobin A1c**, reflecting mean glycemia over the previous 3months
    <u>Correlation of hemoglobin A1c level & plasma glucose level:</u>
    - 6 indicates a mean plasma glucose of 135mg/ dL
    - 7 indicates a mean plasma glucose of 170mg/ dL
    - 8 indicates a mean plasma glucose of 205mg/ dL
    - 9 indicates a mean plasma glucose of 240mg/ dL
    - 10 indicates a mean plasma glucose of 275mg/ dL
    - 11 indicates a mean plasma glucose of 310mg/ dL
    - 12 indicates a mean plasma glucose of 345mg/ dL
  - Pseudohyponatremia, as every 100mg ↑plasma glucose above a baseline of 100mg/ dL→
    - Falsely measured ↓sodium by 1.6mEq/ L→hypertonic hyponatremia, termed factitious hyponatremia (hyperglycemia being the #1 cause)
    ...however, the actual measured sodium concentration should be used to calculate the anion gap in patients with hyperglycemia†, whereas, the corrected sodium concentration should be used to estimate the severity of dehydration

---

†This is because the osmotic movement of water from the intracellular to the extracellular compartment equally dilutes all electrolytes, including chloride & bicarbonate, thereby not requiring a relative correction

DIAGNOSTIC CRITERIA

- **Diabetes mellitus**
  - **Random plasma glucose ≥200mg/ dL w/ hyperglycemic syndrome**
  - **Fasting plasma glucose ≥126mg/ dL X 2**
  - **Glycosylated hemoglobin−HgA1c ≥8%** (normal: 4−6% of the total hemoglobin)

- **Impaired glucose tolerance**
  - **Fasting plasma glucose 100−125mg/ dL X 2**

- **Gestational diabetes mellitus**
  - Test as per the standard diabetes mellitus criteria listed above. If the patient does not meet criteria, perform the following tolerance testing @ >2nd trimester = >24 weeks gestation
  <u>Random oral glucose screening test:</u>
    - 50g glucose PO, being suggestive of gestational diabetes mellitus w/ a plasma glucose ≥130mg/ dL @ 1hour, necessitating fasting oral glucose tolerance testing for diagnosis
  <u>Fasting oral glucose tolerance test:</u>
    - 100g glucose PO, indicating gestational diabetes mellitus w/ ≥2 values being ↑
      - Plasma glucose ≥95mg/ dL @ fasting†
      - Plasma glucose ≥180mg/ dL @ 1hour
      - Plasma glucose ≥155mg/ dL @ 2hours
      - Plasma glucose ≥140mg/ dL @ 3hours
  <u>Statistics:</u>
  - **Gestational diabetes mellitus rule of 15's:**
    - **15%** of pregnant patients will have an abnormal random oral glucose screening test
    - **15%** of pregnant patients w/ a positive random oral glucose screening test, will have an abnormal fasting 3 hour oral glucose tolerance test, indicating gestational diabetes mellitus
    - **15%** of patients w/ gestational diabetes mellitus will require insulin
    - **15%** of patients w/ gestational diabetes mellitus will develop a macrosomic fetus

---

†Blood glucose levels ↓by ~20% during normal pregnancy

- Any **major stress**, such as:
  - ∘**Inflammation**
    - −Infection
    - −Infarction, esp. myocardial or cerebral
  - ∘**Intense pain**, usually being due to inflammation
  - ...→↑counter insulin hormone release (epinephrine, norepinephrine, cortisol, glucagon, & growth hormone)→
    - •↑Hepatic glucose release→
      - ∘Worsening hyperglycemia→
        - −Illness induced ↑insulin requirement, which may lead to either diabetic ketoacidosis−DKA or a hyperosmolar hyperglycemic state−HHS
- **Insulin noncompliance**
  - ∘Esp. w/ a major stress, as patients have ↓appetite→
    - −↓Caloric intake, causing the patient to erroneously ↓insulin amount &/or skip PO meds, when in fact, the patient actually requires ↑insulin
- **Renal failure**→
  - ∘↓Glucose excretion
- **Medications**
  - ∘Dextrose containing intravenous fluids
  - ∘Diuretics (thiazide & loop)
  - ∘Glucocorticoids
  - ∘Protease inhibitors

- **Nephropathy**, via urine albumin testing qyear, being optional once albuminuria is established
- **Retinopathy**, via opthalmologic examination qyear
  - ∘All ♀ planning pregnancy should undergo a baseline examination, w/ repeat during the 1st trimester, & subsequent follow up throughout pregnancy to 1 year postpartum
- **Neuropathy**, via foot examination, including a nylon monofilament test qyear. Once neuropathy is established, the patient should be followed by podiatry

HYPOGLYCEMIA

- Neurons & neuroglia are normally permeable to glucose regardless of the presence of insulin, & rely on glucose as their only energy source, which may be greatly diminished via insulin↑ or oral hypoglycemic treatment. **Whipples triad** is used to diagnose hypoglycemia mediated syndromes, consisting of:
  - ∘The syndrome in question
  - ∘Concurrent hypoglycemia
  - ∘Subsequent relief w/ carbohydrate administration

- **Plasma glucose of 50−70mg/ dL**→
  - ∘Neuronal sensitization→counter insulin hormone release (epinephrine, norepinephrine, cortisol, glucagon, & growth hormone)→↑hepatic glucose release, w/ catecholamines (epinephrine >> norepinephrine)→↑**autonomic sympathetic tone**→
    - −Anxiety
    - −Diaphoresis
    - −Palpitations
    - −Tachycardia
    - −Tremor
    - ...which may be blunted by β receptor blocking medications, or autonomic neuropathy
- **Plasma glucose <50mg/ dL**→
  - ∘↓Neuronal & neuroglial function→
    - −Altered mental status
    - −Blurred vision
    - −Diplopia
    - −Headache
    - −Incoordination=ataxia
    - ...w/ subsequent progression to:
      - •**Coma**
      - •Extensor limb rigidity
      - •Hypothermia
      - •Seizures
      - ...w/ subsequent progression to death

366

†Exogenously administered insulin→
  •↓Plasma & urinary C-peptide level, relative to plasma insulin
  •Injection mark
  •Insulin antibodies

TREATMENT
•**Smoking cessation** via smoking cessation clinic
  ◦Cigarette smoking contributes to 20% of deaths in the U.S., & is the #1 modifiable cause of premature death
•**Exercise**
  ◦An enjoyable form of aerobic exercise on a regular basis (≥3X/ week) for 20–30min., preceded by stretching
•**Emotional stress management**
  ◦Psychological therapy
  ◦Regular exercise
  ◦Biofeedback
  ◦Yoga
  ◦Listening to music
  ◦Gardening
•**Dietician consultation**
•**Hypertension control**
  ◦Systolic blood pressure <120mmHg & diastolic blood pressure <80mmHg
•**Weight loss if overweight/ obese†, via goal daily caloric requirement**
  ◦The caloric total needed to reach & maintain a goal weight depends on physical activity level
  ◦10 calories/ lb of goal weight +
    −33% if sedentary
    −50% if moderately physically active
    −75% if very physically active
  ◦3500 calories are roughly equivalent to 1 lb of body fat
    −Consuming 500calories less/ day X 1week→1 lb weight loss
    −Exercising 500calories/ day X 1week→1 1b weight loss
    …w/ the average human body being able to lose 3.5 lbs/ week maximum, aside from a diuretic effect
•**Nutrient composition**
  ◦Carbohydrate ~60%
  ◦Protein ~15%
    −Protein restriction to 0.7–1g/kg/24h in patients w/ diabetic nephropathy→↓disease progression
    <u>Dose adjustment:</u>
      •Patients w/ ↑catabolic states require ↑amounts
      •If concurrent nephrotic syndrome: 0.8g/kg/24hours + 1g protein/ g proteinuria
  ◦Fat ~25%
    −Mostly polyunsaturated & monounsaturated fats, w/ saturated fats comprising <10% of total caloric intake
•**Meals should be eaten regularly**, & patients should always carry a concentrated sweet‡ in case of hypoglycemic symptoms
•**Med–Alert bracelet** stating that patient is diabetic should be worn
•**Continue diabetic medications when ill**, even if eating less, as the stress of illness→
  ◦↑Insulin requirements
•↓**Concentrated sweet consumption** such as candy, ice cream, & regular sodas
•**Medication caution, as many are contraindicated in pregnancy:**
  ◦Aspirin
  ◦Angiotensin converting enzyme inhibitors–ACEi
  ◦Angiotensin receptor blockers–ARBs
  ◦HMG–CoA reductase inhibitors

---

†For obesity, medical & surgical treatment options may be used (see obesity syndromes section)
‡Patients taking an α–glucosidase inhibitor require milk, containing lactose

DIABETIC TARGET LEVELS

	Normal	Non-pregnant	Pregnant†	All
•Blood glucose				
∘Fasting & pre-prandial	<100mg/dL	90–130mg/dL	60–90mg/dL	
∘1 hour postprandial	<140mg/dL	<160mg/dL	<120mg/dL	
∘Bedtime				110–150mg/dL
∘Hemoglobin A1c (q6months‡)	4–6%			≤7%
•Blood pressure				<120/80mmHg
•Lipid profile (qyear)				
∘LDL cholesterol				<70mg/dL
∘HDL cholesterol				>45mg/dL
∘Triglycerides				<150mg/dL

•In patients w/ ↑hemoglobin A1c levels, who have attained pre-prandial glycemic target levels, check postprandial blood glucose levels
†Blood glucose levels ↓by ~20% during normal pregnancy
‡Check the hemoglobin A1c level q3months in patients:
  •Who have not attained glycemic target levels
  •Whose treatment regimen has changed

HYPOGLYCEMIC MEDICATIONS
Relative glycated hemoglobin effects:
  •Insulin: 1.5–2.5↓
  •Diet & exercise: 0.5–2↓
  •Biguanides: 1–2↓
  •Meglitinides: 1–2↓
  •Sulfonylureas: 1–2↓
  •α glucosidase inhibitors: 0.5–1↓
  •Thiazolinediones: 0.5–1↓

•All the medications, except biguanides (ex. Metformin), have the side effect of **weight gain**

SULFONYLUREAS

Generic (Trade)	M	♀	Start	Max
Glimepiride (Amaryl)	LK	?	1mg PO q24hours	8mg q24hours
Glipizide (Glucotrol)	LK	?	2.5mg PO q24hours	40mg/24hours
•XR formulation			5mg PO q24hours	20mg q24hours
Glyburide (DiaBeta)	LK	P	1.25mg PO q24hours	20mg/24hours
•Micronized form			0.75mg PO q24hours	12mg/24hours

•Administer 30min. prior to breakfast for maximal absorption

Dose adjustment:
  •May double the starting dose (except w/ the Glipizide XR formulation) in non-elderly, well-nourished patients, without hepatic or renal failure

Ideal candidates:
  •Age ≥40years @ disease onset
  •Disease duration <5years prior
  •Fasting plasma glucose <300mg/dL

Mechanism:
  •↑Pancreatic β-islet cell insulin secretion
  •↑Extrapancreatic insulin receptor sensitivity, number, & post-receptor action

BIGUANIDES

Generic	M	♀	Start	Max
Metformin (Glucophage)	K	P	500mg PO q24hours w/ a meal	1.275mg q12hours
•XR formulation			500mg PO q24hours w/ a meal	1g PO q12hours

Mechanism:
  •↓Hepatic gluconeogenesis
  •↑Extrapancreatic insulin receptor sensitivity, esp. in obese patients

Side effects:
  General
    •Anorexia→
      ∘↓Cachexia
  Gastrointestinal
    •Diarrhea
    •Nausea ± vomiting

Hematology
- **Lactic acidemia**–<0.003% of patients treated, but may be fatal

---

- **Does not cause hypoglycemia when used as monotherapy**

Contraindications:
- •Heart failure
- •Liver failure
- •**Renal failure, via creatinine ≥1.5mg/ dL**
- •Pulmonary failure
- •Underlying metabolic acidemia
- •History of alcoholism

- •Hold the medication for 2days prior to, & after any study requiring administration of a hyperosmolar contrast dye which may→
  - ∘Pre–renal &/or intra–renal renal failure

α–GLUCOSIDASE INHIBITORS

Generic (Trade)	M	♀	Start	Max
Acarbose (Precose)	GutK	P	25mg PO q8hours	If ≤60kg: 50mg PO q8hours If >60kg: 100mg PO q8hours
Miglitol (Glyset)	K	P	25mg PO q8hours	100mg q8hours

- •Should be taken at the beginning of each meal
- •<2% of the drug is absorbed

Dose adjustment:
- •Being that gastrointestinal side effects are greatest upon initiation of treatment, consider starting @ 25mg PO q24h to ↓risk, w/ subsequent titration to q8h dosing

Mechanism:
- •Inhibits small intestinal mucosal cell membrane (brush border) α–glucosidase enzymes→
  - ∘↓**Complex carbohydrate digestion**

Side effects:
Gastrointestinal
- •Abdominal discomfort
- •Diarrhea
- •Flatulence
…all of which diminish after 1–2months on the medication

- •**Do not cause hypoglycemia when used as monotherapy**
- •If hypoglycemia occurs, use PO glucose, dextrose, or lactose based products, as **table sugar, comprised of sucrose, will not be well digested**

THIAZOLINEDIONES

Generic (Trade)	M	♀	Start	Max
Pioglitazone (Actos)	L	?	15mg PO q24hours	45mg/ 24hours
Rosiglitazone (Avandia)	L	?	4mg PO q24hours	8mg/ 24hours

Mechanism:
- •↓**Hepatic gluconeogenesis**
- •↑**Glucose uptake in muscle & adipose tissue**
- •↓Fatty acid release from adipose tissue

Side effects:
Cardiovascular
- •**Fluid retention**→
  - ∘Heart failure exacerbation
Gastrointestinal
- •**Idiosyncratic hepatitis**, rarely being fatal

Monitoring:
- •Baseline liver function tests, then
  - ∘q2months during the 1st year, when hepatitis is most common, then
    - −Periodically thereafter, w/ treatment to be withdrawn @ plasma values >3X the upper limit of normal

Contraindications:
- •Patients w/ liver disease or ALT >1.5 X the upper limit of normal

MEGLITINIDES

Generic (Trade)	M ♀	Start	Max
Nateglinide (Starlix)	L ?	60mg PO q8hours	120mg q8hours
Repaglinide (Prandin)	L ?	0.5mg PO q8hours	4mg q8hours

•Administer within 30min. prior to meals

Mechanism:
- •↑Pancreatic β−islet cell insulin secretion, similar to the sulfonylureas, but w/ a faster onset of action, & briefer duration of action

INSULIN: MLK, ♀?

Indications:
- •All patients w/ Type 1 diabetes mellitus
- •Patients w/ Type 2 diabetes mellitus whose blood glucose is uncontrolled on the above medications

Human insulin type (Trade)	Onset	Peak	Duration	Appearance
VERY RAPID ACTING				Clear
Aspart (Novolog)	**15min.**	0.5–1.5h	3–5h	
Lispro (Humalog)	**15min.**	0.5–1.5h	3–5h	

Note: Very rapid acting insulins, & combinations that include them, should be **administered at the beginning of a meal**

	Onset	Peak	Duration	Appearance
RAPID ACTING				Clear
Regular	**0.5–1h**			
•Subcutaneous		2–4h	4–6h	
•Intramuscular		0.5–1h	2–4h	
•Intravenous		10–30min.	1–2h	
Semilente (small zinc crystals)	**0.5–1h**	3–5h	6–8h	

Note: Rapid acting insulins, & combinations that include them, should be **administered 30min. prior to a meal**

	Onset	Peak	Duration	Appearance
INTERMEDIATE ACTING				Cloudy
NPH	**1–2h**	4–12h	14–20h	
•A mixture of regular insulin & protamine zinc insulin				
Lente	**1–2h**	4–12h	18–24h	
•A mixture of semilente−70% & ultralente−30%				

	Onset	Peak	Duration	Appearance
LONG ACTING				
Glargine (Lantus)†	1–2h	**None**	**20–24h**	Clear
Ultralente (large zinc crystals)	4–8h	8–16h	120–36h	Cloudy

†Glargine is a recombinant DNA analog of human insulin, which forms microprecipitates in the subcutaneous tissue→
- •Delayed absorption→
  - ○↑Duration of action, w/ no discernable peak concentration, thus mimicking the continuous infusion of regular insulin via a subcutaneous pump

MIXTURES

NPH & Regular insulin
- •NPH−70% & regular−30%
- •NPH−50% & regular−50%

NPH & Aspart insulin
- •NPH−70% & aspart−30%

Lispro protamine suspension & Lispro insulin (Humalog mix)
- •Lispro protamine suspension−75% & Lispro−25%

SUBCUTANEOUS INSULIN INFUSION PUMP
- •Continuous, long−acting insulin (Ultralente) infusion via subcutaneous infusion catheter (typically in the abdominal wall), w/ bolus doses of short acting insulin (Aspart, Lispro, or Regular) prior to meals.

Dosing:
- •Start 0.3–0.5 units/kg/24h, w/ 10–20units/ 24h considered a safe starting dose→
  - ○2/3^{rds} long acting qam or 2/3^{rds} intermediate acting ÷ bid (2/3^{rds} pre−breakfast & 1/3rd @ bedtime)
  - ○1/3rd very rapid acting ÷ tid (pre−meal) or rapid acting ÷ bid (2/3^{rds} pre−breakfast & 1/3rd pre−dinner)
  - …w/ titration to achieve goal pre & postprandial levels, w/ **the usual amount needed to approach or achieve normoglycemia being ≥0.6 units/kg/24h**

•Premixed combinations are available for ease of use, but require simultaneous pre−dinner administration, whereas intermediate acting insulin is preferably administered at bedtime in order to ↓the occurrence of nocturnal hypoglycemia

Administration:
•All human insulins are prepared @ a concentration of 100units/ mL. Patients may use either a 1mL or 0.5mL, 27–29gauge disposable syringe to draw the correct amount of insulin. Perform a quick subcutaneous injection through clean skin (alcohol wipe not needed), @ 90°, or 45° in a thin patient, in order to avoid deep tissue penetration
•Insulins are administered as subcutaneous only, except regular insulin which may be administered via subcutaneous, intramuscular, or intravenous routes
•Require re–suspension:
  ◦Prior to injection, premixed insulin vials should be gently rolled 20 times between the hands, to evenly re–suspend the components
•Require gentle agitation:
  ◦All cloudy insulins
•May be mixed in the same syringe:
  ◦NPH w/ Aspart, Lispro, or Regular insulin
•May not be mixed in the same syringe:
  ◦**Glargine**, due to its low pH of 4.0
  ◦Lente or ultralente insulins, w/ either rapid or very rapid acting insulins, as their peak effect will be delayed

Absorption:
•Site absorption rate is influenced by the following:
  ◦Injection location†
    –Anterior abdominal wall > posterior arm > anterior thigh, buttocks
  ◦Injection depth
    –Deeper→↑absorption rate
  ◦Injection area blood flow
    –↑W/ exercise or massage

†Administer the medication in the same general area for predictable absorption rates

Side effects:
Mucocutaneous
  •Subcutaneous insulin injections→
    ◦**Lipodystrophy** if frequently injected @ the same site
      –Lipohypertrophy→skin thickening
      –Lipoatrophy→skin depression, occurring w/ impure preparations
Hypersensitivity
  •Animal insulin (bovine > porcine)†→
    ◦Anti–insulin antibody formation→
      –Hypersensitivity reactions
      –Insulin resistance
Hematologic
  •**Hypoglycemia**, which may be severe, requiring assistance to treat

†Patients doing well on animal insulin may remain on it, but upon initiation, human insulin is preferred

Monitoring:
•Uncontrolled
  ◦Pre–prandial & bedtime qday
  ◦1hour postprandial qday for alternating meals
•Controlled†
  ◦Type 1: 1–2X/ day
  ◦Type 2: Several X/ week

†The time of measurement should be alternated so that each (pre–breakfast=fasting, pre–lunch, pre–dinner, bedtime, & 1hour postprandial) is measured during the week

Dose adjustment:
•The insulin adjustment scale is used to cover for deficiencies, by administering that amount of rapid or very rapid acting insulin, in addition to the intended pre–meal dose. If the adjustment is needed several times over the course of a week, then the baseline insulin regimen requires titration

INSULIN DOSAGE ADJUSTMENT SCALE	
Blood glucose (mg/ dL)	Units of rapid/ very rapid acting insulin†
≤60	Eat or drink something sweet promptly & –4units
60–70	–2units
70–140	No change
141–200	+2units
201–250	+4units
251–300	+6units
301–350	+8units & drink plenty of fluids
351–400	+10units & drink plenty of fluids
>400	+12units & drink plenty of fluids

†Subtract 2 for bedtime dose

Differential for morning hyperglycemia:
- **Waning medication level**, being the #1 cause

  Treatment:
  - ↑Evening intermediate or long acting medication dosage

  Caution:
  - The patient may be experiencing the Somogyi effect, in which ↑evening medication dosage→
    - ○Worsened nighttime hypoglycemia, which may→
      - –Death

- **Somogyi effect**

  Pathophysiology:
  - Inappropriately high doses of insulin or oral hypoglycemic medications→
    - ○Nocturnal hypoglycemia→
      - –↑Counter–regulatory hormone release (epinephrine, norepinephrine, cortisol, glucagon, & growth hormone)→↑early morning blood glucose levels

  Treatment:
  - ↓Evening intermediate or long acting medication dosage

- **Dawn phenomenon**

  Pathophysiology:
  - ↑Growth hormone release hours prior to, &/or at the onset of sleep→
    - ○Early morning ↓tissue insulin sensitivity→
      - –↑Early morning blood glucose levels

  Treatment:
  - ↑Evening intermediate or long acting medication dosage

Differentiation:
- Requires the additional measurement of an early am blood glucose level in addition to the pre–bedtime & pre–breakfast levels, for several days, until the diagnosis is established

| Diagnosis | Blood glucose values: | | |
	Pre–bedtime	3AM	Pre–breakfast
Waning medication level	#	↑	↑
Somogyi effect	#	Hypoglycemia	↑
Dawn phenomenon	#	↓ to unchanged	↑

PLATELET INHIBITING MEDICATIONS

Efficacy: Glycoprotein 2b/ 3a inhibitors > thienopyridines > Aspirin
•Do not ↑hemorrhage risk in patients w/ diabetic retinopathy

Generic	M	♀	Dose
Acetylsalicylic acid–ASA=Aspirin	K	U	81mg PO q24hours

Mechanism:
•Aspirin is the only nonsteroidal anti–inflammatory drug–NSAID→
  ◦Irreversible inhibition of both cyclooxygenase–COX enzymes (COX1 & COX2), w/ COX1 being responsible for the production of both thromboxane A_2† & prostacyclin‡→
    −**Near complete inhibition of platelet thromboxane A_2 production within 15 min.**, w/ endothelial & vascular smooth muscle cells producing new enzymes in several hours→ relatively ↑prostacyclin
•Being that platelets lack the enzymatic machinery for protein synthesis, only newly formed platelets (platelet half life=10 days) have the functional enzyme
...this shift in the balance of cytokine production→
    •↓**Thrombus formation**

In Brief:
•**Cyclooxygenase–COX1 enzymes** are found in most cells of the body, being responsible for normal physiologic processes
•**Cyclooxygenase–COX 2 enzymes** are responsible for the production of inflammatory cell prostaglandins

---

•Concomitant NSAID administration→
  ◦Competition for the cyclooxygenase–COX 1 enzyme binding site, w/:
    −Unbound Aspirin being rapidly cleared from plasma
    −Bound NSAID action being reversible & short lived
    ...→↓overall antiplatelet effect, requiring either:
      •Aspirin to be taken @ ≥1hour prior to other NSAIDs
      •Switch to thienopyridine derivative for the antiplatelet effect
†Platelet mediated **thromboxane A_2** release at the site of vascular injury→
  •Platelet aggregation
  •Vasoconstriction
  ...w/ both processes→
    •Thrombus formation
‡Endothelial & vascular smooth muscle cell mediated **prostacyclin** release in the surrounding area→
  •Inhibition of platelet aggregation
  •Vasodilation
  ...w/ both processes→
    •↓Thrombus formation

Side effects:
Gastrointestinal
•Inhibition of the cyclooxygenase–COX1 enzyme→↑peptic inflammatory disease risk→↑**upper gastrointestinal hemorrhage risk** via:
  ◦↓Gastric mucosal prostaglandin synthesis→
    −↓Epithelial cell proliferation
    −↓Mucosal blood flow→↓bicarbonate delivery to the mucosa
    −↓Mucus & bicarbonate secretion from gastric mucosal cells

Indications for peptic inflammatory disease prophylaxis:
•Prophylax w/ proton pump inhibitors–PPI's, histamine 2 selective receptor blockers, or Misoprostol in patients w/ any of the following:
  ◦Age >60 years w/ a history of peptic inflammatory disease
  ◦Anticipated therapy >3 months
  ◦Concurrent glucocorticoid use
  ◦Moderate to high dose NSAID use
Note: Newer NSAIDs (Etodolac, Nabumetone, Salsalate)→
    •↓Risk of NSAID induced peptic inflammation/ ulcer

Genitourinary
- Patients w/ pre-existing bilateral ↓renal perfusion, not necessarily failure:
  - Heart failure
  - Bilateral renal artery stenosis
  - Hypovolemia
  - Renal failure
  ...rely more on the compensatory production of vasodilatory prostaglandins→
  - Afferent arteriole dilation→
    - Maintained glomerular filtration rate–GFR, whereas NSAIDs→
      - ↓Prostaglandin production, which may→renal failure

Pulmonary
- Inhibition of both cyclooxygenase enzymes (COX 1 & COX2)→
  - ↑Lipoxygenase activity→
    - ↑Leukotriene synthesis→symptomatic asthma within 2hours of ingestion in 5% of asthmatics

Rheumatologic
- Acetylsalicylic acid competes w/ uric acid secretion in the renal tubules→
  - ↑Uric acid levels→
    - ↑Risk of uric acid precipitation in the tissues=gout

Pediatric
- **Reye's syndrome**
  - A life threatening fulminant hepatitis→
    - Hepatic encephalopathy in children age ≤16 years w/ a viral infection (esp. influenza or Varicella–zoster virus–VZV)

Overdose:
Pulmonary
- Direct brainstem respiratory center mediated stimulation of pulmonary ventilation→
  - Hyperventilation→
    - **Initial respiratory alkalemia, w/ the subsequent development of an anion gap metabolic acidemia**
- Pulmonary edema

Neurologic
- Altered mental status
- Aseptic meningitis
- Depression
- Hallucinations
- Hyperactivity
- Hyperthermia
- Lightheadedness
- Seizures
- Tinnitus

Gastrointestinal
- Nausea ± vomiting

Mucocutaneous
- Pharyngitis

THIENOPYRIDINE DERIVATIVE

Indications:
- Intolerance to Aspirin

Generic (Trade)	M	♀	Dose
Clopidogrel (Plavix)	LK	P	75mg PO q24hours

Mechanism:
- Inhibits adenosine diphosphate–ADP mediated activation of the glycoprotein 2b/ 3a complex→
  - ↓Platelet activation

- A 300mg loading dose may be used, as maximal effect occurs @ 5hours rather than 5days w/ initiation of the standard 75mg dosage

Side effects:
Gastrointestinal
- Diarrhea

Mucocutaneous
- Dermatitis

Hematologic
- **Thrombotic thrombocytopenic purpura–TTP** within several weeks of initiation

374

LIPID LOWERING MEDICATIONS
•≥20% of Americans have a plasma lipid abnormality→
∘↑Cardiovascular, cerebrovascular, & peripheral vascular disease risk

Indications:
•↓Plasma LDL cholesterol to a goal of <70mg/ dL→
∘↓Atherosclerotic disease progression, w/ some degree of regression

Note: Total & HDL cholesterol levels are more accurate in the non-fasting state, whereas triglyceride levels should only be measured in the fasting state, as they are elevated after a meal. Thus, being as ↑triglycerides→↓calculated LDL level, the LDL cholesterol level may be falsely ↓in the non-fasting state. LDL values cannot be accurately calculated w/ a triglyceride level >400mg/ dL

Relative lipid effects:
•**HMG Co–A reductase inhibitors** correct all lipids, esp. Atorvastatin, Rosuvastatin & Simvastatin
•**Selective cholesterol absorption inhibitors** correct all lipids to half the extent of HMG Co–A reductase inhibitors
•**Niacin** primarily ↓triglyceride levels
•**Fibric acid medications** primarily ↓triglyceride levels
•**Bile acid sequestrants** primarily ↓LDL cholesterol levels
•**Omega–3 fatty acids** primarily ↓VLDL levels
•**Significant dietary lipid restriction** ↓total cholesterol by ~10%

HMG Co–A REDUCTASE INHIBITORS

Generic (Trade)	M ♀	Start	Max
Atorvastatin (Lipitor)	L U	10mg PO qhs	80mg qhs
Fluvastatin (Lescol)	L U	40mg PO qhs	80mg qhs
Lovastatin (Mevacor)	L U	20mg PO qhs	80mg qhs
Pravastatin (Pravachol)	L U	40mg PO qhs	80mg qhs
Rosuvastatin (Crestor)	L U	10mg PO qhs	40mg qhs
Simvastatin (Zocor)	L U	20mg PO qhs	80mg qhs

•These medications are maximally effective if administered in the evening, when the majority of cholesterol synthesis occurs

Mechanisms:
•Inhibit hydroxymethylglutaryl coenzyme A reductase function, being the hepatocyte rate limiting enzyme in cholesterol formation→
∘↓Hepatic cholesterol formation→
  –Feedback ↑hepatocyte LDL receptor formation→↑**plasma LDL cholesterol removal**
•Anti–inflammatory effects→
∘↓Atherosclerotic plaque formation, w/ ↑stability

Side effects:
Gastrointestinal
•**Hepatitis–1.5%**, usually starting within 3months of initial or ↑dose, being:
  ∘Dose related
  ∘Gradual in onset
  ∘Usually benign
•Nausea ± vomiting
Musculoskeletal
•**Myositis–3%**, being:
  ∘Dose related
  ∘Possibly sudden in onset
  ...→muscle pain &/or weakness which progress to **rhabdomyolysis <0.5%**, diagnosed via ↑creatine kinase–CK levels
  Risk factors:
  •↑Age
  •Hypothyroidism
  •Renal failure
  •Small body frame
  •Concomitant administration of:
    ∘Fibric acid medications
    ∘Bile acid sequestrants
    ∘Niacin
Neurologic
•Headaches
•Sleep disturbances
Ophthalmologic
•Minor lens opacities

Interactions

•**Garlic & St. Johns wort**→
  ○↑Hepatocyte cytochrome P450 system activity→
    −↑HMG−CoA reductase inhibitor degradation→↓plasma levels (except pravastatin)
•**Diltiazem & protease inhibitors**→
  ○↓Hepatocyte cytochrome P450 system activity→
    −↓HMG−CoA reductase inhibitor degradation→↑plasma levels (except pravastatin)

Monitoring:
- •Baseline:
  - ○**Liver function tests**, then
    - −3months after dose↑, then periodically thereafter, w/ treatment to be withdrawn @ plasma values >3X the upper limit of normal
  - ○**Creatine kinase** (as an asymptomatic ↑ may be present), then
    - −Prior to dose↑ or adding an interacting medication, in order to compare future possible values, to be obtained if symptomatic, w/ treatment to be discontinued @ either plasma values >10X the upper limit of normal, or lower if class switching fails to relieve the syndrome

SELECTIVE CHOLESTEROL ABSORPTION INHIBITORS: Relatively safe to use in combination w/ HMG−CoA reductase inhibitors

Generic (Trade)	M	♀	Dose
Ezetimibe (Zetia)	L	?	10mg PO q24hours

Mechanism:
- •Acts on the small intestinal brush border membrane enzymes→
  - ○Selectively ↓cholesterol absorption†→
    - −↓Hepatic cholesterol stores→feedback ↑hepatocyte LDL receptor formation→↑**plasma LDL cholesterol removal**

†No significant effects on lipid soluble vitamin absorption (A, D, E, K)

Side effects:
- **Gastrointestinal**
  - •Combination treatment w/ HMG Co−A reductase inhibitors→
    - ○↑**Hepatitis** risk, but **no** ↑**myositis risk**, which makes it the medication of choice for combination treatment

Monitoring:
- •Liver function tests as per concomitant HMG Co−A reductase inhibitor

FIBRIC ACID MEDICATIONS

Generic (Trade)	M	♀	Start	Max
Fenofibrate (Tricor)	LK	?	67mg PO q24hours, w/ a meal	200mg q24hours
Gemfibrozil (Lopid)	LK	?	600mg PO q12hours, prior to meals	1500mg/ 24hours

Side effects:
- **Gastrointestinal**
  - •Nausea

NIACIN

Generic	M	♀	Start	Max
Niacin	K	?	50mg PO q12hours, w/ meals	6g/ 24hours
•XR form			500mg qhs w/ a low fat snack	2g qhs

Mechanism:
- •Inhibits hepatocyte VLDL synthesis & release

Side effects:
- **Gastrointestinal**
  - •Epigastric pain
  - •Hepatitis, esp. w/ the XR form
  - •Nausea
- **Mucocutaneous**
  - •**Cutaneous flushing reaction**, being ↓ w/ NSAID administration 30 min. prior
- **Neurologic**
  - •Headache
- **Hematologic**
  - •**Hyperglycemia**
  - •↑Uric acid

BILE ACID SEQUESTRANTS				
Generic (Trade)	M ♀		Start	Max
Cholestyramine (Questran)	F ?		4g PO q24hours prior to meals	12g q12hours
Colesevelam (Welchol)	F P		3.75g=6tabs q24hours w/ a meal	5.625g=7tabs/ 24hours

Mechanism:
- Bind to intestinal bile acids→
  - ↓Bile acid absorption→
    - −Feedback ↑hepatic conversion of cholesterol to bile acids→↓hepatic cholesterol stores→
      feedback ↑hepatocyte LDL receptor formation→↑plasma LDL cholesterol removal

Side effects:
Gastrointestinal
- ↓Absorption of concomitantly administered medications. Other medications should be taken 1hour prior to, or 5hours after taking a bile acid sequestrant
- Bloating
- Constipation
- Nausea
- High doses→
  - Lipid soluble vitamin deficiencies (A, D, E, K)
  - ↑Stool fat, termed steatorrhea

COMBINATION MEDICATIONS				
Generic (Trade)	M ♀		Start	Max
Lovastatin & niacin (Advicor)	LK U		20mg/ 500mg qhs w/ a low fat snack	20mg/ 1g

DIETARY		
Generic (Trade)	M ♀	Dose
Omega 3−fatty acids (Fish oil)	L ?	A combination dose of EPA + DHA†
•Cardioprotection		1g PO q24hours
•Hypertriglyceridemia		2−4g PO q24hours

†Eicosapentanoic acid−EPA & docosahexanoic acid−DHA
- There are only 2 types of polyunsaturated fatty acids
  - Omega 3−fatty acids, mainly from:
    - **Fish or fish oils**, esp. herring, mackerel, salmon, sardines, trout, & tuna
    - −Beans, esp. soybeans
    - −Green leafy vegetables
    - −Nuts, esp. walnuts
    - −Plant seeds, esp. canola oil & flaxseed
  - Omega 6−fatty acids, mainly from:
    - −Grains
    - −Meats
    - −Nuts, esp. peanuts
    - −Plant seeds, esp. borage oil, corn oil, cottonseed oil, grape seed oil, primrose oil, safflower oil, sesame oil, soybean oil, & sunflower oil
- The Western diet is abundant in omega 6−fatty acids (which are prothrombotic & proinflammatory), w/ humans lacking the necessary enzymes to convert them to omega 3−fatty acids, which therefore need to be obtained from separate dietary sources. However, significant amounts of methylmercury & other environmental toxins may be concentrated in certain fish species (w/ high quality fish oil supplements usually lacking contaminants):
  - King Mackerel
  - Shark
  - Swordfish
  - Tilefish, aka golden bass or golden snapper
  …which are to be avoided by:
  - ♀ who may become or are pregnant
  - ♀ who are breastfeeding
  - Young children

Mechanism:
- Vasodilation→
  - ↓Blood pressure, being dose dependent, w/ a minimal effect of 4/ 2mmHg w/ doses of 3−6g q24h
- ↓Lipid, esp. triglycerides
- Anti−dysrhythmic
- Anti−inflammatory
- ↓Platelet activity

Outcomes:
- •In patients w/ coronary artery disease:
  - ◦↓All cause mortality
  - ◦↓Dysrhythmia mediated sudden death

Side effects:

Cardiovascular
- •↑Bleeding time→
  - ◦Excessive hemorrhage

Gastrointestinal
- •Belching
- •Bloating
- •Fishy aftertaste
- •Nausea ± vomiting

Hematologic
- •Hyperglycemia

Interactions
- •None known, making it safe for use in combination w/ other:
  - ◦Anticoagulant medications
  - ◦Antiplatelet medications
  - ◦Lipid lowering medications

DIETARY

Generic (Trade)	M	♀	Dosage
Garlic (Allium sativum)	?	U	600−900mg PO q24hours

Mechanism:
- •↓Blood pressure
- •↓Lipids
- •↓Platelet activity

RENAL PROTECTION

ANGIOTENSIN CONVERTING ENZYME INHIBITORS−ACEi

Generic (Trade)	M	♀	Start	Max
Benazepril (Lotensin)	LK	U	10mg PO q24hours	40mg/ 24hours
Captopril (Capoten)	LK	U	12.5mg PO q12hours	450mg/ 24hours
Enalapril (Vasotec)	LK	U	5mg PO q24hours	40mg/ 24hours
Fosinopril (Monopril)	LK	U	10mg PO q24hours	40mg/ 24hours
Lisinopril (Prinivil, Zestril)	K	U	10mg PO q24hours	40mg q24hours

Dose adjustment:
- •↓Initial dose by 50% if:
  - ◦Elderly
  - ◦Concomitant diuretic use
  - ◦Renal disease

Mechanism:
- •Reversibly inhibits angiotensin converting enzyme−ACE→
  - ◦↓Bradykinin degradation→
    - −Vasodilation
  - ◦↓Angiotensin 2 formation→
    - −Vasodilation (**arterial** > venous)
    - −↓Renal NaCl & water retention
    - −↓Adrenal cortex aldosterone release→↓renal NaCl & water retention
    - −↓Facilitation of adrenal medullary & presynaptic norepinephrine release→vasodilation
    - −Glomerular efferent arteriole vasodilation→↓intraglomerular hydrostatic pressure→↓filtration→ ↓proteinuria in patients w/ nephropathy
  - ◦↓Cardiovascular remodeling

Outcomes:
- •↓Progression of nephropathies, in part due to anti−proteinuric effects

Side effects:

Cardiovascular
- •Hypotension

Gastrointestinal
- •Altered gustatory sense=dysguesia−3%

378

Genitourinary
- •Acute interstitial nephritis
- •Patients w/ pre-existing bilateral ↓renal perfusion, not necessarily failure:
  - ◦Heart failure
  - ◦Bilateral renal artery stenosis
  - ◦Hypovolemia
  - ◦Renal failure
  - …rely more on the compensatory production of angiotensin 2→
    - •Efferent arteriole constriction→
      - ◦Maintained glomerular filtration rate–GFR, whereas either:
        - –Angiotensin converting enzyme inhibition
        - –Angiotensin 2 receptor blockade
        - …→↓angiotensin 2 production & action respectively, which may→
          - •**Pre-renal renal failure**

Mucocutaneous
- •↓Bradykinin & substance P degradation→↑levels→hypersensitivity–like syndrome→
  - ◦**Angioedema–0.4%**, usually within 2weeks of treatment, but may manifest @ months to years→
    - –Soft tissue edema of the epiglottis, face, lips, oropharynx, &/or tongue
  - ◦**Dermatitis–10%**

Pulmonary
- •↑Bradykinin levels→
  - ◦**Chronic cough–20%**, usually being dry & involuntary

Materno-fetal
- •**Fetal & neonatal morbidity & mortality**

Hematologic
- •↓Aldosterone production ± renal failure→
  - ◦**Hyperkalemia**
- •Neutropenia

Monitoring:
- •Check creatinine & potassium @ 3–10days after initiation or dose↑, then
  - ◦Q3–6months

Contraindications:
Genitourinary
- •Acute renal failure
- •Bilateral renal artery stenosis
- •Unilateral renal artery stenosis of a solitary functioning kidney

Mucocutaneous
- •Angiotensin converting enzyme inhibitor induced angioedema or dermatitis

Materno-fetal
- •Breast feeding
- •**Pregnancy**

Hematologic
- •**Potassium >5mEq/ L**

ANGIOTENSIN 2 RECEPTOR BLOCKERS–ARBs

Generic (Trade)	M	♀	Start	Max
Candesartan (Atacand)	K	?	16mg PO q24hours	32mg q24hours
Eprosartan (Teveten)	F	U	600mg PO q24hours	800mg/ 24hours
Irbesartan (Avapro)	L	U	150mg PO q24hours	300mg q24hours
Olmisartan (Benicar)	K	U	20mg PO q24hours	40mg q24hours
Losartan (Cozaar)	L	U	50mg PO q24hours	100mg/ 24hours
Telmisartan (Micardis)	L	U	40mg PO q24hours	80mg q24hours
Valsartan (Diovan)	L	U	80mg PO q24hours	320mg q24hours

Dose adjustment:
- •↓Initial dose by 50% if:
  - ◦Elderly
  - ◦Concomitant diuretic use
  - ◦Renal disease

Losartan specific:
- •Starting dose is halved if concomitant hepatic disease

Mechanism:
- •Angiotensin 2 receptor blockade→
  - ∘↓Angiotensin 2 action→
    - −Vasodilation (**arterial** > venous)
    - −↓Renal NaCl & water retention
    - −↓Adrenal cortex aldosterone release→↓renal NaCl & water retention
    - −↓Facilitation of adrenal medullary & presynaptic norepinephrine release→vasodilation
    - −Glomerular efferent arteriole vasodilation→↓intraglomerular hydrostatic pressure→↓filtration→
      - ↓proteinuria in patients w/ nephropathy
  - ∘↓Cardiovascular remodeling

Side effects†:
Cardiovascular
- •Hypotension
Gastrointestinal
- •Altered gustatory sense=dysguesia−3%
Genitourinary
- •Acute interstitial nephritis
- •Patients w/ preexisting bilateral ↓renal perfusion, not necessarily failure:
  - ∘Heart failure
  - ∘Bilateral renal artery stenosis
  - ∘Hypovolemia
  - ∘Renal failure
  - …rely more on the compensatory production of angiotensin 2→
    - •Efferent arteriole constriction→
      - ∘Maintained glomerular filtration rate−GFR, whereas either:
        - −Angiotensin converting enzyme inhibition
        - −Angiotensin 2 receptor blockade
        - …→↓angiotensin 2 production & action respectively, which may→
          - **•Pre−renal renal failure**
Materno−fetal
- **•Fetal & neonatal morbidity & mortality**
Hematologic
- •↓Aldosterone production ± renal failure→
  - ∘**Hyperkalemia**
- •Neutropenia

---

†Do not cause the hypersensitivity−like syndrome associated w/ ACE inhibitors, due to lack of bradykinin & substance P elevation

Monitoring:
- •Check creatinine & potassium @ 3−10days after initiation or dose↑, then
  - ∘Q3−6months

Contraindications:
Genitourinary
- •Acute renal failure
- •Bilateral renal artery stenosis
- •Unilateral renal artery stenosis of a solitary functioning kidney
Materno−fetal
- •Breast feeding
- **•Pregnancy**
Hematologic
- **•Potassium >5mEq/ L**

DIABETIC RETINOPATHY ━━━━━━━━━━━━━━━━━━━
- •**Pan−retinal photocoagulation†**
  Indications:
  - •Severe pre−proliferative retinopathy
  - •Proliferative retinopathy
- •**Local photocoagulation†**
  Indications:
  - •Macular edema
- •**Surgery**
  Indications:
  - •Non−clearing vitreous hemorrhage, necessitating a vitrectomy
  - •Retinal tear or detachment
  - •Traction on the macula

380

†Photocoagulation side effects:
- •Destruction of the peripheral retina→
  - ○↓Peripheral & night vision

- •The life expectancy of patients w/ diabetes is ~12years shorter than those without the disease
  - ○**70% of patients w/ diabetes mellitus type 2 will die of cardiovascular disease**

Treatment progression:
- •50% of patients will require the addition of a second medication 3 years after diagnosis
- •75% of patients will require the addition of a second medication 9 years after diagnosis

COMPLICATIONS

DIABETIC KETOACIDOSIS–DKA (Type 1 >> Type 2) ▬▬▬▬▬▬▬▬

Pathophysiology:
- •↓Insulin action→
  - ○↑Activation of adipose cell lipase→
    - –Triglyceride breakdown→↑plasma free fatty acids & glycerol
  - ○↑Fatty acid oxidation→
    - –**Hepatocyte ketone formation** (acetoacetic acid, β hydroxybutyric acid, & acetone) w/ acetoacetic acid being used by peripheral cells for energy (except neurons & neuroglia).

    Unregulated fatty acid oxidation→ketone accumulation in excess of the body's ability to metabolize or excrete them→**ketoacidemia→widened anion gap metabolic acidemia**

Acidemia mediated effects:
Gastrointestinal
- •Nausea ± vomiting

Pulmonary
- •Compensatory ↑respiratory effort→
  - ○Difficulty breathing=**dyspnea**→
    - –Respiratory rate >16/ min.=**tachypnea**
  - …w/ severe acidemia→
    - •**Kussmaul breathing,** being deep, rapid respirations, reflecting major respiratory compensation, w/ acetone being volatile→excretion in expired air→fruity odored breath
    - •Accessory muscle usage (sternocleidomastoid muscles for inspiration & abdominal muscles for expiration)
    - •Speech frequently interrupted by inspiration, termed telegraphic speech
    - •Pursed lip breathing, &/or grunting expirations→positive end–expiratory pressure–PEEP
    - •Paradoxical abdominal motion: Negative intrathoracic pressure→fatigued diaphragm being pulled into the thorax→inspiratory inward motion of the anterior abdominal wall, rather than expected outward motion due to diaphragmatic contraction

Cardiovascular
- •Altered vascular tonicity→
  - ○Vasodilation→**hypotension**→↓perfusion mediated organ failure, esp. involving the:
    - –Central nervous system→altered mental status
    - –Kidneys→renal failure
    - –Lungs→respiratory failure
    - …being termed **distributive shock** if refractory to intravenous fluid infusion

Neurologic
- •**Altered mental status**

Hematologic
- •**Hyperkalemia,** as every 0.1↓ in pH→
  - ○**0.5mEq/ L↑ in potassium** via the H^+/K^+ cell membrane exchange protein→
    - –Potassium extracellular shift
- •Hyperphosphatemia
- •↓Plasma protein–calcium binding→
  - ○↑Free plasma calcium→
    - –**Hypercalcemia,** w/ total plasma calcium being unaffected

Other:
Hematologic
- •Ketone urinary excretion→
  - ○Sodium co–excretion→
    - –Hyponatremia, w/ hydrogen electroneutral replacement→acidemia
- •Stress→
  - ○Neutrophil demargination→
    - –Leukocytosis (be careful to consider infection)

†Plasma anion gap= $[Na^+] - ([Cl^-] + [HCO_3])$
- **Normal value: 8-12 mEq/ L**
- •Equation value: 12 mEq/ L

Correction:
- **Hypoalbuminemia:** For each 1g/ dL ↓in albumin below 4, add 2.5 to the calculated anion gap
- **Acidemia:** Add 2 to the calculated anion gap
- **Alkalemia:** Add 4 to the calculated anion gap

Interpretation:
- •A widened gap indicates the **presence of excess unmeasured anions**, via either:
  - ◦Organic acids
  - ◦Phosphates
  - ◦Sulfates

HYPEROSMOLAR HYPERGLYCEMIC STATE-HHS (Type 2 >> Type1) ▬▬▬▬

Pathophysiology:
- •Tissue insulin resistance→
  - ◦Hyperglycemia, usually without ketoacidemia, as the remaining insulin sensitivity prevents unrestricted fatty acid oxidation→
    - –Dehydration→↑**plasma osmolarity**→↑extracellular osmotic pressure→cellular dehydration, including neuron & neuroglial @ **≥320mOsm/L/kg H_2O** (normal 275-295mOsm/ L)

Neurologic
- •Hyperglycemia→
  - ◦Cerebral dehydration→
    - –**Altered mental status**

Hematologic
- •Hyperglycemia→
  - ◦Dehydration→
    - –↑**Body fluid tonicity, termed osmolarity†**, being predominantly determined by **sodium**, which cannot move freely across cell membranes, thereby inducing transcellular water shifts
  - ◦Pseudohyponatremia, as every 100mg ↑plasma glucose above a baseline of 100mg/ dL→
    - –Falsely measured ↓sodium by 1.6mEq/ L→hypertonic hyponatremia, termed factitious hyponatremia (hyperglycemia being the #1 cause)
    - …however, the actual measured sodium concentration should be used to calculate the anion gap in patients with hyperglycemia‡, whereas, the corrected sodium concentration should be used to estimate the severity of dehydration

---

†The total number of dissolved solutes (in mmol/ kg) in a given solvent, correlates directly w/ the osmotic pressure exerted by the solution across a water permeable, solute impermeable membrane. It may be measured directly via the plasma, or calculated via the following formula:
2 (serum $[Na^+]$) + (blood urea nitrogen/ 2.8) + (serum glucose/ 18), normal being 280-290 mOsm/ kgH_2O
‡This is because the osmotic movement of water from the intracellular to the extracellular compartment equally dilutes all electrolytes, including chloride & bicarbonate, thereby not requiring a relative correction

DIFFERENTIATING AMONG THE COMPLICATIONS			
Factors	Hypoglycemia	DKA	HHS
Type affected	Type 1 > Type 2	Type 1 >> Type 2	Type 2 >> Type 1
Blood glucose	<50mg/ dL	>300mg/ dL	>600mg/ dL
Plasma bicarbonate		<15mEq/ L	>15mEq/ L
Anion gap		Widened	Normal
pH		<7.3	>7.3
Plasma osmolarity			>320
Etiology	Medication induced	Share the same causative etiologies	
Pulmonary acetone excretion	No	Yes	No
Altered mental status→coma→death	Yes	Yes	Yes

TREATMENT

- **Intravenous fluid**, w/ attention to both:
  - **Intravascular volume repletion†** via **Normal saline** (0.9% NaCl) or **lactated Ringer's solution**, as per:
    - −Vital signs
    - −Physical examination
    - −Urine output (normal being ≥0.5mL/kg/h)
    - −Blood urea nitrogen−BUN & creatinine
  - **Intravascular volume maintenance** via ½ **Normal saline** (0.45% NaCl), w/ **5% dextrose added when the plasma glucose is ≤250mg/ dL**, to **maintain a plasma level of 150–200** in order to:
    - −Avoid hypoglycemia
    - −Allow for neuronal adjustment to the ↓extracellular osmolarity→↓cerebral edema risk
    - <u>Adult maintenance fluid:</u>
      - •Weight (kg) + 40= #mL/ hour
    - <u>Additional febrile requirements:</u>
      - •1L/ 24hours for every 1°F >100°F
    - <u>Additional:</u>
      - •Estimate loss for:
        - ◦Diaphoresis
        - ◦Diarrhea
        - ◦Polyuria
        - ◦Tachypnea

<u>Hyperosmolar hyperglycemic state−HHS specific:</u>
- •↓**Plasma sodium @ a rate of ≤0.5mEq/L/hour†** (max 8mEq/L/24h) in order to ↓plasma osmolarity to <295mOsmol/ kg, as an abruptly ↓plasma osmolarity may→
  - ◦**Cerebral edema**→
    - −Altered mental status→death
- •The following formula shows the effect of 1L of any infusate on plasma sodium:

$$\text{Plasma sodium change} = \frac{(\text{infusate sodium} + \text{infusate potassium}) - \text{plasma sodium}}{0.55 \text{ (weight in kg)}}$$

Infusate	Na⁺ (mEq/L)	K⁺ (mEq/L)	Extracellular fluid dist.
5% NaCl in water=hypertonic saline‡	855	0	100%
3% NaCl in water=hypertonic saline‡	513	0	100%
0.9% NaCl in water=normal saline	154	0	100%
0.45% NaCl in water=1/2 normal saline	77	0	73%
0.2% NaCl in 5% dextrose in water=hypotonic saline	34	0	55%
Ringers lactate solution	130	4	97%
5% dextrose in water=free water	0	0	40%

†If plasma sodium is >155mEq/ L or volume overload is a concern, use ½ normal saline
‡Hypertonic solutions must be administered via a central venous line. In addition to their complete distribution in the extracellular compartment, this infusate→
  •Osmosis of water from the intracellular to the extracellular compartment

---

INSULIN
  •**Always measure the plasma potassium prior to initiating insulin treatment**

Generic	Dose
Regular insulin	0.1units/ kg IV bolus (usually 5–7units in adults), then 0.1units/kg/hour IV infusion or IM

INSULIN DOSAGE ADJUSTMENT SCALE

Blood glucose (mg/ dL)	Units of rapid/ very rapid acting insulin†
≤60	1 ampule D50, or eat or drink something sweet promptly, call the house officer, & −4units
60–70	−2units
70–140	**No change**
141–200	+2units
201–250	+4units
251–300	+6units
301–350	+8units
351–400	+10units
>400	+12units & call house officer

†Subtract 2 for bedtime dose

Taper:
- •Intravenous fluid & insulin can be tapered once the patient can tolerate PO intake†, & the following requirements have been met:
  - ∘**Diabetic ketoacidosis–DKA specific:**
    - −The anion gap has closed, w/ hyperglycemia usually resolving prior to ketoacidemia
  - ∘**Hyperosmolar hyperglycemic state–HHS specific:**
    - −Plasma osmolarity ≤295mOsm/ L
    - −Normalized mental status
  - …w/ the subsequent administration of regular insulin via a subcutaneous regimen & sliding scale, **w/ intravenous insulin overlap X 2hours**

Diabetic ketoacidosis–DKA specific:
- •**Why not follow the ketone level?**
  - ∘**Plasma & urine ketone measurements are based on acetoacetic acid level.** The predominant ketone is β–hydroxybutyric acid, which is converted w/ treatment to acetoacetic acid→
    - −Continued ketonemia & ketonuria
- •**Why not follow the pH level?**
  - ∘Fluid repletion→
    - −↑Ketonuria→↑tubular chloride reabsorption→prevention of ↑plasma bicarbonate→ **hyperchloremic non–anion gap metabolic acidemia**

---

†Nausea, vomiting, &/or abdominal pain usually resolve within several hours into treatment

POTASSIUM ▰

- •The typical total body potassium deficit is 3–5mEq/ kg, w/ the plasma potassium typically being normal to ↑ due to **acidemia mediated potassium transcellular shift,** which reverses during insulin & fluid therapy→
  - ∘Hypokalemia→
    - −Dysrhythmia

POTASSIUM
•**Always measure the magnesium level concomitantly**
Indications:
•Ensure a potassium of 4–5mEq/ L
Generic
If concomitant alkalemia:
•Potassium chloride–KCL
If concomitant acidemia:
•Potassium bicarbonate
•Potassium citrate
•Potassium acetate
•Potassium gluconate
•Potassium phosphate
∘Preferred in diabetic ketoacidosis–DKA due to concomitant phosphate depletion

POTASSIUM DOSAGE ADJUSTMENT SCALE†_____

Plasma K⁺ (mEq/ L)	K⁺ repletion (mEq)
≥3.9	None
3.7–3.8	20
3.5–3.6	40
3.3–3.4	60
3.1–3.2	80
≤3	100

†Half all above doses @ a glomerular filtration rate–GFR ≤30mL/ min.

Intravenous repletion guidelines:
- •Use dextrose-free solutions for the initial, repletion as dextrose→
  - ∘↑Insulin secretion→
    - −↑Potassium transcellular shift
- •The hyperosmolar infusion→
  - ∘Vascular irritation/ inflammation. Add 1% lidocaine to the bag to ↓pain
- •**Do not administer >20mEq potassium IV/ hour**
  - ∘≤10mEq/ hour prn via peripheral line. May give via 2 peripheral lines=20mEq/ hour total
  - ∘≤20mEq/ hour prn via central line
  - …as more→

| •Transient right sided heart hyperkalemia→ |
| ◦Dysrhythmias |

Outcomes:
- •Anti–dysrhythmic
- •↑Cardiac contractility in heart failure
- •Modest hypotensive effect in some patients
- •↓Cerebrovascular disease risk, apart from its possible blood pressure lowering effects

MAGNESIUM SULFATE

M ♀	**Dose**
K S	Every 1g IV→0.1mEq/ L ↑in plasma magnesium

Mechanism:
- •Hypomagnesemia→
  - ◦↓Renal tubular potassium reabsorption

PHOSPHATE

•The typical total body phosphate deficit is 1–1.5mmol/ kg, w/ the plasma phosphate typically being normal to ↑ due to **acidemia mediated phosphorous transcellular shift**, which reverses during insulin & fluid therapy→
  - ◦Hypophosphatemia

Monitoring:
- •Measure plasma phosphate 4hours after initiating therapy

Indications for repletion:
- •Plasma phosphate <1mg/ dL

Repletion:
- •7.7mg/ kg IV over 4hours

BICARBONATE

Indications for repletion:
- •pH<7
- •Shock
- •Coma

Repletion:
- •100mEq/ L in ½ Normal saline (0.45% NaCl), being infused until the indications for bicarbonate are no longer present

MONITORING

- •Measure plasma glucose qhour (fingerstick measurements may be used when the plasma glucose is <500mg/ dL), as the plasma glucose level should ↓10% after 1h. If not, ↑the infusion rate by 50–100% (IM insulin by 25–50%) qhour until the desired response is achieved
- •Measure plasma electrolytes q1hour

PROGNOSIS

- •**Diabetic ketoacidosis–DKA:** <5% mortality rate in experienced medical centers
- •**Hyperosmolar hyperglycemic state–HHS:** 15% mortality rate

•Caused by, in order of frequency:
∘↑Production
∘Cellular lysis mediated release
∘Exogenous consumption
...of tetraiodothyronine−T4 (also termed thyroxine) &/or triiodothyronine−T3→
  •Hyperthyroidism→
   ∘↑Cellular metabolism throughout the body
   ∘↑β receptor number & affinity throughout the body

SYNDROMAL CLASSIFICATION ▬▬▬▬▬▬▬
•**Subclinical hyperthyroidism**
∘High normal range thyroid hormone→
 −Feedback mediated ↓thyroid stimulating hormone−TSH
Risk factors:
 •Hypothalamic or pituitary disease
 •Severe disease
 •Medications
  ∘Dopamine
  ∘Glucocorticoids
  ∘Phenytoin
Careful: As this may indicate neoplastic mediated β−human chorionic gonadotropin−βhCG secretion

•**Apathetic hyperthyroidism**
∘Hyperthyroid persons who, for unknown reasons, **lack the typical hyperadrenergic syndrome**
 Risk factors:
 •Elderly
 •Medications
  ∘β receptor blockers

•**Thyroid storm, being a medical emergency**
∘Hyperthyroidism→either:
 −**Altered mental status**
 −**Fever**
 −**High output heart failure**
 ...± nausea, vomiting, &/or diarrhea. This may progress to shock & death if untreated
Risk factors:
 •Hyperthyroidism w:
  ∘Abrupt discontinuation of anti−thyroid hormone medications
  ∘Inflammation
   −Infection
   −Surgery
   −Trauma
  ∘Diabetic ketoacidemia−DKA
  ∘Medications
   −Adrenergic medications
   −Anticholinergic medications
   −Iodine containing medications
   −Thyroid hormone ingestion
  ∘Pregnancy

ETIOLOGIC CLASSIFICATION ▬▬▬▬▬▬▬
•**Autoimmune**
∘**Graves' disease−90%**
 Pathophysiology:
 •**Anti−thyroid stimulating hormone−TSH receptor antibodies**→
  ∘↑Receptor activation (rather than immune mediated destruction)→
   −**Diffuse gland hypertrophy, termed goiter**→hyperthyroidism
 Risk factors:
 •Age: 20−50 years
 •Gender: ♀ > ♂

- **Neoplastic**
  - ∘**Thyroid adenoma**
  - ∘Thyroid adenocarcinoma–rare
  - Risk factors:
    - •Age: ≥40years
    - •History of iodine deficiency
    - •History of neck radiation
  - Other neoplastic causes:
    - •Thyroid stimulating hormone–TSH secreting anterior pituitary adenoma or adenocarcinoma
    - •**Ovarian germ cell neoplasia**, as 10% of teratomas contain functional thyroid tissue, being termed **struma ovarii** if it is the predominant tissue
    - •Neoplastic secretion of β–human chorionic gonadotropin–βhCG, as it is composed of α & β subunits, w/ the α subunit being identical to that of thyroid stimulating hormone–TSH
      - ∘**Testicular germ cell neoplasia**
      - ∘**Trophoblastic tumors**
        - –Hydatidiform mole
        - –Choriocarcinoma
      - ∘**Gestational hyperthyroidism**, via placental β–human chorionic gonadotropin–βhCG secretion, being esp. ↑during the 1ˢᵗ 4 months, also→
        - –Hyperemesis gravidarum, being dangerously excessive vomiting during pregnancy

- **Medications**
  - ∘Iodine containing medications
    - –Amiodarone, also→thyroiditis
    - –Guaifenesin
    - –Iodinated radiocontrast dye
    - ...→↑all phases of thyroid hormone production, termed the Jod–Basedow effect→
  - Risk factors:
    - •Thyroid neoplasia

- **Inflammation=thyroiditis**
  - Pathophysiology:
    - •Thyroiditis→
      - ∘Cell destruction→↑thyroid hormone release→**transient hyperthyroidism** X 2–8 weeks, w/ subsequent:
        - –↓Cellular hormonal store
        - –Feedback mediated anterior pituitary TSH suppression
        - ...→**transient hypothyroidism** X 2–4weeks, w/ subsequent return to a **euthyroid state**
  - Subclassification:
    - •**Viral thyroiditis**, termed subacute, de Quervain's, or granulomatous thyroiditis
    - •**Bacterial thyroiditis**, termed acute, pyogenic, or suppurative thyroiditis, being rare
    - •**Reidel's thyroiditis–rare**, being cause by thyroid gland inflammation→
      - ∘Fibrosis
    - •**Postpartum thyroiditis**, being caused by an autoimmune mediated attack on the thyroid gland, usually occurring @ 2–8 months postpartum in 6% of ♀

- **Other**
  - ∘↑Consumption of thyroid hormone medication, termed **thyrotoxicosis medicamentosa**, usually being due to either:
    - –Psychiatric disease
    - –Desire for weight loss
  - ∘Anterior pituitary resistance to thyroid hormone–very rare

General
- •↑Cellular metabolism→
  - ∘↑**Appetite w/ paradoxical ↓weight**
  - ∘Fatigue
  - ∘Hyperactivity
  - ∘Palpable **thyroid gland enlargement**, being either diffuse, termed goiter, or focal, unless ectopic thyroid hormone secretion→
    - –Feedback mediated inhibition of both the hypothalamus & anterior pituitary gland→↓thryroid stimulating hormone–TSH secretion→thyroid gland atrophy
  - ∘Infectious thyroiditis→
    - –Significant thyroid gland tenderness ± pain radiation to the mandible &/or ears

Cardiovascular
- •↑Cardiac conduction tissue β1 receptor number & affinity→↑cardiac autonomic sympathetic tone→
  - ∘**Tachycardia**
  - ∘↑Cardiac output→
    - –**Systolic hypertension**→↑pulse pressure (systolic – diastolic blood pressure)
  - ∘**Dysrhythmia** (atrial > ventricular)
- •↑Vascular smooth muscle β2 receptor number & affinity→
  - ∘Arteriole vasodilation→
    - –↓Peripheral vascular resistance→↓diastolic blood pressure
- •↑Cellular metabolism→
  - ∘Thyroid bruit, unless ectopic thyroid hormone secretion→
    - –Feedback mediated inhibition of both the hypothalamus & anterior pituitary gland→↓thyroid stimulating hormone–TSH secretion→thyroid gland atrophy

Cutaneous
- •↑Cellular metabolism→
  - ∘↑Heat production→
    - –↑Peripheral vasodilation→**warmth**→**diaphoresis & heat intolerance**
  - ∘↑Sebum production→
    - –**Acne**
  - ...→warm & soft skin
  - ∘Fine hair
  - ∘Gynecomastia, being the ↑development of male mammary glands
  - ∘Onycholysis, being nail loosening, usually incomplete, & at the free border
  - ∘Clubbing of the fingers & toes, termed thyroid acropachy–rare

Gastrointestinal
- •↑Cellular metabolism→
  - ∘↑Gastrointestinal motility→
    - –Borborygmi, being gurgling noises due to the movement of gas in the gastrointestinal tract
    - –Abdominal pain
    - –**Diarrhea**
  - ∘↑Mucous secretion

Genitourinary
- •↑Cellular metabolism→
  - ∘↓Libido, being sexual desire→
    - –Impotence, being the inability to achieve &/or maintain an erection
  - ∘↓Menstrual hemorrhage
  - ∘↑Urine formation→urinary frequency

Musculoskeletal
- •↑Cellular metabolism→
  - ∘↑Myocyte protein catabolism→
    - –**Proximal muscle weakness**
  - ∘↑Osteoclast stimulation→
    - –Osteoporosis

Neurologic
- •↑Somatic motor neuron terminal β2 receptors→
  - ∘**Fine tremor** @ 10–15X/ second, best visualized via:
    - –Placing a sheet of paper on the patients outstretched palms
    - –Tongue fasciculation
    - –Tremor of lightly closed eyelids
- •↑Cellular metabolism→
  - ∘**Hyperreflexia**
  - ∘↑Cerebration→
    - –Alertness, w/ ↓concentration
    - –Anxiety
    - –Emotional lability
    - –Hyperactivity
    - –Irritability
    - –Rapid speech
    - –Insomnia
    - –Delirium
    - –Psychosis
    - –Depression

Pulmonary
- •↑Cellular metabolism→
  - ∘Breathlessness=dyspnea

388

Hematologic
•**Subclinical hyperthyroidism**
　○High normal thyroid hormone, w/ feedback mediated ↓anterior pituitary thyroid stimulating
　hormone–TSH secretion
•**TSH secreting neoplasm, or anterior pituitary thyroid hormone resistance**
　○↑Thyroid stimulating hormone–TSH secretion→
　　–↑Thyroid hormone
•**All others**
　○↑Thyroid hormone, w/ feedback mediated ↓anterior pituitary thyroid stimulating hormone–TSH
　secretion
　Subsyndromes:
　　•**Graves' disease:** Anti–thyroid stimulating hormone–TSH receptor antibodies–80%
　　•**Infectious thyroiditis:** ↑Erythrocyte sedimentation rate–ESR
　　•**βHCG secreting neoplasia:** ↑↑βHCG
　Other findings:
　　•Hypercalcemia
　　•↓Plasma lipids

•Altered plasma thyroxine binding globulin level→
　○Inversely proportional alteration of **active, free thyroid hormone**, without any effect on the total
　plasma content
　↑Plasma thyroxine binding globulin level:
　　•Estrogen containing medications
　　　–Hormone replacement therapy–HRT
　　　–Oral contraceptive pills–OCPs
　　•Hepatitis
　　•Pregnancy

　↓Plasma thyroxine binding globulin level:
　　•Androgens
　　•Cirrhosis
　　•Glucocorticoids
　　•↑Growth hormone→
　　　○Acromegally
　　•Nephritic syndrome
　　•Phenytoin

GRAVES' DISEASE SPECIFIC SYNDROME ▬▬▬▬▬▬▬▬▬▬▬▬▬▬▬▬▬▬▬
Cutaneous
•Local mucopolysaccharide mediated non–pitting edema, termed **circumscribed myxedema**, as
　it usually has sharp, raised borders, w/ an orange peel like appearance
　○Usually forming on the pretibial region, termed **pretibial myxedema–3%**
•Pruritus
•Urticaria
Opthalmologic
•Extraocular myocyte &/or adipocyte autoantibodies→
　○Extraocular muscle inflammation (unilateral or bilateral)→
　　–Intraorbital edema (>90% via magnetic resonance imaging–MRI)
　　–Periorbital edema→eyelid edema
　…w/ lymphocytic infiltration→↑intraorbital pressure→
　　•**Protrusion of the eyeballs, termed exopthalmos**, being apparent in 20–40%, & severe in
　　5% of affected persons→
　　　○Optic nerve compression &/or stretching→
　　　　–↓Visual acuity
　　　　–Altered color vision
　　　　–Diplopia
　　　　…w/ possible progression to blindness
•↑Levator palpebrae muscle tone, w/ concomitant inflammation mediated fibrosis→
　○Eyelid retraction→
　　–**Lid lag**, being observed as the upper eyelids fail to continuously cover the superior limbal
　　margin during descending gaze
　…both→
　　•Stare
　　•↑Corneal exposure→
　　　○Dryness→
　　　　–Conjunctival inflammation=conjunctivitis
　　　　–Corneal inflammation=keratitis→erythema, irritation, photophobia, &/or ulceration

389

Lymphatics
•Lymphadenopathy
•Splenomegally
•Thymus enlargement

IMAGING

•**Radioactive iodine** (I^{123}) **uptake–RAIU scan**
Mechanism:
  •Thyrotrope radioactive iodine uptake→
    ◦Thyroid irradiation, allowing visualization
Findings:
  •**Diffusely ↑thyroid uptake** via either:
    ◦**Graves' disease**
    ◦β–human chorionic gonadotropin–βhCG secreting neoplasm
    ◦Thyroid stimulating hormone–TSH secreting neoplasm
    ◦Anterior pituitary thyroid hormone resistance
  •**Focal or multifocal ↑thyroid uptake** via:
    ◦Thyroid neoplasia (adenoma >> adenocarcinoma)
  •**No thyroid uptake** via:
    ◦Thyroiditis
    ◦Iodine containing medication induced
    ◦Thyrotoxicosis medicamentosa
  •**Ectopic uptake** via either:
    ◦Struma ovarii
    ◦Thyroid cancer metastasis
Outcomes:
  •Being as it is normal in up to 50% of hyperthyroid patients, a normal test does not exclude
  hyperthyroidism

TREATMENT

β1 SELECTIVE RECEPTOR BLOCKERS

Indications:
  •Hypertension (β1)
  •Tachycardia (β1)
  •Tremor (β2)

Generic (Trade)	M	♀	Start	Max
Atenolol (Tenormin)	K	U	25mg PO q24hours	100mg/ 24hours
Metoprolol (Lopressor)	L	?	25mg PO q12hours	225mg q12hours
•XR form (Toprol XL)			50mg PO q24hours	400mg q24hours

α1 & NONSELECTIVE β RECEPTOR BLOCKERS

Generic (Trade)	M	♀	Start	Max
Carvedilol (Coreg)	L	?	6.25mg PO q12hours	25mg q12hours
Labetalol (Normodyne)	LK	?	100mg PO q12hours	1200mg q12hours

Mechanism:
  •Competitive antagonist of the β1 ± β2 receptor→
    ◦↓Sinoatrial & atrioventricular node conduction (β1)→
      –↓Pulse
    ◦Anti–dysrhythmic via nodal effects (β1)
    ◦↓Cardiac muscle contractile strength (β1)
    ◦↓Juxtaglomerular cell renin release (β1)→
      –↓Angiotensin 1, angiotensin 2, & aldosterone formation
    ◦↓Cardiovascular remodeling
    ◦↑Vascular/ organ smooth muscle contraction (β2)→
      –Vasoconstriction
      –Bronchoconstriction
      –Uterine contraction
    ◦↓Tremor (β2)
    ◦↓Hepatocyte glycogenolysis (β2)
  •↓Extrathyroidal tetraiodothyronine–T4 (also termed thyroxine) conversion to the more metabolically
  active triiodothyronine–T3 form

Side effects:
 General
  •Fatigue
  •Malaise
 Cardiovascular
  •Bradycardia ± heart block
  •Hypotension
   ∘Orthostatic hypotension
   ∘Pelvic hypotension→
    −Impotence, being the inability to achieve &/or maintain an erection
  •Initial worsening of systolic heart failure
  •Worsening symptoms of peripheral vascular disease
   ∘Intermittent claudication
   ∘Raynaud's phenomenon
 Pulmonary
  •Bronchoconstriction
 Endocrine
  •↑Risk of developing diabetes mellitus
  •May block catecholamine mediated:
   ∘Physiologic reversal of hypoglycemia via:
    −↓Hepatocyte gluconeogenesis
   ∘↓Hypoglycemic symptoms, termed hypoglycemic unawareness→
    −↓Tachycardia as a warning sign
 Gastrointestinal
  •Diarrhea
  •Nausea ± vomiting
  •Gastroesophageal reflux
 Mucocutaneous
  •Hair thinning
 Neurologic
  •Sedation
  •Sleep alterations
  •↓Libido→
   ∘Impotence
 Psychiatric
  •Depression
 Hematologic
  •↓High density lipoprotein−HDL levels

•Most patients w/ chronic obstructive pulmonary disease−COPD (including asthma), diabetes, &/or peripheral vascular disease can be safely treated w/ **cardioselective β1 receptor blockers,** as they have ↓peripheral effects

Contraindications:
 Cardiovascular
  •**Acutely decompensated heart failure**
  •Hypotension
  •Pulse <50bpm
  •Atrioventricular heart block of any degree
 Pulmonary
  •Moderate to severe chronic obstructive pulmonary disease−COPD, including asthma
 Hyper−catacholamine state
  •Amphetamine use
  •**Cocaine use†**
  •Clonidine withdrawal
  •Monoamine oxidase inhibitor−MAOi mediated tyramine effect
  •Pheochromocytoma
   ...→relatively ↑vascular α1 receptor stimulation="unopposed α effect"→
    •Vasoconstriction→
     ∘Myocardial ischemic syndrome
     ∘Cerebrovascular accident syndrome
     ∘Peripheral vascular ischemic syndrome
   Note: **Carvedilol** & **Labetalol** may be used due to their α1 blocking property

---

†Cocaine use→
  •Varying ischemic syndrome onset per administration route, & may occur @ min. to days (usually within 3hours)

391

ANTIDOTES				
Generic	M	♀	Dose	Max
Glucagon	LK	P	3mg IV slow push over 1min., then 5mg IV slow push over 1 min. if needed	
•Continuous infusion			5mg/ hour	
10% Calcium chloride†			10mL (1 ampule) IV slow push over 3min., q5min. prn	
•Continuous infusion			0.3mEq/ hour	0.7mEq/ h
Onset: 1–2 min., Duration: 30–60 min.				

†Use cautiously in patients taking digoxin, as hypercalcemia→
•Digoxin cardiotoxicity

THIONAMIDE COMPOUNDS				

Indications:
•Temporary treatment, to be used for all patients, as etiology will or may remit
  ◦It may take several weeks for the patient to begin feeling better, as these agents have no effect on previously synthesized thyroid hormone in the form of thyroglobulin. Therefore, allow for administration X 2months prior to beginning titration based on monthly thyroid function tests

Generic (Trade)	M	♀	Dose	Max
Methimazole	L	U	5mg, 10mg, or 20mg PO q8h for mild, moderate, or thyroid storm respectively	120mg/ 24h
Propylthiouracil–PTU	L	U†	100mg, 200mg, or 400mg PO q8h for mild, moderate, or thyroid storm respectively	1200mg/ 24h

†Preferred over Methimazole as it does not cross the placenta as well

Mechanism:
•Inhibit 2 steps essential to thyroid hormone production (but not thyroglobulin production)→
  ◦↓Thyroid hormone production→
    –Feedback mediated ↑thyroid stimulating hormone–TSH secretion→↑thyroglobulin production, being stored intracellularly→**diffuse thyroid gland enlargement, termed goiter**

Additional Propylthiouracil mechanism:
•↓Extrathyroidal tetraiodothyronine–T4 conversion to the more metabolically active triiodothyronine–T3

Outcomes:
•50% breakthrough hyperthyroidism risk @ ≥1year

Side effects:
  Gastrointestinal
    •Hepatitis
  Hematologic
    •**Reversible agranulocytosis <0.1%**

Monitoring:
•Obtain a baseline complete blood count, w/ subsequent periodic monitoring, as indicated via signs of persistent infection, such as persistent pharyngitis &/or fevers

ADDITONAL TREATMENT FOR THYROID STORM ▬▬▬▬▬▬▬▬▬▬
•**Intravenous access** via 2 large bore (≤ #18 gauge) peripheral lines
•**Intravenous fluid,** due to intravascular volume depletion via fever ± vomiting &/or diarrhea
  ◦**Intravascular volume repletion via Normal saline** (0.9% NaCl) or **lactated Ringer's solution,** as per:
    –Vital signs
    –Physical examination
    –Urine output (normal being ≥0.5mL/kg/h)
    –Blood urea nitrogen–BUN & creatinine
  ◦**Intravascular volume maintenance via Normal saline** (0.9% NaCl) or **lactated Ringer's solution**
    Adult maintenance fluid:
      •Weight (kg) + 40= #mL/ hour
    Additional febrile requirements:
      •1L/ 24hours for every 1°F >100°F
    Additional:
      •Estimate loss for:
        ◦Diaphoresis
        ◦Diarrhea
        ◦Polyuria
        ◦Tachypnea

392

...followed by oral rehydration w/ a glucose based electrolyte solution upon both clinical stability & ability to tolerate PO

SYSTEMIC GLUCOCORTICOID TREATMENT			
Generic	M	♀	Dose
Hydrocortisone (Cortef)	L	?	300mg IM/ IV bolus, then 100mg IM/ IV q8hours

•Once disease control is achieved, taper to the lowest effective maintenance dose in order to minimize serious side effects, w/ the goal of discontinuation if possible, w/ attention to relapse

Glucocorticoids	Relative potencies		Duration	Dose equiv.
	Anti-inflammatory	Mineralocorticoid		
Cortisol (physiologic†)	1	1	10hours	20mg
Cortisone (PO)	0.7	2	10hours	25mg
Hydrocortisone (PO, IM, IV)	1	2	10hours	20mg
Methylprednisolone (PO, IM, IA, IV)	5	0.5	15-35hours	5mg
Prednisone (PO)	5	0.5	15-35hours	5mg
Prednisolone (PO, IM, IV)	5	0.8	15-35hours	5mg
Triamcinolone (PO, IM)	5	~0	15-35hours	5mg
Betamethasone (PO, IM, IA)	25	~0	35-70hours	0.75mg
Dexamethasone (PO)	25	~0	35-70hours	0.75mg
Fludrocortisone (PO)	10	125	10hours	

†The physiologic rate of adrenal cortical cortisol production is 20-30mg/ 24hours

Mechanism:
•↓Extrathyroidal tetraiodothyronine−T4 conversion to the more metabolically active triiodothyronine−T3
•Also, thyroid storm→
  ∘↑↑Glucocorticoid metabolism→
    −Relative adrenal insufficiency→hypotension

& EITHER

IODINE: Only to be administered after a thionamide compound, in order to ↓the risk of possible iodine induced hyperthyroidism

Generic	Dose
Lugol's solution	5-10drops (6.3mg iodide/ drop) PO q8h in water or juice
Saturated solution of potassium iodide	1-2drops (38mg iodide/ drop) PO q8h in water or juice
Sodium iodide	500-1000mg IV q12hours

Mechanism:
•Iodine ingested in its typical bound iodide form→
  ∘↓All phases of thyroid hormone production @ 100X the normal plasma level, termed the Wolff Chaikoff effect→
    −↓Thyroid hormone production→feedback mediated ↑anterior pituitary thyroid stimulating hormone−TSH secretion
    −↓Thyroid gland size & vascularity

OR

LITHIUM

Indications:
•Hypersensitivity reaction to iodine

M	♀	Dose
K	U	300mg PO q8hours

Mechanism:
•↓Thyroid hormone release→
  ∘Feedback mediated ↑anterior pituitary thyroid stimulating hormone−TSH secretion

Side effects:
Cardiovascular
  •Dysrhythmias
Endocrine
  •Diffuse thyroid gland enlargement, termed goiter
Gastrointestinal
  •Abdominal pain
  •Diarrhea
  •Nausea ± vomiting

Genitourinary
- •Antidiuretic hormone–ADH receptor antagonism→
  - ∘**Nephrogenic diabetes insipidus**

Mucocutaneous
- •Edema

Neurologic
- •Ataxia
- •↓Communication ability (expression &/or understanding)=aphasia
- •Hyporeflexia
- •Sedation
- •Tremor

Hematologic
- •Leukocytosis

Contraindications:
- •Pregnancy, due to congenital cardiac abnormalities

DEFINATIVE TREATMENT ▄▄▄▄▄▄▄▄▄▄▄▄▄▄▄▄▄▄▄▄▄▄▄▄▄▄▄▄▄▄▄
•**Radioactive iodine (I^{131}) ablation therapy**
  Mechanism:
  - •Thyrotrope radioactive iodine uptake→
    - ∘Thyroid irradiation→
      - –Cellular death, inflammation, & fibrosis
  Outcomes:
  - •Eventual hypothyroidism >75%, which may occur days to decades later

•**Surgery†**
  ∘**Subtotal thyroidectomy for Graves' disease**
    Side effects:
    - •**Immediate onset hypothyroidism–10%**, then 3%qyear afterwards
    - •Hypoparathyroidism
    - •Recurrent hyperthyroidism, even years later
    - •Recurrent laryngeal nerve paralysis→
      - ∘Hoarseness

  ∘**Total thyroidectomy for thyroid cancer**
    Side effects:
    - •**Immediate onset hypothyroidism**, unless metastatic disease is present
    - •Hypoparathyroidism
    - •Recurrent laryngeal nerve paralysis→
      - ∘Hoarseness

---

†Iodine, as above, is given to patients prior to thyroidectomy→
- •↓Thyroid gland size & vascularity→
  - ∘↓Surgical complications

PROGNOSIS
•**Graves' disease:** The course is typically chronic, but spontaneous remission occurs in 25% of patients within several months (usually in patients w/ a mild syndrome)
•**Thyroid storm:**10% mortality w/ treatment, being ~100% without treatment

•Caused by ↓production &/or release of tetraiodothyronine−T4 (also termed thyroxine) &/or triiodothyronine−T3→
  ◦Hypothyroidism→
    −↓Cellular metabolism throughout the body
    −↓β receptor number & affinity throughout the body
Statistics:
  •>99% being caused by either:
    ◦Autoimmune thyroiditis
    ◦Thyroid ablation

CLASSIFICATION/ RISK FACTORS
SYNDROMAL CLASSIFICATION ▬▬▬▬▬▬
•Subclinical hypothyroidism
  ◦Low normal range thyroid hormone→
    −Feedback mediated ↑thyroid stimulating hormone−TSH

•Myxedema coma, being a medical emergency
  ◦Hypothyroidism→either:
    −Altered mental status
    −Hypothermia
Risk factors:
  •Hypothyroidism w:
    ◦Abrupt discontinuation of thyroid hormone medications
    ◦Inflammation
      −Infection
      −Surgery
      −Trauma
    ◦Diabetic ketoacidemia−DKA
    ◦Pregnancy

ETIOLOGIC CLASSIFICATION ▬▬▬▬▬▬▬▬▬▬▬▬▬▬▬▬▬
•Autoimmune thyroiditis, termed Hashimoto's thyroiditis
Pathophysiology:
  •Cellular & antibody mediated thyroid destruction→
    ◦Thyroid gland inflammation=thyroiditis→
      −Cell destruction→↑thyroid hormone release→transient hyperthyroidism
      −Thyroid gland edema→diffuse thyroid gland enlargement, termed goiter
      ...w/ subsequent fibrosis→
        •Hypothyroidism
        •Small contracted thyroid gland
Risk factors:
  •↑Age
  •Gender: ♀7 X ♂
  •Genetic:
    ◦Family history of autoimmune thyroiditis

•Post−ablation hypothyroidism
  ◦May develop days to decades after treatment
Risk factors:
  •Subtotal thyroidectomy, developing immediately after total thyroidectomy for thyroid cancer, unless metastatic disease is present
  •Radioactive iodine (I^{131}) ablation therapy, occurring days to decades later in >75% of patients
  •External beam irradiation involving the neck (ex: neck cancers or Hodgkins lymphoma)

•Medications
  ◦Iodine containing medications
    −Amiodarone
    −Guaifenesin
    −Iodinated radiocontrast dye
    ...→↓all phases of thyroid hormone production, termed the Jod Basedow effect
  ◦Other
    −Aminoglutethimide
    −Interferon α
    ...→reversibly ↓thyroid function

- **Euthyroid sick syndrome**
  - ∘Occurring in 25% of hospitalized patients, due to **severe &/or chronic illness**→inflammatory cytokines→
    - −↓Anterior pituitary thyroid stimulating hormone−TSH secretion
    - −↑Tetraiodothyronine−T4 metabolism
    - ...→↓active free T4, w/ an **inappropriately normal thyroid stimulating hormone−TSH level**, rather than the expected ↑value

Rare etiologies:
- **Central hypothyroidism**
  - ∘**Hypothalamic or pituitary disease**
    - −Infection
    - −Neoplasm
    - −Postpartum pituitary necrosis, termed Sheehan's syndrome
    - −Post−radiation fibrosis
- **Severe dietary iodine deficiency**
  Pathophysiology:
    - •↓↓Dietary iodine (<50mg/ year)→
      - ∘↓Thyroid hormone production, but not the production of thyroglobulin, w/ feedback mediated ↑anterior pituitary thyroid stimulating hormone−TSH secretion→
        - −↑Thyroglobulin production→**diffuse thyroid enlargement, termed goiter**
  Risk factors:
    - •Living in underdeveloped countries
- **Genetic**
  - ∘Defect of thyroid organogenesis
  - ∘Thyroid cell enzyme defect &/or deficit→
    - −↓Thyroid hormone production, but not the production of thyroglobulin, w/ feedback mediated ↑thyroid stimulating hormone−TSH secretion→↑thyroglobulin production→**diffuse thyroid enlargement, termed goiter**
  - ∘Tissue resistance to triiodothyronine−T3, being due to a rare familial genetic mutation of the cellular T3 receptor→
    - −Feedback mediated ↑thyroid stimulating hormone−TSH secretion→↑thyroglobulin production→ **diffuse thyroid enlargement, termed goiter**

DIAGNOSIS

General
- •↓Cellular metabolism→
  - ∘↓**Appetite, w/ paradoxical ↑weight**
  - ∘Fatigue
  - ∘Hypoactivity
  - ∘Palpable **diffuse thyroid gland enlargement**, due to either:
    - −Autoimmune thyroiditis, initially
    - −Iodine deficiency
    - −Tissue resistance to triiodothyronine−T3

Cardiovascular
- •↓Cardiac conduction tissue β1 receptor number & affinity→↓cardiac autonomic sympathetic tone→
  - ∘**Bradycardia**
- •↓Vascular smooth muscle β2 receptor number & affinity→
  - ∘Arteriole vasoconstriction→
    - −↑Peripheral vascular resistance→**diastolic hypertension**

Cutaneous
- •↓Cellular metabolism→
  - ∘↓Heat production→
    - −Peripheral vasoconstriction→**coolness**→↓**sweat, & cold intolerance**
  - ∘↓Sebum production
  - ...→cool, pale, dry, thick, &/or scaly skin
  - ∘Course & brittle hair, w/ hair loss at the lateral eyebrow edges
  - ∘Longituginally ridged nails
  - ∘↑Interstitial fluid albumin→
    - −**Edema, termed myxedema** (laryngeal→hoarseness, tongue→macroglossia)
    - −Effusions (pericardial, pleural, peritoneal, &/or inner ear→↓hearing)

Gastrointestinal
- •↓Cellular metabolism→
  - ∘↓Gastrointestinal motility→
    - −Constipation
  - ∘↓Mucus secretion

396

Genitourinary
- ↓Cellular metabolism→
  - ○↓Libido, being sexual desire→
    - –Impotence, being the inability to achieve &/or maintain an erection
  - ○Altered menstrual hemorrhage, being either ↑ or ↓
  - ○Hyperprolactinemia→
    - –Galactorrhea, being milk–like, persistent nipple discharge

Musculoskeletal
- ↓Cellular metabolism→
  - ○Generalized weakness
  - ○Muscle stiffness
  - ○Myalgias

Neurologic
- ↓Cellular metabolism→
  - ○**Delayed relaxation phase of deep tendon reflexes**
  - ○↓Cerebration→
    - –Anxiety
    - –Coma, termed myxedema coma
    - –Emotional lability
    - –Irritability
    - –Hypokinesis
    - –Delirium
    - –Dementia
    - –↓Memory
    - –Psychosis, termed myxedema madness
    - –Depression

Respiratory
- ↓Central nervous system ventilatory response to ↑$PaCO_2$ &/or ↓PaO_2→
  - ○Hypoventilation

Hematologic
- **Subclinical hypothyroidism**
  - ○Low normal range thyroid hormone, w/ feedback mediated ↑anterior pituitary thyroid stimulating hormone–TSH secretion
- **Euthyroid sick syndrome**
  - ○↓Tetraiodothyronine–T4 w/ a normal triiodothyronine–T3, & inappropriately normal thyroid stimulating hormone–TSH, rather than the expected ↑value
- **All others**, except for the rare etiologies
  - ○↓Thyroid hormone, w/ feedback mediated ↑anterior pituitary thyroid stimulating hormone–TSH secretion

Subsyndromes:
- **Autoimmune thyroiditis:**
  - ○**Anti–thyroid peroxidase antibodies** (previously named anti–microsomal)
  - ○**Anti–thyroglobulin antibodies**
  - ○Anti–thyroid stimulating hormone–TSH antibodies, being destructive, rather than activating as in Graves' disease

Other findings:
- Macrocytic anemia
- Dyslipidemia
- Hyperprolactinemia–1%
- Hyponatremia–2%

- Altered plasma thyroxine binding globulin level→
  - ○Inversely proportional alteration of **active, free thyroid hormone**, without any effect on the total plasma content

↑Plasma thyroxine binding globulin level:
- Estrogen containing medications
  - –Hormone replacement therapy–HRT
  - –Oral contraceptive pills–OCPs
- Hepatitis
- Pregnancy

↓Plasma thyroxine binding globulin level:
- Androgens
- Cirrhosis
- Glucocorticoids
- ↑Growth hormone→
  - Acromegaly
- Nephritic syndrome
- Phenytoin

TREATMENT

THYROID HORMONE

Generic (Trade)	M ♀	Start	Max
Levothyroxine=T4 (Levoxyl, Synthroid)	L S		
•Healthy young adults:		100µg=0.1mg PO q24hours	300µg=0.3mg q24h
•Elderly, or w/ cardiovascular disease:		12.5µg=0.0125mg PO q24h	
...w/ titration q1–2months prn			
•Myxedema coma†		250µg IV bolus, then	
		100µg IV the next day, then	
		50µg IV q24h thereafter, until clinical improvement,	
		w/ subsequent switch to PO treatment	
Liothyronine=T3 (Cytomel)	L S		
•Healthy young adults:		25µg=0.025mg PO q24hours	
•Elderly, or w/ cardiovascular disease:		5µg=0.005mg PO q24hours	
...w/ titration q1–2weeks prn			
Levothyroxine & Liothyronine (Thyrolar)	L S		
•Healthy young adults:		50µg/ 12.5µg PO q24hours	
•Elderly, or w/ cardiovascular disease:		25µg/ 6.25µg PO q24hours	
...w/ titration q2weeks prn			

†Oral thyroid administration is avoided in severe disease due to likely ↓gastrointestinal motility

IRON DEFICIENCY ANEMIA
•Caused by chronic disease→↑iron loss &/or ↓iron absorption→
 ○Anemia
•**All ♂ & postmenopausal ♀ w/ iron deficiency anemia, should be considered to have gastrointestinal cancer until proven otherwise**

IRON PHYSIOLOGY
•Iron is an essential component of hemoglobin, myoglobin, & certain cellular enzymes (ex. catalase, cytochrome oxidase, peroxidase), w/ the total body iron stores being ~5g, 70% of which is bound to hemoglobin
•Most of the iron required for hemoglobin synthesis is provided by erythrocyte catabolism via the monocyte/ macrophage system, w/ subsequent iron recycling. Tissue iron stores act as a reserve in order to maintain hemoglobin synthesis during ↑demand via either ↑erythrocyte loss or ↓iron absorption. Dietary iron serves to replenish normal daily loss via bile, epithelial cell desquamation, urine, & sweat→
 ○1mg iron loss/ 24hours (↑ in ♀ due to menstrual blood loss of 0.7mg iron q24hours), w/ 1000calories containing 7mg of iron in 2 forms:
  −**Heme iron**, being found primarily in meats, w/ absorption in the upper small intestine
  −**Non-heme iron**, usually being in the oxidized ferric form (Fe^{+3}), which is insoluble @ the alkaline pH of the upper small intestine, unless previously chelated by amino acids, carbohydrates, or vitamin C=ascorbic acid in the acidic pH of the stomach→↑upper small intestine absorption
•Gastrointestinal mucosal iron absorption→
 ○Plasma iron release, w/ subsequent binding to apotransferrin→
  −**Transferrin**† formation (which "trans"ports iron in the body), w/ subsequent transferrin receptor mediated endocytosis via all cells, esp. immature erythrocytes, hepatocytes, & monocytes/ macrophages→intracellular iron release w/ subsequent transferrin exocytosis→cycle repetition
•Cytoplasmic iron combines w/ apoferritin→
 ○**Ferritin** formation, which serves as the 1st line of iron storage, which, when stained, can be visualized only via electron microscopy. Apoferritin pool saturation→
  −**Hemosiderin** formation (being large aggregates of denatured ferritin proteins), which serve as the 2nd line of iron storage
•The erythrocyte life span is 4 months, w/ eventual cell membrane fragility→
 ○Altered erythrocyte shape & ↓membrane deformability→
  −Cell rupture in the hepatic sinusoids & splenic trabecular network, termed red pulp→hemoglobin release, w/ subsequent tissue macrophage mediated phagocytosis (esp. in the liver, spleen, & bone marrow)→hemoglobin metabolism→intracellular protein recycling w/ iron & bilirubin release

---

•Inflammation→
 ○Altered macrophage metabolism→
  −↓Iron release
 ○↓Gastrointestinal iron absorption
 ○Altered food preferences→
  −Avoidance of heme iron rich foods, such as meats, w/ preference of foods which→↓non-heme iron absorption, such as tannates (coffee or tea)
 …as the mineral is an essential resource for bacteria, which lack transferrin receptors, & so rely on free body iron which becomes scarce
†Transferrin saturation ≤15%→
 •Inefficient erythrocyte supply
Transferrin saturation >80%→
 •Tissue iron accumulation, esp. within hepatocytes

RISK FACTORS
•**Chronic erythrocyte loss−99%**
 ○**Gastrointestinal hemorrhage**, being the **#1 cause**
 ○Genitourinary hemorrhage
 ○Idiopathic pulmonary hemosiderosis
 ○Intravascular hemolysis†
 ○Phlebotomies
•**Chronic iron malabsorption**
 ○Malabsorption syndromes
 ○Lack of gastric acid via:
  −Achlorhydria
  −Gastrectomy
  …→↓non-heme iron chelation→
   •↓Absorption
 ○Pica, via ingestion of clay or dirt

†Intravascular hemolysis→↑**plasma hemoglobin**→
•Pink/ red colored plasma
•Hemoglobinuria→hematuria
  –Microscopic via positive heme dipstick reaction without erythrocytes
  –Macroscopic, termed gross, via red/ brown colored urine without erythrocytes
…w/ chronic urinary iron loss→
  •Renal tubular cell hemosiderin per Prussian blue staining of the urine sediment
•Iron deficiency anemia, being **microcytic** (MCV <80fL)
•Folic acid deficiency→
  ∘**Macrocytic anemia** (MCV >100fL)
…w/ combination (micro & macrocytic etiologies)→
  •**Normocytic anemia** (MCV 80–100fL)

DIAGNOSIS

•Usually being symptomatic upon either:
  ∘Acute anemia
  ∘Hemoglobin ≤7g/ dL
…w/ no direct correlation between anemia severity & cardiac output

General
  •↓Cellular oxygenation→
    ∘**Fatigue**
    ∘Headache
Cardiovascular
  •The cardiovascular signs are compensatory mechanisms→
    ∘↑Cellular oxygenation, allowing for the patient to possibly be asymptomatic @ rest. However, exertion→
      –↑Tissue O_2 demand→eventual decompensation→symptoms
  •↓Blood viscosity & ↓cellular oxygenation →
    ∘↓Resistance to blood flow & arterial vasodilation respectively, both→↑venous return→↑**cardiac output**→
      –Systolic hypertension→↑pulse pressure (systolic – diastolic blood pressure)
      –Systolic flow murmur
      –Cervical venous hum
  •Acute anemia→
    ∘Thoracic arterial baroreceptor & chemoreceptor activation→
      –↑**Autonomic sympathetic tone**→tachycardia
Mucocutaneous
  •↓Hemoglobin→
    ∘Skin & mucus membrane pallor
      –Extended palmar crease pallor @ a hemoglobin ≤7g/ dL
Gastrointestinal
  •↓Iron→
    ∘Epithelial abnormalities:
      –↓Tongue papillae→smooth, inflammed tongue=**atrophic glossitis**
      –Dry scaling & fissuring at the angles of the lips=angular cheilosis
      –Spooning of the nails=**koilonychia**
  •**Hemorrhage**, which may occur intermittently→
    ∘**Hematemesis:** Vomiting of blood, including very dark, tarry looking blood termed 'coffee ground' emesis
    <u>Lesion localization:</u>
      •Upper gastrointestinal hemorrhage
    ∘**Hematochezia:** Passage of bright red blood per rectum
    <u>Lesion localization:</u>
      •Lower gastrointestinal hemorrhage >> upper gastrointestinal hemorrhage via massive hemorrhage (≥1L) &/or ↑↑peristalsis
    ∘Melena†‡: Passage of sticky, very dark, tarry looking stool, w/ a characteristic odor, requiring ≥50mL of blood, indicating gastrointestinal hemorrhage proximal to ileocecal sphincter >> colonic gastrointestinal hemorrhage via slow hemorrhage &/or ↓peristalsis
    ∘**Fecal occult blood:** Passage of blood detectable only by laboratory testing, requiring ≥20mL of blood. Not helpful in the anatomic determination of the lesion

  •**Digital rectal exam–DRE**
  <u>Indications:</u>
    •To palpate a possible distal rectal tumor
    •Visualization of fecal streaks on glove, in order to identify possible melena &/or hematochezia

•**Fecal occult blood test–FOBT**
Procedure:
◦2 samples are taken from 1 bowel movement/ day X 3 days=6 total samples, which may be stored for <1week
Mechanism:
•Uses the peroxidase activity of hemoglobin to cause a change in the reagent, w/ the patient to avoid the following for ≥3 days prior to, & during testing:
Limitations:
•False positive:
◦Hemoglobin rich foods:
 −Raw red meat
◦Peroxidase rich foods:
 −Uncooked vegetables, esp. broccoli, cauliflower, or turnips
◦Gastrointestinal mucosal irritants:
 −Laxatives
 −Nonsteroidal anti–inflammatory drugs–NSAIDs, including Aspirin
•False negative:
◦↑Dose vitamin C

---

†Iron→
•Melanotic looking stools ± constipation &/or diarrhea
‡Bismuth subsalicylate (Pepto–Bismol)→
•Melanotic looking stools &/or dark tongue

Neurologic
•↓Iron→
◦**Craving for non–nutritional substances (clay, dirt, ice), termed pica**
 −Clay or dirt also→↓intestinal iron absorption
Pulmonary
•Exertion→
◦↑Tissue O_2 demand→
 −Dyspnea=breathlessness
Hematologic
•**Anemia**→
◦↓Hemoglobin (♂ <14g/ dL, ♀ <12g/ dL) & hematocrit (♂ <40%, ♀ <35%)→
 −Compensatory ↑renal **erythropoietin** secretion, w/ paradoxical ↓erythrocyte production→ ↓reticulocytes↑, indicating erythroid hypoproliferation
•↓Bone marrow iron stores, being the first sign→
◦↓**Plasma ferritin** (♂ <30μg/ L, ♀ <10μg/ L), being the most sensitive test. Plasma ferritin has no role in iron metabolism, but is pathognomonic of iron deficiency anemia
 −Plasma ferritin ≤100μg/ L in the presence of inflammation suggests iron deficiency anemia, as it is an acute phase reactant w/ expected ↑levels
•**Thrombocytosis** (>450,000/ μL) of uncertain etiology
Limitations:
•Platelets are acute phase reactants, being ↑w/ inflammation
•↓**Plasma iron** (<65μg/ dL, usually being <30μg/ dL)→
◦Compensatory ↑plasma transferrin→
 −↓Transferrin saturation (<16%)→↑**total iron binding capacity–TIBC** (≥450μg/ dL)
•↓Intra–erythrocyte iron→
◦↓Erythrocyte iron–protoporphyrin conjugation→
 −↑Erythrocyte free protoporphyrin (>61μg/ dL)
◦↓Hemoglobin→
 −↓Mean corpuscular hemoglobin concentration–MCHC (<32g/ dL)→erythrocyte paleness, termed **hypochromia**
•↓**Mean corpuscular volume–MCV** (<80fL), termed **microcytosis**. Microcytic cells, w/ previous normocytic cells→
◦Peripheral erythrocyte size variation, termed anisocytosis→
 −↑**Red cell distribution width–RDW** (>14.5%)

Ratios indicative of iron deficiency anemia:
•Total iron binding capacity–TIBC being >6 X plasma iron
•Mean corpuscular volume–MCV being >13 X erythrocyte count (10^6/ μL)

- Inflammation→
  - ↓Plasma iron
  - ↓Plasma transferrin level & saturation→
    - −Normal to ↑total iron binding capacity−TIBC
  - ↓Reticulocytes
  - ...however,
    - The erythrocyte is usually normocytic & normochromic, w/ a normal red cell distribution width−RDW
    - There is inflammation mediated ↑plasma ferritin
    - The bone marrow iron stores are normal to ↑

†The normal reticulocyte count is ≤2%, which is expected to ↑in anemic states, as a compensatory mechanism of a normally functioning bone marrow. Lack of this compensatory ↑ indicates that there is at least an element of inadequate marrow production as a cause for the anemia. Being that reticulocytes are calculated in relation to erythrocyte number, anemia→
  - Falsely ↑reticulocyte count. In order to correct for this effect, the reticulocyte count should be adjusted for the degree of anemia:

Corrected reticulocyte count= <u>reticulocyte count (hematocrit / 0.45)</u>
$\qquad\qquad$ maturation factor (if hematocrit ≥45%=1, 35%=1.5, 25%=2, 20%=2.5)

INVASIVE PROCEDURES
- **Bone marrow aspiration**
  Findings:
  - ↓Bone marrow iron stores→
    - ↓Hemosiderin formation, being the first sign→
      - −↓Light microscopic observation via Prussian blue staining

TREATMENT
- **Search for the etiologic disease**, esp. gastrointestinal hemorrhage via:
  - Digital rectal examination w/ fecal occult blood testing
  - Endoscopic examination
    - −Colonoscopy
    - −Esophagogastroduodenoscopy−EGD

NON−HEME IRON: Iron replacement is never a treatment, but rather **palliation** until the underlying cause is diagnosed & treated

Indications:
- Symptomatic patients

Generic	M ♀	Dose
Ferrous sulfate	K P	325mg PO q8hours
		&
Vitamin C=ascorbic acid	K ?	

Duration:
- 3months after hematocrit/ hemoglobin normalization, in order to fully replenish body iron stores

Mechanism:
- Concomitant administration of vitamin C=ascorbic acid→
  - ↑Non−heme gastrointestinal absorption→
    - −Progressive syndrome reversal, starting within 2weeks of successful treatment, w/ ↑hematocrit & hemoglobin, being equivalent to a 1unit PRBC transfusion/ week (3%/ 1g/dL respectively) until normalization

Side effects:
- **Gastrointestinal**
  - Melanotic looking stools
  - Constipation &/or diarrhea

•Caused by any chronic disease→↓vitamin B12 or folate→↓thymidine triphosphate formation
  ◦↓DNA synthesis→
    −↓Erythropoiesis
    −Altered cellular maturation→large, immature, & fragile erythrocytes, termed **megaloblasts**, w/
    ↓peripheral survival, being 2 months, rather than the normal 4 months
    ...→anemia

CLASSIFICATION/ RISK FACTORS

VITAMIN B12 DEFICIENCY ANEMIA ▬▬▬▬▬
•Vitamin B12=Cyanocobalamin, is found in all **foods of animal origin** (esp. eggs, milk, kidney, &
liver), w/ tissue stores lasting 2–3years

•**Chronic gastrointestinal malabsorption–>99%**
  ◦**Lack of intrinsic factor, being the #1 cause**
    −Pernicious anemia, a gastric autoimmune disease, being the #1 cause
    −Gastrectomy
    −Inert intrinsic factor
  ◦Ileal resection or disease, as absorption occurs in the proximal 1/3rd of the small intestine
    −Crohn's disease
  ◦Pancreatic failure
    −Chronic, relapsing pancreatitis
    −Pancreatectomy (pancreatico–duodenectomy, termed Whipple's procedure)
    −Pancreatic tumor (cancer, pseudocyst)→pancreatic duct obstruction
  ◦↑Intestinal competition
    −Bacterial overgrowth
    −Diphyllobothrium latum infection, termed Diphyllobothriasis
      Acquisition:
        •A fish tapeworm acquired via the ingestion of raw or undercooked freshwater fish which were
        exposed to human feces containing parasitic eggs. The emerging embryos are eaten by tiny
        copepod crustaceans, w/ the subsequent differentiation into larvae which live in the body
        cavity. The copepod is then eaten by a freshwater fish (ex. perch, pike, trout)→
          ◦Larval muscle infestation, w/ human ingestion→
            −Small intestinal habitation, w/ development into large worms→preferential vitamin B12
            uptake. Fertilized eggs are passed in the feces & must be deposited in fresh water for
            the life cycle to continue
•**Chronic ↓utilization**
  ◦Folic acid deficiency
•**Nutritional deficiency–rare**
  ◦Malnutrition
    −Alcoholics
    −Anorexia nervosa
    −Elderly patients
  ◦Vegan diet, which excludes all animal products

FOLIC ACID DEFICIENCY ANEMIA ▬▬▬▬▬▬▬▬▬▬▬▬▬▬▬▬▬▬▬▬
•Folic acid=vitamin B9, a heat–labile vitamin, is found in **green leafy vegetables**, citrus fruits, kidney,
liver, & yeast, w/ tissue stores lasting 4 months, unless metabolic requirements↑

•**Chronic gastrointestinal malabsorption**
  ◦Ileal resection or disease, as absorption occurs in the proximal 1/3rd of the small intestine
    −Crohn's disease
•**Chronic ↑metabolic requirements**
  ◦Chronic hemodialysis
  ◦Chronic hemolytic anemia
  ◦Hyperthyroidism
  ◦Infancy
  ◦Myeloproliferative disorders
  ◦Pregnancy
  ◦Psoriasis
  ◦Severe exfoliative dermatitis

- **Chronic ↓utilization**
  - ∘Ethanol
  - ∘Medications
    - –Phenytoin
    - –Dihydrofolate reductase inhibitors→↓folic acid metabolism (Methotrexate, Pentamidine, Pyrimethamine, Triamterene, Trimethoprim)
  - ∘Vitamin B12 deficiency
- **Nutritional deficiency**
  - ∘Malnutrition
    - –Alcoholics
    - –Anorexia nervosa
    - –Elderly patients

DIAGNOSIS

- Usually being symptomatic upon either:
  - ∘Acute anemia
  - ∘Hemoglobin ≤7g/ dL
  - …w/ no direct correlation between anemia severity & cardiac output

General
- ↓Cellular oxygenation→
  - ∘**Fatigue**
  - ∘Headache

Cardiovascular
- The cardiovascular signs are compensatory mechanisms→
  - ∘↑Cellular oxygenation, allowing for the patient to possibly be asymptomatic @ rest. However, exertion→
    - –↑Tissue O_2 demand→eventual decompensation→symptoms
- ↓Blood viscosity & ↓cellular oxygenation →
  - ∘↓Resistance to blood flow & arterial vasodilation respectively, both→↑venous return→↑**cardiac output**→
    - –Systolic hypertension→↑pulse pressure (systolic – diastolic blood pressure)
    - –Systolic flow murmur
    - –Cervical venous hum
- Acute anemia→
  - ∘Thoracic arterial baroreceptor & chemoreceptor activation→
    - –↑**Autonomic sympathetic tone**→tachycardia

Mucocutaneous
- ↓Hemoglobin→
  - ∘Skin & mucus membrane pallor
    - –Extended palmar crease pallor @ a hemoglobin ≤7g/ dL

Gastrointestinal
- Epithelial abnormalities:
  - ∘↓Tongue papillae→
    - –Smooth, inflamed tongue=**atrophic glossitis**

Pulmonary
- Exertion→
  - ∘↑Tissue O_2 demand→
    - –Dyspnea=breathlessness

Hematologic
- ↓DNA synthesis→myelosuppression→
  - ∘**Pancytopenia**
    - –**Anemia, w/ oval erythrocytes lacking central pallor.** ↓Hemoglobin (♂ <14g/ dL, ♀ <12g/ dL) & hematocrit (♂ <40%, ♀ <35%)→compensatory ↑renal **erythropoietin** secretion, w/ paradoxical ↓erythrocyte production→↓**reticulocytes**†, indicating erythroid hypoproliferation
    - –Leukopenia, w/ **neutrophil hypersegmentation** (>5 lobes), which persists for several weeks despite appropriate treatment
    - –Thrombocytopenia
  - ∘Altered cellular maturation→
    - –Dissociation of nuclear to cytoplasmic maturation→↑relative cytoplasmic maturation→↑**mean corpuscular volume–MCV (>100fL), termed macrocytosis,** which may precede anemia by ≤1year. Macrocytic cells, w/ previous normocytic cells→peripheral erythrocyte size variation, termed anisocytosis→↑**red cell distribution width–RDW** (>14.5%)
    - –Irregularly shaped cells, termed poikilocytosis, including tear drop cells

404

- Liver function tests
  - Mild extravascular hemolysis→
    - Unconjugated hyperbilirubinemia
- Peripheral blood smear showing Howell-Jolly bodies, being intra-erythrocyte, small, dark staining spherical bodies, also being seen w/ hyposplenism

Vitamin B12 deficiency specific:
Neurologic
- **Subacute combined degeneration**
  Pathophysiology:
    - Myelin degeneration of peripheral nerves & the dorso-lateral columns of the spinal cord→
      - Abnormal sensations, termed paresthesias (numbness, pain, &/or tingling) beginning in the hands & feet (as longer neurons have ↑myelination, & so are affected sooner), w/ proximal progression, as well as ↓fine touch, vibratory, & positional sensation, w/ subsequent:
        - Incoordination=ataxia
        - ↑Muscle tone & tendon reflexes=hyperreflexia
        - Weakness
        ...→clumsiness

Hematologic
- ↓**Plasma vitamin B12 levels**
- W/ **Pernicious anemia, anti-parietal cell antibodies-80%** &/or anti-intrinsic factor antibodies-50%→
  - ↓Intrinsic factor & ↓gastric acid production→
    - Lack of gastric acid=achlorhydria→compensatory ↑gastrin levels
    - ↓Proximal ileal absorption of vitamin B12

Folic acid deficiency specific:
Hematologic
- ↓**Erythrocyte folic acid level**, which remains low for weeks to months despite adequate treatment, whereas plasma folic acid level may rise upon several adequately fortified meals

---

†The normal reticulocyte count is ≤2%, which is expected to ↑in anemic states, as a compensatory mechanism of a normally functioning bone marrow. Lack of this compensatory ↑ indicates that there is at least an element of inadequate marrow production as a cause for the anemia. Being that reticulocytes are calculated in relation to erythrocyte number, anemia→
- Falsely ↑reticulocyte count. In order to correct for this effect, the reticulocyte count should be adjusted for the degree of anemia:

Corrected reticulocyte count= reticulocyte count (hematocrit / 0.45)
                                 maturation factor (if hematocrit ≥45%=1, 35%=1.5, 25%=2, 20%=2.5)

INVASIVE PROCEDURES
- **Bone marrow biopsy**
  Findings:
    - Altered cellular maturation→dissociation of nuclear to cytoplasmic maturation→
      - A relatively immature nucleus, termed a **megaloblast**, seen only on bone marrow biopsy

TREATMENT
- **Treat the etiologic disease**
- **ALWAYS rule out vitamin B12 deficiency before initiating folic acid treatment**, as treatment of vitamin B12 deficiency w/ folic acid→
  - Correction of anemia, but not macrocytosis or neurologic disease

VITAMIN B12 DEFICIENCY ━━━━━━━━━━━━━
- Neurologic abnormalities are reversible if treated within 6 months

VITAMIN B12	
Etiology	**Dose**
Chronic intestinal malabsorption	100µg SC/ IM q24hours X 1week, then qod X 3weeks, then qmonth indefinitely
Nutritional deficiency	
•PO	25-250µg PO q24hours
•Intranasal	500µg intranasal qweek

FOLIC ACID DEFICIENCY ━━━━━━━━━━━━━━━

FOLIC ACID
Dose
1mg PO/ SC/ IM/ IV q24hours until syndrome resolution, then 0.4mg q24hours (0.8mg q24hours in pregnant or lactating ♀)

ETIOLOGIES OF NON-MEGALOBLASTIC MACROCYTIC ANEMIAS

•**Alcoholism**, via myelosuppression→
  ◦Anemia ± macrocytosis, regardless of folate or vitamin B12 deficiency
  ◦Leukopenia
  ◦Thrombocytopenia
•**Hepatic disease**→
  ◦Spur & target cells
•**Hypothyroidism**
•**Medications affecting DNA production**
  ◦Antiretroviral medications
  ◦Chemotherapeutic medications
•**Hemolytic anemia**→↑reticulocyte response
•**Aplastic anemia**
•**Myelodysplastic syndrome**
•**Sideroblastic anemia**, sometimes being microcytic

406

HEMOLYTIC ANEMIA

- Caused by any disease→
  - Erythrocyte destruction, occurring either:
    - Intravascularly
    - Extravascularly, via the monocyte/ macrophage system
  - ...→anemia

CLASSIFICATION/ RISK FACTORS

INTRAVASCULAR HEMOLYSIS
- **Acute hemolytic transfusion reactions**
- **Hemoglobinopathies**
  - Sickle cell anemia
  - Thallasemia (α or β)
- **Hereditary erythrocyte enzyme deficiency**
  - Glucose-6 phosphate dehydrogenase-G6PD deficiency
  - Pyruvate kinase deficiency
- **Infection**
  - Babesiosis
  - Malaria
- **Microangiopathic disease**
  - Severe hypertension
  - Systemic thrombohemorrhagic disease
    - Disseminated intravascular coagulation-DIC
    - Hemolytic uremic syndrome-HUS
    - Thrombotic thrombocytopenic purpura-TTP
  - Vasculitis
- **Paroxysmal nocturnal hemoglobinuria**, via a stem cell defect→
  - Complement mediated erythrocyte lysis
- **Severe & extensive burns**
- **Traumatic**
  - Mechanical heart or heart valve, esp. aortic
- **Hemolytic disease of the newborn, termed erythroblastosis fetalis**

EXTRAVASCULAR HEMOLYSIS
- **Autoimmune hemolytic anemia-AIHA**
  - **Warm autoimmune hemolytic anemia-70%**
    - Idiopathic
    - Autoimmune disease syndromes
    - Human immune deficiency virus-HIV infection
    - Ulcerative colitis
  - **Cold autoimmune hemolytic anemia**, usually @ age >40years
    - Idiopathic
    - Infections: Mycoplasma pneumoniae or Epstein-Barr virus-EBV
    - Neoplasms, esp. Chronic lymphoid leukemia-CLL, Lymphoma, or Waldenstroms macroglobulinemia
- **Delayed hemolytic transfusion reactions**
- **Hereditary erythrocyte cell membrane abnormalities**
  - Spherocytosis >> elliptocytosis, poikilocytosis, stomatocytosis
- **Liver disease**
  - Hepatitis &/or cirrhosis, esp. alcohol related
- **Medications**
  - α-methyldopa
  - Penicillin
  - Quinidine
  - Quinine
- **Splenomegally→**
  - Cellular sequestration, termed hypersplenism

•Usually being symptomatic upon either:
  ○Acute anemia
  ○Hemoglobin ≤7g/ dL
  ...w/ no direct correlation between anemia severity & cardiac output

General
  •↓Cellular oxygenation→
    ○**Fatigue**
    ○Headache
Cardiovascular
  •The cardiovascular signs are compensatory mechanisms→
    ○↑Cellular oxygenation, allowing for the patient to possibly be asymptomatic @ rest. However, exertion→
      –↑Tissue O_2 demand→eventual decompensation→symptoms
  •↓Blood viscosity & ↓cellular oxygenation →
    ○↓Resistance to blood flow & arterial vasodilation respectively, both→↑venous return→↑**cardiac output**→
      –↑Systolic blood pressure→↑pulse pressure (systolic – diastolic blood pressure)
      –Systolic flow murmur
      –Cervical venous hum
  •Acute anemia→
    ○Thoracic arterial baroreceptor & chemoreceptor activation→
      –↑**Autonomic sympathetic tone**→tachycardia
Gastrointestinal
  •Chronic hemolysis→
    ○Unconjugated hyperbilirubinemia→
      –↑Hepatic biliary excretion of conjugated bilirubin→bilirubin gallstone=**cholelithiasis** risk (being black pigmented), occurring in most adults, & usually being asymptomatic
Mucocutaneous
  •↓Hemoglobin→
    ○Skin & mucus membrane pallor
      –Extended palmar crease pallor @ a hemoglobin ≤7g/ dL
  •Hemolysis→
    ○Unconjugated hyperbilirubinemia, w/ a plasma bilirubin >3mg/ dL→yellow staining of tissues:
      –Skin, termed jaundice
      –Sclera, termed scleral icterus
      –Mucus membranes
Pulmonary
  •Exertion→
    ○↑Tissue O_2 demand→
      –Dyspnea=breathlessness
Hematologic
  •Hemolysis→
    ○↓Hemoglobin (♂ <14g/ dL, ♀ <12g/ dL) & hematocrit (♂ <40%, ♀ <35%)→compensatory ↑renal **erythropoietin** secretion→↑**reticulocytes**†, being proportional to the severity of the anemia, provided adequate:
      –Erythropoietin
      –Folic acid
      –Iron
      –Vitamin B12
  •The intramedullary compensatory response
    ○**Reticulocytosis**→
      –↑Mean corpuscular volume–MCV (>100 fL)
      –Retained messenger–RNA→purple coloration per Wright stain, termed polychromatophilia
      –Retained nucleus in severe hemolysis
    ○**Cellular cytoplasm release**→
      –**Hyperkalemia**
      –Hyperphosphatemia→calcium binding→hypocalcemia
      –↑Lactate dehydrogenase–LDH
      –↑Uric acid (> ~7mg/ dL)→gout syndrome
      –Unconjugated hyperbilirubinemia

408

<u>Intravascular specific findings:</u>
Genitourinary
- •Intravascular hemolysis→↑**plasma hemoglobin**→
  - ∘Pink/ red colored plasma
  - ∘Hemoglobinuria→hematuria
    - –Microscopic via positive heme dipstick reaction without erythrocytes
    - –Macroscopic, termed gross, via red/ brown colored urine without erythrocytes
    - …w/ chronic urinary iron loss→
      - •Renal tubular cell hemosiderin per Prussian blue staining of the urine sediment
      - •Iron deficiency anemia, being **microcytic** (MCV <80fL)
      - •Folic acid deficiency→
        - ∘**Macrocytic anemia** (MCV >100fL)
        - …w/ combination (micro & macrocytic etiologies)→
          - •**Normocytic anemia** (MCV 80–100fL)

Hematologic
- •Intravascular hemolysis→↑**plasma hemoglobin**→
  - ∘↓Plasma haptoglobin & hemopexin, being hemoglobin & heme binding proteins, respectively

<u>Extravascular specific findings:</u>
Lymphatics
- •**Splenomegally**

---

†The normal reticulocyte count is ≤2%, which is expected to ↑in anemic states, as a compensatory mechanism of a normally functioning bone marrow. Lack of this compensatory ↑ indicates that there is at least an element of inadequate marrow production as a cause for the anemia. Being that reticulocytes are calculated in relation to erythrocyte number, anemia→
- •Falsely ↑reticulocyte count. In order to correct for this effect, the reticulocyte count should be adjusted for the degree of anemia:

Corrected reticulocyte count= <u>reticulocyte count (hematocrit / 0.45)</u>
                 maturation factor (if hematocrit ≥45%=1, 35%=1.5, 25%=2, 20%=2.5)

INVASIVE PROCEDURES
- •**Bone marrow aspirate**
  <u>Findings:</u>
  - •Erythroid hyperplasia

DIAGNOSIS/ TREATMENT
INTRAVASCULAR HEMOLYSIS ▬▬▬▬
- •**Microangiopathic disease & trauma**
  Hematologic
  - •Peripheral blood smear showing misshapen erythrocytes, termed **schistocytes**, described as:
    - ∘Cell fragments
    - ∘Crescent cells
    - ∘Helmet cells

- •**Glucose 6–phosphate dehydrogenase–G6PD deficiency**
  <u>Pathophysiology:</u>
  - •**X linked metabolic disease**→
    - ∘↑Sensitivity to oxidant stresses:
      - –**Infection**
      - –**Fava beans**
      - –**Oxidant medications** (anti–malarials, Nitrofurantoin, Sulfonamides)
        - …→intermittent, acute **hemolysis**, w/ chronic hemolysis possible depending on the inherited allele
  <u>Risk factors:</u>
  - •**Gender:** ♂ >> ♀, as ♀s are heterozygous, w/ low to normal enzyme levels in most
  - •**Skin color:** Blacks >> whites
  - •**Mediterranean ancestry**
  <u>Diagnosis:</u>
  Hematologic
  - •↓**Erythrocyte enzyme levels**
    <u>Limitations:</u>
    - •May be normal after acute hemolysis, w/ only normal erythrocytes remaining
  - •Peripheral blood smear showing:
    - ∘Bite cells
    - ∘Erythrocyte inclusions, termed Heinz bodies

409

Treatment:
•Avoidance of precipitants

•**Paroxysmal nocturnal hemoglobinuria**
Pathophysiology:
   •**Acquired hematopoietic stem cell mutation→**
      ○**↑Erythrocyte susceptibility to complement mediated lysis→**
         –**Chronic hemolytic anemia,** w/ complement activation→platelet aggregation→
         thrombosis, esp. of the cerebral & intra–abdominal veins
Associated disease syndromes:
   •Aplastic anemia
   •Leukemia
   •Myelodysplastic syndromes–MDS
Diagnostic tests
   •Flow cytometry
   •**Sucrose test**
      Procedure:
         •Erythrocyte incubation w/ sucrose→
            ○Erythrocyte hemolysis
   •**HAM test**
      Indications:
         •Confirmation of a positive sucrose test
      Procedure:
         •Acidified serum→
            ○Erythrocyte hemolysis
Treatment:
   •Supportive

EXTRAVASCULAR HEMOLYSIS
•**Warm autoimmune hemolytic anemia**
Pathophysiology:
   •**Acquired IgG erythrocyte cell membrane autoantibodies→**
      ○Tissue macrophage mediated erythrocyte removal at body temperature (98.6°F=37°C)→
         –Anemia, w/ a hemoglobin usually <7g/ dL
Diagnosis:
   General
      •Fever
   Hematologic
      •**Hepatomegally–35%**
      •**Splenomegally–50%**
      •Positive direct antiglobulin test, termed **Coombs test,** which detects IgG & complement bound to
      the erythrocyte cell membrane
Treatment:
   •First line: Glucocorticoids
   •Second line: Splenectomy

•**Cold autoimmune hemolytic anemia**
Pathophysiology:
   •**Acquired IgM erythrocyte cell membrane autoantibodies→**
      ○Erythrocyte agglutination in capillaries at cold temperatures (<98.6°F=37°C)→
         –Ischemia, which resolves upon re–warming
Diagnosis:
   Mucocutaneous
      •Ischemia→
         ○Skin pallor (usually affecting the ears, fingers, nose, &/or toes) w/ ↑relative mucocutaneous O_2
         extraction→
            –Bluish color, termed cyanosis
   Hematologic
      •Positive direct antiglobulin test, termed **Coombs test,** which detects IgG & complement bound to
      the erythrocyte cell membrane
      •**Cold–reactive IgM autoagglutinins** @ titers >1000, when tested @ 39.2°F=4°C
      •Peripheral blood smear showing spherocytosis
Treatment:
   •Avoidance of extreme cold exposure
   •Wearing warm clothing, as well as gloves & a hat when in cold weather

410

•**Hereditary spherocytosis**
Pathophysiology:
  •**Hereditary cytoskeletal protein defect**→
    ∘Loss of membrane surface area→
      –**Spherocytes**, lacking central pallor, w/ ↓membrane deformability
Diagnosis:
  •Usually diagnosed in the neonate due to jaundice
  Mucocutaneous
    •Chronic leg ulcers
  Hematologic
    •↑Mean corpuscular hemoglobin concentration–MHCH (>36g/ dL)
Diagnostic tests:
  •Peripheral smear showing spherocytes
  •**Osmotic fragility test**
    Procedure:
      •Erythrocyte incubation w/ hypotonic saline→
        ∘↑Susceptibility to lysis due to ↓cell surface area
Complications:
  •Viral infection, esp. **Parvovirus B19, occurring predominantly during childhood**→
    ∘Bone marrow stem cell infection→
      –Pancytopenia, w/ severe anemia
Treatment:
  •Splenectomy

•**Liver disease**
Pathophysiology:
  •Hepatitis &/or cirrhosis→
    ∘↑Cell membrane cholesterol→↑cell membrane surface area→
      –**Target cells**, having a dark center w/ a surrounding light band & dark outermost ring
      …w/ severe cirrhosis or fulminant hepatitis→
        •↑Membrane redundancy→
          ∘**Spur cells**=acanthocytes, being erythrocytes w/ multiple irregular cytoplasmic projections

•**Medications**
Pathophysiology:
  •Medication binds to an erythrocyte cell membrane protein→
    ∘Autoantibody to the medication–protein complex
Diagnosis:
  Hematologic
    •Positive direct antiglobulin test, termed **Coombs test**, which detects IgG & complement bound to
     the erythrocyte cell membrane
Treatment:
  •Discontinuation of the suspected causative medication

411

SICKLE CELL DISEASE

- **Congenitally acquired** amino acid substitution (valine for glutamic acid) within both β chains of the hemoglobin molecule→**hemoglobin S** (S for **sickle**), rather than the normal hemoglobin A (A for adult)→
  - Chronic, intermittently symptomatic, intra–erythrocyte hemoglobin precipitation, w/ subsequent polymerization into long rigid compounds→
    - **Cell lengthening**, forming a "**sickle**" or "crescent" shape, rather than the normal biconcave disc shape→↓cell membrane deformability→**intravascular hemolytic anemia ± vascular occlusion**→ distal ischemia ± infarction↔↑cellular sickling, thus forming a vicious cycle
- Homozygotes usually become symptomatic during childhood or early adolescence (ages 1–17 years), as they are protected during fetal life & early infancy due to the predominance of hemoglobin F (F for fetal)

RISK FACTORS

- **Skin color: Blacks** > whites
- **Ancestry**, esp:
  - Caribbean
  - East Indian
  - Latin American
  - Mediterranean
  - Middle eastern
  - North African

Precipitating factors:
- Acidemia
- Cold or changing weather
- Dehydration
- Hypoxemia via:
  - Cardiac disease
  - Pulmonary disease
  - Severe anemia
  - High altitude exposure
- Infection
- Menstruation
- Stress (mental or physical)

CLASSIFICATION

- **Sickle cell disease–0.5% of black Americans**
  - Both β globin genes contain the mutation, being homozygous for the sickle cell gene→
    - Chronic, low–grade (usually asymptomatic) **sickle cell anemia**, w/ intermittent symptomatic exacerbations, termed **sickle cell crises**

- **Sickle cell trait–10% of black Americans**, only 2% of which ever become symptomatic
  - Only 1 β globin gene contains the mutation, being heterozygous for the sickle cell gene→
    - Carrier state, being **asymptomatic** (w/ most never knowing they are carriers), **without anemia**, except the rare individuals whom experience ≥1 sickle cell crises during their lifetime due to extreme or prolonged precipitating factors (as above)

- **Compound heterozygote hemoglobinopathies**
  - Patients being heterozygous for both sickle cell disease & another hemoglobinopathy (esp. hemoglobin C disease or β–thalassemia disease)→
    - Chronic, low grade (usually asymptomatic) sickle cell anemia, w/ intermittent symptomatic exacerbations, termed sickle cell crises, usually being of ↓frequency & severity than patients affected by sickle cell disease, due to the dilution of hemoglobin S w/ other hemoglobin types

412

VASO-OCCLUSIVE CRISES
•A diagnosis of exclusion. Patients who have had previous crises can often differentiate crisis pain from other pain

General
- •↓Cellular oxygenation→
  - ∘**Fatigue**
  - ∘Headache
- •Inflammatory cytokines→
  - ∘Anorexia→
    - −Cachexia
  - ∘Chills
  - ∘Fatigue
  - ∘**Fever**† ± chills, several days after crisis onset, rarely being >102°F=39°C
  - ∘Headache
  - ∘Malaise
  - ∘Night sweats
  - ∘Weakness

---

†Temperature may be normal in patients w/:
- •Chronic kidney disease, esp. w/ uremia
- •Cirrhosis
- •Heart failure
- •Severe debility
- …or those who are:
  - •Intravenous drug users
  - •Taking certain medications:
    - ∘Acetaminophen
    - ∘Antibiotics
    - ∘Glucocorticoids
    - ∘Nonsteroidal anti-inflammatory drugs−NSAIDs

Cardiovascular
- •**Rigid, sickle shaped erythrocytes**→
  - ∘**Vascular occlusion** (arterioles, capillaries, & venules)→
    - −Organ ischemia ± infarction, usually affecting several organs at once due to the systemic nature of the disease→**pain** & **organ dysfunction**, w/ infarction→inflammation & fibrosis

Gastrointestinal
- •Splenic ischemia ± infarction→
  - ∘Left upper quadrant abdominal pain, w/ infarction→inflammation & fibrosis. Repeated infarctions→splenic fibrosis→**functional asplenia**, wherein the spleen is present, but non-functional. This occurs **predominantly in childhood** over the course of the 1st 10 years of disease→↑infection risk via **encapsulated bacteria:**
    - −Escherichia coli
    - −Haemophilus influenzae
    - −Neisseria meningitides
    - −Pseudomonas aeruginosa
    - −**Salmonella sp.**→**osteomyelitis** (although Staphylococcus aureus is still the #1 cause, regardless of asplenia)
    - −Streptococcus pneumoniae, being the #1 cause of mortality among infants w/ sickle cell disease
    - …all of which may preferentially seed an area of inflammation &/or fibrosis due to ↓immune defenses→
      - •Abscess formation
- •Hepatic ischemia ± infarction→
  - ∘Right upper quadrant abdominal pain, w/ infarction→
    - −Inflammation, termed hepatitis, & fibrosis. Repeated infarctions→cirrhosis
- •Gallbladder ischemia ± infarction→
  - ∘Right upper quadrant abdominal pain, w/ infarction→
    - −Inflammation, termed cholecystitis, & fibrosis
- •Chronic hemolysis→
  - ∘Unconjugated hyperbilirubinemia→
    - −↑Hepatic biliary excretion of conjugated bilirubin→bilirubin gallstone=**cholelithiasis** risk (being black pigmented), occurring in most adults, & usually being asymptomatic

413

Genitourinary
- •Renal ischemia ± infarction→
  - ◦Pain, w/ infarction→
    - −Inflammation, termed aseptic pyelonephritis
    - −Papillary necrosis
    - −Fibrosis
    - …w/ repeated infarctions→intra−renal renal failure
- •Corpus cavernosus occlusion→
  - ◦**Priapism, occurring in 10−40% of** ♂, being an erection lasting ≥24hours, often→
    - −Impotence, being the inability to achieve &/or maintain an erection

Mucocutaneous
- •Mucocutaneous infarction→
  - ◦Ulcerations (sickle cell anemia−20% >> compound heterozygote diseases)
- •Hemolysis→
  - ◦Unconjugated hyperbilirubinemia, w/ a plasma bilirubin >3mg/ dL→yellow staining of tissues:
    - −Skin, termed jaundice
    - −Sclera, termed scleral icterus
    - −Mucus membranes

Musculoskeletal
- •Bone ischemia ± infarction→
  - ◦Pain, w/ infarction→
    - −Inflammation, termed aseptic osteomyelitis
    - −Aseptic necrosis of the femoral heads
    - −Fibrosis
    - −Painful edematous hands & feet, termed the **hand & foot syndrome**, occurring in early infancy
    - …w/ repeated infarction→
      - •Myelofibrosis→
        - −Pancytopenia

Neurologic
- •Central nervous system ischemia ±infarction→
  - ◦Cerebrovascular accident syndromes
  - ◦Seizures

Opthalmologic
- •Retinal ischemia ± infarction→
  - ◦Visual changes, w/ infarction→
    - −Inflammation & fibrosis→retinal disease, termed retinopathy→blindness

Pulmonary
- •Lung ischemia ± infarction→
  - ◦Thoracic pain, w/ infarction→
    - −Inflammation, termed pneumonitis, & fibrosis. Repeated infarctions→emphysema
  - ◦Ventilation/ perfusion mismatch via:
    - −↑Alveolar dead space: Alveolar ventilation through relatively underperfused capillaries
    - −↑Vascular shunting†: Capillary blood flow through relatively underventilated alveoli. Usually occurring, or exacerbated via ↑venous return
    - …→↓diffusion of O_2 & CO_2→
      - •Hypoxemia (SaO_2 ≤ 91% or PaO_2 ≤ 60mmHg‡) on room air, w/ subsequent hypercapnia ($PaCO_2$ ≥45mmHg) due to either:
        - ◦Respiratory muscle fatigue
        - ◦Alveolar hypoventilation
        - …as CO_2 clearance is unimpaired (& may be ↑in the dyspneic patient) as long as adequate ventilation (including lack of diffuse severe ventilation/ perfusion mismatching) is maintained, as:
          - •CO_2 diffuses 20X as rapidly as O_2
          - •Hypercapnia→
            - ◦Immediate brain stem respiratory center mediated stimulation of pulmonary ventilation, which may correct the hypercapnia, but not necessarily the hypoxia
- •Necrotic bone marrow emboli, sickle cell aggregate emboli, &/or venous thromboemboli→
  - ◦Pulmonary infarction

414

<u>Acute chest syndrome-40%:</u>
- •Being that the pulmonary syndrome may be due to either:
- ∘Infection
  - −Assume an infectious in etiology unless proven otherwise, & search for possible concomitant meningitis
- ∘Pulmonary vascular erythrocyte sickling
- ∘Sickle cell aggregate, necrotic bone marrow, or venous thromboemboli
  - …it is termed the **"acute chest syndrome"** until the etiology can be deduced, being formally defined as:
    - •Fever
    - •Cough
    - •New pulmonary infiltrate
    - •Pleurisy, being thoracic pain exacerbated by either:
      - ∘Deep inhalation (including coughing & sneezing)
      - ∘Supine position
      - ∘Thoracic palpation
      - …& being relieved by leaning forward

---

†Being exacerbated by the supine position→
- •↑Systemic venous return→
  - ∘↑Vascular shunting→↑dyspnea, being termed:
    - −Orthopnea, if persistent
    - −Paroxysmal nocturnal dyspnea if intermittent
    - …causing the patient to either use multiple pillows or sleep in a chair
‡Age adjusted normal $PaO_2 = 101 - (0.43 \times age)$

Materno-fetal
- •Placental ischemia ± infarction→
  - ∘Pain
  - ∘Intrauterine growth retardation-IUGR
  - ∘Pre-eclampsia ± eclampsia
  - ∘Spontaneous abortion (sickle cell disease-6% >> compound heterozygote diseases)

Hematologic
- •Intravascular hemolysis→
  - ∘↓Hemoglobin (♂ <14g/ dL, ♀ <12g/ dL) & hematocrit (♂ <40%, ♀ <35%)→compensatory ↑renal **erythropoietin**→↑**reticulocytes**†, being proportional to the severity of the anemia, provided adequate:
    - −Erythropoietin
    - −Folic acid
    - −Iron
    - −Vitamin B12
- •The intramedullary compensatory response
  - ∘**Reticulocytosis**→
    - −↑Mean corpuscular volume-MCV (>100 fL)
    - −Retained messenger-RNA→purple coloration per Wright stain, termed polychromatophilia
    - −Retained nucleus in severe hemolysis
  - ∘**Cellular cytoplasm release**→
    - −**Hyperkalemia**
    - −Hyperphosphatemia→calcium binding→hypocalcemia
    - −↑Lactate dehydrogenase-LDH
    - −↑Uric acid (> ~7mg/ dL)→gout syndrome
    - −Unconjugated hyperbilirubinemia
    - −↓Plasma haptoglobin & hemopexin, being hemoglobin & heme binding proteins, respectively
- •Leukocytosis, rarely >25,000/ μL
- •Peripheral blood smear showing:
  - ∘**Sickle shaped erythrocytes**, w/ hyposplenism→
    - −Howell−Jolly bodies, being intra−erythrocyte, small, dark staining spherical bodies
    - −Target cells

---

†The normal reticulocyte count is ≤2%, which is expected to ↑in anemic states, as a compensatory mechanism of a normally functioning bone marrow. Lack of this compensatory ↑ indicates that there is at least an element of inadequate marrow production as a cause for the anemia. Being that reticulocytes are calculated in relation to erythrocyte number, anemia→
- •Falsely ↑reticulocyte count. In order to correct for this effect, the reticulocyte count should be adjusted for the degree of anemia:

Corrected reticulocyte count= reticulocyte count (hematocrit / 0.45)
maturation factor (if hematocrit ≥45%=1, 35%=1.5, 25%=2, 20%=2.5)

APLASTIC CRISES
Hematologic
- Viral infection, esp. **Parvovirus B19†, occurring predominantly during childhood**→
  - ∘Bone marrow erythroblast infection→
    - −Complete cessation of erythrocyte production→**severe anemia**→pallor & lethargy

---

- Isolation precautions should be undertaken, as any nonimmune pregnant ♀ may become infected→
  - ∘Fetal death if acquired during the 1st trimester
  - ∘Hydrops fetalis if acquired during the 2nd trimester
- †Infection provides lifelong immunocompetent immunity

SEQUESTRATION CRISES
Gastrointestinal
- Altered erythrocyte shape & ↓membrane deformability→**accumulation of sickled erythrocytes** in the hepatic sinusoids & splenic trabecular network, termed red pulp→
  - ∘**Splenomegaly** (prior to predominant splenic fibrosis)→cellular sequestration→pancytopenia, w/ the process termed hypersplenism→
    - −Normocytic, normochromic anemia→fatigue
    - −Leukopenia→immunosuppression→↑infection & neoplasm risk
    - −Thrombocytopenia→↑hemorrhage risk, esp. petechiae
  - ∘Hepatomegaly
  - …being life−threatening in children, but not adults

ELECTRICAL STUDIES
- **Hemoglobin electrophoresis**
  - ∘Detects & differentiates hemoglobin molecule variants based on differing molecule migration rates through an electric field

Findings:
- **Normal adult: HbA >95%, HbA2: 1.5−3.5%, HbF <1%**
- **Sickle cell trait: HbA: 60%, HbS: 40%, HbA2: 1.5−3,5%, HbF <1%**
- **Sickle cell disease: HbS: 85−98%, HbF: 5−15%, HbA2: 1.5−3.5%**

- Fetal hemoglobin−HbF comprises:
  - ∘75% of total hemoglobin @ birth
  - ∘50% @ 6 weeks
  - ∘<1.5% @ 1 year
  - …during which time, adult hemoglobin A normally becomes the predominant form

TREATMENT
CURATIVE INTENT
- **Bone marrow transplantation**
  - Indications, met by 1% of sickle cell disease patients:
    - **Younger patients (usually @ age <16years) w/ severe complications:**
      - ∘Cerebrovascular accident syndrome
      - ∘Recurrent acute chest syndrome
      - ∘Refractory pain
      - …& are healthy enough to tolerate the procedure, w/ appropriate donors available (HLA matched relative >> unrelated donor)

SICKLE CELL CRISIS
- **Oxygen** to maintain PaO_2 >60mmHg or SaO_2 >92%, usually accomplished via nasal cannula @ 2−4L/min.
  - Mechanism:
    - **Oxygenation if required**
    - **Calming effect**→
      - ∘↓Autonomic sympathetic tone→
        - −↓Physical stress
  - Duration:
    - **24−48hours, or longer if needed for oxygenation**

416

•**Vigorous intravenous hydration** via 3–4L/ 24hours, w/ attention to both:
 ◦**Intravascular volume repletion via Normal saline** (0.9% NaCl) or **lactated Ringer's solution**, as
 per:
  –Vital signs
  –Physical examination
  –Urine output (normal being ≥0.5mL/kg/h)
  –Blood urea nitrogen–BUN & creatinine
 ◦**Intravascular volume maintenance via Normal saline** (0.9% NaCl) or **lactated Ringer's solution**
  Adult maintenance fluid:
   •Weight (kg) + 40= #mL/ hour
  Additional febrile requirements:
   •1L/ 24hours for every 1°F >100°F
  Additional:
   •Estimate loss for:
    ◦Diaphoresis
    ◦Diarrhea
    ◦Polyuria
    ◦Tachypnea
  ...followed by oral rehydration w/ a glucose based electrolyte solution upon both clinical stability &
  ability to tolerate PO
•**Type & cross match** the patients blood for possible transfusion of 2–8units of packed red blood cells,
 depending on the clinical severity. O–negative blood may be used if needed emergently
•**Empiric antibiotics**
 Indications:
  •Febrile patient, to treat for possible encapsulated bacterial infection
•**Exchange transfusion**
 Indications:
  •In order to rapidly ↓the proportion of sickled erythrocytes in the situations listed for erythrocyte
  transfusion
 Procedure:
  •Removal of blood, w/ the subsequent infusion of an equivalent volume of erythrocytes & fresh
  frozen plasma–FFP

LEUKOCYTE DEPLETED PACKED RED BLOOD CELLS, as transfusion→
•Alloantibody formation, termed alloimmunization, in 25% of sickle cell disease patients. For this reason, **leukocyte depleted erythrocytes, being phenotypically matched for antigenic determinants that most often elicit an immune response are preferred for transfusion**
Dose
1unit composed of 450mL of blood & 50mL. plasma=500mL total

Indications:
•Hemoglobin <10mg/ dL, in order to rapidly ↓the proportion of sickled erythrocytes in the following situations:
  ◦Symptomatic acute anemia, or severely symptomatic chronic anemia
  ◦Refractory or protracted painful episodes or mucocutaneous ulcerations
  ◦Acute chest syndrome w/ hypoxemia
  ◦Complicated obstetrical problems
  ◦Priapism, when administered early
  ◦Surgery, involving either:
   –The use of general anesthesia
   –The eye
  ◦Primary or secondary cerebrovascular accident syndrome prevention in children
   –Maintain the HbS concentration <30% X 5years, then ≤50% thereafter

Mechanism:
•1unit→
  ◦1g/ dL ↑hemoglobin
  ◦3% ↑hematocrit
  ◦~10% ↑blood volume

Complications: •Every unit of transfused erythrocytes contains 250mg of iron which the body cannot excrete, except via hemorrhage. It initially accumulates in the monocyte/ macrophage system, w/ subsequent organ deposition→   ◦Organ failure via a hemochromatosis–like syndrome
Monitoring: •For patients w/ chronic transfusion requirements, monitor the ferritin level as an indicator of iron overload

> ∘For patients w/ a plasma ferritin >1000ng/ mL, w/ continuing chronic transfusion requirements, who are expected to survive more than several years, treat iron overload w/ the iron chelating agent Desferrioxamine

OPIOID RECEPTOR AGONISTS

Indications:
- •Acute pain

Generic (Trade)	M	♀	Start
Hydromorphone (Dilaudid)	L	?	
•PO form			2mg q4hours
•SC/ IM/ IV forms			0.5mg q4hours
•PR form			3mg q6hours
Morphine sulfate	LK	?	10mg PO/ SC/ IM/ IV q4hours

- •Titrate as high as necessary to relieve pain, w/ tolerable concomitant side effects

Side effects:
Cardiovascular
- •Vasodilation (venous >> arterial)→
  - ∘↓Preload→
    - –↓Cardiac output→**hypotension**
- •**Bradycardia**

Gastrointestinal
- •Central nervous system chemoreceptor trigger zone activation→
  - ∘**Nausea ± vomiting**, exacerbated by ambulation
- •Enteric nervous system opioid receptor activation→
  - ∘↓Gastrointestinal smooth muscle peristalsis→
    - –**Constipation**
- •↑Biliary tract smooth muscle contraction→
  - ∘Biliary colic

Genitourinary
- •↑Ureteral & urinary bladder smooth muscle peristalsis→
  - ∘Prostatic neoplastic syndrome exacerbation
- •↓Uterine muscle tone→
  - ∘Labor prolongation

Neurologic
- •**Altered mental status**
- •Dysphoria
- •Sedation
- •Seizures

Opthalmologic
- •Iris radial smooth muscle relaxation→
  - ∘↓Pupil size=**miosis**, being fixed

Pulmonary
- •Inhibition of medullary respiratory center response to CO_2 concentration→
  - ∘**Respiratory depression**→
    - –Hypercapnic respiratory failure→altered mental status
- •↓Cough reflex

Side effects of chronic use:
- •Development of **tolerance**† to its effects, as the dosage previously sufficient to produce effects progressively fails to do so, as both the central nervous system & liver adapt to its chronic presence by altering:
  - ∘Neuronal membrane constituents
  - ∘Neurotransmitter release & re-uptake
  - ∘Hepatic clearance
  - …which set the stage for the vicious cycle of **dependence** & craving for ever increasing amounts of the medication, regardless of the professional, social, or health risks

---

†Tolerance does not develop to:
- •Constipation
- •Miosis
- •Seizures

418

ANTIDOTE

Generic (Trade)	M	♀	Start	Max
Naloxone (Narcan)	LK	P	2mg IV/ SC/ IM/ ET q2min. prn	10mg total

Mechanism:
- •μ receptor antagonist, which, in the absence of exogenous opioids, have no clinical effect

Duration:
- •1–2hours

Side effects:
- •**Acute opioid withdrawal/ reversal syndrome**
  - ◦Diaphoresis
  - ◦Goose flesh
  - ◦↑Lacrimation
  - ◦Nausea ± vomiting
  - ◦Rhinorrhea
  - ◦Tachypnea
  - …w/ rare:
    - •Hypo or hypertension
    - •Pulmonary edema
    - •Ventricular tachycardia &/or fibrillation

HYDROXYUREA

Indications:
- •Frequent vaso–occlusive crises, reasonably defined as ≥3 crises/ year requiring hospitalization
- •Severe symptomatic anemia

M	♀	Dose	Max
LK	U	500mg PO qam X 2months, then ↑by 500mg q2months to 1,500mg qam	35mg/ kg q24hours

Mechanisms:
- •↑**Hemoglobin F**†, which forms soluble hybrid polymers w/ hemoglobin S→
  - ◦↓Hemoglobin S polymerization→
    - –↓Cellular sickling
- •Mildly ↑total hemoglobin concentration
- •Inhibits ribonucleotide reductase→
  - ◦↓DNA synthesis→
    - –Cytotoxicity to all proliferating cells

---

†10–25% of patients do not experience an ↑hemoglobin F concentration, likely due to genetic factors, including variations in medication metabolism

Side effects:
- •**General**
  - ◦Anorexia→
    - –Cachexia
  - ◦Headache
- •**Gastrointestinal**
  - ◦Constipation
  - ◦Diarrhea
  - ◦Nausea ± vomiting
- •**Genitourinary**
  - ◦Intra–renal renal failure
- •**Mucocutaneous**
  - ◦Alopecia–rare
  - ◦Dermatitis
  - ◦Facial erythema
  - ◦Hyperpigmentation of:
    - –Back
    - –Pressure areas
  - ◦Mucocutaneous ulcerations, esp. oro–labial
  - ◦Nail changes
- •**Myelosuppression→**
  - ◦Macrocytic anemia→
    - –Fatigue
  - ◦Leukopenia→immunosuppression→
    - –↑Infection & neoplasm risk

419

◦Thrombocytopenia→
  –↑Hemorrhage risk, esp. petechiae
•**Neurologic**
  ◦Sedation	

Monitoring:
•Complete blood count q2weeks until a stable dose, w/ acceptable myelotoxicity†, has been
  reached. Then
  ◦q 4–6weeks	

†The following are considered acceptable: •Neutrophils ≥2,000/ μL •Platelets ≥80,000/ μL	

PROGNOSIS

•Patients w/ sickle cell disease have ↓life expectancy, as even w/ **medical treatment, life expectancy averages 45 years of age**, w/ death being due to organ failure. Without medical treatment, 99% die @ age ≤5years, w/ the remainder dying prior to reproductive age

PROPHYLAXIS

•Patients w/ sickle cell trait who are free of cardiovascular disease do not need to restrict daily activity, except for:
  ◦Prolonged or extreme exertion, due to the physical stress, as well as possible concomitant dehydration
  ◦High altitude exposure of >10,000 feet
•All patients of reproductive age should be informed of their risk of having an affected child, w/ **prenatal diagnosis possible via amniocentesis**
  Procedure:
    •Performed in the 2nd trimester, allowing fetal DNA testing via polymerase chain reaction–PCR mediated β globin chain sequence amplification

•Autoimmune or toxin mediated hematopoietic stem cell dysfunction→
 ∘Myelosuppression→
  −**Pancytopenia** (anemia, leukopenia, & thrombocytopenia)

RISK FACTORS
•**Autoimmune mediated**
 ∘**Idiopathic−50%**
 ∘**Viral infection**
  −Cytomegalovirus−CMV
  −Epstein Barr virus−EBV
  −Hepatitis C virus−HCV
  −Human immune deficiency virus−HIV
 ∘**Autoimmune disease**
  −Systemic lupus erythematosus−SLE
 ∘**Pregnancy**

•**Toxin mediated**
 ∘**Medications**
  −Adalimumab
  −Chemotherapeutic medications, being dose dependent
  −Chloramphenicol
  −Cimetidine
  −Felbamate
  −Gold
  −Phenylbutazone
  −Quinacrine
  −Sulfonamides
  −Trimethadione
 ∘**Radiation therapy**
  −Dose dependent, w/ marrow recovery within weeks after final treatment
 ∘**Other toxins**
  −Benzene
  −Insecticides

DIAGNOSIS
General
 •↓Cellular oxygenation→
  ∘**Fatigue**
  ∘Headache
Hematologic
 •**Myelosuppression**→pancytopenia:
  ∘Anemia, being ↓hemoglobin ($\male$ <14g/ dL, $\female$ <12g/ dL) & hematocrit ($\male$ <40%, $\female$ <35%)→
   −Compensatory ↑renal **erythropoietin** secretion, w/ paradoxical ↓erythrocyte production→
   ↓**reticulocytes**†, indicating erythroid hypoproliferation
  ∘Leukopenia→immunosuppression→
   −↑Infection & neoplasm risk
  ∘Thrombocytopenia→
   −↑Hemorrhage risk, esp. petechiae

---

†The normal reticulocyte count is ≤2%, which is expected to ↑in anemic states, as a compensatory mechanism of a normally functioning bone marrow. Lack of this compensatory ↑ indicates that there is at least an element of inadequate marrow production as a cause for the anemia. Being that reticulocytes are calculated in relation to erythrocyte number, anemia→
 •Falsely ↑reticulocyte count. In order to correct for this effect, the reticulocyte count should be adjusted for the degree of anemia:

Corrected reticulocyte count= reticulocyte count (hematocrit / 0.45)
                    maturation factor (if hematocrit ≥45%=1, 35%=1.5, 25%=2, 20%=2.5)

INVASIVE PROCEDURES
•**Bone marrow biopsy**
 Findings:
  •Hypocellular to acellular bone marrow, w/ fat replacement

421

CURATIVE INTENT
•Discontinue possible etiologic medications
•Allogeneic bone marrow or stem cell transplantation
Outcomes:
•Remission–80%, being 55% w/ previous blood transfusion. Thus, blood transfusion should be avoided, if possible, in patients being considered for bone marrow transplantation
Limitations:
•Patients @ age <60 years (being the upper age limit for transplantation @ many centers), who are healthy enough to tolerate the procedure, & for whom appropriate donors are available (HLA matched related donor >> unrelated donor)

SECOND LINE TREATMENT

IMMUNOMODULATING MEDICATIONS
•The following medications usually require 1–6 months for symptomatic improvement, making these medications not useful in the control of acute disease, but rather, useful when prolonged treatment is planned
Generic (Trade)   M ♀
Cyclosporine   L   ?

Mechanism:
•↓Cytokine synthesis (including interleukins & interferons)→
  ○↓T lymphocyte differentiation
  ○↓T lymphocyte activation

Side effects:
General
•Headache
Cardiovascular
•Hypertension
Gastrointestinal
•↓Mucosal cell proliferation→
  ○Mucosal inflammation=mucositis, including inflammation of the oral mucosa=stomatitis→
    –Diarrhea
    –Nausea ± vomiting
•Transient hepatitis
Genitourinary
•Acute tubular necrosis→
  ○Intra–renal renal failure
Mucocutaneous
•Gingival hyperplasia
•Hirsutism
Neurologic
•Seizures
•Tremor
Hematologic
•Myelosuppression→
  ○Macrocytic anemia→
    –Fatigue
  ○Leukopenia→immunosuppression→
    –↑Infection & neoplasm risk
  ○Thrombocytopenia→
    –↑Hemorrhage risk, esp. petechiae
•Hyperkalemia
•Hyperglycemia
•Hyperlipidemia

Monitoring:
•Baseline complete blood count, renal function, & blood pressure. Then,
  ○Renal function & blood pressure qmonth

PACKED RED BLOOD CELLS

Dose

1unit is composed of 450mL of blood & 50mL of plasma=500mL total

Indications:
- **Hemoglobin <10g/ dL** w/:
  - ◦Active hemorrhage
  - ◦Cardiovascular disease
  - ◦Cerebrovascular disease
  - ◦Peripheral vascular disease
  - ◦Pulmonary disease
  - ◦Sepsis
  - ◦Hemoglobinopathy
  - ◦Otherwise critically ill
- **Hemoglobin <7−8g/ dL** otherwise

Mechanism:
- •1unit→
  - ◦1g/ dL ↑hemoglobin
  - ◦3% ↑hematocrit
  - ◦~10% ↑blood volume

Complications:
- •Blood product transfusions→
  - ◦↓**Bone marrow transplantation remission rate**, from 80% to 55%
- •Every unit of transfused erythrocytes contains 250mg of iron which the body cannot excrete, except via hemorrhage. It initially accumulates in the monocyte/ macrophage system, w/ subsequent organ deposition→
  - ◦Organ failure via a hemochromatosis−like syndrome

Monitoring:
- •For patients w/ chronic transfusion requirements, monitor the ferritin level as an indicator of iron overload
  - ◦For patients w/ a plasma ferritin >1000ng/ mL, w/ continuing chronic transfusion requirements, who are expected to survive more than several years, treat iron overload w/ the iron chelating agent Desferrioxamine

RECOMBINANT HUMAN ERYTHROPOIETIN

Generic (Trade)	M	♀	Start
Darbopoetin (Aranesp)	†	?	0.45µg/ kg SC/ IV qweek
Erythropoietin (Epogen, Procrit)	L	?	50−100 units/ kg SC/ IV 3 times/ week

&

Generic	M	♀	Dose
Ferrous sulfate	K	P	325mg PO q8hours
Folic acid	K	S	1mg PO q24hours
Multivitamin			1q24hours

CONVERSION SCALE

Erythropoietin/ week (units)	Darbopoetin qweek† (µg)
<2,500	6.25
2,500−4,999	12.5
5,000−10,999	25
11,000−17,999	40
18,000−33,999	60
34,000−89,999	100
≥90,000	200

- •Administer Darbopoetin q 2weeks in patients receiving Erythropoietin once weekly
- †Darbopoetin is metabolized by cellular enzymes termed sialidases

Goal parameters:
- •Goal hematocrit/ hemoglobin of 33−36%/ 11−12g/dL
  - ◦The ideal hemoglobin level remains a topic of debate, as the current goal parameters were set by the U.S. government to meet Medicare reimbursement goals, rather than to reflect scientific consensus

Dose adjustment:
- ↑Dose by 25% if hemoglobin rises <1g/ dL over 1month
- ↓Dose by 25% if hemoglobin 12–13g/ dL
  - ∘Hold & ↓reinstated dose if hemoglobin >13g/ dL

Mechanism:
- ↑Bone marrow erythrocyte production
- ↑Erythrocyte intravascular survival

Outcomes:
- ↑Hematocrit/ hemoglobin by 6%/ 2g/dL over 1 month

Side effects:
Cardiovascular
- ↑Blood viscosity
- Hypertension

Contraindications:
- Uncontrolled hypertension

Monitoring:
- Blood pressure
- Hemoglobin qweek until stable, then
  - ∘Qmonth

PLATELETS

Indications:
- Platelet count <50,000/ µL w/ either hemorrhage or pre-procedure
- Prophylactically w/ a platelet count <20,000/ µL

Thrombocytopenia mediated hemorrhage risk:
- Platelet count
  - ∘20,000–50,000/ µL w/ minimal trauma
  - ∘10,000–20,000/ µL, possibly spontaneous
  - ∘<10,000/ µL, commonly spontaneous

Dose

6–10 units typically being transfused at a time (50mL/ unit)

Mechanism:
- ↑Platelet count by 5,000–10,000/ µL per unit

MYELOPROLIFERATIVE CYTOKINES

Indications:
- Granulocytopenia, w/ either:
  - ∘Active infection, as a temporizing measure
  - ∘Prophylactically in order to ↓infection incidence & severity

Note: When used in combination w/ erythropoietin, may→
  - Synergistically ↑erythropoiesis

Generic (Trade)	M	♀
Granulocyte colony stimulating factor–GCSF (Filgastrim)	L	U
Granulocyte–monocyte colony stimulating factor GM–CSF (Sargramostim)	L	U

Side effects:
General
- Fever
- Fluid retention
Mucocutaneous
- Dermatitis
Musculoskeletal
- Bone pain
Pulmonary
- Hypoxia

424

MYELODYSPLASTIC SYNDROMES

•Hematopoietic stem cell dysplasia→
  ◦**Ineffective hematopoietic maturation**→
    −↓Cellular maturation mediated release from the bone marrow→cytopenias, w/ the cell lines affected being dependent on the level of stem cell development @ which the dysplasia occurred
•These syndromes are considered **pre−leukemic states** as <20% of nucleated cells are blasts on bone marrow biopsy, thus not fulfilling the criteria for acute leukemia (except for RAEB which is currently a "grey−zone" diagnosis), but having an ↑risk of evolving into an acute leukemia, esp. of the **myeloid** lineage

RISK FACTORS

•↑**Age−#1 risk factor:** Median age @ presentation is 60 years, being rare @ age <30 years
•**Gender:** ♂−60% > ♀
•**Alteration of nucleic acids**
  ◦Benzene
  ◦Chemotherapy, esp:
    −Alkylating medications: Cyclophosphamide, Melphalan
    −Topoisomerase 2 inhibitors: Doxorubicin, Etoposide, Mitoxantrone, Teniposide
  ◦Radiation
•**Genetic**
  ◦Trisomy 21, termed Down's syndrome

CLASSIFICATION/ DIAGNOSIS

The French−American−British FAB classification:
•**Refractory anemia 15−30%**
  Peripheral blood smear findings:
    •Cytopenia of ≥1 lineage(s), w/ <1% of nucleated cells being blasts
  Bone marrow findings:
    •Normal to hypercellular, having dysplastic changes, w/ <5% of nucleated cells being blasts

•**Refractory anemia w/ ringed sideroblasts−13%**
  Peripheral blood smear findings:
    •Cytopenia of ≥1 lineage(s), w/ <1% of nucleated cells being blasts
  Bone marrow findings:
    •Normal to hypercellular, having dysplastic changes, w/ <5% of nucleated cells being blasts (>15% of which are ringed sideroblasts)

•**Refractory anemia w/ excess blasts−RAEB 27%**
  Peripheral blood smear findings:
    •Cytopenia of ≥2 lineages, w/ <5% of nucleated cells being blasts
  Bone marrow findings:
    •Dysplastic changes in all cell lineages, w/ 5−20% of nucleated cells being blasts
  ◦**Refractory anemia w/ excess blasts−RAEB in transformation 20%**
  Peripheral blood smear findings:
    •Cytopenia of ≥2 lineages, w/ >5% of nucleated cells being blasts
  Bone marrow findings:
    •Dysplastic changes in all cell lineages, w/ either:
      ◦20−30% of nucleated cells being blasts
      ◦Blast cells containing Auer rods, being eosinophilic, needle−like cytoplasmic inclusions

•**Chronic myelomonocytic leukemia−15%**
  Peripheral blood smear findings:
    •Monocytes >1,000/ μL, w/ <5% of nucleated cells being blasts
  Bone marrow findings:
    •≤20% of nucleated cells being blasts

---

†Defined as:
  •Hemoglobin <10g/ dL
  •Absolute neutrophil count−ANC <1,500/ μL
  •Platelet count <100,000/ μL

General
  •↓Cellular oxygenation→
    ◦**Fatigue**
    ◦Headache

Cardiovascular
- The cardiovascular signs are compensatory mechanisms→
  - ∘↑Cellular oxygenation, allowing for the patient to possibly be asymptomatic @ rest. However, exertion→
    - −↑Tissue O_2 demand→eventual decompensation→symptoms
- ↓Blood viscosity & ↓cellular oxygenation →
  - ∘↓Resistance to blood flow & arterial vasodilation respectively, both→↑venous return→↑**cardiac output**→
    - −↑Systolic blood pressure→↑pulse pressure (systolic − diastolic blood pressure)
    - −Systolic flow murmur
    - −Cervical venous hum
- Acute anemia→
  - ∘Thoracic arterial baroreceptor & chemoreceptor activation→
    - −↑**Autonomic sympathetic tone**→tachycardia

Mucocutaneous
- ↓Hemoglobin→
  - ∘Skin & mucus membrane pallor
    - −Extended palmar crease pallor @ a hemoglobin ≤7g/ dL

Pulmonary
- Exertion→
  - ∘↑Tissue O_2 demand→
    - −Dyspnea=breathlessness

Hematologic
- Anemia, being ↓hemoglobin (♂ <14g/ dL, ♀ <12g/ dL) & hematocrit (♂ <40%, ♀ <35%), often macrocytic, w/ possible:
  - ∘Size variation, termed anisocytosis
  - ∘Shape irregularity, termed poikilocytosis
  - ∘Compensatory ↑renal **erythropoietin** secretion, w/ paradoxical ↓erythrocyte production→
    ↓**reticulocytes**†, indicating erythroid hypoproliferation
- Leukopenia→
  - ∘↑Infection & neoplasm risk
- Thrombocytopenia→
  - ∘↑Hemorrhage risk, esp. petechiae
- **Hypogranular &/or hyposegmented neutrophils, termed Pelger−Huet cells**
- Large, agranular platelets

---

†The normal reticulocyte count is ≤2%, which is expected to ↑in anemic states, as a compensatory mechanism of a normally functioning bone marrow. Lack of this compensatory ↑ indicates that there is at least an element of inadequate marrow production as a cause for the anemia. Being that reticulocytes are calculated in relation to erythrocyte number, anemia→
- Falsely ↑reticulocyte count. In order to correct for this effect, the reticulocyte count should be adjusted for the degree of anemia:

Corrected reticulocyte count= reticulocyte count (hematocrit / 0.45)
　　　　　　　　　　　　　　　maturation factor (if hematocrit ≥45%=1, 35%=1.5, 25%=2, 20%=2.5)

INVASIVE PROCEDURES
- **Bone marrow biopsy**
  Findings:
  - Normal to hypercellular >> hypocellular
  - Megaloblastic erythroid precursors, w/ either:
    - ∘Dissociation of nuclear to cytoplasmic maturation→
      - −↑Relative cytoplasmic maturation
    - ∘Multiple nuclei
  - Small, hyposegmented megakaryocytes
  - Iron stain may reveal ringed sideroblasts

ADDITIONAL STUDIES
- **Cytogenetic analysis**
  Common chromosomal myelodysplastic abnormalities:
  - Loss of part or all of chromosome 5−13%
  - Loss or part or all of chromosome 7−5%
  - Loss of chromosome X or Y−2%
  - Loss of chromosome 20q−2%
  - Loss of chromosome 17p <1%

•**Curative intent**
  ◦**Allogeneic bone marrow or stem cell transplantation**
   Outcomes:
   •Remission–80%, being 55% w/ previous blood transfusion. Thus, blood transfusion should be avoided if possible, in patients being considered for bone marrow transplantation
   Limitations:
   •Patients @ age <60 years (being the upper age limit for transplantation @ many centers), who are healthy enough to tolerate the procedure, & for whom appropriate donors are available (HLA matched relative donor >> unrelated donor)

PALLIATIVE INTENT

PACKED RED BLOOD CELLS
Dose
1unit is composed of 450mL of blood & 50mL of plasma=500mL total

Indications:
•**Hemoglobin <10g/ dL** w/:
  ◦Active hemorrhage
  ◦Cardiovascular disease
  ◦Cerebrovascular disease
  ◦Peripheral vascular disease
  ◦Pulmonary disease
  ◦Sepsis
  ◦Hemoglobinopathy
  ◦Otherwise critically ill
•**Hemoglobin <7–8g/ dL** otherwise

Mechanism:
•1unit→
  ◦1g/ dL ↑hemoglobin
  ◦3% ↑hematocrit
  ◦~10% ↑blood volume

Complications:
•Blood product transfusions→
  ◦↓**Bone marrow transplantation remission rate**, from 80% to 55%
•Every unit of transfused erythrocytes contains 250mg of iron which the body cannot excrete, except via hemorrhage. It initially accumulates in the monocyte/ macrophage system, w/ subsequent organ deposition→
  ◦Organ failure via a hemochromatosis–like syndrome

Monitoring: •For patients w/ chronic transfusion requirements, monitor the ferritin level as an indicator of iron overload   ◦For patients w/ a plasma ferritin >1000ng/ mL, w/ continuing chronic transfusion requirements, who are expected to survive more than several years, treat iron overload w/ the iron chelating agent Desferrioxamine

RECOMBINANT HUMAN ERYTHROPOIETIN			
Generic (Trade)	M ♀	**Start**	
Darbopoetin (Aranesp)	† ?	0.45µg/ kg SC/ IV qweek	
Erythropoietin (Epogen, Procrit)	L ?	50–100 units/ kg SC/ IV 3 times/ week	
		&	

Generic	M ♀	Dose
Ferrous sulfate	K P	325mg PO q8hours
Folic acid	K S	1mg PO q24hours
Multivitamin		1q24hours

427

CONVERSION SCALE	
Erythropoietin/ week (units)	Darbopoetin qweek† (µg)
<2,500	6.25
2,500–4,999	12.5
5,000–10,999	25
11,000–17,999	40
18,000–33,999	60
34,000–89,999	100
≥90,000	200

•Administer Darbopoetin q 2weeks in patients receiving erythropoietin once weekly
†Darbopoetin is metabolized by cellular enzymes termed sialidases

Goal parameters:
- •Goal hematocrit/ hemoglobin of 33–36%/ 11–12g/dL
  - ∘The ideal hemoglobin level remains a topic of debate, as the current goal parameters were set by the U.S. government to meet Medicare reimbursement goals, rather than to reflect scientific consensus

Dose adjustment:
- •↑Dose by 25% if hemoglobin rises <1g/ dL over 1month
- •↓Dose by 25% if hemoglobin 12–13g/ dL
  - ∘Hold & ↓reinstated dose if hemoglobin >13g/ dL

Mechanism:
- •↑Bone marrow erythrocyte production
- •↑Erythrocyte intravascular survival

Outcomes:
- •↑Hematocrit/ hemoglobin by 6%/ 2g/dL over 1 month

Side effects:
  Cardiovascular
- •↑Blood viscosity
- •Hypertension

Contraindications:
- •Uncontrolled hypertension

Monitoring:
- •Blood pressure
- •Hemoglobin qweek until stable, then
  - ∘Qmonth

PLATELETS

Indications:
- •Platelet count <50,000/ µL w/ either hemorrhage or pre–procedure
- •Prophylactically w/ a platelet count <20,000/ µL

Thrombocytopenia mediated hemorrhage risk:
- •Platelet count
  - ∘20,000–50,000/ µL w/ minimal trauma
  - ∘10,000–20,000/ µL, possibly spontaneous
  - ∘<10,000/ µL, commonly spontaneous

Dose

6–10 units typically being transfused at a time (50mL/ unit)

Mechanism:
- •↑Platelet count by 5,000–10,000/ µL per unit

MYELOPROLIFERATIVE CYTOKINES

Indications:
- •Granulocytopenia, w/ either:
  - ∘Active infection, as a temporizing measure
  - ∘Prophylactically in order to ↓infection incidence & severity

Note: When used in combination w/ erythropoietin, may→
  - •Synergistically ↑erythropoiesis

Generic (Trade)	M ♀
Granulocyte colony stimulating factor-GCSF (Filgastrim)	L U
Granulocyte–monocyte colony stimulating factor GM–CSF (Sargramostim)	L U

428

Side effects:
General
•Fever
•Fluid retention
Mucocutaneous
•Dermatitis
Musculoskeletal
•Bone pain
Pulmonary
•Hypoxia

PROGNOSIS

Progression to acute myeloid leukemia–AML:
- •Refractory anemia–10%
- •Refractory anemia w/ ringed sideroblasts–10%
- •Refractory anemia w/ excess blasts–RAEB 45%
  - ∘Refractory anemia w/ excess blasts–RAEB in transformation–60%
- •Chronic myelomonocytic leukemia–15%

International prognostic scoring system for myelodysplastic syndromes:
- **•0.5 points:**
  - ∘Cytopenia of >1 lineage
  - ∘5–10% of bone marrow nucleated cells being blasts
  - ∘Chromosome abnormalities other than Y-, 5q-, 20q- or those listed below
- **•1 point:**
  - ∘Loss of part or all of chromosome 7
  - ∘≥Any 3 chromosomal abnormalities
- **•1.5 points:**
  - ∘11–20% of bone marrow nucleated cells being blasts
- **•2 points:**
  - ∘21–30% of bone marrow nucleated cells being blasts

Median survival based on point total:
- **•0 points:** 5.7 year median survival
- **•0.5–1 points:** 3.5 year median survival
- **•1.5–2 points:** 1.2 years median survival
- **•≥2.5 points:** 0.4 years median survival

429

POLYCYTHEMIA VERA

•Hematopoietic stem cell dysplasia→
  ◦**Unregulated proliferation of the erythroid lineage** ± other cell lines, dependent on the level of stem cell development @ which the dysplasia occurred→
    –Primary **erythrocytosis**, termed polycythemia vera→↑**blood viscosity, w/ resultant sludging of blood in the microcirculation** (arterioles, capillaries, & venules)→vascular occlusion→distal ischemia ± infarction

RISK FACTORS

•**Age:** 50–60years, w/ 5% diagnosed @ <40 years
•**Gender:** ♂ 1.4 X ♀

DIAGNOSIS

General
•↓Cellular oxygenation→
  ◦**Fatigue**
  ◦Headache
Cardiovascular
•**Erythrocytosis**→
  ◦**Vascular occlusion** (arterioles, capillaries, & venules)→
    –Organ ischemia ± infarction, usually affecting several organs at once due to the systemic nature of the disease→**pain** & **organ dysfunction**, w/ infarction→inflammation & fibrosis
•↑Blood viscosity→
  ◦↓Venous return→
    –↓Jugular venous flow→proximal congestion→sensation of fullness in the head &/or face
  ◦↑Afterload→
    –Compensatory ↑cardiac output→**systolic hypertension–65%**→↑pulse pressure (systolic – diastolic blood pressure)
Gastrointestinal
•Splenic ischemia ± infarction→
  ◦Left upper quadrant abdominal pain, w/ infarction→inflammation & fibrosis. Repeated infarctions→splenic fibrosis→**functional asplenia**, wherein the spleen is present, but non-functional→↑infection risk via **encapsulated bacteria:**
    –Escherichia coli
    –Haemophilus influenzae
    –Neisseria meningitides
    –Pseudomonas aeruginosa
    –Salmonella sp.
    –Streptococcus pneumoniae
    …all of which may preferentially seed an area of inflammation &/or fibrosis due to ↓immune defenses→
      •Abscess formation
•Hepatic ischemia ± infarction→
  ◦Right upper quadrant abdominal pain, w/ infarction→
    –Inflammation, termed hepatitis, & fibrosis. Repeated infarctions→cirrhosis
•Gallbladder ischemia ± infarction→
  ◦Right upper quadrant abdominal pain, w/ infarction→
    –Inflammation, termed cholecystitis, & fibrosis
•Basophil histamine release→
  ◦Peptic inflammatory disease risk
Genitourinary
•Renal ischemia ± infarction→
  ◦Pain, w/ infarction→
    –Inflammation, termed aseptic pyelonephritis
    –Papillary necrosis
    –Fibrosis
    …w/ repeated infarctions→intra–renal renal failure
•Corpus cavernosus occlusion→
  ◦**Priapism**, being an erection lasting ≥24hours, often→
    –Impotence, being the inability to achieve &/or maintain an erection
Lymphatic
•Erythrocyte sequestration→
  ◦**Splenomegally–60%**→
    –Abdominal discomfort

430

Mucocutaneous
- •↑Blood viscosity→
  - ∘↓Mucocutaneous blood flow→
    - –↑O_2 extraction→bluish color=cyanosis
  - ∘Mucocutaneous infarction→
    - –Ulcerations
- •A syndrome of intense burning pain & erythema of the extremities, termed **erythromelalgia**
- •Basophil histamine release→
  - ∘Pruritus, esp. after bathing

Musculoskeletal
- •Bone ischemia ± infarction→
  - ∘Pain, w/ infarction→
    - –Inflammation, termed aseptic osteomyelitis
    - –Aseptic necrosis of the femoral heads
    - –Fibrosis
    - ...w/ repeated infarction→
      - •Myelofibrosis→
        - –Pancytopenia

Neurologic
- •Central nervous system ischemia ±infarction→
  - ∘Cerebrovascular accident syndromes
  - ∘Seizures

Opthalmologic
- •↑Blood viscosity→
  - ∘Engorged & tortuous retinal veins
- •Retinal ischemia ± infarction→
  - ∘Visual changes, w/ infarction→
    - –Inflammation & fibrosis→retinal disease, termed retinopathy→blindness

Pulmonary
- •Lung ischemia ± infarction→
  - ∘Thoracic pain, w/ infarction→
    - –Inflammation, termed pneumonitis, & fibrosis. Repeated infarctions→emphysema
  - ∘Ventilation/ perfusion mismatch via:
    - –↑Alveolar dead space: Alveolar ventilation through relatively underperfused capillaries
    - –↑Vascular shunting†: Capillary blood flow through relatively underventilated alveoli. Usually occurring, or exacerbated via ↑venous return
    - ...→↓diffusion of O_2 & CO_2→
      - •Hypoxemia (SaO_2 ≤ 91% or PaO_2 ≤ 60mmHg‡) on room air, w/ subsequent hypercapnia ($PaCO_2$ ≥45mmHg) due to either:
        - ∘Respiratory muscle fatigue
        - ∘Alveolar hypoventilation
        - ...as CO_2 clearance is unimpaired (& may be ↑in the dyspneic patient) as long as adequate ventilation (including lack of diffuse severe ventilation/ perfusion mismatching) is maintained, as:
          - •CO_2 diffuses 20X as rapidly as O_2
          - •Hypercapnia→
            - ∘Immediate brain stem respiratory center mediated stimulation of pulmonary ventilation, which may correct the hypercapnia, but not necessarily the hypoxia
- •Necrotic bone marrow emboli &/or venous thromboemboli→
  - ∘Pulmonary infarction

---

†Being exacerbated by the supine position→
- •↑Systemic venous return→
  - ∘↑Vascular shunting→↑dyspnea, being termed:
    - –Orthopnea, if persistent
    - –Paroxysmal nocturnal dyspnea if intermittent
    - ...causing the patient to either use multiple pillows or sleep in a chair

‡Age adjusted normal PaO_2 = 101 − (0.43 X age)

Materno–fetal
- •Placental ischemia ± infarction→
  - ∘Pain
  - ∘Intrauterine growth retardation–IUGR
  - ∘Pre–eclampsia ± eclampsia
  - ∘Spontaneous abortion

Hematologic
- **Erythrocytosis**, being ↑hemoglobin (♂ >20g/ dL, ♀ >18g/ dL) & hematocrit (♂ >60%, ♀ >55%) ± leukocytosis &/or thrombocytosis
- Feedback mediated normal to ↓erythropoietin level, as opposed to causes of secondary erythrocytosis which→
  - ↑Erythropoietin
- ↑Leukocyte alkaline phosphatase–LAP, an enzyme produced by functional leukocytes
- ↑Cellular turn over→
  - ↑Uric acid (> ~7mg/ dL)→
    - Gout syndrome
- ↑Vitamin B12 & B12 binding protein
- Peripheral blood smear showing normal erythrocyte morphology

INVASIVE PROCEDURES
- **Bone marrow biopsy**

Findings:
- Hypercellular marrow
- ↓Bone marrow iron stores→
  - ↓Hemosiderin formation, being the first sign→
    - ↓Light microscopic observation via Prussian blue staining
- Myelofibrosis

TREATMENT
- The goal of treatment is to achieve & maintain a hemoglobin level of ♂ 14g/ dL, ♀ 12g/ dL in all patients
- **Phlebotomy**

HYDROXYUREA

Indications:
- Symptomatic erythrocytosis
- Refractory pruritus
- Inability to tolerate phlebotomy

M	♀	Dose	Max
LK	U	500mg PO qam X 2months, then ↑by 500mg q2months to 1,500mg qam	35mg/ kg q24hours

Mechanisms:
- Inhibits ribonucleotide reductase→
  - ↓DNA synthesis→
    - Cytotoxicity to all proliferating cells

Side effects:
- **General**
  - Anorexia→
    - Cachexia
  - Headache
- **Gastrointestinal**
  - Constipation
  - Diarrhea
  - Nausea ± vomiting
- **Genitourinary**
  - Intra–renal renal failure
- **Mucocutaneous**
  - Alopecia–rare
  - Dermatitis
  - Facial erythema
  - Hyperpigmentation of:
    - Back
    - Pressure areas
  - Mucocutaneous ulcerations, esp. oro–labial
  - Nail changes
- **Myelosuppression→**
  - Macrocytic anemia→
    - Fatigue
  - Leukopenia→immunosuppression→
    - ↑Infection & neoplasm risk
  - Thrombocytopenia→
    - ↑Hemorrhage risk, esp. petechiae

- **Neurologic**
  - ∘Sedation

Monitoring:
- •Complete blood count q2weeks until a stable dose, w/ acceptable myelotoxicity†, has been reached. Then
  - ∘q 4–6weeks

---

†The following are considered acceptable:
- •Neutrophils ≥2,000/ µL
- •Platelets ≥80,000/ µL

ERYTHROMELALGIA

NONSTEROIDAL ANTI-INFLAMMATORY DRUGS-NSAIDs

Generic	M ♀	Start	Max
Acetylsalicylic acid–ASA=Aspirin	K U	81mg PO q24hous	325mg q24hours

Mechanism:
- •Aspirin & other anti-inflammatory medications→
  - ∘Respectively to irreversible & reversible inhibition of both cyclooxygenase enzymes (COX–1 & COX–2), being responsible for the production of neural & inflammatory cell prostaglandins respectively→
    - –↓Pain
    - –↓Temperature (antipyretic)
    - –↓Inflammation
- •Aspirin is the only nonsteroidal anti-inflammatory drug–NSAID→
  - ∘Irreversible inhibition of both cyclooxygenase–COX enzymes (COX1 & COX2), w/ COX1 being responsible for the production of both thromboxane A_2 & prostacyclin→
    - **–Near complete inhibition of platelet thromboxane A_2 production within 15 min.**, w/ endothelial & vascular smooth muscle cells producing new enzymes in several hours→ relatively ↑prostacyclin
- •Being that platelets lack the enzymatic machinery for protein synthesis, only newly formed platelets (platelet half life=10 days) have the functional enzyme
  …this shift in the balance of cytokine production→
    - •↓**Thrombus formation**

Background pathophysiology:
- •Inflammatory cell mediated prostaglandins are released at sites of inflammation (in addition to other inflammatory cytokines)→
  - ∘Leukocyte migration→↑inflammation via:
    - –Vasodilation→↑blood flow→erythema, edema, warmth, &/or tenderness/ pain via enhanced neuronal sensitivity
- •Interleukin–IL1→
  - ∘↑Hypothalamic prostaglandin production→
    - –Fever
- •Platelet mediated **thromboxane A_2** release at the site of vascular injury→
  - ∘Platelet aggregation
  - ∘Vasoconstriction
  …w/ both processes→
    - •Thrombus formation
- •Endothelial & vascular smooth muscle cell mediated **prostacyclin** release in the surrounding area→
  - ∘Inhibition of platelet aggregation
  - ∘Vasodilation
  …w/ both processes→
    - •↓Thrombus formation

In Brief:
- •**Cyclooxygenase–COX1 enzymes** are found in most cells of the body, being responsible for normal physiologic processes
- •**Cyclooxygenase–COX 2 enzymes** are responsible for the production of inflammatory cell prostaglandins

---

- •Concomitant NSAID administration→
  - ∘Competition for the cyclooxygenase–COX 1 enzyme binding site, w/:
    - –Unbound Aspirin being rapidly cleared from plasma
    - –Bound NSAID action being reversible & short lived

433

...→↓overall antiplatelet effect, requiring either:
- Aspirin to be taken @ ≥1hour prior to other NSAIDs
- Switch to thienopyridine derivative for the antiplatelet effect

Side effects:
Gastrointestinal
- Inhibition of the cyclooxygenase–COX1 enzyme→↑peptic inflammatory disease risk→↑**upper gastrointestinal hemorrhage risk** via:
  - ↓Gastric mucosal prostaglandin synthesis→
    - ↓Epithelial cell proliferation
    - ↓Mucosal blood flow→↓bicarbonate delivery to the mucosa
    - ↓Mucus & bicarbonate secretion from gastric mucosal cells

Indications for peptic inflammatory disease prophylaxis:
- Prophylax w/ proton pump inhibitors–PPI's, histamine 2 selective receptor blockers, or Misoprostol in patients w/ any of the following:
  - Age >60 years w/ a history of peptic inflammatory disease
  - Anticipated therapy >3 months
  - Concurrent glucocorticoid use
  - Moderate to high dose NSAID use
  Note: Newer NSAIDs (Etodolac, Nabumetone, Salsalate)→
  - ↓Risk of NSAID induced peptic inflammation/ ulcer

Genitourinary
- Patients w/ pre–existing bilateral ↓renal perfusion, not necessarily failure:
  - Heart failure
  - Bilateral renal artery stenosis
  - Hypovolemia
  - Renal failure
  ...rely more on the compensatory production of vasodilatory prostaglandins→
  - Afferent arteriole dilation→
    - Maintained glomerular filtration rate–GFR, whereas NSAIDs→
      - ↓Prostaglandin production, which may→renal failure

Pulmonary
- Inhibition of both cyclooxygenase enzymes (COX 1 & COX2)→
  - ↑Lipoxygenase activity→
    - ↑Leukotriene synthesis→symptomatic asthma within 2hours of ingestion in 5% of asthmatics

Rheumatologic
- Acetylsalicylic acid competes w/ uric acid secretion in the renal tubules→
  - ↑Uric acid levels→
    - ↑Risk of uric acid precipitation in the tissues=gout

Pediatric
- **Reye's syndrome**
  - A life threatening fulminant hepatitis→
    - Hepatic encephalopathy in children age ≤16 years w/ a viral infection (esp. influenza or Varicella–zoster virus–VZV)

Overdose:
Pulmonary
- Direct brainstem respiratory center mediated stimulation of pulmonary ventilation→
  - Hyperventilation→
    - **Initial respiratory alkalemia, w/ the subsequent development of an anion gap metabolic acidemia**
- Pulmonary edema

Neurologic
- Altered mental status
- Aseptic meningitis
- Depression
- Hallucinations
- Hyperactivity
- Hyperthermia
- Lightheadedness
- Seizures
- Tinnitus

Gastrointestinal
- Nausea ± vomiting

Mucocutaneous
•Pharyngitis

HYPERURICEMIA

ALLOPURINOL

M ♀	Start	Titrate	Max
K ?	100mg PO q24hours	qweek to a target uric acid level <6mg/ dL	800mg/ 24hours†

†Doses >300mg should be divided

Dose adjustment:
•Adjust according to renal function

Creatinine clearance	Max dose
10–20mL/ min.	200mg/ 24hours
<10mL/ min.	100mg/ 24hours

Mechanism:
•Inhibits xanthine oxidase→
  ○↓Uric acid production
  ○↑Hypoxanthine & xanthine production, which are much more soluble than uric acid, & readily
    excreted

Side effects:
General
  •**May incite a gout attack during treatment initiation or dosage ↑**
  Risk reduction:
    •Concomitant administration of an anti–inflammatory drugs–NSAIDs, until the target uric acid
      level is reached X ≥6months
Hypersensitivity syndrome†–2% (↑w/ renal failure)
  •Dermatitis
  •Fever
  •Hepatitis
  •Renal failure
  •Vasculitis
  •Eosinophilia
  ...necessitating discontinuation
  Prognosis:
    •20% mortality
Interactions:
  •↓Metabolism of Azathioprine, Mercaptopurine, Theophylline, Warfarin→
    ○↑Plasma concentration

Overdosage:
General
  •Fever
Gastrointestinal
  •Hepatitis
Genitourinary
  •Renal failure

†**Allopurinol desensitization**
  Indication:
    •Mild hypersensitivity syndrome
  Protocol:
    •Start 10μg q24h, then
      ○Double the dose q3–14days until the necessary dosage is reached

435

SECOND LINE

CYTOKINES

Indications:
•Refractory erythrocytosis or pruritus

Generic	M ♀	Start
Interferon−α−2b	K ?	3million units SC/ IM 3X/ week @ bedtime

Mechanism:
•Induces the synthesis of cell encoded enzymes→
　○Selective inhibition of viral messenger RNA translation to protein, without affecting the translation of cellular messenger RNA

Side effects:
General
•Anorexia
•Erythema at the injection site
•Headache
•**Influenze−like syndrome** (fatigue, fever, chills, myalgia) beginning 6−8hours after administration, & lasting ≤12hours
　○Administer w/ antipyretic at bedtime in order to attempt to avoid this syndrome
Cardiovascular
•Dilated cardiomyopathy
Endocrine
•Diabetes mellitus
Gastrointestinal
•Diarrhea
Opthalmologic
•Optic neuritis
•Retinopathy
Neurologic
•Amotivation
•Alopecia
•Altered taste=dysguesia
•↓Concentration
•Depression
•Impaired hearing
•Insomnia
•Irritability
•↓Libido, being sexual desire→
　−Impotence, being the inability to achieve &/or maintain an erection
•Paranoia
•Polyneuropathy
•Seizure
•Suicidal ideation
Hematologic
•Autoantibody induction
•**Leukopenia→**
　○↑Infection &/or neoplasm risk
•**Thrombocytopenia→**
　○↑Hemorrhage risk, esp. petechiae

Absolute contraindications:
Cardiovascular
•Symptomatic cardiac disease
Gastrointestinal
•Decompensated cirrhosis
Neurologic
•Uncontrolled seizure disease
Psychiatric
•Current severe major depression
•History of psychosis
Hematologic
•Neutropenia
•Thrombocytopenia
Other
•Organ transplantation (other than liver)

Relative contraindications:
Rheumatologic
  •Autoimmune disease
Endocrine
  •Uncontrolled diabetes mellitus

PROGNOSIS

•Median survival
  ◦w/ treatment: 11–15years
  ◦Without treatment: 0.5–1.5years
•2% transform into an acute leukemia

AUTOIMMUNE THROMBOCYTOPENIA

•Primary or secondary (via molecular mimicry) mediated antiplatelet antibody (IgG >> IgM)→
∘Macrophage mediated removal & destruction (splenic & hepatic > others)→
−**Thrombocytopenia** (platelet <150,000/ uL)→↑systemic hemorrhage risk

CLASSIFICATION

•**Acute autoimmune thrombocytopenia**, duration ≤6months
∘**Age**
−**Children** >> adults
∘**Infection**, esp.:
−Immediate antecedent **upper respiratory tract infection**

•**Chronic autoimmune thrombocytopenia**, duration >6months
∘**Age**
−Adults (esp. <40 years), comprising >90% of adult cases
∘**Gender:** ♀ 3 X ♂
∘**Autoimmune disease syndromes**
−Antiphospholipid antibody syndrome
−Autoimmune hemolytic anemia–10%, w/ the combination being called **Evans' syndrome**
−Autoimmune thyroid disease (Graves' disease or autoimmune thyroiditis)
−Systemic lupus erythematosus–SLE
∘**Malignancy**
−Lymphoma
−Leukemia, esp. chronic lymphoid leukemia–CLL or large lymphoblastic cell predominance
...→autoantibody production
∘**Viral infection**
−Cytomegalovirus–CMV
−Epstein–Barr virus–EBV
−Hepatitis C virus
−Human immune deficiency virus–HIV
...→autoantibody production

DIAGNOSIS

•The diagnosis of autoimmune thrombocytopenia is one of exclusion

Cardiovascular/ Neurologic
•↑Internal organ hemorrhage risk, most importantly being the central nervous system→
∘**Intracranial hemorrhage, being the #1 cause of death**

Gastrointestinal
•**Hemorrhage**, which may occur intermittently→
∘**Hematemesis:** Vomiting of blood, including very dark, tarry looking blood termed 'coffee ground' emesis
  Lesion localization:
  •Upper gastrointestinal hemorrhage
∘**Hematochezia:** Passage of bright red blood per rectum
  Lesion localization:
  •Lower gastrointestinal hemorrhage >> upper gastrointestinal hemorrhage via massive hemorrhage (≥1L) &/or ↑↑peristalsis
∘**Melena**†‡: Passage of sticky, very dark, tarry looking stool, w/ a characteristic odor, requiring ≥50mL of blood, indicating gastrointestinal hemorrhage proximal to ileocecal sphincter >> colonic gastrointestinal hemorrhage via slow hemorrhage &/or ↓peristalsis
∘**Fecal occult blood:** Passage of blood detectable only by laboratory testing, requiring ≥20mL of blood. Not helpful in the anatomic determination of the lesion
Genitourinary
•Hematuria, being either:
∘Microscopic via positive heme dipstick reaction without erythrocytes
∘Macroscopic, termed gross, via red/ brown colored urine without erythrocytes
•↑Menstrual hemorrhage
Mucocutaneous
•Nasal hemorrhage=epistaxis
•Oro–pharyngeal hemorrhage, esp. the gums upon tooth brushing

- •Skin &/or mucus membrane (nasal, oral, pharyngeal, & or conjunctival) hemorrhage→
  - ○Discoloration which does not blanch upon pressure, termed purpura, being either:
    - –≤3mm=**petechiae**
    - –>3mm=**ecchymoses**
    - …± being palpable due to tumor effect, termed palpable purpura, indicating underlying vascular inflammation, termed vasculitis

Pulmonary
- •Pulmonary hemorrhage→cough, termed hemoptysis

Materno–fetal
- •15% of neonates born to affected mothers have severe thrombocytopenia→
  - ○↑Intracranial hemorrhage risk, esp. during vaginal delivery or w/ invasive fetal blood sampling

Hematologic
- •**Thrombocytopenia** (platelet <150,000/ uL)
- •Antiplatelet antibody positive
  - Outcomes:
    - •Sensitivity–55%, specificity–85%
- •Peripheral blood smear showing **large, immature platelets, termed megathrombocytes**

INVASIVE PROCEDURES

- •**Bone marrow biopsy**
  - Indications:
    - •All patients, in order to rule out possible leukemia, lymphoma, or myelodysplastic disease syndrome
  - Findings:
    - •↑ **to normal megakaryocyte count**

TREATMENT IN THE ADULT

SYSTEMIC GLUCOCORTICOID TREATMENT

Indications:
- •**Hemorrhage**
- •**Platelet count <30,000/ uL**

Generic	M	♀	Dose†
Methylprednisolone	L	?	1–2mg/ kg PO/ IV q24hours X 6weeks
Prednisolone	L	?	1–2mg/ kg PO/ IV q24hours X 6weeks
Prednisone	L	?	1–2mg/ kg PO q24hours X 6weeks

- •Once disease control is achieved, taper to the lowest effective maintenance dose in order to maintain a safe platelet count (>30,000/ uL), while minimizing serious side effects, w/ the goal of discontinuation if possible, w/ attention to relapse syndrome (occurring in the majority of patients) via occasional complete blood count
- •Both the IV & PO routes have equal efficacy
- †If hemorrhage is either:
  - •**Internal**
  - •**Extensive/ progressive mucocutaneous**
  - …administer 1gram IV over 30min., q24hours X 2–5days, w/ platelets & intravenous immune globulin–IVIG

Glucocorticoids	Relative potencies Anti–inflammatory	Mineralocorticoid	Duration	Dose equiv.
Cortisol (physiologic†)	1	1	10hours	20mg
Cortisone (PO)	0.7	2	10hours	25mg
Hydrocortisone (PO, IM, IV)	1	2	10hours	20mg
Methylprednisolone (PO, IM, IA, IV)	5	0.5	15–35hours	5mg
Prednisone (PO)	5	0.5	15–35hours	5mg
Prednisolone (PO, IM, IV)	5	0.8	15–35hours	5mg
Triamcinolone (PO, IM)	5	~0	15–35hours	5mg
Betamethasone (PO, IM, IA)	25	~0	35–70hours	0.75mg
Dexamethasone (PO)	25	~0	35–70hours	0.75mg
Fludrocortisone (PO)	10	125	10hours	

†The physiologic rate of adrenal cortical cortisol production is 20–30mg/ 24hours

Mechanisms:
- •↓Plasma cell anti–platelet antibody production
- •Stabilization of lisosomal & cell membranes→
  - ○↓Macrophage cell membrane Fc receptors→
    - –↓Macrophage mediated platelet phagocytosis

Outcomes:
- Partial or complete short term remission: 50%
- Long term remission: <20%

Side effects of chronic use:
General
- Anorexia→
  - Cachexia
- ↑Perspiration

Cardiovascular
- Mineralocorticoid effects→
  - ↑Renal tubular NaCl & water retention as well as potassium secretion→
    - **Hypertension**
    - **Edema**
    - **Hypokalemia**
- Counter-regulatory=anti-insulin effects→
  - ↑Plasma glucose→
    - **Secondary diabetes mellitus**, which may→ketoacidemia
  - Hyperlipidemia→↑atherosclerosis→
    - **Coronary artery disease**
    - Cerebrovascular disease
    - Peripheral vascular disease

Cutaneous/ subcutaneous
- ↓Fibroblast function→
  - ↓Intercellular matrix production→
    - ↑Bruisability→ecchymoses
    - Poor wound healing
    - Skin striae
- Androgenic effects→
  - Acne
  - ↑Facial hair
  - Thinning scalp hair
- Fat redistribution from the extremities to the:
  - Abdomen→
    - Truncal obesity
  - Shoulders→
    - Supraclavicular fat pads
  - Upper back→
    - Buffalo hump
  - Face→
    - Moon facies
  …w/ concomitant thinning of the arms & legs

Endocrine
- **Adrenal failure** upon abrupt discontinuation after 2weeks

Gastrointestinal
- Inhibition of phospholipase A_2 mediated conversion of cell membrane lipids to arachidonic acid, which is the precursor for both cyclooxygenase-COX enzymes, w/ the cyclooxygenase-COX1 enzyme found in most cells of the body, responsible for normal physiologic function. Inhibition of the cyclooxygenase-COX1 enzyme→↑peptic inflammatory disease risk→↑**upper gastrointestinal hemorrhage risk** via:
  - ↓Gastric mucosal prostaglandin synthesis→
    - ↓Epithelial cell proliferation
    - ↓Mucosal blood flow→↓bicarbonate delivery to the mucosa
    - ↓Mucus & bicarbonate secretion from gastric mucosal cells

Musculoskeletal
- **Avascular necrosis of bone**
- **Osteoporosis**
- Proximal muscle weakness

Neurologic
- Anxiety
- Insomnia
- Psychosis

Opthalmologic
- **Cataracts**

Immunologic
- Inhibition of phospholipase A_2 mediated conversion of cell membrane lipids to arachidonic acid, which is the precursor for both cyclooxygenase–COX enzymes (COX1 & COX2) being responsible for the production of neuronal & inflammatory cell prostaglandins respectively→
  - –↓Pain
  - –↓Temperature (antipyretic)
  - –↓**Inflammation**
- Stabilization of lisosomal & cell membranes→
  - ○↓Cytokine & proteolytic enzyme release
- ↓Lymphocyte & eosinophil production
  ...all→
  - •**Immunosuppression**→
    - –↑**Infection** &/or neoplasm risk

Hematologic
- ↑Erythrocyte production→
  - ○Polycythemia
- ↑Neutrophil demargination→
  - ○Neutrophilia→
    - –**Leukocytosis**

INTRAVENOUS IMMUNE GLOBULIN–IVIG

Indications, being either:
- Hemorrhage, being either internal or extensive/ progressive mucocutaneous
- Platelet count <30,000/ uL, unresponsive to several days of glucocorticoid treatment

Dose

1g/ kg IV q24hours X 2–5days

Outcomes:
- Transient improvement: 70%
- Long term remission: Rare

Mechanism:
- Bind to macrophage IgG Fc receptors→
  - ○Fc receptor downregulation→
    - –↓Macrophage mediated platelet phagocytosis
- Bind to plasma cell IgG Fc receptors→
  - ○Feedback inhibition mediated ↓anti–platelet antibody production

Side effects:
General
- Fever ± chills

Cardiovascular
- Flushing
- Hypotension

Gastrointestinal
- Nausea ± vomiting

Genitourinary
- Acute tubular necrosis, w/ preparations containing sucrose. If used, infuse @ ≤3mg sucrose/kg/min.

Neurologic
- Aseptic meningitis–rare
- Headache

Pulmonary
- Pulmonary failure

Hypersensitivity
- Hypersensitivity reaction if infused rapidly
- **Anaphylaxis** may occur in patients w/ **IgA deficiency** due to varied amounts of IgA, w/ some products being IgA depleted

Contraindications:
- IgA deficiency

INTRAVENOUS ANTI–RhD IMMUNOGLOBULIN (a component of IVIG)

Indications:
- **Rh positive patients** (85% of population) **w/ a functional spleen** (as this is where the majority of erythrocytes are cleared) & either:
  - ◦Hemorrhage, being either internal or extensive/ progressive mucocutaneous
  - ◦Platelet count <30,000/ uL, unresponsive to several days of glucocorticoid treatment

Dose

75ug/ kg IV over 5min. q24hours X 2–5days

Outcomes:
- •Transient improvement: 70%
- •Long term remission: Rare

Mechanism:
- •Bind to the erythrocyte Rh antigen→
  - ◦Antibody coated erythrocytes→
    - –Binding to macrophage IgG Fc receptors→Fc receptor downregulation→↓macrophage mediated platelet phagocytosis
- •Bind to plasma cell IgG Fc receptors→
  - ◦Feedback inhibition mediated ↓anti–platelet antibody production

Side effects:
General
- •Fever ± chills

Genitourinary
- •Renal failure due to intravascular hemolysis→
  - ◦Hemoglobinuria→
    - –Acute tubular necrosis

Neurologic
- •Headache

Hematologic
- •Hemolytic anemia (extravascular >> intravascular)

Hypersensitivity
- •**Anaphylaxis** may occur in patients w/ **IgA deficiency** due to trace amounts of IgA

Contraindications:
- •IgA deficiency

PLATELETS

Indications:
- •Platelet count <50,000/ µL w/ either hemorrhage or pre–procedure
- •Prophylactically w/ a platelet count <20,000/ µL

Thrombocytopenia mediated hemorrhage risk:
- •Platelet count
  - ◦20,000–50,000/ µL w/ minimal trauma
  - ◦10,000–20,000/ µL, possibly spontaneous
  - ◦<10,000/ µL, commonly spontaneous

Dose

6–10 units typically being transfused at a time (50mL/ unit)

Mechanism:
- •↑Platelet count by 5,000–10,000/ µL per unit

ANTIFIBRINOLYTIC MEDICATIONS

Indications:
- •Hemorrhage, being either internal or extensive/ progressive mucocutaneous

Generic (Trade)	M	♀	Dose
Aminocaproic acid (Amicar)	K	U	5g PO or IV over 1hour, then 1g/ hour prn hemorrhage X 8

Onset: <1hour, Duration: 3hours

Mechanism:
- •↓Plasminogen activation→
  - ◦↓Plasmin formation→
    - –↓Thrombolysis

Side effects:
Cardiovascular
- •Thromboembolic disease syndrome
- •Rapid intravenous administration→
  - ∘Bradycardia
  - ∘Dysrhythmia
  - ∘Hypotension

Gastrointestinal
- •Diarrhea
- •Nausea ± vomiting

Musculoskeletal
- •Myositis→
  - ∘Muscle pain &/or weakness, which may→
    - –Rhabdomyolysis, diagnosed via ↑creatine kinase–CK levels

Neurologic
- •Headache
- •Tinnitus

Hematologic
- •Hypercoagulable state when used concomitantly w/ estrogens (oral contraceptive pills–OCPs or hormone replacement therapy–HRT)
- •Hyperkalemia

Contraindications:
- •Active intravascular thrombosis

SECOND LINE TREATMENT ▬▬▬▬▬▬▬▬▬▬▬▬▬▬▬▬▬▬▬
•Splenectomy
Indications:
- •Glucocorticoid dependent patients
- •Platelet count <30,000/ uL, unresponsive to several weeks of glucocorticoid treatment

Outcomes:
- •Response to IVIG or anti–RhD predicts response to splenectomy
- •Long term remission: 65%, w/ failure possibly due to :
  - ∘Accessory spleen†
  - ∘Growth of unremoved splenic tissue†

---

†Splenic remnants can be detected via either:
- •Abdominal magnetic resonance imaging–MRI
- •Radionuclide imaging, using labeled heat–damaged erythrocytes

THIRD LINE TREATMENT ▬▬▬▬▬▬▬▬▬▬▬▬▬▬▬▬▬▬▬
Outcomes:
- •Although used, no large trials proving efficacy exist

IMMUNOMODULATING MEDICATIONS
•The following medications usually require 1–6 months for symptomatic improvement, making these medications not useful in the control of acute disease, but rather, useful when prolonged treatment is planned. Consider combination therapy in patients who have failed 1 medication

Generic (Trade)	M	♀	Start	Max
6–mercaptopurine	L	U	50mg PO q24hours	
Azathioprine†(Imuran)	LK	U	1mg/ kg PO q24hours	2.5mg/kg/24hours
Cyclophosphamide (Cytoxan)			10mg/ kg IV qmonth	2.5mg/kg/24hours

---

†Azathioprine's active metabolite is 6–mercaptopurine

Azathioprine/ 6–mercaptopurine mechanism:
- •Inhibition of enzymes involved in purine metabolism→
  - ∘Cytotoxicity of differentiating lymphocytes (T cell >> B cell)→
    - –↓Anti–platelet antibody production

443

Cyclophosphamide mechanism:
•Forms reactive molecular species which alkylate nucleophilic groups on DNA bases→
  ∘Abnormal base pairing
  ∘Cross−linking of DNA bases
  ∘DNA strand breakage
  ...→cytotoxicity to all proliferating cells→
    •↓Macrophage production→
      ∘↓Macrophage mediated platelet phagocytosis
    •↓Plasma cell production→
      ∘↓Anti−platelet antibody production

Side effects:
Gastrointestinal
  •↓Mucosal cell proliferation→
    ∘Mucosal inflammation=mucositis, including inflammation of the oral mucosa=stomatitis→
      −Diarrhea
      −Nausea ± vomiting
Hematologic
  •**Myelosuppression**→
    ∘Macrocytic anemia→
      −Fatigue
    ∘Leukopenia→immunosuppression→
      −↑Infection & neoplasm risk
    ∘Thrombocytopenia→
      −↑Hemorrhage risk, esp. petechiae

Azathioprine/ 6−mercaptopurine specific:
Gastrointestinal
  •Hepatitis→
    ∘Cirrhosis−rare
Mucocutaneous
  •↓Epithelial cell proliferation→
    ∘Dermatitis
Hematologic
  •Myelosuppression, esp. w/ concomitant:
    ∘Renal failure
    ∘Medications:
      −Allopurinol
      −Angiotensin converting enzyme inhibitor−ACEi

Cyclophosphamide specific:
Genitourinary
  •**Hemorrhagic cystitis**
  •Premature ovarian failure
  •Sterility
Mucocutaneous
  •↓Hair formation→
    ∘Alopecia

Azathioprine/ 6−mercaptopurine specific monitoring:
•Baseline:
  ∘Complete blood count
  ∘Liver function tests
  ...then q2weeks X 2months, then
    •Q2months

Cyclophosphamide specific monitoring:
•Baseline:
  ∘Complete blood count
  ∘Liver function tests
  ∘Renal function
  ∘Urinalysis
  ...then:
    •Complete blood count 1week after dose increase, then
      ∘Q2months
•Urinalysis w/ cytology q6months after medication is discontinued

PLANT ALKALOIDS			
Generic	M ♀	Dose	
Vincristine=Oncovin	L U	100mg PO q24hours	

Mechanism:
•Prevents the assembly of tubulin dimers into microtubules→
  ∘↓Mitotic spindle formation→↓mitosis→
    −↓Macrophage production→↓macrophage mediated platelet phagocytosis
    −↓Macrophage cell membrane Fc receptors→↓macrophage mediated platelet phagocytosis
    −↓Plasma cell production→↓anti−platelet antibody production

Side effects:
Gastrointestinal
  •Constipation
Mucocutaneous
  •↓Hair formation→
    ∘Alopecia, being reversible
Neurologic
  •**Neurotoxicity**→
    ∘Neuropathy→
      −Areflexia
      −Paralytic ileus
      −Peripheral neuritis
Hematologic
  •Mild myelosuppression

PROGNOSIS

•The #1 cause of death from autoimmune thrombocytopenia is **intracranial hemorrhage** (children−1%, adults−5%)
  ∘**Acute autoimmune thrombocytopenia:** Self limited, w/ spontaneous remissions occurring in >90% of patients within 2months
  ∘**Chronic autoimmune thrombocytopenia:** Chronic, w/ only 10% achieving spontaneous remission, usually @ 1−1.5 years

DISSEMINATED INTRAVASCULAR COAGULATION-DIC

•Tissue factor, tissue factor-like substances, bacterial toxins, &/or other procoagulant proteins→
  ∘Systemic coagulation factor XII, termed the Hageman factor, activation→
    -**Systemic microvascular thrombosis** ± embolus→systemic tissue ischemia ± infarction
    -Thrombosis mediated **consumption of platelets & procoagulant proteins**, termed consumption
     coagulopathy→hemorrhage risk

RISK FACTORS

•**Sepsis, being the #1 cause**
  ∘40% of affected patients have either **gram negative or positive bacterial† sepsis**, due to:
    -Bacterial excreted proteins, termed exotoxins
    -Certain bacterial cell wall components, termed endotoxins, such as lipopolysaccharides-LPS found
     in gram negative rods & cocci
  ∘Other much less common causes of sepsis
    -Other bacteria
    -Fungi
    -Protozoa
    -Viruses
•**Acute pancreatitis**, via circulating trypsin
•**Fat embolism**
  ∘Bone fracture→
    -Fat marrow embolus→pulmonary embolism→tissue factor & factor-like substance release
•**Liver disease**, via ↓metabolism of activated procoagulant factors
•**Malignancy‡** Esp.:
  ∘Gastrointestinal mucin-secreting adenocarcinomas
  ∘Pancreatic cancer
  ∘Prostate cancer
  ∘Acute leukemia, occurring in 15% of patients, esp. those w/ **acute promyelocytic leukemia (M3
   subtype)**
  ...all via neoplastic cytokine release→
      •Blood monocyte tissue factor-like substance release
•**Obstetric complications**, esp. during the 3rd trimester
  ∘Placental abruption, occurring in 50% of patients
  ∘Amniotic fluid embolism, occurring in 50% of patients
  ∘Gestational hypertensive syndromes
    -Pre-eclampsia
    -Eclampsia
  ∘Placenta previa
  ∘Retained dead fetus
  ∘Septic abortion
  ...all via uterine tissue factor release
•**Severe hypersensitivity reaction**
•**Severe trauma**, occurring in 60% of persons developing a systemic inflammatory response-SIRS
 syndrome
  ∘Brain injury
  ∘Burns
  ∘Crush injury
  ∘Hypo or hyperthermia
  ∘Surgery
  ...all via tissue factor release
•**Shock**
  ∘Systemic ischemia→
    -Tissue factor release
•**Snake venom**, which may contain procoagulant proteins
•**Transfusion reactions**
•**Vascular disorders**
  ∘Large vascular malformations
    -Large aortic aneurysm-<1%
    -Giant hemangiomas→Kasabach-Merritt syndrome-25%

---

†Contrary to a widely held belief, disseminated intravascular coagulation occurs w/ equal frequency in
both gram negative & positive sepsis
‡10-15% of patients w/ metastatic disease develop disseminated intravascular coagulation

446

Genitourinary
- Intravascular hemolysis→↑**plasma hemoglobin**→
  - Pink/ red colored plasma
  - Hemoglobinuria→hematuria
    - Microscopic via positive heme dipstick reaction without erythrocytes
    - Macroscopic, termed gross, via red/ brown colored urine without erythrocytes

Mucocutaneous
- Hemolysis→
  - Unconjugated hyperbilirubinemia, w/ a plasma bilirubin >3mg/ dL→yellow staining of tissues:
    - Skin, termed jaundice
    - Sclera, termed scleral icterus
    - Mucus membranes

Hematologic
- Systemic microvascular thrombi formation→
  - Turbulent flow
  - Cell membrane shearing effect upon thrombus edges
  - …→**intravascular fragmentation hemolysis**→
    - **Microangiopathic hemolytic anemia–MAHA.** ↓Hemoglobin ($\male$ <14g/ dL, $\female$ <12g/ dL) & hematocrit ($\male$ <40%, $\female$ <35%)→
      - Compensatory ↑renal **erythropoietin** secretion→↑**reticulocytes†**, being proportional to the severity of the anemia, provided adequate:
        - Erythropoietin
        - Folic acid
        - Iron
        - Vitamin B12
    - **Cellular cytoplasm release**, also being due to tissue ischemia ± necrosis→
      - **Hyperkalemia**
      - Hyperphosphatemia→
        - Calcium binding→hypocalcemia
      - ↑Lactate dehydrogenase–LDH
      - ↑Uric acid (> ~7mg/ dL)→
        - Gout syndrome
      - Unconjugated hyperbilirubinemia
    - **Consumption of platelets**→
      - Thrombocytopenia (<150,000/ μL)→↑bleeding time
    - **Consumption of procoagulant proteins**→
      - ↑Activated partial thromboplastin time–aPTT
      - International normalized ration–INR or prothrombin time–PT
      - ↓Fibrinogen† (<150mg/ dL) & ↑fibrinogen degradation products (>10mg/ dL)
      - ↑Fibrin degradation products, termed d-dimers (>0.5μg/ mL)
      - ↓Antithrombin 3
      - Negative direct Coombs test‡
- Intravascular hemolysis→
  - ↓Plasma haptoglobin & hemopexin, being hemoglobin & heme binding proteins, respectively
- The intramedullary compensatory response→
  - Reticulocytosis°→
    - ↑Mean corpuscular volume–MCV (>100 fL)
    - Retained messenger RNA→purple coloration per Wright stain, termed polychromatophilia
    - Retained nucleus in severe hemolysis
- Peripheral blood smear showing misshapen erythrocytes, termed **schistocytes**, described as:
  - Cell fragments
  - Crescent cells
  - Helmet cells

---

†The normal reticulocyte count is ≤2%, which is expected to ↑in anemic states, as a compensatory mechanism of a normally functioning bone marrow. Lack of this compensatory ↑ indicates that there is at least an element of inadequate marrow production as a cause for the anemia. Being that reticulocytes are calculated in relation to erythrocyte number, anemia→
- Falsely ↑reticulocyte count. In order to correct for this effect, the reticulocyte count should be adjusted for the degree of anemia:

Corrected reticulocyte count= reticulocyte count (hematocrit / 0.45)
maturation factor (if hematocrit ≥45%=1, 35%=1.5, 25%=2, 20%=2.5)

‡Fibrinogen is an acute phase reactant, & thus may be normal to elevated
°Detects IgG & complement on erythrocyte cell membranes

•**Bone marrow aspirate**
  Findings:
    •Erythroid hyperplasia

•**Treat the etiologic cause**,if possible, w/ the following supportive measures

PACKED RED BLOOD CELLS
Dose
1unit is composed of 450mL of blood & 50mL of plasma=500mL total

Indications:
•**Hemoglobin <10g/ dL** w/:
  ∘Active hemorrhage
  ∘Cardiovascular disease
  ∘Cerebrovascular disease
  ∘Peripheral vascular disease
  ∘Pulmonary disease
  ∘Sepsis
  ∘Hemoglobinopathy
  ∘Otherwise critically ill
•**Hemoglobin <7–8g/ dL** otherwise

Mechanism:
•1unit→
  ∘1g/ dL ↑hemoglobin
  ∘3% ↑hematocrit
  ∘~10% ↑blood volume

PLATELETS

Indications:
•Platelet count <50,000/ µL w/ either hemorrhage or pre–procedure
•Prophylactically w/ a platelet count <20,000/ µL
 	
Thrombocytopenia mediated hemorrhage risk:
•Platelet count
  ∘20,000–50,000/ µL w/ minimal trauma
  ∘10,000–20,000/ µL, possibly spontaneous
  ∘<10,000/ µL, commonly spontaneous

Dose
6–10 units typically being transfused at a time (50mL/ unit)
Mechanism: •↑Platelet count by 5,000–10,000/ µL per unit

VITAMIN K=Phytonadione
Indications: •To correct the international normalized ratio–INR or prothrombin time–PT
Dose
10mg SC/ IV slow push @ 1mg/ min. in order to ↓anaphylactoid reaction risk
Mechanism: •Requires several hours to days for effect
Side effects: •Avoid intramuscular administration, which may→   ∘Intramuscular hemorrhage

FRESH FROZEN PLASMA–FFP

Indications:
•To correct the international normalized ratio–INR or prothrombin time–PT under the following conditions:
  ∘INR >20
  ∘**Severe hemorrhage**
  ∘**Other need for rapid reversal, such as an emergent procedure**

Dose†
15mL/ kg IV (w/ ~200mL FFP/ unit) q4hours prn

Mechanism:
- •Contains clotting factors 2, 7, 9–13, & heat labile 5 & 7→
  - ∘Immediate onset of action
- •Each unit→
  - ∘8% ↑coagulation factors
  - ∘4% ↑blood volume

FIBRINOGEN

Indications:
- •Fibrinogen level <100mg/ dL, w/ hemorrhage or pre–procedure

Generic	Dose
Cryoprecipitate	10–15 units being transfused at a time (25mL cryoprecipitate/ unit)

Mechanism:
- •Contains factors 8, 13, von Willebrand factor, & fibrinogen
- •Each unit→
  - ∘7mg/ dL ↑plasma fibrinogen

PROGNOSIS

- •Varies per etiology
  - ∘Sepsis or severe trauma mediation→
    - –2X the underlying disease mediated mortality risk

449

•**Thrombotic thrombocytopenic purpura–TTP**
Pathophysiology:
  •Congenital or acquired ↓**ADAMTS 13†** **enzymatic activity** (<5% functional activity) via ↓production, dysfunction, &/or anti–ADAMTS 13 antibodies→
    ○↓Cleavage of large plasma von Willebrand factor multimers‡→**platelet aggregation without concomitant coagulation factor involvement**→
      –**Systemic microvascular thrombosis** ± embolus→systemic tissue ischemia ± infarction
      –Thrombosis mediated **consumption of platelets only** (not involving coagulation factors)→ hemorrhage risk

•**Hemolytic uremic syndrome–HUS**
Pathophysiology:
  •Anti–endothelial antibody mediated microvascular damage→
    ○**Systemic microvascular thrombosis** ± embolus→
      –Systemic tissue ischemia ± infarction
    ○Thrombosis mediated **consumption of platelets only** (not involving coagulation factors)→
      –↑Hemorrhage risk

---

†A metalloprotease produced predominantly by hepatocytes, w/ subsequent plasma release→
  •Endothelial cell membrane receptor binding & activity
‡Multimers of von Willebrand factor (produced by endothelial cells > megakaryocytes), being relatively larger than those normally found in the plasma→
  •Relatively ↑platelet adhesion & subsequent activation

•**Medications**
  ○**Estrogen containing oral contraceptives**
  ○Combination chemotherapy
  ○Immunomodulating medications
    –Cyclosporine
    –Tacrolimus
  ○Quinine
•**Bone marrow, stem cell, or organ transplantation**
•**Total body irradiation**

Thrombotic thrombocytopenic purpura–TTP specific:
•**Age:** 20–50years
•**Gender:** ♀ > ♂
•**Medications**
  ○Thienopyridine derivatives (Ticlopidine > Clopidogrel), within several weeks of initiation
•**Pregnancy**, esp. during both the:
  ○3rd trimester
  ○Postpartum period

Hemolytic uremic syndrome–HUS specific:
•**Age:** <15years
•**Infectious gastroenteritis**, esp:
  ○**Enterohemorrhagic Escherichia coli O157–H7**
  ○Toxigenic strains of Salmonella sp.
  ○Shigella sp.
  ○Viral
  Contraindications to treatments:
    •**Antibiotic treatment**
      ○Suspected or known **Enterohemorrhagic E. Coli O157–H7** (Shiga–toxin producing) mediated diarrheal syndrome, as antibacterial medications (esp. fluoroquinolones & Trimethoprim–Sulfamethoxazole)→
        –↑Shiga–toxin production→↑Hemolytic–uremic syndrome–HUS risk
    •**Anti–motility medications**
      ○Known or suspected **toxin** mediated diarrhea, as anti–motility medications→
        –Toxin retention→↑Hemolytic–uremic syndrome–HUS risk
•**Medications**
  ○A delayed complication of high dose glucocorticoid treatment
•**Postpartum state**

450

•**Genetic**
  ◦Hereditary form→
  −Recurrent episodes

•Syndrome differentiation is made on clinical grounds
  ◦**Hemolytic−uremic syndrome−HUS**, being the triad of:
    −**Microangiopathic hemolytic anemia−MAHA**
    −**Thrombocytopenia**
    −**Renal failure**
  ◦**Thrombotic thrombocytopenic purpura−TTP**, being the triad of hemolytic uremic syndrome−HUS, as well as:
    −**Altered mental status**
    −**Fever**

Genitourinary
  •Intravascular hemolysis→↑**plasma hemoglobin**→
    ◦Pink/ red colored plasma
    ◦Hemoglobinuria→hematuria
      −Microscopic via positive heme dipstick reaction without erythrocytes
      −Macroscopic, termed gross, via red/ brown colored urine without erythrocytes
Mucocutaneous
  •Hemolysis→
    ◦Unconjugated hyperbilirubinemia, w/ a plasma bilirubin >3mg/ dL→yellow staining of tissues:
      −Skin, termed jaundice
      −Sclera, termed scleral icterus
      −Mucus membranes
Hematologic
  •Systemic microvascular thrombi formation→
    ◦Turbulent flow
    ◦Cell membrane shearing effect upon thrombus edges
    ...→**intravascular fragmentation hemolysis**→
        •**Microangiopathic hemolytic anemia−MAHA**. ↓Hemoglobin (♂ <14g/ dL, ♀ <12g/ dL) & hematocrit (♂ <40%, ♀ <35%)→
          ◦Compensatory ↑renal **erythropoietin** secretion→↑**reticulocytes†**, being proportional to the severity of the anemia, provided adequate:
            −Erythropoietin
            −Folic acid
            −Iron
            −Vitamin B12
        •**Cellular cytoplasm release**, also being due to tissue ischemia ± necrosis→
          ◦**Hyperkalemia**
          ◦Hyperphosphatemia→
            −Calcium binding→hypocalcemia
          ◦↑Lactate dehydrogenase−LDH
          ◦↑Uric acid (> ~7mg/ dL)→
            −Gout syndrome
          ◦Unconjugated hyperbilirubinemia
    ◦**Consumption of platelets**→
      −Thrombocytopenia (<150,000/ μL)→↑bleeding time
  •Intravascular hemolysis→
    ◦↓Plasma haptoglobin & hemopexin, being hemoglobin & heme binding proteins, respectively
  •The intramedullary compensatory response→
    ◦Reticulocytosis→
      −↑Mean corpuscular volume−MCV (>100 fL)
      −Retained messenger RNA→purple coloration per Wright stain, termed polychromatophilia
      −Retained nucleus in severe hemolysis
  •Peripheral blood smear showing misshapen erythrocytes, termed **schistocytes**, described as:
    ◦Cell fragments
    ◦Crescent cells
    ◦Helmet cells

---

†The normal reticulocyte count is ≤2%, which is expected to ↑in anemic states, as a compensatory mechanism of a normally functioning bone marrow. Lack of this compensatory ↑ indicates that there is at least an element of inadequate marrow production as a cause for the anemia. Being that reticulocytes are calculated in relation to erythrocyte number, anemia→

•Falsely ↑reticulocyte count. In order to correct for this effect, the reticulocyte count should be adjusted for the degree of anemia:

Corrected reticulocyte count= reticulocyte count (hematocrit / 0.45)
maturation factor (if hematocrit ≥45%=1, 35%=1.5, 25%=2, 20%=2.5)

INVASIVE PROCEDURES

•**Bone marrow aspirate**
Findings:
•Erythroid hyperplasia

TREATMENT

•**Platelet transfusions are contraindicated**, as they may→
∘↑Thrombosis
•**Antibiotic treatment during the hemolytic uremic syndrome may→**
∘↑**Morbidity**
•**Plasmapheresis**
Procedure:
•Removal of blood, w/ the subsequent separation of erythrocytes from the plasma. The plasma is then discarded, containing the causative:
∘In TTP: Large von Willebrand factor multimers ± anti−ADAMTS 13 antibodies
∘In HUS: Anti−endothelial antibodies
…the erythrocytes are then reinfused w/ **fresh frozen plasma−FFP** (containing ADAMTS 13†) until 1.5−2 X the plasma volume‡ has been exchanged q24h, until the patient is in complete remission

---

†A plasma level of ≥5% is sufficient for treatment or prophylaxis
‡1.5−2 X the plasma volume, being ~60−80mL/ kg, as the normal adult plasma volume is:
•♂ 40mL/ kg
•♀ 36mL/ kg

SYSTEMIC GLUCOCORTICOID TREATMENT			
Generic	M ♀	Dose	
Methylprednisolone	L ?	200mg PO/ IV q24hours	
Prednisolone	L ?	200mg PO/ IV q124hours	
Prednisone	L ?	200mg PO q24hours	

•Once disease control is achieved, taper to the lowest effective maintenance dose in order to minimize serious side effects, w/ the goal of discontinuation if possible, w/ attention to a relapse syndrome
•If the total duration of systemic glucocorticoid therapy is ≤2weeks, there is no need to taper
•Both the IV & PO routes have equal efficacy

	Relative potencies			
Glucocorticoids	Anti-inflammatory	Mineralocorticoid	Duration	Dose equiv.
Cortisol (physiologic†)	1	1	10hours	20mg
Cortisone (PO)	0.7	2	10hours	25mg
Hydrocortisone (PO, IM, IV)	1	2	10hours	20mg
Methylprednisolone (PO, IM, IA, IV)	5	0.5	15−35hours	5mg
Prednisone (PO)	5	0.5	15−35hours	5mg
Prednisolone (PO, IM, IV)	5	0.8	15−35hours	5mg
Triamcinolone (PO, IM)	5	~0	115−35hours	5mg
Betamethasone (PO, IM, IA)	25	~0	35−70hours	0.75mg
Dexamethasone (PO)	25	~0	35−70hours	0.75mg
Fludrocortisone (PO)	10	125	10hours	

---

†The physiologic rate of adrenal cortical cortisol production is 20−30mg/ 24hours
Mechanisms:
•↓Plasma cell anti−ADAMTS 13 or anti−endothelial antibodies
Side effects of chronic use:
General
•Anorexia→
∘Cachexia
•↑Perspiration

Cardiovascular
- Mineralocorticoid effects→
  - ↑Renal tubular NaCl & water retention as well as potassium secretion→
    - **-Hypertension**
    - **-Edema**
    - **-Hypokalemia**
- Counter-regulatory=anti-insulin effects→
  - ↑Plasma glucose→
    - **-Secondary diabetes mellitus**, which may→ketoacidemia
  - Hyperlipidemia→↑atherosclerosis→
    - **-Coronary artery disease**
    - -Cerebrovascular disease
    - -Peripheral vascular disease

Cutaneous/ subcutaneous
- ↓Fibroblast function→
  - ↓Intercellular matrix production→
    - -↑Bruisability→ecchymoses
    - -Poor wound healing
    - -Skin striae
- Androgenic effects→
  - Acne
  - ↑Facial hair
  - Thinning scalp hair
- Fat redistribution from the extremities to the:
  - Abdomen→
    - -Truncal obesity
  - Shoulders→
    - -Supraclavicular fat pads
  - Upper back→
    - -Buffalo hump
  - Face→
    - -Moon facies
  - …w/ concomitant thinning of the arms & legs

Endocrine
- **Adrenal failure** upon abrupt discontinuation after 2weeks

Gastrointestinal
- Inhibition of phospholipase A_2 mediated conversion of cell membrane lipids to arachidonic acid, which is the precursor for both cyclooxygenase-COX enzymes, w/ the cyclooxygenase-COX1 enzyme found in most cells of the body, responsible for normal physiologic function. Inhibition of the cyclooxygenase-COX1 enzyme→↑peptic inflammatory disease risk→↑**upper gastrointestinal hemorrhage risk** via:
  - ↓Gastric mucosal prostaglandin synthesis→
    - -↓Epithelial cell proliferation
    - -↓Mucosal blood flow→↓bicarbonate delivery to the mucosa
    - -↓Mucus & bicarbonate secretion from gastric mucosal cells

Musculoskeletal
- **Avascular necrosis of bone**
- **Osteoporosis**
- Proximal muscle weakness

Neurologic
- Anxiety
- Insomnia
- Psychosis

Opthalmologic
- **Cataracts**

Immunologic
- Inhibition of phospholipase A_2 mediated conversion of cell membrane lipids to arachidonic acid, which is the precursor for both cyclooxygenase-COX enzymes (COX1 & COX2) being responsible for the production of neuronal & inflammatory cell prostaglandins respectively→
  - -↓Pain
  - -↓Temperature (antipyretic)
  - -↓**Inflammation**
- Stabilization of lisosomal & cell membranes→
  - ↓Cytokine & proteolytic enzyme release
- ↓Lymphocyte & eosinophil production
- …all→

•**Immunosuppression**→
  −↑**Infection** &/or neoplasm risk
Hematologic
  •↑Erythrocyte production→
    ∘Polycythemia
  •↑Neutrophil demargination→
    ∘Neutrophilia→
      −**Leukocytosis**

PACKED RED BLOOD CELLS
Dose
1 unit is composed of 450mL of blood & 50mL of plasma=500mL total

Indications:
  •**Hemoglobin <10g/ dL** w/:
    ∘Active hemorrhage
    ∘Cardiovascular disease
    ∘Cerebrovascular disease
    ∘Peripheral vascular disease
    ∘Pulmonary disease
    ∘Sepsis
    ∘Hemoglobinopathy
    ∘Otherwise critically ill
  •**Hemoglobin <7−8g/ dL** otherwise

Mechanism:
  •1 unit→
    ∘1g/ dL ↑hemoglobin
    ∘3% ↑hematocrit
    ∘~10% ↑blood volume

PROGNOSIS

•**Thrombotic thrombocytopenic purpura−TTP**
  ∘**10% mortality**
    ∘20% of survivors develop chronic, intermittently symptomatic disease, for which splenectomy &/or chronic immunosuppression should be considered

•**Hemolytic uremic syndrome−HUS**
  ∘<5% mortality in adults

LYMPHOMA

•Caused by the malignant transformation of a **lymphocyte outside the bone marrow,** (atypia→ lymphoma), typically occurring within lymphoid tissue (lymph node, spleen, thymus)→
  ○Infiltration of tissue, w/ spread through lymphatics & blood vessels to other organs=metastases→
    –Extramedullary production→organ enlargement=organomegally & destruction
•All lymphomas are considered metastatic malignancies
•Lymphoma cells, especially undifferentiated cells, do not provide the typical protection against infection or malignancy associated w/ leukocytes

Incidence:
•**Non-Hodgkins lymphoma 6X Hodgkin's lymphoma**

RISK FACTORS

•**Infection**
  ○**Latent viral**
    –Epstein Barr virus–EBV, which in African children→Burkitt's lymphoma
    –Human immune deficiency virus–HIV
    –Human T–cell lymphoma/ leukemia virus–HTLV
  ○**Bacterial**
    –Helicobacter pylori infection→gastric lymphoma
•**Immunosuppression**
  ○Advanced age
  ○Alcoholism
  ○Diabetes mellitus
  ○Hematologic malignancy
  ○HIV infection/ AIDS, w/ 3% developing Non–Hodgkin's lymphoma, esp. Burkitt's lymphoma
  ○Malnutrition
  ○Medications
    –Chemotherapy
    –Chronic glucocorticoid use
    –Immunomodulating medications
  ○Renal dialysis

Hodgkin's lymphoma specific:
•**Age (gender):** 15–45 years (♀ > ♂) & >60 years (♂ > ♀)

Non–Hodgkin's lymphoma specific:
•**Age:** >50 years, except for lymphoblastic @ age 12–40 years
•**Gender:** ♂ > ♀
•**Autoimmune diseases**

CLASSIFICATION

•**Hodgkin's lymphoma**
  ○**Clonal proliferation of a Reed–Sternberg cell,** being bi or multinucleated giant cells of uncertain origination (B–lymphocyte vs. macrophage), w/ large eosinophilic nucleoli. The cells often contain the Epstein–Barr viral–EBV genome, & typically comprise <1% of the cellular elements of the tumor mass

Rye histologic classification:
•Nodular sclerosis–60%
    Gender predominance:
      •Young ♀
•Mixed cellularity–30%, having an intermediate concentration of Reed–Sternberg cells→
  ○Intermediate prognosis
    Usual spread pattern:
      •Disseminated
    Gender predominance:
      •♂ > ♀
•Lymphocyte predominant–5%, having the lowest concentration of Reed–Sternberg cells→
  ○Best prognosis
    Usual spread pattern:
      •Localized
•Lymphocyte depleted–5%, having the highest concentration of Reed–Sternberg cells→
  ○Worst prognosis
    Usual spread pattern:
      •Disseminated

•**Non-Hodgkin's lymphoma**
  ◦**Clonal proliferation of a lymphocyte, usually a B lymphocyte (adults–90%, children–60%)**

Clinical classification according to histology†:
  •**Indolent–80%**, being relapsing
    A. Small lymphocytic
    B. Follicular, predominantly small cleaved cell
    C. Follicular, mixed small cleaved & large cell
    D. Follicular, predominantly large cell
    E. Diffuse, small cleaved cell
    F. Diffuse, mixed small cleaved & large cell
  •**Aggressive–18%**, being **curable**
    G. Diffuse, large cell
    H. Large cell immunoblastic
    I. Lymphoblastic
    J. Small non–cleaved cell
      –Burkitt's lymphoma
      –Non–Burkitt's lymphoma
  •**Other–2%**
    ◦Cutaneous T cell lymphoma, termed mycosis fungoides
    ◦Composite
    ◦Histiocytic
    ◦Extramedullary plasmacytoma
    ◦Unclassifiable

•The higher the histologic grade, the more undifferentiated the cells have become→
  ◦More rapid cell division→
    –**Aggressive neoplasm**→acute course, as death occurs within months if untreated, but are more responsive to treatment due to rapid division
•The lower the histologic grade, the more differentiated the cells have become→
  ◦Less rapid cell division→
    –**Indolent neoplasm**→chronic course, as death occurs within years, but are less responsive to treatment due to slow division
†Lettering refers to the working formulation classification, w/ lymph nodes typically involved in follicular or diffuse patterns

DIAGNOSIS

General†
  •Neoplastic cytokines→
    ◦Anorexia→
      –**Cachexia**
    ◦Chills
    ◦Fatigue
    ◦**Fever**
    ◦Headache
    ◦Malaise
    ◦**Night sweats**
    ◦**Pruritus**
    ◦Weakness

---

†The following are termed **B symptoms**, being poor prognostic signs, occurring in both Hodgkin's lymphoma–35% & Non–Hodgkin's lymphoma–20%
  •**Unexplained weight loss** ≥10% of body weight within 6 months
  •**Unexplained fevers** ≥100.4°F = 38°C for ≥3 consecutive nights, which may be cyclical, occurring q2–4 weeks in Hodgkin's disease, termed Pel–Ebstein fever
  •**Drenching night sweats** requiring either a change of bedclothes &/or sheets for ≥3 consecutive nights

Lymphatics
  •Metastases→
    ◦Extramedullary hematopoeisis→
      –**Lymphadenopathy**, usually being **firm & non–tender**, which may remain stable, or wax & wane in size for many months ± spontaneous regression
      –**Hepatomegally**
      –**Splenomegally**, which may retain a relatively ↑proportion of circulating cells, termed hypersplenism→anemia, leukopenia, &/or thrombocytopenia
      …w/ organ destruction

456

Pattern of lymph node involvement:
- **Hodgkin's lymphoma:** Contiguous
- **Non-Hodgkin's lymphoma:** Non-contiguous

Major lymph node regions:
- **Head & neck**
  - Pharyngeal, forming Waldeyer's ring
  - Cervical
  - Occipital
  - Periauricular
  - Supraclavicular
  - Infraclavicular
- **Arm**
  - Axillary
  - Epitrochlear
  - Brachial
- **Thorax**
  - Pectoral
  - Mediastinal
  - Hilar
- **Abdomen**
  - Splenic
  - Mesenteric
  - Para-aortic
  - Porta-hepatic
- **Pelvis**
  - Iliac
- **Leg**
  - Inguinal
  - Femoral
  - Popliteal

Palpable lymph node characteristics:
- **Size**
  - Those ≥1cm are significant, except for inguinal lymph nodes which may normally be ≤2cm
  - Any size in an unusual location (ex. epitrochlear, periauricular, supraclavicular)
- **Tenderness**
  - Indicative of inflammation
- **Consistency**
  - Stone hard is suggestive of metastatic cancer
  - Rubbery hard is suggestive of lymphoma
- **Matting**
  - Lymph nodes unable to be individualized from the surrounding tissue suggest (listed in descending order of frequency):
    - Metastatic cancer
    - Lymphoma
    - Chronic inflammation
    - Sarcoidosis

Hematologic
- Anemia of chronic disease
- Leukopenia or leukocytosis
- Functional leukopenia→
  - ↑Infection & neoplasm risk
- Thrombocytopenia or thrombocytosis
- Eosinophilia
- Monocytosis
- Inflammatory cytokines→
  - Leukocytosis
  - ↑Acute phase proteins
    - ↑Erythrocyte sedimentation rate-ESR (normal: 5mm/ decade aged + ♂ ≤10mm/h or ♀ ≤20mm/h)
    - ↑C-reactive protein-CRP (normal: <2mg/ L), responding more acutely than ESR, as it rises within several hours, & falls within 3days upon partial resolution
    - ↑Fibrinogen
    - ↑Platelets→thrombocytosis

•Excisional lymph node biopsy
Indications:
•Nodes >1cm for ≥3weeks without explanation
•Nodes of any size in patients w/ a syndrome suggesting the diagnosis
•Histologic classification, as follicular & diffuse architectural features are very difficult to discern via fine needle aspiration–FNA or extranodal biopsy

•Urine & protein electrophoresis
Indications:
•Possible monoclonal immunoglobulin production

Non–Hodgkin's lymphoma specific:
•Fluorescent activated cell sorting–FACS=immunophenotyping, via flow cytometry
Procedure:
•Anti cell–surface protein (ex. clusters of differentiation, immunoglobulin heavy &/or light chain) fluorescent labeled monoclonal antibodies are utilized to segregate the various populations of leukocytes via flow cytometry, as the clonal population may demonstrate a known cell surface protein, allowing for the detection of a predominant monoclonal pattern
Note: Lymphoblasts lack specific morphologic or cytochemical features, w/ diagnosis depending on Immunophenotyping
Immunologic reactivity:
•Common ALL Antigens–CALLA positive: Pre–B cell & B cell
○Being lymphoblast cell surface proteins CD 10 & 19
•Cytoplasmic immunoglobulin–CyIg positive: Pre B cell & B cell
•I antigen–Ia positive: Pre B cell & B cell
•Surface immunoglobulin–SIg positive: B cell
•Terminal deoxynucleotidal transferase–Tdt positive: Pre–B cell & T cell
•T cell markers CD 2, 5, & 7 positive: T cell

•Gene rearrangement analysis=cytogenetics
Findings:
•Burkitt's lymphoma
○Chromosomal translocation→
–Juxtaposition of the c–myc gene on chromosome 8 & an immunoglobulin gene (usually the heavy chain locus on chromosome 14)= t (8;14) > t(2;8), t(8;22)
•Follicular lymphomas
○Most have a chromosomal translocation→
–Juxtaposition of the bcl–2 gene on chromosome 18 & the immunoglobulin heavy chain locus on chromosome 14= t (14;18)

•Possible metastases are assessed via:
○History & physical examination
○Hematologic studies
○Imaging
–**Neck & thoraco–abdomino–pelvic imaging via CT/ MRI** to look for a nodule, mass, infiltrate, lymphadenopathy (esp. the mesenteric, porta–hepatic, splenic hilar, & internal iliac lymph nodes), atelectasis, pleural effusion†, pericardial effusion, &/or osteolytic lesions in affected bones
Limitations:
•Does not reliably visualize the splenic, hepatic, para–aortic, or external iliac lymph nodes
–**Bipedal lymphography**
Indications:
•To visualize the para–aortic & external iliac lymph nodes
Limitations:
•Does not visualize the mesenteric, porta–hepatic, splenic hilar, or internal iliac lymph nodes
–**Positron emission tomographic–PET scanning**
Indications:
•As the computed tomographic–CT scan may remain abnormal long after treatment, a PET scan may help w/ both pre–treatment staging & monitoring treatment response
Mechanism:
•Intravenous radiolabeled glucose is utilized by malignant cells (as well as cells within an inflammatory focus) > normal cells, due to ↑metabolism→
○↑Relative uptake→
–↑Relative visualization

458

-Radionuclide whole body bone scanning
  Indications, being either:
  • ↑Plasma alkaline phosphatase
  • Hypercalcemia
  Procedure:
  • A radioactive agent, termed a tracer, is injected intravenously→
    ◦ Detection of ↑osteoblast activity, indicating new bone formation (as occurs w/ metastases to the bone)
  Agents used:
  • ^{99m}technitium–Tc based agent (99mTc–sestamibi, 99mTc–teboroxime, 99mTc–tetrofosmin)

◦ Invasive procedures:
  -Iliac crest bone marrow biopsy
  -Lumbar puncture
  Indications:
  • Central nervous system disease syndrome for cerebrospinal fluid cytology
  • Lymphoblastic or small non–cleaved cell lymphoma
  -Staging laparotomy‡ for Hodgkin's disease only
  Indications:
  • If the additional information may change treatment, as in indentifying patients who may be able to be treated w/ curative intent via radiation therapy alone (stage ≤2A)
  Procedure:
  • Splenectomy
  • Sampling of the left & right lobes of the liver
  • Sampling of the porta hepatic, splenic hilar, para–aortic, & iliac lymph nodes
  • Sampling of other areas thought to be involved via imaging
  • Bilateral iliac crest bone marrow biopsy if not previously done

---

†Being either:
• Transudative if due to lymph node metastases
• Exudative if due to pleural infiltration
‡If performing a staging laparotomy, administer the streptococcus pneumoniae vaccine prior to the procedure, & q6years thereafter

Thoracic compressive &/or infiltrative syndromes:
• @ **lung apex**=Pancoast tumor→
  ◦ Supraclavicular lymphadenopathy=**Virchow's node**=Sentinal node
  ◦ **Horner's syndrome:** Cervical sympathetic ganglion compression ± infiltration→↓ipsilateral facial autonomic sympathetic tone→
    -↓Iris radial smooth muscle contraction→pupil constriction=**myosis**
    -↓Levator palpebrae smooth muscle contraction→drooping eyelid=**ptosis**
    -↓Sweat gland activation→↓facial sweat=**anhidrosis**→facial dryness
    -↓Ciliary epithelium aqueous humor formation→retracted eyeball, termed "sunken" eye
  ◦ **Pancoasts syndrome:** Horner's syndrome & lower trunk brachial plexopathy→
    -Ipsilateral arm paresis
• @ **Esophagus**→
  ◦ Obstruction→
    -Difficulty swallowing=dysphagia
    -Inflammation=esophagitis→painful swallowing=odynophagia
• @ **Phrenic nerve**→
  ◦ Hiccups
  ◦ Ipsilateral diaphragm paralysis
• @ **Recurrent laryngeal nerve**→
  ◦ Hoarseness
• @ **Superior vena cava**→
  ◦ Obstruction→↑proximal hydrostatic pressure→
    -Dilation of bilateral arm, neck, & head vasculature→facial erythema, edema, &/or bluish color=cyanosis
    -↑Collateral blood flow→dilated abdominal collateral vessels w/ downward flow
    Note: Considered a medical emergency if the patient develops altered mental status
• @ **Thoracic duct**→
  ◦ Chylous pleural effusion=chylothorax, usually being left sided as the thoracic duct ascends to ~T5 on the right side, then on the left thereafter

•@ Tracheobronchial tree→
　◦Cough ± hemoptysis
　◦Wheezing
　◦↓Mucous clearance distal to the obstruction→
　　−Post−obstructive pneumonia

ANN ARBOR STAGING SYSTEM: Used for both lymphoma forms, being far less useful in Non–Hodgkin's lymphoma relative to tumor grade, as >90% are too advanced for curative therapy	
Stage	**Description**
1	•1 lymph node
E	◦Localized disease of 1 extralymphatic organ
2	•2 lymph nodes on the same side of the diaphragm ±
E	◦Localized disease of 1 extralymphatic organ
3	•Lymph node involvement on both sides of the diaphragm ±
E	◦Localized disease of 1extralymphatic organ
S	◦Splenic disease
ES	◦Both
4	•Diffuse involvement of ≥1extralymphatic organ(s) ± lymphatic involvement

†Extralymphatic organs:
　•Pharyngeal, forming Waldeyer's ring
　•Spleen
　•Thymus
Subclassification:
　•A=Absence of constitutional symptoms
　•B symptoms: As above
　•X=Bulky disease, being either:
　　◦>10cm maximal nodal mass diameter
　　◦>1/3 the width of the mediastinum
　•CS=Clinical Staging based on noninvasive tests
　•PS=Pathologic Staging based on tissue biopsy via laparoscopy or staging laparotomy

TREATMENT

HODGKIN'S LYMPHOMA ■■■■■
•Curative intent: All stages
　◦**Stage 1A or 2A:** Radiation therapy (w/ combination chemotherapy for bulky disease)
　◦**Stage 1B or 2B:** Radiation therapy &/or combination chemotherapy (both w/ bulky disease)
　◦**Stage ≥3:** Combination chemotherapy ± radiation therapy
　First line chemotherapy regimen:
　　•ABVD=Doxorubicin (Adriamycin), Bleomycine, Vinblastin, Decarbazine
　　　　　　±
　　•MOPP=Mechlorethamine (Nitrogen mustard), Vincristin (Oncovin), Procarbazine, Prednisone

　Second line chemotherapy regimen:
　　•MOPP=Mechlorethamine (Nitrogen mustard), Vincristin (Oncovin), Procarbazine, Prednisone
　　　　　　&
　　•BAP=Bleomycin, Doxorubicin (Adriamycin), Prednisone

NON–HODGKIN'S LYMPHOMA ■■■■■
INDOLENT LYMPHOMAS_____
•Curative intent
　◦**Localized disease:** Radiation therapy
•Palliative intent
　◦**Diffuse disease– >90%**
　　−Chemotherapy &/or radiation therapy
　　−Interstitial radiation treatment, termed brachytherapy
　　　Procedure:
　　　　•Tissue placement of a radioactive substance
　　−Silastic tube vs. metal stent placement for obstructive lesions
　　−Consider surgical resection for painful &/or obstructive lesions
　　−Bisphosphonates→↓pathologic fracture risk
　　−Surgery for pathologic fractures
　　−Drainage of pleural effusions, w/ subsequent pleurodesis via sclerosing agents (sterile Bleomycin, Doxycycline, Mitoxantrone, Tetracycline, or talc slurry) to prevent reaccumulation

　Single agent chemotherapy, being either:
　　•Chlorambucil, Cladribine, Cyclophosphamide, or Fludrabine

460

Combination chemotherapy regimens:
- **CVP:** Cyclophosphamide, Vincristin (Oncovin), & Prednisone
- **COPP:** Cyclophosphamide, Vincristine (Oncovin), Procarbazine, & Prednisone
- **CHOP ± bleo:** Cyclophosphamide, Doxorubicin (Adriamycin), Vincristin (Oncovin), & Prednisone ± **Bleomycin**

Note: α-interferon may prolong remission duration & overall survival when added to chemotherapy

AGGRESSIVE LYMPHOMAS
- **Curative intent**
  - Combination chemotherapy via:
    - **CHOP ± bleo:** Cyclophosphamide, Doxorubicin (Adriamycin), Vincristin (Oncovin), & Prednisone ± **Bleomycin**
  - Intra-thecal chemotherapy (via Methotrexate) ± cranial radiation therapy
    - Indications:
      - Lymphoblastic or small non-cleaved cell lymphomas
    - Pathophysiology:
      - The central nervous system serves as a sanctuary for leukemic cells (lymphoblasts >> myeloblasts) from systemic chemotherapy, via the blood brain barrier

ADDITIONAL TREATMENT

MONOCLONAL ANTIBODIES
Indications: •Indolent lymphomas   •Diffuse large B cell lymphoma (an aggressive lymphoma)
Generic (Trade)
Rituximab (Rituxan)
Mechanism: •An anti-B lymphocyte CD20 antibody→   ∘Complement mediated cell lysis   ∘Cellular mediated cytotoxicity   ∘Triggering of programmed cell death=apoptosis   †CD20 is expressed on >90% of B cell Non-Hodgkin's lymphomas
Side effects: •Primarily infusion related (usually w/ 1st infusion)→   ∘Fever ± chills   ∘Nausea ± vomiting

PROGNOSIS
- **Hodgkin's lymphoma 5 year survival**
  - Stage 1A, lymphocyte predominant: >90%
  - Stage 1-2: 80%
  - Stage 3-4: 60%
  - Stage 4B, lymphocyte depleted: <40%

- **Non-hodgkin's lymphoma mean survival**
  - Indolent: 7 years
    - **35% eventually evolving into an aggressive lymphoma,** usually diffuse large cell lymphoma
  - Aggressive
    - Without treatment: Weeks to months
    - With treatment: According to the international prognostic index, w/ 35% being cured

  International prognostic index of aggressive lymphomas
  - **Adverse prognostic factors**
    - Age >60 years
    - ↑Lactate dehydrogenase–LDH (>250 IU/ L)
    - Stage ≥3 disease
    - Poor performance status ≥2
    - Involvement of ≥2 extranodal sites
  - Index score:
    - **0-1:** 85% complete remission, w/ a 75% 5 year survival
    - **2:** 65% complete remission, w/ a 50% 5 year survival
    - **3:** 55% complete remission, w/ a 45% 5 year survival
    - **4:** 45% complete remission, w/ a 25% 5 year survival

•Treatment is additive, based on initial treatment. If initial treatment consisted of:
  ∘Radiation therapy, then conventional chemotherapy is used
  ∘Chemotherapy, then ↑dose chemotherapy or total body radiation therapy is used, w/ subsequent:
    –Allogeneic or autologous bone marrow or stem cell transplantation

MONOCLONAL ANTIBODIES
Indications:
•Relapsed, indolent CD20+ B cell Non–Hodgkins lymphoma
Generic (Trade)
Rituximab (Rituxan)

•Caused by the malignant transformation of a **myeloid, erythroid, or lymphoid cell** at any point in its maturation **within the bone marrow** (atypia→leukemia)→
  ∘Infiltration of tissue ± spread through lymphatics & blood vessels to other organs=metastases→
    −Extramedullary production→organ enlargement=organomegaly & destruction
•All leukemias are considered metastatic malignancies
•Leukemic cells, especially undifferentiated cells, do not provide the typical protection against infection or malignancy associated w/ leukocytes

•**Lymphoid leukemias**
  ∘**Acute lymphoid leukemia−ALL**
    −Clonal proliferation of an immature lymphocyte (**B lymphocyte−80%** >> T lymphocyte), being poorly to undifferentiated
    The French−American−British FAB histologic classification of ALL:
      •L1 subtype: Small lymphoblastic cell predominance, being Pre B cell or T cell
      •L2 subtype: Large lymphoblastic cell predominance, being Pre B cell or T cell
      •L3 subtype: Undifferentiated, being B cell
  ∘**Chronic lymphoid leukemia−CLL, being the #1 adult leukemia**
    −Clonal proliferation of a relatively mature lymphocyte (**B lymphocyte−95%** >> T lymphocyte), being moderately to well differentiated
    Subtype:
      •**Hairy cell leukemia**
        ∘Clonal proliferation of a relatively mature **B lymphocyte** w/ unusually **long cytoplasmic projections**, giving it a 'hairy' look

•**Myeloid leukemias**
  ∘**Acute myeloid leukemia−AML**
    −Clonal proliferation of an immature myeloid/ erythroid lineage† cell, being poorly to undifferentiated
    The French−American−British FAB histologic classification of AML:
      •M0 subtype: Acute undifferentiated leukemia−3%
      •M1 subtype: Acute myeloblastic leukemia−20%
      •M2 subtype: Acute myeloblastic leukemia + differentiation−25%
      •M3 subtype: Acute promyelocytic leukemia−10%
      •M4 subtype: Acute myelomonocytic leukemia−25%
        ∘M4E subtype: M4 w/ dysplastic eosinophils
      •M5 subtype: Acute monoblastic leukemia−5%
        ∘M5a subtype: >80% monoblasts
        ∘M5b subtype: >20% promonocytes
      •M6 subtype: Erythroleukemia−5%
      •M7 subtype: Megakaryoblastic leukemia−7%

  ∘**Chronic myeloid leukemia−CML**
    −Clonal proliferation of an relatively mature myeloid/ erythroid lineage† cell, being moderately to well differentiated

---

†The myeloid/ erythroid lineage ultimately produces mature:
  •Monocytes
  •Granulocytes
    ∘Neutrophils
    ∘Basophils
    ∘Eosinophils
  •Platelets
  •Erythrocytes
•The higher the histologic grade, the more undifferentiated the cells have become→
  ∘More rapid cell division→
    −**Acute leukemia**→acute course, as death occurs within months if untreated, but are more responsive to treatment due to rapid division
•The lower the histologic grade, the more differentiated the cells have become→
  ∘Less rapid cell division→
    −**Chronic leukemia**→chronic course, as death occurs within years, but are less responsive to treatment due to slow division

463

- **Age**
  - ○Acute lymphoid leukemia–ALL
    - –20% of adult acute leukemias
    - –85% occur in children→80% of childhood leukemias
  - ○Acute myeloid leukemia–AML
    - –80% of adult acute leukemias
- **Gender:** ♀ > ♂
- **Alteration of nucleic acids**
  - ○Benzene
  - ○Chemotherapy, esp:
    - –Alkylating medications (Cyclophosphamide, Melphalan)
    - –Topoisomerase 2 inhibitors (Doxorubicin, Etoposide, Mitoxantrone, Teniposide)
  - ○Radiation
- **Genetic**
  - ○Any myelodysplastic disorder
    - –Refractory anemia ± ringed sideroblasts or excess blasts ± transformation
  - ○Any myeloproliferative disorder
    - –Chronic myelomonocytic leukemia
    - –Essential thrombocytosis
    - –Myelofibrosis
    - –Polycythemia vera
  - ○Ataxia telangiectasia
  - ○Bloom's syndrome
  - ○Down's syndrome=trisomy 21
  - ○Fanconi's anemia
  - ○Klinefelter's syndrome (47XXY)
  - ○Wiscott–Aldrich syndrome

General
- •Neoplastic cytokines→
  - ○Anorexia→
    - **–Cachexia**
  - ○Chills
  - ○Fatigue
  - ○**Fever**
  - ○Headache
  - ○Malaise
  - ○**Night sweats**
  - ○Weakness

---

†Temperature may be normal in patients w/:
- •Chronic kidney disease, esp. w/ uremia
- •Cirrhosis
- •Heart failure
- •Severe debility
- ...or those who are:
  - •Intravenous drug users
  - •Taking certain medications:
    - ○Acetaminophen
    - ○Antibiotics
    - ○Glucocorticoids
    - ○Nonsteroidal anti–inflammatory drugs–NSAIDs

Lymphatics
- •Metastases→
  - ○Extramedullary hematopoeisis→
    - **–Lymphadenopathy**, usually being **firm & non–tender**, which may remain stable, or wax & wane in size for many months ± spontaneous regression
    - **–Hepatomegally**
    - **–Splenomegally**, which may retain a relatively ↑proportion of circulating cells, termed hypersplenism→anemia, leukopenia, &/or thrombocytopenia
    - ...w/ organ destruction

464

Cardiovascular
- **Blast cell count >100,000/ μL→**
  - ↑Blood viscosity, w/ resultant sludging of blood in the microcirculation, termed **leukostasis**→proximal ischemia ± infarction→
    - −Altered mental status
    - −Cerebrovascular ischemic syndrome
    - −Myocardial ischemic syndrome, also being due to ↑afterload, which may→heart failure syndrome
    - −Peripheral vascular ischemic syndrome
    - −Glomerulonephritis
    - −Headache
    - −Spontaneous hemorrhage, including intraocular hemorrhage→blindness
    - −Mucocutaneous ulcerations
- **Acute promyelocytic leukemia cells, being the M3 subtype, release procoagulant proteins from blast granules→**
  - **Disseminated intravascular coagulation–DIC**

Mucocutaneous
- **Metastases→**
  - Dermatitis
  - Gingival hyperplasia

Musculoskeletal
- **Leukemic cell proliferation→**
  - Destruction of normal marrow→
    - −**Bone pain**
    - −**Pathologic fractures**

Neurologic
- **Leukemic cell metastases→**
  - Cranial nerve palsies
  - Leukemic meningitis

Hematologic
- **Leukemic cell proliferation→**
  - **Leukocytosis, being most common**, due to predominant clonal proliferation
  - Normal leukocyte count, due to equivalent clonal proliferation & marrow destruction
  - Functional leukopenia→
    - −↑Infection & neoplasm risk
  - ↑Blast cell count→
    - −Bandemia in >95% of patients (normal band count being 3–5%)
    - −Reticulocytosis (normal being 1%)
  - Erythrocytosis
  - Thrombocytosis, w/ functional thrombocytopenia
  - **Destruction of normal bone† marrow, which if predominant→**
    - −Normocytic–normochromic anemia→fatigue
    - −Leukopenia→↑infection & neoplasm risk
    - −Thrombocytopenia→↑hemorrhage risk, esp. petechiae
  - ↑Cellular turn over→
    - −Hyperkalemia
    - −Hyperphosphatemia→calcium binding→hypocalcemia
    - −↑Lactate dehydrogenase–LDH
    - −↑Uric acid (> ~7mg/ dL)→gout syndrome
    - …→**tumor lysis syndrome**
- **Inflammatory cytokines→**
  - Leukocytosis
  - ↑Acute phase proteins
    - −↑Erythrocyte sedimentation rate–ESR (normal: 5mm/ decade aged + ♂ ≤10mm/h or ♀ ≤20mm/h)
    - −↑C–reactive protein–CRP (normal: <2mg/ L), responding more acutely than ESR, as it rises within several hours, & falls within 3days upon partial resolution
    - −↑Fibrinogen
    - −↑Platelets→thrombocytosis
- **Leukocyte alkaline phosphatase–LAP, an enzyme produced by functional leukocytes, may be used to differentiate:**
  - A leukemoid reaction (leukocytes >50,000/ μL due to inflammation)→
    - −↑Leukocyte alkaline phosphatase levels
  - Leukemia
    - −↓Leukocyte alkaline phosphatase levels
- ↑Vitamin B12 & B12 binding protein

---

†Tumor replacement of normal bone marrow hematopoietic tissue is termed myelophthisis

•**Bone marrow biopsy**
Findings:
  •Hypercellular marrow, w/ ≥20% of nucleated cells being blasts

Acute lymphoid leukemia–ALL specific:
•**Fluorescent activated cell sorting–FACS=immunophenotyping**, via flow cytometry
Procedure:
  •Anti cell–surface protein (ex. clusters of differentiation, immunoglobulin heavy &/or light chain)
  fluorescent labeled monoclonal antibodies are utilized to segregate the various populations of
  leukocytes via flow cytometry, as the clonal population may demonstrate a known cell surface
  protein, allowing for the detection of a predominant monoclonal pattern
Note: Lymphoblasts lack specific morphologic or cytochemical features, w/ diagnosis depending on
  immunophenotyping
Immunologic reactivity:
  •**Common ALL Antigens–CALLA** positive: Pre–B cell & B cell
  ∘Being lymphoblast cell surface proteins CD 10 & 19
  •**Cytoplasmic immunoglobulin–CyIg** positive: Pre B cell & B cell
  •**I antigen–Ia** positive: Pre B cell & B cell
  •**Surface immunoglobulin–SIg** positive: B cell
  •**Terminal deoxynucleotidal transferase–Tdt** positive: Pre–B cell & T cell
  •**T cell markers CD 2, 5, & 7** positive: T cell

•**Gene rearrangement analysis=cytogenetics**
Findings:
  •Chromosomal translocation→
  ∘Juxtaposition of the breakpoint cluster region–BCR on chromosome 9 & the c–abl oncogene
  on chromosome 22 = t (9;22)→
    –bcr–abl oncogene on the newly formed **Philadelphia chromosome–12%**
Test sensitivity:
  •Chromosome analysis for the detection of the Philadelphia chromosome: 90%
  •Southern blot or polymerase chain reacton–PCR for the detection of gene rearrangements: ~100

Acute myeloid leukemia–AML specific:
•**Cytochemistry**
Staining characteristics:
  •**Blast Auer rods**, being eosinophilic, needle–like cytoplasmic inclusions, indicating myeloid
  lineage, are pathognomonic for AML
  •**Myeloperoxidase** positive, being a phagocyte enzyme: M0–M4(E)
  •**Nonspecific esterase** (α–naphthylacetate or α–naphthylbutyrate) positive: M4(E)–M5(a,b)
  •**Periodic acid Schiff** positive: M5(a,b) & M7

•**Curative intent treatment: All acute leukemias**
  ∘**Chemotherapy**
  –**Induction chemotherapy**, intended to induce remission, not necessarily cure
  Outcomes:
    •Complete remission
    ∘Adults (AML–70% & ALL–60%)
    ∘Children (>90% overall→ALL cure rate of 75%)
  Monitoring post–induction chemotherapy:
    •Complete blood count, peripheral smear, & bone marrow biopsy for possible leukemic
    persistence
  –**Consolidation chemotherapy**, intended to destroy residual leukemic cells
  –**Maintenance chemotherapy**, intended to destroy resistant cells
  Indications:
    •Acute lymphoid leukemia–ALL
  –**Intrathecal chemotherapy** (via Methotrexate or Cytarabine) & **cranial radiation therapy**
  Indications:
    •Acute lymphoid leukemia–ALL
    •Acute myeloid leukemia–AML @ ↑risk for central nervous system recurrence via:
    ∘Leukocyte count >50,000/ µL at presentation
    ∘Acute myelomonocytic–M4 or monoblastic–M5 leukemia
  Pathophysiology:
    •The central nervous system serves as a sanctuary for leukemic cells (lymphoblasts >>
    myeloblasts) from systemic chemotherapy, via the blood brain barrier

466

∘**Allogeneic or autologous bone marrow or stem cell transplantation**
Indications:
- •Acute myeloid leukemia–AML, upon complete remission
- •Acute lymphoid leukemia–ALL, either:
  - ∘Upon initial complete remission in a patient w/ poor prognostic signs, such as the presence of the Philadelphia chromosome
  - ∘Upon relapse w/ subsequent complete remission

Limitations:
- •Patients @ age <60 years (being the upper age limit for transplantation @ many centers), who are healthy enough to tolerate the procedure, & for whom appropriate donors are available (HLA matched relative donor >> unrelated donor)

OTHER
•Leukophoresis
Indications:
- •Leukostasis syndrome
- •↑Leukostasis risk

Procedure:
- •Leukocytes are filtered from the patients blood

ALLOPURINOL

Indications:
- •To be given to all patients, as hyperuricemia (uric acid >7mg/ dL)→
  - ∘Acute tubular necrosis via uric acid mediated:
    - –Direct tubular toxicity
    - –Obstructive tubular casts
    - …→acute intra-renal renal failure

M ♀	Start	Titrate	Max
K ?	100mg PO q24hours	qweek to a target uric acid level <6mg/ dL	800mg/ 24hours†

†Doses >300mg should be divided

Dose adjustment:
- •Adjust according to renal function

Creatinine clearance	Max dose
10–20mL/ min.	200mg/ 24hours
<10mL/ min.	100mg/ 24hours

Mechanism:
- •Inhibits xanthine oxidase→
  - ∘↓**Uric acid production**
  - ∘↑Hypoxanthine & xanthine production, which are much more soluble than uric acid, & readily excreted

Side effects:
General
- •**May incite a gout attack during treatment initiation or dosage ↑**
  Risk reduction:
  - •Concomitant administration of an anti-inflammatory drugs–NSAIDs, until the target uric acid level is reached X ≥6months

Hypersensitivity syndrome†–2% (↑w/ renal failure)
- •Dermatitis
- •Fever
- •Hepatitis
- •Renal failure
- •Vasculitis
- •Eosinophilia
…necessitating discontinuation
Prognosis:
- •20% mortality

Interactions:
- •↓Metabolism of Azathioprine, Mercaptopurine, Theophylline, Warfarin→
  - ∘↑Plasma concentration

Overdosage:
General
- •Fever

Gastrointestinal
 •Hepatitis
Genitourinary
 •Renal failure

†**Allopurinol desensitization**
 Indication:
  •Mild hypersensitivity syndrome
 Protocol:
  •Start 10μg q24hours, then
   ∘Double the dose q3–14days until the necessary dosage is reached

ACUTE MYELOGENOUS LEUKEMIA–M3 SUBTYPE

RETINOIDS

Generic

All–trans retinoic acid

Mechanism:
 •↑Cell line differentiation→
  ∘Improved outcomes

PROGNOSIS

•**Poor prognostic factors**
 ∘Age >60years
 ∘♀ gender
 ∘Poor performance score
 ∘Unfavorable cytogenetics

Acute myeloid leukemia–AML specific:
 •Transformation from myeloproliferative or myelodysplastic disease syndrome
 •Concomitant infection
 •Leukocyte count >20,000/ μL
 •↑Lactate dehydrogenase–LDH

Acute lymphoid leukemia–ALL specific:
 •The absence of a mediastinal mass
 •Leukocyte count >30,000/ μL
 •L2 or 3 subtype
 •B cell immunophenotype
 •Presence of the Philadelphia chromosome

468

CHRONIC MYELOID LEUKEMIA-CML

•**Age:** 20–60 years
•**Alteration of nucleic acids**
 ◦Ionizing radiation

Note: There is no association w/ chemotherapy or heritable disease syndromes

DIAGNOSIS PER DISEASE PHASE
•**40% of patients are asymptomatic during the chronic & accelerated phases**

•**Chronic phase**
 Peripheral blast count:
  •**<10% of nucleated cells**
 Median interval to progression:
  •**3.5–5 years**
 Predominant syndrome:
  General
   •Neoplastic cytokines→
    ◦Anorexia→
     –**Cachexia**
    ◦Chills
    ◦Fatigue
    ◦**Fever**
    ◦Headache
    ◦Malaise
    ◦**Night sweats**
    ◦Weakness
  Lymphatics
   •Metastases→
    ◦Extramedullary hematopoeisis→
     –**Lymphadenopathy**, usually being **firm & non-tender**, which may remain stable, or wax &
      wane in size for many months ± spontaneous regression
     –**Hepatomegally**
     –**Splenomegally**, which may retain a relatively ↑proportion of circulating cells, termed
      hypersplenism→anemia, leukopenia, &/or thrombocytopenia
     …w/ organ destruction
  Hematologic
   •Leukemic cell proliferation→
    ◦**Leukocytosis, usually ≥100,000/ μL**, as cells are mature enough to leave the bone marrow.
     Potentially being millions without causing leukostasis, due to their small size
    ◦Erythrocytosis
    ◦Thrombocytosis w/ functional thrombocytopenia
    ◦**Destruction of normal bone marrow†**, which if predominant→
     –Normocytic–normochromic anemia→fatigue
     –Thrombocytopenia→↑hemorrhage risk, esp. petechiae
   •**Leukocyte alkaline phosphatase–LAP**, an enzyme produced by **functional leukocytes**, may
    be used to differentiate:
    ◦A leukemoid reaction (leukocytes >50,000/ μL due to inflammation)→
     –↑Leukocyte alkaline phosphatase levels
    ◦Leukemia
     –↓Leukocyte alkaline phosphatase levels
   •↑Vitamin B12 & B12 binding protein

•**Accelerated phase**
 Peripheral blast count:
  •**≥15% of nucleated cells**
 Predominant syndrome:
  •Worsening of chronic phase syndrome

- **Acute phase, termed blast crisis**
  - Peripheral & bone marrow blast count:
    - **≥20% of nucleated cells**
  - Predominant syndrome:
    - As for acute leukemia syndromes, but requiring a **blast cell count >200,000/ μL to cause ↑blood viscosity, w/ resultant sludging of blood in the microcirculation, termed leukostasis→** proximal ischemia ± infarction→
      - −Cerebrovascular accident syndromes
      - −Myocardial ischemic syndromes
      - −Glomerulonephritis
      - −Headache
      - −Pulmonary infarction
      - −Visual changes

---

†Tumor replacement of normal bone marrow hematopoietic tissue is termed myelophthisis

INVASIVE PROCEDURES
- **Bone marrow biopsy**
  - Findings:
    - Hypercellular marrow

ADDITIONAL TESTS
- **Gene rearrangement analysis=cytogenetics**
  - Findings:
    - Chromosomal translocation→
      - ○Juxtaposition of the breakpoint cluster region−BCR on chromosome 9 & the c−abl oncogene on chromosome 22 = t (9;22)→
        - −**bcr−abl oncogene** on the newly formed **Philadelphia chromosome−100%**
  - Test sensitivity:
    - Chromosome analysis for the detection of the Philadelphia chromosome: 90%
    - Southern blot or polymerase chain reacton−PCR for the detection of gene rearrangements: ~100

TREATMENT
- **Curative intent**
  - ○All phases

SELECTIVE TYROSINE KINASE INHIBITORS
Generic (Trade)
Imatinib Mesylate (Gleevec)

Mechanism:
• The bcr−abl oncogene→
  ○Oncoprotein w/ aberrant tyrosine kinase activity→
    −Continuous nuclear proliferative signals→eventual malignant transformation
• Selective tyrosine kinase inhibitors→
  ○Inhibition of all tyrosine kinase activity

  - ○**Chronic phase**
    - −**Allogeneic bone marrow or stem cell transplantation**
      - Outcomes:
        - 60% cure rate
      - Limitations:
        - Only 45% of patients w/ chronic myelogenous leukemia−CML are age <60 years, being the upper age limit for transplantation @ many centers. Of these patients, 30% have an acceptable HLA−matched sibling donor, w/ 80% of the remainder having an acceptable HLA−matched unrelated donor, thus making **transplantation an option for only 40% of affected patients**

- **Palliative intent**
  - ○**Chronic phase**
    - −Chemotherapy via Hydroxyurea or Busulfan
    - −Immunomodulating therapy via interferon α→remission of the Philadelphia chromosome
      - Outcomes:
        - Uncertain survival benefit
  - ○**Acute phase, termed blast crisis**
    - −Usually resistant to combination chemotherapy used for acute leukemias

•**Average survival of 3-4 years,** as the clonal cells undergo inevitable transformation to acute leukemia→
  ◦Acute phase, termed blast crisis→
  –Death within months

Poor prognostic factors:
  •Age >60 years
  •Black color
  •Symptomatic disease @ diagnosis
  •Splenomegally or hepatomegally

•↑**Age:** 90% >50years, being rare @age <30years
•**Gender:** ♂ 2X ♀
•**Genetic**
  ◦Relative w/ lymphoid leukemia

Note: There is no association w/ chemotherapy, radiation therapy, or benzene

•**Often asymptomatic**

General
  •Neoplastic cytokines→
    ◦Anorexia→
      –**Cachexia**
    ◦Chills
    ◦Fatigue
    ◦**Fever**
    ◦Headache
    ◦Malaise
    ◦**Night sweats**
    ◦Weakness
Lymphatics
  •Metastases→
    ◦Extramedullary hematopoeisis→
      –**Lymphadenopathy-80%**, usually being **firm & non-tender**, which may remain stable, or wax &
      wane in size for many months ± spontaneous regression
      –**Hepatomegally**
      –**Splenomegally-50%**, which may retain a relatively ↑proportion of circulating cells, termed
      hypersplenism→anemia, leukopenia, &/or thrombocytopenia
      ...w/ organ destruction
Hematologic
  •Leukemic cell proliferation→
    ◦**Leukocytosis†**, as cells are mature enough to leave the bone marrow. **Potentially being millions
    without causing leukostasis, due to their small size**
      –**Lymphocytosis** (>5000/ μL, usually being >15,000/ μL)
    ◦**Destruction of normal bone marrow‡**, which if predominant→
      –Normocytic–normochromic anemia→fatigue
      –Leukopenia→↑infection & neoplasm risk
      –Thrombocytopenia→↑hemorrhage risk, esp. petechiae
  •Deranged B cell activity→
    ◦Autoimmune phenomena
      –**Autoimmune hemolytic anemia**→Coombs test positivity
      –**Autoimmune thrombocytopenia-AITP**→↑splenic macrophage mediated platelet removal→
      thrombocytopenia

---

†Hairy cell leukemia usually→
  •Leukopenia
‡Tumor replacement of normal bone marrow hematopoietic tissue is termed myelophthisis

•**Bone marrow biopsy**
  Findings:
    •**Mature lymphocytic infiltration via small lymphocytes**

•**Microscopy**
  Findings on peripheral smear or tissue section:
    •Ruptured malignant lymphocytes, termed **smudge cells**, due to clonal cell fragility, being
    pathognomonic for chronic lymphoid leukemia–CLL
      ◦**Hairy cell leukemia** lymphocytes
        –Have long cytoplasmic projections, giving it a 'hairy' look
        –Stain tartrate resistant acid phosphatase positive

472

- **Fluorescent activated cell sorting–FACS=immunophenotyping**, via flow cytometry
  - Procedure:
    - Anti cell–surface protein (ex. clusters of differentiation, immunoglobulin heavy &/or light chain) fluorescent labeled monoclonal antibodies are utilized to segregate the various populations of leukocytes via flow cytometry, as the clonal population may demonstrate a known cell surface protein, allowing for the detection of a predominant monoclonal pattern
    - Note: Lymphoblasts lack specific morphologic or cytochemical features, w/ diagnosis depending on immunophenotyping
  - Immunologic reactivity:
    - **Common ALL Antigens–CALLA** positive: Pre–B cell & B cell
      - Being lymphoblast cell surface proteins CD 10 & 19
    - **Cytoplasmic immunoglobulin–CyIg** positive: Pre B cell & B cell
    - **I antigen–Ia** positive: Pre B cell & B cell
    - **Surface immunoglobulin–SIg** positive: B cell
    - **Terminal deoxynucleotidal transferase–Tdt** positive: Pre–B cell & T cell
    - **T cell markers CD 2, 5, & 7** positive: T cell

TREATMENT

- **Curative intent:** Hairy cell leukemia
  - Chemotherapy
- **Palliative intent:** All other forms of chronic lymphoid leukemia–CLL
  - Chemotherapy
    - Indications:
      - Symptomatic adenopathy, splenomegally, anemia, or thrombocytopenia
  - Splenectomy
    - Indications:
      - Symptomatic hypersplenism, autoimmune anemia, or thrombocytopenia

PROGNOSIS

- **Average survival of 3–7 years**, being unaltered by treatment, w/ rare transformation to either:
  - Acute lymphoid leukemia
  - **Diffuse lymphoma**, being termed **Richter's syndrome**

Poor prognostic signs:
- T cell malignancy

RAI prognostic staging system:
- Stage 0: Lymphocytosis only (>15,000/ μL), having a median survival of >10 years
- Stage 1: Lymphocytosis w/ lymphadenopathy, having a median survival of >8 years
- Stage 2: Lymphocytosis w/ either hepatomegally or splenomegally, having a median survival of 6 years
- Stage 3: Lymphocytosis w/ anemia (hemoglobin <11g/ dL not due to AIHA†), having a median survival of 2 years
- Stage 4: Lymphocytosis w/ thrombocytopenia (<100,000/ μL not due to AITP‡)

---

†Autoimmune hemolytic anemia–AIHA
‡Autoimmune thrombocytopenia–AITP

473

MYELOMA

- Caused by the malignant transformation of a **plasma cell** within the bone marrow (atypia→myeloma)→
  - ∘Infiltration of tissue ± spread through lymphatics & blood vessels to other organs=metastases→
    - -Extramedullary production→organ enlargement=organomegally & organ destruction
- Myeloma cells do not provide the typical protection against infection or malignancy associated w/ plasma cells

Statistics:
- Multiple myeloma incidence: 1/ 20,000
- #1 primary bone malignancy→
  - ∘10% of all hematologic cancers→
    - -1% of all cancer mediated deaths in Western countries

CLASSIFICATION

- **Myeloma**

Classification via immunoglobulin production:
- **Monoclonal antibody production†**
  - ∘Production of **IgG–50%** > **IgA–20%** > **IgD–2%** > **IgM–0.5%‡** > **IgE 0.08%** ± unbalanced antibody chain synthesis–25%→
    - -Excess light chain° production
- **Monoclonal light chain production, termed light chain disease–20%**
  - ∘Production of light chain° only
- **Monoclonal altered heavy chain production, termed heavy chain disease–rare**
  - ∘Production of altered heavy chains only, which are 25–50% shorter than their normal counterparts
- **Nonsecretors <5%**

Classification via tumor burden:
- Solitary, termed **plasmacytoma–3%**, indicating the presence of only 1myeloma mass, being either medullary or extramedullary
- Multiple, via the presence of >1myeloma mass, being either medullary or extramedullary
- **Monoclonal gammopathy of undetermined significance–MGUS**
  - ∘A monoclonal gammopathy without clinical effects (tissue destruction, organ dysfunction, or progression) as well as:
    - -**A monoclonal–M component <3g/ dL**
    - -**Bone marrow plasmacytosis <10%**
    - -Lack of urinary light chain proteins°

- **A polyclonal IgG gammopathy** may occur w/ the following:
  - ∘Autoimmune disease syndromes
  - ∘Chronic infection, esp. HIV/ AIDS
  - ∘Liver disease
  - ∘Sarcoidosis
- †Biclonal antibody production occurs in <1% of patients
- ‡Termed **Waldenstrom's macroglobulinemia**
- °Light chains are termed Bence Jones proteins

RISK FACTORS

- **Myeloma**
  - ∘†**Age:** Median age @ diagnosis is 60 years
  - ∘**Gender:** ♂ 1.3 X ♀ (♂2 X ♀ w/ IgM disease)
  - ∘**Skin color†:** Blacks 2X whites, being the #1 hematologic malignancy in blacks
  - ∘**Chemical exposure†**
    - -Asbestos
    - -Pesticides
    - -Petroleum products
  - ∘**Radiation exposure†**

- **Monoclonal gammopathy of undetermined significance–MGUS**
  - ∘†**Age:** Affecting
    - -1% of persons age >50years
    - -10% of persons age >60years

---

†Skin color or chemical/ radiation exposure are not risk factors for IgM disease

Diagnostic criteria for myeloma:
- **Bone marrow plasmacytosis >10%** (or the presence of a plasmacytoma) & either:
  - ∘**Lytic bone lesions**
  - ∘**A plasma or urine electrophoretic monoclonal–M component >3g/ dL** (see below)

General
- •Neoplastic cytokines→
  - ∘Anorexia→
    - −Cachexia
  - ∘Chills
  - ∘Fatigue
  - ∘Fever
  - ∘Headache
  - ∘Malaise
  - ∘Night sweats
  - ∘Weakness

---

†Temperature may be normal in patients w/:
- •Chronic kidney disease, esp. w/ uremia
- •Cirrhosis
- •Heart failure
- •Severe debility
- …or those who are:
  - •Intravenous drug users
  - •Taking certain medications:
    - ∘Acetaminophen
    - ∘Antibiotics
    - ∘Glucocorticoids
    - ∘Nonsteroidal anti–inflammatory drugs–NSAIDs

Cardiovascular
- •Monoclonal cryoglobulinemia, termed Type 1, indicates the presence of monoclonal immunoglobulins (IgG > IgM > IgA) which precipitate in cold temperatures, & solubilize upon rewarming→
  - ∘Microvascular plugging (esp. of the ears, fingers, &/or toes)→
    - −Localized ischemic necrosis
    - −Raynaud's phenomenon

Genitourinary
- •Immunoglobulin light chains & altered heavy chains are readily filtered by the glomerulus. A filtered concentration exceeding renal tubular epithelial cell catabolic capacity→
  - ∘Proteinuria not detected via urine dipstick, which only detects albumin
  - ∘Direct tubular toxicity (lambda > kappa light chains)
  - ∘Obstructive tubular casts
  - …→**acute tubular necrosis–ATN**→
    - •Intrarenal renal failure
- •Renal deposition of immunoglobulin light chains, being termed AL amyloid (lambda > kappa light chains)→
  - ∘**Primary amyloidosis–10%**

Lymphatics
- •Plasma cell metastases (IgM disease > others)→
  - ∘Extramedullary hematopoeisis→
    - −**Lymphadenopathy–80%**, usually being **firm & non–tender**, which may remain stable, or wax & wane in size for many months ± spontaneous regression
    - −**Hepatomegally**
    - −**Splenomegally–50%**, which may retain a relatively ↑proportion of circulating cells, termed hypersplenism→anemia, leukopenia, &/or thrombocytopenia
    - …w/ organ destruction

Musculoskeletal
- •Neoplastic cytokines, esp. interleukin 1β & tumor necrosis factor–TNF→
  - ∘↑Osteoclast activity→surrounding osteolysis (rare w/ IgM disease)→
    - −Surrounding **lytic lesions**
    - −Diffuse demineralization→osteopenia→osteoporosis
    - …→↑**fracture risk ± hypercalcemia**
    - −Bone pain

Neurologic
- •Demineralized vertebral body compression fracture→
  - ∘Sensory nerve root impingement→
    - −Back pain (usually being acute) ± lateral radiation to the flanks & anteriorly, which ↓gradually over several weeks to months
- •Neuronal deposition of immunoglobulin light chains, being termed AL amyloid→
  - ∘Neuropathy
- •Immunoglobulin mediated demyelinating syndrome

Hematologic
- •Monoclonal antibodies do not provide the typical protection against infection associated w/ antibodies, as well as→
  - ∘Feedback mediated ↓production of other immunoglobulin classes→↑infection risk via encapsulated bacteria:
    - −Escherichia coli
    - −Haemophilus influenzae
    - −Neisseria meningitides
    - −Pseudomonas aeruginosa
    - −Salmonella sp.
    - −Streptococcus pneumoniae
- •Myeloma cell proliferation† or autoantibody production→
  - −Normocytic−normochromic anemia→fatigue
  - −Leukopenia→↑infection & neoplasm risk
  - −Thrombocytopenia→↑hemorrhage risk, esp. petechiae
- •Inflammatory cytokines→
  - ∘↑Acute phase proteins
    - −↑Erythrocyte sedimentation rate−ESR (normal: 5mm/ decade aged + ♂ ≤10mm/h or ♀ ≤20mm/h)
    - −↑C−reactive protein−CRP (normal: <2mg/ L), responding more acutely than ESR, as it rises within several hours & falls within 3days upon partial resolution
    - −↑Fibrinogen
    - −↑Platelets→thrombocytosis
- •Osteolysis→
  - •**Hypercalcemia**
- •↑Plasma cell turnover→
  - ∘Hyperkalemia
  - ∘Hyperphosphatemia→
    - −Calcium binding→hypocalcemia
  - ∘↑Lactate dehydrogenase−LDH
  - ∘↑Uric acid (> ~7mg/ dL)→
    - −Gout syndrome
    - ...→**tumor lysis syndrome**
  - ∘↑β_2 microglobulin (normal <0.2mg/ dL), being a portion of the class 2 major histocompatibility−MHC complex proteins on cell surfaces of B/ plasma cells, as well as macrophages
- •↑Angiotensin converting enzyme−ACE levels (>35 U/ L)
- •↓Anion gap w/ cationic IgG immunoglobulin
- •Peripheral smear showing:
  - ∘Erythrocyte stacking, termed **rouleaux formation**
  - ∘Plasmacytosis via a plasma cell count >500/ μL, termed plasma cell leukemia, indicating very aggressive disease, which may occur @ any point in the disease

---

†Tumor replacement of normal bone marrow hematopoietic tissue is termed myelophthisis

ELECTRICAL STUDIES

•**Serum protein electrophoresis−SPEP**
Mechanism:
- •Separates plasma proteins into albumin & non−albumin=globulin (α1, α2, β2, & γ) fractions, w/ hypergammaglobulinemia indicated by an ↑γ fraction, being composed of all plasma immunoglobulins→
  - ∘Electrophoretic **monoclonal−M component >3g/ dL** indicating myeloma, whereas <3g/ dL is required for a diagnosis of monoclonal gammopathy of undetermined significance−MGUS
Limitations:
- •Does not detect light chain disease
Normal values:
- •**Albumin:** 3.3−5.7g/ dL
- •**α1:** 0.1−0.4g/ dL
- •**α2:** 0.3−0.9g/ dL
- •**β:** 0.7−1.5g/ dL
- •**γ:** 0.5−1.4g/ dL

476

- **Urine protein electrophoresis–UPEP**
  - Mechanism:
    - Detects the presence of light chain & altered heavy chain proteins filtered by the glomerulus→
      - Electrophoretic monoclonal–M component

- **Immunofixation electrophoresis–IFE**
  - Mechanism:
    - Determines the primary antibody &/or chain type composing the plasma or urine M component
  - Advantages:
    - May be used to detect a low concentration monoclonal gammopathy of any type, when a high clinical suspicion exists in the face of a normal plasma & urine electrophoresis

ELECTROPHORETIC MONOCLONAL–M COMPONENT FORMATION			
Synthesis type	Antibody size	SPEP	UPEP
Balanced synthesis	Large	+	−
Unbalanced synthesis	Small to large	+	±
Light chain disease	Small	−	±
Heavy chain disease	Intermediate	+	±
Nonsecretors	None	−	−

HYPERVISCOSITY SYNDROME
- Relative plasma viscosity ≥5† (normal being 1.5–1.9 X that of water)→
  - ↑**Blood viscosity** of ≥5 (normal being 1.5–1.9 X that of water), w/ **resultant sludging of blood in the microcirculation**→proximal ischemia ± infarction→
    - Altered mental status
    - Cerebrovascular ischemic syndrome
    - Myocardial ischemic syndrome, also being due to ↑afterload, which may→heart failure syndrome
    - Peripheral vascular ischemic syndrome
    - Glomerulonephritis
    - Headache
    - Spontaneous hemorrhage, including intraocular hemorrhage→blindness
    - Mucocutaneous ulcerations

VALUES ASSOCIATED WITH THE HYPERVISCOSITY SYNDROME		
Immunoglobulin	Normal plasma value	Hyperviscosity via M–spike values
IgM	50–335mg/ dL	>4g/ dL†
IgG‡	580–1760mg/ dL	IgG₃ >5g/ dL
IgA	75–370mg/ dL	>7g/ dL

- The actual level @ which symptoms occur varies from individual, being reasonably reproduceable
- †This syndrome **usually occurs w/ IgM disease–15%**, as IgM is large→
  - 80% being confined to the intravascular space, whereas IgG & IgA are smaller→
    - 80% being extravascular
- ‡85% of total plasma immunoglobulins

IMAGING
- **Whole body x–ray skeletal survey**
  - Findings:
    - **Sharply demarcated, "punched out" bone lytic lesions**, esp @ the pelvis, ribs, skull, & vertebrae
    - Osteopenia

- Lesions will not appear on radionuclide whole body bone scans, which detect ↑osteoblast activity, indicating new bone formation (as occurs w/ metastases to the bone). In myeloma, ↑osteoclast activity→
  - Bone destruction

BIOPSY
- **Bone marrow biopsy**
  - Findings:
    - **Plasmacytosis >10%** indicates myeloma, whereas <10% is required for a diagnosis of monoclonal gammopathy of undetermined significance–MGUS
- **Renal biopsy**
  - Findings:
    - Renal tubular epithelial cell atrophy w/ eosinophilic lamellated casts, termed "myeloma kidney"

477

DURIE–SALMON PROGNOSTIC STAGING SYSTEM				
Finding	Stage 1–All listed	Stage 2	Stage 3A	Stage 3B
Creatinine	<2mg/ dL	Not meeting criteria for stage 1 or 3	<2mg/ dL ± any listed	≥2mg/ dL
Hemoglobin	>10g/ dL		<8.5g/ dL	
Calcium	≤12mg/ dL		>12mg/ dL	
Osteolytic lesions	≤1		>5	
IgG	<5g/ dL		>7g/ dL	
IgA	<3g/ dL		>5g/ dL	
Urine light chain	<4g/ 24hour		>12g/ 24hours	
Median survival without tx:	5years	4.5years	2.5years	15months

β2–microglobulin prognostic staging system:
- •Stage 1: β2 microglobulin <4µg/ mL, indicating a median survival without treatment of 3.5years
- •Stage 2: β2 microglobulin >4µg/ mL, indicating a median survival without treatment of 1year
Limitations:
- •β2 microglobulin may be ↑in patients w/ renal failure, thus complicating the interpretation of an elevated value

TREATMENT
•Monoclonal gammopathy of undetermined significance–MGUS
Outcomes:
- •25% develop either:
  - ◦Malignancy (myeloma, leukemia, or lymphoma)
  - ◦Amyloidosis over a 20 year period
Monitoring:
- •SPEP & UPEP q6months for possible progression, as the disease may covert to any form of myeloma, regardless of initial chain disease type

•Plasmacytoma
- ◦Surgical resection & local radiation therapy
Outcomes:
- •Medullary: Often not truly localized, as myeloma becomes evident in 80% within 10years, w/ the median time for upstaging being 2years
- •Extramedullary: Often truly localized, w/ ↑cure rates

MYELOMA ▬▬
- •The vast majority are incurable

Criteria for partial response:
- •>75%↓ in plasma monoclonal–M component
- •>95%↓ in urine monoclonal–M component
- •Bone marrow plasmacytosis <5%

Criteria for complete response:
- •No plasma or urinary monoclonal–M component
- •No plasmacytosis

•Curative intent
- ◦**Allogeneic or autologous bone marrow or stem cell transplantation**
Indications:
- •Younger patients (usually being age <60 years) who are healthy enough to tolerate the procedure, & for whom appropriate donors are available (HLA matched relative donor >> unrelated donor)
Outcomes:
- •Rarely curative

•Life prolongation intent
- ◦Combination chemotherapy
- –**Myeloma:** Melphalan & Prednisone
- –**IgM disease:** Chlorambucil or Cyclophosphamide, w/ either Cladribine or Fludarabine
Outcomes:
- •Patients who respond w/ a partial remission–70%, have a 3.5year ↑median survival

- **Palliative intent**
  - **Radiation therapy**
    - Indications:
      - Symptomatic osteolytic lesions
  - Silastic tube vs. metal stent placement for obstructive lesions
  - Consider surgical resection for painful &/or obstructive lesions
  - Bisphosphonates→↓pathologic fracture risk
  - Surgery for pathologic fractures
  - Drainage of pleural effusions, w/ subsequent pleurodesis via sclerosing agents (sterile Bleomycin, Doxycycline, Mitoxantrone, Tetracycline, or talc slurry) to prevent reaccumulation

OTHER
- **Plasmapheresis**
  - Indications:
    - Acute renal failure
    - Hyperviscosity syndrome
  - Procedure:
    - Removal of blood, w/ the subsequent separation of erythrocytes from the plasma. The plasma is then discarded, containing the causative immunoglobulins, w/ the erythrocytes being reinfused w/ **fresh frozen plasma−FFP**

ALLOPURINOL

Indications:
- To be given to all patients, as hyperuricemia (uric acid >7mg/ dL)→
  - Acute tubular necrosis via uric acid mediated:
    - −Direct tubular toxicity
    - −Obstructive tubular casts
    - …→acute intra−renal renal failure

M ♀	Start	Titrate	Max
K ?	100mg PO q24hours	qweek to a target uric acid level <6mg/ dL	800mg/ 24hours†

†Doses >300mg should be divided

Dose adjustment:
- Adjust according to renal function

Creatinine clearance	Max dose
10−20mL/ min.	200mg/ 24hour
<10mL/ min.	100mg/ 24hour

Mechanism:
- Inhibits xanthine oxidase→
  - ↓Uric acid production
  - ↑Hypoxanthine & xanthine production, which are much more soluble than uric acid, & readily excreted

Side effects:
General
- **May incite a gout attack during treatment initiation or dosage ↑**
  Risk reduction:
  - Concomitant administration of an anti−inflammatory drugs−NSAIDs, until the target uric acid level is reached X ≥6months
Hypersensitivity syndrome†−2% (↑w/ renal failure)
- Dermatitis
- Fever
- Hepatitis
- Renal failure
- Vasculitis
- Eosinophilia
…necessitating discontinuation
Prognosis:
- 20% mortality
Interactions:
- ↓Metabolism of Azathioprine, Mercaptopurine, Theophylline, Warfarin→
  - ↑Plasma concentration

Overdosage:
General
- Fever

Gastrointestinal
•Hepatitis
Genitourinary
•Renal failure

---

†**Allopurinol desensitization**
Indication:
•Mild hypersensitivity syndrome
Protocol:
•Start 10μg q24h, then
○Double the dose q3–14days until the necessary dosage is reached

INTRAVENOUS IMMUNE GLOBULIN–IVIG

Indications:
•Recurrent infections w/ IgG <400mg/ dL
Dose
1g/ kg IV q24hours X 2–5days
Outcomes:
•Transient improvement: 70%
•Long term remission: Rare
Mechanism:
•Bind to plasma cell IgG Fc receptors→
○Feedback inhibition mediated ↓antibody production
Side effects:
General
•Fever ± chills
Cardiovascular
•Flushing
•Hypotension
Gastrointestinal
•Nausea ± vomiting
Genitourinary
•Acute tubular necrosis, w/ preparations containing sucrose. If used, infuse @ ≤3mg
sucrose/kg/min.
Neurologic
•Aseptic meningitis–rare
•Headache
Pulmonary
•Pulmonary failure
Hypersensitivity
•Hypersensitivity reaction if infused rapidly
•**Anaphylaxis** may occur in patients w/ **IgA deficiency** due to varied amounts of IgA, w/ some
products being IgA depleted
Contraindications:
•IgA deficiency

•Caused by the malignant transformation of a lung cell (hyperplasia→atypia→cancer)→
  ◦Infiltration of tissue ± spread through lymphatics & blood vessels to other organs=metastases
Statistics:
  •**#2 cause of cancer in the the U.S.**
  •**#1 cause of cancer mortality in the U.S.**
    ◦♂-35%, ♀-22% of cancer deaths

•**Bronchogenic cancer-95%**
  Risk factors:
  •**Age:** >40years, w/ the interval from cellular malignant transformation to symptoms being ~5-10
    years
  •**Gender:** ♂ > ♀
  •**Smoking**
    ◦Cigar, cigarette, &/or pipe smoke (active & passive="secondhand")→
      -**85% of lung cancers** (esp. small cell & squamous cell cancers), w/ risk being directly
        proportional to the amount smoked†, not the amount of tar/ cigarette
    ◦Smoking cessation→
      -↓Lung cancer rates, being **nearly equivalent to nonsmokers after 10years**
  •**Genetic**
    ◦Personal or family history of lung cancer
  •**Occupation**
    ◦**Asbestos exposure** via:
      -Construction workers exposed to asbestos insulation
      -Mechanics exposed to asbestos brake linings
      ...→synergistic effect w/ smoking→60X cancer risk
      Mechanism:
        •Macrophage inability to digest asbestos fibers→
          ◦Altered cellular events→
            -Free radical formation→malignancy
    ◦**Radiation exposure** via:
      -Miners exposed to beryllium, radon, or uranium

  Subclassification:
  •**Non-small cell cancer-80%**
    ◦**Adenocarcinoma-40%**, having a weak association w/ smoking, being either:
      -Bronchial
      -Bronchioalveolar, arising from type 2 pneumocytes
    ◦**Squamous cell cancer-30%**
    ◦**Large cell cancer-10%**
  •**Small cell cancer-20%**
  •**Mixed**

•**Mesothelioma**
  ◦Neoplasm of serosal epithelial=mesothelial cells of the:
    -**Pleura**
    -Pericardium
    -Peritoneum
    ...w/ 75% being malignant & 1/3rd of the benign neoplasms transforming to a malignant form
  Risk factors:
  •↑**Age:** Median age @ diagnosis is 60 years, as the interval from asbestos exposure to tumor
    formation is usually 30-40years
  •**Gender:** ♂ 3X ♀
  •**Occupation**
    ◦**Asbestos exposure**, accounting for **75% of malignant pleural mesotheliomas** (not being
      associated w/ benign mesotheliomas), via:
      -Construction workers exposed to asbestos insulation
      -Mechanics exposed to asbestos brake linings
      ...w/ 8% of those working w/ asbestos developing malignant pleural mesothelioma
      Mechanism:
        •Macrophage inability to digest asbestos fibers→
          ◦Altered cellular events→
            -Free radical formation→malignancy
  Note: Although asbestos has a synergistic effect w/ smoking in causing bronchogenic cancer, there
  is **no association between smoking & the development of mesothelioma**

481

- **Other primary lung neoplasia**
  - **Adenoid cystic cancer**=cylindroma, being a tracheal salivary gland neoplasm
  - **Bronchial adenoma**, being a benign or malignant slow growing neoplasm
    Risk factors:
    - Skin color: Whites 25 X blacks
  - **Bronchial carcinoid-2%**, being 90% of adenomas
    - Not associated w/ smoking
    - Rarely produces 5-hydroxyindoleacetic acid-5HIAA
  - **Mucoepidermoid cancer**

- **Secondary lung cancer**, having a **higher incidence than primary cancer**
  - **Metastases from extrapulmonary primary cancer** via:
    - Blood vessels
    - Lymphatics
    - Extension
    ...usually being:
      - Multiple
      - Bilateral
      - Peripherally located

---

†Total cigarettes smoked is expressed as **pack years, being the number of packs smoked/ day X years smoked**

DIAGNOSIS
- **20% of lung cancers are detected incidentally via chest x ray**

General
- Neoplastic cytokines→
  - Anorexia→
    - Cachexia
  - Chills
  - Fatigue
  - Fever†
  - Headache
  - Malaise
  - Night sweats
  - Weakness

---

†Temperature may be normal in patients w/:
- Chronic kidney disease, esp. w/ uremia
- Cirrhosis
- Heart failure
- Severe debility
...or those who are:
  - Intravenous drug users
  - Taking certain medications:
    - Acetaminophen
    - Antibiotics
    - Glucocorticoids
    - Nonsteroidal anti-inflammatory drugs-NSAIDs

Pulmonary
- Lung cancer→
  - **Pulmonary infiltration** ± peritumoral inflammation &/or atelectasis→
    - **Continuous thoracic pain-40%**. However, the malignancy may become large prior to causing pain, as the lung has air spaces & few pain neurons
    - **Cough-75%** ± blood=**hemoptysis-50%**
    ...w/ pleural involvement→
      - Pleurisy, being thoracic pain exacerbated by either:
        - Deep inhalation (including coughing & sneezing)
        - Supine position
        - Thoracic palpation
        ...& being relieved by leaning forward
      - **Pleural effusion, usually being hemorrhagic**
        - Accounting for 20% of all pleural effusions
      - Inflammation of the nearby pericardium=pericarditis

482

•Pulmonary infiltration ± pleural effusion, surrounding atelectasis, &/or bronchial obstruction→
∘Difficulty breathing=**dyspnea–60%**→
  −Respiratory rate >16/ min.=**tachypnea**
  −Accessory muscle usage (sternocleidomastoid muscles for inspiration & abdominal muscles for expiration)
  −Speech frequently interrupted by inspiration=telegraphic speech
  −Pursed lip breathing &/or grunting expirations→positive end−expiratory pressure–PEEP
  −Paradoxical abdominal motion: Negative intrathoracic pressure→fatigued diaphragm being pulled into the thorax→inspiratory inward motion of the anterior abdominal wall, rather than expected outward motion due to diaphragmatic contraction
∘Ventilation/ perfusion mismatch via:
  −↑Alveolar dead space: Alveolar ventilation through relatively underperfused capillaries
  −↑Vascular shunting†: Capillary blood flow through relatively underventilated alveoli. Usually occurring, or exacerbated via ↑venous return
  …→↓diffusion of O_2 & CO_2→
    •Hypoxemia (SaO_2 ≤ 91% or PaO_2 ≤ 60mmHg‡) on room air, w/ subsequent hypercapnia ($PaCO_2$ ≥45mmHg) due to either:
      ∘Respiratory muscle fatigue
      ∘Alveolar hypoventilation
      …as CO_2 clearance is unimpaired (& may be ↑in the dyspneic patient) as long as adequate ventilation (including lack of diffuse severe ventilation/ perfusion mismatching) is maintained, as:
        •CO_2 diffuses 20X as rapidly as O_2
        •Hypercapnia→
          ∘Immediate brain stem respiratory center mediated stimulation of pulmonary

---

†Being exacerbated by the supine position→
•↑Systemic venous return→
  ∘↑Vascular shunting→↑dyspnea, being termed:
    −Orthopnea, if persistent
    −Paroxysmal nocturnal dyspnea if intermittent
    …causing the patient to either use multiple pillows or sleep in a chair
‡Age adjusted normal PaO_2 = 101 − (0.43 X age)

COMPARATIVE THORACIC EXAMINATION FINDINGS			
Physical examination	Consolidation/ empyema	Pleural effusion	Pneumothorax†
Chest expansion	↓	↓	↓‡
Auscultation	↓Breath sounds w/ crackles, rhonchi, wheezes, &/or egophony°		↓Breath sounds
Percussion	↓	↓	↑^
Tactile or auscultatory fremitus	↑ⁿ	↓	↓

Note: Outlining lung compression by all 3 etiologies→
•Atelectasis→
  ∘Signs of consolidation
†If via bronchopleural fistula, may be accompanied by:
•Hemothorax (a pleural effusion)
•Pyothorax=empyema
‡Loss of intrapleural negative pressure→
•Ipsilateral chest wall expansion→
  ∘↑Anteroposterior diameter→
    −↓Respiratory movement
°A patients verbalization of the sound 'E' is heard as 'A'
^Best detected over the midclavicle w/ the patient sitting or standing. The ipsilateral ↓breath sounds should guide you, as otherwise, you may be fooled by the contralateral side being relatively dull to percussion, assuming it to be the diseased lung
ⁿUnless accompanied by a concomitant pleural effusion

Thoracic compressive &/or infiltrative syndromes:
- •@ **lung apex**=Pancoast tumor (esp. w/ squamous cell cancer)→
  - ◦Supraclavicular lymphadenopathy=**Virchow's node**=Sentinal node
  - ◦**Horner's syndrome:** Cervical sympathetic ganglion compression ± infiltration→↓ipsilateral facial autonomic sympathetic tone→
    - −↓Iris radial smooth muscle contraction→pupil constriction=**myosis**
    - −↓Levator palpebrae smooth muscle contraction→drooping eyelid=**ptosis**
    - −↓Sweat gland activation→↓facial sweat=**anhidrosis**→facial dryness
    - −↓Ciliary epithelium aqueous humor formation→retracted eyeball, termed "sunken" eye
  - ◦**Pancoasts syndrome:** Horner's syndrome & lower trunk brachial plexopathy→
    - −**Ipsilateral arm paresis**
- •@ **Esophagus**→
  - ◦Obstruction→
    - −Difficulty swallowing=dysphagia
    - −Inflammation=esophagitis→painful swallowing=odynophagia
- •@ **Phrenic nerve−1%**→
  - ◦Hiccups
  - ◦Ipsilateral diaphragm paralysis
- •@ **Recurrent laryngeal nerve**→
  - ◦Hoarseness−15%
- •@ **Superior vena cava** (esp. w/ small cell cancer)→
  - ◦Obstruction→↑proximal hydrostatic pressure→
    - −Dilation of bilateral arm, neck, & head vasculature→facial erythema, edema, &/or bluish color=cyanosis
    - −↑Collateral blood flow→dilated abdominal collateral vessels w/ downward flow
  - Note: Considered a medical emergency if the patient develops altered mental status
- •@ **Thoracic duct**→
  - ◦Chylous pleural effusion=chylothorax, usually being left sided as the thoracic duct ascends to ~T5 on the right side, then on the left thereafter
- •@ **Tracheobronchial tree**→
  - ◦Cough ± hemoptysis
  - ◦Wheezing
  - ◦↓Mucous clearance distal to the obstruction→
    - −Post−obstructive pneumonia

Paraneoplastic syndromes:
- •Autoimmune mediated:
  - ◦**Lambert−Eaton myasthenic syndrome**
    - −**IgG anti−presynaptic voltage gated calcium ion channels**→↓presynaptic acetylcholine release→**symmetric proximal muscle weakness without atrophy**
    - Risk factors:
      - •**Cancer−70%, esp. small cell lung cancer−50%**
      - •Autoimmune diseases
      - •Idiopathic
    - Outcomes:
      - •Indicates improved prognosis for small cell cancer
- •Neoplastic cytokines→
  - ◦Arterial &/or venous thrombosis ± emboli, termed **Trousseau's syndrome**
  - ◦Digital clubbing
  - ◦**Hypertrophic osteoarthropathy**
    - −Bone inflammation→new periosteal bone formation→**periosteal elevation ± pain upon pressure**
    - Risk factors
      - •**Lung cancer**
- •Hormonal cytokines
  - ◦Small cell cancer→
    - −Adrenocorticotropin hormone−ACTH secretion
    - −Antidiuretic hormone−ADH secretion
    - −Calcitonin secretion
  - ◦Non−small cell cancer
    - −Adenocarcinoma & large cell cancer→growth hormone &/or human chorionic gonadotropin−HCG secretion
    - −Squamous cell cancer→parathyroid hormone related peptide−PTHrp secretion

484

•Chest x ray
Findings:
- •Pulmonary infiltration
  - ∘Interstitial
  - ∘Consolidative, which may be well circumscribed "coin lesions", being termed:
    - –**Nodule if <3cm**
    - –**Mass if ≥3cm**
    - ...± cavitation–5%, esp. w/ squamous cell cancer
- •Pleural effusion
- •Mediastinal lymphadenopathy→
  - ∘Widened mediastinum

•Thoraco–abdomino–pelvic computed tomographic–CT scan
Procedure:
- •Must image the liver & adrenal glands, as the adrenal glands are the only site of metastatic disease in 10% of patients w/ non–small cell cancer
Advantages:
- •↑Visualization of:
  - ∘Parenchymal consolidation, infiltrate, & lymphadenopathy
  - ∘A small pleural effusion
- •Allows for separation of lung, pleural, mediastinal, & chest wall structures

•Positron emission tomographic–PET scan
Mechanism:
- •Intravenous radiolabeled glucose is utilized by malignant cells (as well as cells within an inflammatory focus) > normal cells, due to ↑metabolism→
  - ∘↑Relative uptake→
    - –↑Relative visualization
Outcomes:
- •A lung mass which "lights up", has a 95% chance of being malignant
- •A mass ≥1cm which does not "light up", has a 5% chance of malignancy

Typical cancer location:
- •**Centrally located**, as the following usually arise from a central bronchus
  - ∘Small cell cancer
  - ∘Squamous cell cancer
  - ∘Bronchial carcinoid
- •**Peripherally located**
  - ∘Adenocarcinoma
  - ∘Large cell cancer

Significance of solitary pulmonary nodules†:
- •Noted in 1/ 750 chest x rays, w/:
  - ∘50% being malignant (primary or secondary)
  - ∘50% being benign
    - –80% being granulomas
    - –10% being hamartomas

Benign characteristics of solitary pulmonary nodules:
- •Absence of the above risk factors
- •Smooth, sharp outline
- •Calcifications, suggesting granuloma, being:
  - ∘Central, termed "bulls eye"
  - ∘Diffuse
  - ∘Layered=lamellated
- •Popcorn pattern of calcifications, suggesting hamartoma
- •Computed tomographic–CT density being:
  - ∘High, suggesting granuloma
  - ∘Low, suggesting fat
- •No change @ >2years via repeat computed tomographic–CT scan q3months X 1year, then q6months X 1 year, then qyear X either 2years if low suspicion, or 5years if high suspicion
  - ∘Computed tomographic–CT scan can detect a size change of 0.3mm, whereas x ray requires a 4mm growth to be notable

485

•Doubling time, being either:
  ◦<1month, being very rapid
  ◦>450 days, being very slow
  ...w/ a spherical lesion considered to have doubled in volume w/ a 30%↑diameter

Significance of mediastinal lymphadenopathy‡:
•Node <1cm: 8% malignant
•Node 1–2cm: 30% malignant
•Node >2cm: 60% malignant

Location based differential diagnosis of mediastinal tumors°:
•**Anterior mediastinum**
  ◦Lymphoma
  ◦Substernal thyroid gland
  ◦Thymoma
•**Middle mediastinum**
  ◦**Lymphadenopathy**
  ◦**Metastatic malignancy**
  ◦Aortic aneurysm
  ◦Bronchogenic cyst
  ◦Enlarged pulmonary arteries
  ◦Granulomatous disease (ex: sarcoidosis)
•**Posterior mediastinum**
  ◦Extramedullary hematopoiesis
  ◦Neural tumor
  ◦Paravertebral abscess
  ◦Pheochromocytoma

---

†Masses are often malignant
‡Reactive lymphadenopathy may be due to post–obstructive pneumonia
°The location of a mediastinal mass is the best clue to its cause

CYTOLOGY

•**Sputum cytology**
Procedure:
  •3 early morning specimens†, being either:
    ◦Expectorated
    ◦Induced, via a hypertonic aerosolized saline solution
Outcomes:
  •Sensitivity:
    ◦Adenocarcinoma: <5%
    ◦Squamous cell cancer: 80%

•**Pleural effusion cytology**
Outcomes:
  •Sensitivity being:
    ◦55% w/ 1 sample
    ◦80% w/ 3 samples

•Chest percussion does not improve sensitivity
†If airways obstruction is present, administer bronchodilators prior to collection

INVASIVE PROCEDURES

•**Transthoracic needle biopsy†**
Indications:
  •**Small peripheral lesion**
Outcomes:
  •Sensitivity 80%

•**Transtracheal vs. transbronchial needle biopsy†**
Indications:
  •**Central lesion**
  •**Lymphadenopathy** (mediastinal or paratracheal)
Procedures:
  •Fiberoptic bronchoscopy performed w/ fluoroscopic guidance

486

Outcomes:
- Tumor sensitivity:
  - ∘<2cm: 30%
  - ∘>2cm: 70%

Complications:
- **Pneumothorax**
  - ∘Transthoracic approach: 15%
  - ∘Transtrachial/ bronchial approach: 5%
  - ...both being ↑in patients w/ chronic obstructive pulmonary disease–COPD
- **Pulmonary hemorrhage→**
  - ∘Blood in the pleural space=hemothorax
  - ∘Coughing blood=hematemesis
- **Transient cardiac dysrhythmias** in 5% of elderly patients
- **Bacteremia–2%**
- **Laryngospasm &/or bronchospasm**
- **Low grade fever–15%**
- **Organ perforation**, esp. of the liver or spleen, depending on the side

Contraindications:
- Coagulopathy (INR >1.3 &/or PTT >35seconds) &/or thrombocytopenia (<150,000/ µL)→
  - ∘↑Hemothorax risk
- Ventilator dependent patient, continuous cough &/or hiccups, &/or uncooperative patient→↑risk of:
  - ∘Air embolism
  - ∘Hemothorax
  - ∘Organ perforation, esp. the liver or spleen depending on side
  - ∘Pneumothorax
- Overlying skin infection→
  - ∘↑Deep tissue infection risk

Video assisted thorascopic surgery–VATS
Indications:
- Direct visualization & biopsy of the pleura in patients w/ both:
  - ∘Pleural effusions
  - ∘3 nondiagnostic thoracentesis

Procedure:
1. Administration of general anesthesia via a double lumen endobronchial tube, allowing for the separate mechanical ventilation of each lung
2. Ventilation is then discontinued to the lung w/ the lesion, w/ subsequent insufflation of CO_2→
   - Partial pneumothorax
3. A trocar is then inserted through the 7th intercostal space to create access for the thorascope, w/ subsequent additional trocar insertion being performed if other instruments such as stapling devices &/or lasers need to be used

•Cervical mediastinoscopic biopsy
Indications:
- To biopsy the anterior mediastinal area:
  - ∘Above, or at the carina
  - ∘Right paratracheal lesions
  - ∘Left paratracheal lesions above the aorta
  - ...when inaccessible via transthoracic or transbronchial biopsy

Procedure:
- Performed by inserting a rigid endoscope through a small suprasternal incision

•Open lung biopsy via thoracotomy
Indications:
- A lesion otherwise inaccessible or too small, w/ both:
  - ∘The clinical suspicion of cancer
  - ∘Resection being potentially curative

---

†Due to possible false negatives, if not diagnostic for malignancy, perform:
- Repeat computed tomographic–CT scan q3months X 1year, then q6months X 1 year, then qyear X either 2years if low suspicion, or 5years if high suspicion
  - ∘Computed tomographic–CT scan can detect a size change of 0.3mm, whereas x ray requires a 4mm growth to be notable

487

•Cells usually metastasize to the **regional lymph nodes, bone, central nervous system, liver, & adrenal glands**

•Possible metastases are assessed via:
  ∘History & physical examination
    −Left supraclavicular &/or rarely, retrosternal notch lymphatic metastases→**Virchow's node**= sentinel node
  ∘Hematologic studies
  ∘Imaging
    −**Thoraco−abdomino−pelvic imaging via CT/ MRI** to look for a nodule, mass, infiltrate, lymphadenopathy, atelectasis, pleural effusion, pericardial effusion, &/or osteolytic lesions
      Limitations:
        •Does not reliably visualize the splenic, hepatic, para−aortic, or external iliac lymph nodes
    −**Positron emission tomographic−PET scanning**
      Indications:
        •As the computed tomographic−CT scan may remain abnormal long after treatment, a PET scan may help w/ both pre−treatment staging & monitoring treatment response
      Mechanism:
        •Intravenous radiolabeled glucose is utilized by malignant cells (as well as cells within an inflammatory focus) > normal cells, due to ↑metabolism→
          ∘↑Relative uptake→
            −↑Relative visualization
    −**Radionuclide whole body bone scanning**
      Indications, being either:
        •↑Plasma alkaline phosphatase
        •Hypercalcemia
      Procedure:
        •A radioactive agent, termed a tracer, is injected intravenously→
          ∘Detection of ↑osteoblast activity, indicating new bone formation (as occurs w/ metastases to the bone)
      Agents used:
        •^{99m}technitium−Tc based agent (99mTc−sestamibi, 99mTc−teboroxime, 99mTc−tetrofosmin)

NON−SMALL CELL LUNG CANCER STAGING SYSTEM

Stage	Description	%@ presentation	5year survival
1	•Solitary tumor of any size ± visceral pleural involvement (excluding mediastinal pleura) ≥2cm distal to the carina, without lymphadenopathy	10%	65%
2	•Metastasis confined to ipsilateral peribronchial or hilar lymph nodes	10%	45%
3	•Either: ∘Direct infiltration of any extra−lung parenchymal structure ∘Intrathoracic lymph node metastasis other than ipsilateral peribronchial or hilar lymph nodes		
A	−Resectable	20%	20%
B	−Unresectable	20%	5%
4	•Intra (excluding lymphadenopathy) &/or extra−pulmonary metastasis	40%	1%

SMALL CELL LUNG CANCER STAGING SYSTEM

Stage	Description	%@ presentation	5year survival
Limited	•Confined to a hemithorax & regional lymph nodes (1 radiation port)	33%	20%
Extensive	•Spread beyond a hemithorax (>1 radiation port)	67%	<5%

TREATMENT

•**Cure may be achieved w/ surgical resection >> chemotherapy &/or radiation therapy. However, 75% of all lung cancers are not amenable to surgical resection @ diagnosis**

•**Curative intent**
  ∘**Non−small cell cancer, which may be cured via surgical resection only**
    −Stages 1−2: Neoadjuvant† chemotherapy, followed by either surgical resection‡, or radiation therapy in nonsurgical patients
    −Stage 3A: Neoadjuvant† chemotherapy & radiation therapy, followed by surgical resection‡

- **Life prolongation intent**
  - ◦**Non-small cell cancer**
    - −Stage 3B: Chemotherapy & radiation therapy
    - −Stage 4: A single brain metastasis may be treated via surgical resection, followed by whole brain irradiation
  - ◦**Small cell cancer, being nearly incurable, as it is almost always metastasized @ diagnosis, regardless of the apparent clinical stage.** The disease usually responds to chemotherapy &/or radiation therapy via ↑survival duration, w/ relapse being the rule
    - −Limited: Chemotherapy & radiation therapy ± prophylactic whole brain irradiation
    - −Extensive: Chemotherapy

- **Palliative intent:** Treatment failure or disease relapse
  - ◦Chemotherapy &/or radiation therapy
  - ◦Interstitial radiation treatment, termed brachytherapy
    - Procedure:
      - •Tissue placement of a radioactive substance
  - ◦Silastic tube vs. metal stent placement for obstructive lesions
  - ◦Consider surgical resection for painful &/or obstructive lesions
  - ◦Bisphosphonates→↓pathologic fracture risk
  - ◦Surgery for pathologic fractures
  - ◦Drainage of pleural effusions, w/ subsequent pleurodesis via sclerosing agents (sterile bleomycin, Doxycycline, Mitoxantrone, Tetracycline, or talc slurry) to prevent reaccumulation

---

†Neoadjuvant therapy refers to the use of nonsurgical therapy (chemotherapy &/or radiation therapy) as the initial treatment for cases in which surgery is a suboptimal initial approach. Its purpose is to:
- •↓Tumor size in order to allow for a complete surgical resection
- •Eradicate micrometastatic disease

‡Surgical mortality:
- •Lobectomy: 3%
- •Pneumonectomy: 7%

FOLLOW UP MANAGEMENT
- •Routine cancer prevention via history, physical examination, laboratory studies, & chest x ray qyear, as patients have an ↑risk of both:
  - ◦Relapsed disease
  - ◦Secondary extrapulmonary primary cancer

SCREENING
- •Chest x ray & sputum cytology may be performed qyear
  - Outcomes:
    - •Earlier detection & ↑resectability in heavy cigarette smokers, but **no significant ↓mortality**

PREVENTION
- •**Smoking cessation** via smoking cessation clinic
  - ◦Cigarette smoking contributes to 20% of deaths in the U.S., & is the #1 modifiable cause of premature death

489

BREAST CANCER

•Caused by the malignant transformation of a breast cell (hyperplasia→atypia→cancer)→
  ○Infiltration of tissue ± spread through lymphatics & blood vessels to other organs=metastases
Statistics:
•1 in 8 ♀ develop breast cancer during their lifetime→
  ○**#1 cause of ♀ cancer in the U.S.**
  ...w/ a 35% mortality→
      •#1 cause of cancer related ♀mortality @ age 35-55 years
      •#2 cause of overall cancer related ♀mortality (lung cancer is #1)

RISK FACTORS

•↑**Age**
•**Gender:** ♀ 100X ♂
•**Skin color:** Whites > blacks
•↑**Estrogen exposure**
  ○Nulliparity
  ○Early menarche (age <12years)
  ○Late menopause (age >50years)
  ○Late first pregnancy (age >35years)
  ○Absence of breast feeding
  ○Obesity
  ○Chronic anovulation
  ○**Hormone replacement therapy-HRT**
    −Estrogen @ ≥5years use
    −Progestin without the 5year delay
  Note: No ↑risk w/ oral contraceptive use
•**Genetic**
  ○Personal history of:
    −Endometrial, ovarian, or breast cancer (in situ or infiltrating)
    −Breast atypical hyperplasia ± fibrocystic disease
    −Epitheliosis
    −Papillomatosis
  ○**Family history of breast cancer**, especially
    −1st degree relative-15% of patients
    −Bilateral occurrence
    −Premenopausal diagnosis
  ○**Family history of ovarian cancer**
  ○**Breast cancer=BRCA 1 or BRCA 2 gene mutation-10% of patients**
    −BRCA 1→~50% lifetime ♀ breast cancer risk
          →~30% lifetime ovarian cancer risk
    −BRCA 2→~70% lifetime ♀ breast cancer risk & 6% lifetime ♂ breast cancer risk
          →~15% lifetime ovarian cancer risk
  ○↑**Expression of the HER-2/ neu proto-oncogene-25%**
•**Dietary**
  ○↑Fat
  ○Alcohol
•**Endocrine**
  ○Diabetes mellitus
•**Environment**
  ○↑Socioeconomic status
  ○Urban residence
•**Procedures**
  ○Prior breast biopsy
  ○Thoracic radiation treatment
•**Other**
  ○Tall habitus

490

Histologic classification:
- **Cancer in situ**
  - ○Breast cancer that has not infiltrated the surrounding breast tissue
    - **–Ductal cell cancer**
      - Outcomes:
        - •Ipsilateral infiltrating breast cancer risk of 3%/ year
    - **–Lobular cell cancer**
      - Outcomes:
        - •Infiltrating breast cancer risk (ipsilateral or contralateral) of 1%/ year
- **•Infiltrating cancer**
  - ○**Ductal cell cancer–80%**
  - ○**Lobular cell cancer–10%**
  - ○**Papillary cancer–2%**
  - ○**Medullary cancer**
  - ○**Mucinous cancer**
  - ○**Tubular cancer**

Histologic & infiltrative pattern classification:
- **•Inflammatory cancer–5%**
  - ○Any histologic type w/ infiltration of dermal lymphatic vessels→
    - –Overlying inflammation, indicative of very poor differentiation, being rapidly lethal
- **•Pagets cancer**
  - ○Ductal cell cancer w/ infiltration of the nipple epidermis

Cutaneous/ subcutaneous
- **Breast examination** via a systematic examination of the breast, axillary, & supraclavicular tissue in both the upright & supine positions, w/ the ipsilateral hand placed behind the head→
  - ○Visualization of:
    - –Breast asymmetry
    - –Overlying skin tethering
    - –Nipple eczema, being indicative of Paget's cancer
    - –Skin inflammation, being indicative of inflammatory cancer
    - –Lymphatic obstruction→breast edema, described as peau d'orange, being french for 'orange peel'
  - ○Palpation of a **breast lump** being:
    - **–Hard**
    - **–Irregular**
    - **–Immobile**
    - **–Usually painless**, except w/ inflammatory cancer, w/ pain typically being focal, persistent, & noncyclic
    - **–Unchanged via the menstrual cycle**
    - ...w/ nipple pressure also performed for possible **discharge**, w/ ↑risk features being:
      - •Associated mass
      - •Hemorrhage
      - •Limited to 1 duct
      - •Unilateral
  - ○Palpation of **axillary &/or supraclavicular lymphadenopathy**, typically being
    - –Immobile
    - –Painless
    - ...& having a hard–matted texture, w/ lymphatic obstruction→
      - •Hand/ arm edema

Occurrence of breast cancer via divisible quadrants:
- •Upper–outter: 60%
- •Upper–inner: 15%
- •Lower–outer: 10%
- •Lower–inner: 5%
- •Subareolar: 5%

Most common causes of breast tumor by age:
- •Age 0–25years: Fibroadenoma
- •Age 25–50years: Fibrocystic disease
- •Age >50years: Breast cancer

Hematologic
- •Neoplastic cytokines†
  - ∘CA 15–3 secretion
  - ∘**Carcinoembryonic antigen–CEA** secretion (>2.5ng/ mL)

---

†May be used to monitor for treatment response & possible recurrence, if elevated @ initial diagnosis

IMAGING

•**Breast ultrasound**
  Indications:
  - •To differentiate a cystic vs. solid lesion
  Diagnostic course:
  - •**If cystic**, perform a fine needle aspiration–FNA, w/ fluid sent for cytology
  - •**If solid**, perform a **diagnostic mammography, w/ a fine needle aspiration–FNA of the lesion**

INVASIVE PROCEDURES

•**Fine needle aspiration–FNA**
  Indications:
  - •All breast lesions
  - •The value of a fine needle aspiration–FNA, is that a positive result may lead to the recommendation for mastectomy without the intermediate step of an excisional biopsy
  Diagnostic course:
  - •**If negative for cancer**, perform an excisional biopsy, as fine needle aspiration–FNA cannot rule out cancer
  - •**If positive for cancer**, perform an axillary lymph node biopsy

•**Axillary lymph node biopsy**
  - ∘Lymph node involvement occurs in **40% of patients**
  Procedure:
  - •**Axillary dissection ± sentinel lymph node biopsy** via injection of either a dye or radiolabeled substance into the biopsy cavity &/or around the breast tumor→
    - ∘Substance traveling via lymphatics to the closest draining=sentinel lymph node(s), allowing for biopsy of less lymph nodes for staging→
      - –↓Complication risk
  Outcomes:
  - •**The number of involved lymph nodes is the #1 prognostic factor**
  Complications:
  - •Axillary lymph node removal→
    - ∘Hand/ arm lymphedema→
      - –↓Microbial defense. Avoid blood draws or intravenous lines in the arm
  - •Nerve lesions→
    - ∘Cutaneous numbness
    - ∘Limitations in shoulder mobility
  Diagnostic course:
  - •**If positive for cancer, assume metastatic disease**
  - •**If negative for cancer, assume micrometastatic** disease if the patient has ≥1 of the following high risk factors:
    - ∘**Imaging**
      - –Breast cancer diameter >4cm
    - ∘**Microscopic**
      - –Markers of ↑cell proliferation (↑S phase=dividing fraction, Ki67)
      - –Poorly differentiated
    - ∘**Immunologic**
      - –Estrogen or progesterone receptor negative
      - –Expression of certain cell surface proteins (cathepsin D, EGFR, HER–2/ neu, p53)

METASTATIC SEARCH

•Cells usually metastasize to the **regional lymph nodes**

•Possible metastases are assessed via:
  - ∘History & physical examination
  - ∘Hematologic studies
  - ∘Imaging
    - –**Thoraco–abdomino–pelvic imaging via CT/ MRI** to look for a nodule, mass, infiltrate, lymphadenopathy, atelectasis, pleural effusion, pericardial effusion, &/or osteolytic lesions
      Limitations:
      - •Does not reliably visualize the splenic, hepatic, para–aortic, or external iliac lymph nodes

-Positron emission tomographic-PET scanning
  Indications:
    •As the computed tomographic-CT scan may remain abnormal long after treatment, a PET
    scan may help w/ both pre-treatment staging & monitoring treatment response
  Mechanism:
    •Intravenous radiolabeled glucose is utilized by malignant cells (as well as cells within an
    inflammatory focus) > normal cells, due to ↑metabolism→
      ○↑Relative uptake→
        −↑Relative visualization
-Radionuclide whole body bone scanning
  Indications, being either:
    •↑Plasma alkaline phosphatase
    •Hypercalcemia
  Procedure:
    •A radioactive agent, termed a tracer, is injected intravenously→
      ○Detection of ↑osteoblast activity, indicating new bone formation (as occurs w/ metastases to
      the bone)
  Agents used:
    •[99m]technitium-Tc based agent (99mTc-sestamibi, 99mTc-teboroxime, 99mTc-tetrofosmin)

BREAST CANCER STAGING SYSTEM		
Stage	Characteristics	5 year survival
I	•Tumor ≤2cm in diameter, w/ no lymph node involvement	90%
2A	•Tumor <2cm in diameter, w/ metastases to mobile ipsilateral axillary node(s)→ Tumor >2cm & ≤5cm in diameter, w/ no lymph node involvement	80%
B	•Tumor >2cm & ≤5cm in diameter, w/ metastases to mobile ipsilateral axillary node(s)→tumor >5cm in diameter, w/ no lymph node involvement	65%
3A	•Tumor ≤5cm in diameter, w/ metastases to immobile ipsilateral axillary node(s)→ tumor >5cm in greatest diameter w/ metastases to ipsilateral axillary node(s) (mobile or fixed)	50%
B	•Tumor of any size, w/ direct extension to the skin or chest wall ○Inflammatory cancer ○Skin edema, nodules, or ulcerations …w/ no known distant metastases	45%
C	•Tumor of any size, w/ infraclavicular or supraclavicular lymph node involvement	40%
4	•Distant metastases	15%

TREATMENT

•**Curative intent: Stages 1-3C**
  ○Cancer limited to the breast via either:
    -Lumpectomy
    -Simple mastectomy, being the removal of only the breast
  ○Cancer metastasized to regional lymph nodes, via either:
    -Lumpectomy w/ axillary lymph node removal
    -Modified radical mastectomy, being the removal of the breast & axillary lymph nodes
  …as well as:
    •**Radiation therapy**
    •Systemic adjuvant treatment via both:
      ○**Combination chemotherapy**
      ○**Hormone therapy** if estrogen receptor positive

Additional indications for a modified radical mastectomy:
  •**Cancer ≥5cm in diameter**
  •**Multiple breast cancers**
  •**Small breast**
  •**Contraindications to radiation therapy**
    ○History of prior breast irradiation
    ○Pregnancy

Consideration of neoadjuvant therapy:
  •**Tumors not immediately amenable to lumpectomy or modified radical mastectomy**, either:
    ○Affixed to underlying structures
    ○Involving breast skin (ex: inflammatory breast cancer)

- •Life prolongation intent: Stage 4
  - ◦Combination chemotherapy
    - Indications:
      - •Estrogen receptor negative
  - ◦Hormone therapy
    - Indications:
      - •Estrogen receptor positive
  - ◦Anti-HER-2 monoclonal antibody
    - Indications:
      - •Over expression of the HER-2/ neu gene, encoding a human epidermal growth factor receptor

- •Palliative intent: Treatment failure
  - ◦Chemotherapy &/or radiation therapy
  - ◦Interstitial radiation treatment, termed brachytherapy
    - Procedure:
      - •Tissue placement of a radioactive substance
  - ◦Silastic tube vs. metal stent placement for obstructive lesions
  - ◦Consider surgical resection for painful &/or obstructive lesions
  - ◦Bisphosphonates→↓pathologic fracture risk
  - ◦Surgery for pathologic fractures
  - ◦Drainage of pleural effusions, w/ subsequent pleurodesis via sclerosing agents (sterile Bleomycin, Doxycycline, Mitoxantrone, Tetracycline, or talc slurry) to prevent reaccumulation

---

†Neoadjuvant therapy refers to the use of nonsurgical therapy (chemotherapy, radiation therapy, &/or hormonal therapy) as the initial treatment for cases in which surgery is a suboptimal initial approach. Its purpose is to:
- •↓Tumor size in order to allow for a complete surgical resection
- •Eradicate micrometastatic disease

MIXED ESTROGEN RECEPTOR AGONIST/ ANTAGONIST			
Generic (Trade)	M ♀	Dose	
Tamoxifen (Nolvadex, Tamone) L U		20mg PO q24hours X 5years	

Outcomes:
- •30% respond if estrogen receptor positive
- •70% respond if estrogen & progesterone receptor positive

Side effects in comparison to estrogen:

Positive effects	Estrogen	Tamoxifen
•Breast cancer risk	↑↑	↓↓
•Favorable plasma lipid alteration	+++	++
◦↓LDL & total cholesterol		
•Postmenopausal bone loss prevention	+++	+†

Negative effects	Estrogen	Tamoxifen
•Endometrial cancer risk	↑↑‡	↑ (1.5/ 1000)‡
•Postmenopausal hot flashes	↓↓↓	↑
•Premenopausal hot flashes		↑↑
•Uterine hemorrhage	↑↑↑	↑
•Venous thrombosis risk	↑↑	↑↑
•Hepatocellular cancer risk		↑
•Keratopathy & optic neuritis risk		Rare

†In premenopausal ♀, Tamoxifen→
- •↓Bone mass

‡Combined w/ a progestin in ♀ w/ a uterus to prevent endometrial hyperplasia→
- •Normalized endometrial cancer risk

Contraindications:
- •History of thromboembolic disease

AROMATASE INHIBITORS

Indications:
- •Postmenopausal ♀
- •Consider starting as adjunctive treatment after Tamoxifen

Generic (Trade)
Anastrozole (Arimidex)
Exemestane (Aromasin)
Letrozole (Femara)

Mechanism:
- •Inhibit the function of ovarian & peripheral tissue aromatase activity→
  - ∘↓Conversion of androgens to estrogens (β−estradiol, estriol, & estrone), β−estradiole being the most potent & main estrogen produced

Outcomes:
- •30% respond if estrogen receptor positive
- •70% respond if estrogen & progesterone receptor positive

RECOMBINANT HUMANIZED ANTI−HER−2 MONOCLONAL ANTIBODY

Generic (Trade)
Trastuzumab (Herceptin)

Side effects:
Cardiovascular
- •Synergistic cardiac toxicity when used in combination w/ doxorubicin

SCREENING

- •**Patient performed breast exams qmonth @ age >18years**, performed 1 week after menstruation
  Outcomes:
  - •No proven mortality benefit
- •**Physician performed breast exams qyear @ age >18years**
  Outcomes:
  - •Mortality benefit independent of screening mammography not established
- •**Screening mammography qyear @ age ≥40 years** or magnetic resonance imaging−MRI if either:
  - ∘Age <40 years w/ indication for screening
  - ∘Age ≥40 years w/ dense breast tissue on mammogram
  Findings:
  - •Calcifications
  - •Masses
  - •Tissue distortion
    …necessitating diagnostic mammography w/ a fine needle aspiration−FNA
- •**Genetic testing for the BRCA 1 or 2 gene mutation**
  Indications:
  - •Significant family history of breast cancer

SCREENING IN HIGH RISK PATIENTS
- •**Positive family history**
  - ∘Begin @ age 35years, or 5years prior to the age of youngest relatives' first sign or symptom, whichever is earlier
- •**BRCA 1 or 2 gene carrier**
  - ∘Begin @ age 25 years
- •**History of thoracic radiation**
  - ∘Begin 8 years afterwards

PREVENTION

VITAMINS

Generic	M ♀	Dose
Vitamin D	L ? If >RDA	5−10µg=200−400 IU q24hours

HIGH RISK ♀

MIXED ESTROGEN RECEPTOR AGONIST/ ANTAGONIST

Generic (Trade)	M ♀	Dose
Tamoxifen (Nolvadex, Tamone)	L U	20mg PO q24hours X 5years

Outcomes:
- •50% ↓cancer incidence

- **Prophylactic bilateral oophorectomy**
  - Indications:
    - Consider in BRCA 1 or 2 gene carriers
  - Outcomes:
    - ↓Breast & ovarian cancer incidence
      - ∘↓Breast cancer by 50% in carriers of the BRCA 1 mutation

- **Prophylactic bilateral mastectomy**
  - Indications:
    - Consider in BRCA 1 or 2 gene carriers
    - Consider w/ lobular cell cancer in situ
  - Outcomes:
    - 90%↓ cancer incidence
  - Side effects:
    - Chest wall anesthesia
    - Psychological sequelae
    - The need for multiple reconstructive operations

BENIGN BREAST TUMORS

- **Fibroadenoma**
  - ∘Firm, round, **non-tender** mass, growing by expansion rather than infiltration→
    - –Unaffixed, & thus **mobile** mass, termed "the breast mouse"
- **Fibrocystic disease**
  - ∘Tender/ **painful** mass (esp. during menstruation), often being multiple/ bilateral, w/ **size fluctuation**, being larger during menstruation
  - Note: **May be pre-malignant if contains cellular atypia**
- **Lipoma**
- **Breast abscess**
- **Fat necrosis**

496

•Caused by the malignant transformation of a colonic or rectal mucosal cell (adenomatous polyp formation=colorectal adenoma→atypia→colorectal cancer)→
  ◦Infiltration of tissue ± spread through lymphatics & blood vessels to other organs=metastases
Statistics:
  •#3 cause of cancer & cancer related mortality in the U.S., w/ a lifetime risk of 5%
  •Colon cancer 2.5 X rectal cancer

RISK FACTORS
•↑Age: >40years, w/ 90% of cases @ age >50years
  ◦Median age @ presentation being 67years
•Skin color: Blacks > whites
•Dietary
  ◦Cholesterol
  ◦Low fiber diet→
    −↓Fecal transit time→↑colorectal contact w/ fecal carcinogens
  ◦Red meat
  ◦Saturated fat
•Adenomatous colorectal polyps, esp.:
  ◦Diameter >1cm
    −1−2cm: 10% harbor an adenocarcinoma
    −>2cm: 40% harbor an adenocarcinoma
  ◦Sessile polyp
  ◦Villous or tubulovillous pattern
  ◦High−grade dysplasia
•Inflammatory bowel disease−IBD
  ◦Ulcerative colitis > Crohn's disease, esp. w/ ↑duration &/or ↑colorectal involvement
•Genetic
  ◦First degree relative w/ colorectal cancer
  ◦Previous colorectal cancer
Syndromes:
  •Familial adenomatous polyposis−FAP
    ◦Autosomal dominant inheritance of a mutated adenomatous polyposis coli−APC tumor suppressor gene on the long arm of chromosome 5→
      −100's−1000's of colorectal polyps during childhood &/or young adulthood→~100% lifetime colorectal cancer risk (left > right), as well as ↑gastric, pancreatic, small intestine, & thyroid cancer risk
    Average age of onset: 20's
    Average age of symptom onset: 30's
    Average age of malignancy: 40's
  •Hereditary non−polyposis colorectal cancer−HNPCC=Lynch syndromes
    ◦Autosomal dominant inheritance of mutations in DNA mismatch repair genes→
      −80% lifetime colorectal cancer risk (right > left), as well as ↑endometrial, ovarian, pancreatic, & small intestine cancer risk
    Diagnostic criteria:
      •≥3 family members w/ colorectal cancer, meeting the following criteria:
        ◦1 being a first degree relative of the other two
        ◦1 diagnosed at age <50years of age
        ◦≥2 successive generations affected
  •Peutz−Jegher's syndrome
    ◦Colorectal hamartomatous polyps→
      −↑Colorectal cancer risk
    ◦↑Pancreatic cancer risk
    ◦↑Pigmentation of lips, skin, &/or mucus membranes
  •Juvenile Polyposis
    ◦Colorectal polyps→
      −↑Colorectal cancer risk
    ◦↑Pancreatic cancer risk

CLASSIFICATION
•Colon cancer: Malignancy arising anywhere from the ileocecal valve to the peritoneal reflection, usually located @12cm proximal to the anal verge
•Rectal cancer: Malignancy arising below the peritoneal reflection

497

Histologic classification:
- **Adenocarcinoma–93%**
- **Adenosquamous cancer**
- **Carcinoid tumor**
- **Small cell cancer**
- **Squamous cell cancer**
- **Undifferentiated cancer**
- **Sarcoma**, being extremely rare
- **Lymphoma**, being extremely rare

POLYP CLASSIFICATION

Polyp etiology:
- It is estimated that 10% of colonic polyps are neoplastic, of which, 2% harbor an invasive cancer
- **Adenomatous polyp=colorectal adenoma**
  - Benign neoplasm of exocrine epithelial cells, considered **pre–malignant**, w/ ↑risk of harboring, or subsequent development of, a malignancy
- **Hyperplastic polyp**
  - Non–neoplastic tumor due to hyperplasia of exocrine epithelial cells
- **Inflammatory polyp, termed pseudopolyp**
  - Inflammation mediated mass of granulation tissue, which may become covered w/ regenerating epithelium

Polyp morphology:
- **Sessile polyp:** Having a broad base of attachment
- **Pedunculated polyp:** Having a thin, stalk–like base of attachment
- **Villous polyp:** Either of the above, having finger–like projections, termed microvilli

DIAGNOSIS

General
- Neoplastic cytokines→
  - Anorexia→
    - –Cachexia
  - Chills
  - Fatigue
  - **Fever**†
  - Headache
  - Malaise
  - Night sweats
  - Weakness

---

†Temperature may be normal in patients w/:
- Chronic kidney disease, esp. w/ uremia
- Cirrhosis
- Heart failure
- Severe debility
...or those who are:
  - Intravenous drug users
  - Taking certain medications:
    - Acetaminophen
    - Antibiotics
    - Glucocorticoids
    - Nonsteroidal anti–inflammatory drugs–NSAIDs

Gastrointestinal
Syndrome laterality:
- **Right sided tumor**
  - Palpable abdominal mass
  - Tumor growth→
    - –↓Water absorbtion→flow around the tumor→diarrhea
  - Obstruction is a late sign as feces is predominantly liquid
- **Left sided tumor**
  - Thinned stool caliber
  - Partial obstruction→
    - –Colicky abdominal pain
    - –Alternating constipation & diarrhea

498

Gastrointestinal
- **Hemorrhage**, which may occur intermittently→
  - ◦Mucosal irritation→↑gastrointestinal smooth muscle contraction→↑peristalsis→
    - –**Abdominal pain**, being referred & episodic or "wave like", termed colic
      Areas of reference:
      - •Stomach &/or duodenum: Epigastrium
      - •Small intestine: Periumbilical area
      - •Large intestine: Hypogastrium &/or suprapubic area
      - •Rectum: Suprapubic, sacral, &/or perineal areas
    - –Anorexia
    - –↑Bowel sounds→audible gastrointestinal gurgling, termed borborygmi
    - –Diarrhea
    - –Retrograde peristalsis→nausea ± vomiting
  - ◦**Hematochezia:** Passage of bright red blood per rectum
    Lesion localization:
    - •Lower gastrointestinal hemorrhage >> upper gastrointestinal hemorrhage via massive hemorrhage (≥1L) &/or ↑↑peristalsis
  - ◦**Melena†‡:** Passage of sticky, very dark, tarry looking stool, w/ a characteristic odor, requiring ≥50mL of blood, indicating gastrointestinal hemorrhage proximal to ileocecal sphincter >> colonic gastrointestinal hemorrhage via slow hemorrhage &/or ↓peristalsis
  - ◦**Fecal occult blood:** Passage of blood detectable only by laboratory testing, requiring ≥20mL of blood. Not helpful in the anatomic determination of the lesion

- **Digital rectal exam–DRE**
  Indications:
  - •To palpate a possible distal rectal tumor
  - •Visualization of fecal streaks on glove, in order to identify possible melena &/or hematochezia

- **Fecal occult blood test–FOBT**
  Procedure:
  - ◦2 samples are taken from 1 bowel movement/ day X 3 days=6 total samples, which may be stored for <1week
  Mechanism:
  - •Uses the peroxidase activity of hemoglobin to cause a change in the reagent, w/ the patient to avoid the following for ≥3 days prior to, & during testing:
  Limitations:
  - •False positive:
    - ◦Hemoglobin rich foods:
      - –Raw red meat
    - ◦Peroxidase rich foods:
      - –Uncooked vegetables, esp. broccoli, cauliflower, or turnips
    - ◦Gastrointestinal mucosal irritants:
      - –Laxatives
      - –Nonsteroidal anti–inflammatory drugs–NSAIDs, including Aspirin
  - •False negative:
    - ◦↑Dose vitamin C

---

†Iron→
- •Melanotic looking stools ± constipation &/or diarrhea
‡Bismuth subsalicylate (Pepto–Bismol)→
- •Melanotic looking stools &/or dark tongue

Cutaneous
- •Acanthosis nigricans: Hyperpigmented macules, being rough to the touch, & velvety to sight, associated w/ malignancies, esp. gastrointestinal adenocarcinomas, as well as endocrine diseases & obesity
Hematologic
- •Complete blood count for:
  - ◦**Iron deficiency anemia→**
    - –Microcytic, hypochromic anemia
- •Neoplastic cytokines†:
  - ◦Carcinoembryonic antigen–CEA secretion (>2.5ng/ mL)

Note: Intestinal neoplasia (adenomatous polyp or colorectal cancer) is associated w/:
- •**Streptococcus bovis bacteremia**
- •Clostridium septicum sepsis
†May be used to monitor for treatment response & possible recurrence, if elevated @ initial diagnosis

Barium swallow study
Findings:
•Partial colonic obstruction via a **"napkin ring"** or **"apple–core" sign**
Anatomic colorectal cancer occurrence:
•Colon–75%
  ◦Ascending colon–25%
  ◦Transverse colon–15%
  ◦Descending colon–10%
  ◦Sigmoid colon–25%
•Rectum–25%

•**Colonoscopy**
Indications:
•Visualization to the ileocecal valve, allowing for biopsy ± removal of a lesion via polypectomy
Outcomes:
•Morbidity: 0.4%, being 1.5% w/ polypectomy
•Mortality: 0.02%
•10% of patients w/ colorectal cancer are found to have another colorectal polyp or cancer
Side effects:
•Requires sedating medications
Complications:
•Bacteremia
•**Colonic perforation** (1/ 3,000)
•Major hemorrhage (1/ 1,000)

•Cells usually metastasize to the **regional lymph nodes, liver, lung, bone, & central nervous system**

•Possible metastases are assessed via:
  ◦History & physical examination
  ◦Hematologic studies
  ◦Imaging
    −**Thoraco–abdomino–pelvic imaging via CT/ MRI** to look for a nodule, mass, infiltrate,
    lymphadenopathy, atelectasis, pleural effusion, pericardial effusion, &/or osteolytic lesions
      Limitations:
      •Does not reliably visualize the splenic, hepatic, para–aortic, or external iliac lymph nodes
    −**Positron emission tomographic–PET scanning**
      Indications:
      •As the computed tomographic–CT scan may remain abnormal long after treatment, a PET
      scan may help w/ both pre–treatment staging & monitoring treatment response
      Mechanism:
      •Intravenous radiolabeled glucose is utilized by malignant cells (as well as cells within an
      inflammatory focus) > normal cells, due to ↑metabolism→
        ◦↑Relative uptake→
          −↑Relative visualization
    −**Radionuclide whole body bone scanning**
      Indications, being either:
      •↑Plasma alkaline phosphatase
      •Hypercalcemia
      Procedure:
      •A radioactive agent, termed a tracer, is injected intravenously→
        ◦Detection of ↑osteoblast activity, indicating new bone formation (as occurs w/ metastases to
        the bone)
      Agents used:
      •^{99m}technitium–Tc based agent (99mTc–sestamibi, 99mTc–teboroxime, 99mTc–tetrofosmin)

Stage	Dukes class	Depth of invasion	5 year survival
		Cancer in situ	100%
1	A	To the mucosa/ submucosa	95%
2	B1	To the muscularis propria	90%
	B2	To the serosa	75%
3	C1	≤ 4 positive regional lymph nodes	65%
	C2	> 4 positive regional lymph nodes	35%
4	D	Distant metastases	5%

TREATMENT

•**Curative intent: Stages 1–3**
  ◦Surgical resection
  ◦Systemic adjuvant chemotherapy for stage 3 colorectal
  ◦Adjuvant radiation therapy for stage ≥ 2 rectal cancer

•**Palliative intent: Stage 4**
  ◦Chemotherapy &/or radiation therapy
  ◦Interstitial radiation treatment, termed brachytherapy
    Procedure:
      •Tissue placement of a radioactive substance
  ◦Silastic tube vs. metal stent placement for obstructive lesions
  ◦Consider surgical resection for painful &/or obstructive lesions
  ◦Bisphosphonates→↓pathologic fracture risk
  ◦Surgery for pathologic fractures
  ◦Drainage of pleural effusions, w/ subsequent pleurodesis via sclerosing agents (sterile Bleomycin, Doxycycline, Mitoxantrone, Tetracycline, or talc slurry) to prevent reaccumulation

FOLLOW UP MANAGEMENT

•**History & physical examination** q6months X 3, then
  ◦Qyear X 5years
•**Liver function tests & plasma carcinoembryonic antigen–CEA**, if initially elevated, q6months X 3, then:
  ◦Qyear X 5years
•**Colonoscopy** @1 & 4years, then:
  ◦Q5years thereafter

SCREENING

•**Standard risk patient**
  ◦Beginning @ age 50years
    –**Digital rectal examination–DRE qyear**, as it may detect lesions within 7cm from the anal verge
    –**Fecal occult blood testing–FOBT qyear**, via the take home card system as above
    –**60cm flexible sigmoidoscopy q5years**, w/ visualization to the splenic flexure
      Complications:
        •Colonic perforation: 1/ 7500
        •Major hemorrhage: 0
                                OR
    –**Colonoscopy q10years**, w/ digital rectal exam–DRE @ time of endoscopy, & no need for concomitant yearly fecal occult blood testing

ENDOSCOPIC SCREENING IN HIGH RISK PATIENTS ▬▬▬▬
•**Adenomatous polyp**
  ◦Colonoscopy w/ polypectomy for histology, then:
    –If <1cm, repeat @ 3years, & return to standard guidelines if normal
    –If >1cm repeat q3years X 2, & return to standard guidelines if normal

•**Relative(s) diagnosed w/ a nonhereditary colonic neoplasm† being either:**
  ◦1st degree @ age <60years
  ◦≥Two 1st degree relatives @ any age
    –Colonoscopy q5–10years beginning @ age 40years, or 10years prior to the age of youngest relatives' first sign or symptom, whichever is earlier

501

- •Inflammatory bowel disease–IBD
  - ◦Ulcerative colitis or pancolonic Crohn's disease
    - –Colonoscopy w/ multiple biopsies q1–2years, starting @ 10 years of disease, when risk ↑ 1%/ year
  - ◦Non–pancolonic Crohn's disease
    - –Individualize screening

- •Parent w/ familial adenomatous polyposis–FAP
  - ◦Genotype testing, then:
    - –If positive: Flexible sigmoidoscopy q1–2 years, starting @ 10 years of age
    - –If negative: Flexible sigmoidoscopy @ ages 18 & 35years

- •At risk for hereditary syndrome
  - ◦Genotype testing if available, then:
    - –Colonoscopy qyear @ age ≥ 20years, or 10 years before age of youngest relatives' diagnosis, whichever is soonest

---

†Adenomatous polyp or colorectal cancer

FUTURE POSSIBLE SCREENING TECHNIQUES
- •3–dimensional computed tomographic–CT colography, termed virtual colonoscopy
  Mechanism:
  - •A noninvasive procedure combining the use of computed tomography–CT w/ computer software capable of rendering images of the entire colon meant to simulate an endoscopic view
  Positives:
  - •No sedation required
  - •Less time consuming
  - •Ability to view both sides of bowel folds
  - •Precise lesion localization
  - •Ability to re–examine the images
  Negatives:
  - •? Sensitivity/ specificity
  - •Requires prior colonic cleansing
  - •Requires colonic insufflation
  - •Requires subsequent colonoscopy if a lesion is detected

- •Pill camera
  Mechanism:
  - •An 11mm X 26mm pill, functioning as a camera, allows visualization of the gastrointestinal tract distal to the esophagus (stomach, small intestine, & large intestine), taking 2 images/ second, w/ the images being transmitted to, & stored on, a recording device worn on a belt around the patients abdomen. The study usually lasts ~8hours, after which the recording device is removed, w/ its images loaded into a computer
  Preparation:
  - •12 hour fast prior to capsule ingestion
  - •4 hour fast following capsule ingestion
  Contraindications:
  - •History of intestinal obstruction or major abdominal surgery→
    - ◦↑Capsule enlodgement risk, which may require surgical removal
  - •Automated internal cardioverter–defibrillator–AICD
  - •Pacemaker

- •Fecal DNA testing
  Mechanism:
  - •Fecal DNA is purified & tested via the polymerase chain reaction–PCR for mutations of the adenomatous polyposis coli–APC tumor suppressor gene, which cause polyps & colorectal cancer

PREVENTION			
VITAMINS			
Generic	M ♀		Dose
Vitamin D	L	? If >RDA	5–10μg=200–400 IU q24hours

PROSTATE NEOPLASIA

CLASSIFICATION/ RISK FACTORS

BENIGN PROSTATIC HYPERPLASIA–BPH ▬▬▬▬▬▬▬▬▬▬▬▬▬▬▬▬▬
- •Caused by:
    - ∘↑Prostate epithelial cell division=hyperplasia
    - ∘↑Prostate smooth muscle cell size=hypertrophy
    - ...both of unknown etiology

Risk factors:
- •↑**Age**

AGE RELATED INCIDENCE	
Age (years)	Incidence
30–39	10%
40–49	20%
50–59	40%
60–69	70%
70–79	80%
80–90	90%

PROSTATE CANCER ▬▬▬▬▬▬▬▬▬▬▬▬▬▬▬▬▬▬▬▬▬▬▬▬▬▬▬▬▬▬▬▬▬▬
- •Caused by the malignant transformation of a prostatic epithelial cell (atypia→prostate adenocarcinoma–95%)→
    - ∘Infiltration of tissue ± spread through lymphatics & blood vessels to other organs=metastases

Statistics:
- •#1 ♂ **malignancy in the U.S., affecting 15% of** ♂
- •#2 malignant cause of ♂ mortality in the U.S. (lung cancer is #1)→
    - ∘#7 overall cause of mortality, via 3% of all ♂ deaths (10% of all ♂cancer deaths)

Risk factors†:
- •↑**Age:** >40years
- •**Skin color:** Blacks 2.5 X whites
- •**Genetic:** Family history
- •**Medications**
    - ∘Testosterone

---

†Benign prostatic hyperplasia–BPH is not a risk factor

DIAGNOSIS

- •Both the gastrointestinal & genitourinary syndrome do not reliably distinguish between benign & malignant disease
- •Most patients w/ benign prostatic hyperplasia–BPH are asymptomatic, w/ 35% being symptomatic @ age >65years

Genitourinary
- •Prostate neoplasia ± smooth muscle contraction→
    - ∘Perineal pain
    - ∘**Urethral obstruction**, usually being an:
        - –Early manifestation of benign prostatic hyperplasia–BPH, due to its usual origination in the **transition zone** of the prostate gland
        - –Late manifestation of prostate cancer, due to its usual origination in the **peripheral zone** of the prostate gland
        - ...→↓**urinary stream caliber**→
            - •**Straining**
            - •**Altered urinary bladder function** via:
                - ∘↑Detrusor muscle contraction→
                    - –**Urgency ± incontinence**
                    - –Frequency→nocturia
                - ∘↓Detrusor muscle contraction→↓urinary stream force→
                    - –Delay in starting the urinary stream, termed **hesitancy**
                    - –**Dribbling**
                    - –↑**Residual urine→urinary tract infection risk**
- •Prostate cancer→
    - ∘↓Tissue integrity
    - ∘Vascular invasion
    - ...→hematuria &/or hematospermia

503

Gastrointestinal
•Digital rectal examination–DRE in order to palpate prostate:
  ○Size
  ○Tenderness
  ○Nodularity
    –50% of **firm painless nodules** are malignant, w/ "bony hard" nodules being a late finding of prostate cancer

Benign etiologies of a prostatic nodule:
  •**Benign prostatic hyperplasia–BPH**
    ○Enlarged, rubbery to normal textured lobe, as an inner nodule forces normal tissue outward
  •**Calculi**
  •**Infection, infarction, & post-partial prostatectomy** for benign prostatic hyperplasia–BPH→
    ○Prostate inflammation=prostatitis→
      –Fibrosis

Hematologic
•**Prostate specific antigen–PSA secretion†‡**
  ○Enzyme produced only by prostate epithelial cells, being ↑ w/°:
    –Benign prostatic hyperplasia–BPH
    –Prostate cancer
    –Prostate inflammation=prostatitis via infection, infarction, or prostatic manipulation (biopsy, cystourethroscopy, or transurethral resection of the prostate–TURP)
    –Recent ejaculation
Limitations:
  •**Prostate cancer screening via PSA measurement has no effect on mortality**
Other related tests:
  •**PSA velocity**
    ○The rate of PSA level change, which if **≥0.75ng/ mL @ 6–12 month intervals**, strongly suggests malignancy, as levels ↑faster w/ prostate cancer than benign prostatic hyperplasia–BPH. A PSA doubling time of <2years in patients w/ cancer indicates ↑disease progression risk
  •**PSA form**
    ○Prostate specific antigen–PSA exists in both protein bound & unbound=free forms
      –Patients w/ prostate cancer often have ↓free form (usually <10%), whereas those w/ benign prostatic hyperplasia–BPH usually have >25% in the free form
  •**PSA density**
    ○Total plasma PSA ÷ prostate volume, as estimated via transrectal ultrasound
Age specific PSA thresholds for urology referral:
  •45–49 years: >2.5ng/ mL
  •50–59 years: >3.5ng/ mL
  •60–69 years: >4.5ng/ mL
  •70–79 years: >6.5ng/ mL

---

†May be used to monitor for treatment response & possible recurrence, if elevated @ the initial diagnosis of prostate cancer
‡Finasteride→
  •50%↓total plasma PSA levels (plasma free PSA being unaffected). In order to adjust the measured level, simply multiply it X 2
°Neither rectal examination or instrumentation (ex: transrectal ultrasound) cause false positive elevations in patients w/ benign prostatic enlargement

INVASIVE PROCEDURES
•**Post-void residual–PVR**
  Indications:
    •All patients, for possible urethral obstruction, as >100mL indicates significantly incomplete voiding

•**Transrectal ultrasound–TRUS guided biopsy**
  Indications:
    •All nodules
  Findings:
    •Peripheral hypoechoic lesions comprise 70% of those found, 20% of which are malignant
  Gleason score:
    •Histologic prostate cancer grading via the sum of 2 scores (ranging 2–10), w/ ↑score indicating ↓differentiation→worse prognosis
      ○Primary score (1–5): Based on the epithelial cell pattern of the largest specimen section
      ○Secondary score (1–5): Based on the epithelial cell pattern of the 2nd largest specimen section

504

Gleason score	Histologic description
2 − 4	Well differentiated
5 − 7	Moderately differentiated
8 − 10	Poorly differentiated

METASTATIC SEARCH

•Cells usually metastasize to the **regional lymph nodes & bones−90%**
  ◦The obturator & iliac lymph nodes are usually the first sites of metastases

•Possible metastases are assessed via:
  ◦History & physical examination
  ◦Hematologic studies
  ◦Imaging
   −**Thoraco−abdomino−pelvic imaging via CT/ MRI** to look for a nodule, mass, infiltrate,
    lymphadenopathy, atelectasis, pleural effusion, pericardial effusion, &/or osteolytic lesions
    <u>Limitations:</u>
     •Does not reliably visualize the splenic, hepatic, para−aortic, or external iliac lymph nodes
   −**Positron emission tomographic−PET scanning**
    <u>Indications:</u>
     •As the computed tomographic−CT scan may remain abnormal long after treatment, a PET
      scan may help w/ both pre−treatment staging & monitoring treatment response
    <u>Mechanism:</u>
     •Intravenous radiolabeled glucose is utilized by malignant cells (as well as cells within an
      inflammatory focus) > normal cells, due to ↑metabolism→
      ◦↑Relative uptake→
       −↑Relative visualization
   −**Radionuclide whole body bone scanning**
    <u>Indications, being either:</u>
     •↑Plasma alkaline phosphatase
     •Hypercalcemia
    <u>Procedure:</u>
     •A radioactive agent, termed a tracer, is injected intravenously→
      ◦Detection of ↑osteoblast activity, indicating new bone formation (as occurs w/ metastases to
       the bone)
    <u>Agents used:</u>
     •^{99m}technitium−Tc based agent (99mTc−sestamibi, 99mTc−teboroxime, 99mTc−tetrofosmin)

PROSTATE CANCER STAGING SYSTEM

Stage	Description	% @ diagnosis	5year survival†
A	Incidental histologic finding=subclinical disease	↓	50−80%
B	Tumor limited to the prostate gland	10%	50−90%
C	Prostatic capsular extension without metastases	40%	15−70%
D	Lymph node &/or distant metastases	50%	5−30%

†Overall mortality is 10% @ 6months, w/ 10% surviving >10years

PROSTATE CANCER TREATMENT

•**Curative intent: Stages A−B**
  ◦Radical prostatectomy ± hormonal &/or radiation therapy if high Gleason score
        vs.
  ◦External or interstitial radiation treatment
  <u>Indications:</u>
   •↑Risk for perioperative complications
        vs.
  ◦Close follow up, termed "watchful waiting"
  <u>Indications:</u>
   •Life expectancy <10years & low Gleason score

•**Life prolongation intent: Stage C**
  ◦Radiation therapy &
  ◦Medical or surgical (via bilateral orchiectomy) hormonal treatment

- **Palliative intent: Stage D**
  - ○Medical or surgical (via bilateral orchiectomy) hormonal treatment
  - ○Radiation therapy for painful bone metastases
  - ○Interstitial radiation treatment, termed brachytherapy
    - Procedure:
      - •Tissue placement of a radioactive substance
  - ○Silastic tube vs. metal stent placement for obstructive lesions
  - ○Consider surgical resection for painful &/or obstructive lesions
  - ○Bisphosphonates→↓pathologic fracture risk
  - ○Surgery for pathologic fractures
  - ○Drainage of pleural effusions, w/ subsequent pleurodesis via sclerosing agents (sterile Bleomycin, Doxycycline, Mitoxantrone, Tetracycline, or talc slurry) to prevent reaccumulation

TREATMENT MODALITIES ▬▬▬▬▬▬▬▬▬▬▬▬▬▬▬▬▬▬▬▬▬▬▬▬▬▬▬▬▬▬
- **Radical prostatectomy**
  - Procedure:
    - •Open or laparoscopic removal of the prostate, seminal vesicles, & vas deferens ± limited pelvic lymph node dissection
  - Outcomes:
    - •Overall 10year survival rates are equivalent for both radical prostatectomy & external beam radiation treatment. However, the percentage who die from prostate cancer within 10years is 35% w/ radiation therapy, compared to 15% for radical prostatectomy. Additionally, 35% of patients treated w/ radiation therapy have biopsies showing residual cancer. Therefore, radiation therapy is best reserved for patients who either:
      - ○Refuse radical prostatectomy
      - ○Are @ ↑risk for perioperative complications
  - Complications:
    - •Operative blood loss of 1–2 L
    - •**Impotence–40%**, being the inability to achieve &/or maintain an erection
    - •**Urinary incontinence–10%**
      - ○8% require leak control pads
      - ○2% require correction via either:
        - –An artificial urinary sphincter
        - –Intra–urethral collagen injection
    - •Rectal injury
    - •Urinary bladder neck contracture
    - •Vesicoureteral anastomotic stricture
  - Postoperative:
    - •An indwelling catheter remains in place X 2weeks, w/ most ♂ returning to regular physical activities @ 4–6weeks

- **Radiation treatment**
  - Complications:
    - •Cystitis
    - •Proctitis
    - •Urethral stricture
    - •Urinary incontinence
    - •Impotence, being the inability to achieve &/or maintain an erection

PALLIATIVE TREATMENT_____
- **Hormonal treatment**
  - Mechanism:
    - •**Malignant cell deprivation of circulating androgens→**
      - ○↓Size of both the primary ± metastatic lesions
  - Outcomes:
    - •↓Morbidity, but **no effect on mortality**, w/ medical monotherapy, combination therapy, & orchiectomy being equally efficacious
    - •Most prostatic cancers are hormone dependent, as 75% of patients w/ metastatic disease respond to a form of androgen deprivation treatment. However, **nearly all patients eventually develop hormone resistant disease within 4years, w/ subsequent mean survival being 1year**

GONADOTROPIN RELEASING HORMONE-GnRH ANALOGUES		
Generic (Trade)	M	Dose
Goserelin (Zoladex)	L	3.6mg SC implant qmonth or
		10.8mg SC implant q3months
Leuprolide (Lupron)	L	
•Subcutaneous form		1mg SC q24hours
•Intramuscular form		7.5mg IM qmonth or
		22.5mg IM q3months or
		30mg IM q4months
•Subcutaneous implant		65mg SC implant qyear

Mechanism:
- •Gonadotropin releasing hormone-GnRH is secreted intermittently by the hypothalamus q1-3hours→
  - ◦Anterior pituitary gonadotropin secretion, being leutenizing hormone-LH & follicle stimulating hormone-FSH. When given intermittently, the GnRH analogues mimic physiologic release. However, **steady dose administration→**
    - –↓Leutinizing hormone-LH secretion→↓interstitial cells of Leydig androgens secretion (testosterone, dihydrotestoterone-DHT, & androstenedione), dihydrotestosterone-DHT being the most potent

Outcomes:
- •**35%↓ in prostate volume**

Side effects:
General
- •Initial transiently ↑testosterone levels for ≤1month prior to ↓→
  - ◦**Disease flare during the 1st several weeks of treatment-8%** (ex: ↑urinary symptoms, ↑bone pain, ↑**spinal cord compression if present**)
    - –**Prevented by the concomitant administration of an antiandrogen for 3–6weeks, providing total androgen blockade until the testosterone level falls**
- •Hot flashes
- •↓Libido

Cutaneous/ subcutaneous
- •**Gynecomastia** ± breast tenderness &/or pain

Genitourinary
- •Impotence, being the inability to achieve &/or maintain an erection

Musculoskeletal
- •Osteopenia→
  - ◦**Osteoporosis**

Hematologic
- •Anemia

ANTIANDROGENS		
Generic (Trade)	M	Dose
Bicalutamide (Casodex)	L	50mg PO q24hours
Flutamide (Eulexin)	KL	250mg PO q8hours
Nilutamide (Nilandron)	MK	300mg PO q24hours X 1month, then
		150mg PO q24hours

Mechanism:
- •Nonsteroidal competitive inhibitors of androgens (testosterone, dihydrotestosterone, & androstenedione) at the androgen receptor

Side effects:
General
- •Hot flashes
- •↓Libido

Cutaneous/ subcutaneous
- •**Gynecomastia** ± breast tenderness &/or pain

Gastrointestinal
- •Diarrhea
- •Nausea ± vomiting
- •**Hepatitis**

Genitourinary
- •Impotence, being the inability to achieve &/or maintain an erection

Musculoskeletal
- •Osteopenia→
  - ◦**Osteoporosis**

Hematologic
  •Anemia

Flutamide specific:
Hematologic
  •Methemogobinemia

Nilutamide specific:
Opthalmologic
  •Delayed visual adaptation to darkness
Pulmonary
  •Interstitial pneumonitis
Hematologic
  •Aplastic anemia

Nilutamide specific contraindications:
  •Severe hepatic or pulmonary disease

Monitoring:
  •Periodic liver function tests, w/ treatment to be withdrawn @ plasma values >3X the upper limit of normal

---

5α REDUCTASE INHIBITORS

Generic (Trade)	M	Dose
Dutasteride (Avodart)	L	0.5mg PO q24hours
Finasteride (Proscar)	L	5mg PO q24hours

•Treatment for 6–12months may be needed in order to assess effectiveness

Mechanism:
  •↓5α–reductase activity (a prostatic intracellular enzyme)→
    ○↓Conversion of testosterone to the more potent dihydrotestosterone

Outcomes:
  •20%↓ in prostate volume

Side effects:
General
  •Hot flashes
  •↓Libido
Cutaneous/ subcutaneous
  •Gynecomastia ± breast tenderness &/or pain
Genitourinary
  •Impotence, being the inability to achieve &/or maintain an erection
Interactions
  •50%↓total plasma PSA levels (plasma free PSA being unaffected). In order to adjust the measured level, simply multiply it X 2

•No effect on plasma lipid levels or bone density

RADIOACTIVE MEDICATIONS

Indications:
  •Skeletal metastases mediated pain

Generic (Trade)	Dose
Samarium–153 lexidronam (Quadramet)	1mCi/ kg IV X 1
Strontium–89 (Metastron)	4mCi IV q3months

Mechanism:
  •↓Osteoblastic lesion mediated bone pain

Side effects:
Hematologic
  •Myelosuppression→
    ○Anemia→
      –Fatigue
    ○Leukopenia→immunosuppression→
      –↑Infection & neoplasm risk
    ○Thrombocytopenia→
      –↑Hemorrhage risk

508

SECOND LINE

Generic	M	Dose
Aminoglutethimide		250mg PO q6hours
Ketoconazole (Nizoral)	L	400mg PO q8hours

Side effects:
General
- •Hot flashes
- •↓Libido

Cutaneous/ subcutaneous
- •**Gynecomastia** ± breast tenderness &/or pain

Endocrine
- •Adrenal failure
  - ◦Adrenal crisis being prevented by the concomitant administration of replacement doses of glucocorticoids→
    - −Adrenal gland mineralocorticoid production

Gastrointestinal
- •Diarrhea
- •Nausea ± vomiting

Genitourinary
- •Impotence, being the inability to achieve &/or maintain an erection

Mucocutaneous
- •Dermatitis

Neurologic
- •Ataxia

Musculoskeletal
- •Osteopenia→
  - ◦**Osteoporosis**

Hematologic
- •Anemia

PROSTATE CANCER SCREENING

- •**Digital rectal examination−DRE & Prostate specific antigen−PSA**
  - ◦Qyear @ age 50years, w/ life expectancy ≥10 years, as otherwise, they are likely to die from other disease syndromes

Adjustments:
- •**Black color** or **positive family history** (via a 1st degree relative diagnosed at an early age):
  - ◦The above, starting @ age 45years
- •**Positive family history** via ≥2 first degree relatives diagnosed at an early age:
  - ◦The above, starting @ age 40years

PROSTATE CANCER PREVENTION

- •↑**Plasma levels of the antioxidant carotenoid lycopene**
  - ◦↑Tomato intake

VITAMINS			
Generic	M ♀		Dose
Vitamin D	L	? If >RDA	5−10µg=200−400 IU q24hours

•Both of the following α receptor blockers are equally effective

α1 SELECTIVE RECEPTOR BLOCKERS

Generic (Trade)	M	♀	Start	Max
Alfuzosin (UroXatral)	KL	P	10mg PO qhs	10mg qhs
Doxazosin (Cardura)	L	?	1mg PO qhs	8mg qhs
Terazosin (Hytrin)	LK	?	1mg PO qhs	20mg qhs

Mechanism:
- •Reversible α1 receptor antagonist→
  - ◦Vasodilation (arterial=venous)
  - ◦Organ smooth muscle relaxation→
    - −Bladder trigone relaxation
    - −Prostate relaxation

Side effects:
Cardiovascular
- •Orthostatic hypotension→
  - ◦Presyncope or syncope, being ↓by:
    - −Low starting dose w/ gradual titration. If treatment is interrupted X several days, restart @ low dose w/ gradual titration
    - −Bedtime administration
    - −Continued use
- •Sexual dysfunction
Mucocutaneous
- •Dry mouth
Neurologic
- •Headache
- •Lethargy
- •Nightmares

α1α SELECTIVE RECEPTOR BLOCKERS

Generic (Trade)	M	Start	Max
Tamsulosin (Flomax)	LK	0.4mg q24hours	0.8mg q24hours

Mechanism:
- •Selective α1α receptor antagonist, being limited to prostatic smooth muscle→
  - ◦Selective prostate relaxation

Side effects:
Cardiovascular
- •Relatively ↓orthostatic hypotension risk
  - ◦If treatment is interrupted X several days, restart @ low dose w/ gradual titration
Genitourinary
- •Abnormal ejaculation
Neurologic
- •Dizziness
- •Headache

COMPLEMENTARY TREATMENT

SERENOA REPENS (Saw palmetto)

Dose

320mg PO q24hours w/ food

Mechanism:
- •A lipophilic extract of the saw palmetto berries of the dwarf palm tree→
  - ◦↓5α−reductase activity (a prostatic intracellular enzyme)→
    - −↓Conversion of testosterone to the more potent dihydrotestosterone
  - ◦↓Dihydrotestosterone−DHT binding to the androgen receptor

•Saw palmetto has no effect on the plasma PSA level

PYGEUM AFRICANUM (African Plum Tree)

Dose

100mg PO q24hours of standardized extract containing 14% triterpenes

510

SECOND LINE TREATMENT

5α REDUCTASE INHIBITORS

Generic (Trade)	M	Dose
Dutasteride (Avodart)	L	0.5mg PO q24hours
Finasteride (Proscar)	L	5mg PO q24hours

•Treatment for 6-12months may be needed in order to assess effectiveness

GONADOTROPIN RELEASING HORMONE-GnRH ANALOGUES

Generic (Trade)	M	Dose
Goserelin (Zoladex)	L	3.6mg SC implant qmonth or 10.8mg SC implant q3months
Leuprolide (Lupron) •Subcutaneous form •Intramuscular form •Subcutaneous implant	L	 1mg SC q24hours 7.5mg IM qmonth or 22.5mg IM q3months or 30mg IM q4months 65mg SC implant qyear

ANTIANDROGENS

Generic (Trade)	M	Dose
Bicalutamide (Casodex)	L	50mg PO q24hours
Flutamide (Eulexin)	KL	250mg PO q8hours
Nilutamide (Nilandron)	MK	300mg PO q24hours X 1month, then 150mg PO q24hours

THIRD LINE TREATMENT

•**Transurethral resection of the prostate-TURP**

Statistics:

•2nd most commonly performed surgery in ♂ age >60years in the U.S.

Procedure:

•**Transurethral partial prostatectomy** intended to re-establish prostatic urethral patency, w/ the excised section sent for histologic examination for possible malignancy

Complications:

•The procedure involves opening the bladder neck, w/ likely subsequent inability to contract, which is necessary to produce antegrade ejaculation→

 ◦Ejaculation of semen into the urinary bladder, termed **retrograde ejaculation >95%→functional sterility**

•**Impotence-1%**, being the inability to achieve &/or maintain an erection

•Hemorrhage-10%

•Urethral strictures-10%

•Urinary bladder neck contracture-3%

•**Urinary incontinence-1%**

•Urinary tract infections

•**Transurethral incision of the prostate-TUIP**

Procedure:

•An incision is made through both the bladder neck muscle & through the prostatic adenoma, to the level of the verumontanum

Outcomes:

•Comparable relief to TURP w/ fewer side effects

•**Other**

 ◦Laser therapy

 ◦Thermotherapy

 ◦Open partial prostatectomy

511

CERVICAL CANCER

•Caused by the malignant transformation of a uterine cervical cell (hyperplasia→atypia→cancer)→
  ◦Infiltration of tissue ± spread through lymphatics & blood vessels to other organs=metastases

Statistics:
  •#6 cause of ♀ cancer in the U.S.→
  ◦15,000 cases diagnosed & 5,000 deaths annually

EXPLANATION OF ASSOCIATED CERVICAL ANATOMY

•The vagina & **ectocervix** are comprised of a pink squamous epithelium, while the **endocervix** is comprised of a single layered, mucus secreting (being shiny), red columnar epithelium. The boundary between the 2 epithelium, termed the **squamocolumnar junction, is an area of active squamous cell proliferation, being the #1 site of malignant transformation**
•Prior to menarche & after menopause, the junction is located on the exposed portion of the cervix. However, estrogenic stimulation→
  ◦Squamous cell encroachment into the columnar cell area, via transformation of columnar cells to squamous cells, termed **squamous cell metaplasia**→
    −Inward junctional migration, out of view, within the cervical canal, w/ the area between the original & secondarily formed squamocolumnar junctions termed the **transformation zone**

RISK FACTORS

•**Vaginal sexual intercourse**
  ◦**Multiple sex partners**
    −Unprotected >> protected sex, via the proper use of latex or polyurethane condoms
    −Sex w/ a non−circumsized ♂
    −Sex w/ a ♂ whose previous wife developed cervical cancer
  ◦**History of a sexually transmitted disease−STD**
  ◦Vaginal intercourse at an early age, due to an immature transformation zone→
    −↑Infection risk
  ...all→
    •↑**Human Papillomavirus−HPV** infection risk
      ◦~80 serotypes exist
        −High risk: **16**−55% > **18**−20% > 31, 33, 35, 39, 45, 51, 52, 56, 58, 59, & 68
        −Low risk: 6, 11, 42, 43, & 44
    •↑Herpes simplex virus−HSV type 2 infection risk
•**Personal history of cervical dysplasia or malignancy**
•**Skin color:** Blacks, Hispanics > whites
•**Environment**
  ◦↓Socioeconomic status
•**Immunosuppression**
  ◦Advanced age
  ◦Alcoholism
  ◦Diabetes mellitus
  ◦Hematologic malignancy
  ◦HIV infection/ AIDS
  ◦Malnutrition
  ◦Medications
    −Chemotherapy
    −Chronic glucocorticoid use
    −Immunomodulating medications
  ◦Renal dialysis
•**Cigarette smoke**, via carcinogen secretion through the endocervical glandular mucosa
•**Medications**
  ◦Oral contraceptive pills−OCPs
  ◦**Intrauterine Diethylstilbestrol−DES exposure**→
    −Clear cell cancer, being a type of adenocarcinoma

CLASSIFICATION

CLASSIFICATION SYSTEMS		
Cytologic Bethesda	**Histologic** Dysplasia	CIN†

━━━━━ Within normal limits ━━━━━

| •**Atypical squamous cells** | Inflammation | Inflammation |

Histologic findings:
•Inflammation ± atypia
Outcomes:
•Normal–80%
•Low grade squamous epithelial lesion–LSEL 20%
•Invasive cancer–0.1%

| •**Low grade squamous epithelial lesions–LSEL** | Mild–moderate dysplasia | CIN1–2 |

Histologic findings:
•Epithelial partial thickness dysplasia
Outcomes:
•60% regress spontaneously
•20% remain stable for many years
•20% advance

| •**High grade squamous epithelial lesions–HSEL** | Severe dysplasia | CIN 3 |

Histologic findings:
•Epithelial full thickness dysplasia, termed cancer in situ–CIS
Outcomes:
•40% progress to invasive cancer over an average of 10years

━━━━━ Cervical cancer ━━━━━

◦Squamous cell cancer–80%
◦Adenocarcinoma–19%
◦Lymphoma
◦Sarcoma

---

†Cervical intraepithelial neoplasia–CIN

DIAGNOSIS

Genitourinary
•**Abnormal uterovaginal hemorrhage**
  ◦Prolonged &/or profuse menses, termed menorrhagia
  ◦Hemorrhage between menses, termed metrorrhagia
  …w/ both being termed menometrorrhagia
  ◦Postcoital bleeding
  ◦Postmenopausal (after cessation of menses=amenorrhea X 1year) uterine hemorrhage, which should be considered endometrial cancer until proven otherwise (but also consider cervical cancer)
•Pelvic pain
•Vaginal discharge

Etiologies of postmenopausal hemorrhage, in order of frequency:
  •Atrophic endometritis/ vaginitis
  •Exogenous estrogens
  •Endometrial cancer
  •Uterine polyps
  •Endometrial hyperplasia
  •**Cervical cancer**
  •Trauma
  •Urethral carbuncle

Hematologic
•Complete blood count for:
  ◦Iron deficiency anemia→
    –Microcytic, hypochromic anemia

•**Papanicolaou–PAP smear**
Procedure:
   •Place a **cervical spatula** firmly against the cervix of a non–menstruating ♀, & rotate it 720° in a continuous unidirectional sweep. Then wipe off cervical os mucus, insert a **cervical brush** into the cervical canal, & rotate it 720°. The predominant cell type obtained w/ each biopsy is dependent upon concurrent estrogenic stimulation
Condition specific utensil use:
   •Non–pregnant: Cervical spatula & brush
   •Pregnant: Cervical spatula & moist Q–tip
   •No cervix: Cervical spatula only
Preparations:
   •**Conventional smear**
      ○Smear both specimens together onto a clean microscopic slide, & either immerse into a fixative, or spray fixative onto it to prevent air–drying artifact. It is subsequently stained & examined via light microscopy
      Limitations:
         •Uneven slide cell distribution
         •Improper slide fixation
         •Requires another cervical swab of the transformation zone for Human Papillomavirus–HPV testing
   •**Thin–layer preparation**
      ○Place both specimens into a small bottle containing fixative solution, which is subsequently filtered or centrifuged in order to remove excess blood & debris. The cells are then transferred to a clean microscopic slide in a "mono" layer, which is stained & examined via light microscopy
      Advantages:
         •Avoids uneven slide cell distribution & improper slide fixation
         •Residual material may be used for Human Papillomavirus–HPV testing
Limitations of both techniques:
   •Poor sampling
   •Use of the following within 24hours of testing may interfere w/ accurate cytologic interpretation via cellular alteration &/or removal:
      ○Douch
      ○Lubricants
      ○Tampon use
      ○Vaginal medications

•**Hybrid capture**
Indications:
   •**Atypical squamous cells–ASC** via Papanicolaou–PAP smear
      ○Being that the majority are not clinically significant lesions (via normal histology), this test is used to help in determining whether subsequent referral for colposcopy or close follow up is appropriate
Procedure:
   •Cellular DNA is denatured & mixed w/ RNA probes that bind to the DNA of the 13 high risk serotypes of Human Papillomavirus–HPV. The RNA–DNA complexes, termed hybrids, bind to antibodies coating the tube, w/ the subsequent addition of a certain enzyme→
      ○Light=chemoluminescent reaction. The amount of light detected is used to determine both the presence of Human Papillomavirus–HPV & the viral load
Limitations:
   •False positive via probe cross reactivity w/ low risk serotypes

•**Colposcopy**
Indications:
   •**Atypical squamous cells–ASC w/ a high risk factor:**
      ○Multiple sex partners
      ○History of a sexually transmitted disease–STD
      ○Human Papillomavirus–HPV infection
      ○Personal history of cervical dysplasia or malignancy
      ○Intrauterine Diethylstilbestrol–DES exposure
   •**Atypical squamous cells–ASC consecutively X 2**

514

Procedure:
- •Magnification of the cervix (10–20X), w/ the ability to view the entire lesion & transition zone (so as not to miss a lesion), w/ the subsequent application of either:
  - ◦3–5% acetic acid=vinegar→
    - –Mucus dissolution & cellular dessication=drying→↑visualization→**biopsy of abnormal epithelium which turns white indicating ↑cellular proliferation**
  - ◦**Lugol's solution (an iodine solution)**→
    - –**Staining of normal squamous epithelium** (not of endocervical columnar epithelium)→ **biopsy of unstained epithelium**

INVASIVE PROCEDURES
- •**Lesion biopsy**
  Indications:
  - •All cervical lesions, being required to accurately classify the lesion as malignant or potentially pre–malignant
  Procedure:
  - •**Punch biopsy**, unless colposcopic exam was inadequate in viewing the entirety of the transition zone &/or lesion→
    - ◦**Endocervical curettage–ECC**

METASTATIC SEARCH
- •Possible metastases are assessed via:
  - ◦History & physical examination
    - –Left supraclavicular &/or rarely, retrosternal notch lymphatic metastases→**Virchow's node**= sentinel node
  - ◦Hematologic studies
  - ◦Imaging
    - –**Thoraco–abdomino–pelvic imaging via CT/ MRI** to look for a nodule, mass, infiltrate, lymphadenopathy, atelectasis, pleural effusion, pericardial effusion, &/or osteolytic lesions
      Limitations:
      - •Does not reliably visualize the splenic, hepatic, para–aortic, or external iliac lymph nodes
    - –**Positron emission tomographic–PET scanning**
      Indications:
      - •As the computed tomographic–CT scan may remain abnormal long after treatment, a PET scan may help w/ both pre–treatment staging & monitoring treatment response
      Mechanism:
      - •Intravenous radiolabeled glucose is utilized by malignant cells (as well as cells within an inflammatory focus) > normal cells, due to ↑metabolism→
        - ◦↑Relative uptake→
          - –↑Relative visualization
    - –**Radionuclide whole body bone scanning**
      Indications, being either:
      - •↑Plasma alkaline phosphatase
      - •Hypercalcemia
      Procedure:
      - •A radioactive agent, termed a tracer, is injected intravenously→
        - ◦Detection of ↑osteoblast activity, indicating new bone formation (as occurs w/ metastases to the bone)
      Agents used:
      - •^{99m}technitium–Tc based agent (99mTc–sestamibi, 99mTc–teboroxime, 99mTc–tetrofosmin)

515

FIGO† CLINICAL STAGING OF CERVICAL CANCER		
Stage	**Characteristics**	**5 year survival‡**
0	Cancer confined to the epithelium=Cancer in situ	>99%
I	**Infiltration confined to the cervix**	
A	•Invasion ≤5mm beyond the basement membrane & width ≤7mm	>95%
A1	∘Invasion ≤3mm beyond the basement membrane	
A2	∘Invasion >3mm beyond the basement membrane	
B	•Invasion >1A	85%
II	**Limited extra-cervical infiltration** (no disease of the pelvic wall or lower 1/3 of the vagina)	
A	•No obvious parametrial involvement	85%
B	•Obvious parametrial involvement	65%
III	**Infiltration or metastases limited to the pelvis or lower 1/3 of the vagina**	40%
A	•No pelvic wall disease	
B	•Pelvic wall disease, hydronephrosis, or nonfunctional kidney	
IV	**Infiltration or metastases beyond the true pelvis, or to the mucosa of the bladder or rectum**	20%
A	•Spread to adjacent organs	
B	•Spread to distant organs	

†FIGO=International Federation of Gynecology & Obstetrics
‡Overall 5 year survival rate: White: 70%, black: 55% in the U.S.

TREATMENT
•**Curative intent: All stages**
  ∘**Stage 0:**
    −Small lesion confined to the ectocervix: Carbon dioxide laser or cryotherapy
    −Lesion involving the Endocervix: Loop electrodiathermy excision procedure−LEEP or conization→
      removal of the transformation zone & distal endocervical canal, being sent to pathology to ensure
      adequate surrounding margins
  ∘**Stage 1A1:**
    −Simple total hysterectomy†
  ∘**Stage 1A2:**
    −Extrafascial hysterectomy†
  ∘**Stage 1B−2A**
    −Radical hysterectomy or radiation therapy, both being equally effective
  ∘**Stage 2B−4:**
    −Radiation therapy ± chemotherapy (Cisplatin ± Bleomycin & Doxorubicin)

†For microinvasive disease (1A), cone biopsy is an alternative for patients desiring to preserve fertility

SCREENING
•**Papanicolaou−PAP smear qyear, beginning 3years after the initiation of vaginal sexual activity (but no later than age 21years)**
  ∘3 normal consecutive annual Papanicolaou−PAP smears allow for subsequent q2−3year intervals,
    unless a high risk factor is present
    −Multiple sex partners
    −History of a sexually transmitted disease−STD
    −Human Papillomavirus−HPV infection
    −Personal history of cervical dysplasia or malignancy
    −Intrauterine Diethylstilbestrol−DES exposure
  ∘♀ who have undergone a total hysterectomy for a disease other than cervical neoplasia need no
    longer be screened. However, being that cervical & vaginal cancers share similar risk factors,
    continued screening for vaginal cancer via Papanicolaou−PAP smear testing is indicated
  ∘Consider Papanicolaou−PAP screening cessation in ♀ age ≥70years w/ both:
    −≥3 consecutively normal smears
    −No abnormal smears over the previous 10years
  Outcomes:
    •↓↓Incidence of invasive cervical cancer. However, 35% of ♀ do not have timely screening

PREVENTION
•**Smoking cessation** via smoking cessation clinic
  ∘Cigarette smoking contributes to 20% of deaths in the U.S., & is the #1 modifiable cause of premature
    death

516

ENDOMETRIAL CANCER

•Caused by the malignant transformation of a uterine endometrial mucosal cell (hyperplasia→atypia→ cancer)→
  ◦Infiltration of tissue ± spread through lymphatics &/or blood vessels to other organs=metastases
Statistics:
•**#1 gynecologic neoplasm**→
  ◦#4 ♀ malignancy in the U.S.

RISK FACTORS

•↑**Age:** 70% occur @ age >50years, w/ median age of diagnosis @ 60years
•↑**Estrogen exposure**
  ◦Nulliparity
  ◦Early menarche (age <12years)
  ◦Late menopause (age >50years)
  ◦Late first pregnancy (age >35years)
  ◦Absence of breast feeding
  ◦Obesity
  ◦Chronic anovulation
  ◦Medications:
    −Oral contraceptive−OCP use
    −Tamoxifen
•**Genetic**
  ◦Family history of endometrial cancer
  ◦Personal history of breast, colon, or ovarian cancer
•**Cardiovascular**
  ◦Hypertension
•**Endocrine**
  ◦Diabetes mellitus

CLASSIFICATION

•**Hyperplasia**
  ◦Simple=cystic hyperplasia ± atypia: Proliferation of **both glandular & connective tissue cells** ± cellular atypia†
    Outcomes:
    •Malignant transformation risk being:
      ◦1% without cellular atypia
      ◦10% w/ cellular atypia
  ◦Complex=adenomatous hyperplasia ± atypia: Proliferation of **glandular cells only** ± cellular atypia†
    Outcomes:
    •Malignant transformation risk being:
      ◦5% without cellular atypia
      ◦30% w/ cellular atypia
•**Cancer**
  ◦**Adenocarcinoma−95%**
  ◦**Sarcoma−5%**

---

††Cellular nuclear to cytoplasmic ratio

DIAGNOSIS

Genitourinary
•**Abnormal uterine hemorrhage−90%**
  ◦Prolonged &/or profuse menses, termed menorrhagia
  ◦Hemorrhage between menses, termed metrorrhagia
  …w/ both being termed menometrorrhagia
  ◦Postcoital bleeding
  ◦Postmenopausal (after cessation of menses=amenorrhea X 1year) uterine hemorrhage, which should be considered endometrial cancer until proven otherwise (but also consider cervical cancer)
•Pelvic pain
•Vaginal discharge

Etiologies of postmenopausal hemorrhage, in order of frequency:
- •Atrophic endometritis/ vaginitis
- •Exogenous estrogens
- **•Endometrial cancer**
- •Uterine polyps
- •Endometrial hyperplasia
- •Cervical cancer
- •Trauma
- •Urethral carbuncle

Hematologic
- •Complete blood count for:
  - ∘Iron deficiency anemia→
    - –Microcytic, hypochromic anemia
- •Neoplastic cytokines:
  - ∘α–fetoprotein–AFP 50% secretion (normal: 0–15ng/ mL), also being produced w/:
    - –Other malignancies, esp. colorectal, gastric, hepatocellular, & pancreatic cancers
    - –Liver disease (hepatitis, cirrhosis)
    - –Certain fetal tissues

---

†May be used to monitor for treatment response & possible recurrence, if elevated @ initial diagnosis

•Endometrial biopsy
Outcomes:
- •Sensitivity: 90%

•Papanicolaou–PAP smear
Outcomes:
- •Sensitivity: 35%
      IF BOTH OF THE ABOVE ARE NEGATIVE, PERFORM
•Fractional endocervical dilation & curettage
- ∘**The gold standard** for evaluating postmenopausal hemorrhage
Procedure:
- •The endocervical canal, followed by the uterine cavity endometrium are scraped off=curetted for histologic examination

•Cells usually metastasize to the **regional lymph nodes**

•Possible metastases are assessed via:
- ∘History & physical examination
- ∘Hematologic studies
- ∘Imaging
  - –**Thoraco–abdomino–pelvic imaging via CT/ MRI** to look for a nodule, mass, infiltrate, lymphadenopathy, atelectasis, pleural effusion, pericardial effusion, &/or osteolytic lesions
    Limitations:
    - •Does not reliably visualize the splenic, hepatic, para–aortic, or external iliac lymph nodes
  - –**Positron emission tomographic–PET scanning**
    Indications:
    - •As the computed tomographic–CT scan may remain abnormal long after treatment, a PET scan may help w/ both pre–treatment staging & monitoring treatment response
    Mechanism:
    - •Intravenous radiolabeled glucose is utilized by malignant cells (as well as cells within an inflammatory focus) > normal cells, due to ↑metabolism→
      - ∘↑Relative uptake→
        - –↑Relative visualization
  - –**Radionuclide whole body bone scanning**
    Indications, being either:
    - •↑Plasma alkaline phosphatase
    - •Hypercalcemia
    Procedure:
    - •A radioactive agent, termed a tracer, is injected intravenously→
      - ∘Detection of ↑osteoblast activity, indicating new bone formation (as occurs w/ metastases to the bone)
    Agents used:
    - •99mtechnitium–Tc based agent (99mTc–sestamibi, 99mTc–teboroxime, 99mTc–tetrofosmin)

○Invasive procedures
  −Peritoneal washings, as transtubal migration of malignant cells→omental, ovarian, &/or peritoneal metastases
  −Pelvic & aortic lymph node sampling
  −**Total abdominal hysterectomy−TAH & bilateral salpingo−oophorectomy−BSO**

FIGO† SURGICAL STAGING OF ENDOMETRIAL CANCER		
Stage	**Characteristics**	**5 year survival‡**
I	**Confined to the uterine corpus &/or fundus**	75%
A	•Invasion to <1/2 the myometrium	
B	•Invasion to >1/2 the myometrium	
II	**Limited cervical infiltration**	55%
A	•Endocervical glandular infiltration only	
B	•Cervical stromal infiltration	
III	**Pelvic infiltration &/or metastases**	30%
A	•Serosal/ adnexal disease &/or positive peritoneal cytology	
B	•Vaginal metastases	
C	•Pelvic &/or para−aortic lymph node metastases	
IV	**Other infiltration &/or metastases**	10%
A	•Bowel &/or bladder disease	
B	•All other metastases	

†FIGO=International Federation of Gynecology & Obstetrics
‡65% overall 5 year survival, as most endometrial cancers are diagnosed at stage 1

TREATMENT
•**Curative intent: All stages**
  ○Stages 1−2: Local radiation therapy
  ○Stages 3−4: Local radiation therapy, chemotherapy, & progestin hormonal therapy

•**Palliative intent: Recurrent disease**
  ○Radiation therapy for pelvic disease
  ○Chemotherapy &/or progestin hormonal therapy for extra−pelvic disease
  ○Interstitial radiation treatment, termed brachytherapy
    Procedure:
      •Tissue placement of a radioactive substance
  ○Silastic tube vs. metal stent placement for obstructive lesions
  ○Consider surgical resection for painful &/or obstructive lesions
  ○Bisphosphonates→↓pathologic fracture risk
  ○Surgery for pathologic fractures
  ○Drainage of pleural effusions, w/ subsequent pleurodesis via sclerosing agents (sterile Bleomycin, Doxycycline, Mitoxantrone, Tetracycline, or talc slurry) to prevent reaccumulation

FOLLOW UP MANAGEMENT
•Q3 months X 2 years, as 75% of recurrences occur within 2 years, then
  ○Q6 months X 3 years, as 85% of recurrences occur within 3 years, then
    −Qyear thereafter

SCREENING
•**No effective screening test exists**, including annual Papanicolaou−PAP smears or endometrial biopsies

TREATMENT OF ENDOMETRIAL HYPERPLASIA
•**Nonsurgical candidates, or those who desire fertility preservation**
  ○**Progestin hormonal therapy**→
    −↓Endometrial hyperplasia
    Follow up:
      •Endometrial biopsy @ 3 months
  ○**Endocervical dilation & curettage−D&C**, which may be curative
    Follow up:
      •Endometrial biopsy @ 3 months

•**Surgical candidates who do not desire fertility preservation**
  ○**Total abdominal hysterectomy−TAH**, being the treatment of choice

OVARIAN CANCER

•Caused by the malignant transformation of an ovarian cell (hyperplasia→atypia→cancer)→
  ◦Infiltration of tissue ± spread through lymphatics & blood vessels to other organs=metastases

Statistics:
•Affects 1 in 70 U.S. ♀→
  ◦50% of deaths from gynecologic cancers
  ◦#5 cause of cancer in ♀
  ◦#4 cause of cancer related mortality in ♀

RISK FACTORS

•↑**Age:** Median age 60years
•**Environment**
  ◦↑Socioeconomic status
•↑**Estrogen exposure**
  ◦Nulliparity
  ◦Early menarche (age <12years)
  ◦Late menopause (age >50years)
  ◦Late first pregnancy (age >35years)
  ◦Absence of breast feeding
  ◦Obesity
  ◦Chronic anovulation
•**Genetic**
  ◦Family history of ovarian cancer, esp. a 1st degree relative
  ◦Personal history of breast, colorectal, or endometrial cancer
  ◦**Breast cancer=BRCA 1 or BRCA 2 gene mutation–10% of patients**
    –BRCA 1→~50% lifetime ♀ breast cancer risk
      →~30% lifetime ovarian cancer risk
    –BRCA 2→~70% lifetime ♀ breast cancer risk & 6% lifetime ♂ breast cancer risk
      →~15% lifetime ovarian cancer risk

Syndromes:
•**Hereditary non–polyposis colorectal cancer–HNPCC=Lynch syndromes**
  ◦Autosomal dominant inheritance of mutations in DNA mismatch repair genes→
    –80% lifetime colorectal cancer risk (right > left), as well as ↑endometrial, ovarian, pancreatic,
      & small intestine cancer risk
Diagnostic criteria:
•≥3 family members w/ colorectal cancer, meeting the following criteria:
  ◦1 being a first degree relative of the other two
  ◦1 diagnosed at age <50years of age
  ◦≥2 successive generations affected

•**Other**
  ◦Infertility
  ◦Infertility treatment for >1year

CLASSIFICATION

•**Epithelial cell neoplasia–85%**
  ◦**Serous neoplasia**
    –Serous cystadenoma–60%, 25% being bilateral
    –Serous cystadenocarcinoma–25%, 65% being bilateral
    –Borderline serous tumor–15%, 30% being bilateral
  ◦**Mucinous neoplasia**
    –Mucinous cystadenoma–80%, 5% being bilateral
    –Mucinous cystadenocarcinoma–10%, 20% being bilateral
    –Borderline mucinous tumor–10%, 10% being bilateral
  ◦**Other**
    –Brenner tumor=Transitional tumor†–rare, rarely being malignant, 0% being bilateral
    –Clear cell adenocarcinoma–rare, 40% being bilateral
    –Endometroid cancer‡, 20% being bilateral
    –Undifferentiated cancer, 0% being bilateral

- **Germ cell neoplasia–10%,** 5% being malignant
  - ∘**Teratoma**
    - –Mature–96% (cystic vs. solid=dermoid cyst), being benign, w/ 15% being bilateral
    - –Immature–4%, being malignant & rarely bilateral
    - –Monodermal–rare
  - ∘**Other**
    - –Choriocarcinoma
    - –Dysgerminoma, being malignant, w/ 33% being bilateral
    - –Embryonal cancer
    - –Endodermal sinus tumor=Yolk sac tumor
    - –Mixed cell type
    - –Polyembryona

- **Sex cord stromal neoplasia–5%,** 25% being malignant
  - ∘Granulosa–theca cell neoplasia
    - –Granulosa cell tumor: 20% being malignant, 5% being bilateral
    - –Thecal cell tumor=Thecoma: 1% being malignant, 0% being bilateral
    - –Fibroma°: Rarely malignant, 10% being bilateral
  - ∘Other
    - –Sertoli–Leydig cell tumor: 15% malignant, 0% being bilateral
    - –Gonadoblastoma

- **Metastatic to the ovary–5%,** >50% being bilateral, esp.:
  - ∘Breast cancer
  - ∘Endometrial cancer
  - ∘Gastrointestinal cancer, w/ the ovarian metastases termed **Krukenberg tumors**
  - ∘Leukemia

---

†Resembles transitional epithelium
‡Resembles endometrial cells, w/ endometrial adenocarcinoma coexisting in 25% of patients
°May→
- **Meigs' syndrome,** being a triad of:
  - ∘Ovarian fibroma
  - ∘Hydrothorax (right > left)
  - ∘Ascites
  - ...careful, as a solid ovarian tumor & ascites should be considered malignant until proven otherwise

DIAGNOSIS

- Early disease is often asymptomatic, w/ progression to vague, albeit persistent symptoms→
  - ∘Usual diagnosis @ an advanced stage

Genitourinary
- †intra–abdominal pressure→
  - ∘Abdominal distention
  - ∘Sensation of pelvic &/or abdominal discomfort–50%
- Abdominal mass on examination–30%
- **Adnexal mass on pelvic examination–75%**

Endocrine
- 10% of teratomas contain functional thyroid tissue, being termed **struma ovarii** if it is the predominant tissue→
  - ∘Hyperthyroidism

Gastrointestinal
- Rupture of any mucinous neoplasia→
  - ∘Intra–peritoneal accumulation of thick mucin, termed **Pseudomyxoma peritonei**

Hematologic
- **Epithelial cell neoplasia→**
  - ∘**CA–125** secretion

Abdominal compressive &/or infiltrative syndromes:
- @ Intestine→
  - ∘Constipation–50%
- @ Stomach→
  - ∘Early satiety–50%
- @ Ureter→
  - ∘Hydronephrosis
  - ∘Urinary tract infection

- •@ Urinary bladder→
  - ◦Urinary frequency
- •@ Uterus→
  - ◦Pain w/ vaginal intercourse=dyspareunia

IMAGING

•**Pelvic ultrasonography**
Procedure:
- •Transvaginal & transabdominal ultrasound, which require a distended urinary bladder

•**Pelvic & abdominal computed tomographic–CT scan**

Pelvic mass findings suggestive of malignancy:
- •≥8cm diameter, being most important
- •Solid or semi–solid consistency
- •Septations
- •>3mm wall thickness
- •Bilateral
- •Ascites

INVASIVE PROCEDURES

•**Biopsy**
Procedure:
- •Obtained via surgery (laparoscopy or laparotomy), as transabdominal needle aspiration
  may→
  - ◦Seeding of malignant cells (esp. w/ cystic disease) in the peritoneal cavity & abdominal wall

METASTATIC SEARCH

•Cells usually metastasize to the **regional lymph nodes**

•Possible metastases are assessed via:
- ◦History & physical examination
- ◦Hematologic studies
- ◦Imaging
  - –**Thoraco–abdomino–pelvic imaging via CT/ MRI** to look for a nodule, mass, infiltrate,
    lymphadenopathy, atelectasis, pleural effusion, pericardial effusion, &/or osteolytic lesions
    Limitations:
    - •Does not reliably visualize the splenic, hepatic, para–aortic, or external iliac lymph nodes
  - –**Positron emission tomographic–PET scanning**
    Indications:
    - •As the computed tomographic–CT scan may remain abnormal long after treatment, a PET
      scan may help w/ both pre–treatment staging & monitoring treatment response
    Mechanism:
    - •Intravenous radiolabeled glucose is utilized by malignant cells (as well as cells within an
      inflammatory focus) > normal cells, due to ↑metabolism→
      - ◦↑Relative uptake→
        - –↑Relative visualization
  - –**Radionuclide whole body bone scanning**
    Indications, being either:
    - •↑Plasma alkaline phosphatase
    - •Hypercalcemia
    Procedure:
    - •A radioactive agent, termed a tracer, is injected intravenously→
      - ◦Detection of ↑osteoblast activity, indicating new bone formation (as occurs w/ metastases to
        the bone)
    Agents used:
    - •^{99m}technitium–Tc based agent (99mTc–sestamibi, 99mTc–teboroxime, 99mTc–tetrofosmin)

522

OVARIAN CANCER STAGING SYSTEM

Stage	Description	% @ presentation	5year survival
1	**Cancer confined to the ovaries**	15%	70%
A	•Unilateral disease		
B	•Bilateral disease		
C	•Stage 1A or B w/ either:		
	∘A surface lesion		
	∘A ruptured capsule		
	∘Malignant ascites		
	∘Peritoneal cytology positive for malignant cells		
2	**Pelvic extension**	10%	40%
A	•Extension to the uterus &/or fallopian tubes		
B	•Extension to other pelvic organs (including lymph nodes)		
C	•Stage 2A or B w/ either:		
	∘A surface lesion		
	∘A ruptured capsule		
	∘Malignant ascites		
	∘Peritoneal cytology positive for malignant cells		
3	**Abdominal extension**	65%	15%
A	•Microscopic peritoneal metastasis		
B	•Peritoneal metastases <2cm in diameter		
C	•Peritoneal metastases >2cm in diameter or retroperitoneal or inguinal lymph node metastases		
4	**Distant metastasis**	10%	15%
	•All disease above the diaphragm, or hepatic or splenic non−surface metastases		

TREATMENT

•**Curative intent: All stages**
 ∘**Platinum based chemotherapy** via Paclitaxel & either Cisplatin or Carboplatin
 ∘Surgical resection via:
  −Total abdominal hysterectomy & bilateral salpingo−oophorectomy TAH−BSO
  −Omentectomy
  −Retroperitoneal lymph node sampling

Additional treatment for stages 2−4:
  •Additional surgical debulking
  •"Second look" laparotomy to:
   ∘Evaluate tumor response
   ∘Allow resection of residual cancer

•**Palliative intent: Treatment failure or disease relapse**
 ∘Intraperitoneal platinum based chemotherapy via Paclitaxel & either Cisplatin or Carboplatin
 ∘Silastic tube vs. metal stent placement for obstructive lesions
 ∘Consider surgical resection for painful &/or obstructive lesions
 ∘Bisphosphonates→↓pathologic fracture risk
 ∘Surgery for pathologic fractures
 ∘Drainage of pleural effusions, w/ subsequent pleurodesis via sclerosing agents (sterile Bleomycin, Doxycycline, Mitoxantrone, Tetracycline, or talc slurry) to prevent reaccumulation

SCREENING

•**Asymptomatic w/ no family history**
 ∘No effective screening test exists for the general population (including transvaginal ultrasound & CA−125 measurement)
•**Positive family history**
 ∘**Transvaginal ultrasound & CA−125 measurement qyear**, beginning @ age 35years, or 5years prior to the age of youngest relatives' first sign or symptom, whichever is earlier

PREVENTION

•Breast feeding
•>1 full term pregnancy

ESOPHAGEAL CANCER

- Caused by the malignant transformation of an esophageal cell (hyperplasia→atypia→cancer)→
  - Infiltration of tissue ± spread through lymphatics & blood vessels to other organs=metastases

Statistics:
- 1% of all cancers→
  - #6 cause of cancer mortality in the world (being #7 in U.S. ♂)

RISK FACTORS

- **Age:** >50years, w/ mean age @ diagnosis being 67years
- **Gender:** ♂ 3X ♀
- **Skin color:** Blacks 3X whites
- **Smoking**
  - Cigar, cigarette, &/or pipe smoke (active & passive="secondhand")
- **Environment**
  - Afghanistan, North–central Asia, Northern Iran, & certain areas of Finland, France, Iceland, & South Africa
- **Radiation treatment to the mediastinum**
  - Usually @ ≥10years after exposure

Additional risk factors for squamous cell cancer:
- **Dietary**
  - **Alcohol**
- **Esophageal achalasia**
  - Myenteric plexus ganglion cell degeneration of unknown etiology→
    - −↓Esophageal peristalsis
    - −↑Lower esophageal sphincter–LES tone
    ...→functional obstruction @ the esophagogastric–EG junction→
      - Failure to normally pass food after swallowing→
        - Chronic local inflammation=esophagitis
- **Esophageal diverticula**→
  - Food retention→
    - −Chronic local inflammation=esophagitis
- **Genetic**
  - Congenital tylosis=nonepidermolytic palmoplantar keratoderma–rare, via autosomal dominant inheritance→
    - −Hyperkeratosis of the palms & soles
    - −Thickening of the oral mucosa
    - −↑Esophageal squamous cell cancer risk (up to 95% by age 70years)
- **Plummer–Vinson syndrome**=dysphagia post–cricoid esophageal web syndrome

Additional risk factors for adenocarcinoma:
- **Esophageal metaplasia via chronic gastroesophageal reflux disease–GERD**→
  - Chronic esophageal inflammation=esophagitis→
    - −**Barrett's esophagus–7%** via replacement of the normal squamous epithelium w/ more acid resistant columnar epithelium, resembling gastric epithelium, being salmon colored→**esophageal adenocarcinoma–10%**, esp. those w/ dysplasia

---

Note: Being that both alcohol & smoking also→
- Head & neck cancer, esophageal cancer is discovered incidentally in 1.5% of these patients

CLASSIFICATION

- **Squamous cell cancer–90%**
- **Adenocarcinoma–10%**
- **Other–<1%**
  - Carcinoid
  - Leiomyosarcoma
  - Lymphoma
  - Melanoma

General
- •Neoplastic cytokines→
  - ◦Anorexia→
    - −Cachexia
  - ◦Chills
  - ◦Fatigue
  - ◦Fever†
  - ◦Headache
  - ◦Malaise
  - ◦Night sweats
  - ◦Weakness

---

†Temperature may be normal in patients w/:
- •Chronic kidney disease, esp. w/ uremia
- •Cirrhosis
- •Heart failure
- •Severe debility
- …or those who are:
  - •Intravenous drug users
  - •Taking certain medications:
    - ◦Acetaminophen
    - ◦Antibiotics
    - ◦Glucocorticoids
    - ◦Nonsteroidal anti-inflammatory drugs−NSAIDs

Gastrointestinal
- •Esophageal cancer ± peritumoral inflammation, termed esophagitis→
  - ◦Rapidly progressive esophageal stenosis→
    - −Progressively ↑**difficulty swallowing=dysphagia−75%**, initially for solids, w/ progression to liquids, w/ eventual aspiration of retained food, liquid, & secretions (mucus, saliva)→pneumonia
    - −**Painful swallowing=odynophagia−17%**
    - −Retrosternal chest pain
    - …→cachexia

- •**Hemorrhage**, which may occur intermittently→
  - ◦**Hematemesis:** Vomiting of blood, including very dark, tarry looking blood termed 'coffee ground' emesis
    Lesion localization:
    - •Upper gastrointestinal hemorrhage
  - ◦**Hematochezia:** Passage of bright red blood per rectum
    Lesion localization:
    - •Lower gastrointestinal hemorrhage >> upper gastrointestinal hemorrhage via massive hemorrhage (≥1L) &/or ↑↑peristalsis
  - ◦**Melena†‡:** Passage of sticky, very dark, tarry looking stool, w/ a characteristic odor, requiring ≥50mL of blood, indicating gastrointestinal hemorrhage proximal to ileocecal sphincter >> colonic gastrointestinal hemorrhage via slow hemorrhage &/or ↓peristalsis
  - ◦**Fecal occult blood:** Passage of blood detectable only by laboratory testing, requiring ≥20mL of blood. Not helpful in the anatomic determination of the lesion

- •**Digital rectal exam−DRE**
  Indications:
  - •Visualization of fecal streaks on glove, in order to identify possible melena &/or hematochezia

- •**Fecal occult blood test−FOBT**
  Procedure:
  - ◦2 samples are taken from 1 bowel movement/ day X 3 days=6 total samples, which may be stored for <1week
  Mechanism:
  - •Uses the peroxidase activity of hemoglobin to cause a change in the reagent, w/ the patient to avoid the following for ≥3 days prior to, & during testing:

Limitations:
- •False positive:
  - ◦Hemoglobin rich foods:
    - –Raw red meat
  - ◦Peroxidase rich foods:
    - –Uncooked vegetables, esp. broccoli, cauliflower, or turnips
  - ◦Gastrointestinal mucosal irritants:
    - –Laxatives
    - –Nonsteroidal anti-inflammatory drugs–NSAIDs, including Aspirin
- •False negative:
  - ◦↑Dose vitamin C

---

†Iron→
- •Melanotic looking stools ± constipation &/or diarrhea

‡Bismuth subsalicylate (Pepto-Bismol)→
- •Melanotic looking stools &/or dark tongue

Pulmonary
Thoracic compressive &/or infiltrative syndromes:
- •**@ lung apex**=Pancoast tumor (esp. w/ squamous cell cancer)→
  - ◦Supraclavicular lymphadenopathy=**Virchow's node**=Sentinal node
  - ◦**Horner's syndrome:** Cervical sympathetic ganglion compression ± infiltration→↓ipsilateral facial autonomic sympathetic tone→
    - –↓Iris radial smooth muscle contraction→pupil constriction=**myosis**
    - –↓Levator palpebrae smooth muscle contraction→drooping eyelid=**ptosis**
    - –↓Sweat gland activation→↓facial sweat=**anhidrosis**→facial dryness
    - –↓Ciliary epithelium aqueous humor formation→retracted eyeball, termed "sunken" eye
  - ◦**Pancoasts syndrome:** Horner's syndrome & lower trunk brachial plexopathy→
    - –**Ipsilateral arm paresis**
- •**@ Esophagus**→
  - ◦Obstruction→
    - –Difficulty swallowing=dysphagia
    - –Inflammation=esophagitis→painful swallowing=odynophagia
- •**@ Phrenic nerve**→
  - ◦Hiccups
  - ◦Ipsilateral diaphragm paralysis
- •**@ Recurrent laryngeal nerve**→
  - ◦Hoarseness
- •**@ Aorta**→
  - ◦Aortoesophageal fistula→
    - –Upper gastrointestinal hemorrhage
- •**@ Superior vena cava** (esp. w/ small cell cancer)→
  - ◦Obstruction→↑proximal hydrostatic pressure→
    - –Dilation of bilateral arm, neck, & head vasculature→facial erythema, edema, &/or bluish color=cyanosis
    - –↑Collateral blood flow→dilated abdominal collateral vessels w/ downward flow
  - Note: Considered a medical emergency if the patient develops altered mental status
- •**@ Thoracic duct**→
  - ◦Chylous pleural effusion=chylothorax, usually being left sided as the thoracic duct ascends to ~T5 on the right side, then on the left thereafter
- •**@ Tracheobronchial tree**→
  - ◦Cough ± hemoptysis
  - ◦Wheezing
  - ◦↓Mucous clearance distal to the obstruction→
    - –Post-obstructive pneumonia
  - ◦Esophagotracheal > esophagobronchial fistula formation→
    - –Pneumonia

Cutaneous
- •Acanthosis nigricans: Hyperpigmented macules, being rough to the touch, & velvety to sight, associated w/ malignancies, esp. gastrointestinal adenocarcinomas, as well as endocrine diseases & obesity

•**Barium contrast swallow esophogram**
<u>Indications:</u>
•To look for:
◦A narrowed esophageal lumen
◦Mucosal irregularity
◦Proximal dilation
◦Possible esophagotracheal or bronchial fistula

<u>Anatomic esophageal cancer occurrence:</u>
•Squamous cell cancer
◦Predominant location: Proximal 2/3rds
•Adenocarcinoma
◦Predominant location: Distal 1/3rd

•**Esophagoscopy**
<u>Indications:</u>
•To look for a narrowed esophageal lumen, usually w/ visualization of a friable, ulcerated mass. If the tumor is not directly visible due to esophageal distortion, brushings & washings for cytology should be performed

•Cells usually metastasize to the **regional lymph nodes & lungs**

•Possible metastases are assessed via:
◦History & physical examination
 −Left supraclavicular &/or rarely, retrosternal notch lymphatic metastases→**Virchow's node**= sentinel node
◦Hematologic studies
◦Imaging
 −**Thoraco–abdomino–pelvic imaging via CT/ MRI** to look for a nodule, mass, infiltrate, lymphadenopathy, atelectasis, pleural effusion, pericardial effusion, &/or osteolytic lesions
  <u>Limitations:</u>
  •Does not reliably visualize the splenic, hepatic, para–aortic, or external iliac lymph nodes
 −**Positron emission tomographic–PET scanning**
  <u>Indications:</u>
  •As the computed tomographic–CT scan may remain abnormal long after treatment, a PET scan may help w/ both pre–treatment staging & monitoring treatment response
  <u>Mechanism:</u>
  •Intravenous radiolabeled glucose is utilized by malignant cells (as well as cells within an inflammatory focus) > normal cells, due to ↑metabolism→
   ◦↑Relative uptake→
    −↑Relative visualization
 −**Radionuclide whole body bone scanning**
  <u>Indications, being either:</u>
  •↑Plasma alkaline phosphatase
  •Hypercalcemia
  <u>Procedure:</u>
  •A radioactive agent, termed a tracer, is injected intravenously→
   ◦Detection of ↑osteoblast activity, indicating new bone formation (as occurs w/ metastases to the bone)
  <u>Agents used:</u>
  •^{99m}technitium–Tc based agent (99mTc–sestamibi, 99mTc–teboroxime, 99mTc–tetrofosmin)

ESOPHAGEAL CANCER STAGING SYSTEM

Stage	Invasion depth	5year survival†
0	Confined to the mucosa=cancer in situ‡	>95%
1	<Muscularis propria	65%
2A	Muscularis propria/ adventitia	35%
B	<Adventitia + regional lymph nodes	20%
3	≥Adventitia° + regional lymph nodes	10%
4	Distant metastases	Rare

†Overall 5year survival is 15%, as >50% of patients have either:
- **Unresectable tumors**
- **Radiographically visible metastatic disease**

...at diagnosis, w/ death usually being due to pneumonia
‡Occult invasive is frequently identified in patients w/ suspected cancer in situ who undergo surgical resection
°Infiltration of the aorta or tracheobronchial tree render the tumor inoperable

TREATMENT

- **Curative intent: Stages 0–2B**
  - Neoadjuvant chemotherapy & radiation treatment†
  - Surgical resection & reconstruction‡

  Procedure:
  - Subtotal esophageal resection via both:
    - Laparotomy
    - Either a right transthoracic (right thoracotomy) or transhiatal approach
    ...w/ the residual esophagus being anastamosed to the stomach which is pulled into the chest. If not feasible, then a section of the large intestine is interposed between the residual esophagus & the upper gastrointestinal tract

  Outcomes:
  - Operative mortality 15%, w/ colonic interposition→
    - ↑Morbidity & mortality

- **Palliative intent: Stages 3–4**
  - Chemotherapy &/or radiation therapy
  - Esophageal dilation &/or direct tumor destruction for obstructive lesions
    - Esophageal dilation via peroral bougienage or silastic tube vs. metal stent placement
    - Tumor destruction via endoscopic laser treatment, heat–coagulating probe, or photodynamic therapy
  - Feeding tube placement when needed
    - Percutaneous endoscopic gastrostomy–PEG tube
    - Jejunostomy
  - Silastic tube stent placement for esophagotracheal/ bronchial fistulas
  - Consider surgical resection for painful &/or obstructive lesions
  - Bisphosphonates→↓pathologic fracture risk
  - Surgery for pathologic fractures
  - Drainage of pleural effusions, w/ subsequent pleurodesis via sclerosing agents (sterile Bleomycin, Doxycycline, Mitoxantrone, Tetracycline, or talc slurry) to prevent reaccumulation

†Adenocarcinomas are relatively radio–insensitive.
‡Tumors in the cervical or proximal thoracic area of the esophagus pose surgical difficulties

SCREENING

Indications:
- Barret's esophagus

Procedure:
- Esophagoscopy q1–2years in order to obtain biopsies & cytologic brushings

GASTRIC CANCER

- Caused by the malignant transformation of a gastric cell (hyperplasia→atypia→cancer)→
  - Gastric ulceration, w/ infiltration of tissue ± spread through lymphatics & blood vessels to other organs=metastases

RISK FACTORS

- ↑**Age:** >50years
  - However, diffuse type adenocarcinoma is found more often in younger persons
- **Gender:** ♂ 2X ♀
- **Blood type A**
- ↓**Socioeconomic status**
- **Smoking**
  - Cigar, cigarette, &/or pipe (active & passive="secondhand")
- **Dietary†**
  - Alcohol
  - Hot rice
  - Rice wine
  - Preserved foods
    - Nitrates & nitrites (used as food preservatives), which are converted by gastric bacteria→ nitrosamines & nitrosamides→gastric cancer
    - Salted, smoked, dried, pickled, & cured foods
- **Gastric ulceration↔**
  - Gastric cancer
- ↓**Gastric defenses**
  - Hypochlorhydria
    - Chronic antacid medication use
    - Pernicious anemia
    - ...→bacterial overgrowth→
      - ↑Carcinogen production
- **Helicobacter pylori colonization or infection→**
  - Gastric ulceration
  - Gastric adenocarcinoma
  - Gastric non–Hodgkin's lymphoma
- **Previous gastric surgery**
  - Prior partial gastrectomy for gastric ulceration→
    - ↑Risk of gastric adenocarcinoma @ >20 years

---

†Much of the foods mentioned are eaten by the **Japanese** who have a very high rate of gastric cancer

CLASSIFICATION

- **Adenocarcinoma–90%**
  - Diffuse type: Predominantly infiltrative
  - Intestinal type: Polypoid
- **Non–Hodgkins lymphoma–4%**
- Carcinoid tumor
- Leiomyosarcoma

DIAGNOSIS

General
- Neoplastic cytokines→
  - Anorexia→
    - Cachexia
  - Chills
  - Fatigue
  - **Fever†**
  - Headache
  - Malaise
  - Night sweats
  - Weakness

---

†Temperature may be normal in patients w/:
- Chronic kidney disease, esp. w/ uremia
- Cirrhosis
- Heart failure
- Severe debility

...or those who are:
- •Intravenous drug users
- •Taking certain medications:
  - ◦Acetaminophen
  - ◦Antibiotics
  - ◦Glucocorticoids
  - ◦Nonsteroidal anti-inflammatory drugs–NSAIDs

Gastrointestinal
- •Intermittent epigastric discomfort ±
  - ◦Relief w/ antacid medications
  - ◦Being worsened by eating=dyspepsia
  - ...similar to gastric ulcer syndrome
- •Belching
- •Difficulty swallowing=dysphagia
- •Invasion of the muscular layer→
  - ◦**Early satiety**
  - ◦The subjective sense of abdominal fullness
- •Palpable abdominal mass
- •**Hemorrhage**, which may occur intermittently→
  - ◦**Hematemesis:** Vomiting of blood, including very dark, tarry looking blood termed 'coffee ground' emesis
    - Lesion localization:
      - •Upper gastrointestinal hemorrhage
  - ◦**Hematochezia:** Passage of bright red blood per rectum
    - Lesion localization:
      - •Lower gastrointestinal hemorrhage >> upper gastrointestinal hemorrhage via massive hemorrhage (≥1L) &/or ↑↑peristalsis
  - ◦**Melena†‡:** Passage of sticky, very dark, tarry looking stool, w/ a characteristic odor, requiring ≥50mL of blood, indicating gastrointestinal hemorrhage proximal to ileocecal sphincter >> colonic gastrointestinal hemorrhage via slow hemorrhage &/or ↓peristalsis
  - ◦**Fecal occult blood:** Passage of blood detectable only by laboratory testing, requiring ≥20mL of blood. Not helpful in the anatomic determination of the lesion

- •**Fecal occult blood test–FOBT**
  - Procedure:
    - ◦2 samples are taken from 1 bowel movement/ day X 3 days=6 total samples, which may be stored for <1week
  - Mechanism:
    - •Uses the peroxidase activity of hemoglobin to cause a change in the reagent, w/ the patient to avoid the following for ≥3 days prior to, & during testing:
  - Limitations:
    - •False positive:
      - ◦Hemoglobin rich foods:
        - –Raw red meat
      - ◦Peroxidase rich foods:
        - –Uncooked vegetables, esp. broccoli, cauliflower, or turnips
      - ◦Gastrointestinal mucosal irritants:
        - –Laxatives
        - –Nonsteroidal anti-inflammatory drugs–NSAIDs, including Aspirin
    - •False negative:
      - ◦↑Dose vitamin C

---

†Iron→
- •Melanotic looking stools ± constipation &/or diarrhea

‡Bismuth subsalicylate (Pepto–Bismol)→
- •Melanotic looking stools &/or dark tongue

Cutaneous
- •Acanthosis nigricans: Hyperpigmented macules, being rough to the touch, & velvety to sight, associated w/ malignancies, esp. gastrointestinal adenocarcinomas, as well as endocrine diseases & obesity

Hematologic
- •Complete blood count for:
  - ◦Iron deficiency anemia→
    - –Microcytic, hypochromic anemia

530

•**Barium swallow study**
Findings:
  •Visualization of a **diffuse type lesion**→
  ∘Infiltration of the stomach layers→
    −↓Gastric pliability→**linitis plastica**="leather bottle stomach"

•**Esophagogastroduodenoscopy–EGD**
Indications:
  •Lesion visualization & biopsy
Endoscopic features suggesting malignancy:
  •**Ulceration** w/ either:
    ∘Diameter >1cm
    ∘Mucosal folds not radiating toward the center of the crater
    ∘Shallow mucosal edges

•**Intestinal type** lesions usually present as an ulcer on the lesser curvature or antrum

•**75% of symptomatic patients have metastatic disease**, w/ cells usually metastasizing to the **regional lymph nodes**

•Possible metastases are assessed via:
  ∘History & physical examination
    −Left anterior axillary lymphatic metastases, termed **Irish's node**
    −Left supraclavicular &/or rarely, retrosternal notch lymphatic metastases, termed **Virchow's node**=sentinel node
    −Paraumbilical lymphatic metastases→**Sister Mary Joseph's node**, being palpable through the navel
    −Rectal lymphatic metastases→**rectal shelf of Blumer**, being palpable via rectal exam
    −Ovarian metastases→**Krukenberg's tumor**
  ∘Hematologic studies
  ∘Imaging
    −**Thoraco–abdomino–pelvic imaging via CT/ MRI** to look for a nodule, mass, infiltrate, lymphadenopathy, atelectasis, pleural effusion, pericardial effusion, &/or osteolytic lesions
      Limitations:
      •Does not reliably visualize the splenic, hepatic, para–aortic, or external iliac lymph nodes
    −**Positron emission tomographic–PET scanning**
      Indications:
      •As the computed tomographic–CT scan may remain abnormal long after treatment, a PET scan may help w/ both pre–treatment staging & monitoring treatment response
      Mechanism:
      •Intravenous radiolabeled glucose is utilized by malignant cells (as well as cells within an inflammatory focus) > normal cells, due to ↑metabolism→
        ∘↑Relative uptake→
          −↑Relative visualization
    −**Radionuclide whole body bone scanning**
      Indications, being either:
      •↑Plasma alkaline phosphatase
      •Hypercalcemia
      Procedure:
      •A radioactive agent, termed a tracer, is injected intravenously→
        ∘Detection of ↑osteoblast activity, indicating new bone formation (as occurs w/ metastases to the bone)
      Agents used:
      •^{99m}technitium–Tc based agent (99mTc–sestamibi, 99mTc–teboroxime, 99mTc–tetrofosmin)
  ∘Invasive procedures:
    −Regional lymphadenectomy
      Indications:
      •If the imaging scans are negative for metastases

•**Curative Intent: Disease confined to the stomach**
  ∘Surgical resection (subtotal vs. total gastrectomy) ± chemotherapy

•**Palliative intent: Metastatic disease**
  ∘Chemotherapy
  ∘Feeding tube placement when needed
    −Percutaneous endoscopic gastrostomy−PEG tube
    −Jejunostomy
  ∘Silastic tube stent placement for esophagotracheal/ bronchial fistulas
  ∘Consider surgical resection for painful &/or obstructive lesions
  ∘Bisphosphonates→↓pathologic fracture risk
  ∘Surgery for pathologic fractures
  ∘Drainage of pleural effusions, w/ subsequent pleurodesis via sclerosing agents (sterile Bleomycin, Doxycycline, Mitoxantrone, Tetracycline, or talc slurry) to prevent reaccumulation

•15% overall 5 year survival

•**Dietary**
  ∘Refrigerated foods
  ∘Fruits
  ∘Vegetables
  ∘Vitamin C
  ∘Whole milk

532

PANCREATIC CANCER

•Caused by the malignant transformation of a pancreatic cell (hyperplasia→atypia→cancer)→
  ◦Infiltration of tissue ± spread through lymphatics & blood vessels to other organs=metastases
Statistics:
  •#5 cause of cancer in the U.S.

RISK FACTORS

•↑**Age:** >60 years
•**Gender:** ♂ 2X ♀
•**Skin color:** Blacks > whites
•**Chronic pancreatitis**
•**Smoking**
  ◦Cigar, cigarette, &/or pipe (active & passive="secondhand")
•**Dietary**
  ◦↑Fat diet
•**Endocrine**
  ◦Diabetes mellitus
•**Insecticide–DDT**
•**Genetic**
  Syndromes:
    •**Familial adenomatous polyposis–FAP**
      ◦Autosomal dominant inheritance of a mutated adenomatous polyposis coli–APC tumor suppressor
        gene on the long arm of chromosome 5→
        −100's−1000's of colorectal polyps during childhood &/or young adulthood→~100% lifetime
          colorectal cancer risk (left > right), as well as ↑gastric, pancreatic, small intestine, & thyroid
          cancer risk
      Average age of onset: 20's
      Average age of symptom onset: 30's
      Average age of malignancy: 40's
    •**Hereditary non–polyposis colorectal cancer–HNPCC=Lynch syndromes**
      ◦Autosomal dominant inheritance of mutations in DNA mismatch repair genes→
        −80% lifetime colorectal cancer risk (right > left), as well as ↑endometrial, ovarian, pancreatic,
          & small intestine cancer risk
      Diagnostic criteria:
        •≥3 family members w/ colorectal cancer, meeting the following criteria:
          ◦1 being a first degree relative of the other two
          ◦1 diagnosed at age <50years of age
          ◦≥2 successive generations affected
    •**Peutz–Jegher's syndrome**
      ◦Colorectal hamartomatous polyps→
        −↑Colorectal cancer risk
      ◦↑Pancreatic cancer risk
      ◦↑Pigmentation of lips, skin, &/or mucus membranes
    •**Juvenile Polyposis**
      ◦Colorectal polyps→
        −↑Colorectal cancer risk
      ◦↑Pancreatic cancer risk

CLASSIFICATION

•**Adenocarcinoma–>80%**
  ◦Ductular epithelial cell–85%
  ◦Acinar cell–15%
•**Anaplastic cancer–5%**

DIAGNOSIS

General
  •Neoplastic cytokines→
    ◦Anorexia→
      −Cachexia
    ◦Chills
    ◦Fatigue
    ◦Fever↑
    ◦Headache
    ◦Malaise
    ◦Night sweats
    ◦Weakness

†Temperature may be normal in patients w/:
•Chronic kidney disease, esp. w/ uremia
•Cirrhosis
•Heart failure
•Severe debility
...or those who are:
  •Intravenous drug users
  •Taking certain medications:
    ○Acetaminophen
    ○Antibiotics
    ○Glucocorticoids
    ○Nonsteroidal anti–inflammatory drugs–NSAIDs

Cardiovascular
•Pancreatic body or tail cancers→
  ○Compression ± infiltration of the splenic artery &/or vein ± splenic artery bruit
•Neoplastic cytokines→
  ○Arterial &/or venous thrombosis ± emboli, termed **Trousseau's syndrome–10%**
Gastrointestinal
•**Continuous abdominal pain–90%**, being epigastric &/or periumbilical ± **radiation to the back,**
usually described as "knifelike" or "boring", being relieved by ↓peritoneal stretching, accomplished by
sitting, leaning forward, & or hip flexion
•**Pancreatic head cancer–70%**→compression ± infiltration of the common bile duct→
  ○↓Intestinal bile flow→
    −↓Stool bile→↓stool bilirubin→**light colored/ pale stool, termed acholic stool**
  ○↓Intestinal bile &/or pancreatic lipase flow→↓fat absorption→↑stool fat, termed steatorrhea→
    −Cachexia
    −Diarrhea
    −Floating stools
    −Oily residue on toilet after flushing
    −Vitamins A, D, E, & K malabsorption
  ○↑Bile accumulation in the gallbladder→
    −Gallbladder distention→palpable gallbladder, which if present w/ jaundice, is termed
    Courvoisier's sign†
Mucocutaneous
•**Pancreatic head cancer–70%**→compression ± infiltration of the common bile duct→
cholestasis→↑plasma bilirubin→generalized tissue deposition→congestive hepatitis→↑plasma
bilirubin→subcutaneous deposition→
  ○Yellow staining of tissues @ >3mg/ dL
    −Skin→**jaundice–65%**
    −Sclera→**scleral icterus**
    −Mucus membranes
  ○Pruritis
Hematologic
•↑Amylase &/or lipase–25%
•Neoplastic cytokines:
  ○α–fetoprotein–AFP 23% secretion (normal: 0–20ng/ mL), also being produced by:
    −Other malignancies, esp. colorectal, gastric, hepatocellular, & pancreatic cancers
    −Liver disease (hepatitis, cirrhosis)
    −Certain fetal tissues
  ○**CA 19–9** secretion
  ○Carcinoembryonic antigen–CEA 90% secretion (>2 5ng/ mL)
•Common bile duct obstruction→
  ○Congestive hepatitis→↑liver function tests, w/ the average bilirubin level being 18mg/ mL

---

†Courvoisier's law: If the gallbladder is palpable in the setting of painless jaundice, the etiology will not
be cholelithiasis

IMAGING
•**Abdominal & pelvic computed tomographic–CT scan**
  Findings:
    •Pancreatic tumor ± peri–organ compression &/or infiltration
  Pancreatic cancer location:
    •**Head–70%**
    •Body–20%
    •Tail–10%

•Computed tomographic–CT scan guided percutaneous tumor biopsy

METASTATIC SEARCH
•Cells usually metastasize to the **regional lymph nodes, liver, lungs, bone, & peritoneum**

•Possible metastases are assessed via:
  ∘History & physical examination
    –Left anterior axillary lymphatic metastases, termed **Irish's node**
    –Left supraclavicular &/or rarely, retrosternal notch lymphatic metastases, termed **Virchow's node=**
      sentinel node
    –Paraumbilical lymphatic metastases→**Sister Mary Joseph's node**, being palpable through the
      navel
    –Rectal lymphatic metastases→**rectal shelf of Blumer**, being palpable via rectal exam
    –Ovarian metastases→**Krukenberg's tumor**
  ∘Hematologic studies
  ∘Imaging
    –**Thoraco–abdomino–pelvic imaging via CT/ MRI** to look for a nodule, mass, infiltrate,
      lymphadenopathy, atelectasis, pleural effusion, pericardial effusion, &/or osteolytic lesions
      Limitations:
        •Does not reliably visualize the splenic, hepatic, para–aortic, or external iliac lymph nodes
    –**Positron emission tomographic–PET scanning**
      Indications:
        •As the computed tomographic–CT scan may remain abnormal long after treatment, a PET
          scan may help w/ both pre–treatment staging & monitoring treatment response
      Mechanism:
        •Intravenous radiolabeled glucose is utilized by malignant cells (as well as cells within an
          inflammatory focus) > normal cells, due to ↑metabolism→
          ∘↑Relative uptake→
            –↑Relative visualization
    –**Radionuclide whole body bone scanning**
      Indications, being either:
        •↑Plasma alkaline phosphatase
        •Hypercalcemia
      Procedure:
        •A radioactive agent, termed a tracer, is injected intravenously→
          ∘Detection of ↑osteoblast activity, indicating new bone formation (as occurs w/ metastases to
            the bone)
      Agents used:
        •[99m]technitium–Tc based agent (99mTc–sestamibi, 99mTc–teboroxime, 99mTc–tetrofosmin)

TREATMENT
•**Curative intent: Cancer limited to the pancreas–10%†**
  ∘Surgical resection via **pancreatico–duodenectomy=Whipple's procedure**
    Procedure:
      •Partial or complete resection of the pancreas, as well as resection of the:
        ∘Gastric antrum
        ∘Duodenum
        ∘Proximal jejunum
        ∘Gallbladder
        ∘Distal common bile duct
    Outcomes:
      •20% mortality
      •5 year survival: 5%

•**Palliative intent: Metastasized cancer–90%**
  ∘Chemotherapy &/or radiation therapy
  ∘Silastic tube vs. metal stent placement for obstructive lesions via:
    –Gastrointestinal endoscopy for intestinal stenosis
    –Endoscopic retrograde cholangiopancreatography–ERCP for biliary or pancreatic ductal stenosis
      Outcomes:
        •Pancreatic ductal stricture is visualized in 85% of patients

Side effects:
- •Cholangitis <1%
- •Hemorrhage if sphincterectomy is performed
- •Pancreatitis−1%
- •Peritonitis
- •Death−rare

Contraindications:
- •Pregnancy, due to ionizing radiation
- ∘Pancreatic enzymes for malabsorption
- ∘Narcotics ± neurolytic celiac plexus block w/ lidocaine & alcohol for pain relief
- ∘Consider surgical resection for painful &/or obstructive lesions
- ∘Bisphosphonates→
  - −↓Pathologic fracture risk
- ∘Surgery for pathologic fractures
- ∘Drainage of pleural effusions, w/ subsequent pleurodesis via sclerosing agents (sterile Bleomycin, Doxycycline, Mitoxantrone, Tetracycline, or talc slurry) to prevent reaccumulation

†Head >> body or tail, as pancreatic head cancer is diagnosed earlier due to obstructive syndromes

PROGNOSIS

- •Average survival: 6 months
- •5 year survival: 5%

TESTICULAR CANCER

•Caused by the malignant transformation of a testicular cell (hyperplasia→atypia→cancer)→
  ○Infiltration of tissue ± spread through lymphatics & blood vessels to other organs=metastases
Statistics:
•1% of ♂ cancers
•**The #1 malignancy in ♂ age 20–35years**

RISK FACTORS

•**Age:** 20–40years, w/ a secondary peak incidence @ age >60years
•**Skin color:** Whites 4X blacks
•**Environment**
  ○↑Socioeconomic class
•**History of cryptorchidism–10%**
  ○Undescended testes (intra–abdominal 4X intra–inguinal)→
    –↑Bilateral cancer risk†, even if only 1 testicle was undescended
•**Genetic**
  ○Prior unilateral testicular cancer
  ○Down's syndrome=Trisomy 21
  ○Klinefelter's syndrome (47XXY)

---

†Correction via surgical scrotal placement, termed orchiopexy, does not alter the malignant potential

CLASSIFICATION

•**Germ cell neoplasia–95%**, occurring **predominantly in adults**, except yolk sac neoplasia, which usually occurs during childhood
  ○**Seminoma–33%**
  ○**Non–seminoma**
    –Mixed cell type–40% (may contain seminoma as well)
    –Embryonal cell cancer–20%
    –Teratocarcinoma–5%
    –Choriocarcinoma–1%
    –Yolk sac cancer=endodermal sinus tumor–1%

•**Non–germ cell neoplasia–5%** (only 10% being malignant), occurring **predominantly during childhood**, except sertoli cell neoplasia, which usually occurs during infancy
  ○Leydig cell neoplasia
  ○Sertoli cell neoplasia
  ○Testicular stromal cell neoplasia

DIAGNOSIS

Genitourinary
•Testicular mass, usually being:
  ○**Painless**, w/ acute pain–10% being due to intratesticular hemorrhage
  ○**Solid**, preventing transillumination when a flashlight is placed against the posterior scrotal wall
•A contralateral tumor is found in 5% of affected patients

Germ cell specific:
Subcutaneous
•β–human chorionic gonadotropin–βhCG secretion, being composed of α & β subunits, w/ hCGα being identical to the α subunit of leutinizing hormone–LH→
  ○interstitial cells of Leydig cell estradiol secretion→
    –Gynecomastia–5%
Hematologic
•Neoplastic cytokines:
  ○β–**human chorionic gonadotropin–βHCG** secretion, also being produced by:
    –Other malignancies, esp. colorectal, gastric, liver, lung, & pancreatic cancers
    –Marijuana use
    …w/ non–seminomas (except choriocarcinomas) also→
      •α–**feto protein–AFP** secretion (normal: 0–15ng/ mL), also being produced by:
        ○Other malignancies, esp. colorectal, gastric, hepatocellular, & pancreatic cancers
        ○Liver disease (hepatitis, cirrhosis)
        ○Certain fetal tissues

---

†May be used to monitor for treatment response, & possible recurrence, if elevated @ initial diagnosis

•Scrotal ultrasound
Indications:
•To distinguish between:
◦An intratesticular mass (likely being malignant) from an extra-testicular mass (likely being benign)
◦A solid mass (likely being malignant) from a cystic mass (likely being benign)
Differential diagnosis of findings:
•Intratesticular mass
◦Solid: **Cancer**, granuloma, gumma, orchitis
◦Cystic: Hydrocele
•Extratesticular mass
◦Solid: Epididymitis &/or orchitis†
◦Cystic: Epididymal cyst

---

†Epididymo-orchitis may→
•Obliteration of the normal plane between the testicle & epididymis→
◦A solid mass

•Orchiectomy
Indications:
•All intratesticular solid masses, for histologic diagnosis

•Symptomatic metastatic disease is found in 10% of patients @ presentation, w/ cells usually metastasizing to the **retroperitoneal lymph nodes & lungs**

•Possible metastases are assessed via:
◦History & physical examination
◦Hematologic studies
◦Imaging
–**Thoraco-abdomino-pelvic imaging via CT/ MRI** to look for a nodule, mass, infiltrate, lymphadenopathy, atelectasis, pleural effusion, pericardial effusion, &/or osteolytic lesions
Limitations:
•Does not reliably visualize the splenic, hepatic, para-aortic, or external iliac lymph nodes
–**Positron emission tomographic–PET scanning**
Indications:
•As the computed tomographic–CT scan may remain abnormal long after treatment, a PET scan may help w/ both pre-treatment staging & monitoring treatment response
Mechanism:
•Intravenous radiolabeled glucose is utilized by malignant cells (as well as cells within an inflammatory focus) > normal cells, due to ↑metabolism→
◦↑Relative uptake→
–↑Relative visualization
–**Radionuclide whole body bone scanning**
Indications, being either:
•↑Plasma alkaline phosphatase
•Hypercalcemia
Procedure:
•A radioactive agent, termed a tracer, is injected intravenously→
◦Detection of ↑osteoblast activity, indicating new bone formation (as occurs w/ metastases to the bone)
Agents used:
•[99m]technitium–Tc based agent (99mTc–sestamibi, 99mTc–teboroxime, 99mTc–tetrofosmin)

SIMPLIFIED GERM CELL NEOPLASIA STAGING			
Stage	Description	% @ presentation	5year survival†
1	•Confined to the testis ± spermatic cord‡	40%	≥95%
2	•Retroperitoneal lymph node metastases	40%	
A	◦Largest being <6cm in diameter		≥95%
B	◦Largest being ≥6cm in diameter		70%
3	•Metastatic disease outside the retroperitoneal lymph nodes	20%	70%

†Overall 5year survival rate of 96%
‡Most patients w/ stage 1 disease have microscopic retroperitoneal lymph node metastases

538

- **Germ cell neoplasia**
  - **Seminoma**
    - Stage 1–2A: Radiation therapy
    - Stage 2B–3: Cisplatin based combination chemotherapy w/ Bleomycin & Etoposide
  - **Non-seminoma**
    - Stage 1: Modified template or nerve sparing retroperitoneal lymphadenectomy–RPLND†. If microscopic metastatic disease is found, treat as 2A
    - Stage 2A: Modified template or nerve sparing retroperitoneal lymphadenectomy–RPLND† & Cisplatin based chemotherapy w/ Bleomycin & Etoposide
    - Stage 2B–3: Cisplatin based chemotherapy w/ Bleomycin & Etoposide, as well as residual mass resection via retroperitoneal lymphadenectomy–RPLND if needed

---

†Sparing the T10–L2 sympathetic ganglia→
- Preserved antegrade ejaculation

- Patients are considered cured if disease free @ 2years after remission
- **Physical examination, chest x ray & plasma markers**, if initially elevated, qmonth X 1year, then
  - Q2months X 1year

- Relapsed disease may respond to Cisplatin based chemotherapy, if not administered when originally diagnosed. If the patient has undergone retroperitoneal lymphadenectomy–RPLND, relapsed disease is likely to involve the lungs

RENAL CELL CANCER

•Caused by the malignant transformation of a renal tubular epithelial cell (hyperplasia→atypia→cancer)→
  ◦Infiltration of tissue ± spread through lymphatics & blood vessels to other organs=metastases
Statistics:
  •Comprise 85% of primary renal malignancies, w/ renal pelvic cancer–10% & sarcoma–5% accounting for the remainder

RISK FACTORS

•**Age:** 40–60years
•**Gender:** ♂ 2X ♀
•**Smoking**
  ◦Cigar, cigarette, &/or pipe (active & passive="secondhand")
•**Obesity**
•**Acquired renal cystic disease→**
  ◦Chronic renal failure
•**Exposure**
  ◦Asbestos
  ◦Cadmium
  ◦Leather tanning products
  ◦Petroleum products
•**Hypertension**
•**Genetic†**
  ◦Autosomal dominant polycystic kidney disease
  ◦Chromosome 3p abnormalities, being the location of the von Hippel–Lindau gene
    –Found in 90% of nonhereditary forms of renal cell cancer & those occurring in patients w/ von Hippel–Lindau disease
  ◦Von Hippel–Lindau disease (autosomal dominant inheritance)→
    –Central nervous system hemangioblastomas
    –Endolymphatic sac tumors
    –Epididymal, hepatic, pancreatic, & renal cysts
    –Epididymal papillary cystadenomas
    –Hepatic, renal, & retinal angiomas
    –Pheochromocytomas
    –Renal cell cancer
  ◦Horseshoe kidney

---

†2% of renal cell cancers are associated w/ hereditary syndromes

CLASSIFICATION

Histologic classification:
  •Proximal tubular epithelial cell→
    ◦**Clear cell–78%**
    ◦Chromophilic–13%
  •Cortical collecting duct intercalated cell→
    ◦Chromophobic–5%
    ◦Oncocytic–3%
  •Medullary collecting duct epithelial cell→
    ◦Collecting duct–1%

DIAGNOSIS

General
  •Neoplastic cytokines→
    ◦Anorexia→
      –Cachexia
    ◦Chills
    ◦Fatigue, also being due to possible anemia
    ◦Fever†
    ◦Headache
    ◦Malaise
    ◦Night sweats
    ◦Weakness

---

†Temperature may be normal in patients w/:
  •Chronic kidney disease, esp. w/ uremia
  •Cirrhosis

540

- •Heart failure
- •Severe debility
- ...or those who are:
  - •Intravenous drug users
  - •Taking certain medications:
    - ◦Acetaminophen
    - ◦Antibiotics
    - ◦Glucocorticoids
    - ◦Nonsteroidal anti−inflammatory drugs−NSAIDs

Genitourinary
- •Renal capsule distention ± infiltration→
  - ◦**Flank pain**
  - ◦**Palpable abdominal mass**
- •Collecting system infiltration→
  - ◦**Hematuria−60%**

Cardiovascular
- •Tumor mediated renal ischemia→
  - ◦Compensatory ↑renin production→
    - −Hypertension
- •Inferior vena cava compression &/or infiltration→
  - ◦↑Distal hydrostatic pressure→
    - −Bilateral lower extremity edema
    - −Hemorrhoids
    - −Spermatic venous congestion→bilateral varicocele, which do not reduce when the patient is supine
    - −Vertical abdominal varices w/ upward blood flow as a compensatory mechanism to circumvent the obstruction
- •Left renal vein infiltration→
  - ◦Spermatic venous congestion→
    - −Left varicocele which does not reduce when the patient is supine
- •Vascular compression &/or infiltration→
  - ◦Thrombus formation ± embolus

Gastrointestinal
- •Neoplastic cytokines→
  - ◦Reversible hepatic dysfunction, termed Stauffer's syndrome

Hematologic
- •Parenchymal destruction→
  - ◦↓Erythropoietin production→
    - −Normocytic−normochromic anemia
- •Neoplastic cytokines:
  - ◦Erythropoietin secretion→
    - −Polycythemia−5%
  - ◦Parathyroid hormone related peptide−PTHrP secretion→
    - −Hypercalcemia−10%

IMAGING
- •**Abdominal computed tomographic−CT scan**
  - Findings:
    - •A solid, hypodense renal mass which enhances w/ the administration of intravenous contrast dye
  - Renal mass characteristics suggestive of malignancy:
    - •Any solid component
    - •Loculations
    - •Wall thickness >3mm

METASTATIC SEARCH
- •Cells usually metastasize to the **regional lymph nodes, lungs > bone > adrenal glands, liver, skin, central nervous system**

- •Possible metastases are assessed via:
  - ◦History & physical examination
  - ◦Hematologic studies
  - ◦Imaging
    - −**Thoraco−abdomino−pelvic imaging via CT/ MRI** to look for a nodule, mass, infiltrate, lymphadenopathy, atelectasis, pleural effusion, pericardial effusion, &/or osteolytic lesions
      - Limitations:
        - •Does not reliably visualize the splenic, hepatic, para−aortic, or external iliac lymph nodes

541

-Positron emission tomographic-PET scanning
Indications:
- •As the computed tomographic-CT scan may remain abnormal long after treatment, a PET scan may help w/ both pre-treatment staging & monitoring treatment response
Mechanism:
- •Intravenous radiolabeled glucose is utilized by malignant cells (as well as cells within an inflammatory focus) > normal cells, due to ↑metabolism→
  - ∘↑Relative uptake→
    - -↑Relative visualization

-Radionuclide whole body bone scanning
Indications, being either:
- •↑Plasma alkaline phosphatase
- •Hypercalcemia
Procedure:
- •A radioactive agent, termed a tracer, is injected intravenously→
  - ∘Detection of ↑osteoblast activity, indicating new bone formation (as occurs w/ metastases to the bone)
Agents used:
- •^{99m}technitium-Tc based agent (99mTc-sestamibi, 99mTc-teboroxime, 99mTc-tetrofosmin)

ROBSON STAGING SYSTEM			
Stage	Description	% @ presentation	5year survival
1	•Tumor confined to the kidney		80%
2	•Infiltration of the perinephric fat		60%
3A	•Infiltration of the renal vein or inferior vena cava		35-60%
B	•Regional lymph node metastases	20%	15-30%
4	•Infiltration beyond Gerota's fascia, or distant metastasis	40%	5%

TREATMENT

•**Curative intent: Stages 1-2**
∘**Surgical resection via radical† (preferred) or partial nephrectomy**
Indications for partial nephrectomy:
- •Bilateral renal cell cancer
- •Renal cell cancer in a sole functioning kidney
- •Severe renal failure

•**Survival prolongation intent: Stages 3-4**
∘Chemotherapy &/or immunotherapy, as surgery does not prolong survival
- -Floxuridine or Vinblastine→tumor regression in 15% & 10% of patients respectively
- -Being that malignant cells are antigenic, interferon-α or recombinant human interleukin-2→ tumor regression in 13% of patients, w/ an additional 7% of patients having complete regression to recombinant human interleukin-2

•**Palliative intent: Treatment failure or disease relapse**
∘Chemotherapy &/or immunotherapy
∘Silastic tube stent placement for esophagotracheal/ bronchial fistulas
∘Consider surgical resection for painful &/or obstructive lesions
∘Bisphosphonates→↓pathologic fracture risk
∘Surgery for pathologic fractures
∘Drainage of pleural effusions, w/ subsequent pleurodesis via sclerosing agents (sterile bleomycin, doxycycline, mitoxantrone, tetracycline, or talc slurry) to prevent reaccumulation

---

†Radical nephrectomy involves the removal of the kidney, adrenal gland, regional lymph nodes, surrounding perinephric fat, & Gerota's fascia

PROGNOSIS
•35% of patients who undergo curative intent treatment will have a recurrence

THYROID CANCER

•Caused by the malignant transformation of a thyroid cell (hyperplasia→atypia→cancer)→
  ∘Infiltration of tissue ± spread through lymphatics &/or blood vessels to other organs=metastases
Statistics:
  •Malignancy comprises 5% of thyroid neoplasia

RISK FACTORS

•**Neck irradiation**, esp. during childhood
•**Genetic**
  ∘Family history of multiple endocrine neoplasia–MEN 2:
    –Medullary thyroid cancer
    –Hyperparathyroidism
    –Pheochromocytoma
  ∘Family history of multiple endocrine neoplasia–MEN 3:
    –Medullary thyroid cancer
    –Pheochromocytoma
    –Mucosal neuromas
    –Marfanoid habitus

CLASSIFICATION

•Papillary thyroid cancer–75%
•Follicular thyroid cancer–18%
•Medullary thyroid cancer–2%
•Anaplastic thyroid cancer–5%
•Thyroid lymphoma

DIAGNOSIS

Endocrine
  •Usually presenting as discrete nodules, rather than diffuse infiltration
Hematologic
  •Hyperthyroidism (adenoma >> cancer)
  •Diffuse thyroid infiltration→
    ∘Hypothyrodism
  •Medullary thyroid cancer→
    ∘Calcitonin production

Thoracic compressive &/or infiltrative syndromes:
  •**@ Esophagus→**
    ∘Obstruction→
      –Difficulty swallowing=dysphagia
      –Inflammation=esophagitis→painful swallowing=odynophagia
  •**@ Recurrent laryngeal nerve→**
    ∘Hoarseness
  •**@ Superior vena cava→**
    ∘Obstruction→↑proximal hydrostatic pressure→
      –Dilation of bilateral arm, neck, & head vasculature→facial erythema, edema, &/or bluish
        color=cyanosis
      –↑Collateral blood flow→dilated abdominal collateral vessels w/ downward flow
      Note: Considered a medical emergency if the patient develops altered mental status
  •**@ Tracheobronchial tree→**
    ∘Cough ± hemoptysis
    ∘Wheezing
    ∘↓Mucous clearance distal to the obstruction→
      –Post-obstructive pneumonia

IMAGING

•**Radioactive iodine (I^{123}) uptake–RAIU scan**
  Mechanism:
    •Thyrotrope radioactive iodine uptake→
      ∘Thyroid irradiation, allowing visualization
  Findings:
    •**Diffusely ↑thyroid uptake** via either:
      ∘**Graves' disease**
      ∘β–human chorionic gonadotropin–βhCG secreting neoplasm
      ∘Thyroid stimulating hormone–TSH secreting neoplasm
      ∘Anterior pituitary thyroid hormone resistance

- **Focal or multifocal ↑thyroid uptake** via:
  - ○Thyroid neoplasia (adenoma >> adenocarcinoma)
- **No thyroid uptake** via:
  - ○Thyroiditis
  - ○Iodine containing medication induced
  - ○Thyrotoxicosis medicamentosa
- **Ectopic uptake** via either:
  - ○Struma ovarii
  - ○Thyroid cancer metastasis

Outcomes:
- Being as it is normal in up to 50% of hyperthyroid patients, a normal test does not exclude hyperthyroidism

INVASIVE PROCEDURES

- **Fine needle aspiration–FNA**

Indications:
- Radioactive iodine (I^{123}) uptake–RAIU scan showing either:
  - ○↓Area tracer uptake
  - ○Ectopic iodine uptake
- Syndrome suggestive of cancer

Neoplastic findings:
- **Benign–75%**
  - ○Observation
- **Malignant–5%**
  - ○Total thyroidectomy, w/ lifelong thyroid hormone replacement in order to both:
    - –Prevent hypothyroidism
    - –Suppress thyroid stimulating hormone–TSH secretion→↓recurrence risk
- **Indeterminate–20%** (20% of which are malignant):
  - ○Total thyroidectomy if having ↓area tracer uptake

TREATMENT

- **Total thyroidectomy†**

Side effects:
- **Immediate onset hypothyroidism**, unless metastatic disease is present
- Hypoparathyroidism
- Recurrent laryngeal nerve paralysis→
  - ○Hoarseness

- **Post–surgical radioactive iodine (I^{131}) ablation therapy**

Mechanism:
- Thyrotrope radioactive iodine uptake→
  - ○Thyroid irradiation→
    - –Cellular death, inflammation, & fibrosis

---

†Iodine is given to patients prior to thyroidectomy→
- ↓Thyroid gland size & vascularity→
  - ○↓Surgical complications

MELANOMA

•Caused by the **malignant transformation of a skin melanocyte**, usually located in the basal layer of the epidermis (hyperplasia→atypia→melanoma)→
  ◦Infiltration of tissue ± spread through lymphatics & blood vessels to other organs=metastases
Statistics:
  •5% of skin cancers→
    ◦#1 cause of skin cancer related mortality
  •3% of cancers→
    ◦#6 cause of ♂cancer, #7 cause of ♀cancer

RISK FACTORS

•**Gender:** ♀ 1.5 X ♂
•**Benign melanocyte neoplasms**
  ◦Freckles
  ◦Moles=nevi
    −30% of malignant melanomas develop from previously existing moles, w/ the remainder developing from normal skin
•**Ultraviolet light (UVA & UVB)**
  ◦Extensive sun exposure, esp. during adolescence & young adulthood
  ◦History of severe or frequent sunburns
  ◦Living close to the equator
Mechanism:
  •UVA†→
    ◦Deep dermal penetration→
      −Connective tissue damage→wrinkles & leathery textured skin
  •UVB→
    ◦Melanocyte stimulation→
      −↑Melanin production, w/ excessive exposure→sunburn
•↓**Ultraviolet light defenses**
  ◦Difficulty tanning
  ◦↓Pigmentation
    −Fair skin (white >> black)
    −Light colored hair
    −Blue eyes
•**Immunosuppression**
  ◦Advanced age
  ◦Alcoholism
  ◦Diabetes mellitus
  ◦Hematologic malignancy
  ◦HIV infection/ AIDS
  ◦Malnutrition
  ◦Medications
    −Chemotherapy
    −Chronic glucocorticoid use
    −Immunomodulating medications
  ◦Renal dialysis
•**Genetic**
  ◦Personal or family history of any skin cancer
  ◦Xeroderma pigmentosa: Autosomal recessive disease→
    −Defective DNA repair

---

†Lights used in tanning beds & sun lamps emit mainly UVA radiation→
  •↓Sunburn, but continued skin cancer risk

CLASSIFICATION

•**Superficial spreading–70%**
  ◦**Found anywhere**, often the upper back or lower legs, w/ a usual age of 40−50years
•**Nodular–15%†**
  ◦**Found anywhere**
•**Lentigo maligna–5%**
  ◦**Found in sun exposed areas**, w/ a usual age of 50−70years
•**Acral lentiginous melanoma <5%‡**
  ◦Found in the palms, soles, subungual°, & mucus membranes (vulva > anus, pharynx, sinuses)

†**Nodular melanoma's** growth is predominantly vertical→
•Early malignant potential, w/ usual lack of the typical ABCD signs (see below). The other forms have predominantly horizontal growth
‡**Acral lentiginous melanoma** usually occurs in blacks & Asians
°Pigment extension from the nail bed to the skin is referred to as Hutchinson's sign

DIAGNOSIS

Cutaneous
•Skin lesion (macule, papule, or nodule), esp. one newly formed in an adult, usually being pigmented†, w/ colors representing combinations of blacks, blues, browns, reds &/or whites ± hemorrhage, crusting, paresthesia, &/or pruritus

The ABCDE'S of suspicious lesions termed atypical moles:
•**Asymmetry**
•**Border irregularity**
•**Color variation**, representing different depths of melanocyte invasion, w/ inflammation & immunologic response
•**Diameter >6mm**
•**Elevation above the skin surface**
•**Size &/or shape change**

---

†Rarely, a melanoma may be **amelanotic**, indicating a lack of dark pigmentation→
•Predominance of reds & whites

INVASIVE PROCEDURES

•**Excisional biopsy**
Indications:
•To allow for:
  ○Determination of invasion depth
  ○Possible removal
Findings:
•Melanocytes w/ marked cellular atypia via:
  ○Hyperchromatic nuclei w/ prominent nucleoli
  ○Vacuolated cytoplasm in various morphologic forms=polymorphism
  ...± dermal invasion

METASTATIC SEARCH

•Cells usually metastasize to the **regional lymph nodes, central nervous system, liver, lungs > bone pleura**

•Possible metastases are assessed via:
  ○History & physical examination
  ○Hematologic studies
  ○Imaging
    −**Thoraco−abdomino−pelvic imaging via CT/ MRI** to look for a nodule, mass, infiltrate, lymphadenopathy, atelectasis, pleural effusion, pericardial effusion, &/or osteolytic lesions
    Limitations:
      •Does not reliably visualize the splenic, hepatic, para−aortic, or external iliac lymph nodes
    −**Positron emission tomographic−PET scanning**
    Indications:
      •As the computed tomographic−CT scan may remain abnormal long after treatment, a PET scan may help w/ both pre−treatment staging & monitoring treatment response
    Mechanism:
      •Intravenous radiolabeled glucose is utilized by malignant cells (as well as cells within an inflammatory focus) > normal cells, due to ↑metabolism→
        ○↑Relative uptake→
          −↑Relative visualization
    −**Radionuclide whole body bone scanning**
    Indications, being either:
      •↑Plasma alkaline phosphatase
      •Hypercalcemia
    Procedure:
      •A radioactive agent, termed a tracer, is injected intravenously→
        ○Detection of ↑osteoblast activity, indicating new bone formation (as occurs w/ metastases to the bone)
    Agents used:
      •^{99m}technitium−Tc based agent (99mTc−sestamibi, 99mTc−teboroxime, 99mTc−tetrofosmin)

546

∘Invasive procedures
  −Regional lymph node dissection or
  −Sentinal lymph node biopsy
    Procedure:
    •Injection of either a dye or radiolabeled substance into the biopsy cavity &/or around the tumor→
      ∘Substance traveling via lymphatics to the closest draining=sentinel lymph node(s), allowing for biopsy of less lymph nodes for staging→
        −↓Complication risk

MELANOMA STAGING SYSTEMS

Stage	Description				
1	Tumor limited to the skin ± subcutaneous tissue, being further categorized via **invasion depth**, being the #1 prognostic factor				
	Breslow thickness	**Clark level**	**Distal location**	**5year survival**	**%Metastases**
	In situ	I	Epidermis	98%	Extremely rare
	<0.76mm	II	Papillary dermis	98%	2.5%
	0.76–1.5mm	III	Deep papillary dermis	90%	20%
	1.51–4mm	IV	Reticular dermis	72%	40%
	>4mm	V	Subcutaneous tissue	<50%	70%
2	**Regional lymph node metastases**			<30%	
3	**Distant metastases**, indicating a median survival of 6 months				

TREATMENT

•**Curative intent: Stages 1–2**
  ∘**Re–excision**
    Indications:
    •Appropriate cancer free margins, if not obtained via excisional biopsy
      ∘**In situ** requiring 0.5cm margins
      ∘**Invasive** requiring 2–3cm margins
        −There is no evidence that excising margins >3cm affects mortality
      ∘**Subungual lesions** requiring amputation of either the:
        −Distal interphalangeal–DIP joint for finger primaries
        −Interphalangeal joint for thumb primaries

CYTOKINES

Indications:
  •Stage 1, Breslow thickness >1.5mm
  •Stage 2

Generic	M	♀	Dose
Interferon–α–2b	K	?	20million units/ m² IV q24hours 5days/ week X 1month, then 10million units SC 3X/ week X 11months

Mechanism:
  •Induces the synthesis of cell encoded enzymes→
    ∘Selective inhibition of viral messenger RNA translation to protein, without affecting the translation of cellular messenger RNA

Side effects:
  General
    •Anorexia
    •Erythema at the injection site
    •Headache
    •**Influenze–like syndrome** (fatigue, fever, chills, myalgia) beginning 6–8hours after administration, & lasting ≤12hours
      ∘Administer w/ antipyretic at bedtime in order to attempt to avoid this syndrome
  Cardiovascular
    •Dilated cardiomyopathy
  Endocrine
    •Diabetes mellitus
  Gastrointestinal
    •Diarrhea
  Opthalmologic
    •Optic neuritis
    •Retinopathy

Neurologic
- •Amotivation
- •Alopecia
- •Altered taste=dysguesia
- •↓Concentration
- •Depression
- •Impaired hearing
- •Insomnia
- •Irritability
- •↓Libido, being sexual desire→
  - −Impotence, being the inability to achieve &/or maintain an erection
- •Paranoia
- •Polyneuropathy
- •Seizure
- •Suicidal ideation

Hematologic
- •Autoantibody induction
- •**Leukopenia→**
  - ∘↑Infection &/or neoplasm risk
- •**Thrombocytopenia→**
  - ∘↑Hemorrhage risk, esp. petechiae

Absolute contraindications:
Cardiovascular
- •Symptomatic cardiac disease

Gastrointestinal
- •Decompensated cirrhosis

Neurologic
- •Uncontrolled seizure disease

Psychiatric
- •Current severe major depression
- •History of psychosis

Hematologic
- •Neutropenia
- •Thrombocytopenia

Other
- •Organ transplantation (other than liver)

Relative contraindications:
Rheumatologic
- •Autoimmune disease

Endocrine
- •Uncontrolled diabetes mellitus

•**Palliative intent: Stage 3**
  Note: Patients w/ 1 metastatic lesion may benefit from surgical resection. Otherwise, palliative
        treatment via the following:
  - ∘Chemotherapy
  - ∘Silastic tube stent placement for esophagotracheal/ bronchial fistulas
  - ∘Consider radiation therapy &/or surgical resection for painful &/or obstructive lesions
  - ∘Bisphosphonates→↓pathologic fracture risk
  - ∘Surgery for pathologic fractures
  - ∘Drainage of pleural effusions, w/ subsequent pleurodesis via sclerosing agents (sterile bleomycin,
    doxycycline, mitoxantrone, tetracycline, or talc slurry) to prevent reaccumulation

PREVENTION

•**Avoidance of sun exposure**
  - ∘When exposed, use:
    - −UVA & UVB sunscreen, w/ a sun protection factor–SPF ≥15†
    - −Wide brim hat to shade your face, ears, & neck
    - −Long sleeved shirt & pants
•**Excisional biopsy of all changing or atypical moles**

---

†The sun protection factor–SPF number indicates the relative length of time skin can be exposed to
UVB rays w/ little sunburn risk. Protection time is calculated as (SPF#) X (usual exposure time causing
burn). However, sweating & water→
  •↓Protection time, necessitating more frequent applications

548

TUMOR LYSIS SYNDROME

•Rapid cell death→
  ◦Rapid release of intracellular contents→
    –Electrolyte abnormalities
    –Acute renal failure

RISK FACTORS

•**Rapidly proliferating** malignancy, esp.:
  ◦Acute leukemias
  ◦Aggressive non–Hodgkin's lymphomas
  ◦Myeloma
•**Chemotherapy** of either:
  ◦Rapidly proliferating malignancies (as above)
  ◦Patients w/ a large tumor burden

DIAGNOSIS

Genitourinary
•↑Uric acid & calcium phosphate→
  ◦Acute tubular necrosis–ATN via both:
    –Direct tubular toxicity
    –Obstructive tubular casts
    …→**acute intra–renal renal failure**
Hematologic
•**Cellular cytoplasm release**, also being due to tissue ischemia ± necrosis→
  ◦**Hyperkalemia**, necessitating a baseline electrocardiogram–ECG in patients w/ the above risk
   factors
  ◦Hyperphosphatemia→
    –Calcium binding→hypocalcemia
  ◦↑Lactate dehydrogenase–LDH
  ◦↑Uric acid (> ~7mg/ dL)→
    –Gout syndrome

TREATMENT

•**Vigorous intravenous hydration** to achieve a urine output of 100–200mL/ h→↑electrolyte & uric acid
excretion, w/ attention to both:
  ◦**Intravascular volume repletion via Normal saline (0.9% NaCl)** or **lactated Ringer's solution**, as
   per:
    –Vital signs
    –Physical examination
    –Urine output (normal being ≥0.5mL/kg/h)
    –Blood urea nitrogen–BUN & creatinine
  ◦**Intravascular volume maintenance via Normal saline (0.9% NaCl)** or **lactated Ringer's solution**
   Adult maintenance fluid:
    •Weight (kg) + 40= #mL/ hour
   Additional febrile requirements:
    •1L/ 24hours for every 1°F >100°F
   Additional:
    •Estimate loss for:
      ◦Diaphoresis
      ◦Diarrhea
      ◦Polyuria
      ◦Tachypnea
…followed by oral rehydration w/ a glucose based electrolyte solution upon both clinical stability &
ability to tolerate PO

•**Urinary alkalinization**
  Mechanism:
    •↑Intravascular volume
    •Urinary alkalinization to a pH >7→
      ◦↑Uric acid (as it is a weak acid) solubility→
        –↓Nephropathy risk
  Caution:
    •Urinary alkalinization→
      ◦↑Xanthine & calcium phosphate precipitation, which may→
        –Crystal formation→tubular toxicity→acute tubular necrosis–ATN→intrarenal renal failure
      …so avoid urinary alkalinization in patients w/ hyperphosphatemia

549

SODIUM BICARBONATE

M ♀	Dose
K ?	75mEq/ 1L of 1/2 normal saline IV, in order to maintain an isoosmolar solution

±

CARBONIC ANHYDRASE INHIBITOR

Generic (Trade)	M ♀	Dose
Acetazolamide (Diamox) LK	?	250mg PO q24–12hours X several days

Mechanism:
- ↓Carbonic anhydrase activity→
  - ↓Renal tubular bicarbonate ion reabsorption→
    - –Bicarbonate diuresis→urinary alkalinization. However, compensatory ↓NaHCO3 renal excretion→a limited bicarbonate diuresis, lasting ≤3 days

Side effects:
Hematologic
- ↓Renal tubular bicarbonate ion reabsorption→
  - ◦Hyperchloremic, non–anion gap metabolic acidemia

PREVENTION OF CHEMOTHERAPY MEDIATED TUMOR LYSIS SYNDROME

- For patients w/ risk factors, hospital admission w/ prophylactic medication is indicated, w/ monitoring of:
  - ◦Blood urea nitrogen–BUN
  - ◦Creatinine
  - ◦Electrolytes
  - ◦Uric acid measurement
  …w/ the following medications started the day prior to chemotherapy
- **Intravenous fluid**, as above

ALLOPURINOL

M ♀	Start	Titrate	Max
K ?	250mg PO q12hours X 1day, then 300mg PO q24hours	To a target uric acid level <6mg/ dL	800mg/ 24hours

†Doses >300mg should be divided

Dose adjustment:
- Adjust according to renal function

Creatinine clearance	Max dose
10–20mL/ min.	200mg/ 24hours
<10mL/ min.	100mg/ 24hours

Mechanism:
- Inhibits xanthine oxidase→
  - ◦↓**Uric acid production**
  - ◦↑Hypoxanthine & xanthine production, which are much more soluble than uric acid, & readily excreted

Side effects:
General
- **May incite a gout attack during treatment initiation or dosage ↑**
  Risk reduction:
  - Concomitant administration of an anti–inflammatory drugs–NSAIDs, until the target uric acid level is reached X ≥6months
Hypersensitivity syndrome†–2% (↑w/ renal failure)
- Dermatitis
- Fever
- Hepatitis
- Renal failure
- Vasculitis
- Eosinophilia
…necessitating discontinuation
  Prognosis:
  - 20% mortality
Interactions:
- ↓Metabolism of Azathioprine, Mercaptopurine, Theophylline, Warfarin→
  - ◦↑Plasma concentration

550

Overdosage:
General
  •Fever
Gastrointestinal
  •Hepatitis
Genitourinary
  •Renal failure

---

†**Allopurinol desensitization**
Indication:
  •Mild hypersensitivity syndrome
Protocol:
  •Start 10μg q24hours, then
    ∘Double the dose q3–14days until the necessary dosage is reached

•Caused by the ascending >95% vs. hematogenous spread of a microorganism to the genitourinary tract→
  ◦Inflammation
•All ascending infections begin by the organism colonizing the perineum→
  ◦Ascension of any of the mucous membrane tracts:
    –Urethra
    –Rectum
    –Vagina
    ...esp. via a foreign body, such as a catheter
•As an organism ascends, it may cause inflammation in all the areas distal to its farthest location
  ◦**Sexually transmitted organisms do not cause infection proximal to the urethra**, rather they infect the:
    –Urethra & peri–urethral structures (prostate, epididymis, &/or testicle)
    –Entire female genital tract
    ...as well as the:
      •Pharynx
      •Rectum
Statistics:
  •Urinary tract infections–UTI's are the #1 bacterial infections worldwide

•**Anatomic classification**
  ◦**Lower tract**
    –Urethritis
    –Periurethral infections: prostatitis &/or epididymitis
    –Cystitis
  ◦**Upper tract**
    –Pyelonephritis
    –Intrarenal or perinephric abscess
    –Ureteritis
  ◦**Vaginitis:** Inflammation of the vagina ± the ectocervix=ectocervicitis
  ◦**Pelvic inflammatory disease–PID:** Infection proximal to the ectocervix:
    –Endocervix=endocervicitis
    –Endometrium=endometritis
    –Fallopian tubes=salpingitis
    –Ovaries=oophoritis
    –Tubo–ovarian abscess
    –Adnexa=parametritis
    –Peritoneum=peritonitis

•**Clinical classification**
  ◦**Uncomplicated urinary tract infections**
    –Cystitis in a non–pregnant ♀ patient w/ a structurally (no congenital or acquired abnormality) & functionally (no neurologic dysfunction) normal urinary tract
  ◦**Complicated urinary tract infections**
    –All other urinary tract infections
  ◦**Asymptomatic bacteriuria**
    –≥1,000 colony forming units–CFU/ mL in the urine of an asymptomatic ♂
    –≥100,000 colony forming units–CFU/ mL in the urine of an asymptomatic ♀

•**Enterobacteriaceal urinary tract infection**
  ◦**Age**
    –<1year: ♂ > ♀, due to the ↑prevalence of ♂ congenital genitourinary abnormalities
    –1–50years: ♀ >> ♂, due to ♀ shorter urethra
    –>50years: ♀ > ♂, w/ ↑♂ risk due to benign prostatic hyperplasia–BPH
  ◦♀ **Gender–# 1 risk factor**
    –**Short urethra**
    –Sexual intercourse, via urethral reverberations
    –Delayed postcoital micturition
    –Use of a diaphragm w/ a spermicide→altered vaginal pH→altered vaginal/ perineal flora
    –↓Estrogen, as during perimenopause & menopause
    –Obstruction via pregnancy or gynecologic abnormalities (ex: leiomyomas)
    –"Non–secretor" Lewis blood group
    –P1 blood group phenotype

∘♂ **Gender**
  -Obstruction via **benign prostatic hyperplasia–BPH** or prostate cancer
  -Lack of circumcision→colonization of the glans & prepuce
  -Insertive anal intercourse
  -Delayed postcoital micturition
  -♀ sexual partner w/ vaginal enterobacteriaceae colonization
∘**Other obstruction**
  -Autonomic neuropathy
  -Nephrolithiasis
  -Posterior urethral valves
  -Strictures
  -Ureterovesicular reflux
  Mechanism:
    •Obstruction of urine flow→
      ∘Inadequate urination→stagnant urine proximal to the obstruction→
        -↑Bacterial growth
        -Hydronephrosis
        ...→urinary tract infection
∘**Urinary tract instrumentation**
  -Urinary catheterization (indwelling catheters > external catheters, intermittent catheterization). All catheters should be replaced q2–3 weeks. Urinary catheter obstruction or infrequent intermittent catheterization→obstruction of urine flow
∘**Immunosuppression**
  -Advanced age
  -Alcoholism
  -Diabetes mellitus
  -Hematologic malignancy
  -HIV infection/ AIDS
  -Malnutrition
  -Medications (chemotherapy, chronic glucocorticoid use, immunomodulating medications)
  -Renal dialysis

•**Candidal sp. genitourinary tract infection**
  ∘Antibiotic use
  ∘Alteration of the vaginal flora via antibiotics or diaphragm w/ a spermicide
  ∘Diabetes mellitus
  ∘Frequent sexual intercourse, esp. fellatio
  ∘Fungemia
  ∘Immunosuppression (as listed above)
  ∘Obesity
  ∘Pregnancy
  ∘Previous candidal vaginitis
  ∘Urinary catheterization (indwelling catheters > external catheters, intermittent catheterization)

•**Bacterial vaginitis via ? organism**
  ∘Alteration of the vaginal flora via antibiotics or diaphragm w/ a spermicide
  ∘Sexual intercourse
  ∘Use of an intrauterine device–IUD

•**Sexually transmitted infections of the genitourinary tract**
  ∘**Pelvic inflammatory disease–PID**
    Additional risk factors:
      •Age <25years–75%
      •Nulliparity–75%
      •Intrauterine device–IUD
      •Prior pelvic inflammatory disease–PID
  ∘**Other**
    -**Proctitis**, via anal intercourse or spread from a colonized perineum
    -**Pharyngitis**, via deep kissing, fellatio, anilingus, or cunilingus, depending on the partner's primary site of infection

553

- **Predominantly enterobacteriaceae**
  - ○Cystitis, ureteritis, & pyelonephritis
    - Organisms:
    - **Enterobacteriaceae**
      - ○**Escherichia coli–80% of all UTI's**
      - ○Enterobacter cloacae
      - ○Klebsiella pneumoniae
      - ○Proteus mirabilis & vulgaris
      - ○Providencia rettgeri
      - ○Pseudomonas aeruginosa, esp. in:
        - –Hospital acquired UTI's
        - –Ill patients
      - ○Serratia marcescens
    - **Enterococcus faecalis
    - **Staphylococcus saprophyticus**, esp. in ♀
    - **Fungi**
    - **Mycobacterium tuberculosis**, via either:
      - ○Progressive primary extrapulmonary disease
      - ○Reactivation of latent disease
      - ...→**sterile pyuria**
    - **Adenovirus**→
      - ○**Hemorrhagic cystitis**

- **Predominantly sexually transmitted organisms**
  - ○Urethritis, prostatitis, & epididymitis
    - Organisms:
    - **Sexually transmitted organisms**
      - ○**Chlamydia trachomatis–#1 sexually transmitted bacterium in developed countries**
      - ○Herpes simplex virus–HSV 2–90% > HSV 1
      - ○Mycoplasma hominis
      - ○Neisseria gonorrhoeae
      - ○Trichomonas vaginalis
      - ○Ureaplasma urealyticum
    - **Enterobacteriaceae**
      - ○**Escherichia coli–80% of all UTI's**
      - ○Enterobacter cloacae
      - ○Klebsiella pneumoniae
      - ○Proteus mirabilis & vulgaris
      - ○Providencia rettgeri
      - ○Pseudomonas aeruginosa, esp. in:
        - –Hospital acquired UTI's
        - –Ill patients
      - ○Serratia marcescens
    - **Enterococcus faecalis

- **Vaginitis**
  - ○Sexually transmitted organisms
    - –Trichomonas vaginalis–25%
    - –Chlamydia trachomatis
    - –Neisseria gonorrhoeae
  - ○**Bacterial vaginosis–40%** via unknown organism
  - ○**Candida sp.–25%**
    - –Candida albicans–90% >> C. glabrata, C. krusei, C. tropicalis, C. pseudotropicalis

- **Pelvic inflammatory disease–PID**
  - ○Sexually transmitted organisms
    - –Chlamydia trachomatis
    - –Mycoplasma hominis
    - –Neisseria gonorrhoeae
    - ...w/ subsequent **superinfection** via both:
      - **Facultative anaerobes**
        - ○Enterobacteriaceae
        - ○Haemophilus sp.
        - ○Streptococcus sp.
        - ○Staphylococcus sp.

554

- **Anaerobes**
  - ∘Bacteroides sp., esp. fragilis
  - ∘Clostridium sp.
  - ∘Peptococcus sp.
  - ∘Peptostreptococcus sp.

- **Proctitis/ pharyngitis**
  - ∘**Sexually transmitted organisms**
    - −Chlamydia trachomatis
    - −Herpes simplex virus−HSV 1 or 2
    - −Neisseria gonorrhoeae
    - −Treponema pallidum

DIAGNOSIS

- •Urethritis, vaginitis, pelvic inflammatory disease−PID, & proctitis are usually asymptomatic
- •Patients w/ an indwelling urinary catheter or neurogenic bladder may lack the syndrome of a lower urinary tract infection

Syndrome of a urinary tract infection:
Genitourinary
- •Burning pain on urination=dysuria
- •Urinary frequency, urgency, &/or hesitancy
- •Foul smelling urine
- •Meatal purulence
- •Urethral pruritus

Hematologic
- •Blood chemistry for possible:
  - ∘Renal failure via:
    - −Bilateral hydronephrosis
    - −Unilateral hydronephrosis if only 1 functional kidney
    - −Septic shock→pre−renal renal failure

Cystitis specific:
Genitourinary
- •Low back &/or **suprapubic pain**

Ureteritis/ pyelonephritis specific:
General
- •Inflammatory cytokines→
  - ∘Anorexia→
    - −Cachexia
  - ∘Chills
  - ∘Fatigue
  - ∘**Fever**
  - ∘Headache
  - ∘Malaise
  - ∘Night sweats
  - ∘Weakness

Gastrointestinal
- •Diarrhea
- •**Nausea ± vomiting**

Genitourinary
- •**Costovertebral angle−CVA tenderness to percussion**

Prostatitis specific:
Genitourinary
- •**Warm, tender, & enlarged prostate via digital rectal examination−DRE**
- •Perianal &/or suprapubic pain

<u>Epididymitis specific:</u>
General
- Inflammatory cytokines→
  - Anorexia→
    - −Cachexia
  - Chills
  - Fatigue
  - **Fever**
  - Headache
  - Malaise
  - Night sweats
  - Weakness

Genitourinary
- **Painful, erythematous, & edematous scrotum**

<u>Vaginitis specific:</u>
Genitourinary
- **Vaginal discharge ± foul odor**, being rare w/ Neisseria gonorrhoeae or Chlamydia trachomatis
- Vulvar & vaginal erythema, edema, &/or pruritus

<u>Pelvic inflammatory disease−PID specific:</u>
General
- Inflammatory cytokines→
  - Anorexia→
    - −Cachexia
  - Chills
  - Fatigue
  - **Fever**
  - Headache
  - Malaise
  - Night sweats
  - Weakness

Gastrointestinal
- **Abdomino−pelvic pain &/or discomfort−95%**, usually being:
  - Bilateral
  - Dull
  - Subacute in onset
  - …± radiation down the legs
- Diarrhea
- Nausea ± vomiting
- Ascension of organisms out of the fallopian tubes→
  - Peritoneal inflammation=**peritonitis**
  - Liver capsule=Glisson's capsule inflammation=**perihepatitis, termed the Fitz−Hugh−Curtis syndrome**→
    - −Right upper quadrant abdominal pain ± radiation to the right shoulder
    - −String−like adhesions from the liver capsule to the visceral peritoneum

Genitourinary
- **Mucopurulent vaginal discharge−55%** &/or hemorrhage−35%, both originating from the external os
- **Pain on vaginal sexual intercourse=dyspareunia**

<u>Proctitis specific:</u>
Gastrointestinal
- **Rectal pain**, esp. on defecation
- Anal erythema, edema, &/or pruritus
- Mucopurulent discharge
- Constipation
- Tenesmus, being a painful contraction of the anal sphincter→
  - Urgent desire to defecate &/or urinate, w/ the resultant passage of little feces or urine respectively

Indications for various physical examinations:
- **Digital rectal examination–DRE:**
  - ∘Possible prostate enlargement via:
    - –Benign prostatic hyperplasia–BPH
    - –Prostatitis
    - –Prostate cancer
  - ∘Rectal pain
- **Prostate massage†**
  - ∘Possible prostatitis
- **Post-void residual–PVR**
  - ∘Possible urethral obstruction or autonomic neuropathy
- **Pelvic examination:**
  - ∘Possible vaginitis‡ or pelvic inflammatory disease–PID°

---

†Performed in order to obtain both a:
- •Prostatic expressate for gram stain & culture
- •Post–prostatic massage urine specimen for gram stain, culture, & ligase/ polymerase chain reaction testing

‡If vaginitis is suspected, obtain a specimen from the lateral vaginal walls

°Often accompanied by:
- •Adnexal tenderness &/or mass
- •**Cervical motion tenderness, termed the chandelier sign**, as manipulation of the cervix→
  - ∘The patient jumping in pain as though to grab a chandelier

URINE STUDIES

URINE ACQUISITION

•Midstream urine collection

Indications:
- •Suspected urinary tract infection

Procedure:
- •Obtained after the patient has cleaned the urethral meatus w/ sterile soapy gauze pads:
  - ∘1 for ♂, w/ foreskin retracted
  - ∘4 for ♀, wiping front to back
  - ...followed by warm water gauze pads, again, 1 for ♂, 4 for ♀

•Initial urine stream or any swab collection

Indications:
- •Suspected sexually transmitted organisms for DNA testing via the ligase/ polymerase chain reaction

•Urethral catheterization vs. suprapubic catheterization–rarely necessary

Indications:
- •Patients unable to provide a urine specimen

Side effects:
- •**Decompression hemorrhagic cystitis**, due to overly rapid urinary bladder decompression (esp. after prolonged expansion) via the rapid removal of >1L of urine

Limitations:
- •↑↑Bacterial counts due to either:
  - ∘Urine @ room temp >1hour
  - ∘Urine refrigerated >48hours

URINE SCREENING

URINE DIPSTICK EXAMINATION	
Component	**Normal values**
Specific gravity	1.001–1.035
pH	5–9
Protein	0–**Measures albumin only**, not hemoglobin, myoglobin, or immunoglobulins
Glucose	0
Ketones	0–**Measures acetoacetate only**, not acetone or β–hydroxybutyric acid
Bilirubin	0–**Measures conjugated bilirubin** indicative of hepatitis
Blood	0–**Measures hemoglobin** (both within erythrocytes & free) & **myoglobin**
Nitrite†	0
Leukocyte esterase‡	0

---

†Normally, the urine does not contain nitrites. However, many gram negative bacteria convert urinary nitrate (derived from the diet) to nitrite, indicating bacteriuria. However, this finding is of low sensitivity as several criteria in addition to gram negative bacteriuria must be met:

•Adequate numbers of the bacteria (≥100,000 organisms/ mL) must be present within the urinary tract, & be in contact w/ the urine for a sufficient amount of time (usually >4hours) for adequate nitrate conversion to occur. Therefore, the early morning urine sample is preferred
‡A leukocyte enzyme w/ a sensitivity of ~85% for urinary tract infections

URINE MICROSCOPIC EXAMINATION
•**Diagnosis of bacteriuria via gram stain**
Findings:
  •**Uncentrifuged urine**
    ◦≥1 bacterium/ hpf, being equivalent to ≥100,000 CFU/ mL urine
    ◦1 bacterium/ several hpf, being equivalent to 10,000–100,000 CFU/ mL urine

•**Diagnosis of asymptomatic bacteriuria**
Findings:
  •**Asymptomatic** patient w/:
    ◦≥1000 CFU/ mL in ♂
    ◦≥100,000 CFU/ mL in ♀
    ...of a single or predominant organism

•**Diagnosis of a urinary tract infection via gram stain**
Findings:
  •**Centrifuged urine**
    ◦≥10 leukocytes/ hpf=**pyuria** in a **symptomatic** patient
Outcomes:
  •Sensitivity: 95%

•**Diagnosis of a urinary tract infection via culture**
Findings:
  •**≥100 CFU/ mL in a symptomatic patient**

•**Diagnosis of Candidal sp. urinary tract infection via fungal stain**
  ◦Although Candida sp. can cause cystitis, ureteritis, &/or pyelonephritis, candiduria usually indicates urethral &/or urinary bladder colonization, esp. in the presence of an indwelling urinary catheter
Findings:
  •>10,000 CFU/ mL in the absence of an indwelling urinary catheter, usually indicates infection

Differential diagnosis of sterile pyuria†:
•Appendicitis
•Fastidious organisms
  ◦Sexually transmitted organisms
  ◦Mycobacteria
•Genitourinary tumor
•Inadequately treated urinary tract infection
•Interstitial cystitis
•Intrarenal renal disease
  ◦Acute tubular necrosis
  ◦Acute glomerulonephritis
  ◦Acute interstitial nephritis
  ◦Polycystic kidney disease
•Medication mediated cystitis
  ◦Chemotherapy
•Nephrolithiasis
•Papillary necrosis
•Prostatitis
•Reiter's syndrome
•Transplant rejection
•Transurethral resection of the prostate–TURP, for ≤several months

---

†≥10 leukocytes/ hpf of centrifuged urine
•hpf=high power field=oil immersion field
•CFU=colony forming units=organisms

DIAGNOSIS OF A SEXUALLY TRANSMITTED INFECTION ▬▬▬▬

•Diagnosis of Neisseria gonorrhoeae infection

Microscopic findings:
- **A gram negative diplococcus, usually found within polymorphonuclear leukocytes†**

Culture mediums used‡:
- •Martin–Lewis
- •NYC
- •Theyer–Martin

Other tests:
- •Ligase or polymerase chain reaction°

•Diagnosis of Chlamydia trachomatis infection

Microscopic findings:
- **•Polymorphonuclear leukocytes without intracellular diplococci**

Culture medium used‡:
- •Tissue culture

Other tests:
- •Ligase or polymerase chain reaction°
- •Culture media DNA probe
- •Direct fluorescent Chlamydia test
- •Enzyme immunoassay

---

†Sensitivities are as follows:
- •Symptomatic ♂ urethritis–90%
- •Pelvic inflammatory disease–PID 50%
- •Proctitis–40%

‡Culture of urethral, ectocervical, rectal, or pharyngeal mucous membrane specimens onto a selective media

Procedure:
- •The urethral swab sample should be taken via either:
  - ◦Visible meatal discharge
  - ◦Following insertion of the swab 2–4cm into the urethra & rotated unidirectionally for 5 seconds

°Use either:
- •Any swab collection
- •First void urine

DIAGNOSIS OF INFECTIOUS VAGINITIS ▬▬▬▬▬▬▬▬

•Candida sp. vaginitis

Statistics:
- •Occurs in 75% of ♀ during their lifetime, w/ 50% having ≥2 episodes

Discharge characteristics:
- •Appearance: **Thick–curdy white**
- •Odor: None
- •pH: <4.5

Microscopic characteristics:
- •10% KOH solution showing **hyphae or mycelia**

•Trichomonas vaginalis vaginitis

Statistics:
- •Found in the prostatic secretions of 70% of ♂ partners of infected ♀

Discharge characteristics:
- •Appearance: Grey–yellow–green, being profuse
- •Odor: Foul
- •pH: >4.5

Microscopic characteristics:
- •Wet saline mount showing:
  - ◦**Motile flagellated protozoa**
  - ◦**Many neutrophils**

Complications:
- •↑Bacterial vaginitis risk
- •During pregnancy→↑risk of:
  - ◦Chorioamnionitis
  - ◦Premature rupture of membranes–PROM
  - ◦Pre–term ↓birth weight

559

•**Bacterial vaginitis**–via unknown organism
  Discharge characteristics:
    •Appearance: White/ clear, being thin
    •Odor: **Fishy** on KOH prep
    •pH: >4.5
  Microscopic characteristics:
    •**Clue cells**, being vaginal epithelial cells w/ adherent bacteria
  Complications:
    •During pregnancy→↑risk of:
      ○Chorioamnionitis
      ○Premature rupture of membranes–PROM
      ○Pre–term ↓birth weight

OTHER STUDIES

•**Blood cultures**
  Indications:
    •**Severe infection**
      –Pyelonephritis
      –Sepsis
    •**Immunosuppression**
      ○Advanced age
      ○Alcoholism
      ○Diabetes mellitus
      ○Hematologic malignancy
      ○HIV infection/ AIDS
      ○Malnutrition
      ○Medications
        –Chemotherapy
        –Chronic glucocorticoid use
        –Immunomodulating medications
      ○Renal dialysis
    •"Sick" looking patients
  Procedure:
    •2 sets of aerobic & anaerobic culture mediums, w/ each bottle inoculated w/ ≥10mL of fluid
  Limitations:
    •Careful, as source may be contaminated via:
      ○Concomitant infection
      ○Intravascular line/ catheter, or the lack of aseptic technique→
        –Skin organism contamination

IMAGING

•**Abdominal computed tomographic–CT scan or ultrasound**
  Indications:
    •Suspected abscess
      ○Febrile despite 72hours of antibiotic treatment
    •Suspected hydronephrosis
    •Suspected nephrolithiasis

•**Vaginal ultrasound**
  Indications:
    •Suspected pelvic inflammatory disease–PID, to look for possible abscess:
      ○Adnexal abscess
      ○Tubo–ovarian abscess–TOA
      …&/or fluid in the cul de sac

TREATMENT

•**Cure, in a catheter associated urinary tract infection is unlikely unless it is removed**

•**Empiric antibiotic treatment**
  ○If treatment is initially begun w/ intravenous medication, the switch to PO medication should be
    attempted upon clinical improvement (fever resolution & clinical stabilization) X 24hours, if an
    acceptable PO medication is available, & the patient is able to take PO medication
  ○**Organism–narrowed therapy** should be initiated promptly upon stain, culture, & sensitivities results

560

∘The following antibiotics achieve equivalent plasma levels via PO or intravenous administration in persons w/ a functioning gastrointestinal tract:
  −Chloramphenicol
  −Doxycycline
  −Minocycline
  −Most fluoroquinolones
  −Trimethoprim/ Sulfamethoxazole
Bactericidal antibiotics
  •**Cell wall synthesis inhibitors**
    ∘β lactam medications:
      −Carbapenems
      −Cephalosporins
      −Monobactams
      −Penicillins
    ∘Vancomycin
  •**DNA synthesis inhibitors**
    ∘Fluoroquinolones
    ∘Linezolid
    ∘Metronidazole
    ∘Rifampin
    ∘Quinupristin & dalfopristin
  •**Aminoglycosides**

ASYMPTOMATIC BACTERIURIA

Indications to treat:
  •Pregnancy
  •Patients scheduled to undergo urologic surgery
Treatment:
  •As for uncomplicated cystitis
Screening/ outcomes:
  •All pregnant ♀ should be screened & treated for asymptomatic bacteriuria during the 1st trimester→
    ∘↓Pyelonephritis risk, as it develops in 25% of patients otherwise
  •All preoperative urologic surgical patients should also be screened & treated for asymptomatic bacteriuria→
    ∘↓Intra & postoperative bacteremia risk

DYSURIA

Treatment duration:
  •**2days** only, so as not to mask refractory symptoms indicating possible medication resistance or complication

PHENAZOPYRIDINE (Pyridium)		
M ♀	**Dose**	
K P	200mg PO tid after meals	
Side effects:		
General		
•**Orange discoloration** of body fluids, including sweat, tears, & urine, which stain clothing & contact lenses		
Contraindications:		
•Hepatitis		
•Renal failure		

METHYLENE BLUE		
M ♀	**Dose**	
GutK ?	65−130mg PO tid after meals, w/ a liberal amount of water	
Side effects:		
General		
•**Blue−green discoloration** of body fluids, including sweat, tears, & urine, which stain clothing & contact lenses		

BACTERIAL CYSTITIS

•Up to 35% of cases have "silent" upper urinary tract involvement

Treatment duration:
•Uncomplicated cystitis: 3days
•Complicated cystitis: 10days

TRIMETHOPRIM–SULFAMETHOXAZOLE TMP–SMX (Bactrim, Septra)		
M ♀	**Dose**	
K U	1 double strength–DS tab (160mg TMP/ 800mg SMX) PO q12hours	

Trimethoprim specific mechanism:
•↓Dihydrofolate reductase action→
  ○↓Tetrahydrofolate, being required as a methyl donor for the synthesis of purines & pyrimidines→
   −↓Nucleotide synthesis

Sulfonamide specific mechanism:
•A P–aminobenzoic acid–PABA analogue→
  ○Competitive inhibition of dihydropteroate synthetase mediated PABA conversion to dihydrofolate→
   −↓Tetrahydrofolate, being required as a methyl donor for the synthesis of purines &
    pyrimidines→ ↓nucleotide synthesis

Side effects:
Mucocutaneous
•**Dermatitis** via maculopapular rash, urticaria >> exfoliative dermatitis, photosensitivity, Stevens–
 Johnson syndrome, or toxic epidermal necrolysis
Genitourinary
•Acute interstitial nephritis
Neurologic
•Aseptic meningitis
Pulmonary
•The sulfite component of the combination medication→
  ○Asthma exacerbation in sensitive patients
Hematologic
•**Myelosuppression**→
  ○Anemia→
   −Fatigue
  ○Leukopenia→immunosuppression→
   −↑Infection & neoplasm risk
  ○Thrombocytopenia→
   −↑Hemorrhage risk

Trimethoprim specific:
Genitourinary
•Blocks distal renal tubule Na^+/K^+ exchange→
  ○**Hyperkalemia**
•Competes w/ creatinine for tubular secretion→
  ○↑Creatinine, without concomitantly ↑blood urea nitrogen–BUN
Hematologic
•↑Homocysteine levels

Sulfamethoxazole specific:
General
•Anorexia
•Drug fever via hypersensitivity syndrome
Gastrointestinal
•Nausea ± vomiting
Genitourinary
•Crystalluria→
  ○Acute tubular necrosis
•Hepatitis
Hematologic
•**G6PD deficiency mediated hemolytic anemia**

Contraindications:
•Neonates or near term ♀s, as sulfamethoxazole competitively binds to albumin, thus displacing
 bilirubin→
  ○↑Kernicterus risk

FLUOROQUINOLONES

Generic (Trade)	M	♀	Dose
Ciprofloxacin (Cipro)	LK	?	250mg PO q12hours
Gatifloxacin (Tequin)	K	?	400mg PO q24hours
Levofloxacin (Levaquin)	KL	?	250mg PO q24hours
Moxifloxacin (Avelox)	LK	?	400mg PO q24hours
Norfloxacin (Noroxin)	LK	?	400mg PO q12hours
Ofloxacin (Floxin)	LK	?	200mg PO q12hours

Mechanism:
- ↓DNA gyrase=topoisomerase action→
  - ↓Bacterial DNA synthesis

Side effects:
General
- •Hypersensitivity reactions

Gastrointestinal
- •Gastroenteritis→
  - ◦Diarrhea
  - ◦Nausea ± vomiting

Mucocutaneous
- •Phototoxicity

Neurologic
- •Dizziness
- •Drowsiness
- •Headache
- •Restlessness

Materno–fetal
- •Fetal & child tendon malformation (including breast fed)→
  - ◦↑Tendon rupture risk

OR

TETRACYCLINES

Generic (Trade)	M	♀	Dose
Doxycycline (Adoxa)	LK	?	100mg PO q12hours
Tetracycline (Sumycin)	LK	U	500mg PO q12hours

Mechanism:
- •Affects the ribosomal 30S subunit→
  - ◦↓Ribosomal binding to transfer RNA

Side effects:
Gastrointestinal
- •Acute hepatic fatty necrosis
- •Gastroenteritis→
  - ◦Abdominal pain

Genitourinary
- •Acute tubular necrosis

Mucocutaneous
- •Photosensitivity

Neurologic
- •Pseudotumor cerebri

Materno–fetal
- •Fetus to age 10 years→
  - ◦Tooth staining
  - ◦↓Bone growth

563

•The following are less effective, but safe during pregnancy

CEPHALOSPORINS: 1ˢᵗ generation			

CEPHALOSPORINS: 1st generation

Generic (Trade)	M	♀	Dose
Cephalexin (Keflex)	K	P	500mg PO q12hours

Mechanism:
•A β–lactam ring structure which binds to bacterial transpeptidase→
  ◦↓Transpeptidase function→
    –↓Bacterial cell wall peptidoglycan cross–linking→↓cell wall synthesis→osmotic influx of
      extracellular fluid→↑intracellular hydrostatic pressure→cell rupture→cell death=bactericidal
•↑Bacterial autolytic enzymes→
  ◦Peptidoglycan degradation

•Certain bacteria produce β–lactamase→
  ◦Cleavage of this essential structural component of cephalosporins & certain penicillins (as the
    other β–lactam medications differ sufficiently to prevent ring cleavage)→
    –Antibiotic inactivation. This process may be antagonized by the concomitant administration of
      β–lactamase inhibitors (Clavulanic acid=clavulanate, Sulbactam, or Tazobactam)→renewed
      susceptibility

Side effects:
General
•**Hypersensitivity reactions ≤10%**
  ◦Anaphylaxis–0.5%→
    –Death–0.002% (1:50,000)
  ◦Acute interstitial nephritis
  ◦Dermatitis
  ◦Drug fever
  ◦Hemolytic anemia
  …having cross–hypersensitivity to other β lactam medications (penicillins, carbapenems), except
    monobactams (ex. Aztreonam)
Gastrointestinal
•Clostridium dificile pseudomembraneous colitis (3ʳᵈ generation > others)

OR

PENICILLINS			

PENICILLINS

Generic (Trade)	M	♀	Dose
Amoxicillin–clavulanic acid (Augmentin)	K	P	500mg PO q8hours

Mechanism:
•A β–lactam ring structure which binds to bacterial transpeptidase→
  ◦↓Transpeptidase function→
    –↓Bacterial cell wall peptidoglycan cross–linking→↓cell wall synthesis→osmotic influx of
      extracellular fluid→↑intracellular hydrostatic pressure→cell rupture→cell death=bactericidal
•↑Bacterial autolytic enzymes→
  ◦Peptidoglycan degradation

•Certain bacteria produce β–lactamase→
  ◦Cleavage of this essential structural component of cephalosporins & certain penicillins (as the
    other β–lactam medications differ sufficiently to prevent ring cleavage)→
    –Antibiotic inactivation. This process may be antagonized by the concomitant administration of
      β–lactamase inhibitors (Clavulanic acid=clavulanate, Sulbactam, or Tazobactam)→renewed
      susceptibility

Side effects:
General
•**Hypersensitivity reactions ≤10%**
  ◦Anaphylaxis–0.5%→
    –Death–0.002% (1:50,000)
  ◦Acute interstitial nephritis
  ◦Dermatitis
  ◦Drug fever
  ◦Hemolytic anemia
  …having cross–hypersensitivity to other β lactam medications (cephalosporins, carbapenems),
    except monobactams (ex. Aztreonam)

CANDIDAL CYSTITIS ▬▬▬▬▬▬▬▬▬▬▬▬▬▬▬▬▬▬▬▬▬▬▬▬▬▬▬▬▬▬▬

AZOLE ANTIFUNGAL MEDICATIONS

Generic (Trade)	M	♀	Dose
Fluconazole (Diflucan)	K	?	200mg PO/ IV on day 1, then 100mg PO/ IV q24hours X 4days

Mechanism:
- •Inhibition of ergosterol† synthesis→
  - ∘Fungal cell membrane disruption, w/ no clinically significant resistance

---

†Ergosterol is not found on human or bacterial cell membranes, thus allowing for selective toxicity

SECOND LINE

AMPHOTERICIN B

Generic (Trade)	M	♀	Dose
Non–lipid Amphotericin B (Fungizone)	C	P	0.3mg/ kg IV infusion over 2hours X 1dose

AMPHOTERICIN B LIPID FORMULATIONS

Indications, being either:
- •Creatinine >2.5mg/ dL
- •Refractory or intolerant of the non–lipid formulation

Generic (Trade)	M	♀	Dose
Amphotericin B cholesteryl complex† (Amphotec)	?	P	4mg/ kg IV infusion over 2hours X 1
Amphotericin B lipid complex (Abelcet)	?	P	5mg/ kg IV infusion over 2hours X 1
Liposomal Amphotericin B (AmBisome)	?	P	3mg/ kg IV infusion over 2hours X 1

- •The lipid preparations preferentially accumulate in the organs of the reticuloendothelial system–RES as opposed to the kidneys, thus allowing for ↑dosing w/ concomitantly ↓nephrotoxicity risk. Although the lipid formulations allow for ↑tissue concentrations & distribution volume, none of them have been shown to have ↑efficacy
- †Also named Amphotericin B colloidal dispersion–ABCD

Non–lipid specific dosage adjustment:
- •Should renal failure occur w/ the non–lipid formulation, either:
  - ∘Administer q48hours
  - ∘↓Dosage by 50%
  - ∘Switch to a lipid formulation

Mechanism:
- •Bonding to ergosterol†→
  - ∘Fungal cell membrane disruption, w/ no clinically significant resistance

---

†Ergosterol is not found on human or bacterial cell membranes, thus allowing for selective toxicity

Side effects: **Non–lipid > Lipid formulations†**
General
- •Inflammatory cytokine release→
  - ∘Anorexia
  - ∘**Chills**
    - –Treated w/ Meperidine 25–50mg IV, followed by dantrolene if intractable
  - ∘**Fevers**, w/ ↓frequency & severity w/ repeated doses
  - ∘Metallic taste
Cardiovascular
- •Bradycardia
- •Hypotension–rare
- •**Thrombophlebitis**
  - ∘Improved w/ the addition of 1,000 units of Heparin to the infusion
Gastrointestinal
- •Nausea ± vomiting
Genitourinary
- •Tubular toxicity (which may be avoided w/ hydration via 500mL of normal saline prior to, & after infusion)→
  - ∘Acute tubular necrosis→
    - –**Intra–renal renal failure**
  - ∘**Hypokalemia**
    - –May be treated w/ a potassium sparing diuretic added throughout treatment
Mucocutaneous
- •Flushing

565

Musculoskeletal
- •Inflammatory cytokine release→
  - ◦Myalgia

Neurologic
- •Seizures

Hematologic
- •↓Erythropoietin→
  - −Normocytic−normochromic anemia
- •Hypocapnia
- •Hypomagnesemia
- •**Myelosuppression**→
  - ◦Anemia→
    - −Fatigue
  - ◦Leukopenia→immunosuppression→
    - −↑Infection & neoplasm risk
  - ◦Thrombocytopenia→
    - −↑Hemorrhage risk, esp. petechiae

---

†Ampho B cholesteryl complex > Ampho B lipid complex > Liposomal ampho B

URETHRITIS &/OR CERVICITIS ▀▀▀▀▀▀▀▀▀
GONOCOCCAL: Neisseria gonorrhoeae

CEPHALOSPORINS: 3rd generation

Generic (Trade)	M	♀	Dose
Ceftriaxone (Rocephin)	KB	P	125mg IM X1dose

OR

FLUOROQUINOLONES

Generic (Trade)	M	♀	Dose
Ciprofloxacin (Cipro)	LK	?	500mg PO X1dose
Levofloxacin (Levaquin)	KL	?	500mg PO X1dose
Ofloxacin (Floxin)	LK	?	400mg PO X1dose

OR

MACROLIDES

Generic (Trade)	M	♀	Dose
Azithromycin (Zithromax)	L	P	2g PO X 1dose

Mechanism:
- •Affects the ribosomal 50S subunit→
  - ◦↓Transfer RNA translocation

Side effects:
- **Hematologic**
  - •Eosinophilia
- **Gastrointestinal**
  - •Gastroenteritis→
    - ◦Diarrhea
    - ◦Nausea ± vomiting
  - •Hepatitis
- **Neurologic**
  - •Transient deafness

NONGONOCOCCAL: Chlamydia trachomatis, Ureaplasma urealyticum

MACROLIDES

Generic (Trade)	M	♀	Dose
Azithromycin (Zithromax)	L	P	1g PO X 1dose

OR

TETRACYCLINES

Generic (Trade)	M	♀	Dose
Doxycycline (Adoxa)	LK	?	100mg PO q12hours X 1week

OR

FLUOROQUINOLONES

Generic (Trade)	M	♀	Dose
Ciprofloxacin (Cipro)	LK	?	500mg PO q24hours X 1week
Ofloxacin (Floxin)	LK	?	300mg PO q12hours X 1week

566

NONGONOCOCCAL: Trichomonas vaginalis

METRONIDAZOLE (Flagyl)	
M ♀	**Dose**
KL P-U in 1st trimester	2g PO X 1dose

Mechanism:
- •DNA binding→
  - ◦DNA strand breakage

Side effects:

General
- **•Disulfuram-like reaction to alcohol**
  - ◦Avoid alcoholic beverages during, & for 48hours after completion of treatment

Gastrointestinal
- •Nausea ± vomiting-10%
- •Taste changes=dysgeusia (esp. metallic taste)

Genitourinary
- •Dark urine, being common, but harmless

Neurological
- •Peripheral neuropathy
- •Seizures

Hematologic
- •Transient neutropenia-8%

PROSTATITIS

Treatment duration:
- •Acute prostatitis: 1month
- •Chronic prostatitis: 1-3months

FLUOROQUINOLONES			
Generic (Trade)	**M**	**♀**	**Dose**
Ciprofloxacin (Cipro)	LK	?	500mg PO q12hours
Levofloxacin (Levaquin)	KL	?	750mg PO q24hours

OR

TRIMETHOPRIM-SULFAMETHOXAZOLE TMP-SMX (Bactrim, Septra)		
M	**♀**	**Dose**
K	U	1 double strength-DS tablet (160mg TMP & 800mg SMX/ tab) PO q12hours

EPIDIDYMITIS &/OR PROCTITIS

CEPHALOSPORINS: 3rd generation			
Generic (Trade)	**M**	**♀**	**Dose**
Ceftriaxone (Rocephin)	KB	P	250mg IM X 1dose

&

TETRACYCLINES			
Generic (Trade)	**M**	**♀**	**Dose**
Doxycycline (Adoxa)	LK	?	100mg PO q12hours X 1week

BACTERIAL PYELONEPHRITIS

•After blood cultures have been obtained, begin intravenous-IV treatment promptly

Treatment duration:
- **•2weeks**

FLUOROQUINOLONES			
Generic (Trade)	**M**	**♀**	**Dose**
Ciprofloxacin (Cipro)	LK	?	500mg IV/ PO q12hours
Gatifloxacin (Tequin)	K	?	400mg IV/ PO q24hours
Levofloxacin (Levaquin)	KL	?	750mg IV/ PO q24hours

FUNGAL PYELONEPHRITIS OR DISSEMINATED CANDIDIASIS ▬▬▬▬
Treatment duration:
•Until clinical improvement, including 2weeks after last positive blood culture

•**AMPHOTERICIN B** as above

±

FLUCYTOSINE (Ancobon)			
M ♀ Dose		**Peak**	**Trough**
K ? 12.5–37.5mg/ kg PO q6hours		70–90mg/ L	30–40mg/ L

Mechanism:
•A nucleoside analogue metabolized to fluorouracil→
  ◦Inhibition of thymidylate synthetase→
    −↓Thymidine synthesis→↓DNA synthesis→cytotoxicity to all proliferating cells
•Not used alone, as resistance emerges rapidly

SECOND LINE

AZOLE ANTIFUNGAL MEDICATIONS		
Generic (Trade)	**M ♀ Dose**	
Fluconazole (Diflucan) K ? 400mg IV/ PO q24hours		

VAGINITIS ▬▬▬▬
Candida sp. vaginitis

AZOLE ANTIFUNGAL MEDICATIONS			
Generic (Trade)	**M**	**♀**	**Dose**
Butoconazole (Gynazole, Mycelex–3)	LK	?	
•Intravaginal cream			2%–5g qhs X 3days
Clotrimazole (Mycelex)	LK	P	
•Intravaginal cream			2%–5g qhs X 3days
•Intravaginal tab			500mg X 1 dose
Fluconazole (Diflucan)	K	?	150mg PO X 1dose
Itraconazole (Sporanox)	L	?	200mg PO q12hours X 1day
Miconazole (Monistat, Monazole)	LK	P	
•Intravaginal cream			2%–5g qhs X 7days
•Intravaginal suppository			400mg qhs X 3days
•Vaginal insert			1.2g X 1dose
Nystatin (Mycostatin)	Ø	S	
•Intravaginal tab			100,000 units qhs X 2weeks
Terconazole (Terazol)	LK	?	
•Intravaginal cream			0.8%–5g qhs X 3days
•Vaginal suppository			80mg qhs X 3days
Tioconazole (Monistat 1–Day, Vagistat–1)	Ø	?	
•Intravaginal ointment			6.5%–4.6g X 1dose

Bacterial vaginitis

CLINDAMYCIN (Cleocin)	
M ♀	**Dose**
L P	
•PO form	300mg q12hours X 1week
•Intravaginal cream	2%–5g qhs X 1week

Mechanism:
•Affects the ribosomal 50S subunit→
  ◦↓Peptide bond formation

Side effects:
  Gastrointestinal
    •**Clostridium dificile pseudomembraneous colitis**
    •Gastroenteritis→
      ◦Diarrhea
      ◦Nausea ± vomiting
  Mucocutaneous
    •Dermatitis

568

METRONIDAZOLE (Flagyl)		
M ♀		Dose
KL P–U in 1st trimester		
•PO form		2g X 1 dose
•Intravaginal gel		0.75%–5g qhs X 5days

Trichomonas vaginalis vaginitis

METRONIDAZOLE (Flagyl)		
M ♀		Dose
KL P–U in 1st trimester		2g PO X 1dose, for both the patient & sexual partners

PELVIC INFLAMMATORY DISEASE–PID ▬▬▬▬▬▬▬▬
•After blood cultures have been obtained, begin intravenous–IV treatment promptly
Complications:
  •**Associated abscess**, treated via laparoscopy/ laparotomy for drainage/ removal
Treatment duration:
  •**2weeks**
Outcomes:
  •Pelvic inflammatory disease–PID→
    ∘Fibrosis=adhesions→
      –↑Ectopic pregnancy risk
      –↑Infertility risk (20% after 1 episode, 35% after 2 episodes, 75% after ≥3 episodes)

TETRACYCLINES			
Generic (Trade)	M	♀	Dose
Doxycycline (Adoxa)	LK	?	100mg IV/ PO q12hours

&

CEPHALOSPORINS: 2nd generation			
Generic (Trade)	M	♀	Dose
Cefotetan (Cefotan)	KB	P	2g IV q12hours
Cefoxitin (Mefoxin)	K	P	2g IV q6hours

DIARRHEA SYNDROMES

•Caused by either:
  ◦Microorganisms†
  ◦Noninfectious gastrointestinal disease or dysfunction
  ...→↑**stool water concentration** ± ↑**frequency of bowel movements**→
    •≥3 semisolid or liquid bowel movements/ day X ≥2 consecutive days
Statistics:
  •**#2 Cause of mortality worldwide** (#1 is cardiovascular disease), accounting for >2million deaths/ year
  •In regards to children in the developing countries of Asia, Africa, & Latin America, diarrhea→
  ◦#1 Cause of childhood mortality
  ◦↓Physical & cognitive development

---

†In the U.S., most cases of infectious diarrhea syndromes occur during the winter months

CLASSIFICATION/ RISK FACTORS

Subclassifications:
  •**Acute diarrhea syndrome:** Symptoms begin suddenly, & last ≤1month (95% lasting <1week), usually being infectious
  •**Chronic diarrhea syndrome:** Symptoms usually begin insidiously, & last >1month

ABNORMAL MOTILITY DIARRHEA ▬▬▬▬▬▬▬▬▬▬▬▬▬▬▬▬▬▬▬▬▬▬▬▬▬▬▬▬
Mechanism:
  •↑Transit→
  ◦↓Nutrient, electrolyte, & water absorption
Etiologies:
  •**Antibiotics,** via a direct effect on the intestinal mucosa
  ◦Erythromycin→
    −Motilin receptor agonism→↑gastric emptying rate
  ◦Clavulanic acid→
    −↑Small intestinal motility
  •**Endocrine**
  ◦Diabetic autonomic neuropathy
  ◦Hyperthyroidism
  •**Gastrointestinal hemorrhage**
  •**Irritable bowel syndrome−IBS**
  •**Post−surgical**
  ◦Blind bowel loop w/ bacterial overgrowth
  ◦Partial or total gastrectomy
  ◦Vagotomy
  •**Scleroderma**

INFLAMMATORY DIARRHEA ▬▬▬▬▬▬▬▬▬▬▬▬▬▬▬▬▬▬▬▬▬▬▬▬▬▬▬▬▬▬▬
Mechanism:
  •Gastrointestinal inflammation=gastroenteritis→
    −↑Mucus production ± purulence ± hemorrhage
    −↑Gastrointestinal motility
    ...→↓nutrient, electrolyte, & water absorption
Etiologies:
  •**Collagen vascular disease**
  •**Hypersensitivity syndrome** via allergy to a digested allergen
  •**Infectious**
  ◦**Invasive** microbial gastroenteritis, being viral, bacterial, or parasitic
  ◦**Cytotoxin−**mediated gastroenteritis
  •**Inflammatory bowel disease−IBD**
  ◦Crohn's disease
  ◦Ulcerative colitis
  •**Intestinal ischemia**

- **Medications**, possibly up to several months after discontinuation
  - ○**Antibiotics**, esp.:
    - −Clindamycin−20%
    - −Ampicillin−10%
    - −Cephalosporins−8%
    - −Tetracyclines−6%
    - ...→endogenous organism overgrowth, esp.:
      - •**Clostridium difficile−25%**
      - •Candida albicans
      - •Clostridium perfringens type A
      - •Salmonella sp.
      - •Staphylococcus aureus
      - ...± cytotoxin production
  - ○Chemotherapeutic medications→
    - −Mucositis
- •**Radiation therapy**

OSMOTIC DIARRHEA

- •All diarrhea has an osmotic component

Mechanism:
- •Malabsorbed intestinal nutrients→
  - ○↓Nutrient, electrolyte, & water absorption via osmotic pressure

Etiologies:
- •**Antibiotics** via their direct effect on the intestinal flora→
  - ○↓Anaerobic bacterial concentrations→
    - −↓Carbohydrate metabolism
- •↓**Digestion**
  - ○↓Bile
  - ○↓Pancreatic enzymes
  - ○Disaccharidase deficiency
  - ○Lactase deficiency
  - ○Extensive bowel resections
- •**Mucosal transport defects**
  - ○Intestinal lymphoma
  - ○Small intestinal mucosal sprue
    - −Celiac
    - −Tropical
  - ○Whipples disease
- •**Neoplasm:**
  - ○Colorectal cancer (right sided > left sided)
- •**Poorly absorbed solutes**
  - ○Laxative medications
  - ○Magnesium containing medications
  - ○Mannitol
  - ○Sorbitol
  - ○Hyperosmolar enteral solutions

SECRETORY DIARRHEA

Mechanism:
- •↑Electrolyte secretion into the bowel lumen→
  - ○↑Water via osmotic pressure→
    - −↓Nutrient, electrolyte, & water absorption

Etiologies:
- •**Antibiotics** via their direct effect on the intestinal flora→
  - ○↓Anaerobic bacterial concentrations→
    - −↓Metabolism of bile acids, which are potent colonic secretory agents
- •**Dietary**
  - ○Caffeine
- •**Endocrine**
  - ○Hyperthyroidism
- •**Infectious**
  - ○Bacterial **enterotoxin** mediated
- •**Medications**
  - ○Laxative abuse

- **Neoplastic**
  - ∘Carcinoid tumor→
    - –Serotonin secretion
  - ∘Gastrinoma→
    - –Gastrin secretion
  - ∘Glucagonoma→
    - –Glucagon secretion
  - ∘Intestinal villous adenomatous polyps
  - ∘Medullary thyroid cancer→
    - –Calcitonin secretion
  - ∘VIPoma→
    - –Vasoactive intestinal peptide–VIP secretion

PSYCHOGENIC DIARRHEA ▬▬▬▬▬▬▬▬▬▬▬▬▬▬▬▬▬▬▬▬▬▬

Mechanism:
- •↑Parasympathetic autonomic nervous system tone→
  - ∘↑Gastrointestinal motility & mucus secretion→
    - –↓Nutrient, electrolyte, & water absorption.

Etiologies:
- **Nervousness**

OTHER MEDICATIONS ASSOCIATED WITH DIARRHEA ▬▬▬▬▬▬▬▬▬▬▬

- •Alcohol
- •Bumetanide
- •Colchicine
- •Digitalis
- •Ethacrynic acid
- •Furosemide
- •Hydralazine
- •Guanethedine
- •Methyldopa
- •Propranolol
- •Quinidine
- •Reserpine

DIAGNOSIS

- •Most cases of acute infectious diarrhea syndromes are self limited, w/ 50% lasting <1day

Cardiovascular
- •Diarrhea, which along w/ vomiting & anorexia→↓intravascular volume→
  - ∘≥10% blood volume loss→
    - –↑Autonomic sympathetic tone→↑pulse
  - ∘≥20% blood volume loss→
    - –Orthostatic hypotension (supine to standing→↑20 pulse, ↓20 SBP, &/or ↓10 DBP)→ lightheadedness upon standing
    - –Urine output 20–30mL/ hour (normal being >30mL/ hour)
  - ∘≥30% blood volume loss→
    - –Recumbent hypotension &/or tachycardia
  - ∘≥40% blood volume loss→
    - –Altered mental status &/or urine output <20mL/ hour
    - –Hypovolemic shock, being hypotension + organ failure, unresponsive to fluid resuscitation

Gastrointestinal
- •Mucosal irritation→
  - ∘↑Gastrointestinal smooth muscle contraction→↑peristalsis→
    - –**Abdominal pain**, being referred & episodic or "wave like", termed colic
      - Areas of reference:
        - •Stomach &/or duodenum: Epigastrium
        - •Small intestine: Periumbilical area
        - •Large intestine: Hypogastrium &/or suprapubic area
        - •Rectum: Suprapubic, sacral, &/or perineal areas
    - –Anorexia
    - –↑Bowel sounds→audible gastrointestinal gurgling, termed borborygmi
    - –Diarrhea
    - –Retrograde peristalsis→nausea ± vomiting

Mucocutaneous
- Hypovolemia→
  - ◦Dry mucous membranes
  - ◦Dry skin→
    - –↓Skin turgor→skin tenting

Hematologic
- ↓Fluid & electrolyte absorption→
  - ◦Intravascular volume loss→
    - –↑Creatinine & blood urea nitrogen–BUN, indicating pre–renal renal failure
  - ◦Hypochloremia
  - ◦Hypokalemia
  - ◦Hyponatremia
- Diarrhea→
  - ◦Bicarbonate loss→
    - –Non–anion gap, hyperchloremic metabolic acidemia
- Vomitus→
  - ◦Hydrogen loss→
    - –Metabolic alkalemia

INFECTIOUS DIARRHEA

SMALL INTESTINAL DISEASE
- Infrequent, large volume, watery bowel movements

Organism	Mechanism	Source
Bacteria:		
•Enterotoxigenic E. coli	Enterotoxin mediated	Fecal–oral
•Enteroaggregative E. coli	Enterotoxin mediated	Fecal–oral
•Enteropathogenic E. coli	Enterotoxin mediated	Fecal–oral
•Vibrio cholera	Enterotoxin mediated	Fecal–oral
Bacteria responsible for "food poisoning†":		
•Bacillus cereus	Enterotoxin mediated	Grains‡ (esp. rice)
•Clostridium perfringens type A	Enterotoxin mediated	Soil contamination of food°
•Staphylococcus aureus	Preformed enterotoxin mediated	Human mucocutaneous contamination of food
Parasites:		
•Cryptosporidium parvum	Cellular attachment	Fecal–oral
•Giardia lamblia	Cellular attachment	Fecal–oral
•Isospora belli	Mucosal invasion	Fecal–oral
Viruses:		
•Adenovirus	Mucosal cellular invasion	Fecal–oral
•Norwalk virus	Mucosal cellular invasion	Fecal–oral
•Rotavirus	Mucosal cellular invasion	Fecal–oral

†Consumption of food contaminated w/ an enterotoxin producing bacteria→
- Noninflammatory acute diarrhea syndrome lasting <24hours
  - ◦Sufficient pre–formed toxin→
    - –Incubation period of 1–6hours
    - –Vomiting > diarrhea
  - ◦Insufficient pre–formed toxin→
    - –Incubation period >6hours
    - –Diarrhea > vomiting

‡Spores on grains (esp. rice) may survive cooking temperatures→
- Germination after many hours, if kept warm→
  - ◦Enterotoxin production

°Spores in the soil contaminate food & may survive cooking temperatures→
- Germination after several hours if kept warm→
  - ◦Enterotoxin production

LARGE INTESTINAL DISEASE
•Frequent, small volume, watery bowel movements

Organism	Mechanism	Source
Bacteria:		
•Clostridium difficile†	Colonic enterotoxin (toxin A) & cytotoxin (toxin B)	Overgrowth
Parasites:		
•Entamoeba histolytica	Colonic mucosal invasion	Fecal–oral

†The #1 identifiable cause of both antibiotic associated & hospital acquired diarrhea syndromes

Risk factors for Clostridium difficile colitis:
•**Antibiotics**, esp.:
 ◦Clindamycin
 ◦Ampicillin
 ◦Cephalosporins
 ◦Tetracyclines
•**Immunosuppression**
 ◦Advanced age
 ◦Alcoholism
 ◦Diabetes mellitus
 ◦Hematologic malignancy
 ◦HIV infection/ AIDS
 ◦Malnutrition
 ◦Medications
   −Chemotherapy
   −Chronic glucocorticoid use
   −Immunomodulating medications
 ◦Renal dialysis
•**Hospitalization**, as bacterial spores can be isolated from the:
 ◦Hospital facilities in general (fomites & surfaces)
 ◦Skin of healthcare workers
Complications of Clostridium difficile colitis:
•Protein losing enteropathy→
 ◦Hypoalbuminemia→
   −Anasarca
•**Complete loss of intestinal smooth muscle tone→**
 ◦Abdominal pain, tenderness, & **massive dilation, termed toxic megacolon→**
   −Intraluminal air accumulation→↑intraluminal pressure→↓colonic vascular flow (venous > arterial)→congestive ischemia→necrosis→**perforation & hemorrhage**→generalized peritonitis
   Iatrogenic precipitants: Induced in patients w/ severe colitis by:
   •**Anticholinergic medications→**
     ◦↓Gastrointestinal tone
   •**Opiates→**
     ◦↓Gastrointestinal tone
   •Barium enema preparation
   •Lower endoscopy preparation

BIMODAL DISEASE
•Affecting the small intestine, then the large intestine

Organism	Mechanism	Source
Bacteria:		
•Campylobacter jejuni	Small intestine enterotoxin & colonic mucosal invasion	Fecal-oral
•Enterohemorrhagic E. coli 0157−H7	Small intestine enterotoxin & colonic cytotoxin	Fecal-oral
•Enteroinvasive E. coli−EIEC	Small intestine enterotoxin & colonic mucosal invasion	Fecal-oral
•Salmonella sp.	Small & large intestinal mucosal invasion	Fecal-oral
•Shigella sp.	Small intestine enterotoxin & colonic mucosal invasion	Fecal-oral
•Vibrio parahemolyticus	Small intestine enterotoxin ± colonic mucosal invasion	Seafood

574

"TRAVELER'S DIARRHEA"

•Diarrhea occurring in travelers to another country (usually being a **developing country** in Asia, Africa, or Latin America) due to fecal–oral organism transmission

Organisms, in order of frequency:
- **Enterotoxigenic Escherichia coli**
- Campylobacter jejuni
- Shigella sp.
- Aeromonas sp.
- Entamoeba histolytica
- Giardia lamblia
- Salmonella sp.
- Non-cholera vibrios

Prevention:
- Ingestion of:
  - Previously boiled water or bottled beverage
  - Freshly prepared, thoroughly cooked food
  - Fruit that must be peeled
  - Vegetables that have been washed in previously boiled or bottled water

STOOL EVALUATION

Indications:
- Fever
- Severe dehydration
- Gross fecal blood, mucus, &/or pus
- Recent antibiotic use
- Immunodeficiency
- Recent outbreak
- Duration ≥5 days

Fecal studies for suspected infectious diarrhea:
- **Bacterial culture**
- **Ova & parasites** X 3 samples
- **Shiga toxin**
  Indications:
  - Acute onset hemorrhagic diarrhea (esp. those being afebrile) as they may be infected w/ Enterohemorrhagic E. coli–ETEC O157–H7
- **Microscopic examination for leukocytes**
  Procedure:
  1. Place fecal mucus &/or feces on a glass slide
  2. Add 2 drops of Methylene blue solution & mix
  3. Place a cover slip & allow 3 min. for polymorphonuclear & mononuclear cell nuclei to take up the stain→
     - Blue nuclei
  Outcomes:
  - Sensitivity–75%, specificity–85%

Studies for suspected Clostridium Difficile colitis:
- **Fecal Clostridium difficile toxins A &/or B**
  Procedure:
  - Detected via either:
    - Cell culture cytopathic effect (toxin B > toxin A)
    - Enzyme linked immunosorbent assay–ELISA
  Limitations:
  - Must be tested within 12hours after collection, as toxin B is labile
  - Toxigenic &/or non-toxigenic strains of Clostridium difficile are found in the colonic flora of:
    - 3% of the general population
    - 25% of hospitalized patients
  Outcomes:
  - Repeating the test slightly ↑diagnostic yield
  Note: The presence of IgG antibody to toxin A is protective against infection & relapse
- **Sigmoidoscopy**
  Findings:
  - Cytotoxin (toxin B) production→
    - Mucosal inflammatory, 1–5mm, raised yellow–white plaques, termed **pseudomembraneous colitis**

<u>Fecal studies for suspected osmotic diarrhea:</u>
- Osmotic diarrhea is indicated via either:
  - Osmotic gap >50mOsm/ L†
  - Syndrome relief upon fasting
  - Malalabsorption→↑fecal fat measured via:
    - Qualitative testing
      <u>Procedure:</u>
      - Sudan staining of feces→
        - >60 fat droplets/ high power field
      <u>Outcomes:</u>
      - Clinically useful only if positive. Regardless of the outcome, perform the quantitative test which has relatively ↑sensitivity & specificity
    - Quantitative testing:
      <u>Indications:</u>
      - Diagnosis
      - To follow treatment response
      <u>Procedure:</u>
      - The patient's dietary fat should be ≥50g/ d X 2 days prior to stool collection for 72hours (which should be refrigerated)

---

†Osmotic gap=measured stool osmolarity (usually ~290mOsm) − calculated stool osmolarity: 2 (stool sodium + stool potassium)

TREATMENT

MILD–MODERATE DIARRHEA ▬▬▬▬
- **Avoidance of milk products,** as mucosal inflammation→
  - Transient lactase deficiency
- **Oral fluids if tolerated,** w/ a glucose based electrolyte solution. Intravenous normal saline or lactated Ringer's solution if not

SEVERE DIARRHEA ▬▬▬▬
- **Intravenous fluid,** w/ attention to both:
  - **Intravascular volume repletion via Normal saline** (0.9% NaCl) or **lactated Ringer's solution,** as per:
    - Vital signs
    - Physical examination
    - Urine output (normal being ≥0.5mL/kg/h)
    - Blood urea nitrogen-BUN & creatinine
  - **Intravascular volume maintenance via Normal saline** (0.9% NaCl) or **lactated Ringer's solution**
    <u>Adult maintenance fluid:</u>
    - Weight (kg) + 40= #mL/ hour
    <u>Additional febrile requirements:</u>
    - 1L/ 24hours for every 1°F >100°F
    <u>Additional:</u>
    - Estimate loss for:
      - Diaphoresis
      - Diarrhea
      - Polyuria
      - Tachypnea
  ...followed by oral rehydration w/ a glucose based electrolyte solution upon both clinical stability & ability to tolerate PO

ANTIPERISTALSIS MEDICATIONS			
Generic	M ♀	**Start**	**Max**
<u>First line:</u>			
Bismuth subsalicylate (Pepto–Bismol)	K U	2tabs or 30mL PO q30–60min.	16tabs or 240mL/ d
Loperamide (Imodium)†	L P	4mg PO initially, then 2mg PO prn loose stool	16mg/ 24hours
<u>Second line:</u>			
Attapulgite (Kaopectate)	Ø P	1.5g PO prn loose stool	6doses=9g/ 24h
Difenoxin & atropine (Motofen)	L ?	2tabs PO initially, then 1tab prn loose stool	8tabs/ 24hours
Diphenoxylate‡ & atropine (Lomotil)	L ?	2tabs or 10mL PO q6hours	
Opium‡	L P, U	w/ long–term use	
• Opium tincture:		0.3–0.6mL PO q6hours	
• Paregoric:		5–10mL PO q24h–q6hours	

†Unlike the other opioid based anti−motility medications (diphenoxylate, opium), loperamide does not penetrate the central nervous system, & so has no significant addiction potential
‡Opioids→
  •↑Toxic megacolon risk w/ colitis

Bismuth subsalicylate specific side effects:
  Gastrointestinal
    •Blackening of the tongue &/or stool

Contraindications:
  •**Suspected or known toxin mediated diarrhea, as anti−motility medications→**
    ∘**Toxin retention→**
      −†**Hemolytic uremic syndrome−HUS risk**

ANTIEMETIC MEDICATIONS

Generic	M	♀	Start	Max
Prochlorperazine (Compazine)	LK	?	5mg PO/ IM/ IV q8hours	10mg q6hours
•PR form			25mg PR q12hours	
•XR form			15mg PO q24hours	30mg q24hours
Promethazine (Phenergan)	LK	?	12.5mg PO/ IM/ PR/ IV q6hours	25mg q4hours
Thiethylperazine (Torecan)	L	?	10mg PO/ IM q24hours	10mg q8hours
Trimethobenzamide (Tigan)	LK	?	200mg PO/ IM/ PR q6hours	

Prochlorperazine specific side effects:
  Cardiovascular
    •Dysrhythmias
    •Hypotension w/ IV administration
  Mucocutaneous
    •Gynecomastia
  Neurologic
    •Anticholinergic effects
    •Extrapyramidal dysfunction
    •Sedation
    •Seizures
  Hematologic
    •Leukopenia
    •Thrombocytopenia

Promethazine specific side effects:
  Cardiovascular
    •Hypotension w/ IV administration
  Neurologic
    •Anticholinergic effects
    •Extrapyramidal dysfunction
    •Sedation

Trimethobenzamde specific side effects:
  Neurologic
    •Sedation

•**Empiric antibiotic treatment**
  Indications:
    •**If stool evaluation is indicated, as above**
  Contraindications:
    •Suspected or known **Enterohemorrhagic E. Coli O157−H7** (Shiga−toxin producing) mediated diarrhea syndrome, as antibacterial medications (esp. fluoroquinolones & Trimethoprim−Sulfamethoxazole)→
      ∘↑Shiga−toxin production→
        −↑**Hemolytic−uremic syndrome−HUS risk**

    ∘If treatment is initially begun w/ intravenous medication, the switch to PO medication should be attempted upon clinical improvement (fever resolution & clinical stabilization) X 24hours, if an acceptable PO medication is available, & the patient is able to take PO medication
    ∘**Organism−narrowed therapy** should be initiated promptly upon stain, culture, & sensitivities results

∘The following antibiotics achieve equivalent plasma levels via PO or intravenous administration in persons w/ a functioning gastrointestinal tract:
  −Chloramphenicol
  −Doxycycline
  −Minocycline
  −Most fluoroquinolones
  −Trimethoprim/ sulfamethoxazole
Bactericidal antibiotics
  •Cell wall synthesis inhibitors
    ∘β lactam medications:
      −Carbapenems
      −Cephalosporins
      −Monobactams
      −Penicillins
    ∘Vancomycin
  •DNA synthesis inhibitors
    ∘Fluoroquinolones
    ∘Linezolid
    ∘Metronidazole
    ∘Rifampin
    ∘Quinupristin & dalfopristin
  •Aminoglycosides

Treatment duration:
  •5days. See below for suspected Clostridium difficile colitis

FLUOROQUINOLONES			
Generic (Trade)	M	♀	Dose
Ciprofloxacin (Cipro)	LK	?	500mg PO q12hours
Gatifloxacin (Tequin)	K	?	400mg PO q24hours
Levofloxacin (Levaquin)	KL	?	250mg PO q24hours
Moxifloxacin (Avelox)	LK	?	400mg PO q24hours
Norfloxacin (Noroxin)	LK	?	400mg PO q12hours
Ofloxacin (Floxin)	LK	?	300mg PO q12hours

Mechanism:
  •↓DNA gyrase=topoisomerase action→
    ∘↓Bacterial DNA synthesis

Side effects:
  General
    •Hypersensitivity reactions
  Gastrointestinal
    •Gastroenteritis→
      ∘Diarrhea
      ∘Nausea ± vomiting
  Mucocutaneous
    •Phototoxicity
  Neurologic
    •Dizziness
    •Drowsiness
    •Headache
    •Restlessness
  Materno−fetal
    •Fetal & child tendon malformation (including breast fed)→
      ∘↑Tendon rupture risk

CLOSTRIDIUM DIFFICILE COLITIS ▬▬▬▬▬▬▬▬
•Anti-motility medications are contraindicated as they→
  ∘Toxin retention→
    −↑Hemolytic uremic syndrome−HUS risk

Treatment duration:
  •10days, w/ the anticipated response being resolution of:
    ∘Fever within 1day
    ∘Diarrhea @ 4−5days

METRONIDAZOLE (Flagyl)		
M ♀	**Dose**	
KL P–U in 1ˢᵗ trimester	500mg PO (preferred over IV) q8hours	

Mechanism:
- •DNA binding→
  - ◦DNA strand breakage

Side effects:
General
- •**Disulfuram–like reaction to alcohol**
  - ◦Avoid alcoholic beverages during, & for 48hours after completion of treatment

Gastrointestinal
- •Nausea ± vomiting–10%
- •Taste changes=dysgeusia (esp. metallic taste)

Genitourinary
- •Dark urine, being common, but harmless

Neurological
- •Peripheral neuropathy
- •Seizures

Hematologic
- •Transient neutropenia–8%

OR

VANCOMYCIN (Vanco)

Indications:
- •Intolerance or refractoriness† to Metronidazole
- •Pregnancy
- •Lactation

†Indicated by failure to respond @3–5days of treatment

M ♀	**Dose**
K ?	125–500mg PO q6hours, as IV administration is ineffective

Mechanism:
- •Direct cell wall peptidoglycan binding→
  - ◦↓Transpeptidase function→
    - –↓Bacterial cell wall peptidoglycan cross–linking→↓cell wall synthesis→osmotic influx of extracellular fluid→↑intracellular hydrostatic pressure→cell rupture→cell death=bactericidal

- •Vancomycin resistant enterococci–VRE & staphylococci–VRS have developed

Side effects:
Otolaryngology
- •Ototoxicity

PREVENTION/ TREATMENT

PROBIOTICS: Living microorganisms being beneficial upon ingestion	

Indications:
- •All patients at risk for, or experiencing diarrhea from any etiology

Name	Dose
Lactobacillus GG	500mg of a lyophilized (freeze dried) bacterial preparation PO q24hours
Saccharomyces boulardii	1g of a lyophilized (freeze dried) yeast preparation PO q24hours

Mechanism:
- •Alter the intestinal microflora→
  - ◦↓Growth of pathogenic bacteria
  - ◦Improved digestion

Saccharomyces boulardii specific†:
- •The organism produces a protease→
  - ◦Destruction of the receptor site of the Clostridium difficile colonic cytotoxin (toxin B)

†The organism is eliminated from the intestine within several days of discontinuation

S. boulardii specific outcomes:
- •50% ↓incidence of antibiotic associated diarrhea

579

•Caused by the inhalation or aspiration (as there is an average of 1billion bacteria/ mL saliva) >> hematogenous spread, of microorganisms to the bronchoalveolar units of the lungs→
  ◦Inflammation=pneumonia, being either primary, or due to reactivation disease

Statistics:
  •**#6 cause of mortality in the U.S.:** Pneumonia
  •**#1 lethal infectious disease in the U.S.:** Pneumonia
  •**#1 lethal infectious disease in the world:** Mycobacterium tuberculosis→tuberculosis
  •**#1 lethal infectious disease in HIV patients:** Pneumocystis carinii pneumonia–PCP
  •**#1 AIDS defining illness:** Pneumocystis carinii pneumonia–PCP
  •**#1 lethal nosocomial infectious disease:** Hospital–acquired pneumonia–HAP
  •**#1 Intensive care unit–ICU infection:** Hospital acquired pneumonia–HAP

CLASSIFICATION/ RISK FACTORS/ ORGANISMS

COMMUNITY ACQUIRED PNEUMONIA–CAP ▬▬▬▬▬▬▬▬▬▬

•Pneumonia developing in a **relatively healthy person,** either:
  ◦**Out in the community**
  ◦**Within 48hours of hospital or nursing home admission**

Risk factors:
  •**Cigarette smoking**
  •**Immunosuppression**
  ◦Advanced age
  ◦Alcoholism
  ◦Diabetes mellitus
  ◦Hematologic malignancy
  ◦HIV infection/ AIDS
  ◦Malnutrition
  ◦Medications
    −Chronic glucocorticoid use
    −Chemotherapy
    −Immunomodulating medications
  ◦Renal dialysis
  •**Splenectomy or deficiency of the terminal complement components (C5–C8)**→
  ◦↑Infection risk via encapsulated bacteria:
    −Escherichia coli
    −Haemophilus influenzae
    −Neisseria meningitides
    −Pseudomonas aeruginosa
    −Salmonella sp.
    −Streptococcus pneumoneae

Statistics:
  •4million cases/ year in the U.S.→
  ◦1million hospitalizations

Organisms:
  •**No organism identified in >50% of cases**
  •**Bacterial pneumonia**
  ◦**Streptococcus pneumoneae–40%**
  ◦**Haemophilus influenzae–15%,** esp. in COPD patients
  ◦Atypical organisms (see below)
  ◦Anaerobes, esp. in alcoholics & others at ↑aspiration risk
  ◦Enterobacteriaceae, esp. in alcoholics & others at ↑aspiration risk
    −Escherichia coli
    −Enterobacter cloacae
    −Klebsiella pneumoniae
    −Proteus mirabilis & vulgaris
    −Providencia rettgeri
    −Pseudomonas aeruginosa
    −Serratia marcescens
  ◦Moraxella catarrhalis, esp. in COPD patients
  ◦Staphylococcus aureus, esp. as a post–viral superinfection
  •**Viral pneumonia**
  ◦Adenovirus
  ◦Influenza virus
  ◦Parainfluenza virus

580

•Pneumonia developing @ >48hours of either **hospital or nursing home admission**
  Pathophysiology:
    •Actually a misnomer as the microorganisms typically responsible for hospital acquired
    pneumonia-HAP, cause pneumonia in **moderate to severely ill patients, regardless of location**
    due to an illness-induced loss of the protective fibronectin coating of the oropharynx→
      ◦Oropharyngeal colonization by the organisms typically responsible for hospital acquired
      pneumonia-HAP
  Additional risk factors:
    •↑**Gastric pH**
      ◦Medications
        −Antacids
        −Histamine 2 selective receptor blockers
        −Proton pump inhibitors
      ◦Pernicious anemia
      ...→loss of the protective gastric acid coating→
        •Gastroesophageal colonization by the organisms typically responsible for hospital acquired
        pneumonia-HAP
  Organisms:
    •**Bacterial pneumonia-95%**
      ◦**Enterobacteriaceae** (esp. Klebsiella sp., & Enterobacter sp.)
        −Escherichia coli
        −Enterobacter cloacae
        −Klebsiella pneumoniae
        −Proteus mirabilis & vulgaris
        −Providencia rettgeri
        −**Pseudomonas aeruginosa**
        −Serratia marcescens
      ◦Atypical organisms (see below)
      ◦Haemophilus influenzae
      ◦Staphylococcus aureus
      ◦Streptococcus pneumoneae
    •**Viral pneumonia**
      ◦Cytomegalovirus-CMV
      ◦Influenza virus
      ◦Parainfluenza virus
    •**Fungal pneumonia**, esp. Aspergillus sp.

SUBCLASSIFICATIONS
•**Aspiration pneumonia**
  ◦Pneumonia developing in patients w/ a condition that predisposes to aspiration
    −Altered mental status
    −Dysphagia
    −Intubation
    −Neurologic deficits
    ...→↓cough reflex→
      •Aspiration

•**Atypical pneumonia**
  ◦A subacute form of pneumonia w/ a patchy interstitial infiltrate, for which no microorganism can be
  isolated using conventional sputum staining & cultures
  Organisms:
    •**Atypical organisms**
      ◦Chlamydia pneumoniae
      ◦Mycoplasma pneumoneae
      ◦Legionella sp. (pneumophilia > bozemanii, micdadei)→
        −Legionnaires' disease
        Acquisition:
          •The organisms are associated w/ **contaminated water supplies** via vapor
            ◦Community sources
              −Air conditioners
              −Water cooling towers
            ◦Hospital sources
              −Showers
              −Sinks

- **Atypical zoonotic bacteria—rare**
  - ○Chlamydia psittaci→
    - −Psittacosis
    - Acquisition:
      - •**The organism infects birds & many mammals**→
        - ○**High fecal concentrations**, which when dried→
          - −Human infection via aerosol inhalation of organisms
  - ○Coxiella burnetti→
    - −Q fever
    - Acquisition:
      - •The organism **infects cattle, goats, & sheep**→
        - ○High concentrations in **feces, urine, unpasteurized milk, placental, & amniotic fluid,** which when dried→
          - −Human infection via aerosol inhalation of organisms
      - Note: The organism can also be acquired via **direct contact w/ carcasses in slaughterhouses**

- **Opportunistic pneumonia**
  - ○Pneumonia caused by a **normally nonpathogenic microorganism** (including latent organisms) in immunosuppressed patients

DIAGNOSIS

•Respiratory isolation w/ purified protein derivative—PPD placement if mycobacterial tuberculosis infection is suspected. Respiratory isolation is not needed for suspected mycobacteria other than tuberculosis—MOTT infection

General
- •Inflammatory cytokines→
  - ○Anorexia→
    - −Cachexia
  - ○Chills
  - ○Fatigue
  - ○**Fever—75%**
  - ○Headache
  - ○Malaise
  - ○Night sweats
  - ○Weakness

---

†Temperature may be normal in patients w/:
- •Chronic kidney disease, esp. w/ uremia
- •Cirrhosis
- •Heart failure
- •Severe debility
- …or those who are:
  - •Intravenous drug users
  - •Taking certain medications:
    - ○Acetaminophen
    - ○Antibiotics
    - ○Glucocorticoids
    - ○Nonsteroidal anti−inflammatory drugs—NSAIDs

Pulmonary
- •Bronchoalveolar inflammation→
  - ○**Cough—85%** ± **sputum production—65%**
  - ○Pleurisy—30%, being thoracic pain exacerbated by either:
    - −Deep inhalation (including coughing & sneezing)
    - −Supine position
    - −Thoracic palpation
    - …& being relieved by leaning forward
  - ○Difficulty breathing=**dyspnea—60%**→
    - −Respiratory rate >16/ min.=**tachypnea**
    - −Accessory muscle usage (sternocleidomastoid muscles for inspiration & abdominal muscles for expiration)
    - −Speech frequently interrupted by inspiration=telegraphic speech
    - −Pursed lip breathing &/or grunting expirations→positive end−expiratory pressure—PEEP
    - −Paradoxical abdominal motion: Negative intrathoracic pressure→fatigued diaphragm being pulled into the thorax→inspiratory inward motion of the anterior abdominal wall, rather than expected outward motion due to diaphragmatic contraction

582

∘Ventilation/ perfusion mismatch via:
  –↑Alveolar dead space: Alveolar ventilation through relatively underperfused capillaries
  –↑Vascular shunting†: Capillary blood flow through relatively underventilated alveoli. Usually
    occurring, or exacerbated via ↑venous return
  …→↓diffusion of O_2 & CO_2→
    •Hypoxemia (SaO_2 ≤ 91% or PaO_2 ≤ 60mmHg‡) on room air, w/ subsequent hypercapnia
      ($PaCO_2$ ≥45mmHg) due to either:
      ∘Respiratory muscle fatigue
      ∘Alveolar hypoventilation
      …as CO_2 clearance is unimpaired (& may be ↑in the dyspneic patient) as long as
        adequate ventilation (including lack of diffuse severe ventilation/ perfusion
        mismatching) is maintained, as:
        •CO_2 diffuses 20X as rapidly as O_2
        •Hypercapnia→
          ∘Immediate brain stem respiratory center mediated stimulation of pulmonary
            ventilation, which may correct the hypercapnia, but not necessarily the hypoxia

Suggestive sputum findings:
  •Anaerobic sp.→
    ∘Putrid odor due to the amines & fatty acids they produce
  •Streptococcus pneumoneae→
    ∘Blood tinged sputum, termed "rusty sputum"
  •Klebsiella sp.→
    ∘Thickened consistency w/ mucus & blood, termed "currant jelly sputum"

---

†Being exacerbated by the supine position→
  •↑Systemic venous return→
    ∘↑Vascular shunting→↑dyspnea, being termed:
      –Orthopnea, if persistent
      –Paroxysmal nocturnal dyspnea if intermittent
      …causing the patient to either use multiple pillows or sleep in a chair
‡Age adjusted normal PaO_2 = 101 − (0.43 X age)

COMPARATIVE THORACIC EXAMINATION FINDINGS			
Physical examination	**Consolidation/ empyema**	**Pleural effusion**	**Pneumothorax†**
Chest expansion	↓	↓	↓‡
Auscultation	↓Breath sounds w/ crackles, rhonchi, wheezes, &/or egophony°		↓Breath sounds
Percussion	↓	↓	↕^
Tactile or auscultatory fremitus	↑n	↓	↕

Note: Outlining lung compression by all 3 etiologies→
      •Atelectasis→
        ∘Signs of consolidation
†If via bronchopleural fistula, may be accompanied by:
  •Hemothorax (a pleural effusion)
  •Pyothorax=empyema
‡Loss of intrapleural negative pressure→
  •Ipsilateral chest wall expansion→
    ∘↑Anteroposterior diameter→
      –↓Respiratory movement
°A patients verbalization of the sound 'E' is heard as 'A'
^Best detected over the midclavicle w/ the patient sitting or standing. The ipsilateral ↓breath sounds
should guide you, as otherwise, you may be fooled by the contralateral side being relatively dull to
percussion, assuming it to be the diseased lung
nUnless accompanied by a concomitant pleural effusion

Cardiovascular
  •**Relative bradycardia w/ viral & atypical organisms (except Mycoplasma pneumoneae)**
    Appropriate temperature–pulse relationship:
      •102°F→110bpm. Thereafter, every 1°F ↑→10bpm↑ (ex. 103°F→120bpm, 104°F→130bpm, etc…)
    Inclusion criteria:
      •The patient must be an adult w/ a temperature ≥102°F, w/ both the pulse & temperature taken at
        the same time

Exclusion criteria:
- •Dysrhythmia
- •Cardiac rate altering medication
- •Pacemaker mediated rhythm

Hematologic
- •Inflammatory cytokines→
  - ◦Leukocytosis
  - ◦Leukopenia w/ either:
    - –Viral infection
    - –Severe Streptococcus pneumoneae infection
    - –Pneumonia secondary to a cause of neutropenia
  - ◦↑Acute phase proteins
    - –↑Erythrocyte sedimentation rate–ESR (normal: 5mm/ decade aged + ♂ ≤10mm/h or ♀ ≤20mm/h)
    - –↑C–reactive protein–CRP (normal: <2mg/ L), responding more acutely than ESR, as it rises within several hours & falls within 3days upon partial resolution
    - –↑Fibrinogen
    - –↑Platelets→thrombocytosis
- •↑Lactate dehydrogenase–LDH, indicative of pneumonitis, being ↑↑ w/ Pneumocystis carinii pneumonia–PCP

Suggestive extrapulmonary findings of atypical organisms:
- •**Legionella sp.**
  - –Cardiovascular: Relative bradycardia
  - –Gastrointestinal: Abdominal pain, diarrhea, nausea ± vomiting
  - –Hematologic: Hyponatremia
- •**Mycoplasma pneumoneae**
  - –Cardiovascular: Myopericarditis
  - –Gastrointestinal: Hepatitis
  - –Mucocutaneous: Erythema multiforme
  - –Neurologic: Aseptic meningitis, encephalitis, peripheral neuropathy
  - –Outer ear: Bullous myringitis
  - –Hematologic: Hemolytic anemia, **cold agglutinins–50%**†
- •**Coxiella burnetti**
  - –Cardiovascular: Relative bradycardia
  - –Gastrointestinal: Hepatitis

---

†Cold agglutinins are acquired IgM erythrocyte cell membrane autoantibodies→
- •Erythrocyte agglutination in capillaries at cold temperatures (<98.6°F=37°C)→
  - ◦Extravascular hemolytic anemia
  - ◦Ischemia (usually affecting the ears, fingers, nose, &/or toes), which resolves upon re–warming
Etiologies:
- •Idiopathic
- •Infections: Mycoplasma pneumoneae or Epstein–Barr virus–EBV
- •Neoplasms, esp. chronic lymphoid leukemia–CLL, lymphoma, or Waldenstroms macroglobulinemia

•**Chest x ray**

Findings:

•**A new infiltrate** is the gold standard for the diagnosis of acute pneumonia, being either:
- ∘Interstitial
- ∘Lobar
- ∘Multilobar

•Pleural effusion (bacterial & mycoplasmal > viral), which if present, should undergo diagnostic ± therapeutic thoracentesis
- ∘Requires ≥300mL of fluid to be visualized via posteroanterior chest x ray
  - –Posteroanterior view: Blunting of the costophrenic angle
  - –Lateral view: Blunting of the posterior diaphragm
  - …w/ fluid usually tapering slightly up the lateral pleural wall, forming a **meniscus**, unless the effusion is accompanied by either:
    - •Fluid loculation

    Pathophysiology:
    - •Current &/or previous pleural inflammation→
      - ∘Outlining pleural layer fibrosis→**loculation of effusion** ± bulging into the lung
        - –**Interpleural effusion:** Between the lung & chest wall
        - –**Infrapulmonary effusion:** Between the lung & diaphragm
        - –**Interlobular effusion:** Between 2 lung lobes, esp. the horizontal fissure
    - •Pneumothorax, being almost always due to a bronchopleural fistula
    - …→loss of the meniscus
- ∘Requires ≥15mL of fluid to be visualized via decubitus CXR

  Indications:
  - •Pleural effusion present on posteroanterior CXR, in order to check for loculation

•Hilar &/or mediastinal lymphadenopathy

•Cavitary lesions, usually via:
- ∘Bacteria, esp. anaerobes, Klebsiella sp., Pseudomonas aeruginosa, or Staphylococcus aureus
- ∘Mycobacterial sp.
- …w/ air fluid levels occurring mostly in those caused by bacteria

Suggestive radiographic findings:

•**Bacterial pneumonia:** Dense & asymmetric infiltrate

•**Viral & Pneumocystis carinii pneumonia:** Diffuse, symmetric, interstitial infiltrate

•**Aspiration pneumonia:** Infiltrate in a lung lobe that is dependent in the recumbent position
- ∘Supine position→
  - –Superior segment of the right lower lobe
  - –Posterior segment of the right upper lobe

•**Post–obstructive pneumonia:** The right middle lobe is the most common site of obstruction
- ∘Being that a right middle lobe pneumonia may signify a post–obstructive process, radiographic resolution must be ensured via repeat imaging @ 6weeks after treatment completion

Outcomes:

•Radiographic resolution upon adequate treatment
- ∘50% within 2weeks
- ∘25% @ 2–6weeks
- ∘25% @ >6weeks

Limitations:

•False negative chest x ray is possible in the following circumstances:
- ∘**Within 24hours of infection**
- ∘**Within 48hours of Pneumocystis carinii pneumonia–PCP infection–30%**
- ∘**Severe neutropenia**
- ∘**Severe dehydration**

•Sputum must be transported to the laboratory for testing within 2hours

•If tuberculosis is suspected, **3 consecutive early morning sputum samples** must be obtained for acid fast bacillus staining

SPUTUM ACQUISITION

•**Induced sputum**

Indications:

•Nonproductive cough

•Suspected Pneumocystis carinii pneumonia–PCP, as the presence of neutrophils in expectorated sputum prevents the detection of typical cysts

Procedure:

•A nebulized hypertonic saline solution is inhaled by the patient in order to induce a deep cough

•Procedure acquired sputum
Indications:
- •Immunosuppressed patients
- •Poor response to medical treatment
- •Possible Pneumocystis carinii pneumonia–PCP
- •Possible mycobacterial infection not otherwise diagnosed
- •Unable to produce useful sputum

◦**Protected bronchoalveolar lavage–BAL**
Procedure:
1. A bronchoscope is passed through the upper respiratory tract & wedged into a distal airway. In order to prevent upper airways contamination, the bronchoscope contains a dual catheter device in which one catheter is housed within a larger outer catheter, which is plugged at its distal end w/ a dissolvable material such as gelatin
2. The inner catheter is advanced, knocking off the distal plug, allowing for advancement into the lower airways, w/ subsequent lavage w/ ≥120mL of isotonic saline
3. ≤25% of the instilled volume is aspirated back into the catheter, which is retracted into the outer catheter, w/ the entire device retracted through the bronchoscope

Threshold for a positive culture result
- •10^4 CFU/ mL

◦**Protected specimen brushings–PSB**
Procedure:
1. A bronchoscope is passed through the upper respiratory tract & wedged into a distal airway. In order to prevent upper airways contamination, the bronchoscope contains a dual catheter device in which one catheter is housed within a larger outer catheter, which is plugged at its distal end w/ a dissolvable material such as gelatin
2. The inner catheter is advanced, knocking off the distal plug, allowing for advancement of a brush into the lower airways
3. Once the brushing is obtained, the brush is retracted into the inner catheter, which is retracted into the outer catheter, w/ the entire device retracted through the bronchoscope
4. The brush is then placed in 1mL transport medium

Threshold for a positive culture result
- •10^3 CFU/ mL

•CFU=colony forming units=organisms

SPUTUM SCREENING ▬▬▬▬▬▬▬▬▬▬▬▬▬▬▬▬▬▬▬▬▬▬▬▬▬▬▬▬▬▬▬▬▬▬▬▬▬▬
Criteria for an appropriate sputum sample:
- •**Indicating derivation from the lower airways:**
  - ◦<10 epithelial cells/ lpf (X100)
  - ◦≥1 macrophage on any magnification
- •**Indicating derivation from an inflammatory area**
  - ◦>25 neutrophils/ lpf (X100)
- •**Indicating necrotizing pneumonia**
  - ◦Elastin fibers on a 40% KOH preparation

•lpf=low power field

SPUTUM & PLEURAL FLUID STUDIES ▬▬▬▬▬▬▬▬▬▬▬▬▬▬▬▬▬▬▬▬▬▬▬▬▬▬
•For pleural fluid cultures, 2 sets of aerobic & anaerobic culture mediums are recommended, w/ each bottle inoculated w/ ≥10mL of pleural fluid

•Gram stain & culture
Indications:
- •Possible bacterial infection (all patients)

•Fungal stains & cultures
Indications:
- •Possible fungal infection (including Pneumocystis carinii)
Visualized Pneumocystis carinii†
- •Trophic forms, being 1–4μm in diameter, within foamy exudates via:
  - ◦Gram–Weigert stain
  - ◦Modified Papanicolaou stain
  - ◦Wright–Giemsa stain

586

- Cystic forms, being 8μm in diameter, w/ intracystic bodies via:
  - Calcofluor white
  - Cresyl echt violet stain
  - **Gomori methenamine silver stain**
  - Toluidine blue O

- **Acid fast bacillus–AFB stain**
  Indications:
  - Suspected Mycobacterium tuberculosis infection
  Mechanism:
  - Auramine stained mycobacteria, visualized by fluorescence microscopy, resist acid/ alcohol decolorization=acid/ alcohol fast bacilli–AFB
  Outcomes/ limitations:
  - Stain positive indicates possible active disease, as **M. kansasii & M. avium intracellulare–MAI look identical to M. tuberculosis**

- **Mycobacterial culture**
  Indications:
  - Definitive proof of active tuberculosis & infectivity, as 50% of culture positive patients are AFB stain negative
  - To test for antimicrobial susceptibilities
  Outcomes:
  - **Culture negative indicates latent or no infection**
  - **Culture positive (which may require 2months) is definitive proof of active tuberculosis & infectivity**, being greatly ↑ if concomitantly stain positive

- **Sputum polymerase chain reaction–PCR**
  Indications:
  - To identify the mycobacterial species found via either acid-fast bacillus–AFB stain &/or culture
  - Suspected Chlamydia pneumoniae pneumonia
  - Suspected Pneumocystis carinii pneumonia–PCP
  Outcomes:
  - Mycobacteria:
    - Stain positive samples: Sensitivity & specificity >95%
    - Stain negative samples: Specificity >95%, sensitivity 40–77%

- **Direct fluorescent antibody–DFA staining**
  Procedure:
  - The patients sputum, serum, or cerebrospinal fluid is incubated w/ fluorescent dye (fluorescein or rhodamine)–labeled IgG antibodies against organism surface antigens, w/ subsequent washing. Matching serum antigens→
    - Post-wash trophozoite or cyst visualization via an ultraviolet light microscope
  - Being termed "direct" as the antibody binds directly to the antigen
  Indications:
  - Suspected Legionella pneumophilia
  - Suspected Pneumocystis carinii pneumonia–PCP
    - Stains both trophic & cystic forms
  Outcomes:
  - Legionella pneumophilia
    - Sensitivity: 20–80%
    - Specificity: 98%
  Limitations:
  - False positive:
    - Anti-Legionella sp. antibodies may cross react w/ Pseudomonas aeruginosa & Francisella tularensis

- **Cytology**
  Indications:
  - Suspected malignancy mediated post-obstructive pneumonia

---

†There is no serologic test for Pneumocystis carinii, & the organism has not been grown in culture

•**Cultures**
Indications:
  •All patients requiring hospital admission
Procedure:
  •2 sets of aerobic & anaerobic culture mediums, w/ each bottle inoculated w/ ≥10mL of fluid
Outcomes:
  •Community acquired pneumonia–CAP sensitivity
    ∘Streptococcus pneumoneae: 5–20%
    ∘Others: 10–45%
  •Hospital acquired pneumonia–HAP sensitivity: 10%
Limitations:
  •Careful, as source may be contaminated via:
    ∘Concomitant infection
    ∘Intravascular line/ catheter, or lack of aseptic technique→
      –Skin organism contamination

•**Urine antigen assay**
Indications:
  •Suspected atypical pneumonia
Mechanism:
  •Detects **Legionella pneumophila serogroup 1 antigen**, accounting for 70% of Legionellla sp. infections
Outcomes:
  •Sensitivity 65% during week 1 & 100% by week 2
  •Specificity 100%

•**Human Immune Deficiency virus–HIV serology**
Indications:
  •Ages 15–55years

COMMUNITY ACQUIRED PNEUMONIA PROGNOSIS & TRIAGE SCORE		
Score†	30 day mortality	Suggested Triage
≤70	<1%	Outpatient
71–90	3%	Brief inpatient–general medicine ward
91–130	8%	Inpatient–general medicine ward
>130	30%	Inpatient–intensive care unit–ICU

•25% of patients will require hospitalization, w/ an overall 25% inpatient mortality rate
Indications to admit regardless of score:
  •**Altered mental status**
  •**Hypotension**
  •**Hypoxemic respiratory failure**
  •**Suppurative disease** (empyema, lung abscess)
  •**Metastatic disease** (endocarditis, meningitis, osteomyelitis)

Point calculation:
  •**Gender:** ♂age, ♀age **−10**
  •10: Nursing home resident
  •**Comorbidities**
    ∘10: Heart failure
    ∘10: Cerebrovascular disease
    ∘10: Renal failure
    ∘20: Chronic liver disease (hepatitis, cirrhosis)
    ∘30: Malignancy†
  •**Physical examination**
    ∘10: Tachycardia ≥125
    ∘15: Temperature ≤35°C or ≥104°F=40°C
    ∘20: Altered mental status
    ∘20: Tachypnea of ≥30/ min.
  •**Hematologic**
    ∘10: Glucose ≥250mg/ dL
    ∘10: Hematocrit <30%
    ∘10: Hypoxemic respiratory failure

    ○20: Blood urea nitrogen–BUN ≥30mg/ dL
    ○20: Sodium <130mEq/ L
    ○30: Arterial pH <7.35
•**Other**
    ○10: Pleural effusion

---

†Active or in remission, being diagnosed within 1 year to the pneumonia (except basal or squamous cell cancers)

TREATMENT

•**Empiric intravenous antibiotics**
  ○If treatment is initially begun w/ intravenous medication, the switch to PO medication should be attempted upon clinical improvement (fever resolution & clinical stabilization) X 24hours, if an acceptable PO medication is available, & the patient is able to take PO medication
  ○**Organism–narrowed therapy** should be initiated promptly upon stain, culture, & sensitivities results
  ○The following antibiotics achieve equivalent plasma levels via PO or intravenous administration in persons w/ a functioning gastrointestinal tract:
    –Chloramphenicol
    –Doxycycline
    –Minocycline
    –Most fluoroquinolones
    –Trimethoprim/ Sulfamethoxazole

Bactericidal antibiotics
  •**Cell wall synthesis inhibitors**
    ○β lactam medications:
      –Carbapenems
      –Cephalosporins
      –Monobactams
      –Penicillins
    ○Vancomycin
  •**DNA synthesis inhibitors**
    ○Fluoroquinolones
    ○Linezolid
    ○Metronidazole
    ○Rifampin
    ○Quinupristin & dalfopristin
  •**Aminoglycosides**

  ○**Consider treating for possible Pneumocystis carinii pneumonia–PCP** in patients w/ either:
    –HIV/ AIDS
    –Chronic glucocorticoid or immunomodulating medication treatment

Treatment duration:
  •Community & hospital acquired pneumonia: 2 weeks
  •Pneumocystis carinii pneumonia–PCP: 3 weeks
  •Tuberculosis: See section

•Azithromycin X 5 days can be considered equivalent to a 2 week course due to its prolonged biological half–life

COMMUNITY ACQUIRED PNEUMONIA ▬▬▬
OUTPATIENT TREATMENT

MACROLIDES			
Generic (Trade)	**M** ♀	**Dose**	
Azithromycin (Zithromax)	L P	500mg PO q24hours	
Mechanism: •Affects the ribosomal 50S subunit→ ○↓Transfer RNA translocation			

Side effects:
  Hematologic
    •Eosinophilia
  Gastrointestinal
    •Gastroenteritis→
      ○Diarrhea
      ○Nausea ± vomiting			

- •Hepatitis
Neurologic
- •Transient deafness

OR

TETRACYCLINES

Generic (Trade)	M	♀	Dose
Doxycycline (Adoxa)	LK	?	200mg PO q12hours X 3 days loading dose, then 100mg PO q12hours

Mechanism:
- •Affects the ribosomal 30S subunit→
  - ∘↓Ribosomal binding to transfer RNA

Side effects:
Gastrointestinal
- •Acute hepatic fatty necrosis
- •Gastroenteritis→
  - ∘Abdominal pain
Genitourinary
- •Acute tubular necrosis
Mucocutaneous
- •Photosensitivity
Neurologic
- •Pseudotumor cerebri
Materno−fetal
- •Fetus to age 10 years→
  - ∘Tooth staining
  - ∘↓Bone growth

OR

FLUOROQUINOLONES

Generic (Trade)	M	♀	Dose
Gatifloxacin (Tequin)	K	?	400mg PO q24hours
Levofloxacin (Levaquin)	KL	?	500mg PO q24hours
Moxifloxacin (Avelox)	LK	?	400mg PO q24hours

Mechanism:
- •↓DNA gyrase=topoisomerase action→
  - ∘↓Bacterial DNA synthesis

Side effects:
General
- •Hypersensitivity reactions
Gastrointestinal
- •Gastroenteritis→
  - ∘Diarrhea
  - ∘Nausea ± vomiting
Mucocutaneous
- •Phototoxicity
Neurologic
- •Dizziness
- •Drowsiness
- •Headache
- •Restlessness
Materno−fetal
- •Fetal & child tendon malformation (including breast fed)→
  - ∘↑Tendon rupture risk

INPATIENT TREATMENT

FLUOROQUINOLONES

Generic (Trade)	M	♀	Dose
Gatifloxacin (Tequin)	K	?	400mg PO/ IV q24hours
Levofloxacin (Levaquin)	KL	?	500mg PO/ IV q24hours
Moxifloxacin (Avelox)	LK	?	400mg PO/ IV q24hours

OR THE COMBINATON OF

590

CEPHALOSPORINS: 3rd–4th generation			
Generic (Trade)	**M** ♀		**Dose**
Cefotaxime (Claforan)	KL	P	2g IV/ IM q12hours
Ceftriaxone (Rocephin)	KB	P	2g IV/ IM q24hours

Mechanism:
- •A β−lactam ring structure which binds to bacterial transpeptidase→
  - ∘↓Transpeptidase function→
    - −↓Bacterial cell wall peptidoglycan cross−linking→↓cell wall synthesis→osmotic influx of extracellular fluid→↑intracellular hydrostatic pressure→cell rupture→cell death=bactericidal
- •↑Bacterial autolytic enzymes→
  - ∘Peptidoglycan degradation

- •Certain bacteria produce β−lactamase→
  - ∘Cleavage of this essential structural component of cephalosporins & certain penicillins (as the other β−lactam medications differ sufficiently to prevent ring cleavage)→
    - −Antibiotic inactivation. This process may be antagonized by the concomitant administration of **β−lactamase inhibitors** (Clavulanic acid=clavulanate, Sulbactam, or Tazobactam)→renewed susceptibility

Side effects:
General
- •**Hypersensitivity reactions ≤10%**
  - ∘Anaphylaxis−0.5%→
    - −Death−0.002% (1:50,000)
  - ∘Acute interstitial nephritis
  - ∘Dermatitis
  - ∘Drug fever
  - ∘Hemolytic anemia
  - …having cross−hypersensitivity to other β lactam medications (penicillins, carbapenems), except monobactams (ex. Aztreonam)

Gastrointestinal
- •Clostridium dificile pseudomembraneous colitis (3rd generation > others)

&

MACROLIDES			
Generic (Trade)	**M** ♀		**Dose**
Azithromycin (Zithromax)	L	P	500mg PO/ IV q24hours

HOSPITAL ACQUIRED PNEUMONIA−HAP, BRONCHIECTASIS, OR CYSTIC FIBROSIS ▬▬▬
- •**ANY 2 OF THE FOLLOWING** in order to provide double coverage for possible Pseudomonas aeruginosa infection

AMINOGLYCOSIDES					
Generic (Trade)	**M** ♀		**Dosing†**	**Peak**	**Trough**
Amikacin (Amikin)	K	U	15mg/ kg IV q24hours	>30µg/ mL	<5µg/ mL
Gentamycin (Garamycin)	K	U	7mg/ kg IV q24hours	>6µg/ mL	<2µg/ mL
Tobramycin (Nebcin)	K	U	7mg/ kg IV q24hours	>6µg/ mL	<2µg/ mL

- •Peak levels are obtained 30minutes after the dose, w/ trough levels being obtained at the end of the dosing interval. Plasma peak & trough levels are directly related to clinical efficacy & toxicity respectively
- †Patients receiving an aminoglycoside for synergy w/ a β−lactam medication versus Enterococcus sp. should receive thrice daily dosing

Dose adjustment based on creatinine clearance (mL/ min.)
- •40−59: q36hours
- •20−39: q48hours

Obesity dosage adjustment:
- •Ideal weight† + 0.4 (actual weight − ideal weight)=adjusted weight

---

†♂: 50kg + 2.3kg per inch > 5'
♀: 45.5kg + 2.3kg per inch > 5'

Mechanism:
- •Affects the ribosomal 30S subunit→
  - ∘↓Initiation complex function
  - ∘Misreading of messenger RNA

Side effects:
Genitourinary
•**Nephrotoxicity†** (Gentamicin > Tobramycin > Amikacin > Neomycin), w/ renal failure usually @ ≥1week via acute tubular necrosis
  Risk factors:
    •↑Age
    •Cirrhosis
    •Hypovolemia
    •Hypokalemia
    •Hypomagnesemia
    •Renal failure
Neurologic
•**Ototoxicity**, being dose related & irreversible→
  ∘High frequency sound loss
    Risk factors:
      •Concomitant use w/ other ototoxic medications such as loop diuretics
      •Renal failure
      •Use >2weeks
•Neuromuscular blockade via:
  ∘↓Presynaptic acetylcholine release
  ∘↓Postsynaptic sensitivity to acetylcholine

---

†Early signs of nephrotoxicity include:
  •↓Ability to concentrate the urine (noted via ↓specific gravity)
  •Cylindrical urinary casts
  •Proteinuria
‡Audiometry is required to document ototoxicity, as the hearing loss occurs above the frequency range of normal human conversation

Monitoring:
  •Obtain baseline & serial audiometry w/ treatment >2weeks

CARBAPENEMS			
Generic (Trade)	M	♀	**Dose**
Imipinem−Cilastatin (Primaxin)	K	?	500mg IV q6hours
Meropenem (Merrem)	K	P	1g IV q8hours

Mechanism:
  •A β−lactam ring structure which binds to bacterial transpeptidase→
    ∘↓Transpeptidase function→
      −↓Bacterial cell wall peptidoglycan cross−linking→↓cell wall synthesis→osmotic influx of extracellular fluid→↑intracellular hydrostatic pressure→cell rupture→cell death=bactericidal

Side effects:
General
•Hypersensitivity reactions
  ∘Anaphylaxis
  ∘Acute interstitial nephritis
  ∘Dermatitis
  ∘Drug fever
  ∘Hemolytic anemia
  …having **cross−hypersensitivity to other β−lactam medications** (penicillins, cephalosporins), except monobactams (ex. Aztreonam)
Cardiovascular
•Venous inflammation=phlebitis
Gastrointestinal
•Gastroenteritis→
  ∘Diarrhea
  ∘Nausea ± vomiting
•Clostridium dificile pseudomembraneous colitis
Neurologic
•**Seizures** (Imipenem > Meropenem), esp. w/
  ∘↑Age
  ∘Renal failure
  ∘Seizure history

Imipenem dosage	Seizure occurrence
500mg q6h	0.2−1%
1g q6h	10%

592

PENICILLINS

Generic (Trade)	M	♀	Dose
Piperacillin–Tazobactam (Zosyn)	K	P	4.5g IV q6hours
Ticarcillin–clavulanic acid (Timentin)	K	P	50mg/ kg IV q4hours

Mechanism:
- •A β–lactam ring structure which binds to bacterial transpeptidase→
  - ◦↓Transpeptidase function→
    - –↓Bacterial cell wall peptidoglycan cross–linking→↓cell wall synthesis→osmotic influx of extracellular fluid→↑intracellular hydrostatic pressure→cell rupture→cell death=bactericidal
- •↑Bacterial autolytic enzymes→
  - ◦Peptidoglycan degradation

- •Certain bacteria produce β–lactamase→
  - ◦Cleavage of this essential structural component of cephalosporins & certain penicillins (as the other β–lactam medications differ sufficiently to prevent ring cleavage)→
    - –Antibiotic inactivation. This process may be antagonized by the concomitant administration of β–lactamase inhibitors (Clavulanic acid=clavulanate, Sulbactam, or Tazobactam)→renewed susceptibility

Side effects:
General
- •**Hypersensitivity reactions ≤10%**
  - ◦Anaphylaxis–0.5%→
    - –Death–0.002% (1:50,000)
  - ◦Acute interstitial nephritis
  - ◦Dermatitis
  - ◦Drug fever
  - ◦Hemolytic anemia
  - …having cross–hypersensitivity to other β lactam medications (cephalosporins, carbapenems), except monobactams (ex. Aztreonam)

CEPHALOSPORINS: 3rd–4th generation

Generic (Trade)	M	♀	Dose
Cefipime (Maxipime)	K	P	2g IV q8hours
Ceftazidime (Ceptaz, Fortaz)	K	P	2g IV q8hours

FLUOROQUINOLONES

Generic (Trade)	M	♀	Dose
Levofloxacin (Levaquin)	KL	?	750mg IV q24hours

ADDITIIONAL TREATMENT

VANCOMYCIN

Indications:
- •Suspected **methicillin resistant Staphylococcus aureus–MRSA** via:
  - ◦History of colonization/ infection
  - ◦Recent hospitalization or nursing home residence
  - ◦Recent invasive procedure
  - ◦Severe mucositis

M	♀	Dose	Peak	Trough
K	?	1g IV q12hours, to be administered over 1 hour	30–40µg/ mL	>5µg/ mL

- •Peak levels are obtained 30minutes after the dose, w/ trough levels being obtained at the end of the dosing interval. Plasma peak & trough levels are directly related to toxicity & clinical efficacy respectively

Mechanism:
- •Direct cell wall peptidoglycan binding→
  - ◦↓Transpeptidase function→
    - –↓Bacterial cell wall peptidoglycan cross–linking→↓cell wall synthesis→osmotic influx of extracellular fluid→↑intracellular hydrostatic pressure→cell rupture→cell death=bactericidal

---

- •Vancomycin resistant enterococci-VRE & staphylococci-VRS have developed

Side effects:
General
- •Rapid intravenous administration (over <1hour)→
  - ◦Intrinsic hypersensitivity syndrome→

–Face, neck, &/or upper thoracic angioedema, termed "red man syndrome". Occurrence does not prevent continued use, unless accompanied by an anaphylactoid reaction
Cardiovascular
•Venous inflammation=phlebitis ± thrombus formation
Otolaryngology
•Ototoxicity

CLINDAMYCIN (Cleocin)

Indications:
•Suspected:
  ∘Aspiration pneumonia
  ∘Lung abscess
  ∘Empyema

M	♀	Dose
L	P	900mg IV q8hours or 450mg PO q6hours

Mechanism:
•Affects the ribosomal 50S subunit→
  ∘↓Peptide bond formation

Side effects:
Gastrointestinal
  •**Clostridium deficile pseudomembraneous colitis**
  •Gastroenteritis→
    ∘Diarrhea
    ∘Nausea ± vomiting
Mucocutaneous
  •Dermatitis

PREVENTION

HOSPITAL ACQUIRED PNEUMONIA ▰▰▰▰▰▰▰
Prophylaxis:
•Staff hand washing
•Adequate nutritional support
•Early removal of nasal & oral tubes
•**Severe illness induced gastric inflammation/ ulceration prophylaxis**
  Mechanism:
  •↓Mucosal blood flow→
    ∘↓Bicarbonate delivery to the mucosa
    ∘↓Mucus & bicarbonate secretion from gastric mucosal cells
    ∘↓Epithelial proliferation
  Indications:
  •Emergent or major surgery
  •**Severe illness**
  •Severe trauma, esp. head injury
  Prophylaxis:
  •Proton pump inhibitors, histamine 2 selective receptor blockers, antacids, or pernicious anemia→
    ∘Loss of the protective gastic acid coating→gastroesophageal colonization by oropharyngeal organisms→
      –↑**Hospital acquired pneumonia risk via aspiration**
      –↑**Stress erosion/ ulceration mediated organism translocation risk**→bacteremia
      ...all being ↓risk w/ the use of **sucralfate**, which typically does not ↑gastric pH
•**Selective digestive decontamination**
  ∘Moderate to severe illness–induced loss of the protective fibronectin coating of the oropharynx→
    –Oropharyngeal colonization by the organisms typically responsible for hospital acquired pneumonia

---

MUCOSAL COATING MEDICATIONS

Generic (Trade)	M	♀	Dose
Sucralfate (Carafate)	Ø	P	2g PO q12hours (1hours prior to meals &/or qhs)

•Do not administer concomitantly w/ other acid suppressing medications, as ↑gastric pH→
  ∘↓Efficacy, as this medication requires an acidic environment

Mechanism:
- •An aluminum hydroxide complex of sucrose that:
  - ◦Forms a protective coating over the inflammatory/ ulcerated area
  - ◦↑Prostaglandin synthesis
  - ◦Binds to bile salts
  - ...and does not ↑gastric pH

Side effects:
Gastrointestinal
- •Constipation

Genitourinary
- •Aluminum toxicity, in the presence of renal failure

Hematologic
- •Aluminum binding to intestinal phosphate→
  - ◦↓Intestinal phosphate absorption which may→
    - −Hypophosphatemia

SELECTIVE DIGESTIVE DECONTAMINATION

Location	Prophylaxis
Oropharynx	A methylcellulose paste† containing •2% Amphotericin •2% Polymyxin E •2% Tobramycin ...applied to the buccal mucosa & tongue via a gloved finger q6hours
Distal gastrointestinal tract	A solution containing •500mg Amphotericin •100mg Polymyxin E •80mg Tobramycin ...administered via nasogastric tube q6hours

†The hospital pharmacy will make the paste

Mechanism:
- •**Eradication of Pseudomonas aeruginosa, as well as most gastrointestinal fungi & enterobacteriaceae @ 1week**
- •The normal gastrointestinal bacterial flora, composed mostly of anaerobes, is relatively unaffected
- ...→treatment & prevention of gastrointestinal colonization by the organisms typically responsible for hospital acquired:
  - •Pneumonia
  - •Urinary tract infections
  - •Bacteremia/ fungemia via mucocutaneous routes:
    - ◦Cutaneous lesion
    - ◦Gastrointestinal translocation
    - ◦Intravascular catheter

Side effects:
- •The antimicrobials used are nonabsorbable, & thus do not cause systemic toxicity

VENTILATOR ASSOCIATED PNEUMONIA−1%/ 24hours ▬▬▬▬▬▬

Pathophysiology:
- •Due to pericuff microaspiration of:
  - ◦Esophagogastric mucus
  - ◦Saliva
  - ◦Tube feedings

Outcomes:
- •30% mortality

Additional prophylaxis:
- •Avoidance of gastric distention
- •Routine orotracheal suctioning w/ continuous subglottic suctioning
- •Semirecumbent positioning of the patient

INFLUENZA VACCINE_____

Indications:
- **Age ≥50years**
- **Chronic disease**, including alcoholism
- **Close residential contact**
  - ○Chronic care facilities
    - –Board & care housing
    - –Nursing home care housing
  - ○Homeless shelters
  - ○Military personnel
  - ○Jails
- **Healthcare workers**
  - ○Including home care workers & household members
- **Children ages†:**
  - ○**6months–2years**, as the vaccine is not FDA approved for children age <6months
  - ○**2years–18years if on chronic Aspirin therapy** in order to ↓Reye's syndrome risk
  - …w/ those age <13years requiring the fractionated virus vaccine
- **Household contacts of non–immunized children ages:**
  - ○**≤2years**
  - ○**≤18years if on chronic Aspirin therapy** in order to ↓Reye's syndrome risk
- **Pregnancy**
  - ○Pregnancy is associated w/ ↑**influenza severity & complication risk**. There is also an association between influenza infection during the 2nd & 3rd trimesters & the subsequent development of schizophrenia in the child
    - –Being that spontaneous abortions=miscarriages occur predominantly in the 1st trimester of pregnancy, the vaccine has traditionally not been given during this time in order to avoid a coincidental association, unless the pregnancy will extend into the influenza season, in which case, earlier administration is preferred

Dose:
- **0.5mL IM injection qyear**
  - ○Best given within 2months prior to the **winter=influenza season**
    - –**Northern hemisphere: December to March**
    - –Southern Hemisphere: April to September
    - –Tropics: All year

Mechanism:
- Inactivated virus (whole or fractionated) or surface antigens, w/ the strains being determined annually in the U.S. by the FDA

Outcomes:
- 75% efficacious for ages 6months–60years, being ↓@ age >60years

Contraindications:
- Hypersensitivity syndrome to eggs, as the vaccine is prepared from virus grown in chick embryos

Complications:
General
- •Fever
- •Malaise
- •Myalgia
- …from 6hours–2days post–vaccination

Mucocutaneous
- •Mild local inflammation ± soreness–30%

Other
- •Hypersensitivity reaction–rare
- •Neurologic reaction

STEPTOCOCCUS PNEUMONIAE VACCINE _____

Indications:
- **Age ≥50years**
- **Chronic disease**, including alcoholism
- **Close residential contact**
  - ○Chronic care facilities
    - –Board & care housing
    - –Nursing home care housing
  - ○Homeless shelters
  - ○Military personnel
  - ○Jails
- **Prior Streptococcal pneumonia infection**

- **Children** of all ages, w/ those age <2years requiring the conjugate heptavalent pneumococcal vaccine (Prevnar), w/ doses & timing varying by age
- **Asplenia**
  - Anatomic
  - Functional
  …being best if administered prior to asplenia, w/ repeat q6years
- **2 weeks prior to immunosuppressive treatment**
  - Chemotherapy
  - Immunomodulating medications

Dose
- **0.5mL SC/ IM X 1, w/ a booster @ 5 years**

Mechanism:
- Bacterial capsular polysaccharides of 23 serotypes

Outcomes:
- 70% efficacious for 10years
  - ↓For immunosuppressed or age <2years

HAEMOPHILUS INFLUENZAE TYPE B VACCINE _____

Indications:
- **Asplenia**
  - Anatomic
  - Functional
  …being best if administered prior to asplenia

Dose
- **0.5mL IM X1**

Mechanism:
- Bacterial capsular polysaccharide conjugated to protein

Contraindications:
- **Pregnancy**

PNEUMOCYSTIS CARINII PNEUMONIA–PCP
A pneumonia supplement

•Caused by the primary seeding or reactivation of latent Pneumocystis carinii in an organ
•Pneumocystis carinii is now considered a fungus (rather than a protozoan as previously thought) based on mitochondrial DNA analysis, although it:
  ◦Does not grow on fungal media
  ◦Is not affected by antifungal medications
Statistics:
  •Being transmitted via inhalation, it is distributed throughout the world, w/ 70% of the worlds population being infected

RISK FACTORS

•**Immunosuppression**
  ◦HIV infection/ AIDS, esp. @ a **helper (CD4+) T–lymphocyte count <200/ μL**
  ◦Medications
    –Chemotherapy
    –Chronic glucocorticoid use
    –Immunomodulating medications

CLASSIFICATION

•**Primary infection**
  ◦Typically asymptomatic
Pathophysiology:
  •Pneumocystis carinii reaches the alveoli of the lungs→
    ◦Replication & dissemination throughout the body, via blood & lymphatic vessels→
      –Localized inflammation→macrophage engulfment, which cannot contain the infection→fibrotic walling off of the remaining organisms, termed granuloma formation, occurring throughout the body→subclinical infection, w/ low level replication within the granulomas, termed latent infection, which may persist a lifetime
Outcomes:
  •Immunosuppression→
    ◦↑Progressive primary infection & reactivation disease risk

•**Progressive primary infection**
Pathophysiology:
  •Inappropriate granuloma formation & organism containment→either:
    ◦**Localized disease**
      –Pulmonary
      –Extrapulmonary
    ◦**Systemic disease**

•**Reactivation of latent infection**
  ◦**Localized disease**
    –Pulmonary
    –Extrapulmonary, usually of the bone marrow, liver, lymph nodes, &/or spleen
  ◦**Systemic disease**

IMAGING

•**Chest x ray**
Finding:
  •Typically shows **bilateral "batwing" perihilar, diffuse, symmetric, interstitial infiltrates** which:
    ◦May require 48hours to become apparent
    ◦Become increasingly homogenous & diffuse as the disease progresses

•**Thoracic computed tomographic–CT scan**
Indications:
  •Normal chest x ray w/ a high clinical suspicion
Findings:
  •Extensive ground–glass attenuation
  •Cystic lesions

TRIMETHOPRIM–SULFAMETHOXAZOLE TMP–SMX (Bactrim, Septra)

M ♀	Dose
K U	PO: 2 double strength–DS tab (160mg TMP/ 800mg SMX) PO q6hours
	IV: 5mg/ kg TMP q6hours

•Ensure that the patient is receiving 20mg TMP/kg/24hours

Trimethoprim specific mechanism:
- •↓Dihydrofolate reductase action→
  - ∘↓Tetrahydrofolate, being required as a methyl donor for the synthesis of purines & pyrimidines→
    - −↓Nucleotide synthesis

Sulfonamide specific mechanism:
- •A P–aminobenzoic acid–PABA analogue→
  - ∘Competitive inhibition of dihydropteroate synthetase mediated PABA conversion to dihydrofolate→
    - −↓Tetrahydrofolate, being required as a methyl donor for the synthesis of purines & pyrimidines→ ↓nucleotide synthesis

Side effects:
Mucocutaneous
- •**Dermatitis** via maculopapular rash, urticaria >> exfoliative dermatitis, photosensitivity, Stevens–Johnson syndrome, or toxic epidermal necrolysis

Genitourinary
- •Acute interstitial nephritis

Neurologic
- •Aseptic meningitis

Pulmonary
- •The sulfite component of the combination medication→
  - ∘Asthma exacerbation in sensitive patients

Hematologic
- •**Myelosuppression**→
  - ∘Anemia→
    - −Fatigue
  - ∘Leukopenia→immunosuppression→
    - −↑Infection & neoplasm risk
  - ∘Thrombocytopenia→
    - −↑Hemorrhage risk

Trimethoprim specific:
Genitourinary
- •Blocks distal renal tubule Na^+/K^+ exchange→
  - ∘**Hyperkalemia**
- •Competes w/ creatinine for tubular secretion→
  - ∘↑Creatinine, without concomitantly ↑blood urea nitrogen–BUN

Hematologic
- •↑Homocysteine levels

Sulfamethoxazole specific:
General
- •Anorexia
- •Drug fever via hypersensitivity syndrome

Gastrointestinal
- •Nausea ± vomiting

Genitourinary
- •Crystalluria→
  - ∘Acute tubular necrosis
- •Hepatitis

Hematologic
- •**G6PD deficiency mediated hemolytic anemia**

Contraindications:
- •Neonates or near term ♀s, as sulfamethoxazole competitively binds to albumin, thus displacing bilirubin→
  - ∘↑Kernicterus risk

PENTAMIDINE (Pentam)

M ♀	Dose
K ?	IM/ IV: 4mg/ kg q24hours Nebulized: 600mg q24hours

Outcomes:
- If improvement is not evident after 5days of treatment, indicating organism resistance to the medication, treatment is considered a failure–35%

Side effects:
Cardiovascular
- Dysrhythmia (esp. w/ IM/ IV administration)
  - Prolonged QT interval→
    - ↑Torsades de pointes risk
- Hypotension (esp. w/ IM/ IV administration)

Gastrointestinal
- Nausea ± vomiting
- Pancreatitis

Genitourinary
- Acute tubular necrosis

Mucocutaneous
- Sterile abscesses w/ IM injection

Pulmonary
- Bronchospasm w/ inhalation

Hematologic
- Neutropenia–15%
- Thrombocytopenia
- Hypocalcemia
- Hypoglycemia (esp. w/ IM/ IV administration) &/or hyperglycemia

ADDITIONAL TREATMENT

SYSTEMIC GLUCOCORTICOID TREATMENT

Indications:
- **To be given w/ or just prior to 1st antibiotic dose† w/ either a:**
  - PaO_2 <70mmHg or SaO_2 <90%
  - Alveolar–arterial gradient >35

†Treatment delay of ≥72hours after antimicrobial treatment has been initiated, offers no benefit

Generic	M ♀	Dose
Methylprednisolone	L ?	40mg PO/ IV q12hours X 5days, then 40mg PO/ IV q24hours X 5 days, then 20mg PO/ IV q24hours X 11 days
Prednisolone	L ?	40mg PO/ IV q12hours X 5days, then 40mg PO/ IV q24hours X 5 days, then 20mg PO/ IV q24hours X 11 days
Prednisone	L ?	40mg PO q12hours X 5 days, then 40mg PO q24hours X 5 days, then 20mg PO q24hours X 11 days

- Both the IV & PO routes have equal efficacy

Glucocorticoids	Relative potencies		Duration	Dose equiv.
	Anti–inflammatory	Mineralocorticoid		
Cortisol (physiologic†)	1	1	10hours	20mg
Cortisone (PO)	0.7	2	10hours	25mg
Hydrocortisone (PO, IM, IV)	1	2	10hours	20mg
Methylprednisolone (PO, IM, IA, IV)	5	0.5	15–35hours	5mg
Prednisone (PO)	5	0.5	15–35hours	5mg
Prednisolone (PO, IM, IV)	5	0.8	15–35hours	5mg
Triamcinolone (PO, IM)	5	~0	15–35hours	5mg
Betamethasone (PO, IM, IA)	25	~0	35–70hours	0.75mg
Dexamethasone (PO)	25	~0	35–70hours	0.75mg
Fludrocortisone (PO)	10	125	10hours	

†The physiologic rate of adrenal cortical cortisol production is 20–30mg/ 24hours

<u>Mechanism:</u>
- •Appropriate antibiotic treatment→
  - ◦Fungal death & lysis→
    - –Antigenemia→↑**pneumonitis** within 24hours (usually within 2hours) after initial treatment
- •Glucocorticoids→
  - ◦↓Pulmonary inflammation→
    - –↓Pneumonitis

<u>Side effects of chronic use:</u>
General
- •Anorexia→
  - ◦Cachexia
- •↑Perspiration

Cardiovascular
- •Mineralocorticoid effects→
  - ◦↑Renal tubular NaCl & water retention as well as potassium secretion→
    - –**Hypertension**
    - –**Edema**
    - –**Hypokalemia**
- •Counter–regulatory=anti–insulin effects→
  - ◦↑Plasma glucose→
    - –**Secondary diabetes mellitus,** which may→ketoacidemia
  - ◦Hyperlipidemia→↑atherosclerosis→
    - –**Coronary artery disease**
    - –Cerebrovascular disease
    - –Peripheral vascular disease

Cutaneous/ subcutaneous
- •↓Fibroblast function→
  - ◦↓Intercellular matrix production→
    - –↑Bruisability→ecchymoses
    - –Poor wound healing
    - –Skin striae
- •Androgenic effects→
  - ◦Acne
  - ◦↑Facial hair
  - ◦Thinning scalp hair
- •Fat redistribution from the extremities to the:
  - ◦Abdomen→
    - –Truncal obesity
  - ◦Shoulders→
    - –Supraclavicular fat pads
  - ◦Upper back→
    - –Buffalo hump
  - ◦Face→
    - –Moon facies
  - …w/ concomitant thinning of the arms & legs

Endocrine
- •**Adrenal failure** upon abrupt discontinuation after 2weeks

Gastrointestinal
- •Inhibition of phospholipase A_2 mediated conversion of cell membrane lipids to arachidonic acid, which is the precursor for both cyclooxygenase–COX enzymes, w/ the cyclooxygenase–COX1 enzyme found in most cells of the body, responsible for normal physiologic function. Inhibition of the cyclooxygenase–COX1 enzyme→↑peptic inflammatory disease risk→↑**upper gastrointestinal hemorrhage risk** via:
  - ◦↓Gastric mucosal prostaglandin synthesis→
    - –↓Epithelial cell proliferation
    - –↓Mucosal blood flow→↓bicarbonate delivery to the mucosa
    - –↓Mucus & bicarbonate secretion from gastric mucosal cells

Musculoskeletal
- •**Avascular necrosis of bone**
- •**Osteoporosis**
- •Proximal muscle weakness

Neurologic
- •Anxiety
- •Insomnia
- •Psychosis

601

Opthalmologic
- Cataracts

Immunologic
- Inhibition of phospholipase A_2 mediated conversion of cell membrane lipids to arachidonic acid, which is the precursor for both cyclooxygenase–COX enzymes (COX1 & COX2) being responsible for the production of neuronal & inflammatory cell prostaglandins respectively→
  - ↓Pain
  - ↓Temperature (antipyretic)
  - **↓Inflammation**
- Stabilization of lisosomal & cell membranes→
  - ○↓Cytokine & proteolytic enzyme release
- ↓Lymphocyte & eosinophil production
  ...all→
  - **Immunosuppression→**
    - **↑Infection** &/or neoplasm risk

Hematologic
- ↑Erythrocyte production→
  - ○Polycythemia
- ↑Neutrophil demargination→
  - ○Neutrophilia→
    - **Leukocytosis**

PREVENTION

Indications in HIV+/ AIDS patients:
- **HIV/ AIDS patients w/ either:**
  - ○Helper (CD4+) T lymphocyte count <200/ μL
  - ○**Fever of unknown origin–FUO**
  - ○**Oropharyngeal candidiasis**
- **Patients w/, or anticipated to have a severe &/or prolonged neutropenic course**

First line:
- Trimethoprim–Sulfamethoxazole–TMP/SMX–DS tab PO q24h

Second line:
- Dapsone 100mg PO q24hours

Third line:
- Atovaquone 1.5g PO q24hours w/ meals
- Aerosolized Pentamidine 300mg/ 6mL sterile water via nebulizer qmonth
- Dapsone 200mg PO qweek + Pyrimethamine 75mg PO qweek + Leukovorin 25mg PO qweek

Indications to discontinue prophylaxis:
- HIV/ AIDS patients: CD4+ count >200/ μL X 3months, regardless of previous infection
- Neutropenic patients: Resolved neutropenia

PROGNOSIS

- Without appropriate antibiotic treatment: ~100% mortality
- With appropriate antibiotic treatment: 50% survive the first episode

602

•Caused by the primary seeding or reactivation of latent Mycobacterium tuberculosis in an organ

Statistics:
- •Infects 35% of the world's population→
  - ◦**#1 lethal infectious disease in the world**→
    - −~3million deaths/ year

RISK FACTORS

- •**Immunosuppression**
  - ◦Advanced age
  - ◦Alcoholism
  - ◦Diabetes mellitus
  - ◦Hematologic malignancy
  - ◦HIV infection/ AIDS
  - ◦Malnutrition
  - ◦Medications
    - −Chemotherapy
    - −Chronic glucocorticoid use
    - −Immunomodulating medications
  - ◦Renal dialysis
- •**Crowded living conditions**
  - ◦Homeless shelters
  - ◦Jails
  - ◦Military barracks
  - ◦Nursing homes
- •**Residency in underdeveloped nations**
  - ◦Africa
  - ◦Asia
  - ◦Latin America
- •**Other**
  - ◦Healthcare workers (including mycobacteriology lab personnel)
  - ◦Intravenous drug users
  - ◦Silicosis

CLASSIFICATION

- •**Primary infection**
  - ◦Typically asymptomatic

  Pathophysiology:
  - •Infection is acquired from persons w/ active pulmonary or laryngeal infection→
    - ◦Airways inflammation→
      - −**Cough→carriage on aerosol droplets→inhalation by others** (typically requiring several hours of exposure to cause infection)
  - •Mycobacterium tuberculosis reaches the alveoli of the lungs→
    - ◦Replication & dissemination throughout the body via blood & lymphatic vessels→
      - −Localized inflammation→macrophage engulfment, which cannot contain the infection→fibrotic walling off of the remaining organisms, termed granuloma formation, occurring throughout the body→subclinical infection, w/ low level replication within the granulomas, termed latent infection, which may persist a lifetime

  Outcomes:
  - •95% of immunocompetent patients develop latent infection
  - •Immunosuppression→
    - ◦↑Progressive primary infection & reactivation disease risk

- •**Progressive primary infection**

  Pathophysiology:
  - •Inappropriate granuloma formation & organism containment→either:
    - ◦**Localized disease**
      - −HIV negative: 85% pulmonary, 15% extrapulmonary
      - −HIV positive: 35% pulmonary, 65% extrapulmonary
    - ◦**Systemic disease=miliary tuberculosis**

603

•**Reactivation of latent infection**
   ◦HIV negative: 5% within 2years, & another 5% over the remainder of their lifetime
   ◦HIV positive: 10% annual risk
   ...→
   ◦**Localized disease**
   –Pulmonary–95%
   –Extrapulmonary
   ◦**Systemic disease=miliary tuberculosis**

•Respiratory isolation w/ purified protein derivative–PPD placement if mycobacterial tuberculosis infection is suspected. Respiratory isolation is not needed for suspected mycobacteria other than tuberculosis–MOTT infection

Lymphatic
   •Lymphatic tuberculosis→
   ◦Inflammation→
   –Lymphadenopathy
   –Lymphadenitis
   ...usually in the cervical region, termed scrofula
Gastrointestinal
   •May involve the gastrointestinal tract @ any level, esp. the:
   ◦**Ileocecal area**, which may mimic appendicitis
Genitourinary
   •May involve the genitourinary tract @ any level→
   ◦Urinary tract infection w/ **sterile pyuria†** wherein the urine culture is negative for typical pathogens
   ◦Pelvic inflammatory disease–PID
Neurologic
   •Inflammation→
   ◦Meningoencephalitis
Rheumatologic
   •May involve any bone or joint→
   ◦Inflammation→
   –Arthritis, usually monoarticular
   –Osteomyelitis, usually of the **vertebral bodies**, termed **Pott's disease**→back pain, gibbus spinal deformity, paraspinal abscess, spinal cord compression, &/or nerve root compression

†≥10 leukocytes/ hpf of centrifuged urine

•**Blood cultures** via 2 sets of aerobic & anaerobic culture mediums, w/ each bottle inoculated w/ ≥10mL of pleural fluid
   Indications:
   •HIV positive patients, rarely being positive in HIV negative patients

•**Urine analysis w/ acid fast bacillus–AFB stain & culture** via 3 consecutive morning urine samples should be obtained
   Indications:
   •Suspected urinary tract infection

•**Bone marrow biopsy w/ acid fast bacillus–AFB stain & culture**
   Indications:
   •Suspected osteomyelitis

•**Cerebrospinal fluid w/ acid–fast bacillus–AFB stain & culture** on ≥4 occasions
   Indications:
   •Suspected central nervous system infection

•**Gastrointestinal endoscopic mediated biopsy w/ acid–fast bacillus–AFB stain & culture**
   Indications:
   •Suspected gastrointestinal infection, as the presence of acid fast bacilli–AFB in the feces does not indicate intestinal disease

•**Excisional biopsy of an enlarged lymph node w/ acid–fast bacillus–AFB stain & culture**

PURIFIED PROTEIN DERIVATIVE–PPD=MANTOUX TEST ▬▬▬▬▬▬▬▬▬▬▬▬

Indications:
- •Likely recent infection
- •Risk factor for the development of active disease (as listed above)

Procedure:
- •A concentrated filtrate from heat killed cultures of M. tuberculosis is administered by intradermal injection of 5 tuberculin units in a 0.1mL diluent on the volar surface of the forearm, to be read for delayed type hypersensitivity mediated **induration (not erythema) @ 48–72hours** (although a reading obtained within 1week is accurate)

Outcomes:
- •Induration indicates latent or active mycobacterial infection

Limitations:
- •False positive:
  - ◦Previous **Bacillus Calmette–Guerin–BCG vaccination**
    - –However, being that the BCG vaccine is frequently administered in countries w/ ↑tuberculosis transmission risk, as well as its inadequate protection against the disease, it is recommended that a history of BCG vaccination be ignored in the interpretation of a tuberculin skin test
  - ◦Previous mycobacterial infection other than tuberculosis–MOTT
- •False negative:
  - ◦**Recent infection,** as it usually requires 1.5–3months to develop adequate cellular immunity
  - ◦**Anergy** (esp. w/ immunosuppressed patients)
    - –15% of infected immunocompetent persons will have a false negative reaction
    - –Administer the test w/ controls (mumps &/or candida proteins), which should be positive unless the patient is anergic
  - ◦Skin test reversion from positive to negative may indicate immunosuppression
  - ◦Waning immunity
    - –Over time, delayed hypersensitivity resulting from infection may wane→false negative reaction, which may become positive if retested within 1year, as the initial test may serve to boost a latent positive, termed the "booster" phenomenon. Thus, persons who are to have yearly testing should undergo a two–step testing procedure, w/ retesting @ 2weeks after a negative initial test, so as to avoid future confusion as to weather a positive result is due to a booster phenomenon versus interval acquired infection

PPD induration	Positive reaction
Any	•HIV positive & anergic or •Recent contact w/ patient w/ active disease
≥5mm	•Immunosuppressed patients or •Chest x ray w/ fibrotic lesions consistent w/ old healed TB lesions
≥10mm	•Non–immunosuppressed patients w/ risk factors or •Children & adolescents exposed to adults w/ risk factors
≥15mm	•All others†

†Persons without any risk factors should not be screened, as this population is likely to generate false positive results in most cases

Chest x ray
Findings:
- •Typically shows interstitial, lobar, &/or multilobar infiltrates†, usually being:
  - ◦**Apical w/ reactivation disease**
  - ◦**Non–apical w/ progressive primary disease**
  - ◦Possible **miliary pattern** via diffusely scattered 1–5mm "millet seed size" nodules

- •In patients diagnosed w/ active tuberculosis, a repeat imaging study should be obtained at the end of treatment to serve as a baseline for future reference
†AIDS patients may have atypical infiltrative patterns, such as:
- •**Diffuse interstitial infiltrates**
- •**Sole lymphadenopathy**

- •**Biopsy**
  Findings:
  - •**Granulomata w/ caseation necrosis, termed tubercles,** which heal by calcification & fibrosis

605

•The organism replicates slowly, w/ a doubling time of 20hours, w/ long periods of dormancy necessitating prolonged antituberculous treatment for both:
  ◦Active infection, to induce latency
  ◦Latent infection, to ↓potential future reactivation by 70%
  ...as only dividing organisms are killed

Mycobactericidal medications:
  •Isoniazid–INH
  •Rifampin–RIF

ACTIVE TUBERCULOSIS
•All states require that cases of active tuberculosis be **reported to public health authorities** in order to:
  ◦Provide patient education
  ◦Ensure compliance, thus preventing the emergence of drug–resistant organisms
  ◦Coordinate the evaluation of contacts
  ◦Monitor patterns of drug resistance
  ◦Identify possible outbreaks
•Empiric therapy consists of 4 medications†, being easily remembered w/ the acronym **RIPE:**
  ◦Rifampin, Isoniazid, Pyrazinamide, & Ethambutol

Risk factors for drug resistance:
  •Previous Mycobacterium tuberculosis treatment for either latent or active disease
  •Contact w/ persons known or suspected to have active drug–resistant Mycobacterium tuberculosis
  •Immigration from a developing country or other areas w/ ↑prevalence of resistance
  •HIV positive
  •Homelessness
  •Institutionalized
  •Intravenous drug user

Treatment duration:
  •**Non–meningeal tuberculosis**
    If sensitive to Isoniazid & Rifampin
      •Discontinue Ethambutol
      •Continue Pyrazinamide for a total of 2 months
      •Continue Isoniazid & Rifampin for a total of 6 months (9–12 months if HIV co–infected w/ either slow clinical or microbiologic response)
    If resistant to Isoniazid
      •Continue Rifampin, Pyrazinamide, & Ethambutol X 6–9months (9–12months if HIV co–infected)
    If multiple drug resistance (resistant to ≥2 medications)
      •Treat w/ ≥3 medications to which the organism is sensitive X 18–24months

  •**Meningeal tuberculosis**
    If sensitive to Isoniazid & Rifampin:
      •Discontinue Ethambutol
      •Continue Pyrazinamide for a total of 2months
      •Continue Isoniazid & Rifampin for a total of 1 year, w/ the addition of glucocorticoids→
        ◦↓Meningeal inflammation

ISONIAZID–INH		
M ♀	**Dose**	
LK ?	300mg PO q24hours	

Side effects:
  Gastrointestinal
    •**Hepatitis–15%,** usually being asymptomatic
    Risk factors:
      •Age ≥35years

Age	Incidence of severe hepatitis
<20years	Rare
20–34years	1.2%
≥35years	1.8%

      •Alcoholism
      •Postpartum state
      •Underlying liver disease
  Mucocutaneous
    •Dermatitis

Neurologic
- **Peripheral neuropathy−≤2%**
  - ∘Prevented by the concomitant administration of **vitamin B6=Pyridoxine**
  - Risk factors:
    - •Alcoholism
    - •Children
    - •Malnourishment
    - …all of whom may be or become Pyridoxine deficient
    - •Diabetes mellitus, which predisposes to peripheral neuropathy

Contraindications:
- •Active liver disease
- •Pregnancy

Monitoring:
- •Liver function test if symptomatic for possible hepatitis
- •Obtain baseline & monthly liver function tests in persons w/ risk factors for hepatitis
- …w/ discontinuation if severe hepatitis occurs, defined as either:
  - **•Symptomatic**
  - **•Having a plasma aminotransferase level ≥5 X normal values**

&

VITAMIN B6=Pyridoxine

Indications:
- •Peripheral neuropathy prophylaxis

M ♀	Dose
K S	25mg PO q24hours

&

RIFAMPIN

M ♀	Dose
L ?	600mg PO q24hours

Dose adjustment:
- •Body weight <50kg: 450mg PO q24hours

Side effects:
General
- •Flu−like syndrome w/ fevers, chills, headache, bone pain, &/or dyspnea
- **•Orange discoloration** of body fluids, including sweat, tears, & urine†, which stain clothing & contact lenses

Gastrointestinal
- **•Hepatitis**, usually asymptomatic
  - Risk factors:
    - •Age ≥35years
    - •Alcoholism
    - •Postpartum state
    - •Underlying liver disease

Mucocutaneous
- •Dermatitis

Hematologic
- •Thrombocytopenia

Interactions
- •The concomitant administration of Rifampin w/ either:
  - ∘**Protease inhibitors** or
  - ∘**Nonnucleoside reverse transcriptase inhibitors−NNRTIs**
  - …→↓Plasma antiretroviral medication levels, w/ concomitantly ↑Rifampin levels. To avoid this, replace Rifampin w/ Rifabutin which has ↓interactions w/ protease inhibitors (except Ritonavir) & nonnucleoside reverse transcriptase inhibitors−NNRTIs (except Delavirdine)

†Compliance can be assessed via urine evaluation for orange discoloration

Monitoring:
- •Liver function test if symptomatic for possible hepatitis
- •Obtain baseline & monthly liver function tests in persons w/ risk factors for hepatitis w/ discontinuation if severe hepatitis occurs defined as either:
  - ∘**Symptomatic**
  - ∘**Plasma aminotransferase levels ≥5 X normal values**

&

PYRAZINAMIDE			
M	♀	Dose	Max
LK	?	25mg/ kg PO q24hours	2g PO q24hours

Side effects:
Musculoskeletal
  •Arthralgia
Hematologic
  •Hyperuricemia†

---

†Compliance can be assessed via ↑uric acid levels

Monitoring:
  •Obtain baseline uric acid level

Contraindications:
  •Gout

&

ETHAMBUTOL			
M	♀	Dose	Max
LK	P	15–25mg/ kg PO q24hours X 2months, then If needed: 15mg/ kg PO q24hours	2.5g q24hours

Side effects:
Opthalmologic
  •**Optic neuropathy** (optic neuritis or retrobulbar neuritis)→either:
    ◦Unilateral or bilateral ↓visual acuity
    ◦Central scotomata, being an area of ↓vision of varying shape & size
    ◦Loss of red–green color vision
    …w/ toxicity being related to both dose & treatment duration, w/ most cases occurring @
    >2months of treatment, & resolving upon discontinuation

Dose	Incidence of optic neuropathy
>15mg/ kg	1%
>25mg/ kg	6%
>35mg/ kg	15%

Monitoring:
  •Obtain a baseline eye examination via ophthalmology, to include:
    ◦Visual acuity via Snellen chart
    ◦Color discrimination
    ◦Finger perimetry
    ◦Opthalmoscopy

Contraindications:
  •Children too young to report visual changes

SECOND LINE TREATMENT OPTIONS

AMINOGLYCOSIDES				
Generic (Trade)	M	♀	Dose	Max
Amikacin (Amikin)	K	U	7.5–10mg/ kg IM/ IV q24hours	1500mg/ 24hours

Dose adjustment based on creatinine clearance (mL/ min.)
  •40–59: q36hours
  •20–39: q48hours

Obesity dosage adjustment:
  •Ideal weight†† + 0.4 (actual weight – ideal weight)=adjusted weight

---

†♂: 50kg + 2.3kg per inch > 5'
  ♀: 45.5kg + 2.3kg per inch > 5'

Mechanism:
  •Affects the ribosomal 30S subunit→
    ◦↓Initiation complex function
    ◦Misreading of messenger RNA

608

Side effects:
  Genitourinary
    •**Nephrotoxicity†** (Gentamicin > Tobramycin > Amikacin > Neomycin), w/ renal failure usually @ ≥1week via acute tubular necrosis
      Risk factors:
        •↑Age
        •Cirrhosis
        •Hypovolemia
        •Hypokalemia
        •Hypomagnesemia
        •Renal failure
  Neurologic
    •**Ototoxicity**, being dose related & irreversible→
      ∘High frequency sound loss
      Risk factors:
        •Concomitant use w/ other ototoxic medications such as loop diuretics
        •Renal failure
        •Use >2weeks
    •Neuromuscular blockade via:
      ∘↓Presynaptic acetylcholine release
      ∘↓Postsynaptic sensitivity to acetylcholine

---

†Early signs of nephrotoxicity include:
  •↓Ability to concentrate the urine (noted via ↓specific gravity)
  •Cylindrical urinary casts
  •Proteinuria
‡Audiometry is required to document ototoxicity, as the hearing loss occurs above the frequency range of normal human conversation

Monitoring:
  •Obtain baseline & serial audiometry w/ treatment >2weeks

FLUOROQUINOLONES

Generic (Trade)	M	♀	Dose
Ciprofloxacin (Cipro)	LK	?	750mg PO/ IV q12hours
Ofloxacin (Floxin)	LK	?	400mg PO/ IV q12hours

Mechanism:
  •↓DNA gyrase=topoisomerase action→
    ∘↓Bacterial DNA synthesis

Side effects:
  General
    •Hypersensitivity reactions
  Gastrointestinal
    •Gastroenteritis→
      ∘Diarrhea
      ∘Nausea ± vomiting
  Mucocutaneous
    •Phototoxicity
  Neurologic
    •Dizziness
    •Drowsiness
    •Headache
    •Restlessness
  Materno-fetal
    •Fetal & child tendon malformation (including breast fed)→
      ∘↑Tendon rupture risk

RIFABUTIN (Mycobutin)

M	♀	Dose
L	P	300mg PO q24hours

CLOFAZIMINE (Lamprene)

M	♀	Dose
F	?	100mg PO q24hours

LATENT TUBERCULOSIS

Duration:
- 9 months vs.
- 12months if either:
  - Radiographic evidence of previous active tuberculosis
  - HIV co-infection

ISONIAZID-INH		
M ♀	**Dose**	
LK ?	300mg PO q24hours	

&

VITAMIN B6=Pyridoxine		
Indications:		
• Peripheral neuropathy prophylaxis		
M ♀	**Dose**	
K S	25mg PO q24hours	

SECOND LINE

RIFAMPIN-RIF		
Indications:		
• Isoniazid resistance		
M ♀	**Dose**	
L ?	600mg PO q24hours	
Dose adjustment:		
• Body weight <50kg: 450mg PO q24hours		

TREATMENT MONITORING

- Monitor all patients w/ monthly:
  - Sputum acid fast bacillus-AFB stains & cultures, which should be negative by within 3 months. If not, consider either:
    - Drug resistance: Recheck susceptibilities
    - Medical noncompliance: Directly observed therapy
    - Drug malabsorption
- Compliance can be assessed via:
  - Pill counts
  - Urine evaluation for orange discoloration in patients taking Rifampin
  - ↑Uric acid levels in patients taking Pyrazinamide

PREVENTION

- **Bacillus Calmette Gurin-BCG vaccine**
  Mechanism:
  - Live, attenuated Mycobacterium bovis vaccine→
    - ↓Risk of active tuberculosis (esp. in children), but does not prevent infection
  Side effects:
  - Not used in the U.S. as it may cause a **false positive PPD skin test induration of <10mm**, w/ a larger induration possible if recently administered
  Contraindications:
  - Immunosuppression, which may→
    - Disseminated Mycobacterium bovis disease

610

FUNGAL INFECTIOUS SYNDROMES
A pneumonia supplement

•Caused by fungal inhalation, wound contamination, &/or ingestion (depending on the fungus)→
  ○Primary seeding or subsequent reactivation of a latent fungal infection in an organ
•Most fungi are:
  ○Biphasic, having 2 forms:
    –Environmental temperature form: **Mold, being the only transmissible form**
    –Human tissue temperature form: Yeast
  ○Nucleus containing organisms=eukaryotic, which produce sexually &/or asexually
  ...w/ fungal infection=mycotic infection=mycoses

RISK FACTORS

•**Immunosuppression**
  ○Advanced age
  ○Alcoholism
  ○Diabetes mellitus
  ○Hematologic malignancy
  ○HIV infection/ AIDS
  ○Malnutrition
  ○Medications
    –Chemotherapy
    –Chronic glucocorticoid use
    –Immunomodulating medications
  ○Renal dialysis
•**Construction sites**→
  ○Fungal spore aerosolization

PATHOPHYSIOLOGY

•**Primary infection**
  ○Typically asymptomatic
  Pathophysiology:
    •Fungal spores reach the alveoli of the lungs→
      ○Replication & dissemination throughout the body via blood & lymphatic vessels→
        –Localized inflammation→macrophage engulfment, which cannot contain the infection→fibrotic
         walling off of the remaining organisms, termed granuloma formation, occurring throughout the
         body→subclinical infection, w/ low level replication within the granulomas, termed latent
         infection, which may persist a lifetime
  Outcomes:
    •95% of immunocompetent patients develop latent infection
    •Symptomatic primary pulmonary mycosis may→
      ○Chronic pulmonary mycosis→
        –Chronic syndrome, esp. in patients w/ chronic obstructive pulmonary disease–COPD, usually
         being ≤4months, w/ 20% progressing to respiratory failure
    •Immunosuppression†→
      ○↑Progressive primary infection &/or reactivation disease risk

•**Progressive primary infection**
  Pathophysiology:
    •Inappropriate granuloma formation & organism containment→either:
      ○**Localized disease**
        –HIV positive: 35% pulmonary, 65% extrapulmonary
      ○**Systemic disease**

•**Reactivation of latent infection**
  ○HIV negative: 5% lifetime risk
  ○HIV positive: 5% annual risk
  ...→
      ○**Localized disease**
        –Pulmonary
        –Extrapulmonary
      ○**Systemic disease**

---

†Unlike other pathogenic fungi, most cases of extrapulmonary or disseminated Blastomyces
dermatitides occur in immunocompetent persons

611

Mucocutaneous
- •Erythema multiforme
- •Fungal antigens→
  - ◦Delayed (cell mediated) hypersensitivity response→
    - –Red tender nodules on extensor surfaces, termed **erythema nodosum**, not being a sign of extrapulmonary disease, as the lesions contain no organisms

PATHOGENIC FUNGI ▬▬▬▬▬▬▬
- •Cause disease in both healthy & immunosuppressed patients

- •**Blastomyces dermatitides**
  - Acquisition:
    - •Inhalation
  - Distribution:
    - •**Eastern U.S.**, esp.:
      - ◦Mississippi
      - ◦Ohio
      - ◦The great lakes region
    - •Central & south America
    - •Central Africa
    - •The middle east
  - Likely extrapulmonary sites of infection:
    - •Bones
    - •Joints
    - •Prostate
    - •Skin
    - •Subcutaneous tissue
  - Preferred stains:
    - •KOH wet mount
  - Environmental form:
    - •Mycelia
  - Host form:
    - •Big (7–15µm), thick walled yeast w/ a single broad based bud
  - Host response:
    - •Granulomatous
  - Culture:
    - •Sabouraud's medium

- •**Coccidioides immitis**
  - Additional risk factors:
    - •**Gender:** ♂ > ♀
    - •**Color: Blacks** > whites
    - •**Ethnicity:** Filipino > others
    - •**3rd trimester of pregnancy**
  - Acquisition:
    - •Inhalation
  - Distribution:
    - •**Southwestern U.S.**, esp.:
      - ◦Arizona
      - ◦California, esp.:
        - –The San Joaquin valley, termed "Valley fever"
      - ◦New Mexico
      - ◦Texas
    - •Northern Mexico
    - •Central & south America
  - Likely extrapulmonary sites of infection:
    - •Bones
    - •Joints
    - •Lymph nodes
    - •Meninges
    - •Skin
    - •Subcutaneous tissue
    - ...w/ extrapulmonary disease occurring in:
      - •1% of infected persons
      - •10% of infected Blacks & Filipinos

Preferred stains:
- •Calcofluor
- •Hematoxylin–eosin
- •KOH wet mount
- •Methenamine silver
- •Periodic acid–schiff PAS

Environmental form:
- •Mycelia

Host form:
- •**Large spherule** (10–75µm) **filled w/ endospores**

Host response:
- •Granulomatous

Culture:
- •Difficult to culture
- •Cerebrospinal fluid sensitivity: 40%

- •**Cryptococcus neoformans**

  Acquisition:
  - •Inhalation

  Distribution:
  - •Ubiquitous, esp. in **bird feces (pigeon** > others)

  Likely extrapulmonary sites of infection:
  - •**Meninges**, being the:
    - ◦#1 site of extrapulmonary disease
    - ◦**#1 cause of meningitis in AIDS patients**, which may present w/ normal CSF findings=aseptic meningitis
    - ◦**50% of cases occur in immunocompetent patients**
  - •Bones
  - •Mucous membranes
  - •Prostate
  - •Skin

  Preferred stains:
  - •**India ink**
    - ◦Cerebrospinal fluid sensitivity: 50%

  Environmental & host form (**not dimorphic**):
  - •Ovoid yeast (4–7µm) w/ a **thick polysaccharide capsule ± budding cells**

  Host response:
  - •**Non–granulomatous**

  Culture:
  - •Cerebrospinal fluid sensitivity: 75%

- •**Histoplasma capsulatum**

  Acquisition:
  - •Inhalation

  Distribution:
  - •Central & eastern U.S., esp.:
    - ◦**The river valleys** of:
      - –Mississippi
      - –Ohio
      - –Tennessee
    - ◦**Bird or bat habitats** via fungal contamination of feces=guano
      - –Attics
      - –Aviaries
      - –Caves
      - –Coups
      - –Silos

  Likely extrapulmonary sites of infection:
  - •Adrenal glands
  - •Bones
  - •Liver
  - •Lymph nodes
  - •Spleen

  Preferred stains:
  - •Giemsa
  - •Methenamine silver
  - •Periodic acid–schiff PAS

Environmental form:
- •Mycelia

Host form:
- •Ovoid yeast (2–4μm), usually being **within macrophages**

Host response:
- •Granulomatous

Culture:
- •Cerebrospinal fluid sensitivity: 25–65%

OPPORTUNISTIC FUNGI ▬▬▬▬▬▬▬▬▬▬▬▬▬▬▬▬▬▬▬▬▬▬
- •Infection is usually **limited to immunosuppressed patients**

- •**Aspergillus sp.†** (**fumigatus** > fluvus, niger, terreus)

  Acquisition:
  - •Inhalation
  - •Wound contamination, esp. **burns**

  Distribution:
  - •Ubiquitous

  Likely extrapulmonary sites of infection:
  - •Brain
  - •Kidneys
  - •Liver
  - •Lymph nodes
  - •Paranasal sinuses, being the #1 cause of fungal sinusitis

  Preferred stains:
  - •KOH wet mount

  Environmental & host form (**not dimorphic**):
  - •**Septate hyphae** (2–5μm) w/ **45° angle branching**

  Host response:
  - •Granulomatous

  Culture:
  - •Difficult to culture
    - ∘Careful as may be a colonizer

  Disease forms:
  - •**Aspergilloma** (fungus ball):
    - ∘A hyphal mass within a pulmonary cavity formed via:
      - −A previous cavitary disease (ex: tuberculosis)
      - −Chronic obstructive pulmonary disease−COPD bullae
      - ...± pulmonary infiltration
  - •**Allergic bronchopulmonary aspergillosis–ABPA**
    - ∘Aspergillus sp. bronchial colonization→
      - −Extrinsic allergic asthma
      - −Pulmonary infiltrate w/ eosinophilia–PIE syndrome
  - •**Invasive pulmonary aspergillosis**
  - •**Disseminated aspergillosis**

- •**Candida sp.** (**albicans** > glabrata, krusei, parapsilosis, tropicalis)

  Acquisition:
  - •Endogenous floral overgrowth

  Distribution:
  - •Normal mucocutaneous flora of the:
    - ∘Skin
    - ∘Gastrointestinal tract
    - ∘Respiratory tract
    - ∘Vagina
  - •Food
  - •Soil

  Additional risk factors:
  - •Antibiotic exposure

  Likely sites of infection:
  - •Eyes
  - •Gastrointestinal tract
  - •Genitourinary tract
  - •Skin

  Preferred stains:
  - •KOH wet mount

614

Uninfected tissue form:
- Ovoid yeast ± 1bud

Infected tissue form:
- Chains of elongated yeasts (4–6µm), resembling hyphae, termed **pseudohyphae**
- C. albicans forms germ tubes & chlamydospores which differentiates it

Culture:
- Candida sp. are the only fungi often grown from blood culture
  - Careful as may be normal flora or a colonizer
- Disseminated disease sensitivity: 45%

Disease forms:
- **Mucocutaneous candidiasis→**
  - Dermatitis, esp. between juxtaposed skin surfaces, termed intertriginous areas (ex. abdominal folds, buttocks, thigh–scrotum interface, breast–underskin interface), as friction, sweat, warmth, & moisture→
    - Candidal floral overgrowth→inflammation, termed intertrigo
  - Enteritis
  - Esophagitis
  - Oropharyngeal candidiasis
  - Vulvovaginitis

  Appearance:
  - **Pseudomembranous candidiasis‡, being the most common form**
    - White curd–like lesions >1cm in diameter=plaques throughout the affected mucous membranes, being **easily removable** (thus termed pseudomembrane)→
      - Exposure of underlying erythematous mucous membranes ± hemorrhage
  - **Candidal leukoplakia**
    - Squamous cell hyperkeratosis→
      - **White lesions which cannot be wiped off**
  - **Erythematous candidiasis**
    - Erythematous, smooth, non-palpable lesions, termed patches
  - **Disseminated candidiasis**
    - **Candida sp. isolation from ≥3 separate sites** (ex: sputum, urine, vascular catheter) is presumptive for disseminated candidiasis
    - Inflammation of the tissues within the eyeball=**endophthalmitis→**
      - Raised white lesions, which may be visible via fundoscopic examination, being mandatory upon suspicion of disseminated candidiasis as it is pathognomonic

- **Phycomycosis†** (Absidia, Cunninghamella, **Mucor**, Rhizopus)

  Acquisition:
  - Inhalation
  - Ingestion
  - Wound contamination, esp. **burns**

  Distribution:
  - Ubiquitous

  Additional risk factors:
  - **Diabetes mellitus w/ ketoacidemia**

  Likely extrapulmonary sites of infection:
  - Gastrointestinal tract
  - Paranasal sinuses

  Preferred stains:
  - KOH wet mount
  - Hematoxylin–eosin stain useful for Mucor

  Environmental & host form (**not dimorphic**):
  - **Non–septate hyphae** (10–15µm) w/ **90° angle branching**

  Culture:
  - Difficult to culture

  Forms:
  - **Rhinocerebral mucormycosis**
    - Infection occurring in the upper respiratory tract→subsequent contiguous structure invasion:
      - Carotid artery
      - Cranial nerves
      - Meninges
      - Cavernous sinuses
      - Cerebrum
      - Cerebellum
  - **Pulmonary mucormycosis**
    - Infection occurring in the lungs→
      - Inflammation, termed pneumonia→contiguous structure invasion ± pulmonary embolism

•Disseminated mucormycosis, being rare

•**Pneumocystis carinii** (see section)

•Branching tubular yeast cells, termed **hyphae**, intercommunicate→
  ◦A visible fungal colony=**mycelium**
•The reproductive (sexual or asexual) body of a fungus is the **spore**
†Both Aspergillus sp. & Phycomycetes organisms have the tendency to infiltrate surrounding tissue via branching hyphae→
  ◦Contiguous spread
  ◦**Vascular infiltration**→
    −**Hemorrhage**
    −**Thrombosis** ± embolism→distal infection ± ischemia ± infarction
‡Termed thrush if oropharyngeal

SEROLOGY

ANTIBODY DETECTION ▬▬▬▬▬▬▬▬▬▬▬▬▬▬▬▬▬▬▬▬▬▬▬▬▬▬▬▬▬▬

•**Complement fixation test**
  Indications:
  •To test for antibodies to both:
    ◦**Coccidioides immitis**
    ◦**Histoplasma capsulatum**
    ...being more accurate than enzyme linked immunosorbent assay−ELISA or latex particle agglutination
  Timing:
  •Primary infection→
    ◦Measurable antibody within 1 month w/:
      −Titers <1:4 being normal
      −Titers >1:16 indicating infection (active vs. latent)
      −Titers >1:32 indicating active infection
    ◦Antibody titers measured @ ≤1 & 2 weeks of syndrome onset, showing a 4−fold↑ indicates active infection
  Procedure:
  •The patient's **plasma or cerebrospinal fluid:**
    1. Is heated to 56°C X 30 min. to inactivate complement
    2. Is then placed into a series of tubes containing successive 2−fold dilutions of the plasma (ex: 10µg/ mL, 5µg/ mL, 2.5 µg/ mL, 1.25 µg/ mL)
    3. A fixed amount of the mycelial or yeast−phase antigen (yeast having ↑sensitivity) in question is then placed in each tube, followed by a fixed amount of complement, w/ the subsequent addition of erythrocytes & anti−erythrocyte antibodies
  •Anti−fungal antibody→
    ◦Complement fixation→
      −↓↓Free complement→↓↓complement mediated erythrocyte lysis, w/ the highest dilution lacking visible erythrocyte lysis being used to determine the concentration of plasma antibody
  Limitations:
  •False positive:
    ◦Cross reaction w/ antibodies to other pathogenic fungal antigens

•**Latex particle agglutination test**
  Indications:
  •To test for antibodies to **Cryptococcus neoformans**
  Procedure:
  •The patient's **plasma or cerebrospinal fluid** is added to latex beads coated w/ anti−C. neoformans capsular polysaccharide antibody
  •Matching plasma antigen→
    ◦Visible latex bead clumping=agglutination, necessitating a mandatory lumbar puncture for possible C. neoformans meningitis
  Outcomes:
  •Cerebrospinal fluid sensitivity in meningitis: 98% in AIDS patients, 85% in others
  Limitations:
  •False positive:
    ◦Rheumatoid factor

•**Fungal skin test**
Indications:
 •To test for a delayed type hypersensitivity reaction to:
  ○**Candida albicans**
  ○**Coccidioides immitis**
  ○**Histoplasma capsulatum†**
Timing:
 •May become positive @ 2–4 weeks after infection
Procedure:
 •Similar to the purified protein derivative–PPD skin test, w/ an intradermal injection of fungal protein
  to be read for induration (not erythema) @ 48–72hours, w/ a positive result (≥5mm induration)
  indicating infection (active vs. latent)
Limitations:
 •False negative:
  ○**Recent infection**, as it usually requires 2–4weeks to develop adequate cellular immunity
  ○**Anergy** (esp. w/ immunosuppressed patients)
   –Administer the test w/ controls (mumps &/or candida proteins), which should be positive unless
    the patient is anergic
  ○Skin test reversion from positive to negative may indicate immunosuppression
  ○Waning immunity
   –Over time, delayed hypersensitivity resulting from infection may wane→false negative reaction,
    which may become positive if retested within 1year, as the initial test may serve to boost a
    latent positive, termed the "booster" phenomenon

---

†Careful as the histoplasmin skin test→
 •Anti–H. capsulatum antibody production→
  ○Uninterpretable future serologic tests

TREATMENT
•Prophylaxis, if used, is to be administered for the duration of an immunosuppressed state

H. CAPSULATUM, C. IMMITIS, B. DERMATITIDIS

AMPHOTERICIN B			
Generic (Trade)	M	♀	Dose
Non-lipid Amphotericin B (Fungizone)	C	P	1–1.5mg/ kg IV infusion over 2hours q24hours

AMPHOTERICIN B LIPID FORMULATIONS			

Indications, being either:
 •Creatinine >2.5mg/ dL
 •Refractory or intolerant of the non–lipid formulation

Generic (Trade)	M	♀	Dose
Amphotericin B cholesteryl complex† (Amphotec)	?	P	4mg/ kg IV infusion over 2hours q24h
Amphotericin B lipid complex (Abelcet)	?	P	5mg/ kg IV infusion over 2hours q24h
Liposomal Amphotericin B (AmBisome)	?	P	3mg/ kg IV infusion over 2hours q24h

---

•The lipid preparations preferentially accumulate in the organs of the reticuloendothelial system–RES
as opposed to the kidneys, thus allowing for ↑dosing w/ concomitantly ↓nephrotoxicity risk. Although
the lipid formulations allow for ↑tissue concentrations & distribution volume, none of them have been
shown to have ↑efficacy
†Also named Amphotericin B colloidal dispersion–ABCD

Non–lipid specific dosage adjustment:
 •Should renal failure occur w/ the non–lipid formulation, either:
  ○Administer q48h
  ○↓Dosage by 50%
  ○Switch to a lipid formulation

Mechanism:
 •Bonding to ergosterol†→
  ○Fungal cell membrane disruption, w/ no clinically significant resistance

---

†Ergosterol is not found on human or bacterial cell membranes, thus allowing for selective toxicity
Side effects: **Non–lipid > Lipid formulations†**
 General
  •Inflammatory cytokine release→
   ○Anorexia

  ◦Chills
   −Treated w/ Meperidine 25−50mg IV, followed by dantrolene if intractable
  ◦**Fevers**, w/ ↓frequency & severity w/ repeated doses
  ◦Metallic taste
Cardiovascular
 •Bradycardia
 •Hypotension−rare
 •**Thrombophlebitis**
  ◦Improved w/ the addition of 1,000 units of Heparin to the infusion
Gastrointestinal
 •Nausea ± vomiting
Genitourinary
 •Tubular toxicity (which may be avoided w/ hydration via 500mL of normal saline prior to, & after infusion)→
  ◦Acute tubular necrosis→
   −**Intra−renal renal failure**
  ◦**Hypokalemia**
   −May be treated w/ a potassium sparing diuretic added throughout treatment
Mucocutaneous
 •Flushing
Musculoskeletal
 •Inflammatory cytokine release→
  ◦Myalgia
Neurologic
 •Seizures
Hematologic
 •↓Erythropoietin→
  −Normocytic−normochromic anemia
 •Hypocapnia
 •Hypomagnesemia
 •**Myelosuppression**→
  ◦Anemia→
   −Fatigue
  ◦Leukopenia→immunosuppression→
   −↑Infection & neoplasm risk
  ◦Thrombocytopenia→
   −↑Hemorrhage risk, esp. petechiae

---

†Ampho B cholesteryl complex > Ampho B lipid complex > Liposomal ampho B

OR

AZOLE ANTIFUNGAL MEDICATIONS

Generic (Trade)	M ♀	Dose
Itraconazole (Sporanox)	L ?	200mg IV over 1 hour or PO q12hours X 2days, then 200mg IV/ PO q24hours
Ketoconazole (Nizoral)	L ?	200−400mg PO q24hours

Mechanism:
 •Inhibition of ergosterol† synthesis→
  ◦Fungal cell membrane disruption, w/ no clinically significant resistance

---

†Ergosterol is not found on human or bacterial cell membranes, thus allowing for selective toxicity

618

CRYPTOCOCCUS NEOFORMANS ▬▬▬▬▬▬▬▬▬▬▬▬▬▬▬▬▬▬▬▬

Treatment duration:
- **•Cryptococcal meningitis:** 3months after cerebrospinal fluid culture is negative
  - ∘Cryptococcal meningitis prophylaxis is required in all HIV infection/ AIDS patients after initial treatment of any cryptococcal infection, via Fluconazole @ half the treatment dose

•AMPHOTERICIN B as above

±

FLUCYTOSINE (Ancobon)				
M ♀	Dose		Peak	Trough
K ?	12.5-37.5mg/ kg PO q6hours		70-90mg/ L	30-40mg/ L

Mechanism:
- •A nucleoside analogue metabolized to fluorouracil→
  - ∘Inhibition of thymidylate synthetase→
    - −↓Thymidine synthesis→↓DNA synthesis→cytotoxicity to all proliferating cells
- •Not used alone, as resistance emerges rapidly

SECOND LINE TREATMENT

AZOLE ANTIFUNGAL MEDICATIONS			
Generic (Trade)	M ♀	Dose	
Fluconazole (Diflucan)	K ?	400mg IV/ PO q24hours	

PHYCOMYCOSIS ▬▬▬▬▬▬▬▬▬▬▬▬▬▬▬▬▬▬▬▬
- **•Attempt to re-establish normal host defense mechanisms**
- **•AMPHOTERICIN B** as above
- **•Surgical debridement**

ASPERGILLUS SP. ▬▬▬▬▬▬▬▬▬
- **•Aspergilloma** (fungus ball): Generally observed rather than treated
- **•Allergic bronchopulmonary aspergillosis:** Glucocorticoid treatment

INVASIVE OR DISSEMINATED DISEASE_____
- **•Attempt to re-establish normal host defense mechanisms**
- **•AMPHOTERICIN B** as above
- **•Surgical debridement**

SECOND LINE TREATMENT

AZOLE ANTIFUNGAL MEDICATIONS			
Generic (Trade)	M ♀	Dose	Max
Itraconazole (Sporanox)	L ?	200mg IV over 1hour or PO q12hours X 2days, then 200mg PO/ IV q24hours	
Voriconazole (Vfend)	L U	400mg PO†/ IV q12hours X 2doses, then 200mg PO†/ IV q12hours	300mg q12h

†Administer PO dosing on an empty stomach, being 1hour prior to, or 2hours after a meal

OR

CASPOFUNGIN (Cancidas)		
M ♀	Dose	
KL ?	70mg IV loading dose over 1hour on day 1, then 50mg IV over 1hour q24hours, w/ subsequent titration to 70mg IV q24hours if unresponsive	

CANDIDA SP. ▬▬▬▬▬▬

MUCOCUTANEOUS CANDIDIASIS

Treatment duration:
- **Oropharyngeal candidiasis: ≥2weeks**
- **Esophageal candidiasis:** ≥3weeks, to include 2weeks after syndrome resolution

NYSTATIN (Mycostatin)		
Indications:		
•Oropharyngeal candidiasis		
M ♀ Dose		
Ø P 4–6mL PO swish & swallow solution q6hours or		
1–2 troches slowly dissolved in the mouth 5X/ 24hours		

Mechanism:
- •Binding to ergosterol†→
  ◦Fungal cell membrane disruption, w/ no clinically significant resistance

†Ergosterol is not found on human or bacterial cell membranes, thus allowing for selective toxicity

Side effects:
General
- •Bad taste, which is why most patients prefer Clotrimazole (see below)

Gastrointestinal
- •Diarrhea
- •Nausea ± vomiting

OR

AZOLE ANTIFUNGAL MEDICATIONS			
Indications:			
•Oropharyngeal candidiasis			
Generic (Trade)	**M ♀**	**Dose**	
Clotrimazole (Mycelex)	L ?	1 troche slowly dissolved in the mouth 5X/ 24hours	
•Prophylaxis		1 troche slowly dissolved in the mouth q8hours	

OR

AZOLE ANTIFUNGAL MEDICATIONS		
Generic (Trade)	**M ♀**	**Treatment & prophylactic dose**
Itraconazole (Sporanox)	L ?	200mg PO/ IV q24hours
Fluconazole (Diflucan)	K ?	200mg PO/ IV on day 1, then
		100mg PO/ IV q24hours
Ketoconazole (Nizoral)	L ?	200 PO q24hours

INTRAVASCULAR LINE ASOCIATED CANDIDEMIA

Treatment duration:
- •Until clinical improvement, to include 2weeks after last positive blood culture

•Removal of all intravascular lines/ catheters

&

AZOLE ANTIFUNGAL MEDICATIONS		
Generic (Trade)	**M ♀**	**Dose**
Fluconazole (Diflucan)	K ?	200mg PO/ IV on day 1, then
		100mg PO/ IV q24hours
Ketoconazole (Nizoral)	L ?	200 PO q24hours

INVASIVE OR DISSEMINATED DISEASE

- •For genitourinary tract infection, see section
- **•Endocarditis requires valve replacement**

Treatment duration:
- •Until clinical improvement, to include 2weeks after last positive blood culture

•AMPHOTERICIN B as above

±

FLUCYTOSINE (Ancobon)			
M ♀ Dose		**Peak**	**Trough**
K ? 12.5–37.5mg/ kg PO q6hours		70–90mg/ L	30–40mg/ L

SECOND LINE TREATMENT

AZOLE ANTIFUNGAL MEDICATIONS			
Generic (Trade)	**M**	**♀**	**Dose**
Fluconazole (Diflucan)	K	?	400mg IV/ PO q24hours

•Caused by the hematogenous spread of microorganisms, which adhere to the cardiac endothelium= endocardium (both valvular &/or chamber wall)→
  ◦Inflammation=endocarditis
•Any organism, except viruses, can cause endocarditis, w/ certain organisms having a propensity to infect either native or prosthetic heart valves

RISK FACTORS

•**Gender:** ♂ 1.7 X ♀
•**Immunosuppression**
  ◦Advanced age
  ◦Alcoholism
  ◦Diabetes mellitus
  ◦Hematologic malignancy
  ◦HIV infection/ AIDS
  ◦Malnutrition
  ◦Medications
    –Chronic glucocorticoid use
    –Chemotherapy
    –Immunomodulating medications
  ◦Renal dialysis
•**Previously damaged/ abnormal endocardium–50%→**
  ◦**Left sided endocarditis** >> right sided endocarditis, as the mitral & aortic valves are much more often damaged &/or abnormal via:
    –Calcific degeneration
    –Congenital malformation
    –Mitral valve prolapse–MVP†, esp. w/ mitral regurgitation or thickened leaflets
    –Myxoma
    –Previous endocarditis
    –Primary hypertrophic cardiomyopathy, due to altered endocardial shear forces
    –Prosthetic valve
    –Rheumatic fever→rheumatic heart disease
    …all→depositon of thrombin & platelets→
      •↑Hospitability to infection by circulating organisms via:
        ◦Infection, esp.:
          –Poor dental hygiene→gingivitis
          –Upper respiratory tract infection
        ◦Mucocutaneous procedures, esp:
          –Dental procedures
          –Surgical procedures
•**Repetitive bacteremia**
  ◦Chronic bacterial infection, esp. poor dental hygiene→gingivitis
  ◦**Right sided endocarditis** > left sided endocarditis
    –Intravenous line/ catheter, including chronic hemodialysis
    –Intravenous drug use‡ ± "skin popping," wherein the drug is injected directly into the subcutaneous tissue when previously accessible veins have sclerosed

---

†Mitral valve prolapse–MVP & rheumatic heart disease are the #1 predisposing cardiac lesions in developed & developing countries respectively, due to their large incidence within the general population
‡Some IV drug users lick the needle prior to injection, thus making oral flora a consideration

The following cardiac conditions are not considered risk factors:
  •**Congenital**
    ◦Isolated secundum atrial septal defect
  •**Cardiac procedures**
    ◦Coronary artery bypass grafts–CABG
    ◦Implanted cardiac pacemaker &/or cardioverter/ defibrillator

NATIVE VALVE ENDOCARDITIS ▬▬▬▬▬▬▬▬▬▬▬▬▬▬▬▬▬▬
•**Non–intravenous drug user**
  Organisms, listed in order of frequency:
  •**Viridans Streptococci–50%**
    ∘Streptococcus mitis, mutans, & sanguis
  •**Staphylococcus aureus–20%**
  •Other Streptococcus sp., esp:
    ∘Streptococcus pneumoniae
    ∘Streptococcus bovis
  •Enterococcus sp.
    ∘Enterococcus faecalis
    ∘Enterococcus faecium
  •Staphylococcus epidermidis
  •Enterobacteriaceae, esp:
    ∘Pseudomonas sp.
    ∘Salmonella sp.
    ∘Serratia sp.
  •Anaerobes, esp:
    ∘Bacteroides sp.

•**Intravenous drug user†**
  Organisms, listed in order of frequency:
  •**Staphylococcus aureus–60%**
  •**Enterobacteriaceae–20%**
    ∘Escherichia coli
    ∘Enterobacter cloacae
    ∘Klebsiella pneumoniae
    ∘Proteus mirabilis & vulgaris
    ∘Providencia rettgeri
    ∘Pseudomonas aeruginosa
    ∘Serratia marcescens
  •Viridans streptococci
    ∘Streptococcus mitis, mutans, & sanguis
  •Enterococcus sp.
    ∘Enterococcus faecalis
    ∘Enterococcus faecium
  •Fungi
  •Staphylococcus epidermidis
  •Other Streptococcus sp.

PROSTHETIC VALVE ENDOCARDITIS ▬▬▬▬▬▬▬▬▬▬▬▬▬▬▬
•**Early:** <2months after surgery, indicating acquisition @ implantation
  Organisms, listed in order of frequency:
  •**Staphylococcus epidermidis–40%**
  •**Staphylococcus aureus–20%**
  •**Enterobacteriaceae–20%**
    ∘Escherichia coli
    ∘Enterobacter cloacae
    ∘Klebsiella pneumoniae
    ∘Proteus mirabilis & vulgaris
    ∘Providencia rettgeri
    ∘Pseudomonas aeruginosa
    ∘Serratia marcescens
  •Fungi
  •Diptheroids
  •Viridans streptococci
    ∘Streptococcus mitis, mutans, & sanguis
  •Other Streptococcus sp.
  •Enterococcus sp.
    ∘Enterococcus faecalis
    ∘Enterococcus faecium

623

- **Late:** >2months after surgery, indicating hematogenous acquisition
  Organisms, listed in order of frequency:
  - **Viridans Streptococci−25%**
    - ∘Streptococcus mitis, mutans, & sanguis
  - **Staphylococcus epidermidis−20%**
  - **Staphylococcus aureus**
  - **Enterococcus sp.**
    - ∘Enterococcus faecalis
    - ∘Enterococcus faecium
  - **Enterobacteriaceae**
    - ∘Escherichia coli
    - ∘Enterobacter cloacae
    - ∘Klebsiella pneumoniae
    - ∘Proteus mirabilis & vulgaris
    - ∘Providencia rettgeri
    - ∘Pseudomonas aeruginosa
    - ∘Serratia marcescens
  - **Other Streptococcus sp.**

SUBCLASSIFICATION

- **Acute bacterial endocarditis**
  - ∘Caused by more virulent organisms, esp. **Staphylococcus sp.**, tending to cause acute disease, being a syndrome <1month
- **Subacute bacterial endocarditis**
  - ∘Caused by less virulent organisms, esp.:
    - **−Streptococcus sp.**
    - −Enterococcus faecalis
    - −Coagulase−negative Staphylococcus sp.
    - −Enterobacteriaceae
    - −Fungi
    ...which tend to cause subacute disease, being a syndrome >1month

- **Culture negative endocarditis <5%**
  - ∘**Recent antimicrobial exposure−#1 cause**
    - −However, >90% of blood cultures are positive for organisms even after several antibiotic doses have been administered
  - ∘**HACEK group infection:** Oxacillin resistant, fastidious, gram negative, non−enteric organisms which typically produce a syndrome of chronic disease, being composed of:
    - −Haemophilus sp. (aphrophilus, parainfluenzae, paraphrophilus)
    - −Actinobacillus actinomycetemcomitans
    - −Cardiobacterium hominis
    - −Eikenella corrodens
    - −Kingella kingae
  - ∘**Other organisms**
    - −Abiotrophia sp. (previously classified as nutritionally deficient streptococci)
    - −Bartonella sp. (esp. henselae & quintana)
    - −Brucella sp. (esp. abortus & melitensis)
    - −Chlamydia psittaci & trachomatis
    - −Coxiella burnetti
    - −Legionella sp.
    - −Rickettsiae sp.
    - −Tropheryma whipplei

---

†Although polymicrobial infective endocarditis is uncommon, it is encountered most often in association w/ intravenous drug use

General
- •Inflammatory cytokines→
  - ◦Anorexia→
    - –Cachexia
  - ◦Chills
  - ◦Fatigue
  - ◦**Fever–85%†**, being intermittent & low grade @ 101–102°F
    - –Endocarditis accounts for 8% of cases of fever of unknown origin–FUO, as untreated subacute bacterial endocarditis may continue undetected for up to 1.5years
  - ◦Headache
  - ◦Malaise
  - ◦Night sweats
  - ◦Weakness

---

†Temperature may be normal in patients w/:
- •Chronic kidney disease, esp. w/ uremia
- •Cirrhosis
- •Heart failure
- •Severe debility
- …or those who are:
  - •Intravenous drug users
  - •Taking certain medications:
    - ◦Acetaminophen
    - ◦Antibiotics
    - ◦Glucocorticoids
    - ◦Nonsteroidal anti–inflammatory drugs–NSAIDs

Cardiovascular
- •Valve damage→
  - ◦**New or changing regurgitant murmur–85%**
  - ◦**Heart failure**, w/ aortic valve > mitral valve > other valve infection
- •Intracardiac extension of infection→
  - ◦Conduction abnormalities=dysrhythmias

Gastrointestinal
- •Splenomegally (subacute disease–50% > acute disease–20%)
- •Hepatitis
- •**Septic thromboemboli**, having a propensity to travel to the spleen & mesentery→
  - ◦Abscess formation
  - ◦Distal infarction
    - –**Splenic infarct**→left upper quadrant abdominal pain, friction rub, &/or splenic abscess
    - …both of which should be considered if the patient remains febrile despite appropriate antibiotics

Genitourinary
- •Septic thromboemboli &/or immune complex deposition→
  - ◦**Glomerulonephritis**→
    - –Proteinuria
    - –Hematuria (>5 erythrocytes/ hpf)
    - –Pyuria (>5 leukocytes/ hpf)
    - –Erythrocyte casts
    - …w/ the subsequent development of:
      - •Intra–renal renal failure

Mucocutaneous
- •**Septic thromboemboli**→
  - ◦**Janeway lesions: Non–tender** red macules & papules on the palms & soles
- •**Circulating immune complexes**→
  - ◦**Osler's nodes: Tender**, raised subcutaneous lesions (usually being red @ ≤3days & brownish thereafter) in the:
    - –Pads of the fingers & toes
    - –Thenar eminence
    - …occurring in subacute disease–25% >> acute disease
  - ◦**Splinter hemorrhages: Non–tender** linear lesions (usually being red @ ≤3days & brownish thereafter) in the proximal nail beds, being parallel to the long axis of the finger or toe

- ∘**Mucocutaneous petechiae**, esp involving the:
  - −Conjunctiva
  - −Distal extremities
  - −Oral mucosa
  - −Retina w/ central pallor, termed **Roth's spots**
  - −Upper chest

Musculoskeletal
- •Septic thromboemboli &/or immune complex deposition→
  - ∘Arthritis
- •Subacute endocarditis→
  - ∘Clubbing of the digits (fingers &/or toes)

Neurologic−30%
- •Septic thromboemboli→
  - ∘**Cerebrovascular accident syndrome**, esp. involving the middle cerebral arterial system
- •Hematogenous organism spread, septic thromboemboli, &/or immune complex deposition→
  - ∘Endothelial &/or vasa vasorum impaction, esp. @ arterial branch points→
    - −Central nervous system abscess
    - −Encephalitis
    - −Meningitis
    - −**Mycotic aneurysm formation**, being asymptomatic until rupture→subarachnoid hemorrhage→severe headache ± coma

Pulmonary
- •Pulmonary disease is due to either:
  - ∘Right sided endocarditis
  - ∘Left sided w/ either:
    - −Atrial septal defect−ASD
    - −Ventricular septal defect−VSD
    - −Patent ductus arteriosus−PDA
    - …w/ septic thromboemboli→
      - •Pulmonary infarction
    - …w/ both septic thromboemboli &/or immune complex deposition→
      - •Multiple pulmonary abscesses, esp. @ the lung periphery
      - •Pneumonia

Hematologic
- •Inflammatory cytokines→
  - ∘Leukocytosis (acute > subacute endocarditis)
  - ∘↑Acute phase proteins
    - −↑Erythrocyte sedimentation rate−ESR (normal: 5mm/ decade aged + ♂ ≤10mm/h or ♀ ≤20mm/h)
    - −↑C−reactive protein−CRP (normal: <2mg/ L), responding more acutely than ESR, as it rises within several hours & falls within 3days upon partial resolution
    - −↑Fibrinogen
    - −↑Platelets→thrombocytosis
- •Anemia via:
  - ∘Vegetation mediated hemolysis
  - ∘Subacute endocarditis→
    - −Anemia of chronic inflammatory disease, being normocytic & normochromic
- •↑Antibody production→
  - ∘Polyclonal hypergammaglobulinemia→hypocomplementemia, esp. of C3 & C4→↑infection risk via encapsulated bacteria:
    - −Escherichia coli
    - −Haemophilus influenzae
    - −Neisseria meningitides
    - −Pseudomonas aeruginosa
    - −Salmonella sp.
    - −Streptococcus pneumoniae
  - ∘Antinuclear antibody−ANA production
  - ∘Rheumatoid factor production (subacute > acute endocarditis), being positive w/ a titer of ≥1:80
    - −Antibody towards the Fc portion of IgG, being either IgA, IgE, IgG, or IgM, w/ standard tests best at detecting IgM
    - <u>Limitations:</u>
      - •Titer does not correlate w/ disease activity
      - •False negative:
        - ∘Other Ig types

- •False positive:
  - ○Autoimmune diseases
  - ○Interstitial pulmonary fibrosis
  - ○Liver disease
  - ○5−10% of healthy adults

MODIFIED DUKE UNIVERSITY CRITERIA FOR INFECTIVE ENDOCARDITIS:
- •The presence of either:
  - ○2 major criteria
  - ○1 major & 3 minor criteria
  - ○5 minor criteria
  - ...indicate an 80% likelihood

Major criteria	Minor criteria
•**Sustained bacteremia** via either: ○Positive blood cultures X 2sets by a typical organism ○1 positive blood culture for Coxiella burnetti •**Antiphase1 IgG antibody titer >1:800** •**Endocardial involvement** per echocardiogram, via either: ○Vegetations seen as a discrete, echogenic, oscillating, intracardiac mass ○Valve perforation ○Abscess ○Prosthetic valve dehiscence ○New valvular regurgitation −Changes in a pre−existing murmur are not sufficient	•**Presence of a risk factor** (see above) •**Fever** >100.4°F = 38°C •**Vascular phenomenon** via either: ○Septic arterial or pulmonary emboli ○Mycotic aneurysm ○Intracranial hemorrhage ○Conjunctival hemorrhage ○Janeway lesions •**Immune complex deposition** via either: ○Glomerulonephritis ○Osler's nodes ○Roth's spots •**Autoantibody production** via: ○Rheumatoid factor positivity •**Positive blood cultures not meeting major criteria** •**Serologic evidence of active infection by a typical organism**

BLOOD CULTURES

Procedure:
- •3 sets of aerobic & anaerobic culture mediums, w/:
  - ○Each set drawn from a different site, ideally spaced ≥1 hour apart (5min. apart if hemodynamically unstable)
  - ○Each bottle inoculated w/ ≥10mL of blood

Outcomes:
- •Typical pathogens can be isolated within days, whereas the HACEK group may take several weeks.
  - ○If negative, or if fastidious organisms are suspected, ask the laboratory to hold the cultures for several weeks

Limitations:
- •Careful, as source may be contaminated via:
  - ○Concomitant infection
  - ○Intravascular line/ catheter, or lack of aseptic technique→
    - −Skin organism contamination

Staphylococcal sp. laboratory features:
- •All are:
  - ○**Gram positive cocci in clusters**
  - ○Catalase enzyme production positive
- •Only Staphylococcus aureus
  - ○Is coagulase enzyme production positive
  - ○Produces a beta erythrocyte hemolytic pattern, whereas the others are gamma hemolytic

Streptococcal sp. laboratory features:
- •All are:
  - ○**Gram positive cocci in chains**
  - ○Catalase enzyme production negative
- •Hemolysis pattern:
  - ○Alpha
    - −Streptococcus pneumoniae
    - −Viridan's streptococci
  - ○Beta
    - −Streptococcus agalactiae & pyogenes

627

○Alpha or gamma
  –Streptococcus bovis†
○Alpha, beta, or gamma
  –All other streptococci

•Alpha hemolysis is indicated by incomplete enzyme mediated erythrocyte lysis→
  ○Peri–colony green zone
•Beta homolysis is indicated by complete enzyme mediated erythrocyte lysis→
  ○Peri–colony clear zone
•Gamma hemolysis is indicated by lack of erythrocyte lysis
†**Streptococcus bovis** bacteremia or endocarditis requires a colonoscopy to search for a possible colorectal neoplasm (cancer or polyp), being found in 20% of patients

IMAGING

•**Transthoracic echocardiography–TTE**
  Procedure:
  •A 2 dimensional ultrasonographic image, allowing real time visualization of:
    ○Ventricular wall thickness
    ○Cavity size (both atrial & ventricular)
    ○Myocardial & valve function, allowing ejection fraction–EF estimation (% of end diastolic volume ejected during ventricular systole)
    ○The pericardial space
  •Doppler ultrasonography uses Doppler shift to detect vessel flow velocity→
    ○Valve regurgitation visualization
    ○Estimation of valve pressure gradients
  Findings:
  •Vegetations† (fungi & HACEK organisms causing large vegetations), which occur on the:
    ○Valves, being the #1 site→
      –Valve damage ± regurgitation
    ○Mural endocardium
    ○Chordae tendineae→
      –Rupture
    ○Septal defect
  •Prosthetic valve dehiscence
  •Heart failure
  Limitations:
  •↓Visualization in obese or emphysematous patients
  •May not allow adequate:
    ○Visualization of the anterior aspect of a prosthetic aortic valve
    ○Functional assessment of a prosthetic aortic valve
  •Transesophageal echocardiography–TEE is more sensitive in detecting:
    ○Thrombotic ± infectious vegetations
    ○Abscesses
    ○Valve damage
    …esp. in a patient w/ a prosthetic heart valve. However, transthoracic echocardiography is the initial test of choice due to its noninvasive nature, as transesophageal echocardiography may→
      •Pharyngeal swallow receptor mediated reflex:
        ○Bradycardia
        ○Hypotension

---

†Vegetations may persist unchanged for several years after clinical cure

ELECTRICAL STUDIES

•**Electrocardiography–ECG**
  Indications:
  •A baseline & subsequent surveillance electrocardiography–ECG should be performed q24h while the patient is febrile. Then, periodically during treatment w/ particular attention to the **PR interval†**, as prolongation may signify the development of a valvular ring abscess

---

†**PR interval:** Beginning of the P wave to the beginning of the QRS wave, representing the time it takes for atrial depolarization to reach the ventricles (normal: 0.12–0.2 sec=3–5small boxes)

628

•**Empiric intravenous antibiotics**
  ◦After blood cultures have been obtained, begin intravenous treatment promptly w/ bactericidal antibiotics, as the organism must be killed by the antibiotic alone, without help from neutrophils, which have great difficulty infiltrating the vegetation. Antibiotic treatment also→
    −↓Septic thromboembolic phenomena†
  ◦**Gentamycin** is added to all the treatment regimens due to its synergistic bactericidal effect w/ penicillins→
    −↑Killing
    −↓Resistance emergence
  ◦Anticoagulation treatment in patients w/ prosthetic valves should be continued unless cerebral thromboembolization occurs, w/ reinstitution @ 72hours if there is no evidence of intracerebral hemorrhage
  ◦**Surveillance blood cultures** of ≥2sets should be obtained after 48hours of appropriate antibiotic treatment in order to document organism clearance, w/ repeat cultures every 24−48hours until negative (which should occur within 2−5days of appropriate treatment)
  ◦The switch to PO medication should be attempted upon clinical improvement via fever resolution (usually within 1week, but may persist for 3weeks) & clinical stabilization X 24hours, if an acceptable PO medication is available, & the patient is able to take PO medication
  ◦**Organism−narrowed therapy** should be initiated promptly upon stain, culture, & sensitivities results
  ◦The following antibiotics achieve equivalent plasma levels via PO or intravenous administration in persons w/ a functioning gastrointestinal tract:
    −Chloramphenicol
    −Doxycycline
    −Minocycline
    −Most fluoroquinolones
    −Trimethoprim/ Sulfamethoxazole

Bactericidal antibiotics
  •**Cell wall synthesis inhibitors**
    ◦β lactam medications:
      −Carbapenems
      −Cephalosporins
      −Monobactams
      −Penicillins
    ◦Vancomycin
  •**DNA synthesis inhibitors**
    ◦Fluoroquinolones
    ◦Linezolid
    ◦Metronidazole
    ◦Rifampin
    ◦Quinupristin & dalfopristin
  •**Aminoglycosides**

Treatment duration:
  •**All forms: 4−6weeks‡**, w/ the aminoglycoside used for the initial 2weeks, except w/ enterococcal sp. or HACEK organism endocarditis, for which it is used the entire duration of treatment
  •Cure can only be confirmed upon antimicrobial cessation, w/ subsequent passage of 2months without recurrence of organisemia
    ◦Obtain blood cultures @ 1, 2, 4, & 8 weeks post−treatment to monitor for recurrence

---

†Anticoagulant therapy→
  •†Intracranial hemorrhage risk, & has not been shown to prevent vegetative embolic phenomenon. In the presence of intracranial hemorrhage or mycotic aneurysm formation, chronic anticoagulation therapy should be discontinued until the complications have been treated
‡Uncomplicated Staphylococcus sp. mediated right sided endocarditis may be treated via a 2week course

AMINOGLYCOSIDES

Generic (Trade)	M	♀	Dosing†	Peak	Trough
Gentamycin (Garamycin)	K	U	7mg/ kg IV q24hours	>6μg/ mL	<2μg/ mL

•Peak levels are obtained 30minutes after the dose, w/ trough levels being obtained at the end of the dosing interval. Plasma peak & trough levels are directly related to clinical efficacy & toxicity respectively
†Patients receiving an aminoglycoside for synergy w/ a β−lactam medication versus Enterococcus sp. should receive thrice daily dosing

Dose adjustment based on creatinine clearance (mL/ min.)
  •40−59: q36hours
  •20−39: q48hours

Obesity dosage adjustment:
  •Ideal weight† + 0.4 (actual weight − ideal weight)=adjusted weight

†♂: 50kg + 2.3kg per inch > 5'
  ♀: 45.5kg + 2.3kg per inch > 5'

Mechanism:
  •Affects the ribosomal 30S subunit→
    ○↓Initiation complex function
    ○Misreading of messenger RNA

Side effects:
  Genitourinary
  •**Nephrotoxicity†** (Gentamicin > Tobramycin > Amikacin > Neomycin), w/ renal failure usually @ ≥1week via acute tubular necrosis
    Risk factors:
      •↑Age
      •Cirrhosis
      •Hypovolemia
      •Hypokalemia
      •Hypomagnesemia
      •Renal failure
  Neurologic
  •**Ototoxicity,** being dose related & irreversible→
    ○High frequency sound loss
    Risk factors:
      •Concomitant use w/ other ototoxic medications such as loop diuretics
      •Renal failure
      •Use >2weeks
  •Neuromuscular blockade via:
    ○↓Presynaptic acetylcholine release
    ○↓Postsynaptic sensitivity to acetylcholine

†Early signs of nephrotoxicity include:
  •↓Ability to concentrate the urine (noted via ↓specific gravity)
  •Cylindrical urinary casts
  •Proteinuria
‡Audiometry is required to document ototoxicity, as the hearing loss occurs above the frequency range of normal human conversation

Monitoring:
  •Obtain baseline & serial audiometry w/ treatment >2weeks

PENICILLINS: To ensure adequate coverage of Enterococcus sp.

Generic (Trade)	M	♀	Dose
Ampicillin (Principen)	K	P	12g/ 24hours via continuous IV infusion or 3g IV q4hours

Mechanism:
- •A β-lactam ring structure which binds to bacterial transpeptidase→
  - ○↓Transpeptidase function→
    - −↓Bacterial cell wall peptidoglycan cross-linking→↓cell wall synthesis→osmotic influx of extracellular fluid→↑intracellular hydrostatic pressure→cell rupture→cell death=bactericidal
- •↑Bacterial autolytic enzymes→
  - ○Peptidoglycan degradation

- •Certain bacteria produce β-lactamase→
  - ○Cleavage of this essential structural component of cephalosporins & certain penicillins (as the other β-lactam medications differ sufficiently to prevent ring cleavage)→
    - −Antibiotic inactivation. This process may be antagonized by the concomitant administration of β-lactamase inhibitors (Clavulanic acid=clavulanate, Sulbactam, or Tazobactam)→renewed susceptibility

Side effects:
General
- •**Hypersensitivity reactions ≤10%**
  - ○Anaphylaxis−0.5%→
    - −Death−0.002% (1:50,000)
  - ○Acute interstitial nephritis
  - ○Dermatitis
  - ○Drug fever
  - ○Hemolytic anemia
  - …having cross−hypersensitivity to other β lactam medications (cephalosporins, carbapenems), except monobactams (ex. Aztreonam)

& EITHER

PENICILLINS

Generic (Trade)	M	♀	Dose
Nafcillin (Nallpen)	L	P	2g IV q4hours
Oxacillin (Bactocill)	KL	P	2g IV q4hours

OR

VANCOMYCIN

Indications:
- •Suspected **methicillin resistant Staphylococcus aureus−MRSA** via:
  - ○History of colonization/ infection
  - ○Intravascular line mediated infection
  - ○Recent hospitalization or nursing home residence
  - ○Recent invasive procedure
  - ○Severe mucositis

M	♀	Dose	Peak	Trough
K	?	1g IV q12hours, to be administered over 1hour	30−40µg/ mL	>5µg/ mL

- •Peak levels are obtained 30minutes after the dose, w/ trough levels being obtained at the end of the dosing interval. Plasma peak & trough levels are directly related to toxicity & clinical efficacy respectively

Mechanism:
- •Direct cell wall peptidoglycan binding→
  - ○↓Transpeptidase function→
    - −↓Bacterial cell wall peptidoglycan cross-linking→↓cell wall synthesis→osmotic influx of extracellular fluid→↑intracellular hydrostatic pressure→cell rupture→cell death=bactericidal

---

- •Vancomycin resistant enterococci−VRE & staphylococci−VRS have developed

Side effects:
General
- •Rapid intravenous administration (over <1hour)→
  - ○Intrinsic hypersensitivity syndrome→
    - −Face, neck, &/or upper thoracic angioedema, termed "red man syndrome". Occurrence does not prevent continued use, unless accompanied by an anaphylactoid reaction

631

Cardiovascular
•Venous inflammation=phlebitis ± thrombus formation
Otolaryngology
•Ototoxicity

ADDITIONAL TREATMENT FOR PROSTHETIC VALVE ENDOCARDITIS

VANCOMYCIN

M ♀	Dose	Peak	Trough
K ?	1g IV q12hours, to be administered over 1 hour	30–40µg/ mL	>5µg/ mL

&

RIFAMPIN

M ♀	Dose
L ?	300mg PO q8hours

Side effects:
General
•Flu–like syndrome w/ fevers, chills, headache, bone pain, &/or dyspnea
•**Orange discoloration** of body fluids, including sweat, tears, & urine†, which stain clothing &
  contact lenses
Gastrointestinal
•**Hepatitis,** usually asymptomatic
  Risk factors:
    •Age ≥35years
    •Alcoholism
    •Postpartum state
    •Underlying liver disease
Mucocutaneous
•Dermatitis
Hematologic
•Thrombocytopenia
Interactions
•The concomitant administration of Rifampin w/ either:
  ∘**Protease inhibitors** or
  ∘**Nonnucleoside reverse transcriptase inhibitors–NNRTIs**
  ...→↓Plasma antiretroviral medication levels, w/ concomitantly ↑Rifampin levels. To avoid this,
    replace Rifampin w/ Rifabutin which has ↓interactions w/ protease inhibitors (except
    Ritonavir) & nonnucleoside reverse transcriptase inhibitors–NNRTIs (except Delavirdine)

†Compliance can be assessed via urine evaluation for orange discoloration

Monitoring:
•Liver function test if symptomatic for possible hepatitis
•Obtain baseline & monthly liver function tests in persons w/ risk factors for hepatitis w/
  discontinuation if severe hepatitis occurs defined as either:
  ∘**Symptomatic**
  ∘**Plasma aminotransferase levels ≥5 X normal values**

INDICATIONS FOR SURGICAL TREATMENT ▬▬▬▬▬

•Prior to surgery, administer as many days of medication as reasonably possible, in order to:
  ∘↓Prosthetic infection risk
  ∘↑Peri–prosthetic tissue integrity
  ...→↓prosthetic dehiscence risk

Indications:
•**Heart failure, being the #1 cause of death,** occurring w/ aortic > mitral regurgitation
•Prosthetic valve involvement†
•Poor response to medical treatment, such as:
  ∘Positive blood culture @ >1week of appropriate antibiotic treatment
•Lack of effective medical treatment:
  ∘Brucella sp.
  ∘Pseudomonas sp.
  ∘Fungal infection
•Intracardiac extension of infection→
  ∘Abscess requiring drainage
  ∘Conduction abnormalities
•Recurrent septic thromboemboli‡
•Large (>1cm) vegetations

632

- Rupture of the chordae tendineae or papillary muscles
- Large or symptomatic mycotic aneurysms

---

†~50% of patients w/ Streptococcal sp. prosthetic valve endocarditis are cured by intravenous antibacterial treatment. In this situation, surgery is indicated w/ either:
- A poor response to medical treatment
- Recurrent infection after treatment cessation

‡Cerebral septic thromboembolism is often considered a contraindication to immediate cardiac surgery, as the risk of hemorrhagic conversion of the distal ischemic/ infarcted tissue during cardiopulmonary bypass is ↑ within 2weeks

PROGNOSIS

- **Overall mortality:**
  - 100% without appropriate antibiotic treatment
  - With appropriate antibiotic treatment:
    - −50% w/ either enterobacteriaceae or fungi
    - −10% for right sided endocarditis in intravenous drug users
    - −25% in all others
    - …w/ death usually due to either:
      - Central nervous system septic thromboembolism
      - Septic shock

PROPHYLAXIS

Indications:
- All procedures involving mucous membranes in patients w/ a previously damaged/ abnormal endocardium
- All patients w/ a history of rheumatic heart disease require endocarditis prophylaxis to age ≥40years

Administration:
- All PO medications should be taken 1hour prior to the procedure
- All IM & IV medications should be administered (w/ any infusions being completed) within 30min. prior to the procedure

PENICILLINS			
Generic (Trade)	M	♀	**Dose**
Amoxicillin (Amoxil)	K	P	2g PO
Ampicillin (Principen)	K	P	2g IM/ IV

ALTERNATIVE OPTONS FOR BETA LACTAM HYPERSENSITIVITY ▬▬▬▬▬▬▬
PROCEDURES ABOVE THE DIAPHRAGM_____
- In order to cover the **Streptococcus viridans group**

CLINDAMYCIN (Cleocin)		
M	♀	**Dose**
L	P	600mg PO/ IV

Mechanism:
- Affects the ribosomal 50S subunit→
  - ↓Peptide bond formation

OR

MACROLIDES			
Generic (Trade)	M	♀	**Dose**
Azithromycin (Zithromax)	L	P	500mg PO
Clarithromycin (Biaxin)	KL	?	500mg PO

Mechanism:
- Affects the ribosomal 50S subunit→
  - ↓Transfer RNA translocation

PROCEDURES BELOW THE DIAPHRAGM_____
- In order to cover **Enterococcus sp.**

VANCOMYCIN		
M	♀	**Dose**
K	?	1g IV over 1 hour

633

NONGONOCOCCAL SEPTIC ARTHRITIS

•Caused by the hematogenous spread to, or direct seeding of a joint by bacteria other than Neisseria gonorrhoeae→
   ◦Inflammation=septic arthritis→
     –Abscess formation, which if not adequately treated→permanent joint destruction

RISK FACTORS

•**Immunosuppression** via:
   ◦Advanced age
   ◦Alcoholism
   ◦Diabetes mellitus
   ◦Hematologic malignancy
   ◦HIV infection/ AIDS
   ◦Malnutrition
   ◦Medications
     –Chronic glucocorticoid use
     –Chemotherapy
     –Immunomodulating medications
   ◦Renal dialysis
•**Abnormal joint anatomy**
   ◦Previous joint trauma via:
     –Accident
     –Joint aspiration
     –Previous or current arthritis (ex. gout, osteoarthritis, rheumatoid arthritis)
     –Prosthesis
     –Surgery
•**Contiguous spread from nearby infection** via:
   ◦Abscess
   ◦Cellulitis
   ◦Osteomyelitis
   ◦Septic bursitis
•**Repetitive bacteremia** via:
   ◦Chronic bacterial infection, esp. poor dental hygiene→gingivitis
   ◦Bacterial endocarditis
   ◦Intravenous drug use
   ◦Intravenous line/ catheter

ORGANISMS

•**Nonprosthetic joint**
   ◦**Staphylococcus aureus–55%**
   ◦Streptococcal sp.–25%
   ◦Enterobacteriaceae–15%
     –Escherichia coli
     –Enterobacter cloacae
     –Klebsiella pneumoniae
     –Proteus mirabilis & vulgaris
     –Providencia rettgeri
     –Pseudomonas aeruginosa
     –Serratia marcescens
   ◦Staphylococcus epidermidis

•**Prosthetic joint**
   ◦Staphylococcus aureus–25%
   ◦Staphylococcus epidermidis–25%
   ◦Streptococcal sp.–20%
   ◦Enterobacteriaceae–20%
     –Escherichia coli
     –Enterobacter cloacae
     –Klebsiella pneumoniae
     –Proteus mirabilis & vulgaris
     –Providencia rettgeri
     –Pseudomonas aeruginosa
     –Serratia marcescens
   ◦Anaerobes

- **Penetrating trauma**
  - ◦Polymicrobial infection

- **Dog or cat bite**
  - ◦**Pasteurella multocida–50%**

General
- •Inflammatory cytokines→
  - ◦Anorexia→
    - –Cachexia
  - ◦Chills
  - ◦Fatigue
  - ◦Fever, however, >50% of patients are afebrile†
  - ◦Headache
  - ◦Malaise
  - ◦Night sweats
  - ◦Weakness

---

†Temperature may be normal in patients w/:
- •Chronic kidney disease, esp. w/ uremia
- •Cirrhosis
- •Heart failure
- •Severe debility
- …or those who are:
  - •Intravenous drug users
  - •Taking certain medications:
    - ◦Acetaminophen
    - ◦Antibiotics
    - ◦Glucocorticoids
    - ◦Nonsteroidal anti–inflammatory drugs–NSAIDs

Musculoskeletal
- •Joint infection→
  - ◦**Acute monoarthritis–90%†** >> polyarthritis–10%→
    - –Edematous, erythematous, warm, & painful joints‡, bursae°, tendon sheaths, &/or periarticular tissue
    - –↓Range of motion
    - –Inability to bear weight on the affected joint
    - …all being more pronounced in native joints

Commonly affected joints:
- •Joints distal to, and including the hip
  - ◦**Knee–55%**
  - ◦Hip–15%
    - –Pain is usually felt in the groin area, w/ ↓range of motion→difficulty putting on pants, socks, & shoes
    - –When supine, the patient prefers the affected hip rotated externally (lateral knee), w/ ↑pain upon internal rotation (medial knee). If the hip is flexed, suspect a psoas abscess
- •Joints distal to, and including the shoulder

Rarely affected joints, except in intravenous drug users:
- •Manubriosternal joint
- •Sacroiliac joint
  - ◦Pain usually felt in the sacral &/or buttock region ± radiation down the posterior thigh to the knee
- •Sternoclavicular joint
  - ◦Inflammation may be visualized, but the pain is usually felt in the shoulders
- •Symphysis pubis
- •Vertebral joints

---

†**Acute monoarthritis should be considered infectious in etiology until proven otherwise**
‡Deeply situated joints prevent the visualization of inflammation
- ◦Hip joints
- ◦Shoulder joints
- ◦Sacroiliac joints
°Presenting as joint pain on range of motion, w/ preserved ability to bear weight

635

Mucocutaneous
- Infection may track→
  - Abscess
  - Fistula

Hematologic
- Inflammatory cytokines→
  - Leukocytosis
  - ↑Acute phase proteins
    - ↑Erythrocyte sedimentation rate-ESR (normal: 5mm/ decade aged + ♂ ≤10mm/h or ♀ ≤20mm/h)
    - ↑C-reactive protein-CRP (normal: <2mg/ L), responding more acutely than ESR, as it rises within several hours & falls within 3days upon partial resolution
    - ↑Fibrinogen
    - ↑Platelets→thrombocytosis

BLOOD CULTURES

Procedure:
- 2 sets of aerobic & anaerobic culture mediums, w/ each bottle inoculated w/ ≥10mL of blood
- Typical pathogens can be isolated within days, w/ a sensitivity of 50%

Limitations:
- Careful, as source may be contaminated via:
  - Concomitant infection
  - Intravascular line/ catheter, or lack of aseptic technique→
    - Skin organism contamination

Staphylococcal sp. laboratory features:
- All are:
  - **Gram positive cocci in clusters**
  - Catalase enzyme production positive
- Only Staphylococcus aureus
  - Is coagulase enzyme production positive
  - Produces a beta erythrocyte hemolytic pattern, whereas the others are gamma hemolytic

Streptococcal sp. laboratory features:
- All are:
  - **Gram positive cocci in chains**
  - Catalase enzyme production negative
- Hemolysis pattern:
  - Alpha
    - Streptococcus pneumoniae
    - Viridan's streptococci
  - Beta
    - Streptococcus agalactiae & pyogenes
  - Alpha or gamma
    - Streptococcus bovis
  - Alpha, beta, or gamma
    - All other streptococci

- Alpha hemolysis is indicated by incomplete enzyme mediated erythrocyte lysis→
  - Peri-colony green zone
- Beta homolysis is indicated by complete enzyme mediated erythrocyte lysis→
  - Peri-colony clear zone
- Gamma hemolysis is indicated by lack of erythrocyte lysis

IMAGING

- **X rays**
  Indications:
  - All patients w/ suspected disease
  Appropriate views:
  - Hand joints: Single anteroposterior-AP view†
  - Hip joints: Single anteroposterior-AP view of the pelvis†
  - Knee joints: Anteroposterior & lateral views
  - Spine: Anteroposterior, lateral, & oblique views
  Findings:
  - Joint effusion
  - Periarticular soft tissue edema

†Lateral & oblique views should be obtained if either:
- An abnormality is detected
- Findings do not correlate w/ the clinical picture

INVASIVE PROCEDURES

- **Arthrocentesis**
  Indications:
  - All affected joints should be aspirated & examined
  Contraindications:
  - Through infected soft tissue →
    - Organism introduction into the synovial space
  Synovial studies:
  - Gross appearance:
    - >3.5mL of fluid (normal being <3.5mL), being turbid=cloudy, dark yellow or purulent (normal being clear straw colored)
  - Leukocyte count:
    - >3,000/ μL, usually being >50,000/ μL, w/ neutrophil predominance (normal being <180/ μL w/ a mononuclear predominance)
    - >100,000/ μL w/ Staphylococcal or Streptococcal sp. infection
  - Glucose level:
    - <20 (normal being ~plasma level)
  - Protein level:
    - >3.5g/ dL
  - Bacterial gram stain & culture: Positive

TREATMENT

- **Joint rest**
  - Begin passive range of motion exercises upon clinical improvement, in order to preserve joint function
- **Joint drainage** via:
  - Arthrocentesis
    - Repeat as often as necessary to control effusion
  - Open surgical drainage & debridement for:
    - Joints difficult to aspirate
    - Joints showing no improvement within several days after arthrocentesis
    - Prosthetic joint infections, necessitating removal of the prosthesis
- **Empiric intravenous antibiotics**, w/ initial treatment guided by gram stain
  - The switch to PO medication should be attempted upon clinical improvement via fever resolution & clinical stabilization X 24hours, if an acceptable PO medication is available, & the patient is able to take PO medication
  - **Organism-narrowed therapy** should be initiated promptly upon stain, culture, & sensitivities results
  - The following antibiotics achieve equivalent plasma levels via PO or intravenous administration in persons w/ a functioning gastrointestinal tract:
    - Chloramphenicol
    - Doxycycline
    - Minocycline
    - Most fluoroquinolones
    - Trimethoprim/ Sulfamethoxazole

Bactericidal antibiotics
- **Cell wall synthesis inhibitors**
  - β lactam medications:
    - Carbapenems
    - Cephalosporins
    - Monobactams
    - Penicillins
  - Vancomycin
- **DNA synthesis inhibitors**
  - Fluoroquinolones
  - Linezolid
  - Metronidazole
  - Rifampin
  - Quinupristin & dalfopristin
- **Aminoglycosides**

637

Treatment duration:
- **Staphylococcus aureus:** 1 month
- **All other organisms:** 3 weeks
- **Prosthetic joint:** Intravenous treatment X 1 month after prosthesis removal†, then
  PO X 2–4 months, followed by the implantation of a new prosthesis

---

†If the prosthesis cannot be removed due to the patient being a poor surgical candidate, antibiotic treatment should be continued for ≥6months, depending on whether the infection can be cured or simply suppressed

GRAM POSITIVE COCCI

PENICILLINS

Generic (Trade)	M	♀	Dose
Nafcillin (Nallpen)	L	P	2g IV q4hours
Oxacillin (Bactocill)	KL	P	2g IV q4hours

Mechanism:
- A β–lactam ring structure which binds to bacterial transpeptidase→
  - ↓Transpeptidase function→
    - ↓Bacterial cell wall peptidoglycan cross–linking→↓cell wall synthesis→osmotic influx of extracellular fluid→↑intracellular hydrostatic pressure→cell rupture→cell death=bactericidal
- ↑Bacterial autolytic enzymes→
  - Peptidoglycan degradation

- Certain bacteria produce β–lactamase→
  - Cleavage of this essential structural component of cephalosporins & certain penicillins (as the other β–lactam medications differ sufficiently to prevent ring cleavage)→
    - Antibiotic inactivation. This process may be antagonized by the concomitant administration of **β–lactamase inhibitors** (Clavulanic acid=clavulanate, Sulbactam, or Tazobactam)→renewed susceptibility

Side effects:
General
- **Hypersensitivity reactions ≤10%**
  - Anaphylaxis–0.5%→
    - Death–0.002% (1:50,000)
  - Acute interstitial nephritis
  - Dermatitis
  - Drug fever
  - Hemolytic anemia
  ...having cross–hypersensitivity to other β lactam medications (cephalosporins, carbapenems), except monobactams (ex. Aztreonam)

VANCOMYCIN

Indications:
- Suspected **methicillin resistant Staphylococcus aureus–MRSA** via:
  - History of colonization/ infection
  - Intravascular line mediated infection
  - Recent hospitalization or nursing home residence
  - Recent invasive procedure
  - Severe mucositis

M	♀	Dose	Peak	Trough
K	?	1g IV q12hours, to be administered over 1hour	30–40µg/ mL	>5µg/ mL

- Peak levels are obtained 30minutes after the dose, w/ trough levels being obtained at the end of the dosing interval. Plasma peak & trough levels are directly related to toxicity & clinical efficacy respectively

Mechanism:
- Direct cell wall peptidoglycan binding→
  - ↓Transpeptidase function→
    - ↓Bacterial cell wall peptidoglycan cross–linking→↓cell wall synthesis→osmotic influx of extracellular fluid→↑intracellular hydrostatic pressure→cell rupture→cell death=bactericidal

- Vancomycin resistant enterococci–VRE & staphylococci–VRS have developed

Side effects:
General
- •Rapid intravenous administration (over <1hour)→
  - ∘Intrinsic hypersensitivity syndrome→
    - −Face, neck, &/or upper thoracic angioedema, termed "red man syndrome". Occurrence does not prevent continued use, unless accompanied by an anaphylactoid reaction

Cardiovascular
- •Venous inflammation=phlebitis ± thrombus formation

Otolaryngology
- •Ototoxicity

GRAM NEGATIVE BACTERIA/ NO ORGANISMS

CEPHALOSPORINS: 3rd–4th generation

Generic (Trade)	M	♀	Dose
Cefotaxime (Claforan)	KL	P	2g IV/ IM q12hours
Ceftriaxone (Rocephin)	KB	P	2g IV/ IM q24hours

Mechanism:
- •A β–lactam ring structure which binds to bacterial transpeptidase→
  - ∘↓Transpeptidase function→
    - −↓Bacterial cell wall peptidoglycan cross–linking→↓cell wall synthesis→osmotic influx of extracellular fluid→↑intracellular hydrostatic pressure→cell rupture→cell death=bactericidal
- •↑Bacterial autolytic enzymes→
  - ∘Peptidoglycan degradation

- •Certain bacteria produce β–lactamase→
  - ∘Cleavage of this essential structural component of cephalosporins & certain penicillins (as the other β–lactam medications differ sufficiently to prevent ring cleavage)→
    - −Antibiotic inactivation. This process may be antagonized by the concomitant administration of β–lactamase inhibitors (Clavulanic acid=clavulanate, Sulbactam, or Tazobactam)→renewed susceptibility

Side effects:
General
- •**Hypersensitivity reactions ≤10%**
  - ∘Anaphylaxis−0.5%→
    - −Death−0.002% (1:50,000)
  - ∘Acute interstitial nephritis
  - ∘Dermatitis
  - ∘Drug fever
  - ∘Hemolytic anemia
  - …having cross–hypersensitivity to other β lactam medications (penicillins, carbapenems), except monobactams (ex. Aztreonam)

Gastrointestinal
- •Clostridium dificile pseudomembraneous colitis (3rd generation > others)

ANIMAL BITE

PENICILLINS

Generic (Trade)	M	♀	Dose
Ampicillin–Sulbactam (Unasyn)	K	P	3g IM/ IV q6hours
Piperacillin–Tazobactam (Zosyn)	K	P	3.375g IV q6hours
Ticarcillin–Clavulanic acid (Timentin)	K	P	3.1g IV q6hours

PROGNOSIS

- •**10% mortality due to acute respiratory distress syndrome–ARDS**
- •30% of patients have permanent joint destruction

Poor prognostic indicators:
- •Age >65 years
- •Polyarticular infection
- •Delay in initiating appropriate treatment
- •Other form of arthritis in the affected joint (especially rheumatoid arthritis)

PREVENTION

- •**Prophylactic antibiotics**

Indications:
- •Prior to prosthetic implant surgery
- •Prior to any surgical procedure involving mucous membranes in patients w/ prosthetic implants

639

GONOCOCCAL SEPTIC ARTHRITIS

•Caused by the hematogenous spread of **Neisseria gonorrhoeae**→
◦Inflammation=septic arthritis

Statistics:
•**95% of septic arthritis &/or tenosynovitis in adults age <40years**

RISK FACTORS

•**Patient must be sexually active**
◦All forms of sexual intercourse, as the organism originates from sites of sexually transmitted infections, w/ few patients being symptomatic at the initial site.**Sexually transmitted organisms do not cause infection proximal to the urethra**, rather they infect the:
–Urethra & peri–urethral structures (prostate, epididymis, &/or testicle)
–Entire female genital tract
...as well as the:
•Pharynx
•Rectum

•**Age <45years**
◦? ↑Host resistance vs. ↓sexual activity @ older ages
•**Gender**
◦♀ 4X ♂, w/ ↑risk during:
–Menstruation
–Pregnancy
–Postpartum period
•**Homosexual ♂**
•**Complement deficiency, being rare**
◦Especially C3–C8

ORGANISM

•**Neisseria gonorrhoeae**
◦A gram negative diplococcus, usually found within polymorphonuclear leukocytes→hematogenous dissemination in <1% of all infections→arthritis via either:
–Direct joint infection
–Immune complex deposition
–Deposition of cell wall fragments of dead bacteria

DIAGNOSIS

General
•Inflammatory cytokines→
◦Anorexia→
–Cachexia
◦Chills
◦Fatigue
◦Fever, however, >50% of patients are afebrile†
◦Headache
◦Malaise
◦Night sweats
◦Weakness

---

†Temperature may be normal in patients w/:
•Chronic kidney disease, esp. w/ uremia
•Cirrhosis
•Heart failure
•Severe debility
...or those who are:
•Intravenous drug users
•Taking certain medications:
◦Acetaminophen
◦Antibiotics
◦Glucocorticoids
◦Nonsteroidal anti–inflammatory drugs–NSAIDs

640

Musculoskeletal
- Joint infection→
  - ○**Acute polyarthritis–70%** (migratory or additive) > monoarthritis–30%†→
    - –Edematous, erythematous, warm, & painful joints‡, bursae°, tendon sheaths, &/or periarticular tissue
    - –↓Range of motion
    - –Inability to bear weight on the affected joint
    - …all being more pronounced in native joints
  - ○Inflammation along a tendon=**tenosynovitis–70%**→
    - –"Sausage–like" tendon distention
    - –Pain on flexion of the tendon against resistance

Commonly affected joints:
- Joints distal to the hip
  - ○The knee being most common in monoarthritis
- Joints distal to the shoulder

---

†**Acute monoarthritis should be considered infectious in etiology until proven otherwise**
- Patients w/ monoarthritis are unlikely to develop tenosynovitis or cutaneous lesions

‡Deeply situated joints prevent the visualization of inflammation
- ○Hip joints
- ○Shoulder joints
- ○Sacroiliac joints

°Presenting as joint pain on range of motion, w/ preserved ability to bear weight

Cutaneous–70%
- Lesions (usually on the trunk & extensor surface of the distal extremities) beginning as red papules→
  - ○Hemorrhagic pustules on a necrotic base being:
    - –Asymptomatic
    - –Often <20
    - –<Several mm diameter

Hematologic
- Inflammatory cytokines→
  - ○Leukocytosis
  - ○↑Acute phase proteins
    - –↑Erythrocyte sedimentation rate–ESR (normal: 5mm/ decade aged + ♂ ≤10mm/h or ♀ ≤20mm/h)
    - –↑C–reactive protein–CRP (normal: <2mg/ L), responding more acutely than ESR, as it rises within several hours & falls within 3days upon partial resolution
    - –↑Fibrinogen
    - –↑Platelets→thrombocytosis
- Complement deficiency, being rare: ↓CH50

IMAGING
- **X rays**
  Indications:
  - All patients w/ suspected disease
  Appropriate views:
  - Hand joints: Single anteroposterior–AP view†
  - Hip joints: Single anteroposterior–AP view of the pelvis†
  - Knee joints: Anteroposterior & lateral views
  - Spine: Anteroposterior, lateral, & oblique views
  Findings:
  - Joint effusion
  - Periarticular soft tissue edema

---

†Lateral & oblique views should be obtained if either:
- An abnormality is detected
- Findings do not correlate w/ the clinical picture

INVASIVE PROCEDURES
- **Arthrocentesis**
  Indications:
  - All affected joints should be aspirated & examined
  Contraindications:
  - Through infected soft tissue→
    - ○Organism introduction into the synovial space

<u>Synovial studies:</u>
- Gross appearance:
  - >3.5mL of fluid (normal being <3.5mL), being turbid=cloudy, dark yellow or purulent (normal being clear straw colored)
- Leukocyte count:
  - **>50,000/ µL**, w/ neutrophil predominance (normal being <180/ µL w/ a mononuclear predominance)
- Glucose level:
  - <20, also being seen w/ empyema (normal being ~plasma level)
- Protein level:
  - >3.5g/ dL
- Bacterial gram stain sensitivity: 20%
- Bacterial culture sensitivity: 50% when inoculated onto Theyer–Martin media
- Neisseria gonorrhoeae PCR: Positive

OTHER STUDIES

•**Diagnosis of Neisseria gonorrhoeae infection**
<u>Microscopic findings:</u>
- **A gram negative diplococcus, usually found within polymorphonuclear leukocytes†**
<u>Culture mediums used‡:</u>
- **Martin–Lewis**
- **NYC**
- **Theyer–Martin**
<u>Other tests:</u>
- **Ligase or polymerase chain reaction°**

---

†Sensitivities are as follows:
- Symptomatic ♂ urethritis–90%
- Pelvic inflammatory disease–PID 50%
- Proctitis–40%

‡Culture of urethral, ectocervical, rectal, or pharyngeal mucous membrane specimens onto a selective media
<u>Procedure:</u>
- The urethral swab sample should be taken via either:
  - Visible meatal discharge
  - Following insertion of the swab 2–4cm into the urethra & rotated unidirectionally for 5 seconds
°Use either:
- Any swab collection
- First void urine

TREATMENT

•**Joint rest**
  - Unlike nongonococcal septic arthritis, physical therapy is unnecessary, as the inflammation resolves quickly
•**Joint drainage** via:
  - Arthrocentesis
    - Rarely requiring repeat arthrocentesis in order to control effusion
  - Rarely requiring open surgical drainage & debridement for:
    - Joints difficult to aspirate
•**Test for other sexually transmitted infections**
  - Human Immune Deficiency Virus–HIV
  - Treponema pallidum
  - Chronic hepatitis B &/or C infection
•**Treat empirically for Chlamydia trachomatis co–infection**, based on primary clinical, or suspected site of infection
•**Intravenous antibiotics**
  - The switch to PO medication should be attempted upon clinical improvement via fever resolution & clinical stabilization X 24hours, if an acceptable PO medication is available, & the patient is able to take PO medication
  - **Organism–narrowed therapy** should be initiated promptly upon stain, culture, & sensitivities results
  - The following antibiotics achieve equivalent plasma levels via PO or intravenous administration in persons w/ a functioning gastrointestinal tract:
    - Chloramphenicol
    - Doxycycline
    - Minocycline
    - Most fluoroquinolones
    - Trimethoprim/ Sulfamethoxazole

642

Bactericidal antibiotics
- **Cell wall synthesis inhibitors**
  - ∘β lactam medications:
    - −Carbapenems
    - −Cephalosporins
    - −Monobactams
    - −Penicillins
  - ∘Vancomycin
- **DNA synthesis inhibitors**
  - ∘Fluoroquinolones
  - ∘Linezolid
  - ∘Metronidazole
  - ∘Rifampin
  - ∘Quinupristin & dalfopristin
- **Aminoglycosides**

Treatment duration:
- •1week

CEPHALOSPORINS: 3rd–4th generation			
Generic (Trade)	M	♀	Dose
Ceftriaxone (Rocephin)	KB	P	2g IV/ IM q24hours

Mechanism:
- •A β−lactam ring structure which binds to bacterial transpeptidase→
  - ∘↓Transpeptidase function→
    - −↓Bacterial cell wall peptidoglycan cross−linking→↓cell wall synthesis→osmotic influx of extracellular fluid→↑intracellular hydrostatic pressure→cell rupture→cell death=bactericidal
- •↑Bacterial autolytic enzymes→
  - ∘Peptidoglycan degradation

- •Certain bacteria produce β−lactamase→
  - ∘Cleavage of this essential structural component of cephalosporins & certain penicillins (as the other β−lactam medications differ sufficiently to prevent ring cleavage)→
    - −Antibiotic inactivation. This process may be antagonized by the concomitant administration of **β−lactamase inhibitors** (Clavulanic acid=clavulanate, Sulbactam, or Tazobactam)→renewed susceptibility

Side effects:
General
- •**Hypersensitivity reactions ≤10%**
  - ∘Anaphylaxis−0.5%→
    - −Death−0.002% (1:50,000)
  - ∘Acute interstitial nephritis
  - ∘Dermatitis
  - ∘Drug fever
  - ∘Hemolytic anemia
  - …having cross−hypersensitivity to other β lactam medications (penicillins, carbapenems), except monobactams (ex. Aztreonam)
Gastrointestinal
- •Clostridium dificile pseudomembraneous colitis (3rd generation > others)

FOLLOWED BY

FLUOROQUINOLONES			
Generic (Trade)	M	♀	Dose
Ciprofloxacin (Cipro)	LK	?	500mg PO q12hours
Levofloxacin (Levaquin)	KL	?	500mg PO q24hours

Mechanism:
- •↓DNA gyrase=topoisomerase action→
  - ∘↓Bacterial DNA synthesis

Side effects:
General
- •Hypersensitivity reactions
Gastrointestinal
- •Gastroenteritis→
  - ∘Diarrhea
  - ∘Nausea ± vomiting

643

Mucocutaneous
- •Phototoxicity

Neurologic
- •Dizziness
- •Drowsiness
- •Headache
- •Restlessness

Materno-fetal
- •Fetal & child tendon malformation (including breast fed)→
  - ∘↑Tendon rupture risk

PROGNOSIS

- •0% mortality
- •<5% of patients have permanent joint destruction

644

•Caused by the hematogenous spread of viruses to the liver→
  ◦Hepatocyte death via:
    −Cytopathic effect
    −Immune mediated attack
    ...→inflammation=hepatitis
Statistics:
  •The hepatitis B virus is the #1 worldwide cause:
    ◦Chronic hepatitis
    ◦Cirrhosis
    ◦Hepatocellular cancer

RISK FACTORS

HEPATITIS A OR E VIRUS INFECTION ▬▬▬▬▬▬▬▬▬
•Fecal−mucosal transmission
  ◦Certain sexual acts
    −Anilingus
    −Insertive anal intercourse
  ◦Contaminated water supplies†
    −Raw or partially cooked shellfish from sewage contaminated water may harbor Hepatitis A virus
  ◦Crowded living conditions
    −Childrens day care centers
    −Jails
    −Military barracks
    −Nursing homes
  ◦Poor handwashing

---

†Hepatitis E is a major cause of water−borne epidemics in Africa, Asia, India, & Mexico

HEPATITIS B, C, &/OR D VIRUS INFECTION ▬▬▬▬▬▬▬
•All forms of sexual intercourse (hepatitis B >> C virus)
  ◦Vaginal (esp. during menstruation), anal, or oral sex, esp. w/:
    −Unprotected sexual intercourse. Protection is achieved via the proper use of latex or
    polyurethane condoms, as well as rubber or latex dams for cunniligus
    −Sex w/ an uncircumsized > circumsized ♂
  Note: In any act, the person in contact w/ infected semen is at ↑relative risk

•Materno−fetal/ child transmission (hepatitis B >> C virus)
  ◦Transplacentally to the fetus
  ◦During birth via infected vaginal fluid & blood
  ◦Breast milk
  Outcomes:
    •↑↑Risk of chronic hepatitis B virus infection

•Intravenous drug use w/ needle sharing
  ◦Unsterilized > sterilized syringes
  Needle sterilization:
    1. Draw full strength household alcohol or bleach up the syringe, through the needle until full
    2. Completely immerse the needle & syringe for >2min.
    3. Discharge the alcohol/ bleach
    4. Repeat the process, then rinse by filling & discharging the syringe w/ water X3

•Inadvertent needle stick w/ used needle
  ◦Healthcare employees
  ◦Police officers during body or bag checks

  Percutaneous infection risk
    •Hepatitis B virus: 1/ 3
    •Hepatitis C virus: 1/ 33

•Infected blood contact w/ mucus membranes (eyes or mouth)−rare
  ◦Accident victims
  ◦Healthcare employees

- **Infection via infected blood, blood products, or transplanted organs†, being rare**
  - ○Donated blood began to be screened for hepatitis C virus in 1990

  <u>Screened blood transfusion risk</u>
  - •Hepatitis B virus: 1/ 63,000 units
  - •Hepatitis C virus: 1/ 103,000 units

- **Child–maternal transmission, being rare**
  - ○Breast feeding an infected infant

- **Idiopathic–50% of hepatitis C cases**

- **All patients w/ chronic hepatitis should be considered infectious** & refrain from:
  - ○Unprotected sex
  - ○Blood or organ donation
  - ○Sharing tooth brushes or razors
  - †Including semen used for artificial insemination

CLASSIFICATION

- **Acute hepatitis**
  - ○Hepatic inflammation <6 months
- **Chronic hepatitis**
  - ○Hepatic inflammation ≥6 months→
    - –Fibrosis=cirrhosis ± hepatocellular cancer–HCC, being the #2 cause of cancer deaths worldwide
- **Fulminant hepatitis**
  - ○Hepatic encephalopathy within 2weeks of the presenting syndrome of acute hepatitis

ORGANISMS

Virus	Transmission†	U.S. cases	Incubation	% Fulminant
Hepatitis A	Fecal–mucosal	45%	2–6 weeks	0.1%‡
Hepatitis E	Fecal–mucosal	<1%	2–6 weeks	1% (15% if pregnant)
Hepatitis B	S–50% >P >M	35%	1–6 months	0.1%
Hepatitis C	P >S >M	15%	1–6 months	0.1%
Hepatitis D	S >P >M	2%	?	30% w/ concomitant hepatitis B

- **Hepatitis D virus** is a passenger virus which is **pathogenic only w/ hepatitis B viral co–infection** (simultaneously or w/ hepatitis D viral superinfection)→
  - ○Severe hepatitis, w/ hepatitis D viral infection clearance occurring only w/ the clearance of hepatitis B viral infection, as anti–HDV antibody does not clear the infection
- **Hepatitis E virus** is usually found in Africa, Asia, India, & Mexico
- †PSM=Parenteral, Sexual, Materno–fetal
- ‡Patients w/ chronic liver disease are at ↑risk for fulminant hepatitis A

DIAGNOSIS

General
- •Inflammatory cytokines→
  - ○Anorexia→
    - –Cachexia
  - ○Chills
  - ○Fatigue
  - ○Fever, usually being low grade†
  - ○Headache
  - ○Malaise
  - ○Night sweats
  - ○Weakness

---

†Temperature may be normal in patients w/:
- •Chronic kidney disease, esp. w/ uremia
- •Cirrhosis
- •Heart failure
- •Severe debility

...or those who are:
- •Intravenous drug users
- •Taking certain medications:
  - ∘Acetaminophen
  - ∘Antibiotics
  - ∘Glucocorticoids
  - ∘Nonsteroidal anti−inflammatory drugs−NSAIDs

Gastrointestinal
- •Diarrhea
- •Nausea ± vomiting
- •Hepatomegaly→liver capsule (Glisson's capsule) distention→
  - ∘Continuous right upper quadrant abdominal pain ±
    - −Tenderness to palpation, which may be worsened by bending, sleeping on the right side, &/or eating
    - −Radiation to the right scapular area
- •Hepatocyte destruction→↓bile formation→
  - ∘↓Stool bilirubin→**light colored/ pale stool, termed acholic stool**
  - ∘↓Fat absorption→
    - −↑Stool fat, termed steatorrhea→**foul smelling, floating stools,** leaving an oily residue on the toilet
    - −Cachexia
    - −Diarrhea
    - −Vitamin A, D, E, & K malabsorption

Genitourinary
- •Hepatocyte destruction→↑plasma conjugated bilirubin→
  - ∘↑Urine bilirubin→
    - −**Dark "coca−cola" colored urine**

Lymphatic
- •Lymphadenopathy, being posterior cervical w/ hepatitis B virus

Mucocutaneous
- •↑Plasma bilirubin→subcutaneous deposition→
  - ∘Yellow staining of tissues @ >3mg/ dL
    - −Skin→**jaundice−30%**
    - −Sclera→**scleral icterus**
    - −Mucus membranes
  - ∘Pruritis

Hematologic
- •Inflammatory cytokines→
  - ∘Leukocytosis
  - ∘↑Acute phase proteins
    - −↑Erythrocyte sedimentation rate−ESR (normal: 5mm/ decade aged + ♂ ≤10mm/h or ♀ ≤20mm/h)
    - −↑C−reactive protein−CRP (normal: <2mg/ L), responding more acutely than ESR, as it rises within several hours & falls within 3days, upon partial resolution
    - −↑Fibrinogen
    - −↑Platelets→thrombocytosis
- •Hepatocyte lysis→
  - ∘↑Hepatic enzyme levels
    - −↑Alkaline phosphatase
    - −↑**Aminotransferases**† (alanine aminotransferase−ALT & aspartate aminotransferase−AST), being detectable @ ≥2months, unless the infection is cleared or latent
    - −↑γ glutamyl transpeptidase−GGT
    - −↑5' nucleotidase−5NT
  - ∘↑**Bilirubin** (conjugated=direct & unconjugated=indirect)
- •Autoantibody formation
  - ∘Antinuclear antibodies−ANA
  - ∘Anti−thyroglobulin A
  - ∘Rheumatoid factor
- •Thrombocytopenia, being cytokine mediated

---

†Alcoholic hepatitis→
- •**Aspartate aminotransferase−AST 2−3 X alanine aminotransferase−ALT,** (normal being 1:1) w/ the AST usually <500 U/ L

Immune mediated extra-hepatic manifestations:
- Hepatitis B virus→
  - Immune complex deposition→
    - Arthralgias
    - Glomerulonephritis
    - Urticaria
- Hepatitis C virus→
  - Immune mediated illness→
    - Type 2 cryoglobulinemia
    - Mooren's corneal ulcers
    - Membranous glomerulonephritis
    - Focal lymphocytic sialadenitis
    - ?Autoimmune thyroiditis
    - ...& rarely (♂ > ♀):
      - Agranulocytosis
      - Aplastic anemia
      - Hemolytic anemia

SEROLOGIC MARKERS OF DISEASE STAGE

Hepatitis A	IgM anti-HAV	IgG anti-HAV
Acute	+	±
Previous	−	+
Vaccinated	−	+

Hepatitis B	HBsAg	Anti-HBsAg	HBeAg	Anti-HBeAg	Anti-HBcAg	HBV DNA	Anti-HDV†
Acute	+	−	+	−	IgM, IgG	−	−
Chronic							
•Low infectivity	+	−	−	+	IgG	+	−
•High infectivity	+	−	+	−	IgG	+	−
Previous	−	+	−	+	±IgG	−	−
Vaccinated	−	+	−	−	−	−	−
Acute hepatitis D	+	−	+	−	IgM, IgG	−	IgM
Chronic hepatitis D	+	−	+	−	IgG	±	IgG

Hepatitis C	Anti-HCAg	HCV RNA	RIBA‡
Acute	±		+
Chronic	+	+	
Previous	+°	−	+

Hepatitis E	IgM anti-HEV
Acute	+

†Antibodies are detected @3weeks, w/ IgM lasting 3weeks & IgG lasting indefinitely
‡A positive Anti-HCAg via ELISA (the standard screening test), but negative HCV RNA via PCR could be the result of either a:
- Cleared infection
- False positive ELISA
...which can be distinguished via radioimmunoblot assay-RIBA, being a much more sensitive test for Anti-HCVAg
°Anti-HCAg levels gradually decline over time in patients without chronic infection, & may be undetectable @ >15years

HEPATITIS B SEROLOGIC MARKER DESCRIPTION

Marker	Description
HBsAg	•A protein expressed on circulating viral particles (the intact virus, a spherical particle, & tubular particle) **indicating active infection & infectivity** •Used to screen blood donors Plasma detection: •@1month, lasting 6months if cleared, being found indefinitely w/ chronic disease
Anti-HBsAg	•Indicates previously cleared infection or vaccination, w/ subsequent immunity to re-infection •Is the only viral marker present post-vaccination •May eventually become undetectable in recovered patients Plasma detection: •@6months if cleared, lasting indefinitely
HBeAg	•Derived from intracellular viral protein cleavage during viral replication, **indicating active infection, being either acute or chronic w/ ↑infectivity** Plasma detection: •@5weeks, lasting 3months if cleared, being found indefinitely w/ chronic active disease
Anti-HBeAg	•Indicates HBeAg clearance & lack of replication Plasma detection: •@3.5months, lasting indefinitely
HBcAg	•A non-circulating protein found only in the nuclei of infected hepatocytes→ ∘Cell surface expression of derived peptides
Anti-HBcAg	•IgM: The first antibody to appear, indicating acute infection or possible flare of chronic hepatitis B •IgG: Indicates previous or chronic infection ...w/ **neither antibody being protective** Plasma detection: •@2months, lasting 1year vs. indefinitely
HBV DNA	•Indicates chronic active infection

INDICATORS OF LIVER FAILURE

Indicating the presence of either:
•Fulminant hepatitis
•Chronic disease→cirrhosis→portal hypertension syndrome
...both→
  •Liver failure→
    ∘↓Metabolism of:
      −Nitrogenous waste products (**ammonia**, uric acid), which are the end-products of protein catabolism
      −Biogenic amines (ex. gamma aminobutyric acid-GABA)
      −Endogenous benzodiazepine-like substances via GABA-ergic neurotransmission
      −Medications
      −Mercaptans derived from methionine metabolism
      −Toxic intestinal products
      ...as blood bypasses hepatic filtration via portal-systemic anastomoses→
        •Direct flow into the systemic circulation→
          ∘**Central nervous system dysfunction, termed hepatic encephalopathy→**
            −**Altered mental status**
            −Altered neuromuscular function
    ∘↓Hepatocyte protein synthesis→**hypoalbuminemia**→↓intravascular osmotic pressure→systemic fluid transudation→interstitial edema→
      −↑Weight (1L fluid=1kg=2.2 lbs)
      −**Pitting edema**, requiring ≥3L of fluid, usually beginning in the most dependent body part (feet & ankles=pedal edema &/or sacral edema in bed-bound patients)→eventual generalized edema=**anasarca**
      −Transudative peritoneal (**ascites**), pleural, pericardial, &/or synovial effusions
    ∘↓Hepatocyte protein synthesis→
      −↓Formation of procoagulant proteins (except von Willebrand factor-vWF†) & anticoagulant proteins→overall **coagulopathy** via an ↑international normalized ratio-INR‡ & activated partial thromboplastin time-aPTT→↑hemorrhage risk

†von Willebrand factor–vWF is synthesized by endothelial cells, w/ subsequent release & binding to factor 8c in order to produce the compete factor 8 protein

‡↓Vitamin K absorption via an edematous intestine→
   •↑INR, w/ prolongation that persists despite parenteral administration of vitamin K, indicating hepatic synthetic failure

IMAGING

•**Abdominal ultrasound**
Indications:
   •All patients w/ hepatitis, as it allows for visualization of the hepatic anatomy, as well as the measurement of portal venous pressures

INVASIVE PROCEDURES

•**Liver biopsy**
Indications:
   •All patients w/ chronic hepatitis & ↑aminotransferase levels, to determine hepatitis severity in terms of inflammation (mild, moderate, or severe, which may change over time) & fibrosis. It is not, however, mandatory prior to the initiation of treatment, w/ some authorities recommending biopsy only if treatment does not result in a sustained remission

TREATMENT

FULMINANT HEPATITIS ▬▬▬▬▬▬▬▬▬▬▬▬▬▬▬▬▬▬▬▬▬▬▬▬▬▬▬▬
•Sepsis prophylaxis via antibiotics
•Peptic inflammatory disease prophylaxis via proton pump inhibitors–PPIs or histamine–2 selective receptor blockers˙
•Mannitol for cerebral edema
•**Liver transplantation**
Outcomes:
   •100% re–infected, but usually w/ milder disease
   •Max 1 year survival: 90%
   •Max 5 year survival: 80%
Contraindications:
   •Active substance abuse
   •Extra–hepatic malignancy
   •HIV infection
   •Sepsis
   •Severe comorbidity

CHRONIC HEPATITIS B ▬▬▬▬▬▬▬▬▬▬▬▬▬▬▬▬▬▬▬▬▬▬▬▬▬▬▬

CYTOKINES			
Generic	M	♀	Start
Interferon–α–2b	K	?	5million units SC q24hours X 4months or 10million units SC 3X/ week X 4months

Mechanism:
   •Induces the synthesis of cell encoded enzymes→
      ∘Selective inhibition of viral messenger RNA translation to protein, without affecting the translation of cellular messenger RNA

Outcomes:
   •Sustained loss of viral markers of replication
   •Normalization of plasma aminotransferases–35%

Side effects:
   General
      •Anorexia
      •Erythema at the injection site
      •Headache
      •**Influenze–like syndrome** (fatigue, fever, chills, myalgia) beginning 6–8hours after administration, & lasting ≤12hours
         ∘Administer w/ antipyretic at bedtime in order to attempt to avoid this syndrome
   Cardiovascular
      •Dilated cardiomyopathy
   Endocrine
      •Diabetes mellitus
   Gastrointestinal
      •Diarrhea

650

Opthalmologic
- Optic neuritis
- Retinopathy

Neurologic
- Amotivation
- Alopecia
- Altered taste=dysguesia
- ↓Concentration
- Depression
- Impaired hearing
- Insomnia
- Irritability
- ↓Libido, being sexual desire→
  - −Impotence, being the inability to achieve &/or maintain an erection
- Paranoia
- Polyneuropathy
- Seizure
- Suicidal ideation

Hematologic
- Autoantibody induction
- **Leukopenia→**
  - ○↑Infection &/or neoplasm risk
- **Thrombocytopenia→**
  - ○↑Hemorrhage risk, esp. petechiae

Absolute contraindications:
Cardiovascular
- Symptomatic cardiac disease

Gastrointestinal
- Decompensated cirrhosis

Neurologic
- Uncontrolled seizure disease

Psychiatric
- Current severe major depression
- History of psychosis

Hematologic
- Neutropenia
- Thrombocytopenia

Other
- Organ transplantation (other than liver)

Relative contraindications:
Rheumatologic
- Autoimmune disease

Endocrine
- Uncontrolled diabetes mellitus

SECOND LINE

ANTIVIRAL

Generic (Trade)	M	♀	Dose
Famciclovir (Famvir)	K	P	500mg PO q8hours X 13months

OR

NUCLEOSIDE REVERSE TRANSCRIPTASE INHIBITOR−NRTI

Generic	M	♀	Dose
Lamivudine−3TC (Epivir)	K	?	100mg PO q24hours X 13months

Outcomes:
- 20% sustained response rate

COMPLEMENTARY TREATMENT

MILK THISTLE

♀	Dose
?	100−200mg PO q8hours of standardized extract w/ 70−80% silymarin

Treatment duration:
- •Treatment duration for hepatitis C is dependent on the viral genotype
  - ∘Genotype 1: 1year
  - ∘Genotypes 2 or 3: 6months
  - …w/ treatment failure defined by the presence of viral RNA @ 6months of treatment, whereas lack of viral RNA @ 6months after treatment cessation is usually indicative of a durable remission

NUCLEOSIDE ANALOGUE			
Generic	M	♀	Dose
Ribavirin	CK	U	400mg PO q12hours

Side effects:
General
- •Nasal congestion
- •Pruritus

Rheumatologic
- •Gout

Hematologic
- •**Anemia**
- •Hemolysis

Absolute contraindications:
Genitourinary
- •End stage renal disease

Cardiovascular
- •Severe cardiac disease

Materno–fetal
- •Pregnancy, or the absence of a reliable form of contraception

Hematologic
- •Anemia
- •Hemoglobinopathies

Relative contraindications:
General
- •Elderly

Cardiovascular
- •Uncontrolled hypertension

&

CYTOKINES			
Generic	M	♀	Dose
Pegylated interferon α–2b†	K	?	Weight based, SC qweek at bedtime

Weight (lb / kg)	Dose
<88 lbs / <40kg	50µg
88–111 lbs / 40–50kg	64µg
112–133 lbs / 51–60kg	80µg
134–166 lbs / 61–75kg	96µg
167–187 lbs / 76–85kg	120µg
>187 lbs / 86kg	150µg

†Formed by the attachment of polyethylene glycol to interferon α–2b

Outcomes:
- •**Chronic hepatitis C:**
  - ∘30% overall sustained response rate, being 55% if combined w/ Ribavirin

SECOND LINE TREATMENT

NUCLEOSIDE ANALOGUE			
Generic	M	♀	Dose
Ribavirin	CK	U	If ≤75kg: 400mg qam & 600mg qpm
			If >75kg: 600mg PO q12hours

CYTOKINES			
Generic	M	♀	Dose
Interferon–α–2b	K	?	3million units 3X/ week SC/ IM qhs

Outcomes:
•**Chronic hepatitis C:**
  ○20% sustained response rate, being 45% if combined w/ Ribavirin

THIRD LINE TREATMENT

Indications:
•Monotherapy for patients w/ contraindications or intolerable side effects to combination therapy

CYTOKINES			
Generic	M	♀	Dose
Pegylated interferon α–2b†	K	?	Weight based, SC qweek at bedtime

Weight (lb / kg)	Dose
<88 lbs / <40kg	50µg
88–111 lbs / 40–50kg	64µg
112–133 lbs / 51–60kg	80µg
134–166 lbs / 61–75kg	96µg
167–187 lbs / 76–85kg	120µg
>187 lbs / 86kg	150µg

†Formed by the attachment of polyethylene glycol to interferon α–2b
Outcomes:
•**Chronic hepatitis C:**
  ○30% overall sustained response rate

COMPLEMENTARY TREATMENT

MILK THISTLE	
♀	Dose
?	100–200mg PO q8hours of standardized extract w/ 70–80% silymarin

PROGNOSIS

Fulminant hepatitis outcomes:
•Mortality >80% w/ medical treatment alone, being ~100% @ age >45 years w/ other serious medical disease

Hepatitis virus	Chronic disease†	Cirrhosis	Hepatocellular cancer‡
A & E	0%	0%	0%
B	10% (90% in neonates)————→	25–50%——→	10%

Progression to cirrhosis:
  •5–10years avg., w/ subsequent progression to hepatocellular cancer @ 25years avg.

C	80%--------------------------→	25%———→	1–5%/ year

Progression to cirrhosis:
  •20 years avg., w/ subsequent progression to hepatocellular cancer @ 30 years avg.

D	As per hepatitis B		

†% of U.S. population w/ chronic hepatitis:
  •A & E: 0%
  •B: 0.1%
  •C: 1.8%
  •D: <<0.1%
‡It is rare for hepatocellular cancer to occur in the absence of cirrhosis. Monitor for occurrence via α–fetoprotein–AFP (normal 0–15ng/ mL), w/ serious concern @ >200
Limitations:
  •Falsely ↑ via:
    ○Hepatitis
    ○Non–seminomatous testicular neoplasms (except choriocarcinomas)
    ○Pregnancy

653

•It is extremely important that all patients w/ chronic liver disease be immunized to hepatitis A & B if they lack the appropriate protective antibodies (via prior exposure or vaccination), especially as **patients w/ chronic liver disease are at ↑risk for fulminant hepatitis A**

•**Hepatitis A**
Dose:
•**1mL IM @ 0 & 6–12months**
Mechanism:
•Inactivated whole virus vaccine
Indications:
•All persons
Postexposure prophylaxis:
•Administer hepatitis A immunoglobulin–HAIG & vaccine

•**Hepatitis B ± D**
Dose:
•**1mL IM @ 0, 1, & 7 months**
Mechanism:
•Recombinant HBsAg vaccine
Indications:
•All persons
Outcomes:
•Neutralizing anti–HBsAg in 95% of patients†, being ↓in immunosuppressed patients
Postexposure prophylaxis:
•Administer hepatitis B immunoglobulin–HBIG & vaccine
  ◦All pregnant ♀ should be screened for HBsAg, as newborns of positive mothers should receive the vaccine within 12hours of birth

•**Hepatitis C or E**
  ◦No effective medical prophylaxis is currently available, other than avoidance of risk factors

•**Combination vaccines**
  ◦Hepatitis A & B combination vaccine (Twinrex)
    Dose:
    •**1mL IM @ 0, 1, & 6months**

---

†Patients not developing protective anti–HBsAg titers (≤10mIU/ mL) should receive 1vaccine dose q month, w/ subsequent titer measurements until either:
•Protective levels are obtained
•The max of 3 subsequent doses are administered

654

•Caused by the hematogenous or direct spread of microorganisms to the subarachnoid space→
  ○Inflammation of the pia & arachnoid mater=meningitis

RISK FACTORS

•**Age**
  ○70% of cases of bacterial meningitis occur in children age <5years
  ○**>80% of all cases of meningitis occur in patients age <15years**
•**Immunosuppression**
  ○Advanced age
  ○Alcoholism
  ○Diabetes mellitus
  ○Hematologic malignancy
  ○HIV infection/ AIDS
  ○Malnutrition
  ○Medications
    −Chemotherapy
    −Chronic glucocorticoid use
    −Immunomodulating medications
  ○Renal dialysis
•**Splenectomy or deficiency of the terminal complement components (C5−C8)→**
  ○↑Infection risk via encapsulated bacteria:
    −Escherichia coli
    −Haemophilus influenzae
    −Neisseria meningitides
    −Pseudomonas aeruginosa
    −Salmonella sp.
    −Streptococcus pneumoneae
•**Cranial or spinal trauma, surgery, or congenital malformation**
  ○Spina bifida cystica + myelocele or meningomyelocele→
    −↑Infection risk via skin organisms (diptheroids, enterobacteriaceae, Propionibacterium acnes, Staphylococcus sp.)
  ○Oropharyngeal trauma
    −Streptococcus pneumoneae > others
•**Infection of the:**
  ○**Upper respiratory tract**
    −Mastoiditis
    −Otitis media
    −Sinusitis
  ○**Head/ neck**
    −Cellulitis
    −Orbital infection
    −Osteomyelitis
  ○**Dura mater**
    −Epidural abscess

CLASSIFICATION/ ORGANISMS

•**Bacterial meningitis**
  ○**Encapsulated bacteria**
    −Streptococcus pneumoneae, being most common
    −Neisseria meningitides
    −Haemophilus influenzae
  ○Enterobacteriaceae, accounting for 25% of all central nervous system infections in patient's age >65 years
    −Listeria sp.
    −Staphylococcus sp.

•**Fungal meningitis**
  ○Cryptococcus neoformans, being most common
  ○Blastomyces dermatitides
  ○Coccidiodes immitis
  ○Histoplasma capsulatum

- **Mycobacterial meningitis**
  - Mycobacterium tuberculosis, being either:
    - –Progressive primary infection
    - –Reactivation disease

- **Protozoal meningitis**
  - Toxoplasma gondii

- **Viral meningitis**
  - **Enteroviruses–50%**
    - –Coxsackievirus
    - –Echovirus
    - –Poliovirus
  - Adenovirus
  - Herpes simplex virus type 2 > 1
  - Human immune deficiency virus–HIV
  - Mumps virus
  - Arthropod borne viruses
    - –Eastern equine encephalitis virus
    - –Western equine encephalitis virus
    - –California encephalitis virus
    - –St. Louis encephalitis virus
  - Cytomegalovirus–CMV
  - Epstein–Barr virus–EBV

ASEPTIC MENINGITIS

- Causes for which no microorganism can be isolated using conventional staining & cultures

- **Infectious**
  - Fungal meningitis
  - Mycoplasma pneumoniae
  - Rickettsial meningitis
    - –Coxiella sp.
    - –Ehrlichia sp.
  - Spirochetal meningitis
    - –Borrelia burgdorferi
    - –Leptospira sp.
    - –Treponema pallidum
  - Viral meningitis
  - Parameningeal infection
    - –Brain abscess
    - –Epidural abscess
    - –Subdural abscess
    - –Septic thrombophlebitis of the dural venous sinuses

- **Noninfectious**
  - Medications
    - –Isoniazid
    - –Nonsteroidal anti–inflammatory drugs–NSAIDs
    - –Penicillin
    - –Sulfamethoxazole
    - –Trimethoprim
  - Neoplastic disease
    - –Carcinomatous meningitis
  - Rheumatic diseases
    - –Behcet's syndrome
    - –Systemic lupus erythematosus–SLE
  - Other
    - –Mollaret's meningitis
    - –Sarcoidosis
    - –Vogt–Koyanagi–Harada syndrome

General
- Inflammatory cytokines→
  - Anorexia→
    - Cachexia
  - Chills
  - Fatigue
  - **Fever–95%**
  - Headache
  - Malaise
  - Night sweats
  - Weakness
- Meningeal inflammation→
  - **Headache**
  - Opisthotonic posture: Head hyperextended w/ the body bowed forward
  - **Stiff neck=nuchal rigidity=meningismus–90%**
    - **Brudzinski's sign–50%** (think "Brudzinski's bend"): Manual head flexion in the supine position→leg flexion
    - **Kernig's sign–50%** (think "Kernig's kick"): Inability to flex the leg in the supine position due to stiffness of the hamstring muscles
    - Bulging fontanelles in neonates/ infants

---

†Temperature may be normal in patients w/:
- Chronic kidney disease, esp. w/ uremia
- Cirrhosis
- Heart failure
- Severe debility
...or those who are:
  - Intravenous drug users
  - Taking certain medications:
    - Acetaminophen
    - Antibiotics
    - Glucocorticoids
    - Nonsteroidal anti–inflammatory drugs–NSAIDs

Neurologic
- Meningeal ± cerebral inflammation=encephalitis &/or intracranial abscess→
  - **Altered mental status–80%**
    - Confusion
    - Clumsiness
    - Lethargy
    - Delirium
    - Coma
  - **↑Intracranial pressure†→**
    - Altered mental status
    - Cushing reaction‡
    - Headache
    - Nausea ± vomiting
  - Communicating hydrocephalus via arachnoid villi obstruction w/ cellular debris→
    - ↑Intracranial pressure
  - Focal deficits
    - Cranial nerve palsies
    - ↓Communication ability (expression &/or understanding)=aphasia
    - Hemiparesis
    - Impaired voluntary movement=ataxia
    - Visual field deficits
  - Seizures

Pediatrics:
- **Sensorineural hearing loss**, being the #1 complication in neonates
  - ↑Risk w/ Streptococcus pneumoneae infection

---

†The ophthalmologic exam in a patient w/ ↑intracranial pressure may show **papilledema**, identified via either:
- Blurring of the normally sharp optic disk margins
- Bulging of the optic disk

657

○Congestion &/or hemorrhage of the peripapillary veins→
  –Loss of normal venous pulsation
‡↑Intracranial pressure→
  •Vascular compression→
    ○↓Cerebral blood flow→
      –Cerebral ischemia→reflex hypertension→↑cerebral arterial pressure in order to overcome
      intracerebral pressure→↑cerebral blood flow. If intracerebral pressure cannot be overcome by
      ↑↑systemic blood pressure, ischemia→↓vasomotor center sympathetic tone→hypotension→
      distributive shock→death

Cutaneous–70%
•Disseminated gonococcal infection, occurring in <1% of Neisseria gonorhoeae infections→
  ○Lesions (usually on the trunk & extensor surface of the distal extremities) beginning as red
  papules→hemorrhagic pustules on a necrotic base being:
    –Asymptomatic
    –Often <20
    –<Several mm diameter
•Herpes simplex virus mediated vesicular skin lesions

Hematologic
•Inflammatory cytokines→
  ○Leukocytosis
  ○↑Acute phase proteins
    –↑Erythrocyte sedimentation rate–ESR (normal: 5mm/ decade aged + ♂ ≤10mm/h or ♀ ≤20mm/h)
    –↑C–reactive protein–CRP (normal: <2mg/ L), responding more acutely than ESR, as it rises
    within several hours & falls within 3days upon partial resolution
    –↑Fibrinogen
    –↑Platelets→thrombocytosis

IMAGING
•**Brain computed tomographic–CT scan** without & w/ contrast
Indications:
  •All patients w/ suspected central nervous system infection, for a possible mass lesion
    ○Epidural abscess/ hematoma
    ○Subdural abscess/ hematoma
    ○Intraparenchymal abscess/ hematoma
  •**If the patient has focal neurologic signs or papilledema**, promptly obtain a head computed
  tomographic–CT scan without & w/ contrast **prior to lumbar puncture**, as when cerebrospinal
  fluid is removed in the presence of a tumor, the ↑intracranial pressure produced may shift the brain
  downward=herniation through the tentorial notch &/or foramen magnum→
    ○Death. However, the generalized inflammation occurring w/ meningitis rarely has this effect

INVASIVE PROCEDURES
•**Lumbar puncture**
Procedure:
  •Performed through the **L3–L4/ L4–L5 interspace** (typically found via an imaginary line connecting
  the iliac crests) as the spinal cord ends at ~L1–L2
Side effects:
  •**Post–lumbar puncture headache 10–40%**
    ○Cerebrospinal fluid aspiration w/ continued leak via the lumbar puncture dural rent→
      –↓Cerebrospinal fluid, w/ loss of ≥20mL→↓intracranial pressure→non–nervous tissue tugging→
      upright postural headache, w/ usual onset within 48hours ± tinnitus &/or ↓hearing. Relieved
      upon recumbency, w/ resolution occurring gradually over hours to 2weeks
Prevention of headache:
  •Use the smallest gauge needle practical, while aligning the bevel parallel to the dural fibers which
  run longitudinally, in order to separate, not cut, the fibers
  •The following have not been shown to be risk factors:
    ○Position or hydration before, during, or after the procedure
Treatment of headache:
  •For severe &/or prolonged headaches, ask an anesthesiologist to place an epidural blood patch,
  consisting of 20mL of autologous venous blood injected into the epidural space previously
  punctured→
    ○Immediate relief in 95% of patients

658

Contraindications:
- Infection involving the path of the spinal needle
  - Cellulitis
  - Epidural abscess
- Coagulopathy (INR >1.3 &/or PTT >35seconds) &/or thrombocytopenia (<50,000/ μL)→
- ↑Intracranial pressure due to a localized lesion
  - Abscess
  - Localized edema
  - Localized hemorrhage
  - Neoplasm
  ...which may→
  - **Focal neurologic deficits**

CEREBROSPINAL FLUID ANALYSIS

Lab studies:
- **Tube 1:** Protein & glucose
- **Tube 2:** Cell count & differential
- **Tube 3:** Gram stain & culture
- **Tube 4:** Other studies as clinically indicated
  - Acid fast bacillus stain–AFB stain & culture
  - Complement fixation test for:
    - Anti–Coccidiodes immitis antibodies
    - Anti–Histoplasma capsulatum antibodies
  - Fungal staining
    - India ink staining for Cryptococcus neoformans
  - Latex particle agglutination test for:
    - Cryptococcal neoformans antigen
  - Polymerase chain reaction test for:
    - Herpes simplex viral DNA
    - Varicella–zoster viral DNA
  - Venereal disease research laboratory–VDRL test for:
    - Anti–cardiolipin–cholesterol–lecithin antibodies, produced when Treponema pallidum interacts w/ host tissues

CEREBROSPINAL FLUID CHARACTERISTICS

Studies	Differential findings				
Opening CSF pressure Normal: 18cm=180mmH$_2$0 Inflammation: Normal–↑	**>18cm H$_2$O** Meningitis Encephalitis Mass lesions				
Protein Normal: <45mg/ dL Inflammation: ↑	**45–100mg/ dL** Bacterial Viral Aseptic	**>200mg/ dL** Bacterial Fungal Mycobacterial Abscess			
Glucose Normal: >50% of plasma Inflammation: Normal–↓	**Low** Bacterial Fungal Mycobacterial	**Normal** Viral Abscess Aseptic			
Cells Normal: ≤4 cells/ μL Inflammation: ↑	**>1000 cells** Bacterial	**<500 cells** Early bacterial Viral Fungal Spirochetal Abscess Aseptic	**>50% PMN's** Bacterial Early viral Amebic	**>50% Mono's** Viral Fungal Mycobacterial Spirochetal	**Erythrocytes** HSV–1 Mycobacterial Traumatic tap

PMNs= polymorphonuclear leukocytes
Mono's= monocytes

659

•**If the patient lacks focal neurologic signs & papilledema:**
  ◦After blood cultures & cerebrospinal fluid have been obtained, begin empiric intravenous treatment promptly w/ bactericidal antibiotics, as the organism must be killed by the antibiotic alone, without help from neutrophils, which, along w/ immunoglobulin & complement proteins, have great difficulty infiltrating the central nervous system

•**If either focal neurologic signs or papilledema exist:**
  ◦After blood cultures have been obtained, begin empiric intravenous treatment promptly & obtain a head computed tomographic–CT scan to rule out a mass lesion prior to performing a lumbar puncture
    –Cerebrospinal fluid yield is unlikely to be reduced if obtained within 4hours of antibiotic administration

•**Empiric intravenous antibiotics**
  ◦The switch to PO medication should be attempted upon clinical improvement via fever resolution & clinical stabilization X 24hours, if an acceptable PO medication is available, & the patient is able to take PO medication
  ◦**Organism–narrowed therapy** should be initiated promptly upon stain, culture, & sensitivities results
  ◦The following antibiotics achieve equivalent plasma levels via PO or intravenous administration in persons w/ a functioning gastrointestinal tract:
    –Chloramphenicol
    –Doxycycline
    –Minocycline
    –Most fluoroquinolones
    –Trimethoprim/ Sulfamethoxazole

Bactericidal antibiotics
  •**Cell wall synthesis inhibitors**
    ◦β lactam medications:
      –Carbapenems
      –Cephalosporins
      –Monobactams
      –Penicillins
    ◦Vancomycin
  •**DNA synthesis inhibitors**
    ◦Fluoroquinolones
    ◦Linezolid
    ◦Metronidazole
    ◦Rifampin
    ◦Quinupristin & dalfopristin
  •**Aminoglycosides**

Treatment duration:
  •Bacterial meningitis: 3weeks
  •Fungal meningitis: 6weeks
  •Encephalitis: 3weeks
  •Abscess: 6weeks

CEPHALOSPORINS: 3rd–4th generation, to cover Haemophilus influenzae, Neisseria meningitides, & Streptococcus pneumoneae

Generic (Trade)	M	♀	Dose
Cefotaxime (Claforan)	KL	P	2g IV/ IM q12hours
Ceftriaxone (Rocephin)	KB	P	2g IV/ IM q24hours

Mechanism:
  •A β–lactam ring structure which binds to bacterial transpeptidase→
    ◦↓Transpeptidase function→
      –↓Bacterial cell wall peptidoglycan cross–linking→↓cell wall synthesis→osmotic influx of extracellular fluid→↑intracellular hydrostatic pressure→cell rupture→cell death=bactericidal
  •↑Bacterial autolytic enzymes→
    ◦Peptidoglycan degradation

  •Certain bacteria produce β–lactamase→
    ◦Cleavage of this essential structural component of cephalosporins & certain penicillins (as the other β–lactam medications differ sufficiently to prevent ring cleavage)→
      –Antibiotic inactivation. This process may be antagonized by the concomitant administration of **β–lactamase inhibitors** (Clavulanic acid=clavulanate, Sulbactam, or Tazobactam)→renewed susceptibility

660

Side effects:
General
- **Hypersensitivity reactions ≤10%**
  - ∘Anaphylaxis−0.5%→
    - −Death−0.002% (1:50,000)
  - ∘Acute interstitial nephritis
  - ∘Dermatitis
  - ∘Drug fever
  - ∘Hemolytic anemia
  - …having cross−hypersensitivity to other β lactam medications (penicillins, carbapenems), except monobactams (ex. Aztreonam)
Gastrointestinal
- •Clostridium dificile pseudomembraneous colitis (3rd generation > others)

&

VANCOMYCIN: To cover β−lactam resistant Streptococcus pneumoneae

M ♀	Dose	Peak	Trough
K ?	1g IV q12hours, to be administered over 1hour	30−40µg/ mL	>5µg/ mL

- •Peak levels are obtained 30minutes after the dose, w/ trough levels being obtained at the end of the dosing interval. Plasma peak & trough levels are directly related to toxicity & clinical efficacy respectively

Mechanism:
- •Direct cell wall peptidoglycan binding→
  - ∘↓Transpeptidase function→
    - −↓Bacterial cell wall peptidoglycan cross−linking→↓cell wall synthesis→osmotic influx of extracellular fluid→↑intracellular hydrostatic pressure→cell rupture→cell death=bactericidal

- •Vancomycin resistant enterococci−VRE & staphylococci−VRS have developed

Side effects:
General
- •Rapid intravenous administration (over <1hour)→
  - ∘Intrinsic hypersensitivity syndrome→
    - −Face, neck, &/or upper thoracic angioedema, termed "red man syndrome". Occurrence does not prevent continued use, unless accompanied by an anaphylactoid reaction
Cardiovascular
- •Venous inflammation=phlebitis ± thrombus formation
Otolaryngology
- •Ototoxicity

&

PENICILLINS: To cover Listeria sp.

Generic (Trade)	M ♀	Dose
Ampicillin (Principen)	K P	2g IV q4hours

Mechanism:
- •A β−lactam ring structure which binds to bacterial transpeptidase→
  - ∘↓Transpeptidase function→
    - −↓Bacterial cell wall peptidoglycan cross−linking→↓cell wall synthesis→osmotic influx of extracellular fluid→↑intracellular hydrostatic pressure→cell rupture→cell death=bactericidal
- •↑Bacterial autolytic enzymes→
  - ∘Peptidoglycan degradation

- •Certain bacteria produce β−lactamase→
  - ∘Cleavage of this essential structural component of cephalosporins & certain penicillins (as the other β−lactam medications differ sufficiently to prevent ring cleavage)→
    - −Antibiotic inactivation. This process may be antagonized by the concomitant administration of **β−lactamase inhibitors** (Clavulanic acid=clavulanate, Sulbactam, or Tazobactam)→renewed susceptibility

Side effects:
General
- **Hypersensitivity reactions ≤10%**
  - ∘Anaphylaxis−0.5%→
    - −Death−0.002% (1:50,000)
  - ∘Acute interstitial nephritis
  - ∘Dermatitis
  - ∘Drug fever

○Hemolytic anemia
...having cross−hypersensitivity to other β lactam medications (cephalosporins, carbapenems), except monobactams (ex. Aztreonam)

IF HYPERSENSITIVITY TO β−LACTAM MEDICATIONS

CHLORAMPHENICOL (Chloromycetin): To cover Neisseria meningitides

M	♀	Dose
LK	?	15mg/ kg IV q6hours

Mechanism:
•Affects the ribosomal 50S subunit→
  ○↓Peptidyltransferase function→
    −↓Peptide bond formation

Side effects:
Hematologic
•Irreversible, idiosyncratic, aplastic anemia 1/ 25,000
•Reversible, dose related myelosuppression
Materno−fetal
•Gray baby syndrome in newborns

&

VANCOMYCIN: To cover Streptococcus pneumoneae

M	♀	Dose	Peak	Trough
K	?	1g IV q12hours, to be administered over 1hour	30−40µg/ mL	>5µg/ mL

&

TRIMETHOPRIM−SULFAMETHOXAZOLE TMP−SMX (Bactrim, Septra): To cover Listeria sp.

M	♀	Dose
K	U	PO: 2 double strength−DS tabs (160mg TMP/ 800mg SMX) PO q6hours
		IV: 5mg/ kg TMP q6hours

•Ensure that the patient is receiving 20mg TMP/kg/24hours

Trimethoprim specific mechanism:
•↓Dihydrofolate reductase action→
  ○↓Tetrahydrofolate, being required as a methyl donor for the synthesis of purines & pyrimidines→
    −↓Nucleotide synthesis

Sulfonamide specific mechanism:
•A P−aminobenzoic acid−PABA analogue→
  ○Competitive inhibition of dihydropteroate synthetase mediated PABA conversion to dihydrofolate→
    −↓Tetrahydrofolate, being required as a methyl donor for the synthesis of purines &
      pyrimidines→ ↓nucleotide synthesis

Side effects:
Mucocutaneous
•Dermatitis via maculopapular rash, urticaria >> exfoliative dermatitis, photosensitivity, Stevens−Johnson syndrome, or toxic epidermal necrolysis
Genitourinary
•Acute interstitial nephritis
Neurologic
•Aseptic meningitis
Pulmonary
•The sulfite component of the combination medication→
  ○Asthma exacerbation in sensitive patients
Hematologic
•Myelosuppression→
  ○Anemia→
    −Fatigue
  ○Leukopenia→immunosuppression→
    −↑Infection & neoplasm risk
  ○Thrombocytopenia→
    −↑Hemorrhage risk

Trimethoprim specific:
Genitourinary
•Blocks distal renal tubule Na^+/K^+ exchange→
  ○**Hyperkalemia**

662

- •Competes w/ creatinine for tubular secretion→
  - ∘↑Creatinine, without concomitantly ↑blood urea nitrogen–BUN
- **Hematologic**
  - •↑Homocysteine levels

Sulfamethoxazole specific:
- **General**
  - •Anorexia
  - •Drug fever via hypersensitivity syndrome
- **Gastrointestinal**
  - •Nausea ± vomiting
- **Genitourinary**
  - •Crystalluria→
    - ∘Acute tubular necrosis
  - •Hepatitis
- **Hematologic**
  - **•G6PD deficiency mediated hemolytic anemia**

Contraindications:
- •Neonates or near term ♀s, as sulfamethoxazole competitively binds to albumin, thus displacing bilirubin→
  - ∘↑Kernicterus risk

CSF SHUNT, RECENT HEAD TRAUMA (including neurosurgery)

CEPHALOSPORINS: 3rd–4th generation, to cover Pseudomonas aeruginosa

Generic (Trade)	M	♀	Dose
Ceftazidime (Ceptaz, Fortaz)	K	P	2g IV q8hours

&

VANCOMYCIN: To cover methicillin resistant Staphylococcus aureus–MRSA

M	♀	Dose	Peak	Trough
K	?	1g IV q12hours, to be administered over 1hour	30–40µg/ mL	>5µg/ mL

VIRAL MENINGITIS
HERPES SIMPLEX VIRUS–HSV 1 OR 2

ANTIVIRAL MEDICATIONS

Generic (Trade)	M	♀	Dose
Acyclovir (Zovirax)	K	P	10mg/ kg IV q8hours

OTHER THERAPEUTIC MEASURES

SYSTEMIC GLUCOCORTICOID TREATMENT

Indications:
- **•To be given w/ or just prior to the 1st antibiotic dose†** in patients w/ suspected bacterial meningitis

†Treatment delay of ≥72hours after antimicrobial treatment has been initiated, offers no benefit

Generic	M	♀	Dose
Dexamethasone (Decadron)	L	?	0.4mg/ kg IV q12hours X 2days

- •Both the IV & PO routes have equal efficacy
- •Being that the total duration of systemic glucocorticoid therapy is ≤2weeks, there is no need to taper

Glucocorticoids	Relative potencies Anti-inflammatory	Mineralocorticoid	Duration	Dose equiv.
Cortisol (physiologic†)	1	1	10hours	20mg
Cortisone (PO)	0.7	2	10hours	25mg
Hydrocortisone (PO, IM, IV)	1	2	10hours	20mg
Methylprednisolone (PO, IM, IA, IV)	5	0.5	15–35hours	5mg
Prednisone (PO)	5	0.5	15–35hours	5mg
Prednisolone (PO, IM, IV)	5	0.8	15–35hours	5mg
Triamcinolone (PO, IM)	5	~0	15–35hours	5mg
Betamethasone (PO, IM, IA)	25	~0	35–70hours	0.75mg
Dexamethasone (PO)	25	~0	35–70hours	0.75mg
Fludrocortisone (PO)	10	125	10hours	

†The physiologic rate of adrenal cortical cortisol production is 20–30mg/ 24hours

Mechanism:
- •Appropriate antibiotic treatment→
  - ◦Organism death & lysis→
    - –Antigenemia→↑**meningitis** within 24hours (usually within 2hours) after initial treatment
- •Glucocorticoids→
  - ◦↓Meningeal inflammation→
    - –↓Intracranial pressure
    - –↓Possible mass effect

Outcomes:
- •↓Morbidity (including neurologic sequelae) & mortality, esp. w/ infection via either:
  - ◦Haemophilus influenza
  - ◦Neisseria meningitides
  - ◦Streptococcus pneumoneae

±

RIFAMPIN

Indications:
- •Any regimen which includes Vancomycin, for the duration of Dexamethasone use, as Dexamethasone→
  - ◦↓Cerebrospinal Vancomycin levels

M ♀	Dose
L ?	600mg PO q24hours

Dose adjustment:
- •Body weight <50kg: 450mg PO q24hours

Side effects:
General
- •Flu–like syndrome w/ fevers, chills, headache, bone pain, &/or dyspnea
- •**Orange discoloration** of body fluids, including sweat, tears, & urine†, which stain clothing & contact lenses

Gastrointestinal
- •**Hepatitis**, usually asymptomatic
  - Risk factors:
    - •Age ≥35years
    - •Alcoholism
    - •Postpartum state
    - •Underlying liver disease

Mucocutaneous
- •Dermatitis

Hematologic
- •Thrombocytopenia

Interactions
- •The concomitant administration of Rifampin w/ either:
  - ◦**Protease inhibitors** or
  - ◦**Nonnucleoside reverse transcriptase inhibitors–NNRTIs**
  - …→↓Plasma antiretroviral medication levels, w/ concomitantly ↑Rifampin levels. To avoid this, replace Rifampin w/ Rifabutin which has ↓interactions w/ protease inhibitors (except Ritonavir) & nonnucleoside reverse transcriptase inhibitors–NNRTIs (except Delavirdine)

†Compliance can be assessed via urine evaluation for orange discoloration

Monitoring:
- •Liver function test if symptomatic for possible hepatitis
- •Obtain baseline & monthly liver function tests in persons w/ risk factors for hepatitis w/ discontinuation if severe hepatitis occurs defined as either:
  - ◦**Symptomatic**
  - ◦**Plasma aminotransferase levels ≥5 X normal values**

PROGNOSIS

- •In hospital mortality is:
  - ◦25% for community acquired meningitis
  - ◦35% for hospital acquired meningitis

664

PRE-EXPOSURE PROPHYLAXIS ▬▬▬▬
STEPTOCOCCUS PNEUMONIAE VACCINE _____
Indications:
- **Age ≥50years**
- **Chronic disease**, including alcoholism
- **Close residential contact**
  ○ Chronic care facilities
    – Board & care housing
    – Nursing home care housing
  ○ Homeless shelters
  ○ Military personnel
  ○ Jails
- **Prior Streptococcal pneumonia infection**
- **Children** of all ages, w/ those age <2years requiring the conjugate heptavalent pneumococcal vaccine (Prevnar), w/ doses & timing varying by age
- **Asplenia**
  ○ Anatomic
  ○ Functional
  …being best if administered prior to asplenia, w/ repeat q6years
- **2 weeks prior to immunosuppressive treatment**
  ○ Chemotherapy
  ○ Immunomodulating medications

Dose
- **0.5mL SC/ IM X 1, w/ a booster @ 5 years**
Mechanism:
- Bacterial capsular polysaccharides of 23 serotypes
Outcomes:
- **70% efficacious for 10years**
  ○ ↓For immunosuppressed or age <2years

HAEMOPHILUS INFLUENZAE TYPE B VACCINE _____
Indications:
- **Asplenia**
  ○ Anatomic
  ○ Functional
  …being best if administered prior to asplenia
Dose
- **0.5mL IM X1**
Mechanism:
- Bacterial capsular polysaccharide conjugated to protein
Contraindications:
- **Pregnancy**

NEISSERIA MENINGITIDES VACCINE_____
Indications:
- **College students living in dormitories**
Dose:
- **0.5mL SC X 1**
Mechanism:
- Bacterial polysaccharides of serotypes A, C, Y, & W–135, but not B

POSTEXPOSURE PROPHYLAXIS ▬▬▬▬▬▬▬▬
Indications:
- Close contacts

HAEMOPHILUS INFLUENZAE

RIFAMPIN		
M ♀	**Dose**	
L ?	600mg PO q24hours X 4days	

665

NEISSERIA MENINGITIDES

FLUOROQUINOLONES

Generic (Trade)	M	♀	Dose
Ciprofloxacin (Cipro)	LK	?	500mg PO X 1
Levofloxacin (Levaquin)	KL	?	500mg PO X 1

Mechanism:
- ↓DNA gyrase=topoisomerase action→
  - ↓Bacterial DNA synthesis

OR

MACROLIDES

Generic (Trade)	M	♀	Dose
Azithromycin (Zithromax)	L	P	500mg PO X 1

Mechanism:
- Affects the ribosomal 50S subunit→
  - ↓Transfer RNA translocation

OR

CEPHALOSPORINS: 4th generation

Generic (Trade)	M	♀	Dose
Ceftriaxone (Rocephin)	KB	P	250mg IM X 1

666

•Caused by **Human immune deficiency virus-HIV infection** (HIV-1 or HIV-2)→
  ◦↓Helper (CD4+) T lymphocyte count, normal being 1,000cells/ μL→
    −Immunosuppression→↑autoimmune, infectious, & malignant disease risk
Statistics:
•~1 million Americans are infected w/ the HIV, w/ ~30 million persons being infected worldwide, esp. in underdeveloped countries:
  ◦Africa-70%
  ◦Asia-20%
  ◦Latin America
•16,000 persons are infected q24hours worldwide
•7,000 persons die q24hours worldwide due to complications

RISK FACTORS

•Viral transmission occurs via either:
  ◦Infected helper (CD4+) T lymphocytes
  ◦Direct viral transmission
  ...through mucous membranes (esp. w/ a lesion) or torn skin, w/ fluid viral concentrations being highest in **blood, semen, vaginal secretions, & breast milk**. Although found in all body fluids, transmission via feces, saliva, sweat, urine, & mosquitoes is not known to occur

•**All forms of sexual intercourse-60%**
  ◦Vaginal (esp. during menstruation), anal, or oral sex, esp. w/:
    −Unprotected sexual intercourse. Protection is achieved via the proper use of latex or polyurethane condoms, as well as rubber or latex dams for cunnilingus
    −Sex w/ an uncircumsized > circumsized ♂
  Note: In any act, the person in contact w/ infected semen is at ↑relative risk

Transmission risk:
  •Receptive anal intercourse: 1/ 100
  •Insertive anal intercourse: 1/ 1,000
  •Receptive vaginal intercourse: 1/ 1,000
  •Insertive vaginal intercourse: 1/ 10,000
  •Receptive fellatio w/ ejaculation: 1/ 1,000

•**Materno-fetal/ child transmission-25%**
  ◦Transplacentally to the fetus-25%
  ◦During birth via infected vaginal fluid & blood-50%
  ◦Breast milk-25%

Transmission risk: 1/4 w/ an untreated mother, 1/ 12-20 w/ a treated mother

•**Intravenous drug use w/ needle sharing-15%**
  ◦Unsterilized > sterilized syringes
  Needle sterilization:
    1. Draw full strength household alcohol or bleach up the syringe, through the needle until full
    2. Completely immerse the needle & syringe for >2min.
    3. Discharge the alcohol/ bleach
    4. Repeat the process, then rinse by filling & discharging the syringe w/ water X3

Transmission risk: 1/ 150

•**Inadvertent needle stick, being rare**
  ◦Healthcare employees
  ◦Police officers during body or bag checks

Transmission risk: 1/ 300

•**Infected blood contact w/ mucus membranes (eyes or mouth)-rare**
  ◦Accident victims
  ◦Healthcare employees

667

- **Infection via infected blood, blood products, or transplanted organs†, being rare**
  - ∘Donated blood began to be screened for HIV in 1985, becoming a very rare form of transmission

Transmission risk:
  - •Screened blood transfusion: 1/ 1,000,000

- **Child–maternal transmission, being rare**
  - ∘Breast feeding an infected infant

---

†Including semen used for artificial insemination

INFECTIOUS LIFE CYCLE

- •Infection→
  - ∘Systemic viral membrane glycoprotein interaction w/ helper (CD4+) T lymphocyte, monocyte, & macrophage membrane receptors→
    1. Cell binding, entry, & viral uncoating→
       - •Viral **reverse transcriptase** mediated viral RNA transcription to DNA, w/ subsequent:
    2. Nuclear entrance→
       - •Viral **integrase** mediated viral DNA integration into cellular DNA→
         - ∘Cellular RNA polymerase mediated viral DNA transcription→
           - –Viral messenger RNA, w/ subsequent:
    3. Cytoplasmic entrance→
       - •Cellular ribosome mediated viral protein production:
         - ∘Structural, core, & matrix proteins
         - ∘Enzymes
           - –Integrase
           - –Protease
           - –Reverse transcriptase
         - ...→viral formation, w/ viral **protease** mediated intra–viral protein cleavage→
           - •A mature, infectious virus, w/ subsequent:
    4. Cell membrane attachment & budding, occurring only in helper (CD4+) T lymphocytes→
       - •Helper (CD4+) T lymphocyte inactivation ± death
       - •Monocyte & macrophage infection, w/ subsequent:
         - ∘Tissue infiltration
         - ∘↓Cellular function
         - ∘Inter–cell membrane attachment→
           - –Multinucleated giant cells w/ eventual death

  - ∘Immune response via:
    - –Cytotoxic T cells @ ~3 weeks
    - –Anti–HIV IgA, IgM, & IgG antibodies @ 1.5–3months, termed seroconversion
    - ...→↓↓blood viral concentration=**viral load**. However, there is continued:
      - •Low–level lymphoid tissue (lymph nodes, spleen) viral production→
        - ∘Low–level helper (CD4+) T lymphocyte dysfunction & death→
          - –Gradual Immunosuppression
      - •Latent viral infection via nuclear genomic incorporation

- •Immunosuppression↔
  - ∘↓Viral suppression & containment↔↑viral replication↔↓helper (CD4+) T lymphocyte count, w/ an average loss of 25–50cells/µL/year X 8 years, during which the patient is asymptomatic & likely to unknowingly transmit the virus. Subsequently, the average loss becomes 50–100 cells/µL/year, indicating progression to AIDS within 2 years via significant immune dysregulation→
    - –↑**Autoimmune, infectious, & malignancy risk**, w/ the median time from untreated infection to the development of AIDS being 11 years, w/ peak incidence @ ages 30–40years (11% of cases being diagnosed @ age >50years)→death @ an average of 1.3 years without treatment

668

HIV INFECTION ▬▬▬▬▬

•Enzyme linked immunosorbent assay–ELISA
Indications:
- •Primary screening test for the detection of anti–HIV 1 antibodies

Procedure:
- •HIV antigens affixed to a plastic plate are incubated w/ the patient's plasma. If the patient is infected & has produced antibodies, then the addition of enzymatically labeled (horseradish peroxidase) anti–human IgG allows for color visualization via a spectrophotometer

Outcomes:
- •Sensitivity 99.5% @ ≥4 months after infection
- •Specificity 99%, w/ a positive result necessitating confirmation via Western blot testing

Limitations:
- •False negative:
  - ◦Premature testing
- •False positive:
  - ◦Autoimmune diseases

•Western blot
Indications:
- •A positive ELISA result

Procedure:
- •Acrylamide gel electrophoresis mediated HIV-1 protein separation→
  - ◦Discrete protein bands consisting of:
    - –Core proteins (p17, p24, p55)
    - –Polymerase proteins (p31, p51, p66)
    - –Envelope proteins (gp41, gp120, gp160)
    - …which are transferred ("blotted") onto filter paper, w/ the subsequent addition of the patients plasma. If the patient is infected & has produced antibodies, then the addition of either radioactively labeled or enzymatically labeled (horseradish peroxidase) anti–human IgG allows for Geiger counter detection or color visualization via a spectrophotometer respectively

Interpretation:
- •Positive: HIV–1 band pattern consisting of (gp41 or p24) + (gp120 or gp160)
- •Indeterminate: Any HIV–1 band pattern not meeting the criteria for positive results, necessitating confirmation via polymerase chain reaction–PCR testing
- •Negative: No HIV–1 bands

•Polymerase chain reaction–PCR
Indications:
- •Detection of HIV-1 viral RNA in patients within 4months after suspected exposure, as antibody production may not have reached a level sufficient for adequate ELISA sensitivity
- •An indeterminate Western blot result
- •To determine blood viral concentration, termed viral load (viral RNA/ mL plasma)

Mechanism:
- •Either qualitative or quantitative via viral load measurement of HIV-1 viral RNA

Disease progression as indicated via viral load:
- •Slow
  - ◦Branched chain–b DNA: <10,000/ mL
  - ◦Reverse transcriptase–RT PCR: <20,000/ mL
- •Moderate
  - ◦Branched chain–b DNA: 10,000–30,000/ mL
  - ◦Reverse transcriptase–RT PCR: 20,000–60,000/ mL
- •Fast
  - ◦Branched chain–b DNA: >30,000/ mL
  - ◦Reverse transcriptase–RT PCR: >60,000/ mL

•HIV–1 p24 antigen assay
Indications:
- •Used to screen all donated blood
- •Diagnosis of the Acute Retroviral Syndrome, as antibody production has likely not begun

Mechanism:
- •Detects the HIV–1 core protein p24

Outcomes:
- Sensitivity depends on disease stage
  - Acute retroviral syndrome: 100%
  - Helper (CD4+) T lymphocyte count of:
    - 200–500 cells/ µL: 45–70%
    - <200 cells/ µL: 75–100%

Limitations:
- After seroconversion, the antigen is bound by anti–p24 antibodies, and may become undetectable

•HIV viral culture

- There are both **saliva & urine tests** available which use ELISA, w/ Western blot confirmation if necessary
- Both the plasma helper (CD4+) T lymphocyte & HIV RNA levels may be acutely affected by immune stimulation, & thus, generally should not be measured within 1 month after either:
  - Resolution of inflammation
  - Immunization

Why measure both helper (CD4+) T lymphocytes & viral load?
- Consider HIV as a train going through your town. The helper (CD4+) T lymphocyte count informs you of the train's position at a given time, while the viral load informs you of the train's speed (↓amount indicating a slower rate of progression). Once the train reaches it's destination, the patient dies. Therefore, both are necessary to make an informed prognosis

ACQUIRED IMMUNE DEFICIENCY SYNDROME–AIDS ▬▬▬▬▬▬▬
- HIV infection w/ either:
  - **Helper (CD4+) T lymphocyte count** being either:
    - <200cells/ µL
    - <14% of the total lymphocyte count
  - **Certain opportunistic diseases**, termed AIDS defining diseases:

Infection (reactivation of latent infection >> newly acquired infection):
- **Pneumocystis carinii pneumonia–PCP 40%**, being both the:
  - #1 lethal infectious disease in HIV patients
  - #1 AIDS defining illness
- **Non genitourinary or oral Candidal sp. infection–15%**
- **Mycobacterium tuberculosis infection**
  - Pulmonary–7%
  - Extrapulmonary–2%
- **Cytomegalovirus–CMV** infection other than liver, lymph nodes, or spleen
  - Eye–7%
- **Disseminated Mycobacterium avium intracellulare complex–MAI infection 5%**
- **Extrapulmonary Cryptococcus neoformans infection–5%**
- **Herpes simplex virus–HSV infection–5%**→either:
  - Mucocutaneous ulcer >1month
  - Esophagitis
  - Bronchitis
  - Pneumonitis
- **Pneumonia**, being ≥2 episodes within 1year–5%
- **Toxoplasma gondii infection–1%**
- **Cryptosporidium parvum→**
  - Diarrhea >1month–1%
- **Extrapulmonary Histoplasma capsulatum infection–1%**
- **Progressive multifocal leukoencephalopathy–PML–1%**
- **Extrapulmonary Coccidioides immitis infection–0.2%**
- **Isospora belli→**
  - Diarrhea >1month–0.2%
- **Non–typhoid Salmonella sp. infection–0.2%**

Malignancy:
- **Kaposi's sarcoma–7%, being the most common cancer in AIDS patients**
- **Invasive cervical cancer–0.6%**
- **Lymphoma**
  - Burkitt's–0.7%
  - Large cell immunoblastic–2.3%
  - Primary of the central nervous system–0.7%

670

<u>Other:</u>
- **HIV wasting syndrome–18%**, comprised of:
  - ○Fever of unknown origin–FUO X ≥1month
  - ○Involuntary weight loss >10% of baseline
  - ○Chronic diarrhea (≥2 loose stools/ 24h X ≥1month) &/or chronic weakness
- **HIV encephalopathy→**
  - ○Dementia→
    - –Disabling cognitive &/or other dysfunction interfering w/ occupation &/or activities of daily living–5%

- Once a patient is diagnosed w/ AIDS, they are forever considered an AIDS patient regardless of future clinical or serologic improvement
- †The percentages total >100%, as some patients have a dual diagnosis
ACUTE RETROVIRAL SYNDROME–60% ▬▬▬▬▬▬▬
- Systemic viremia→
  - ○Mononucleosis–like syndrome beginning 2–6 weeks after infection, & lasting ≤1month

General
- Inflammatory cytokines→
  - ○Anorexia→
    - –Cachexia
  - ○Chills
  - ○Fatigue
  - ○**Fever–95%**
  - ○Headache
  - ○Malaise
  - ○Night sweats
  - ○Weakness

---

†Temperature may be normal in patients w/:
- Chronic kidney disease, esp. w/ uremia
- Cirrhosis
- Heart failure
- Severe debility
…or those who are:
- Intravenous drug users
- Taking certain medications:
  - ○Acetaminophen
  - ○Antibiotics
  - ○Glucocorticoids
  - ○Nonsteroidal anti–inflammatory drugs–NSAIDs

Gastrointestinal
- Gastroenteritis→
  - ○Diarrhea
  - ○Nausea ± vomiting
- Hepatitis
Lymphatics
  - ○†Leukocyte replication→
    - –**Lymphadenopathy–75%**
    - –**Hepatomegally**
    - –**Splenomegally**, which may retain a relatively †proportion of circulating cells. termed hypersplenism→anemia, granulocytopenia, &/or thrombocytopenia
Mucocutaneous
- **Pharyngitis without exudative effusion–70%→**
  - ○Sore throat
  - ○Pain on swallowing=odynophagia
- **Erythematous maculopapular rash–70%**, usually being symmetric, esp. affecting the face, thorax, palms, &/or soles
- Mucosal ulcerations of the mouth, pharynx, esophagus, &/or genitalia
- Oropharyngeal candidiasis=thrush–12%
Neurologic–10%
- Meningitis
- Encephalitis
- Peripheral neuropathy
- Facial palsy
- Guillan–Barre syndrome

671

- Brachial neuritis
- Radiculopathy
- Psychosis

Hematologic
- Leukocytosis

TREATMENT

- Use a 3–4 medication combination, termed "cocktail", thereby:
  - Acting at different viral life cycle stages
  - ↓Viral resistance
- Treatment does not eradicate HIV infection

Indications for the initiation of antiretroviral treatment†:
- Absolute indications:
  - **Acquired immune deficiency syndrome–AIDS**
  - **Symptomatic HIV Infection, including the acute retroviral syndrome**
- Relative indications:
  - Helper (CD4+) T lymphocyte count <350cells/ μL
  - HIV RNA
    - Branched chain–b DNA: >30,000/ mL
    - Reverse transcriptase–RT PCR: >60,000/ mL

Risks of early antiretroviral treatment:
- ↓Quality of life from both:
  - Medication side effects
  - The persistent need for multi–daily administration
- Earlier development of medication resistance→
  - Future limitation of efficacious medication combinations
  - ↑Risk of medication resistant virus dissemination

Benefits of early antiretroviral treatment:
- Delay or prevent the onset of a severe immunocompromised state
- Complete suppression of viral replication→
  - ↓Medication resistance risk
- ↓Transmission risk

Assessment of antiretroviral therapeutic response:
- **@ 1month:** ≥0.5 log titer reduction from pre–treatment value
  - Calculation: 5 (initial viral load ÷ 10)
- **@ 2 months:** ≥1 log titer reduction from pre–treatment value
  - Calculation: Initial viral load ÷ 10
- **@ 4–6 months & thereafter:** Undetectable, being ≤50 copies of RNA/ mL

Differential of a poor antiretroviral therapeutic response:
- Noncompliance, being the #1 cause of treatment failure
- Medication resistance
- Medication malabsorption
- Medication–medication interaction

Action to a poor antiretroviral therapeutic response:
- Regardless of the cause, the patient should stop all antiretroviral medications & undergo viral genotyping or phenotyping assays in order to detect possible resistance conferring mutations, prior to reinstitution of antiretroviral treatment

Effects of discontinuing antiretroviral treatment‡:
- Discontinuation of antiretroviral treatment→
  - Re–emergence of the "wild–type" HIV, as the dominant viral strain @ ~2weeks, as it is more "fit"→
    - ↓Helper (CD4+) T lymphocyte count beginning @ 2–4weeks
- These "wild–type" strains are typically sensitive to most, if not all the medications to which resistance had previously been demonstrated→
  - Virologic response to the re–introduction of previously used anti–retroviral treatment. However, resistant viral strains, which remained as a minority species, will eventually re–emerge as the dominant species upon the re–imposed selective pressure

---

†Initiation of antiretroviral treatment may worsen concomitant infections for several weeks, due to immune stimulation, being termed the **immune reconstitution syndrome**

672

‡If antiretroviral treatment must be interrupted for some reason, stop all the antiretroviral medications together in order to ↓resistance formation

NUCLEOSIDE REVERSE TRANSCRIPTASE INHIBITORS–NRTIs

Generic (Trade)	M	♀	Dose
Abacavir–ABC (Ziagen)	ML	?	300mg PO q12hours
Didanosine–ddI (Videx)	LK	P	If >60kg: 400mg PO q24hours on an empty stomach
			If <60kg: 250mg PO q24hours on an empty stomach
Emtricitabine–FTC† (Emtriva)	K	P	200mg PO q24hours
Lamivudine–3TC (Epivir)	K	?	If >50kg: 150mg PO q12hours
			If <50kg: 2mg/ kg PO q12hours
Stavudine–d4T (Zerit)	LK	?	If >60kg: 40mg PO q12hours
			If <60kg: 30mg PO q12hours
Zalcitabine–ddC (Hivid)	K	?	0.75mg PO q8hours on an empty stomach
Zidovudine–AZT,ZDV (Retrovir)	LK	?	300mg PO q12hours

†A 5–fluorinated derivative of Lamivudine

Generic combination (Trade)	M	♀	Dose
Zidovudine–ZDV & Lamivudine–3TC (Combivir)	LK	?	1tab PO q12hours
Zidovudine–ZDV, Lamuvudine–3TC, & Abacavir (Trizivir)	LK	?	1tab PO q12hours

Mechanism:
- •Selectively inhibit Human immune deficiency virus–HIV reverse transcriptase mediated DNA synthesis

Lamivudine specific:
- •→Human immune deficiency–HIV reverse transcriptase mutation→
  - ∘↑Zidovudine susceptibility

Side effects:
General
- •Headache
- •Hypersensitivity reaction

Musculoskeletal
- •**Lipodystrophy syndrome**
  - ∘Fat redistribution from the extremities & face→
    - –Thin arms, legs, & face, w/ collapsed cheeks
    - –↑Fat deposition in the breasts, neck, thorax (esp. supraclavicular fat pads or dorsocervical fat pad, termed "buffalo hump") &/or abdomen
    - …w/ discontinuation→
      - •Resolution in some patients

Gastrointestinal
- •**Pancreatitis** via:
  - ∘Didanosine–5%
  - ∘Stavudine–1%

Neurologic
- •**Peripheral neuropathy** via:
  - ∘Didanosine–20%
  - ∘Stavudine–17%
  - ∘Zalcitabine–30%

Hematologic
- •**Dyslipidemia**
- •Lactic acidemia w/ hepatic steatosis & hepatomegally, being rare

Abacavir specific:
General
- •**Abacavir hypersensitivity reaction–5%**
  - ∘A severe, potentially fatal, hypersensitivity reaction, usually **occurring within 1.5months**, being characterized by:
    - –A flu–like syndrome
    - –Dermatitis
    - –Gastrointestinal distress
    - …all of which worsen w/ successive doses. If suspected, **discontinue the medication immediately, w/ re–challenge being contraindicated as it may cause anaphylaxis**
  Risk factors:
    - •Color: Whites > blacks

Emtricitabine specific:
Mucocutaneous
•Hyperpigmentation of the palms & soles, esp. in darker colored persons

Zidovudine specific:
Hematologic
•**Myelosuppression–3%**→
◦Anemia→
−Fatigue
◦Leukopenia→immunosuppression→
−↑Infection & neoplasm risk
◦Thrombocytopenia→
−↑Hemorrhage risk, esp. petechiae

Zidovudine specific monitoring:
•Complete blood count w/ differential @ baseline, then
◦Q3months

NUCLEOTIDE REVERSE TRANSCRIPTASE INHIBITOR–NtRTs

Generic (Trade)	M	♀	Dose
Tenofovir (Viread)	K	P	300mg PO q24hours w/ food

Mechanism:
•Selectively inhibit Human immune deficiency virus–HIV reverse transcriptase mediated DNA synthesis

Side effects:
Gastrointestinal
•Diarrhea
•Nausea ± vomiting
Musculoskeletal
•Osteoporosis
Hematologic
•Lactic acidemia w/ hepatic steatosis & hepatomegally, being rare

---

NONNUCLEOSIDE REVERSE TRANSCRIPTASE INHIBITORS–NNRTIs

Generic (Trade)	M	♀	Dose
Delavirdine–DLV (Rescriptor)	L	?	400mg PO q8hours
Efavirenz–EFV (Sustiva)	L	?	600mg PO qhs
Nevirapine–NVP (Viramune)	LK	?	200mg PO q24hours X 2weeks, then
			200mg PO q12hours

Mechanism:
•Selectively inhibit Human immune deficiency virus–HIV reverse transcriptase mediated DNA synthesis

Side effects:
Mucocutaneous
•Dermatitis
Hematologic
•Hypertriglyceridemia
Interactions
•False positive 9–tetrahydrocannabinol–THC testing for marijuana
•The concomitant administration of Rifampin w/ either:
◦**Protease inhibitors** or
◦**Nonnucleoside reverse transcriptase inhibitors–NNRTIs**
…→↓plasma antiretroviral medication levels, w/ concomitantly ↑Rifampin levels. To avoid this, replace Rifampin w/ Rifabutin, which has ↓interactions w/ protease inhibitors (except Ritonavir) & nonnucleoside reverse transcriptase inhibitors (except Delavirdine)

Efavirenz specific:
Neurologic–50%
•↓Concentration
•Daytime somnolence
•Dizziness
•Insomnia
•Nightmares
•Hallucinations
…upon treatment initiation, which usually resolve w/ continued treatment

674

Nevirapine specific:
Gastrointestinal
•**Hepatitis–1%,** which may be severe=fulminant
Mucocutaneous
•**Severe skin reaction** via either:
 ∘Stevens–Johnson syndrome
 ∘Toxic epidermal necrolysis

Nevirapine specific monitoring:
•Liver function tests @ baseline, then
 ∘Q2weeks X 2, then
  –Qmonth X 3, then q3months

PROTEASE INHIBITORS

Generic (Trade)	M	♀	Dose
Amprenavir–APV (Agenerase)	L	?	1.2g PO q12hours = **16pills/ 24h.** Avoid w/ ↑fat meal
Atazanavir–ATV (Reyataz)	L	P	400mg q24hours w/ food
Fosamprenavir† (Lexiva)			1.4g q12hours
Indinavir–IDV (Crixivan)	LK	?	800mg PO q8hours on an empty stomach‡
Nelfinavir–NFV (Viracept)	L	P	1.25g PO q12hours w/ meals
Ritonavir–RTV (Norvir)	L	?	Start 300mg PO q12hours w/ meals & titrate by 100mg/ dose q3days→600mg PO q12hours
Saquinavir–SQV	L	P	
•Invirase			600mg PO q8hours w/ meals = **9pills/ 24hours**
•Fortovase			1.2g PO q8hours w/ meals = **18pills/ 24hours**

†A prodrug of Amprenavir
‡1hour before, or 2hours after a meal

Generic combination (Trade)	M	♀	Dose
Ritonavir & Amprenavir	L	?	200mg & 1200mg PO q24hours
Ritonavir & Atazanavir	L	?	100mg & 300mg PO q24hours
Ritonavir & Fosamprenavir			PI naïve: 200mg & 1400mg PO q24hours
			PI non–naïve: 100mg & 700mg PO q12hours
			W/ Efavirenze: 300mg & 1400mg PO q24hours
Ritonavir & Lopinavir (Kaletra)	L	U	3tabs (33.3mg & 133.3mg per tab) PO q12hours w/ food
Ritonavir & Saquinavir	L	?	400mg & 400mg Invirase PO q12hours
Ritonavir & Indinavir	LK	?	PI naïve: 100mg & 800mg tab PO q12hours
			PI non–naive: 200mg & 800mg

Mechanism:
•Selectively inhibit Human immune deficiency virus–HIV protease function

Side effects:
General
 •Headache
Endocrine
 •**Insulin resistance→**
  ∘Diabetes mellitus, usually occurring @ 2months of therapy, w/ a range of 2days–13months. Most authorities recommend continuing antiretroviral treatment, unless severe complications occur. Resolution w/ discontinuation is unknown.
Gastrointestinal
 •Diarrhea
 •Nausea ± vomiting
Mucocutaneous
 •Circumoral paresthesia via:
  ∘Amprenavir
  ∘Ritonavir–5%
Musculoskeletal
 •**Lipodystrophy syndrome**
  ∘Fat redistribution from the extremities & face→
   –Thin arms, legs, & face, w/ collapsed cheeks
   –↑Fat deposition in the breasts, neck, thorax (esp. supraclavicular fat pads or dorsocervical fat pad, termed "buffalo hump") &/or abdomen
   …w/ discontinuation→
    •Resolution in some patients

Hematologic
- **Dyslipidemia.** Consider continuing antiretroviral treatment unless risk–benefit analysis indicates otherwise. Discontinuation→
  - ∘Resolution in some patients
- **Unconjugated hyperbilirubinemia** via:
  - ∘Atazanavir
  - ∘Indinavir
- •↑**Hemorrhage risk in Hemophilia A or B patients**

Interactions
- •↑**Sildenafil** (Viagra) **effect.** Use a max dose of 25mg PO q48h
- •Protease inhibitors→
  - ∘↓Hepatocyte cytochrome P450 system activity→
    - –↓HMG–CoA reductase inhibitor metabolism→↑plasma levels (except Pravastatin). So, patients who are dyslipidemic & do not respond to dietary interventions, may be started only on Pravastatin
- •The concomitant administration of Rifampin w/ either:
  - ∘**Protease inhibitors** or
  - ∘**Nonnucleoside reverse transcriptase inhibitors–NNRTIs**
  - ...→↓plasma antiretroviral medication levels, w/ concomitantly ↑Rifampin levels. To avoid this, replace Rifampin w/ Rifabutin, which has ↓interactions w/ protease inhibitors (except Ritonavir) & nonnucleoside reverse transcriptase inhibitors (except Delavirdine)
- •**Garlic & St. Johns wort**→
  - ∘↑Hepatocyte cytochrome P450 system activity→
    - –↑**Protease inhibitor metabolism**→↓plasma levels

Amprenavir specific:
Mucocutaneous
- •**Dermatitis–30%,** w/ 1% being severe via either:
  - ∘Stevens–Johnson syndrome
  - ∘Toxic epidermal necrolysis

Indinavir specific:
Genitourinary
- •**Nephrolithiasis–7%**

Monitoring:
- •Fasting blood glucose @ baseline, then
  - ∘Q4 months
- •Fasting lipid profile @ baseline, then
  - ∘Q4 months

Indinavir specific:
- •Urinalysis & renal function @ baseline, then
  - ∘Qyear

VIRAL CELL MEMBRANE FUSION INHIBITORS

Generic (Trade)	M	♀	Dose
Enfuvirtide=Peptide T–20 (Fuzeon)	S	P	90mg SC q12hours, alternating doses among the upper arm, anterior thigh, & abdomen

Mechanism:
- •Inhibits viral gp41 mediated cell fusion

Side effects:
Mucocutaneous
- •Injection site inflammation→
  - ∘Erythema, cysts, nodules, &/or pain
Hematologic
- •Eosinophilia

HIGHLY ACTIVE ANTIRETROVIRAL THERAPY–HAART† ▬▬▬▬▬▬
Preferred combination regimens:
- •**2 NRTIs:** (Zidovudine–ZDV or Stavudine–d4T) + (Lamivudine–3TC or Didanosine–ddI)
  & EITHER
- •**2 PIs:** Ritonavir‡ & (Indinavir, NIfinavir, or Saquinavir)
  OR
- •**1 NNRTI:** Nevirapine or Efavirenz

676

Alternative combination regimens:
- **2 NRTIs:** Didanosine–ddI + Lamivudine–3TC
  ### & EITHER
- **1–2 PIs:** (Lopinavir + Ritonavir), (Nelfinavir + Saquinavir), Amprenavir, Ritonavir, or Saquinavir SGL°
  ### OR
- **1 NNRTI:** Delavirdine
  ### OR
- **Another NRTI:** Abacavir

Mechanism:
- $\uparrow$Helper (CD4+) T lymphocyte count
- $\downarrow$Plasma HIV RNA

Outcomes:
- $\downarrow$Opportunistic infections, malignancies, & autoimmune syndromes$\rightarrow$
  - $\uparrow$Life span & quality of life
- Treatment of the acute retroviral syndrome X $\geq$2 years$\rightarrow$
  - $\downarrow$Viral setpoint$\rightarrow$
    - $\downarrow$Disease progression

Complications:
- HIV infected patients treated w/ combination antiretroviral regimens experience $\uparrow$**atherosclerosis** via:
  - HIV &/or antiretroviral mediated endothelial inflammation
  - HIV &/or antiretroviral mediated dyslipidemia
  - Antiretroviral mediated insulin resistance
  ...$\rightarrow$
    - $\uparrow$Myocardial ischemic syndrome risk
    - $\uparrow$Cerebrovascular accident syndrome risk
    - $\uparrow$Peripheral vascular ischemic syndrome risk

Combinations not recommended:
- Due to possible resistance, overlapping toxicity, or other evidence against use
  - < Triple therapy
  - Zalcitibine–ddC + (Didanosine–ddI, Lamivudine–3TC, or Stavudine–d4T)
  - Zidovudine–ZDV + Stavudine–d4T
  - Abacavir–ABC + (Didanosine–ddI + Stavudine–d4T) or (Lamivudine–3TC + Tenofovir–TDF)
  - Hydroxyurea w/ any of the above
  - Rifampin + protease inhibitors or nonnucleoside reverse transcriptase inhibitors–NNRTIs
  - **In pregnancy:**
    - Efavirenze–EFV, due to fetal abnormalities which have occurred in pregnant monkeys
    - The combination of Stavudine–d4T & Didanosine–ddI, due to fatal lactic acidemia

---

†Termed mega–HAART if $\geq$5 medications are used
‡Ritonavir is included in the above regimens primarily because it$\rightarrow$
- $\downarrow$Hepatocyte cytochrome P450 system function more than other protease inhibitors$\rightarrow$
  - $\downarrow$Hepatic antiretroviral metabolism$\rightarrow$
    - Prolongation of viricidal plasma levels, being termed the **"protease inhibitor boost"**$\rightarrow$$\downarrow$dosage frequency of the accompanying medications$\rightarrow$$\uparrow$patient compliance & quality of life
°Soft gel capsule, as the use of Saquinavir hard gel capsule is not recommended, except in combination w/ Ritonavir

TREATMENT DURING PREGNANCY ▬▬▬▬▬▬▬▬
- All pregnant ♀ should be screened for HIV infection
- Report cases of exposure to antiretroviral medications during pregnancy to the Antiretroviral Pregnancy Registry @ 1–800–258–4263 or www.apregistry.com in order to assist in monitoring patients for possible teratogenic effects

- **Start or continue highly active antiretroviral treatment–HAART** as for non–pregnant patients
- **Needed vaccinations should be administered upon viral load undetectability,** in order to $\downarrow$transmission risk due to immune response mediated transiently $\uparrow$plasma viral load
- **Avoid the use of invasive:**
  - **Testing:** Amniocentesis
  - **Monitoring:** Fetal scalp electrodes or blood sampling
  - **Instruments to assist delivery**
- **Scheduled cesarean section delivery @ 38weeks** if the viral load is likely to be >1,000/ µL, based on the viral load @ 34–36 weeks of gestation. This will $\downarrow$possible viral transmission via infected vaginal fluid & blood. There is no evidence of a benefit after the onset of labor, rupture of membranes, or w/ a viral load <1,000cells/ µL
- **Avoid a prolonged interval between the rupture of the membranes & delivery**

- **During vaginal delivery, avoid an episiotomy** which→
  - ○↑Neonatal exposure to maternal blood
- **The infant should be washed before any percutaneous procedure** (blood drawing or injections) **is performed**
- **The mother must not breast feed her infant**

&

NUCLEOSIDE REVERSE TRANSCRIPTASE INHIBITORS-NRTIs			
Generic (Trade)	M	♀	Dose
Zidovudine–AZT, ZDV (Retrovir)	LK	?	
•During pregnancy:			300mg PO q12hours during the 2nd & 3rd trimesters only, due to ? safety during 1st trimester organogenesis
•During labor:			2mg/ kg IV loading dose, then 1mg/kg/hour
•Neonate:			2mg/ kg q6hours starting 8–12hours after birth & continued X 6 weeks

Treatment outcomes:
- •No treatment→25% transmission risk
- •Zidovudine→8% transmission risk
- •Highly active antiretroviral treatment–HAART→1.5% transmission risk

Monitoring:
- **Assess neonatal HIV infection status** via testing @ 1 day, 1 month, & 3–6months

INFECTION PROPHYLAXIS

- **Safer sex practices**
- **Stop any illicit drug use**, as all→
  - ○↓Inhibitions→
    - −↑Risk of unsafe sex &/or sharing intravenous drug needles. If the patient is unwilling to stop using intravenous drugs, then they must not share needles, or at the very least sterilize the syringe & needle between use w/ the other person

PROPHYLAXIS BASED ON CD4 COUNT		
CD4 count	Organism	Prophylaxis

Any	Mycobacterium tuberculosis	•Recent contact w/ patient w/ active disease
		•PPD induration of:
		  ○Any size if anergic
		  ○≥5mm induration

	Streptococcus pneumoniae	•If age ≥2 years:
		  ○Pneumococcal vaccine series
		    −Best when CD4 >350/ μL

	Haemophilus influenza	•Haemophilus influenza type b vaccine
	Hepatitis A virus	•If anti–HAV negative ○Vaccination series
	Hepatitis B virus	•If anti–HBSab negative ○Vaccination series
	Influenza A virus	•P: Vaccination qyear, prior to the influenza season •A: Rimantadine 100mg PO q12hours or Amantadine 100mg PO q12hours

	Varicella–zoster virus	•If naive exposure:
		  ○Varicella–zoster immune globulin–VZIG: 5vials
		  (1.25mL/ vial) IM within 96hours postexposure
		    −Best if within 48hours postexposure
		•A: Acyclovir 800mg PO 5X/ 24hours X 1week

<200
or fever of unknown origin–FUO
or oropharyngeal candidiasis
	Pneumocystis carinii	•P: Trimethoprim sulfamethoxazole DS tab PO q24hours
		•A: Dapsone 100mg q24hours or
		  Atovaquone 1.5g q24hours w/ meals or
		  Aerosolized Pentamidine 300mg/ 6mL sterile water
		  via nebulizer q1month or
		  Dapsone 200mg qwk + Pyrimethamine 75mg qwk +
		  Leukovorin 25mg qwk

Discontinue @ a helper (CD4+) T lymphocyte count > 200 cells/ μL X 3months

678

CD4 count	Organism	Prophylaxis
<100 or <200 if previous infection	Toxoplasma gondii	•If IgG+: Trimethoprim sulfamethoxazole DS tab PO q24hours •A: Dapsone 50mg q24h + Pyrimethamine 50mg qwk + folinic acid 25mg qwk or Atovaquone 1.5g q24h

Discontinue @ a helper (CD4+) T lymphocyte count >200 cells/ μL X 3months, or X 6 months if previous infection

<75 or <100 if previous infection	Mycobacterium avium complex	•P: Azithromycin 1.2g qwk •A: Rifabutin 300mg q24hours

Discontinue @ a helper (CD4+) T lymphocyte count >100 cells/ μL X 3months, or X 6months if previous infection

<50 or <100 if previous infection	Cytomegalovirus	•If CMV PCR positive ∘Gancyclovir 1g PO q8hours w/ meals

Discontinue @ a helper (CD4+) T lymphocyte count >150 cells/ μL X 6months

---

P=Preferred treatment
A=Alternative treatment
•Patients immunized while having a helper (CD4+) T lymphocytes count <200 cells/ μL should be reimmunized if the count increases to >200 cells/ μL
Note: Prior to initiating **Trimethoprim–Sulfamethoxazole** or **Dapsone** treatment, measure plasma glucose–6–phosphate dehydrogenase–G6PD levels, as both→
•**Hemolytic anemia** in enzyme deficient patients

MONITORING

Hematology:
•Helper (CD4+) T lymphocyte count @
  ∘Baseline, then q3months (q6 months if >600 cells/ μL)
•PCR quantitative plasma HIV RNA=viral load
  ∘As for T lymphocyte count
•Complete blood count w/ differential
  ∘Baseline, then q6 months
•Liver function tests
  ∘Baseline, then as needed
•Blood chemistry
  ∘Baseline, then as needed
•Syphilis serology via RPR or VDRL
  ∘Baseline, then qyear if negative
•Cytomegalovirus–CMV IgG serology via PCR
  ∘Baseline
•Toxoplasma gondii IgG serology
  ∘Baseline
•Measles antibody if born >1957
Cytology:
•Papanicolaou smear in ♀ w/ a uterus
  ∘Baseline, then qyear
•Consider anal swabs for cytologic evaluation of patients w/ a history of receptive anal intercourse
  ∘Baseline, then qyear
Imaging:
•Posteroanterior & lateral chest x ray
  ∘Baseline, then as deemed necessary
Other:
•Tuberculosis screening via PPD skin test
  ∘Baseline, then qyear if negative
•Opthalmologic examination for CMV retinitis
  ∘Q6months if helper (CD4+) T lymphocyte count <100cells/ μL

679

•Consult an infectious disease physician

Indications:
- **Best when started within 2hours after potential exposure**, w/ minimal effect if started @ >24hours, & no effect if started @ >72hours

NUCLEOSIDE REVERSE TRANSCRIPTASE INHIBITORS-NRTIs			
Generic (Trade)	M ♀	**Dose**	
Zidovudine-AZT, ZDV (Retrovir) LK ?		300mg PO q12hours	

&

NUCLEOSIDE REVERSE TRANSCRIPTASE INHIBITORS-NRTIs			
Generic (Generic)	M ♀	**Dose**	
Lamivudine-3TC (Epivir) K ?		150mg PO q12hours	
Mechanism:			
•→Human immune deficiency-HIV reverse transcriptase mutation→			
०↑Zidovudine susceptibility			

±

PROTEASE INHIBITORS			
Generic (Generic)	M ♀	**Dose**	
Indinavir-IDV (Crixivan) LK ?		800mg PO q8hours	

Monitoring:
- **If exposure was shown to be from an HIV infected person, or is unknown, assess HIV infection status** via enzyme linked immunosorbent assay-ELISA @ exposure, 3 months (95% specificity), & 6 months (>99% specificity)

- Any infection→
  - Inflammation→
    - Cytokine release→systemic (rather than solely localized) syndrome
- Common sites of primary infection, listed on order of frequency:
  - **Lungs**
  - Gastrointestinal/ biliary tract
  - Urinary tract
  - ...w/ a primary site of infection not found in 25% of patients

Statistics:
- Sepsis develops in >500,000 patients/ year→
  - 20% mortality/ organ failure→
    - 40% overall mortality

CLASSIFICATION/ DIAGNOSIS

SEPSIS

- Diagnostic criteria, requiring ≥2 of the following, being due to an infectious organism†:
  - **Temperature** >100.4°F=38°C (fever) or <96.8°F=36°C (hypothermia)
  - **Pulse** >90/ min.
  - **Respiratory rate** >20/ min.
  - **Hyperventilation**→
    - $PaCO_2$ <32mmHg
  - **Leukocyte count** >12,000/ µL (leukocytosis) or <4,000/ µL (leukopenia)
  - **Immature neutrophils, termed bands** >10%

Etiologic organisms, listed in order of frequency:
- **Gram negative bacteria**
- Gram positive bacteria
- Fungi

SEVERE SEPSIS

- Sepsis→
  - Newly developed or worsened organ failure, esp. involving the:
    - Cardiovascular system→hypotension, lactic acidemia, disseminated intravascular coagulation
    - Central nervous system→altered mental status
    - Kidneys→renal failure
    - Lungs→respiratory failure
  - **Multiple organ failure syndrome–MOFS** if ≥2 organ systems are affected

SEPTIC SHOCK

- Severe sepsis→
  - hypotension **refractory to intravenous fluid bolus infusion** w/ ↓**perfusion mediated organ failure**

Central venous pressure–CVP monitoring

- The pressure obtained from the large central veins (venae cavae, common iliac veins) or right atrium (normal 1–6mm Hg†), w/ spontaneous intravascular variation usually being ≤4mmHg, but as high as 7mmHg), being equivalent to the right ventricular end diastolic pressure when there is no obstruction between the right atrium & ventricle
- A calibrated transducer is connected to the catheter, & placed at the zero reference point for central venous pressure, being the midaxillary 4th intercostal space, corresponding to the position of the atria in the supine position
- Intravascular pressure is the pressure in the vessel lumen relative to atmospheric pressure (zero). However, respiratory mediated intrathoracic & intra–abdominal pressure changes are transmitted into the lumen of the vasculature, w/ extravascular pressure being close to zero at the end of a spontaneous expiration‡. Thus, the intravascular pressure is the:
  - Highest pressure recorded during spontaneous respiration
  - Lowest pressure recorded during positive pressure ventilation
- An ↑value indicates heart failure, whereas a normal pressure in the setting of hypotension indicates either hypovolemic or distributive hypotension (septic or anaphylactic)

---

†CVP in mmHg X 1.36 = CVP in cm H_2O

681

‡Unless either:
  • Positive end expiratory pressure–PEEP, which should be subtracted from the end expiratory pressure value
  • ↑intra–abdominal pressure
  ...are being produced

PATHOPHYSIOLOGY OF THE SEPSIS SYNDROME

• Localized microbial cell wall proteins, endotoxin, &/or exotoxin release→
  ◦ Monocyte/ macrophage activation
  ◦ Neutrophil activation
  ◦ Complement activation
  ◦ Coagulation protein activation
  ...→localized inflammation & procoagulant state→
    • Localized tissue destruction, w/ the severity being determined predominantly by the hosts immune response to the infectious organism, rather than the organism itself
• ↑Severity→↑inflammation→
  ◦ ↑Plasma levels of microbial cell wall proteins, endotoxins, &/or exotoxins
  ◦ ↑Plasma levels of leukocytes & products including:
    – Cytokines, esp. interferon–IFN γ, interleukins–IL 1, 2, 6, & 8; tumor necrosis factors–TNF α & β, leukotrienes, myocardial depressant factors, nitric oxide, platelet activating factor, prostaglandins, proteases, & thromboxane A_2
    – Complement components, esp. C3a & C5a
    ...→systemic inflammation & procoagulant state which may→
      • Disseminated intravascular coagulation–DIC

Cardiovascular

• Diffuse cardiovascular inflammation & intravascular coagulation→
  ◦ Systemic vasodilation
  ◦ ↑Vascular permeability
  ...→**altered autoregulatory blood flow distribution**→
    • **Hypotension**
    • Interstitial edema, also being due to vascular permeability mediated hypoalbuminemia
    ...→↓tissue perfusion & venous return→
      • Compensatory ↑autonomic sympathetic tone→
        ◦ Tachycardia, tachypnea (>16/ min.), & vasoconstriction→
          – **Normal to supranormal cardiac output**
          – Improved, although suboptimal, tissue perfusion
          ...which can be augmented via administration of intravenous fluids
• ↓Tissue perfusion→
  ◦ ↑Plasma lactic acid
  ...indicating oxygen deprivation of metabolically active tissues→
    • **Subsequent organ failure**. Inadequate treatment at this early phase, eventually (usually within hours to days)→
      ◦ Cardiovascular failure via:
        – ↑Cytokine concentration, including various myocardial depressant factors
        – Cardiovascular acidemia, edema, & ischemia
        ...w/ gradually ↓compensatory autonomic sympathetic tone→
          • **↓Renal perfusion**→
            ◦ Pre–renal renal failure→
              – Acute tubular necrosis
          • **↓Central nervous system perfusion**→
            ◦ Altered mental status
          • **↓Gastrointestinal perfusion**→
            ◦ ↓Ability to retain enteric bacteria & their byproducts↔↑sepsis severity
            ◦ ↓Nutrient absorption
          • **↓Myocardial perfusion**→
            ◦ Myocardial ischemic syndromes
          • **↓Pulmonary perfusion**→
            ◦ ↑Respiratory effort→difficulty breathing=**dyspnea**→
              – Respiratory rate >16/ min.=**tachypnea**
              – Accessory muscle usage (sternocleidomastoid muscles for inspiration & abdominal muscles for expiration)
              – Speech frequently interrupted by inspiration=telegraphic speech
              – Pursed lip breathing &/or grunting expirations→positive end–expiratory pressure–PEEP

682

−Paradoxical abdominal motion: Negative intrathoracic pressure→fatigued diaphragm being pulled into the thorax→inspiratory inward motion of the anterior abdominal wall, rather than expected outward motion due to diaphragmatic contraction
∘Ventilation/ perfusion mismatch via:
  −↑Alveolar dead space: Alveolar ventilation through relatively underperfused capillaries
  −↑Vascular shunting†: Capillary blood flow through relatively underventilated alveoli. usually occurring, or exacerbated via via ↑venous return
∘↑Pulmonary vascular permeability→
  −Interstitial & alveolar effusion→**acute respiratory distress syndrome−ARDS**
  ...→↓diffusion of O_2 & CO_2→
      •Hypoxemia (SaO_2 ≤ 91% or PaO_2 ≤ 60mmHg‡) on room air, w/ subsequent hypercapnia ($PaCO_2$ ≥45mmHg) due to either:
        ∘Respiratory muscle fatigue
        ∘Alveolar hypoventilation
      ...as CO_2 clearance is unimpaired (& may be ↑in the dyspneic patient) as long as adequate ventilation (including lack of diffuse severe ventilation/ perfusion mismatching) is maintained, as:
      •CO_2 diffuses 20X as rapidly as O_2
      •Hypercapnia→
        ∘Immediate brain stem respiratory center mediated stimulation of pulmonary ventilation, which may correct the hypercapnia, but not necessarily the hypoxia

---

†Being exacerbated by the supine position→
  •↑Systemic venous return→
    ∘↑Vascular shunting→↑dyspnea, being termed:
      −**Orthopnea**, if persistent
      −**Paroxysmal nocturnal dyspnea** if intermittent
      ...causing the patient to either use multiple pillows or sleep in a chair
‡Age adjusted normal PaO_2 = 101 − (0.43 X age)

DIAGNOSIS OF SEPSIS

•**Stains & cultures**
  ∘Blood
  ∘All intravascular catheter tips should be obtained
  ∘All suspected sites of infection:
    −Sputum
    −Stool
    −Urine
    −Effusions (pericardial, peritoneal, pleural, synovial)
    −Cerebrospinal fluid
    ...w/ concomitant drainage (abscess, empyema) or debridement if necessary
•Examine the:
  ∘Oropharynx, including dentition
  ∘Middle ears
  ∘Sinuses (ethmoid, frontal, maxillary, & sphenoid) via computed tomographic−CT or magnetic resonance imaging−MRI scan, as x−rays are not sensitive enough to detect either:
    −Sphenoid sinusitis
    −Early frontal or maxillary sinusitis
  ...esp. in patients w/ a nasogastric or orogastric tube

INTRAVASCULAR CATHETER TIP STUDIES
•**Quantitative blood culture method**
  Procedure:
    •2 sets of aerobic & anaerobic culture mediums are recommended for all patients, w/ each bottle inoculated w/ ≥10mL of blood
      ∘**1 set from blood drawn through the indwelling vascular catheter**
      ∘**1 set from blood drawn from the periphery**
      ...w/ subsequent placement of a fixed volume of culture fluid onto a culture plate
  Diagnosis of catheter related sepsis:
    •Catheter blood culture growing either:
    ∘**>100 CFU/ mL**
    ∘**>10 X peripheral blood CFU/ mL**

Outcomes:
- •Sensitivity: 80%
- •Specificity: 100%

•**Semiquantitative catheter tip culture method**
Indications:
- •Erythema &/or purulence @ the catheter insertion site, thus requiring catheter removal
Procedure:
- •Involves the removal of the suspected catheter, w/ subsequent culturing of the intravascular segment (distal 5cm) via directly rolling the catheter tip across the surface of a culture plate
- •At the time of catheter removal, 1 set of aerobic & anaerobic culture mediums must also be obtained, w/ each bottle being inoculated w/ ≥10mL of blood drawn from the periphery
Diagnosis of catheter related sepsis:
- •Catheter culture growing:
  - ◦**>15 CFU**, w/ the same or no organism grown from the peripheral blood
Outcomes:
- •55% of catheters removed for suspected catheter related sepsis show little to no growth on culture mediums
- •Sensitivity: 35%
- •Specificity: 100%
Advantages:
- •Allows for concomitant gram staining via submitting a portion of the distal segment, which is slit longitudinally, thus exposing the inner lumen, & allowing both the inner & outer surfaces to be stained
Limitations:
- •↓Sensitivity, which can be ↑ w/ bedside culture immediately upon removal
- •Requires catheter removal & insertion of a replacement catheter

TREATMENT
•**Empiric intravenous antibiotics as per neutropenic fever**
- ◦If treatment is initially begun w/ intravenous medication, the switch to PO medication should be attempted upon clinical improvement (fever resolution & clinical stabilization) X 24hours, if an acceptable PO medication is available, & the patient is able to take PO medication
- ◦**Organism-narrowed therapy** should be initiated promptly upon stain, culture, & sensitivities results
- ◦The following antibiotics achieve equivalent plasma levels via PO or intravenous administration in persons w/ a functioning gastrointestinal tract:
  - –Chloramphenicol
  - –Doxycycline
  - –Minocycline
  - –Most fluoroquinolones
  - –Trimethoprim/ Sulfamethoxazole
Bactericidal antibiotics
- •**Cell wall synthesis inhibitors**
  - ◦β lactam medications:
    - –Carbapenems
    - –Cephalosporins
    - –Monobactams
    - –Penicillins
  - ◦Vancomycin
- •**DNA synthesis inhibitors**
  - ◦Fluoroquinolones
  - ◦Linezolid
  - ◦Metronidazole
  - ◦Rifampin
  - ◦Quinupristin & Dalfopristin
- •**Aminoglycosides**

•**Intravenous fluid,** w/ attention to both:
- ◦**Intravascular volume repletion† via Normal saline** (0.9% NaCl) or **lactated Ringer's solution,** as per:
  - –Vital signs
  - –Physical examination
  - –Urine output (normal being ≥0.5mL/kg/h)
  - –Blood urea nitrogen–BUN & creatinine
  - ...**ensuring a central venous pressure–CVP of 8–12mmHg** (after any PEEP is subtracted) within 6hours of diagnosis

684

Adult maintenance fluid:
  •Weight (kg) + 40= #mL/ hour
Additional febrile requirements:
  •1L/ 24hours for every 1°F >100°F
Additional:
  •Estimate loss for:
    ◦Diaphoresis
    ◦Diarrhea
    ◦Polyuria
    ◦Tachypnea

INTENSIVE INSULIN TREATMENT: 100units regular insulin/ 100mL normal saline
•**Always measure the plasma potassium prior to initiating insulin treatment**

Generic	Plasma glucose	Start
Regular insulin	<110	No need
	110–220	2units/ hour IV infusion
	>220	4units/ hour IV infusion

Goal:
  •To maintain blood glucose @ **80–110mg/ dL**

Dose adjustment:
  •1/2 all doses @ a glomerular filtration rate–GFR ≤30mL/ min.

Blood glucose (mg/ dL)	Action
≤60	1 ampule D50, discontinue infusion, call house officer, recheck q15 min. until blood glucose >100. Then restart infusion at half the previous rate
61–70	Hold for 1 hour, then –2units/ hour
71–80	–1unit/ hour
81–110	No change
111–200	+1unit/ hour
201–300	+2units/ hour
>300	Call house officer

•**Ensure an intravenous glucose source if enteral glucose is interrupted**
•Infusion should be **halved** upon the discontinuation/ tapering of:
  ◦Glucocorticoids
  ◦Catecholamine infusion (epinephrine, norepinephrine)
•Infusion should be **discontinued** upon:
  ◦Patient leaving the intensive care unit:
    –Imaging
    –Procedure
    –Surgery

Mechanisms:
  •Hyperglycemia→
    ◦↓Neutrophil function→
      –Immunosuppression→↑disease severity risk, whereas maintenance of normoglycemia prevents this phenomenon
  •Insulin→
    ◦↓Cellular apoptosis

Outcomes:
  •↓Morbidity & mortality regardless of a history of diabetes mellitus when compared to conventional treatment which maintained blood glucose @180–200mg/ dL

Limitations:
  •It has yet to be determined whether less intensive treatment of blood glucose (ex: 110–160mg/ dL) provides similar benefits

Monitoring:
  •Measure plasma glucose qhour (fingerstick measurements may be used when the plasma glucose is <500mg/ dL) until goal is met X 3 consecutive hours, after which, monitor q2hours. If either the insulin dose or glucose source change, return to monitoring q1hour

685

POTASSIUM	
•Always measure the magnesium level concomitantly	

Indications:
•Ensure a potassium of 4–5mEq/ L

Generic

If concomitant alkalemia:
•Potassium chloride–KCL
If concomitant acidemia:
•Potassium bicarbonate
•Potassium citrate
•Potassium acetate
•Potassium gluconate
•Potassium phosphate
　◦Preferred in diabetic ketoacidosis–DKA due to concomitant phosphate depletion
POTASSIUM DOSAGE ADJUSTMENT SCALE†_____

Plasma K^+ (mEq/ L)	K^+ repletion (mEq)
≥3.9	None
3.7–3.8	20
3.5–3.6	40
3.3–3.4	60
3.1–3.2	80
≤3	100

†Half all above doses @ a glomerular filtration rate–GFR ≤30mL/ min.

Intravenous repletion guidelines:
•The hyperosmolar infusion→
　◦Vascular irritation/ inflammation. Add 1% Lidocaine to the bag to ↓pain
•**Do not administer >20mEq potassium IV/ hour**
　◦≤10mEq/ hour prn via peripheral line. May give via 2 peripheral lines=20mEq/ hour total
　◦≤20mEq/ hour prn via central line
　…as more→
　　•Transient right sided heart hyperkalemia→
　　◦Dysrhythmias

Outcomes:
•Anti–dysrhythmic
•↑Cardiac contractility in heart failure
•Modest hypotensive effect in some patients
•↓Cerebrovascular disease risk, apart from its possible blood pressure lowering effects

MAGNESIUM SULFATE	
M ♀	**Dose**
K S	Every 1g IV→0.1mEq/ L ↑in plasma magnesium

Mechanism:
•Hypomagnesemia→
　◦↓Renal tubular potassium reabsorption

ADDITIONAL TREATMENT FOR SEVERE SEPSIS ▬▬▬▬▬▬

SYSTEMIC GLUCOCORTICOID TREATMENT

Indications:
•**Known adrenal failure**
　◦Primary, due to adrenal dysfunction=Addison's disease
　◦Secondary, due to central nervous system dysfunction, including:
　　–**Chronic glucocorticoid administration**→hypothalamic & pituitary negative feedback
　　mediated ↓corticotropin releasing hormone–CRH & adrenocorticotropin hormone–ACTH
　　production respectively
•**Otherwise, begin empirically & continue if found to have absolute or relative hypoadrenalism**
via the cosyntropin stimulation test

The Cosyntropin stimulation test:
1. Administration of Cosyntropin 250µg=0.25mg IV
2. Measurement of plasma cortisol levels @ 0 & 1hour after Cosyntropin administration
3. **Adrenal failure during an acute severe illness**, being either:
　•**Absolute:** Random cortisol level <20µg/ dL (normal 5–20µg/ dL)
　•**Relative:** 1hour level increase of <9µg/ dL (being unlikely w/ a random cortisol level >34µg/ dL)

†Cosyntropin is a synthetic peptide consisting of the first 24 amino acids of adrenocorticotropin hormone—ACTH

Generic (Trade)	M ♀	Dose

INITIAL EMPIRIC TREATMENT

Generic (Trade)	M ♀	Dose
Dexamethasone (Decadron)	L ?	4mg IM/ IV X 1 during the test, as Dexamethasone will not interfere w/ the plasma cortisol assay **& IF SHOCK**
Fludricortisone (Florinef)	L ?	50µg PO X 1

CONTINUED TREATMENT

Generic (Trade)	M ♀	Dose
Hydrocortisone (Cortef)	L ?	100mg IM/ IV q8hours X 1week replaces Dexamethasone once the diagnosis is made, as this medication has ↑mineralocorticoid activity **& IF SHOCK**
Fludricortisone (Florinef)	L ?	50µg PO q24hours X 1week

•In patients w/ known adrenal insufficiency, once disease control is achieved, taper after 1 week to the lowest effective maintenance dose in order to minimize serious side effects

	Relative potencies			
Glucocorticoids	**Anti-inflammatory**	**Mineralocorticoid**	**Duration**	**Dose equiv.**
Cortisol (physiologic†)	1	1	10hours	20mg
Cortisone (PO)	0.7	2	10hours	25mg
Hydrocortisone (PO, IM, IV)	1	2	10hours	20mg
Methylprednisolone (PO, IM, IA, IV)	5	0.5	15–35hours	5mg
Prednisone (PO)	5	0.5	15–35hours	5mg
Prednisolone (PO, IM, IV)	5	0.8	15–35hours	5mg
Triamcinolone (PO, IM)	5	~0	15–35hours	5mg
Betamethasone (PO, IM, IA)	25	~0	35–70hours	0.75mg
Dexamethasone (PO)	25	~0	35–70hours	0.75mg
Fludrocortisone (PO)	10	125	10hours	

†The physiologic rate of adrenal cortical cortisol production is 20–30mg/ 24hours

Outcomes:
•↓Morbidity & mortality

ANTICOAGULANTS

Indications:
•Patients w/ severe sepsis who have a ↑mortality risk as indicated by an **APACHE 2† score of ≥25** (being of greatest benefit), as activated protein C was not effective in patients w/ a score <20, being associated w/ ↑hemorrhage risk

†Acute Physiology and Chronic Health Evaluation—APACHE 2 severity of illness scoring system, which utilizes patient age, physiologic data, & chronic disease in order to predict intensive care unit death risk. The scoring system was designed & validated for patients who have been in the intensive care unit for 24hours

Generic (Trade)	M ♀	Dose
Recombinant human activated protein C=Drotrecogin α (Xigris)	P ?	24µg/kg/h X 96hours†

•Do not expose to heat or direct sunlight
†If the infusion is interrupted, it should be restarted & continued to complete 96hours

Mechanisms:
•Protein C→
  ◦Factors 5 & 8 inactivation→
    –↓Thrombin formation→↓localized thrombosis mediated ischemia & inflammation→↓systemic inflammation
  ◦↓Leukocyte cytokine production & cellular adhesion→
    –↓Systemic inflammation
  ◦↓Cellular apoptosis

Outcomes:
•↓Mortality

Side effects:
Cardiovascular
•↑**Hemorrhage risk**, being potentially life threatening in 3.5% of patients
  ◦**Percutaneous procedure:** Stop infusion 1hour prior, & restart infusion 1hour after
  ◦**Major surgery:** Stop infusion 1hour prior, & restart infusion 12hours after

Hematologic
- •↑Activated partial thromboplastin time–aPTT

Contraindications:
- •Conditions & medications which→
  - ∘↑Hemorrhage risk
- •Active hemorrhage, not including menses
- •Severe bleeding diathesis
- •Severe thrombocytopenia (platelet count ≤20,000/ μL)
- •Recent significant trauma
- •Hemorrhagic stroke within 3months
- •Intracranial &/or spinal
  - ∘Aneurysm
  - ∘Arteriovenous malformation–AVM
  - ∘Neoplasm
- •Evidence of cerebral herniation
- •Presence of an epidural catheter
- •Prior hypersensitivity reaction to Drotrecogin α

ADDITIONAL TREATMENT FOR SEPTIC SHOCK

INOTROPIC & PRESSOR MEDICATIONS: The following medications must be administered via a central line, & should be titrated based on blood pressure response to keep the systolic blood pressure >90mmHg

Medication	Receptor activation	Clinical effects†
Dopamine	Low dose: D1 & 2 effects predominate	•Renal & other splanchnic **vasodilation**
	Med dose: β1 & 2 effects predominate	•↑Chronotropy, inotropy, & vasodilation
	High dose: α1 effects predominate	•Vasoconstriction
Low: 1–5µg/kg/min.; Medium: 5–10µg/kg/min.; High: 10–20µg/kg/min.		
Epinephrine	α1, α2, β1, β2	•↑Chronotropy, inotropy, & vasoconstriction
Start @ 1µg/ min. (max 20µg/ min.)		
Norepinephrine	α1, α2 > β1	•↑Chronotropy, inotropy, & vasoconstriction
Start @ 1µg/ min. (max 30µg/ min.)		
Phenylephrine	α1	•**Vasoconstriction‡**
Start @ 10µg/ min. (max 300µg/ min.)		
Vasopressin	V1$_A$	•Vasoconstriction°
	V1$_B$	•↑Anterior pituitary ACTH secretion
	V2	•↑Distal convoluted tubule & collecting duct water reabsorption=antidiuretic effect
Low dose: Start 0.01 units/ min. (max 0.05units/ min.)		

Note: Dobutamine is not listed, as it is the preferred inotrope in patients w/ heart failure mediated shock, & has no role in septic shock as it can ↑hypotension

†Chronotropy=rate of contraction; Inotropy=strength of muscular contractility

‡Making Phenylephrine the preferred pressor in tachycardic patients

°During shock, plasma vasopressin levels initially ↑in order to attempt to maintain adequate perfusion pressure. However, within hours, pituitary vasopressin stores may become depleted, w/ levels rapidly↓ to normal (<5pg/ ml)→relative vasopressin deficiency
- •Patients w/ vasodilatory shock are usually very sensitive to the effects of low doses of vasopressin (much more than those w/ other forms of shock), w/ little to no vasoconstrictive effect in normal subjects

688

•Fever ≥100°F=37.8°C occurring in a neutropenic patient, defined as having an **absolute neutrophil count–ANC†** <500cells/ μL
•Most significant cases are due to **malignancy or its treatment**

---

†Absolute neutrophil count–ANC=Neutrophils + band cells (immature polymorphonuclear cells)

RISK FACTORS FOR THE DEVELOPMENT OF NEUTROPENIA

•Any of the following may cause isolated neutropenia→
  ◦Leukocytopenia

•**↓Bone marrow production**
  ◦**Neoplastic**
    –Leukemia
    –Myeloma
    –Bone metastases
  ◦**Neoplastic treatment**
    –Bone marrow or stem cell transplantation
    –Chemotherapeutic medications→neutrophil count nadir 2 weeks after last administered dose
    –Large radiation treatment field
  ◦**Benign chronic neutropenia**
    –Mild, chronically ↓neutrophil count
  ◦**Chemicals**
    –Arsenic
    –Benzene
    –Bismuth
    –Dichlorodiphenyltrichloroethane–DDT
    –Dinitrophenol
    –Nitrous oxide
  ◦**Folate or vitamin B12 deficiency**, as both are needed for DNA synthesis
  ◦**Genetic**
    –Cyclic neutropenia, being a rare autosomal dominant disease→cyclic ↓neutrophil count (usually q3–4 weeks) lasting <1 week
  ◦**Infections**, esp:
    –Human immune deficiency virus–HIV
    –Mycobacterium tuberculosis
    –Viruses
    …via either:
        •Bone marrow cellular infection
        •Secondary immune mediated process via:
          ◦Antibody–antigen deposition
          ◦Leukocyte dysfunction→autoimmune disease
          ◦Molecular mimicry→autoimmune disease
  ◦**Medications**, via a hypersensitivity syndrome
    –Diuretic medications: Acetazolamide, Chlorthalidone, Hydrochlorothiazide
    –Hypoglycemics: Sulfonylureas (Chlorpropamide, Tolbutamide)
    –Anti–dysrhythmic medications: Procainamide, Propranolol, Tocainide, Quinidine
    –Anti–bacterial medications: Chloramphenicol, Isoniazid–INH, Nitrofurantoin, Penicillins, Rifampin, Sulfonamides, Vancomycin
    –Anti–parasitic medications: Dapsone, Pyrimethamine, Quinine
    –Anti–viral medications: Ganciclovir, Valganciclovir
    –Anti–hypertensive medications: Captopril, Methyldopa
    –Anti–inflammatory medications: Aminopyrine, Ibuprofen, Gold salts, Indomethacin, Phenylbutazone
    –Anti–psychotic medications: Chlorpromazine, Prochlorperazine, Promazine
    –Anti–seizure medications: Carbemazepine, Ethosuximide, Phenytoin, Trimethadione
    –Anti–thyroid medications: Methimazole, Propylthiouracil, Thiouracil
  ◦**Myelodysplastic syndromes**
  ◦**Stem cell disease**
    –Paroxysmal nocturnal hemoglobinuria

•**↓Neutrophil survival**
  ◦**Autoimmune disease**, via antineutrophil antibody production, esp. w/:
    –Autoimmune neutropenia
    –Sjogren's syndrome
    –Systemic lupus erythematosus

689

- **Abnormal cell distribution**
  - Splenomegally→
    - −Hypersplenism
  - Severe inflammation→
    - −↑Neutrophil extravasation

ETIOLOGIES OF FEVER IN NEUTROPENIC PATIENTS
INFECTION-50%
- Bacteremia of uncertain source−15%
- HEENT infection (Head, Ears, Eyes, Nose, Throat)−10%
- Pneumonia−10%
- Cutaneous
- Gastrointestinal
- Genitourinary
- Other
...w/ infection risk being directly proportional to neutropenia severity & duration

Pathophysiology:
- Neutropenia > lymphopenia→
  - Immunosuppresion→↑risk of:
    - −Mucocutaneous microorganism tissue invasion, noting that the mucocutaneous flora may rapidly change within the hospital
    - −Microorganism reactivation disease

Infection risk relative to absolute neutrophil count
- >1,500 cells/ μL→normal risk
- 1,000−1,500 cells/ μL→mildly ↑risk
- 500−1,000 cells/ μL→50% ↑risk
- 100−500 cells/ μL→100% ↑risk
- <100 cells/ μL→200% ↑risk

Organisms, listed in order of frequency:
- **Bacteria**
  - **Gram positive aerobic bacteria−60%**
    - −Staphylococcus aureus
    - −Staphylococcus epidermidis
    - −Enterococcus sp. (faecalis, faecium)
    - −Viridans streptococci (S. mitis, mutans, & sanguis)
    - −Bacillus sp.
    - −Corynebacterium jeikeium
  - **Gram negative aerobic bacteria−30%**
    - −Enterobacteriaceae: Escherichia coli, Enterobacter cloacae, Klebsiella pneumoniae, Proteus mirabilis & vulgaris, Providencia rettgeri, Pseudomonas aeruginosa, Serratia marcescens
    - −Acinetobacter sp.
    - −Citrobacter freundii
    - −Legionella sp.
    - −Serratia marcescens
  - **Anaerobic bacteria−4%**
    - −Clostridium sp.
    - −Stenotrophomonas maltophilia
  - **Mycobacteria**
    - −Mycobacterium tuberculosis, avium−intracellulare, cheloneae, or fortuitum
- **Fungi−2%**
  - Aspergillus sp. (fumigatus, flavis, niger, & terreus)
  - Candida sp., esp: albicans, glabrata, lusitaniae, kruzei, parapsilosis, & tropicalis
  - Pneumocystis carinii
  - Cryptococcus neoformans
  - Fusarium
  - Malassezia furfur
  - Phycomycosis (Mucor, Rhizopus, Absidia, Cuninghamella)
  - Pseudoallescheria boydii
  - Trichosporon
- **Viruses**
  - Cytomegalovirus−CMV
  - Epstein−Barr virus−EBV
  - Herpes simplex viruses−HSV 1 or 2
  - Varicella−zoster virus−VZV

690

- **Parasites**
  - ∘Strongyloides stercoralis
  - ∘Toxoplasma gondii

UNKNOWN-50% ▄▄
- •Via possible:
  - ∘Occult infection
  - ∘Medications via hypersensitivity syndrome, termed a drug fever
    - −Chemotherapeutic medications: Bleomycin & Arabinoside 2−CDA, usually being transient, & occurring prior to the development of neutropenia
    - −Histamine−2 selective receptor blockers: Cimetidine
    - −Thrombolytic medications: Streptokinase
    - −Anti−dysrhythmic medications: Procainamide, Quinidine
    - −Anti−bacterial medications: Cephalosporins, Penicillins, Rifampin, Vancomycin
    - −Anti−fungal medications: Amphotericin
    - −Anti−viral medications: Ganciclovir, Valganciclovir
    - −Anti−hypertensive medications: Hydralazine
    - −Anti−seizure medications: Carbemazepine, Phenytoin
  - ∘Chemotherapy mediated mucositis
  - ∘Neoplastic mediated tissue necrosis
  - ∘Paraneoplastic syndrome, esp.:
    - −Hepatocellular cancer
    - −Leukemia
    - −Lymphoma
    - −Renal cell cancer

DIAGNOSIS OF MEDICATION INDUCED HYPERSENSITIVITY SYNDROME
- •**A diagnosis of exclusion**, confirmed by withdrawing the suspected causative medication, w/ subsequent defervescence
- •**General**
  - •**Fever−50%** ± chills
- •**Cardiovascular**
  - ∘Hypotension−18%
- •**Mucocutaneous**
  - ∘**Dermatitis−18%**
- •**Musculoskeletal**
  - ∘Muscle pain=myalgias−25%
- •**Hematologic**
  - ∘**Eosinophilia−22%**
  - ∘Leukocytosis−22%

DIAGNOSIS OF SEPSIS
- •**Stains & cultures**
  - ∘Blood
  - ∘All intravascular catheter tips should be obtained
  - ∘All suspected sites of infection:
    - −Sputum
    - −Stool
    - −Urine
    - −Effusions (pericardial, peritoneal, pleural, synovial)
    - −Cerebrospinal fluid
    - …w/ concomitant drainage (abscess, empyema) or debridement if necessary
- •Examine the:
  - ∘Oropharynx, including dentition
  - ∘Middle ears
  - ∘Sinuses (ethmoid, frontal, maxillary, & sphenoid) via computed tomographic−CT or magnetic resonance imaging−MRI scan, as x−rays are not sensitive enough to detect either:
    - −Sphenoid sinusitis
    - −Early frontal or maxillary sinusitis
    - …esp. in patients w/ a nasogastric or orogastric tube

•**Quantitative blood culture method**
Procedure:
  •2 sets of aerobic & anaerobic culture mediums are recommended for all patients, w/ each bottle inoculated w/ ≥10mL of blood
    ○**1 set from blood drawn through the indwelling vascular catheter**
    ○**1 set from blood drawn from the periphery**
    …w/ subsequent placement of a fixed volume of culture fluid onto a culture plate
Diagnosis of catheter related sepsis:
  •Catheter blood culture growing either:
    ○**>100 CFU/ mL**
    ○**>10 X peripheral blood CFU/ mL**
Outcomes:
  •Sensitivity: 80%
  •Specificity: 100%

•**Semiquantitative catheter tip culture method**
Indications:
  •Erythema &/or purulence @ the catheter insertion site, thus requiring catheter removal
Procedure:
  •Involves the removal of the suspected catheter, w/ subsequent culturing of the intravascular segment (distal 5cm) via directly rolling the catheter tip across the surface of a culture plate
  •At the time of catheter removal, 1 set of aerobic & anaerobic culture mediums must also be obtained, w/ each bottle being inoculated w/ ≥10mL of blood drawn from the periphery
Diagnosis of catheter related sepsis:
  •Catheter culture growing:
    ○**>15 CFU**, w/ the same or no organism grown from the peripheral blood
Outcomes:
  •55% of catheters removed for suspected catheter related sepsis show little to no growth on culture mediums
  •Sensitivity: 35%
  •Specificity: 100%
Advantages:
  •Allows for concomitant gram staining via submitting a portion of the distal segment, which is slit longitudinally, thus exposing the inner lumen. & allowing both the inner & outer surfaces to be stained
Limitations:
  •↓Sensitivity, which can be ↑ w/ bedside culture immediately upon removal
  •Requires catheter removal & insertion of a replacement catheter

INFECTION PROPHYLAXIS
•**Standard neutropenic precautions**
Indications:
  •At all times, in order to ↓transmission of microorganisms to the neutropenic patient
Precautions
  •**Patient isolation**
  •Handwashing immediately prior to entering the room
  •All persons w/ a known transmissible respiratory tract infection should not enter the patient's room. If this is a health care provider which needs to enter the room, then a face mask must be worn
  •The patient should wear a face mask upon exiting the room in order to ↓transmission of respiratory pathogens
  •The patient's room should remain free of:
    ○Live flowers
    ○Raw foods, including fruits & vegetables
    ○Soil
    …as they are a source of gram negative bacteria
  •The patient's food should be free of spices due to potential contamination w/ fungal spores
  •Avoid all rectal temperatures & examinations which→
    ○Enterobacteriaceael & anaerobic bacteremia
  •Avoid intramuscular injections which→
    ○Cutaneous organism penetration
    ○Hematoma formation w/ ↑infection risk
  •Water purification in order to ↓nosocomial Legionella sp. infection risk
  •Use of high−efficiency particulate air−HEPA filters, as nearby construction→
    ○Aerosolization of Aspergillus sp. spores

692

•Additional neutropenic precautions
  Indications:
    •Patients w/, or anticipated to have, a severe or prolonged neutropenic course
  Precautions:
    •Oropharyngeal, esophageal, & vaginal candidiasis prophylaxis: Fluconazole
    •Cytomegalovirus–CMV reactivation prophylaxis: Gancyclovir
    •Herpes–simplex virus–HSV 1 & 2 reactivation prophylaxis: Acyclovir
    •Mycobacterium tuberculosis reactivation prophylaxis: Isoniazid–INH
    •Pneumocystis carinii reactivation prophylaxis: Trimethoprim–Sulfamethoxazole, also being
    recommended for either:
      ◦Bone marrow transplant recipients
      ◦Febrile patients receiving ↑dose glucocorticoids
    •Selective digestive decontamination
      ◦Moderate to severe illness–induced loss of the protective fibronectin coating of the
      oropharynx→
        –Oropharyngeal colonization by the organisms typically responsible for hospital acquired
        pneumonia

SELECTIVE DIGESTIVE DECONTAMINATION	
Location	**Prophylaxis**
Oropharynx	A methylcellulose paste† containing •2% Amphotericin •2% Polymyxin E •2% Tobramycin …applied to the buccal mucosa & tongue via a gloved finger q6hours
Distal gastrointestinal tract	A solution containing •500mg Amphotericin •100mg Polymyxin E •80mg Tobramycin …administered via nasogastric tube q6hours

†The hospital pharmacy will make the paste

Mechanism:
  •Eradication of Pseudomonas aeruginosa, as well as most gastrointestinal fungi &
    enterobacteriaceae @ 1week
  •The normal gastrointestinal bacterial flora, composed mostly of anaerobes, is relatively
  unaffected
  …→treatment & prevention of gastrointestinal colonization by the organisms typically
    responsible for hospital acquired:
      •Pneumonia
      •Urinary tract infections
      •Bacteremia/ fungemia via mucocutaneous routes:
        ◦Cutaneous lesion
        ◦Gastrointestinal translocation
        ◦Intravascular catheter

Side effects:
  •The antimicrobials used are nonabsorbable, & thus do not cause systemic toxicity

693

•**Assume an infectious cause of febrile neutropenia, & begin empiric antibiotic treatment as below within 1hour**
  ◦**Organism–narrowed therapy** should be initiated promptly upon stain, culture, & sensitivities results
  Bactericidal antibiotics
    •**Cell wall synthesis inhibitors**
      ◦β lactam medications:
        −Carbapenems
        −Cephalosporins
        −Monobactams
        −Penicillins
      ◦Vancomycin
    •**DNA synthesis inhibitors**
      ◦Fluoroquinolones
      ◦Linezolid
      ◦Metronidazole
      ◦Rifampin
      ◦Quinupristin & dalfopristin
    •**Aminoglycosides**

•**ANY 2 OF THE FOLLOWING** in order to provide double coverage for possible Pseudomonas aeruginosa infection

AMINOGLYCOSIDES					
Generic (Trade)	M	♀	**Dosing†**	**Peak**	**Trough**
Amikacin (Amikin)	K	U	15mg/ kg IV q24hours	>30µg/ mL	<5µg/ mL
Gentamycin (Garamycin)	K	U	7mg/ kg IV q24hours	>6µg/ mL	<2µg/ mL
Tobramycin (Nebcin)	K	U	7mg/ kg IV q24hours	>6µg/ mL	<2µg/ mL

•Peak levels are obtained 30minutes after the dose, w/ trough levels being obtained at the end of the dosing interval. Plasma peak & trough levels are directly related to clinical efficacy & toxicity respectively
†Patients receiving an aminoglycoside for synergy w/ a β–lactam medication versus Enterococcus sp. should receive thrice daily dosing

Dose adjustment based on creatinine clearance (mL/ min.)
  •40–59: q36hours
  •20–39: q48hours

Obesity dosage adjustment:
  •Ideal weight† + 0.4 (actual weight − ideal weight)=adjusted weight

†♂: 50kg + 2.3kg per inch > 5'
  ♀: 45.5kg + 2.3kg per inch > 5'

Mechanism:
  •Affects the ribosomal 30S subunit→
    ◦↓Initiation complex function
    ◦Misreading of messenger RNA

Side effects:
  Genitourinary
    •**Nephrotoxicity†** (Gentamicin > Tobramycin > Amikacin > Neomycin), w/ renal failure usually @ ≥1week via acute tubular necrosis
      Risk factors:
        •↑Age
        •Cirrhosis
        •Hypovolemia
        •Hypokalemia
        •Hypomagnesemia
        •Renal failure
  Neurologic
    •**Ototoxicity**, being dose related & irreversible→
      ◦High frequency sound loss
      Risk factors:
        •Concomitant use w/ other ototoxic medications such as loop diuretics
        •Renal failure
        •Use >2weeks

694

•Neuromuscular blockade via:
  ◦↓Presynaptic acetylcholine release
  ◦↓Postsynaptic sensitivity to acetylcholine

---

†Early signs of nephrotoxicity include:
•↓Ability to concentrate the urine (noted via ↓specific gravity)
•Cylindrical urinary casts
•Proteinuria
‡Audiometry is required to document ototoxicity, as the hearing loss occurs above the frequency range of normal human conversation

Monitoring:
•Obtain baseline & serial audiometry w/ treatment >2weeks

CARBAPENEMS

Generic (Trade)	M	♀	Dose
Imipinem-Cilastatin (Primaxin)	K	?	500mg IV q6hours
Meropenem (Merrem)	K	P	1g IV q8hours

Mechanism:
•A β-lactam ring structure which binds to bacterial transpeptidase→
  ◦↓Transpeptidase function→
    −↓Bacterial cell wall peptidoglycan cross-linking→↓cell wall synthesis→osmotic influx of extracellular fluid→↑intracellular hydrostatic pressure→cell rupture→cell death=bactericidal

Side effects:
General
•Hypersensitivity reactions
  ◦Anaphylaxis
  ◦Acute interstitial nephritis
  ◦Dermatitis
  ◦Drug fever
  ◦Hemolytic anemia
  …having **cross-hypersensitivity to other β-lactam medications** (penicillins, cephalosporins), except monobactams (ex. Aztreonam)
Cardiovascular
•Venous inflammation=phlebitis
Gastrointestinal
•Gastroenteritis→
  ◦Diarrhea
  ◦Nausea ± vomiting
•Clostridium dificile pseudomembraneous colitis
Neurologic
•**Seizures** (Imipenem > Meropenem), esp. w/
  ◦↑Age
  ◦Renal failure
  ◦Seizure history

Imipenem dosage	Seizure occurrence
500mg q6hours	0.2–1%
1g q6hours	10%

Generic (Trade)	M	♀	Dose
Piperacillin–Tazobactam (Zosyn)	K	P	4.5g IV q6hours
Ticarcillin–Clavulanic acid (Timentin)	K	P	50mg/ kg IV q4hours

Mechanism:
- A β–lactam ring structure which binds to bacterial transpeptidase→
  - ↓Transpeptidase function→
    - –↓Bacterial cell wall peptidoglycan cross–linking→↓cell wall synthesis→osmotic influx of extracellular fluid→↑intracellular hydrostatic pressure→cell rupture→cell death=bactericidal
- ↑Bacterial autolytic enzymes→
  - Peptidoglycan degradation

- Certain bacteria produce β–lactamase→
  - Cleavage of this essential structural component of cephalosporins & certain penicillins (as the other β–lactam medications differ sufficiently to prevent ring cleavage)→
    - –Antibiotic inactivation. This process may be antagonized by the concomitant administration of β–lactamase inhibitors (Clavulanic acid=Clavulanate, Sulbactam, or Tazobactam)→renewed susceptibility

Side effects:
General
- **Hypersensitivity reactions ≤10%**
  - Anaphylaxis–0.5%→
    - –Death–0.002% (1:50,000)
  - Acute interstitial nephritis
  - Dermatitis
  - Drug fever
  - Hemolytic anemia
  …having cross–hypersensitivity to other β lactam medications (cephalosporins, carbapenems), except monobactams (ex. Aztreonam)

CEPHALOSPORINS: $3^{rd}-4^{th}$ generation			
Generic (Trade)	M	♀	Dose
Cefipime (Maxipime)	K	P	2g IV q8hours
Ceftazidime (Ceptaz, Fortaz)	K	P	2g IV q8hours

Mechanism:
- A β–lactam ring structure which binds to bacterial transpeptidase→
  - ↓Transpeptidase function→
    - –↓Bacterial cell wall peptidoglycan cross–linking→↓cell wall synthesis→osmotic influx of extracellular fluid→↑intracellular hydrostatic pressure→cell rupture→cell death=bactericidal
- ↑Bacterial autolytic enzymes→
  - Peptidoglycan degradation

- Certain bacteria produce β–lactamase→
  - Cleavage of this essential structural component of cephalosporins & certain penicillins (as the other β–lactam medications differ sufficiently to prevent ring cleavage)→
    - –Antibiotic inactivation. This process may be antagonized by the concomitant administration of β–lactamase inhibitors (Clavulanic acid=clavulanate, Sulbactam, or Tazobactam)→renewed susceptibility

Side effects:
General
- **Hypersensitivity reactions ≤10%**
  - Anaphylaxis–0.5%→
    - –Death–0.002% (1:50,000)
  - Acute interstitial nephritis
  - Dermatitis
  - Drug fever
  - Hemolytic anemia
  …having cross–hypersensitivity to other β lactam medications (penicillins, carbapenems), except monobactams (ex. Aztreonam)
Gastrointestinal
- Clostridium dificile pseudomembranous colitis (3rd generation > others)

696

FLUOROQUINOLONES

Generic (Trade)	M	♀	Dose
Levofloxacin (Levaquin)	KL	?	750mg IV q24hours

Mechanism:
- •↓DNA gyrase=topoisomerase action→
  - ○↓Bacterial DNA synthesis

Side effects:
General
- •Hypersensitivity reactions

Gastrointestinal
- •Gastroenteritis→
  - ○Diarrhea
  - ○Nausea ± vomiting

Mucocutaneous
- •Phototoxicity

Neurologic
- •Dizziness
- •Drowsiness
- •Headache
- •Restlessness

Materno−fetal
- •Fetal & child tendon malformation (including breast fed)→
  - ○↑Tendon rupture risk

ADDITIONAL TREATMENT ▬▬▬▬▬▬
- •**Consider treating for possible Pneumocystis carinii pneumonia−PCP** in patients w/ either:
  - ○HIV/ AIDS
  - ○Chronic glucocorticoid or immunomodulating medication treatment

MONOBACTAMS

Indications:
- •To be included in the initial regiman for patients w/ hypersensitivity to beta lactam medications

Generic (Trade)	M	♀	Dose
Aztreonam (Azactam)	K	P	2g IV q6hours

- •The only β-lactam based medication which can be administered to patients w/ hypersensitivity syndrome to the the β-lactam structure

Mechanism:
- •A β−lactam ring structure which binds to bacterial transpeptidase→
  - ○↓Transpeptidase function→
    - −↓Bacterial cell wall peptidoglycan cross−linking→↓cell wall synthesis→osmotic influx of extracellular fluid→↑intracellular hydrostatic pressure→cell rupture→cell death=bactericidal
- •↑Bacterial autolytic enzymes→
  - ○Peptidoglycan degradation

MYELOPROLIFERATIVE CYTOKINES

Generic (Trade)	M	♀
Granulocyte colony stimulating factor−GCSF (Filgastrim)	L	U
Granulocyte−monocyte colony stimulating factor GM−CSF (Sargramostim)	L	U

Outcomes:
- •↓Duration of neutropenia, but most studies show that cytokine treatment does not ↓duration of hospitalization or mortality

Side effects:
General
- •Fever
- •Fluid retention

Mucocutaneous
- •Dermatitis

Musculoskeletal
- •Bone pain

Pulmonary
- •Hypoxia

VANCOMYCIN

Indications:
- •Suspected **methicillin resistant Staphylococcus aureus–MRSA** via:
  - ◦History of colonization/ infection
  - ◦Intravascular line mediated infection
  - ◦Recent hospitalization or nursing home residence
  - ◦Recent invasive procedure
  - ◦Severe mucositis
  - ◦**Inadequate response to treatment @ 48hours**

M ♀	Dose	Peak	Trough
K ?	1g IV q12hours, to be administered over 1hour	30–40µg/ mL	>5µg/ mL

- •Peak levels are obtained 30minutes after the dose, w/ trough levels being obtained at the end of the dosing interval. Plasma peak & trough levels are directly related to toxicity & clinical efficacy respectively

Mechanism:
- •Direct cell wall peptidoglycan binding→
  - ◦↓Transpeptidase function→
    - –↓Bacterial cell wall peptidoglycan cross–linking→↓cell wall synthesis→osmotic influx of extracellular fluid→↑intracellular hydrostatic pressure→cell rupture→cell death=bactericidal

- •Vancomycin resistant enterococci–VRE & staphylococci–VRS have developed

Side effects:
General
- •Rapid intravenous administration (over <1hour)→
  - ◦Intrinsic hypersensitivity syndrome→
    - –Face, neck, &/or upper thoracic angioedema, termed "red man syndrome". Occurrence does not prevent continued use, unless accompanied by an anaphylactoid reaction

Cardiovascular
- •Venous inflammation=phlebitis ± thrombus formation

Otolaryngology
- •Ototoxicity

AMPHOTERICIN B

Indications:
- •Suspected fungal infection
  - ◦Patient w/ oropharyngeal candidiasis
- •**Inadequate response to treatment @ 96hours**

Generic (Trade)		M ♀	Dose
Non–lipid Amphotericin B (Fungizone)		C P	1–1.5mg/ kg IV infusion over 2hours q24hours

AMPHOTERICIN B LIPID FORMULATIONS

Indications, being either:
- •Creatinine >2.5mg/ dL
- •Refractory or intolerant of the non–lipid formulation

Generic (Trade)	M ♀	Dose
Amphotericin B cholesteryl complex† (Amphotec)	? P	4mg/ kg IV infusion over 2hours q24h
Amphotericin B lipid complex (Abelcet)	? P	5mg/ kg IV infusion over 2hours q24h
Liposomal amphotericin B (AmBisome)	? P	3mg/ kg IV infusion over 2hours q24h

- •The lipid preparations preferentially accumulate in the organs of the reticuloendothelial system–RES as opposed to the kidneys, thus allowing for ↑dosing w/ concomitantly ↓nephrotoxicity risk. Although the lipid formulations allow for ↑tissue concentrations & distribution volume, none of them have been shown to have ↑efficacy
†Also named Amphotericin B colloidal dispersion–ABCD

Non–lipid specific dosage adjustment:
- •Should renal failure occur w/ the non–lipid formulation, either:
  - ◦Administer q48h
  - ◦↓Dosage by 50%
  - ◦Switch to a lipid formulation

Mechanism:
- •Bonding to ergosterol†→
  - ◦Fungal cell membrane disruption, w/ no clinically significant resistance

†Ergosterol is not found on human or bacterial cell membranes, thus allowing for selective toxicity

698

Side effects: **Non-lipid > Lipid formulations†**
  General
    •Inflammatory cytokine release→
      ◦Anorexia
      ◦**Chills**
        −Treated w/ Meperidine 25−50mg IV, followed by Dantrolene if intractable
      ◦**Fevers,** w/ ↓frequency & severity w/ repeated doses
      ◦Metallic taste
  Cardiovascular
    •Bradycardia
    •Hypotension−rare
    •**Thrombophlebitis**
      ◦Improved w/ the addition of 1,000 units of Heparin to the infusion
  Gastrointestinal
    •Nausea ± vomiting
  Genitourinary
    •Tubular toxicity (which may be avoided w/ hydration via 500mL of normal saline prior to, & after infusion)→
      ◦Acute tubular necrosis→
        −**Intra−renal renal failure**
      ◦**Hypokalemia**
        −May be treated w/ a potassium sparing diuretic added throughout treatment
  Mucocutaneous
    •Flushing
  Musculoskeletal
    •Inflammatory cytokine release→
      ◦Myalgia
  Neurologic
    •Seizures
  Hematologic
    •↓Erythropoietin→
      −Normocytic−normochromic anemia
    •Hypocapnia
    •Hypomagnesemia
    •**Myelosuppression→**
      ◦Anemia→
        −Fatigue
      ◦Leukopenia→immunosuppression→
        −↑Infection & neoplasm risk
      ◦Thrombocytopenia→
        −↑Hemorrhage risk, esp. petechiae

†Ampho B cholesteryl complex > Ampho B lipid complex > Liposomal ampho B

ANTIVIRAL MEDICATIONS

Indications:
  •Suspected Cytomegalovirus infection
  •**Inadequate response to treatment @ 96hours**

Generic (Trade)	M	♀	Dose
Gancyclovir (Cytovene, DHPG)	K	U	5mg/ kg IV q12hours

Side effects:
  General
    •Headache
    •**Fever−50%**
  Cardiovascular
    •Phlebitis @ infusion site
  Mucocutaneous
    •Dermatitis
  Opthalmologic
    •**Retinal detachment−10%**
  Gastrointestinal
    •Nausea ± vomiting
  Neurologic
    •Seizures
  Hematologic
    •**Myelosuppression** @ plasma level >100mg/ mL, esp. w/ renal failure→

∘Anemia→
  −Fatigue
∘Leukopenia→immunosuppression→
  −↑Infection & neoplasm risk
∘Thrombocytopenia→
  −↑Hemorrhage risk, esp. petechiae

- Caused by ↓osteoblast activity→
  - Relatively ↑osteoclast activity→
    - Bone demineralization (calcium & phosphate)
    - ↓Bone matrix formation
    ...→↓**bone density**, being > than the age expected norm→
      - Diffuse osteopenia→
        - Osteoporosis (regional or generalized)→
          - Bone weakening→↑**fracture risk**

Statistics:
- #1 bone disease in adults, w/ type 1 affecting 25million Americans→
  - 1.5 million fractures in the U.S./ year
- 55% of white postmenopausal ♀ have osteopenia, & 30% have osteoporosis, w/ 50% of those w/ osteoporosis experiencing ≥1 fracture

CLASSIFICATION/ RISK FACTORS
PRIMARY OSTEOPOROSIS ■■■■
- **Type 1, termed postmenopausal/ postclimacteric osteoporosis**
  - ↓**Estrogen or testosterone**→↓osteoblast activity→↓bone density:
    - 2–5%/ year of trabecular bone
    - 1–2%/ year of cortical bone X 5 years, w/ subsequent equalization to that of trabecular bone
    ...→diffuse osteopenia→
      - Osteoporosis, w/ **most bone loss occurring within 5–10 years post–hormonal decline**

- **Type 2, termed senile osteoporosis**
  - ↑**Age**→
    - ↓Osteoblast activity
    - ↓Renal production of 1,25 dihydroxycholecalciferol→↓intestinal calcium absorption→secondary hyperparathyroidism
    ...→↓bone density (trabecular bone=cortical bone)

Risk factors:
- **Age:** ≥30years→net bone loss (♀–1%/ year > ♂), which accelerates w/:
  - **Type 1: ♀ @ age ≥45 years**
  - **Type 2: @ age ≥70 years**
  Age related osteoporosis prevalence:
  - 50–59 years: 15%
  - 60–69 years: 20%
  - 70–79 years: 40%
  - ≥80 years: 70%
- **Gender**
  - Type 1: ♀ >> ♂
  - Type 2: ♀ 2 X ♂
- **Skin color/ ethnicity:** White & Asian ♀ > black ♀, due to the formers' relatively ↓peak bone density
- **Genetics**
  - Family history of osteoporosis
- **Body morphology**
  - Slender body structure→
    - ↓Peak bone density
- **Endocrine**
  - Diabetes mellitus
- **Lifestyle**
  - Alcohol→
    - ↓Osteoblast function
  - Caffeine→
    - ↑Urinary calcium excretion
  - ↓**Calcium or vitamin D intake**
  - ↓Sun exposure→
    - ↓Vitamin D production
  - **Cigarette smoking** & high altitude residence→earlier onset estrogen deficiency syndromes (perimenopause & menopause)
  - Sedentary lifestyle
- **Nulliparity**

•**Osteoporosis secondary to a disease or medication**

Risk factors:
•**Autoimmune disease syndromes**
  ∘Rheumatoid arthritis
•**Chronic liver disease**
•**Chronic renal disease**
•**Endocrine**
  ∘Hyperparathyroidism
  ∘Hyperthyroidism
  ∘Hypogonadism
  ∘↑Glucocorticoids→
    −Cushings disease or syndrome
  ∘↑Growth hormone→
    −Acromegally
•**Malnutrition**
•**Medications**
  ∘**Androgen deprivation treatment**
    −Gonadotropin releasing hormone−GnRH analogues: Goserelin, Leuprolide
    −Antiandrogens: Bicalutamide, Flutamide, NIlutamide
    −Androgen synthesis inhibitors: Aminoglutethimide, Ketoconazole
  ∘Chemotherapy medications
  ∘Chronic use (≥3 months) of antiseizure medications
  ∘Cyclosporine→
    −↑Osteoclast mediated bone resorption
  ∘Glucocorticoids
  ∘Heparin→
    −↑Osteoclast mediated bone resorption, esp. w/ high molecular weight Heparin, usually w/ use
     ≥1month
  ∘Lithium
  ∘Thyroid hormone replacement, if causing hyperthyroidism
•**Neoplastic**
  ∘Malignancy, esp. myeloma & disease metastatic to the bone
•**Osteogenesis imperfecta**

DIAGNOSIS

Musculoskeletal
•**Fractures** via:
  ∘Cortical bone loss, esp. **long bones**→
    −Distal radial fracture, termed Colles' fracture
    −Proximal femoral, humerus, or tibial fracture
  ∘Trabecular bone loss, esp. **vertebrae**

Femoral fractures:
  •Femoral neck &/or intertrochanteric region fractures, either cause, or are caused by a fall, esp.
   falling to the side, due to ↓soft tissue available to dissipate the force of impact

Vertebral fractures:
  •Occur in 35% of ♀ by age 65years, often w/ minimal stress, such as w/:
    −Bending
    −Coughing
    −Lifting a light object
    −Sneezing
    ...→predominant mid−thoracic to upper lumbar vertebral:
        •**Complete compression** (predominating in Type 1)→
          ∘↓Height
        •**Anterior wedging** (predominating in Type 2)→
          ∘↓Height
        ∘Dorsal kyphosis & cervical lordosis→
          −Stooped posture, termed Dowager's hump
        ...both→
          •Sensory nerve root impingement→
            ∘Back pain, usually being acute ± lateral radiation to the flanks & anteriorly, which ↓
             gradually over several weeks to months

702

- •Mandibular bone resorption→
  - ∘↑Tooth loss

Genitourinary
- •↑Urinary calcium, being either:
  - ∘>7.5mmol/ 24hour collection
  - ∘>3.3mmol/ 12 hour overnight collection
- •↑Urinary collagen breakdown products:
  - ∘Pyridinium cross−links
  - ∘N−telopeptides

Biochemical markers of bone turnover†:
- •The following are indicative of **bone resorption:**
  - ∘Urinary excretion of:
    - −Galactosyl hydroxylysine
    - −Hydroxyproline
    - −Pyridium cross−links of collagen (ex. deoxypyridinoline)
    - −C & N−telopeptides of collagen

Hematologic
- •↓Plasma 1,25−dihydroxycholecalciferol (<20pg/ mL), the most potent form of vitamin D

Biochemical markers of bone turnover†:
- •The following are indicative of **bone formation:**
  - ∘Plasma alkaline phosphatase, a bone isoenzyme
  - ∘Plasma osteocalcin
  - ∘Plasma C & N−propeptides of type 1 collagen

---

†As turnover marker levels fluctuate on a daily basis, several measurements should be made prior to & during treatment, in order to calculate an average that will be helpful in monitoring treatment response
- •**Why measure both bone density & bone turnover markers?**
  - ∘Consider bone loss as a train going through your town. The bone mass informs you of the train's position at a given time, while the turnover markers inform you of the train's speed (↓amount indicating a slower rate of progression). Once the train reaches it's destination, the patient has a fracture. However, although theoretically useful in order to make an informed prognosis, the appropriate use of turnover markers is controversial

BONE DENSITY IMAGING

Indications:
- •♀ **age ≥60years not receiving osteoporosis treatment**
- •Patients w/ a syndrome of possible ↓bone mass
- •Patients who are chronically taking ↑risk medications
- •Patients w/ asymptomatic primary hyperparathyroidism, in whom a diagnosis of ↓bone mass indicates the need for surgery

- •**X rays**
  - Findings of vertebral osteoporosis:
    - •↓Trabecular bone density→
      - ∘↑**Prominence of the surrounding cortical bone**, termed "picture frame" vertebral bodies
      - ∘Weakened vertebral body→
        - −Intervertebral disk expansion→**biconcave "codfish" vertebrae**
        - −Intervertebral disk intrusion into the vertebral body→Schmorl's nodules
      - ∘Vertebral fractures via either:
        - −Complete compression→↓anterior & posterior height
        - −Anterior wedging→↓anterior height only
  - Limitations:
    - •**≥30% bone density loss** is required for disease to be visualized

- •**Bone densitometry**
  - ∘Allows for bone mineral density−BMD measurements, w/ the recommended sites being:
    - −The **hip** via the femoral neck or total hip score, whichever is lower
    - −The **lumbar spine** (L1−L4)
  - Imaging modalities (listed via ↑radiation exposure):
    - •Dual energy X−ray absorptiometry−DEXA, which scans the entire skeleton
    - •Dual photon absorptiometry−DPA, which scans the entire skeleton
    - •Single photon absorptiometry−SPA, which scans the calcaneous bone & radius
    - •Quantitative computed tomography−QCAT, which scans the lumbar spine & radius

703

<u>Bone density scores:</u>
- The **T score** represents the deviation of a patients bone density score from the **normal populations mean lifetime peak bone mass** in standard units
  - ○Fracture risk doubles for every 1 standard deviation below peak bone density
    - −**Normal**, indicated by a T score <1 standard deviation below peak bone mass
    - −**Osteopenia**, indicated by a T score of 1−2.4 standard deviation(s) below peak bone mass
    - −**Osteoporosis**, indicated by a T score ≥2.5 standard deviations below peak bone mass
- The **Z score** represents the deviation of a patients bone density score from **age−matched individuals** in order to determine whether the patient's bone mass is unexpectedly low, indicated by ≥2 standard deviations below the age matched norm. If so, assess for causes of secondary osteoporosis

<u>Limitations:</u>
- Different manufacturers of bone densitometers use different reference populations & calibrations→
  - ○Bone mass difference of ≤12% among different machines. Thus, optimal management involves the use of the same manufacturer's bone densitometer

TREATMENT & PREVENTION
- **The goal of medical treatment is fracture prevention**

PRIMARY OSTEOPOROSIS TREATMENT & FRACTURE PREVENTION ▰▰▰▰▰▰▰
- **Smoking cessation** via smoking cessation clinic
  - ○Cigarette smoking contributes to 20% of deaths in the U.S. & is the #1 modifiable cause of premature death
- **Exercise**
  - ○An enjoyable form of weight bearing exercise, such as walking or jogging, on a regular basis (≥3X/ week) for 20−30min., preceded by stretching→
    - −↑Bone formation→reversal of bone loss
    - −↑Muscle mass
    - …→↓fall risk
- **↓Caffeine intake**
  - ○≤2 drinks/ 24hours
- **↓Alcohol consumption**
  - ○Only 1drink (8−12 ounces of beer, 3−5 ounces of wine, or 1 ounce of liquor) q24hours in patients without a history of drug abuse
  - ○≥2 drinks/ 24hours→
    - −↑Abuse risk
    - −Hepatitis (♀ > ♂)
    - −Hypertension

VITAMINS & MINERALS			
Generic	M	♀	Dose
Vitamin D	L	? If >RDA	20µg=800 IU q24hours
&			
Calcium carbonate	K	P	500mg PO q8hours w/ meals

ADDITIONAL PRIMARY OSTEOPOROSIS TREATMENT ▰▰▰▰▰▰▰▰
<u>Indications:</u>
- History of a fragility fracture
- T score > 2 standard deviations below peak bone mass

- There is no evidence that any of the following medications reduce fractures in ♀ who do not meet the indications stated above
- There is also no evidence that the use of combination therapy is more effective than monotherapy

BISPHOSPHONATES			
Generic (Trade)	M	♀	Dose
Alendronate (Fosamax)	K	?	70mg PO qweek
Risedronate (Actonel)	K	?	35mg PO qweek
Zoledronic acid (Zometa)	K	?	4mg IV qyear
• Should be taken 30min. prior to breakfast, as <10% is absorbed in the presence of food			
<u>Mechanism:</u>
• Binds to hydroxyapatite crystals→
○↓Bone turnover			

Side effects:
Gastrointestinal
  •**Esophagitis,** esp. w/ qd dosing, usually beginning within 1 month after treatment is started
    Risk reduction:
      ∘Take w/ ≥8oz of water & remain upright for ≥30min.

Absolute Contraindications:
  •Achalasia
  •Esophageal stricture

Relative contraindications:
  •Gastroesophageal reflux disease–GERD

SECOND LINE TREATMENT

SALMON CALCITONIN (Calcimar)		
M ♀		Dose

Plasma ?
  •SC/ IM forms   100 units q24hours
  •Intranasal form   200 units q24hours w/ alternating nostrils

Mechanism:
  •Hormone normally produced by thyroid interstitial parafollicular cells→
    ∘Inhibition of osteoclast function & formation

Contraindications:
  •Hypersensitivity to salmon protein or gelatin diluent

MIXED ESTROGEN RECEPTOR AGONIST/ ANTAGONIST				

Indications:
  •Postmenopausal ♀

Generic (Trade)	M ♀	Dose
Raloxifene (Evista)	L U	60mg PO q24hours

Side effects in comparison to estrogen:

Positive effects	Estrogen	Raloxifene
•Breast cancer risk	↑↑	↓↓
•Favorable plasma lipid alteration	+++	+
∘↓LDL & total cholesterol		
•Postmenopausal bone loss prevention	+++	++†
Negative effects		
•Endometrial cancer risk	↑↑‡	Ø
•Postmenopausal hot flashes	↓↓↓	↑
•Premenopausal hot flashes		↑↑
•Uterine hemorrhage	↑↑↑	Ø
•**Venous thrombosis risk**	↑↑	↑↑

†Being more than any other medication in this class

Contraindications:
  •History of thromboembolic disease

THIRD LINE TREATMENT

ESTROGEN REPLACEMENT THERAPY–ERT†				

Indications:
  •Postmenopausal ♀

Generic (Trade)	M ♀	Start	Max
Conjugated equine estrogens (Premarin)	L U	0.3mg PO q24hours	1.25mg q24
Conjugated synthetic estrogens (Cenestin)	L U	0.3mg PO q24hours	1.25mg q24h
Esterified estrogens (Menest)	L U	0.3mg PO q24hours	Same
Estradiole (Estrace, Estradiol, Gynodiol)	L U	0.5mg PO q24hours	2mg q24hours
Estradiole cypionate (Depo–Estradiol)	L U	1mg IM qmonth	5mg qmonth
Estradiole valerate (Delestrogen)	L U	10mg IM qmonth	20mg qmonth
Estrone (Estrone 5, EstraGyn 5)	L U	0.1mg IM qweek	1mg qweek
Transdermal estradiol (Climara, FemPatch)	L U	0.025mg/ 24h patch qweek†	0.1mg/ 24hours

•The above formulations are given in their continuous as opposed to cyclic schedule, for ease of adherence
†Rotate application sites

705

Mechanism:
- Estrogen→
  - ↓Cortical & trabecular bone resorption, esp. if initiated within 5years postmenopause

Outcomes:
- 50% ↓fracture risk of:
  - Forearm
  - Hip
  - Pelvis
  - Vertebrae
- Many patients experience a 2–4%/ year ↑bone mass X several years, w/ significant bone loss being rare in compliant patients

Positive effects:
- Favorable plasma lipid alteration
  - ↓LDL & total cholesterol
- ↓Postmenopausal bone loss
- ↓Postmenopausal hot flashes
- ↓Vulvar & vaginal atrophy

Negative effects:
- **↑Breast cancer** risk w/ treatment X ≥5years
- **↑Endometrial cancer**† in 0.5% of patients receiving unopposed estrogen X ≥10years
- **↑Cerebrovascular accident syndrome** risk
- **↑Thromboembolic syndrome risk**
  - Deep venous thrombosis ± pulmonary embolism
- Breast tenderness
- Cholelithiasis→
  - ↑Cholecystitis risk
- Headaches
- Uterine hemorrhage w/ cyclic progestin co–treatment
- Weight gain

†Previously combined w/ a progestin in s w/ a uterus to prevent endometrial hyperplasia→
- Normalized estrogen mediated endometrial cancer risk. However, the estrogen–progestin combination has been shown to:
  - **↑Breast cancer risk** without the 5year delay
  - **↑Thromboembolic syndrome risk** more than estrogen alone
  - **↑Myocardial ischemic syndrome risk**, which is why the combination is no longer recommended

Contraindications:
- History of breast cancer or thromboembolic disease

SECONDARY OSTEOPOROSIS TREATMENT

BISPHOSPONATES

Generic (Trade)	M	♀	Dose
Alendronate (Fosamax)	K	?	70mg PO qweek
Risedronate (Actonel)	K	?	35mg PO qweek
Zoledronic acid (Zometa)	K	?	4mg IV qyear

- Should be taken 30min. prior to breakfast, as <10% is absorbed in the presence of food

FALL RISK ASSESSMENT & PROPHYLAXIS

- Being that **the majority of fractures in the elderly are a result of falling,** fall prevention is of major importance

Fall risk factors:
- Altered mental status
- Arthritis
- Cerebrovascular accident
- Deconditioning
- Orthostatic hypotension
- Peripheral neuropathy
- Polypharmacy
- ↓Visual acuity
- …via either:
  - Lower extremity weakness
  - Impaired balance or gait

706

<u>Fall risk assessment:</u>
- **One leg balance test**
  - <u>Procedure:</u>
    - Ask the patient to stand unassisted on one leg X 5seconds, repeating w/ the other leg. Inability to perform this task indicates ↑fall risk

<u>Fall risk prophylaxis:</u>
- **Review medications** to determine possible cause/ contributor
- **Vision & hearing assessment**
- **Occupational therapy**
  - To teach the patient how to better perform activities of daily living–ADLs ± assistive devices if necessary:
    - Braces, crutches, &/or walkers→↑stability & ↑mobility
    - Strategically placed rails, such as along stairwells, by the toilet, & in the bath &/or shower
- **Physical therapy**
  - For gait training
  - To teach the patient:
    - Joint protective maneuvers
    - Energy conserving maneuvers
    - The therapeutic use of heat & massage, w/ heat treatment via baths, towels, electric heating pads, &/or paraffin wax baths→↓peri–articular muscle spasm→↓joint pain
  - To provide an individualized exercise program incorporating range of motion–ROM & muscle strengthening→
    - ↑Stability of weight bearing joints
- **Home safety** evaluation to ensure:
  - Adequate lighting, including night lights in bedrooms, hallways, & bathrooms
  - Uncluttered walkways
  - Securely fastened stairway handrails
  - Bathroom grab bars in the shower/ bathtub & by the toilet
  - Raised toilet seats
  - Nonslip rubber suction mats in the shower/ bathtub & slick bathroom floors
  - Throw rugs are either fastened to the floor or removed

HIP FRACTURE PROGNOSIS
- **15% mortality within 3 months** due to surgical complications, esp.:
  - Pulmonary thromboembolism
  - Nosocomial infections

<u>Age based 1 year mortality:</u>
- **<70 years: 20%**
- **70–79 years: 30%**
- **80–89 years: 40%**

•Slow, chronically progressive, mildly inflammatory, osteocartilagenous joint destruction without accompanying systemic symptoms

Statistics:
  •**The #1 form of arthritis**

•↑**Age–#1 risk factor:** >45 years
  ◦35% of persons age >65 years have symptomatic osteoarthritis
  ◦85% of persons age ≥75 years have either clinical or radiographic evidence of osteoarthritis
•**Gender:** ♀ > ♂
•**Skin color:** Blacks > whites
•**Joint abnormality**
  ◦Excessive joint stress
    −Any exercise involving running or jumping†, esp. w/ concomitant neuropathy
    −Obesity
    −Repetitive fine motor tasks
  ◦Joint damage
    −Prior arthritis, esp. w/ concomitant neuropathy
    −Trauma
  ◦Endocrine‡
    −Diabetes mellitus
    −↑Growth hormone→acromegaly
    −Hyperparathyroidism
  ◦Genetic‡
    −Autosomal dominant type II procollagen gene (COL2A1) mutation→mild chondrodysplasia→ premature osteoarthritis
  ◦Metabolic disorder‡
    −Amyloidosis
    −Crystal deposition disease (gout, calcium pyrophosphate dihydrate deposition disease–CPPD)
    −Hemochromatosis
    −Ochronosis
    −Paget's disease
    −Wilson's disease
  ◦Nutritional
    −Trace element deficiency→Kashin–Bek disease
  ◦Postural or developmental defects
    −Hyperlaxity syndromes
    −Legg–Calve–Perthes disease
    −Scoliosis
    −Slipped capital femoral epiphyses

---

†Jogging→
  •Oscillating joint movement→
    −↓Risk relative to running & jumping
‡Premature osteoarthritis, which occurs @ age <45 years, should lead to the consideration of underlying endocrine, metabolic, or genetic disease

Musculoskeletal
  •↓Articular cartilage proteoglycan concentration (responsible for tensile strength) & ↑water content→
    ◦Weakened articular cartilage→
      −**Irregular cartilage fragmentation & ulceration**→cartilage cell=chondrocyte repair, which is eventually overwhelmed→subchondral bone microfractures, w/ bone compression & reactive proliferation→**sclerosis** & ↑water content→↑intraosseous pressure→↓blood flow→bone ischemia

  Affected joints:
    •Large weight bearing joints, being the most commonly affected
      ◦Hip
      ◦Knee

- •Small joints
  - ○**Vertebral joints**, esp. the movable lower cervical & lumbar spine
  - ○Hands
    - –Proximal interphalangeal joints–PIPs
    - –Distal interphalangeal joints–DIPs
  - ○Wrist
    - –1st Carpometacarpal joints→lateral wrist pain
  - ○Feet
    - –Metatarsophalangeal joints–MTPs, esp. the 1st, causing big toe base pain
  - ○Acromioclavicular joint→
    - –Shoulder pain

Rare involvement:
- •Hand & arm joints proximal to the proximal interphalangeal–PIP joints
  - ○Metacarpophalangeal–MCP joints (finger bases)
  - ○2nd–5th Carpometacarpal joints (wrists)
  - ○Elbows
- •Ankles
- •Opposing cartilage surface irregularity→
  - ○**Crepitance**, occurring in 90% of knee osteoarthritis, being a sound or sensation likened to crunching potato chips upon joint range of motion. It is an early sign of osteoarthritis, & may be palpable &/or audible to the examiner

Effects of chronic, inadequately controlled disease:
- •Joint locking during range of motion indicates likely synovial cartilage &/or bone detritus
- •The body's attempt to compensate & stabilize the joint→
  - ○**Periarticular muscle spasm**
  - ○Subchondral bone cysts, termed geodes
  - ○Proliferation of bone @ the joint margin→**osteophytes, termed "bone spurs"**
    - –Proximal interphalangeal–PIP joint osteophytes form **Bouchard's nodes**
    - –Distal interphalangeal–DIP osteophytes form **Heberden's nodes**
  - ...→synovial, joint capsule, &/or periosteal stretching ± inflammation→
    - •Gradually worsening **joint pain**, being:
      - ○↑By use ± palpation
      - ○↑By ↓barometric pressure during cold or rainy weather→
        - –↑Intra-articular pressure→↑joint pain
      - ○↓By rest, w/ eventual ↑severity→
        - –Rest pain
      - ...w/ minimal to no edema, erythema, or warmth, unless joint debris→
        - •Inflammation
    - •**Gradually worsening stiffness lasting <30min., esp. after prolonged inactivity (even several hours), being termed the gel phenomenon**
    - •Irregular articular cartilage loss→
      - ○Joint malalignment, termed subluxation→
        - –Finger "broken staff" appearance
        - –Varus (bow-legged) > valgus limb deformity, being due to medial or lateral knee articular cartilage loss respectively
      - ...w/ pain, stiffness, & malalignment→
        - •↓Function
          - ○Hip or knee arthritis→
            - –↓Ambulation
        - •Finger arthritis→
          - ○Inability to use the hands
          - ...→periarticular muscle atrophy↔
            - •Muscle weakness
              - ○Hip abductor weakness→
                - –Classic waddling, termed Trendelenburg gait

Neurologic
- •Spinal osteoarthritis→
  - ○Motor &/or sensory neural compression→
    - –Weakness
    - –Abnormal sensations, termed paresthesias, esp. pain &/or numbness

709

•**X rays**
Indications:
  •All patients w/ suspected disease, in order for both diagnosis & staging
Appropriate views:
  •Hand joints: Single anteroposterior–AP view of both hands†
  •Hip joints: Single anteroposterior–AP view of the pelvis†
  •Knee joints: Anteroposterior & lateral views
  •Spine: Anteroposterior, lateral, & oblique views
Findings:
  •Early disease:
    ◦Normal or irregular loss of radiolucent cartilage→
      –Irregular joint space narrowing
  •Moderate disease:
    ◦Joint margin proliferation→
      –Osteophyte, termed "bone spur"
    ◦Progressive joint space narrowing
  •Late disease:
    ◦Bone malalignment
    ◦Significant joint space narrowing
    ◦Subchondral bone compression & reactive proliferation→
      –Sclerosis→↑bone density
    ◦Subchondral cyst formation

---

†Lateral & oblique views should be obtained if either:
  •An abnormality is detected
  •Findings do not correlate w/ the clinical picture

•**Arthrocentesis**
Contraindications:
  •Through infected soft tissue→
    ◦Organism introduction into the synovial space
Synovial studies:
  •Gross appearance:
    ◦>3.5mL of fluid (normal being <3.5mL), being the normal clear straw colored
  •Leukocyte count:
    ◦<3,000/ μL, being neutrophil depleted (<25% neutrophils). Normal being <180/ μL w/ a mononuclear predominance
  •Glucose level:
    ◦Normal, being ~plasma level
  •Protein level:
    ◦2–3.5g/ dL
  •Bacterial gram stain & culture: Negative

•**Weight loss if overweight/ obese†, via goal daily caloric requirement**
  ◦The caloric total needed to reach & maintain a goal weight depends on physical activity level
  ◦10 calories/ lb of goal weight +
    –33% if sedentary
    –50% if moderately physically active
    –75% if very physically active
  ◦3500 calories are roughly equivalent to 1 lb of body fat
    –Consuming 500calories less/ day X 1week→1 lb weight loss
    –Exercising 500calories/ day X 1week→1 lb weight loss
  …w/ the average human body being able to lose 3.5 lbs/ week maximum, aside from a diuretic effect
•**Joint rest**
  ◦Being that joint pain is often exacerbated by use, short periods of joint rest throughout the day, during active synovitis→
    –↓Pain
•**Occupational therapy**
  ◦To teach the patient how to better perform activities of daily living–ADLs ± assistive devices if necessary:
    –Splints to rest finger joints
    –Braces, crutches, &/or walkers to ↓weight on affected joints→↓pain, ↑stability, & ↑mobility
    –Eating utensils w/ large handles

710

-Nonslip rubber table & bathroom mats (including for the shower &/or bath)
-Strategically placed rails, such as along stairwells, by the toilet, & in the bath &/or shower
•**Physical therapy**
  ◦For gait training
  ◦To teach the patient:
    -Joint protective maneuvers
    -Energy conserving maneuvers
    -The therapeutic use of heat & massage, w/ heat treatment via baths, towels, electric heating pads,
     &/or paraffin wax baths→↓peri–articular muscle spasm→↓joint pain
  ◦To provide an individualized exercise program incorporating range of motion–ROM & muscle
   strengthening→
    -↑Stability of weight bearing joints

---

†For obesity, medical & surgical treatment options may be used (see obesity syndromes section)

ACETAMINOPHEN			
M ♀	Dose		Max
LK P	650mg PO q6hours prn		4g/ 24hours

Mechanism:
•Reversible inhibition of the cyclooxygenase–COX 1 enzyme in the central nervous system >>
 peripheral tissues→
  ◦Predominantly ↓central nervous system prostaglandin synthesis→
    -↓Pain
    -↓Temperature (antipyretic)
    ...w/ minimal effects on inflammatory cell mediated inflammation

Background physiology:
•Presynaptic neuronal mediated prostaglandins are released in response to afferent signals,
 indicating peripheral inflammation→
  ◦Enhanced sensitivity of pain neurons (but not direct excitement)→
    -Pain
•Interleukin–IL1→
  ◦↑Hypothalamic prostaglandin production→
    -Fever

Side effects:
 Gastrointestinal
  •**Hepatitis**
   Mechanism:
    •90% of Acetaminophen undergoes either hepatocyte mediated:
      ◦Glucoronidation→
        -Nontoxic glucorinides
      ◦Sulfation→
        -Nontoxic sulfates
    •10% of Acetaminophen undergoes hepatocyte mediated oxidation by the cytochrome P450
     enzyme complex→
      ◦A potentially toxic reactive electrophilic compound, which then undergoes either:
        -Conjugation w/ cellular glutathione→nontoxic compound
        -Reaction w/ cellular proteins→cellular toxicity ± death→**hepatitis**
    •Normally, glutathione depletion occurs w/ ingestion of >10g of Acetaminophen. However, any
     substance which ↑cytochrome P450 function (such as ethanol) causes relatively more
     Acetaminophen to be diverted to the formation of the toxic compound→
      ◦More rapid hepatocyte depletion of glutathione→
        -Cell toxicity at lower ingested Acetaminophen doses

Contraindications:
 •**Do not administer Acetaminophen to chronic heavy ethanol drinkers**

CYCLOOXYGENASE–COX 2 SELECTIVE INHIBITING NSAIDS			
Generic (Trade)	**M**	**♀**	**Dose**
Celecoxib (Celebrex)	L	U	200mg PO q12hours

Mechanism:
- •Selective, reversible inhibition of the cyclooxygenase–COX 2 enzyme, being responsible for the production of inflammatory cell prostaglandins→
  - ∘↓Pain
  - ∘↓Inflammation
  - …w/ minimal cyclooxygenase–COX 1 mediated effects

Background pathophysiology:
- •Inflammatory cell mediated prostaglandins are released at sites of inflammation (in addition to other inflammatory cytokines)→
  - ∘Leukocyte migration→↑inflammation via:
    - –Vasodilation→↑blood flow→erythema, edema, warmth, &/or tenderness/ pain via enhanced neuronal sensitivity

In Brief:
- •**Cyclooxygenase–COX1 enzymes** are found in most cells of the body, being responsible for normal physiologic processes
- •**Cyclooxygenase–COX 2 enzymes** are responsible for the production of inflammatory cell prostaglandins

Cyclooxyegenase–COX 1 mediated effects	Effects of relatively ↓inhibition
Hypothalamic prostaglandin synthesis	No antipyretic effect
Platelet thromboxane A$_2$ synthesis	No antiplatelet effect
Gastric mucosal cell prostaglandin synthesis	↓Peptic inflammatory disease risk
Glomerular afferent arteriole prostaglandin synthesis	↓Renal failure risk

Side effects:
Cardiovascular
- •Hypertension

Gastrointestinal
- •Inhibition of the cyclooxygenase–COX1 enzyme→↑peptic inflammatory disease risk→↑**upper gastrointestinal hemorrhage risk** via:
  - ∘↓Gastric mucosal prostaglandin synthesis→
    - –↓Epithelial proliferation
    - –↓Mucosal blood flow→↓bicarbonate delivery to the mucosa
    - –↓Mucus & bicarbonate secretion from gastric mucosal cells

Genitourinary
- •Patients w/ pre-existing bilateral ↓renal perfusion, not necessarily failure:
  - ∘Heart failure
  - ∘Bilateral renal artery stenosis
  - ∘Hypovolemia
  - ∘Renal failure
  - …rely more on the compensatory production of vasodilatory prostaglandins→
    - •Afferent arteriole dilation→
      - ∘Maintained glomerular filtration rate–GFR, whereas NSAIDs→
        - –↓Prostaglandin production, which may→renal failure

Pulmonary
- •Inhibition of both cyclooxygenase enzymes (COX 1 & COX2)→
  - ∘↑Lipoxygenase activity→
    - –↑Leukotriene synthesis→symptomatic asthma within 2hours of ingestion in 5% of asthmatics

Caution:
- •Minimal inhibition of COX–1→
  - ∘↓Endothelial & vascular smooth muscle cell prostacyclin† production relative to platelet thromboxane‡ production→cytokine imbalance in favor of vasoconstriction→
    - –Hypertension
    - –↑Cerebrovascular accident syndrome risk
    - –↑Myocardial ischemic syndrome risk

Contraindications:
- •Sulfa hypersensitivity due to a sulfa moiety

NONSTEROIDAL ANTI-INFLAMMATORY DRUGS-NSAIDs			
Generic	M ♀	Start	Max
Ibuprofen	L P in 1st & 2nd, U in 3rd trimester	600mg PO q8hours	3.2g/ 24hours
Indomethacin	L P in 1st & 2nd, U in 3rd trimester	50mg PO/ PR q8hours	
Naproxen •XR form	L P in 1st & 2nd, U in 3rd trimester	375mg PO q12hours 750mg PO q24hours	

•One cannot predict which NSAID a patient will respond to
•Attempt to eventually ↓dosage &/or limit use to exacerbations in order to ↓side effect risk

Mechanism:
•Aspirin & other anti-inflammatory medications→
  ∘Respectively to irreversible & reversible inhibition of both cyclooxygenase enzymes (COX-1 & COX-2), being responsible for the production of neural & inflammatory cell prostaglandins respectively→
    −↓Pain
    −↓Temperature (antipyretic)
    −↓Inflammation

Background pathophysiology:
•Inflammatory cell mediated prostaglandins are released at sites of inflammation (in addition to other inflammatory cytokines)→
  ∘Leukocyte migration→↑inflammation via:
    −Vasodilation→↑blood flow→erythema, edema, warmth, &/or tenderness/ pain via enhanced neuronal sensitivity
•Interleukin-IL1→
  ∘↑Hypothalamic prostaglandin production→
    −Fever

In Brief:
•**Cyclooxygenase-COX1 enzymes** are found in most cells of the body, being responsible for normal physiologic processes
•**Cyclooxygenase-COX 2 enzymes** are responsible for the production of inflammatory cell prostaglandins

Side effects:
Gastrointestinal
•Inhibition of the cyclooxygenase-COX1 enzyme→↑peptic inflammatory disease risk→↑**upper gastrointestinal hemorrhage risk** via:
  ∘↓Gastric mucosal prostaglandin synthesis→
    −↓Epithelial cell proliferation
    −↓Mucosal blood flow→↓bicarbonate delivery to the mucosa
    −↓Mucus & bicarbonate secretion from gastric mucosal cells

Indications for peptic inflammatory disease prophylaxis:
•Prophylax w/ proton pump inhibitors-PPI's, histamine 2 selective receptor blockers, or Misoprostol in patients w/ any of the following:
  ∘Age >60 years w/ a history of peptic inflammatory disease
  ∘Anticipated therapy >3 months
  ∘Concurrent glucocorticoid use
  ∘Moderate to high dose NSAID use
  Note: Newer NSAIDs (Etodolac, Nabumetone, Salsalate)→
    •↓Risk of NSAID induced peptic inflammation/ ulcer

Genitourinary
•Patients w/ pre-existing bilateral ↓renal perfusion, not necessarily failure:
  ∘Heart failure
  ∘Bilateral renal artery stenosis
  ∘Hypovolemia
  ∘Renal failure
  …rely more on the compensatory production of vasodilatory prostaglandins→
    •Afferent arteriole dilation→
      ∘Maintained glomerular filtration rate-GFR, whereas NSAIDs→
        −↓Prostaglandin production, which may→renal failure

Pulmonary
- •Inhibition of both cyclooxygenase enzymes (COX 1 & COX2)→
  - ∘↑Lipoxygenase activity→
    - −↑Leukotriene synthesis→symptomatic asthma within 2hours of ingestion in 5% of asthmatics

CAPSAICIN		
M ♀	**Dose**	
? ?	0.025%–0.075% applied to the affected area ≤qid, w/ prompt handwashing after application	

- •Continued application for 2–4 weeks is necessary to achieve benefit

Mechanism:
- •Substance P antagonism

Side effects:
Cutaneous
- •Burning pain–>30%, being ↓w/ continued use

COMPLEMENTARY TREATMENT
- •There is no evidence of ↑benefit via combination Glucosamine–Chondroitin treatment over monotherapy

GLUCOSAMINE	
♀	**Dose**
U	500mg PO q8hours

Side effects:
Hematologic
- •↓Glucose tolerance

Contraindications:
- •Shellfish hypersensitivity

CHONDROITIN	
♀	**Dose**
?	200–400mg PO q12–8hours or 1.2g PO q24hours

SECOND LINE TREATMENT

INTRA–ARTICULAR GLUCOCORTICOID INJECTION			
Generic	M ♀	**Dose**	
Trimacinolone	L ?		
•Intra–articular form			
∘Finger:		2mg IA	
∘Knee:		40mg IA	
∘Shoulder:		20mg IA	

Outcomes:
- •Variable & short–lasting effects. If pain relief is not achieved for several months w/ 1–2 injections, then abandon this treatment as ≥3 intra–articular injections/ year may→
  - ∘↑Tissue breakdown→
    - −↑Disease severity

INTRA–ARTICULAR HYALURONIC ACID INJECTION			
Generic (Trade)	M ♀	**Treatment cycle**	
Sodium hyaluronate	KL ?		
Hyalgan		2mL IA qweek X 3–5weeks	
Supartz		2.5mL IA qweek X 5weeks	
Hylan G–F 20 (Synvisc)	KL ?	2mL IA qweek X 3wees	

Outcomes:
- •Intra–articular injections typically lead to variable & short–lasting effects (possibly several months)

Side effects:
- •Joint inflammation→
  - ∘Pain & swelling

714

THIRD LINE TREATMENT ▬▬▬▬▬▬▬▬▬▬▬▬▬▬▬▬▬▬▬
•Arthroscopic surgery
  <u>Procedure:</u>
    •Removal of meniscal fragments, cartilage debris, &/or osteophytes, termed bone spurs

•Total joint arthroplasty
  <u>Indications:</u>
    •Disabling pain
  <u>Procedure:</u>
    •Total joint replacement
  <u>Outcomes:</u>
    •The prosthesis usually require replacement @ 10–15 years

FOURTH LINE TREATMENT ▬▬▬▬▬▬▬▬▬▬▬▬▬▬▬▬▬
•Arthrodesis
  <u>Procedure:</u>
    •Surgical joint fusion

RHEUMATOID ARTHRITIS

•**A chronic, intermittently symptomatic autoimmune disease** of unknown etiology→
  ◦Cellular & autoantibody mediated attack of tendons & serosal membranes:
    –Joints
    –Bursae
    –Tendon sheaths
    –Pericardium
    –Pleura
    ...→direct damage & immune complex deposition→
        •Systemic inflammation
Statistics:
  •2nd most common arthritis, affecting 1% of adults (osteoarthritis is #1)→
    ◦#1 chronic inflammatory arthritis

RISK FACTORS

•**Age:** Usual onset of 25–40years, but ranges from infancy to age 90years
•**Gender**
  ◦♀ 3X ♂ @ age <60years
  ◦♀=♂ @ age ≥60years
•**Genetics**
  ◦Family history
  ◦MHC class II DR1 or DR4
•**Ethnicity**
  ◦Native Americans

CLASSIFICATION/ DIAGNOSIS

Diagnostic criteria for Rheumatoid arthritis:
  •≥6 weeks of ≥4 of the following are required:
    ◦Arthritis of ≥3 joints simultaneously
    ◦Hand or wrist arthritis
    ◦Symmetric arthritis
    ◦Morning stiffness >1hour
    ◦Rheumatoid nodules
    ◦Positive Rheumatoid factor
    ◦Imaging showing hand or wrist erosions or osteopenia
Outcomes:
  •90% sensitivity & specificity

Common concomitant autoimmune disease syndromes:
  •Keratoconjunctivitis sicca, termed Sjogren's syndrome–12% (♀ > ♂)
  •Polymyalgia rheumatica
  •Raynaud's phenomenon

Subsyndromes of Rheumatoid arthritis:
  •**Felty's syndrome**
    ◦Rheumatoid arthritis & massive splenomegaly→selective granulocytopenia→
      –↑Infection risk
      –Refractory leg ulcers
  •**Juvenile rheumatoid arthritis–JRA**
    ◦Age ≤16 years w/ arthritis of ≥1 joint(s) lasting ≥6weeks, w/ exclusion of other causes
      –**Oligoarthritis–50%**, affecting <5 joints (esp. large weight bearing joints) & associated w/
        concomitant **chronic anterior uveitis†–20%**
      –**Polyarthritis–20%**, affecting >5 joints (esp. large weight bearing joints) & associated w/
        concomitant chronic anterior uveitis–5%
      –**Systemic disease, termed Still's disease–10%:** May occur to age ≤50years
        Syndrome:
          •Diaphoresis
          •**Intermittent high fevers** (up to 106°F) ± chills
          •Facial flushing
          •Non–pruritic, macular (<1cm diameter non–palpable lesions) **salmon colored rash–80%**,
            esp. affecting the thorax, being difficult to see in blacks, & usually:
              ◦Occurring w/ febrile episodes
              ◦Lasting ≤1 hour
            ...all usually @ night, & may precede arthritis by several months

716

†**Chronic uveitis:** Inflammation of the eye chamber, associated w/ anti−nuclear antibodies−ANAs
Monitoring:
  •Patients w/ oligoarthritis & antinuclear antibodies−ANAs should be screened q3−4 months via
  slit−lamp examination

General
•Inflammatory cytokines→
  ∘Anorexia→
    −Cachexia
  ∘Chills
  ∘Fatigue
  ∘**Fever,** being infrequent & low grade (<101°F)
  ∘Headache
  ∘Malaise
  ∘Night sweats
  ∘Weakness
  ...which may precede the onset of joint symptoms by several weeks

---

†Temperature may be normal in patients w/:
•Chronic kidney disease, esp. w/ uremia
•Cirrhosis
•Heart failure
•Severe debility
...or those who are:
  •Intravenous drug users
  •Taking certain medications:
    ∘Acetaminophen
    ∘Antibiotics
    ∘Glucocorticoids
    ∘Nonsteroidal anti−inflammatory drugs−NSAIDs

Musculoskeletal
•Serosal inflammatory cell infiltration of:
  ∘Joints→
    −**Arthritis,** usually being **polyarticular,** additive, & symmetric; whereas monoarticular disease
    affects the knee > other joints

    Affected joints:
      •Small joints > large weight bearing joints
        ∘Hands
          −Metacarpophalangeal joints−MCPs
          −Proximal interphalangeal joints−PIPs
        ∘Wrist
          −Carpometacarpal joints
        ∘Elbows
        ∘Feet
        ∘Cricoarytenoid joints
        ∘Sternoclavicular joints
        ∘Temporomandibular joints−TMJs
        ∘**Cervical vertebrae 1 & 2−50%,** being the atlas & axis respectively→
          −Transverse ligament laxity→**atlantoaxial subluxation**→↑cervical cord compression risk

        Indications for radiographic imaging of the atlantoaxial joint:
          •Cervical fusion may be needed in order to prevent catastrophic compressive myelopathy
          in the following:
            ∘Atlantoaxial subluxation must be ruled out prior to neck manipulation, as in
            endotracheal intubation
            ∘Patients who develop:
              −Neck pain
              −Weakness
              −Gait disturbance
              −Spinal or upper extremity paresthesias

        Rare involvement:
          •**Distal interphalangeal joints−DIPs**
          •Sacroiliac joints
          •Thoraco−lumbar spine

717

∘Bursae (olecranon, popliteal, subacromial, retrocalcaneal)→
  −Bursitis
∘Tendon sheaths→
  −Tenosynovitis
∘Tendons→
  −Tendonitis
∘Skin→
  −Cellulitis
...→edematous, erythematous, warm, & extremely painful joints, bursae, tendon sheaths, &/or periarticular tissue, usually **being worse in the morning, w/ joint stiffness lasting >1hour after prolonged inactivity (even several hours), being termed the gel phenomenon**

Effects of chronic, inadequately controlled disease:
• Progressive inflammation→
  ∘Inflammatory hypertrophied synovial mass, termed pannus, extending to overlie the articular cartilage→
    −**Osteo−cartilagenous erosions, termed "rat−bite" or "punched out" erosions, beginning at the joint margins** where bone is not protected by cartilage
  ∘Knee synovitis→synovial cyst formation, esp. popliteal &/or sub−popliteal, termed Baker's cyst→
    −Venous &/or lymphatic compression→distal lower extremity pitting edema
    −Rupture→calf dissection→deep venous thrombosis−like=pseudothrombophlebitis syndrome
  ∘Periarticular osteopenia→
    −Osteoporosis→↑fracture risk
  ∘↓Ligament attachment→
    −Damaged joint structure→bone malalignment, termed subluxation
  ∘Tenosynovitis→palpable tendon synovial sheath (esp. the wrist), w/ the inflamed, edematous synovium & surrounding tissue→
    −Median nerve compression→carpal tunnel syndrome→finger paresthesia, esp. numbness &/or tingling
  ∘Tendinitis→fibrosis→contracture→
    −**Boutonniere deformity:** Flexion of proximal interphalangeal joint−PIP & hyperextension of distal interphalangeal joint−DIP
    −**Swan neck deformity:** Extension of the proximal interphalangeal joint−PIP & flexion of the distal interphalangeal joint−DIP
    −**Ulnar deviation of the phalanges**
    −Tendon rupture, esp. the 4th &/or 5th extensor tendons→tendon displacement & inability to extend the involved digits
    ...w/ pain, stiffness, & malalignment→
      •↓Function
        ∘Hip or knee arthritis→
          −↓Ambulation
        ∘Finger arthritis→
          −Inability to use the hands
        ...→periarticular muscle atrophy↔
          •Muscle weakness

Cardiovascular
• Serosal inflammatory cell infiltration of the pericardium→
  ∘Pericarditis
• Immune complex deposition→focal arteriolitis→
  ∘Myocardial ischemia ± infarction
  ∘Myocardial rheumatoid nodules→
    −Dysrhythmia
    −Valvular regurgitation
Gastrointestinal
• ↑Peptic inflammatory disease risk, apart from the treating medications
Mucocutaneous
• Immune complex deposition→**dermal & subcutaneous vasculitis 10−25%**→
  ∘Hemorrhage→
    −Skin &/or mucus membrane (nasal, oral, pharyngeal, &/or conjunctival) discoloration which does not blanch upon pressure, termed purpura (≤3mm=petechiae or >3mm=ecchymoses) ± being palpable due to tumor effect, termed palpable purpura, indicating vascular inflammaton
    −Nailbed splinter hemorrhages
  ∘Ulcerations, esp. of the distal leg & ankles→
    −Necrotizing ulcerations w/ diffuse dermal neutrophil infiltration, termed **pyoderma gangrenosum**
  ∘Infarcts surrounding the nails, termed periungual infarcts

718

    ◦Vascular stasis &/or hyalinization→
     –Capillary & venule dilation→a net–like pattern of macular, purple–blue skin discoloration, termed
      livedo reticularis
    ◦Patchy or diffuse alopecia
    ◦Focal arteriolitis→
     –Granuloma formation w/ central necrosis, termed a **rheumatoid nodule**
      Rheumatod nodule locations:
       •**Subcutaneous–25%**→
        ◦Nodules, usually near inflamed joints or pressure–exposed areas:
         –Achilles tendon
         –Infrapatellar tendon
         –Extensor surface of elbow &/or forearm
       •Synovial→
        ◦Intra–articular mass
        ◦Bursal mass
       •Other organs, esp:
        ◦Lungs
        ◦Myocardium
        ◦Sclera

Opthalmologic
•Serosal inflammatory cell infiltration of the sclera &/or episclera→
  ◦Scleritis &/or episcleritis respectively
Pulmonary
•Serosal inflammatory cell infiltration of the pleura→pleuritis–50%→
  ◦Pleurisy, being thoracic pain exacerbated by either:
   –Deep inhalation (including coughing & sneezing)
   –Supine position
   –Thoracic palpation
   ...& being relieved by leaning forward
  ◦Exudative pleural effusion w/ **glucose <20mg/ dL** (careful as this may also indicate an empyema)
•Serosal inflammatory cell infiltration of the cricoarytenoid joints→
  ◦Vocal cord dysfunction→
   –Airways obstruction
   –Hoarseness
•Immune complex deposition→pulmonary vasculitis→
  ◦Diffuse interstitial fibrosis <5%→
   –Pulmonary hypertension
  ◦Focal arteriolitis→
   –Rheumatoid nodules
Lymphatics
•Inflammation→↑leukocyte replication→
  ◦Lymphadenopathy (local or generalized)–20%
  ◦Splenomegally–8%
Neurologic
•Immune complex deposition within the vasa nervosum, being the vasculature supplying nerves→
  ◦Neuronal ischemia ± infarction→
   –Autonomic neuropathy
   –Peripheral neuropathy (motor &/or sensory)
Hematologic
•Chronic disease→
  ◦Anemia of chronic inflammatory disease, being normocytic & normochromic–50%
  ◦Secondary amyloidosis 5–25%, w/ rheumatoid arthritis being the #1 cause (osteomyelitis being #2)
•Active disease→inflammatory cytokines→
  ◦Leukocytosis
  ◦↑Acute phase proteins, being useful in monitoring disease activity
   –↑Erythrocyte sedimentation rate–ESR (normal: 5mm/ decade aged + ♂ ≤10mm/h or ♀ ≤20mm/h)
   –↑C–reactive protein–CRP (normal: <2mg/ L), responding more acutely than ESR, as it rises
    within several hours & falls within 3days upon partial resolution
   –↑Fibrinogen
   –↑Platelets→thrombocytosis
•Felty' syndrome→
  ◦Massive splenomegaly→
   –Selective granulocytopenia

•↑Antibody production→
　　∘Polyclonal hypergammaglobulinemia→hypocomplementemia, esp. of C3 & C4→↑infection risk via encapsulated bacteria:
　　　　–Escherichia coli
　　　　–Haemophilus influenzae
　　　　–Neisseria meningitides
　　　　–Pseudomonas aeruginosa
　　　　–Salmonella sp.
　　　　–Streptococcus pneumoniae
　　∘Antinuclear antibody–ANA production–30–60%, being positive w/ a titer >1:160
　　　　–Anti–histone–15%
　　　　–Anti–ribonucleoprotein–RNP 10%
　　　　–Anti–dsDNA–≤5%
　　　　–Anti–Ro=SS–A ≤5%
　　　　–Anti–La=SS–B ≤2%
　　Limitations:
　　　　•Titer does not correlate w/ disease activity
　　　　•False positive:
　　　　　∘Other autoimmune diseases
　　　　　∘Certain medication reactions
　　　　　∘Viral infections
　　　　　∘General population–2%
　　∘**Rheumatoid factor production–80%**, being positive w/ a titer of ≥1:80
　　　　–Antibody towards the Fc portion of IgG, being either IgA, IgE, IgG, or IgM, w/ standard tests best at detecting IgM
　　Limitations:
　　　　•Titer does not correlate w/ disease activity
　　　　•False negative:
　　　　　∘Other Ig types
　　　　•False positive:
　　　　　∘Autoimmune diseases
　　　　　∘Endocarditis
　　　　　∘Interstitial pulmonary fibrosis
　　　　　∘Liver disease
　　　　　∘5–10% of healthy adults
　　•Antiphospholipid antibody production
　　　　∘False positive plasma VDRL or RPR test
•Positive Lupus erythematosus–LE cell prep–25%
　　Procedure:
　　　　•In–vitro testing of plasma allows for the visualization of neutrophils w/ the formation of a round body composed of:
　　　　　∘Antinuclear antibodies
　　　　　∘Complement
　　　　　∘Phagocytosed nucleus of another cell

IMAGING

•**X rays**
　　Indications:
　　　　•All patients w/ suspected disease, in order for both diagnosis & staging
　　Appropriate views:
　　　　•Hand joints: Single anteroposterior–AP view of both hands†
　　　　•Hip joints: Single anteroposterior–AP view of the pelvis†
　　　　•Knee joints: Anteroposterior & lateral views
　　　　•Spine: Anteroposterior, lateral, & oblique views
　　Findings:
　　　　•Early disease:
　　　　　∘Normal, or periarticular soft tissue edema
　　　　•Moderate disease:
　　　　　∘Periarticular osteopenia
　　　　　∘Irregular loss of radiolucent cartilage→
　　　　　　–Irregular joint space narrowing
　　　　•Late disease, w/ progressively↑:
　　　　　∘Osteopenia
　　　　　∘Joint space narrowing
　　　　　∘Bone malalignment
　　　　　∘Joint margin "punched–out" erosions

†Lateral & oblique views should be obtained if either:
- An abnormality is detected
- Findings do not correlate w/ the clinical picture

INVASIVE PROCEDURES

- **Arthrocentesis**
  Indications:
  - All initial affected joints should be aspirated & examined for:
    - ◦Possible crystal deposition disease
    - ◦**Possible infection**
  Contraindications:
  - Through infected soft tissue→
    - ◦Organism introduction into the synovial space
  Synovial studies:
  - Gross appearance:
    - ◦>3.5mL of fluid (normal being <3.5mL), being turbid=cloudy, dark yellow (normal being clear straw colored)
  - Leukocyte count:
    - ◦>3,000/ μL w/ neutrophil predominance (normal being <180/ μL w/ a mononuclear predominance)
  - Glucose level:
    - ◦<20, also being seen w/ empyema (normal being ~plasma level)
  - Protein level:
    - ◦>3.5g/ dL
  - Bacterial stain & culture: Negative

TREATMENT

- Because significant joint destruction can occur within 2years of disease onset, it is important to initiate treatment w/ medications intended to modify the disease course before irreversible joint damage occurs

- **Joint rest**
  - ◦Being that joint pain is often exacerbated by use, short periods of joint rest throughout the day, during active synovitis→
    - −↓Pain
- **Occupational therapy**
  - ◦To teach the patient how to better perform activities of daily living–ADLs ± assistive devices if necessary:
    - −Splints to rest finger joints
    - −Braces, crutches, &/or walkers to ↓weight on affected joints→↓pain, ↑stability, & ↑mobility
    - −Eating utensils w/ large handles
    - −Nonslip rubber table & bathroom mats (including for the shower &/or bath)
    - −Strategically placed rails, such as along stairwells, by the toilet, & in the bath &/or shower
- **Physical therapy**
  - ◦For gait training
  - ◦To teach the patient:
    - −Joint protective maneuvers
    - −Energy conserving maneuvers
    - −The therapeutic use of heat & massage, w/ heat treatment via baths, towels, electric heating pads, &/or paraffin wax baths→↓peri−articular muscle spasm→↓joint pain
  - ◦To provide an individualized exercise program incorporating range of motion–ROM & muscle strengthening→
    - −↑Stability of weight bearing joints
- **Felty's syndrome:** Splenectomy

Indications:
- •Severe systemic disease
- •↓Inflammation while an immunomodulating medication is taking effect

Generic	M	♀	Dose
Methylprednisolone	L	?	5–10mg PO q24hours
Prednisolone	L	?	5–10mg PO q24hours
Prednisone	L	?	5–10mg PO q24hours
Trimacinolone	L	?	

- •Intra–articular–IA form†
  - ∘Finger: 2mg IA
  - ∘Knee: 40mg IA
  - ∘Shoulder: 20mg IA

- •Once disease control is achieved, taper to the lowest effective maintenance dose in order to minimize serious side effects, w/ the goal of discontinuation if possible, w/ attention to relapse syndrome

†Outcomes:
- •Variable & short–lasting effects. If pain relief is not achieved for several months w/ 1–2 injections, then abandon this treatment, as ≥3 intra–articular injections/ year may→
  - ∘↑Tissue breakdown→
    - –↑Disease severity

Glucocorticoids	Relative potencies Anti–inflammatory	Mineralocorticoid	Duration	Dose equiv.
Cortisol (physiologic†)	1	1	10hours	20mg
Cortisone (PO)	0.7	2	10hours	25mg
Hydrocortisone (PO, IM, IV)	1	2	10hours	20mg
Methylprednisolone (PO, IM, IA, IV)	5	0.5	15–35hours	5mg
Prednisone (PO)	5	0.5	15–35hours	5mg
Prednisolone (PO, IM, IV)	5	0.8	15–35hours	5mg
Triamcinolone (PO, IM)	5	~0	15–35hours	5mg
Betamethasone (PO, IM, IA)	25	~0	35–70hours	0.75mg
Dexamethasone (PO)	25	~0	35–70hours	0.75mg
Fludrocortisone (PO)	10	125	10hours	

†The physiologic rate of adrenal cortical cortisol production is 20–30mg/ 24hours

Side effects of chronic use:
General
- •Anorexia→
  - ∘Cachexia
- •↑Perspiration

Cardiovascular
- •Mineralocorticoid effects→
  - ∘↑Renal tubular NaCl & water retention as well as potassium secretion→
    - **–Hypertension**
    - **–Edema**
    - **–Hypokalemia**
- •Counter–regulatory=anti–insulin effects→
  - ∘↑Plasma glucose→
    - **–Secondary diabetes mellitus**, which may→ketoacidemia
  - ∘Hyperlipidemia→↑atherosclerosis→
    - **–Coronary artery disease**
    - –Cerebrovascular disease
    - –Peripheral vascular disease

Cutaneous/ subcutaneous
- •↓Fibroblast function→
  - ∘↓Intercellular matrix production→
    - –↑Bruisability→ecchymoses
    - –Poor wound healing
    - –Skin striae
- •Androgenic effects→
  - ∘Acne
  - ∘↑Facial hair
  - ∘Thinning scalp hair

•Fat redistribution from the extremities to the:
  ◦Abdomen→
    –Truncal obesity
  ◦Shoulders→
    –Supraclavicular fat pads
  ◦Upper back→
    –Buffalo hump
  ◦Face→
    –Moon facies
  …w/ concomitant thinning of the arms & legs
Endocrine
•**Adrenal failure** upon abrupt discontinuation after 2weeks
Gastrointestinal
•Inhibition of phospholipase A$_2$ mediated conversion of cell membrane lipids to arachidonic acid, which is the precursor for both cyclooxygenase–COX enzymes, w/ the cyclooxygenase–COX1 enzyme found in most cells of the body, responsible for normal physiologic function. Inhibition of the cyclooxygenase–COX1 enzyme→↑peptic inflammatory disease risk→↑**upper gastrointestinal hemorrhage risk** via:
  ◦↓Gastric mucosal prostaglandin synthesis→
    –↓Epithelial cell proliferation
    –↓Mucosal blood flow→↓bicarbonate delivery to the mucosa
    –↓Mucus & bicarbonate secretion from gastric mucosal cells
Musculoskeletal
•**Avascular necrosis of bone**
•**Osteoporosis**
•Proximal muscle weakness
Neurologic
•Anxiety
•Insomnia
•Psychosis
Opthalmologic
•**Cataracts**
Immunologic
•Inhibition of phospholipase A$_2$ mediated conversion of cell membrane lipids to arachidonic acid, which is the precursor for both cyclooxygenase–COX enzymes (COX1 & COX2) being responsible for the production of neuronal & inflammatory cell prostaglandins respectively→
    –↓Pain
    –↓Temperature (antipyretic)
    –↓**Inflammation**
•Stabilization of lisosomal & cell membranes→
  ◦↓Cytokine & proteolytic enzyme release
•↓Lymphocyte & eosinophil production
  …all→
    •**Immunosuppression**→
      –↑**Infection** &/or neoplasm risk
Hematologic
•↑Erythrocyte production→
  ◦Polycythemia
•↑Neutrophil demargination→
  ◦Neutrophilia→
    –**Leukocytosis**

•The following medications usually require 1–6 months for symptomatic improvement, making these medications not useful in the control of acute disease, but rather, useful when prolonged treatment is planned. Consider combination therapy in patients who have failed 1 medication

Generic (Trade)	M	♀	Dose	Max
Hydroxychloroquine (Plaquenil)	K	?	400–600mg PO q24hours w/ a meal, then 200–400mg q24hours upon clinical response	
Methotrexate (Rheumatrex, Trexall)	LK	U	7.5mg PO qweek	20mg qweek
Sulfasalazine (Azulfidine)	L	P	500mg PO q24hours, then titrate to 1g PO q12hours	

•Once disease control is achieved, taper to the lowest effective maintenance dose in order to minimize serious side effects

Hydroxychloroquine mechanism: Unknown

Methotrexate mechanism:
•Folate analog→
 ◦Dihydrofolate reductase inhibition→
  –↓DNA synthesis→cytotoxicity to all proliferating cells

Sulfasalazine mechanism: Unknown

Side effects:
Gastrointestinal
•↓Mucosal cell proliferation→
 ◦Mucosal inflammation=mucositis, including inflammation of the oral mucosa=stomatitis→
  –Diarrhea
  –Nausea ± vomiting
Hematologic
•**Myelosuppression**→
 ◦Macrocytic anemia→
  –Fatigue
 ◦Leukopenia→immunosuppression→
  –↑Infection & neoplasm risk
 ◦Thrombocytopenia→
  –↑Hemorrhage risk, esp. petechiae

Hydroxychloroquine specific:
Opthalmologic
•Accommodation defects
•Blurred visual scotomas
•Corneal deposits
•Extraocular muscle weakness
•Night blindness
•**Retinopathy–rare**, being related to cumulative dose, which may→
 ◦Irreversible visual loss
Mucocutaneous
•↓Hair formation→
 ◦Alopecia
•↓Epithelial cell proliferation→
 ◦Dermatitis
•Skin pigmentation
•Stevens–Johnson syndrome
Musculoskeletal
•Myopathy
Neurologic
•Headache
•Insomnia
•Neuropathy
•Tinnitus
•Vertigo

<u>Methotrexate specific:</u>
•Concomitant use of **folic acid** 1mg PO q24h may ↓side effects without ↓efficacy

Gastrointestinal
•Dyspepsia
•Hepatitis→
  ∘Cirrhosis−rare
Genitourinary
•Bladder cancer
•Hemorrhagic cystitis
•Infertility
•Miscarriage
Lymphatic
•Lymphadenopathy
Mucocutaneous
•↓Hair formation→
  ∘Alopecia
Pulmonary
•Interstitial fibrosis→
  ∘Pulmonary hypertension
•**Interstitial pneumonitis−2%** (noninfectious lung inflammation), not being dose related→
  ∘Dyspnea
  ∘Nonproductive cough
  ∘Pulmonary hemorrhage→
  −Hemoptysis
•Pleuritis→
  ∘Pleuritic thoracic pain
  ∘Pleural effusions

<u>Sulfasalazine specific:</u>
General
•Orange−yellow discoloration of body fluids, including sweat, tears, & urine, which stain clothing & contact lenses
Cutaneous
•Photosensitivity
Gastrointestinal
•Hepatitis
•Oral ulcerations
Genitourinary
•↓Sperm count

<u>Hydroxychloroquine monitoring:</u>
•Baseline ophthalmologic examination, then
  ∘Q6months

<u>Methotrexate monitoring:</u>
•Baseline:
  ∘Complete blood count
  ∘Liver function tests
  ∘Albumin
  ∘Renal function
  ∘Hepatitis B & C serologies
  ∘Chest x ray
  …then q2month:
    •Complete blood count
    •Liver function tests, w/ treatment to be withdrawn @ plasma values >3 X the upper limit of normal
    •Albumin
    •Renal function

<u>Sulfasalazine monitoring:</u>
•Baseline:
  ∘Complete blood count
  ∘Liver function tests, w/ treatment to be withdrawn @ plasma values >3 X the upper limit of normal
  …then qweek X 1month, then
    •Q2months

725

CYCLOOXYGENASE–COX 2 SELECTIVE INHIBITING NSAIDS

Generic (Trade)	M	♀	Dose
Celecoxib (Celebrex)	L	U	200mg PO q12hours

Mechanism:
- Selective, reversible inhibition of the cyclooxygenase–COX 2 enzyme, being responsible for the production of inflammatory cell prostaglandins→
  - ↓Pain
  - ↓Inflammation
  ...w/ **minimal cyclooxygenase–COX 1 mediated effects**

Background pathophysiology:
- Inflammatory cell mediated prostaglandins are released at sites of inflammation (in addition to other inflammatory cytokines)→
  - Leukocyte migration→↑inflammation via:
    - Vasodilation→↑blood flow→erythema, edema, warmth, &/or tenderness/ pain via enhanced neuronal sensitivity

In Brief:
- **Cyclooxygenase–COX1 enzymes** are found in most cells of the body, being responsible for normal physiologic processes
- **Cyclooxygenase–COX 2 enzymes** are responsible for the production of inflammatory cell prostaglandins

Cyclooxyegenase–COX 1 mediated effects	Effects of relatively ↓inhibition
Hypothalamic prostaglandin synthesis	No antipyretic effect
Platelet thromboxane A_2 synthesis	No antiplatelet effect
Gastric mucosal cell prostaglandin synthesis	↓Peptic inflammatory disease risk
Glomerular afferent arteriole prostaglandin synthesis	↓Renal failure risk

Side effects:
Cardiovascular
- Hypertension

Gastrointestinal
- Inhibition of the cyclooxygenase–COX1 enzyme→↑peptic inflammatory disease risk→↑**upper gastrointestinal hemorrhage risk** via:
  - ↓Gastric mucosal prostaglandin synthesis→
    - ↓Epithelial proliferation
    - ↓Mucosal blood flow→↓bicarbonate delivery to the mucosa
    - ↓Mucus & bicarbonate secretion from gastric mucosal cells

Genitourinary
- Patients w/ pre-existing bilateral ↓renal perfusion, not necessarily failure:
  - Heart failure
  - Bilateral renal artery stenosis
  - Hypovolemia
  - Renal failure
  ...rely more on the compensatory production of vasodilatory prostaglandins→
  - Afferent arteriole dilation→
    - Maintained glomerular filtration rate–GFR, whereas NSAIDs→
      - ↓Prostaglandin production, which may→renal failure

Pulmonary
- Inhibition of both cyclooxygenase enzymes (COX 1 & COX2)→
  - ↑Lipoxygenase activity→
    - ↑Leukotriene synthesis→symptomatic asthma within 2hours of ingestion in 5% of asthmatics

Caution:
- Minimal inhibition of COX–1→
  - ↓Endothelial & vascular smooth muscle cell prostacyclin† production relative to platelet thromboxane‡ production→cytokine imbalance in favor of vasoconstriction→
    - Hypertension
    - ↑Cerebrovascular accident syndrome risk
    - ↑Myocardial ischemic syndrome risk

Contraindications:
- Sulfa hypersensitivity due to a sulfa moiety

726

NONSTEROIDAL ANTI-INFLAMMATORY DRUGS-NSAIDs

Generic	M ♀	Start	Max
Ibuprofen	L P in 1st & 2nd, U in 3rd trimester	600mg PO q8hours	3.2g/ 24hours
Indomethacin	L P in 1st & 2nd, U in 3rd trimester	50mg PO/ PR q8hours	
Naproxen •XR form	L P in 1st & 2nd, U in 3rd trimester	375mg PO q12hours 750mg PO q24hours	

•One cannot predict which NSAID a patient will respond to
•Attempt to eventually ↓dosage &/or limit use to exacerbations in order to ↓side effect risk

Mechanism:
•Aspirin & other anti-inflammatory medications→
  ○Respectively to irreversible & reversible inhibition of both cyclooxygenase enzymes (COX-1 & COX-2), being responsible for the production of neural & inflammatory cell prostaglandins respectively→
    −↓Pain
    −↓Temperature (antipyretic)
    −↓Inflammation

Background pathophysiology:
•Inflammatory cell mediated prostaglandins are released at sites of inflammation (in addition to other inflammatory cytokines)→
  ○Leukocyte migration→↑inflammation via:
    −Vasodilation→↑blood flow→erythema, edema, warmth, &/or tenderness/ pain via enhanced neuronal sensitivity
•Interleukin–IL1→
  ○↑Hypothalamic prostaglandin production→
    −Fever

In Brief:
•**Cyclooxygenase–COX1 enzymes** are found in most cells of the body, being responsible for normal physiologic processes
•**Cyclooxygenase–COX 2 enzymes** are responsible for the production of inflammatory cell prostaglandins

Side effects:
Gastrointestinal
•Inhibition of the cyclooxygenase–COX1 enzyme→↑peptic inflammatory disease risk→↑**upper gastrointestinal hemorrhage risk** via:
  ○↓Gastric mucosal prostaglandin synthesis→
    −↓Epithelial cell proliferation
    −↓Mucosal blood flow→↓bicarbonate delivery to the mucosa
    −↓Mucus & bicarbonate secretion from gastric mucosal cells

Indications for peptic inflammatory disease prophylaxis:
•Prophylax w/ proton pump inhibitors–PPI's, histamine 2 selective receptor blockers, or Misoprostol in patients w/ any of the following:
  ○Age >60 years w/ a history of peptic inflammatory disease
  ○Anticipated therapy >3 months
  ○Concurrent glucocorticoid use
  ○Moderate to high dose NSAID use
  Note: Newer NSAIDs (Etodolac, Nabumetone, Salsalate)→
    •↓Risk of NSAID induced peptic inflammation/ ulcer

Genitourinary
•Patients w/ pre-existing bilateral ↓renal perfusion, not necessarily failure:
  ○Heart failure
  ○Bilateral renal artery stenosis
  ○Hypovolemia
  ○Renal failure
  …rely more on the compensatory production of vasodilatory prostaglandins→
    •Afferent arteriole dilation→
      ○Maintained glomerular filtration rate–GFR, whereas NSAIDs→
        −↓Prostaglandin production, which may→renal failure

Pulmonary
- •Inhibition of both cyclooxygenase enzymes (COX 1 & COX2)→
  - ∘↑Lipoxygenase activity→
    - −↑Leukotriene synthesis→symptomatic asthma within 2hours of ingestion in 5% of asthmatics

---

CAPSAICIN

M	♀	Dose
?	?	0.025%−0.075% applied to the affected area ≤qid, w/ prompt handwashing after application

- •Continued application for 2−4 weeks is necessary to achieve benefit

Mechanism:
- •Substance P antagonism

Side effects:
Cutaneous
- •Burning pain−>30%, being ↓w/ continued use

SECOND LINE TREATMENT ■■■■■■

IMMUNOMODULATING MEDICATIONS
- •The following medications usually require 1−6 months for symptomatic improvement, making these medications not useful in the control of acute disease, but rather, useful when prolonged treatment is planned. Consider combination therapy in patients who have failed 1medication

Generic (Trade)	M	♀	Dose
Leflunomide (Arava)	LK	U	100mg PO q24hours X 3days, then 10−20mg PO q24hours

Mechanism:
- •Inhibits dihydroorotate dehydrogenase†→
  - ∘Arrest of activated lymphocytes
- •Inhibits NF−kappa B activation→
  - ∘Downregulation of several pro−inflammatory genes

---

†Rate limiting enzyme responsible for de novo pyrimidine synthesis. Inactive lymphocytes can synthesize pyrimidines via salvage pathways, but active lymphocytes are dependent on de novo synthesis

Side effects:
General
- •Cachexia

Cardiovascular
- •Hypertension

Gastrointestinal
- •Hepatitis
- •↓Mucosal cell proliferation→
  - ∘Mucosal inflammation=mucositis, including inflammation of the oral mucosa=stomatitis→
    - −Diarrhea
    - −Nausea ± vomiting

Genitourinary
- •↑Proximal renal tubule uric acid excretion→
  - ∘↓Uric acid

Mucocutaneous
- •↓Hair formation→
  - ∘Alopecia
- •↓Epithelial cell proliferation→
  - ∘Dermatitis

Neurologic
- •Peripheral neuropathy

Pulmonary
- •Interstitial pneumonitis

Hematologic
- •**Myelosuppression→**
  - ∘Macrocytic anemia→
    - −Fatigue
  - ∘Leukopenia→immunosuppression→
    - −↑Infection & neoplasm risk

728

  ∘Thrombocytopenia→
   −↑Hemorrhage risk, esp. petechiae
Materno−fetal
 •Teratogenic→
  ∘Fetal malformation
  ∘Fetal death

Contraindications:
 •Underlying hepatic disease, or history of either:
  ∘↑Ethanol intake
  ∘Viral hepatitis

Monitoring:
 •Baseline:
  ∘Complete blood count
  ∘Liver function tests
  ∘Renal function
  ∘Hepatitis B & C serologies
  …then
   •Complete blood count
   •Liver function tests
   •Renal function
   …q2weeks X 2, then
    •Qmonth

ANTICYTOKINE MEDICATIONS				
Generic (Trade)	M	♀	**Dose**	**Max**
Adalimumab (Humira)	P	P	40mg SC qoweek	40mg qweek
Etanercept (Enbrel)	P	P	25mg SC 2X/ week	
Infliximab† (Remicade)	P	P	3mg/ kg IV over 2hours @ 0, 2, & 6weeks, then q2months	10mg/ kg
Anakinra (Kineret)	K	P	100mg SC q24hours	

†Ensure concomitant use w/ Methotrexate due to the frequent development of anti−infliximab antibodies

Adalimumab mechanism:
 •A human monoclonal antibody which binds to:
  ∘Plasma tumor necrosis factor−TNF α, thus:
   −Preventing its interaction w/ cell membrane TNF−α receptors
   −↑Plasma clearance
  ∘Cell membrane receptor bound TNF α→
   −Antibody & cytokine dependent cytotoxicity

Etanercept mechanism:
 •A recombinant tumor necrosis factor−TNF receptor/ human IgG1 Fc domain† fusion protein, which binds to plasma TNF α & β, thus:
  ∘Preventing their interaction w/ cell membrane TNF receptors
  ∘↑Plasma clearance

Infliximab mechanism:
 •A chimeric IgG1 monoclonal antibody which binds to:
  ∘Plasma tumor necrosis factor−TNF α, thus:
   −Preventing its interaction w/ cell membrane TNF−α receptors
   −↑Plasma clearance
  ∘Cell membrane receptor bound TNF−α→
   −Antibody & cytokine dependent cytotoxicity

Anakinra mechanism:
 •Recombinant human interleukin IL−1 receptor antagonist−ILra

†Used to extend the in vivo half life of the receptor

Side effects:
 General
  •Hypersensitivity syndrome
 Gastrointestinal
  •Hepatitis−rare

Immunologic
- Tumor necrosis factors & interleukins are required for appropriate granuloma formation & maintenance, for the prevention of progressive primary & **reactivation fungal & mycobacterial disease**, w/ suppression→
  - ○Severe infections (primary & reactivation)
    - –Tuberculosis (reactivation >> primary), usually occurring within 5months of treatment, w/ extrapulmonary & widespread systemic disease, termed miliary tuberculosis, being common

Mucocutaneous
- Mild injection site reactions

Neurologic–rare
- Aseptic meningitis
- Multiple sclerosis
- Myelitis
- Optic neuritis
- Peripheral neuropathy

Hematologic
- Aplastic anemia–rare
- **Lymphoma**
- Systemic lupus erythematosus–SLE–rare
- Vasculitis
- **Development of anti–medication antibodies→**
  - ○↑Plasma clearance→
    - –↓Efficacy
  - ○↑Infusion reactions

Adalimumab specific:
Interactions
- Concomitant administration of Methotrexate→
  - ○45% ↓plasma clearance

Infliximab specific:
General
- **"Cytokine release syndrome"→**
  - ○Fevers ± chills
  - ○Headache
  - ○Nausea ± vomiting
  - …associated w/ monoclonal antibody infusion
  - Risk reduction:
    - Slower infusion rates
    - Antihistamine administration
    - Antibodies containing less mouse sequence

Cardiovascular
- **Heart failure**

Anakinra specific:
Hematologic
- ↓Neutrophil count→
  - ○Severe neutropenia–0.3%
- Thrombocytopenia→
  - ○↑Hemorrhage risk, esp. petechiae

Monitoring:
- Obtain a **purified protein derivative–PPD test** @ baseline
  - ○Positive responders who have not previously been treated should receive appropriate treatment prior to initiation of anti–cytokine treatment

Infliximab specific:
- Heart failure

Anakinra specific monitoring:
- Complete blood count @ baseline, then
  - ○Qmonth X 3, then
  - ○Q3months

Contraindications:
- **Active infection**

> Anakinra specific:
> •Do not use concomitantly w/ anti−TNFα medications, due to the possibility of marked immunosuppression

THIRD LINE TREATMENT
•Arthroscopic surgery
Procedure:
•Removal of meniscal fragments, cartilage debris, &/or osteophytes, termed bone spurs

•Total joint arthroplasty
Indications:
•Disabling pain
Procedure:
•Total joint replacement
Outcomes:
•The prosthesis usually require replacement @ 10−15 years

FOURTH LINE TREATMENT
•Arthrodesis
Procedure:
•Surgical joint fusion

PROGNOSIS
•On average, patients w/ rheumatoid arthritis die ~10years earlier than people without the disease

•Caused by the deposition of crystals throughout the body→
  ◦Intermittently symptomatic inflammation, usually restricted to the musculoskeletal & urinary systems
Statistics:
  •Gout is the #1 inflammatory arthritis in ♂ @ age >30years, affecting 1% of ♂ in Western countries
  •Calcium pyrophosphate dihydrate–CPPD deposition disease is half as common as gout

CRYSTAL PATHOPHYSIOLOGY

Gout:
  •Uric acid is a metabolic byproduct of purine metabolism (which are essential components of DNA
  synthesis) as well as directly synthesized from 5–phosphoribosyl–1–pyrophosphate (5–PRPP) &
  glutamine. Being that humans lack the mammalian enzyme uricase, which metabolizes uric acid to
  allantoin, humans are the only mammals in which gout develops spontaneously via the plasma uric
  acid level rising above its saturation point @ body temperature (~7mg/ dL)†→
    ◦Precipitation→
      –Diffuse deposition, esp. in the joints & periarticular tissues, where the crystals are phagocytosed
      by neutrophils & macrophages→inflammatory cytokine release, w/ subsequent leukocyte death↔
      uric acid crystal & proteolytic enzyme release, w/ the crystals becoming progressively less
      inflammatory after several cycles of ingestion & release

Calcium pyrophosphate dihydrate–CPPD deposition disease:
  •Joint cartilage calcium pyrophosphate crystals are shed into the synovial fluid where the crystals are
  phagocytosed by neutrophils & macrophages→
    ◦Inflammatory cytokine release, w/ subsequent leukocyte death↔
      –Calcium pyrophosphate crystal & proteolytic enzyme release, w/ the crystals becoming
      progressively less inflammatory after several cycles of ingestion & release

---

†Most patients w/ hyperuricemia do not develop gout

CLASSIFICATION/ RISK FACTORS

GOUT ━━━━━━━━━━━━━━━━━━━━━━━━━━━━━━━
•**Age:** ♂ >30years, ♀ >45years
•**Gender:** ♂ 8X premenopausal & 3X postmenopausal ♀, as estrogen→
  ◦Renal uric acid excretion
•**Endocrine**
  ◦Diabetes mellitus
•**Environment**
  ◦Pacific Islanders (Filipinos & Samoans)
•**Hypertension**
•**Hypertriglyceridemia**
•**Obesity**

•↓**Renal uric acid excretion–85%**
  ◦**Acidemia**
  ◦**Dehydration**
  ◦**Lifestyle:**
    –**Alcohol**
  ◦**Medications**
    –**Aspirin**
    –**Diuretics** (all classes)
    –Cyclosporine
    –Anti–mycobacterial medications: Ethambutol, Pyrazinamide
    –Theophylline
  ◦**Renal failure**
  ◦**Toxins**
    –Lead (also→↓synovial fluid uric acid solubility)→"saturnine gout" developing in drinkers of illegal
    "moonshine" whiskey distilled through lead lined stills
  ◦**Idiopathic**

- •↑**Uric acid production–10%**
  - ◦**Lifestyle:**
    - –**Alcohol**
  - ◦↑**Cell turnover**
    - –Metastatic cancer, hematologic malignancy, or tumor lysis syndrome
    - –Chronic hemolytic anemia
    - –Polycythemia vera
    - –Psoriasis
  - ◦↑**ATP degradation**
    - –Severe muscle exertion
    - –Status epilepticus
  - ◦**Congenital purine metabolism enzyme defects–rare**
    - –Glycogen storage disease type 1
    - –Lesch–Nyhan syndrome, being an X–linked hypoxanthine–guanine phosphoribosyltransferase–GPRT deficiency
    - –5–phosphoribosyl–1–pyrophosphate reductase–PRPPR overactivity

- •↑**Uric acid intake**
  - ◦↑**Purine food content**
    - –**Beer**
    - –**Meats**
    - –**Seafood**

CALCIUM PYROPHOSPHATE DIHYDRATE–CPPD DEPOSITION DISEASE ▬▬▬▬▬

- •**Age:** >50years
- •**Any form of arthritis**
- •**Chronic renal failure**
- •**Dehydration**
- •**Endocrine**
  - ◦↑Growth hormone→
    - –Acromegaly
  - ◦Diabetes mellitus
  - ◦**Hyperparathyroidism**
  - ◦Hypothyroidism
- •**Genetic**
  - ◦Autosomal dominant inherited defects of pyrophosphate production
- •**Inflammation**
- •**Metabolic**
  - ◦Amyloidosis
  - ◦**Hemochromatosis**
  - ◦Hypercalcemia
  - ◦Hypomagnesemia
  - ◦Hypophosphatemia
  - ◦Ochronosis
  - ◦Paget's disease
  - ◦Wilson's disease

Subclassification according to the syndrome it most resembles:
- •**Pseudo–gout–20%**, esp. affecting the knees, shoulders, & wrists
- •**Pseudo–osteoarthritis**, esp. affecting the knees & shoulders
- •**Pseudo–rheumatoid arthritis**, esp. affecting the wrists & metacarpophalangeal–MCP joints

DIAGNOSIS OF GOUT

General
- •Inflammatory cytokines→
  - ◦Fever, usually being low–grade (<101°F)

---

†Temperature may be normal in patients w/:
- •Chronic kidney disease, esp. w/ uremia
- •Cirrhosis
- •Heart failure
- •Severe debility

...or those who are:
- •Intravenous drug users
- •Taking certain medications:
  - ◦Acetaminophen
  - ◦Antibiotics
  - ◦Glucocorticoids
  - ◦Nonsteroidal anti–inflammatory drugs–NSAIDs

Musculoskeletal
- •Hyperuricemia→crystal deposition within:
  - ◦Joints→
    - –**Arthritis (monoarticular–90%** >> polyarticular)

  Affected joints:
  - •Small joints > large weight bearing joints
    - ◦Feet, esp the **1ˢᵗ metatarsophalangeal–MTP joint, termed podagra,** being the most common
      - –55% initially, 80% overall
      - –Thought to be most susceptible as it is very prone to trauma & cooling
    - ◦Ankles
    - ◦Knees
    - ◦Hands
    - ◦Wrists
    - ◦Elbows

  Rare involvement:
  - •Hips
  - •Shoulders
  - •Vertebral joints

  Precipitating factors:
  - •**Rapid plasma uric acid level fluctuations**
  - •**Fasting**
  - •**↓Temperature**
  - •**Inflammation**
    ...→↓uric acid solubility

  - ◦Bursae (olecranon, popliteal, subacromial, retrocalcaneal)→
    - –Bursitis
  - ◦Tendon sheaths→
    - –Tenosynovitis
  - ◦Tendons→
    - –Tendonitis
  - ◦Skin→
    - –Cellulitis
    ...→edematous, erythematous, warm, & extremely painful joints, bursae, tendon sheaths, &/or periarticular tissue X days to weeks ± desquamation & pruritus overlying the affected area

Effects of chronic, inadequately controlled disease:
- •Progressive crystal accumulation→
  - ◦Crystal macroaggregates, termed **tophi–20%,** usually occurring @ ≥10years
    - –The diagnosis is confirmed via either needle aspiration or spontaneous rupture of a tophus, eliciting a white, chalky material shown to be composed of uric acid crystals via microscopy
    Tophi locations:
    - •Subcutaneous→
      - ◦Nodules, usually near inflamed joints or pressure–exposed areas:
        - –Achilles tendon
        - –Infrapatellar tendon
        - –Extensor surface of elbow &/or forearm
    - •Synovial→
      - ◦Intra–articular mass
      - ◦Bursal mass, esp. the olecranon bursa

- •Other organs, esp:
  - ○Cornea
  - ○Lungs
  - ○Myocardium
  - ○Nasal cartilage
  - ○Pinna of the ear
  - ○Sclera

- •A rheumatoid arthritis–like syndrome, w/ progressive inflammation→
  - ○**Joint stiffness, esp. after prolonged inactivity (even several hours), being termed the gel phenomenon**
  - ○Inflammatory hypertrophied synovial mass, termed pannus, extending to overlie the articular cartilage→
    - –**Osteo–cartilagenous erosions, termed "rat–bite" or "punched out" erosions, beginning at the joint margins** where bone is not protected by cartilage, ± intra–erosion tophi
  - ○Periarticular osteopenia→
    - –Osteoporosis→↑fracture risk
  - ○↓Ligament attachment→
    - –Damaged joint structure→bone malalignment, termed subluxation
  - ○Tenosynovitis→palpable tendon synovial sheath (esp. the wrist), w/ the inflamed, edematous synovium & surrounding tissue→
    - –Median nerve compression→carpal tunnel syndrome→finger paresthesia, esp. numbness &/or tingling
  - ○Tendinitis→fibrosis→contracture→
    - –**Boutonniere deformity:** Flexion of proximal interphalangeal joint–PIP & hyperextension of distal interphalangeal joint–DIP
    - –**Swan neck deformity:** Extension of the proximal interphalangeal joint–PIP & flexion of the distal interphalangeal joint–DIP
    - –**Ulnar deviation of the phalanges**
    - –Tendon rupture, esp. the 4th &/or 5th extensor tendons→tendon displacement & inability to extend the involved digits
    - …w/ pain, stiffness, & malalignment→
      - •↓Function
        - ○Hip or knee arthritis→
          - –↓Ambulation
        - ○Finger arthritis→
          - –Inability to use the hands
      - …→periarticular muscle atrophy↔
        - •Muscle weakness

Genitourinary
- •Hyperuricemia→
  - ○↑Renal excretion→↑urinary uric acid concentration→↑precipitation risk→
    - –**Uric acid stones**, being 7% of all renal stones
    - –Uric acid nidi, around which **calcium stones** form
- •Tumor lysis syndrome→↑uric acid & calcium phosphate→
  - ○Acute tubular necrosis via both:
    - –Direct tubular toxicity
    - –Obstructive tubular casts
    - …→**acute intra–renal renal failure**

24 hour urine uric acid
Indications:
- •To determine if the patient is under–excreting or overproducing uric acid

Procedure:
- •24hour urine collection while on usual diet

Limitations:
- •Cannot reliably identify uric acid overproduction in patients w/ moderate renal failure, defined by either:
  - ○Glomerular filtration rate–GFR <60mL/ min.
  - ○Biochemical evidence of renal failure

Results:
- •<700mg/ 24h indicates under–excretion
- •>1000mg/ 24h indicates overproduction
- •700–1000mg/ 24h being indeterminate

Effects of chronic, inadequately controlled disease:
•Chronic renal interstitial deposition of uric acid, as well as tubule exposure→
∘Progressive intra-renal renal failure-rare

Hematologic
•↑**Uric acid,** w/ normal (2-7mg/ dL) to ↓levels possible during an acute exacerbation
•Active disease→
∘Leukocytosis
∘↑Acute phase proteins, being useful in monitoring disease activity
-↑Erythrocyte sedimentation rate-ESR (normal: 5mm/ decade aged + ♂ ≤10mm/h or ♀ ≤20mm/h)
-↑C-reactive protein-CRP (normal: <2mg/ L), responding more acutely than ESR, as it rises
within several hours & falls within 3days upon partial resolution
-↑Fibrinogen
-↑Platelets→thrombocytosis

IMAGING STUDIES

•**X rays**
Indications:
•All patients w/ suspected disease, for staging
Appropriate views:
•Hand joints: Single anteroposterior-AP view of both hands†
•Hip joints: Single anteroposterior-AP view of the pelvis†
•Knee joints: Anteroposterior & lateral views
•Spine: Anteroposterior, lateral, & oblique views
Findings:
•Early disease‡:
∘Normal, or periarticular soft tissue edema
•Moderate disease:
∘Periarticular osteopenia
∘Irregular loss of radiolucent cartilage→
-Irregular joint space narrowing
•Late disease, w/ progressively↑:
∘Osteopenia
∘Joint space narrowing
∘Bone malalignment
∘Joint margin "punched-out" erosions

---

†Lateral & oblique views should be obtained if either:
•An abnormality is detected
•Findings do not correlate w/ the clinical picture
‡Additional early findings w/ calcium pyrophosphate deposition-CPPD disease include:
•**Punctate &/or linear tissue calcification, termed chondrocalcinosis, in the joint cartilage,
capsule, &/or ligaments** (esp. the knees, triangular ligament of the wrist, & pubic ramus). However,
most patients w/ chondrocalcinosis do not develop CPPD

INVASIVE PROCEDURES

Arthrocentesis
Indications:
•All initial affected joints should be aspirated & examined for:
∘Possible crystal deposition disease
∘**Possible infection**, which may precipitate a disease flare
Contraindications:
•Through infected soft tissue→
∘Organism introduction into the synovial space
Synovial studies:
•Gross appearance:
∘>3.5mL of fluid (normal being <3.5mL), being turbid=cloudy, dark yellow (normal being clear straw
colored)
•Leukocyte count:
∘2,000-100,000/ μL w/ neutrophil predominance (normal being <180/ μL w/ a mononuclear
predominance)
•Glucose level:
∘>25, but < plasma (normal being ~plasma level)
•Protein level:
∘>3.5g/ dL
•Bacterial stain & culture: Negative

- •Microscopic examination†:
  - ○**Uric acid crystals**, being:
    - −Intracellular & extracellular **needle shaped** crystals 3−20µm long
    - −**Negatively birefringent**, being yellow when parallel, & blue when perpendicular to the axis of the red compensator on a polarizing microscope
  - ○**Calcium pyrophosphate crystals**, being:
    - −Intracellular & extracellular **rhomboid shaped** crystals
    - −**Weakly positively birefringent**, being yellow when perpendicular, & blue when parallel to the axis of the red compensator on a polarizing microscope

---

†Crystals may also be present during the intervals between flares

TREATMENT

GOUT
- •Acute treatment is focused on ↓inflammation, whereas chronic treatment is focused on ↓plasma uric acid levels. However, if the patient is taking a uric acid lowering medication, continue the medication during a flare, as discontinuation→
  - ○Plasma uric acid level fluctuation→
    - −↑Exacerbation severity
- •**Discontinue alcohol consumption**
- •**Discontinue possible causative medications**
- •↓**Intake of hyperuricemic foods**

ACUTE TREATMENT

CYCLOOXYGENASE−COX 2 SELECTIVE INHIBITING NSAIDS

Generic (Trade)	M	♀	Dose
Celecoxib (Celebrex)	L	U	200mg PO q12hours

Mechanism:
- •Selective, reversible inhibition of the cyclooxygenase−COX 2 enzyme, being responsible for the production of inflammatory cell prostaglandins→
  - ○↓Pain
  - ○↓Inflammation
  - ...w/ **minimal cyclooxygenase−COX 1 mediated effects**

Background pathophysiology:
- •Inflammatory cell mediated prostaglandins are released at sites of inflammation (in addition to other inflammatory cytokines)→
  - ○Leukocyte migration→↑inflammation via:
    - −Vasodilation→↑blood flow→erythema, edema, warmth, &/or tenderness/ pain via enhanced neuronal sensitivity

In Brief:
- •**Cyclooxygenase−COX1 enzymes** are found in most cells of the body, being responsible for normal physiologic processes
- •**Cyclooxygenase−COX 2 enzymes** are responsible for the production of inflammatory cell prostaglandins

Cyclooxyegenase−COX 1 mediated effects	Effects of relatively ↓inhibition
Hypothalamic prostaglandin synthesis	No antipyretic effect
Platelet thromboxane A_2 synthesis	No antiplatelet effect
Gastric mucosal cell prostaglandin synthesis	↓Peptic inflammatory disease risk
Glomerular afferent arteriole prostaglandin synthesis	↓Renal failure risk

Side effects:
Cardiovascular
- •Hypertension

Gastrointestinal
- •Inhibition of the cyclooxygenase−COX1 enzyme→↑peptic inflammatory disease risk→↑**upper gastrointestinal hemorrhage risk** via:
  - ○↓Gastric mucosal prostaglandin synthesis→
    - −↓Epithelial proliferation
    - −↓Mucosal blood flow→↓bicarbonate delivery to the mucosa
    - −↓Mucus & bicarbonate secretion from gastric mucosal cells

Genitourinary
- •Patients w/ pre-existing bilateral ↓renal perfusion, not necessarily failure:
  - ◦Heart failure
  - ◦Bilateral renal artery stenosis
  - ◦Hypovolemia
  - ◦Renal failure
  - …rely more on the compensatory production of vasodilatory prostaglandins→
    - •Afferent arteriole dilation→
      - ◦Maintained glomerular filtration rate–GFR, whereas NSAIDs→
        - –↓Prostaglandin production, which may→renal failure

Pulmonary
- •Inhibition of both cyclooxygenase enzymes (COX 1 & COX2)→
  - ◦↑Lipoxygenase activity→
    - –↑Leukotriene synthesis→symptomatic asthma within 2hours of ingestion in 5% of asthmatics

Caution:
- •Minimal inhibition of COX–1→
  - ◦↓Endothelial & vascular smooth muscle cell prostacyclin† production relative to platelet thromboxane‡ production→cytokine imbalance in favor of vasoconstriction→
    - –Hypertension
    - –↑Cerebrovascular accident syndrome risk
    - –↑Myocardial ischemic syndrome risk

Contraindications:
- •Sulfa hypersensitivity due to a sulfa moiety

NONSTEROIDAL ANTI–INFLAMMATORY DRUGS–NSAIDs

Generic	M ♀		Start	Max
Ibuprofen	L	P in 1st & 2nd, U in 3rd trimester	600mg PO q8hours	3.2g/ 24hours
Indomethacin	L	P in 1st & 2nd, U in 3rd trimester	50mg PO/ PR q8hours	
Naproxen	L	P in 1st & 2nd, U in 3rd trimester	375mg PO q12hours	
•XR form			750mg PO q24hours	

- •One cannot predict which NSAID a patient will respond to
- •Attempt to eventually ↓dosage &/or limit use to exacerbations in order to ↓side effect risk

Mechanism:
- •Aspirin & other anti–inflammatory medications→
  - ◦Respectively to irreversible & reversible inhibition of both cyclooxygenase enzymes (COX–1 & COX–2), being responsible for the production of neural & inflammatory cell prostaglandins respectively→
    - –↓Pain
    - –↓Temperature (antipyretic)
    - –↓Inflammation

Background pathophysiology:
- •Inflammatory cell mediated prostaglandins are released at sites of inflammation (in addition to other inflammatory cytokines)→
  - ◦Leukocyte migration→↑inflammation via:
    - –Vasodilation→↑blood flow→erythema, edema, warmth, &/or tenderness/ pain via enhanced neuronal sensitivity
- •Interleukin–IL1→
  - ◦↑Hypothalamic prostaglandin production→
    - –Fever

In Brief:
- •**Cyclooxygenase–COX1 enzymes** are found in most cells of the body, being responsible for normal physiologic processes
- •**Cyclooxygenase–COX 2 enzymes** are responsible for the production of inflammatory cell prostaglandins

Side effects:

Gastrointestinal
- Inhibition of the cyclooxygenase–COX1 enzyme→↑peptic inflammatory disease risk→↑**upper gastrointestinal hemorrhage risk** via:
  - ↓Gastric mucosal prostaglandin synthesis→
    - ↓Epithelial cell proliferation
    - ↓Mucosal blood flow→↓bicarbonate delivery to the mucosa
    - ↓Mucus & bicarbonate secretion from gastric mucosal cells

Indications for peptic inflammatory disease prophylaxis:
- Prophylax w/ proton pump inhibitors–PPI's, histamine 2 selective receptor blockers, or Misoprostol in patients w/ any of the following:
  - Age >60 years w/ a history of peptic inflammatory disease
  - Anticipated therapy >3 months
  - Concurrent glucocorticoid use
  - Moderate to high dose NSAID use
Note: Newer NSAIDs (Etodolac, Nabumetone, Salsalate)→
- ↓Risk of NSAID induced peptic inflammation/ ulcer

Genitourinary
- Patients w/ pre-existing bilateral ↓renal perfusion, not necessarily failure:
  - Heart failure
  - Bilateral renal artery stenosis
  - Hypovolemia
  - Renal failure
  ...rely more on the compensatory production of vasodilatory prostaglandins→
    - Afferent arteriole dilation→
      - Maintained glomerular filtration rate–GFR, whereas NSAIDs→
        - ↓Prostaglandin production, which may→renal failure

Pulmonary
- Inhibition of both cyclooxygenase enzymes (COX 1 & COX2)→
  - ↑Lipoxygenase activity→
    - ↑Leukotriene synthesis→symptomatic asthma within 2hours of ingestion in 5% of asthmatics

ACUTE SECOND LINE TREATMENT

COLCHICINE

M	♀	Dose	Max
L	?	1.2mg PO, then 0.6mg q1–2hours until either: •Syndrome relief •Unacceptable side effects ...then administer as per renal function	8mg/ 24hours

- Although available, intravenous administration is discouraged due to:
  - Possible lethal side effects
  - Teratogenicity

Dose adjustment:
- Adjust according to renal function, w/ further dose↓ by 50% in patients age ≥70years

Creatinine clearance	Max dose
≥50mL/ min.	0.6mg q12hours
35–49ml/ min.	0.6mg q24hours
10–34ml/ min.	0.6mg q2–3days

Mechanism:
- Binds to tubulin (a microtubular protein)→
  - ↓Mitotic spindle & microtubular formation→
    - ↓Inflammatory cell division, chemotaxis, & phagocytosis→↓inflammation

Limitations:
- Most effective if administered within 48hours of syndrome onset. Not effective if administered once the inflammatory process if fully established

Side effects:
Gastrointestinal
•**Diarrhea**
•Nausea ± vomiting
Mucocutaneous
•Alopecia

Overdose (IV >> PO):
Gastrointestinal
•Hemorrhagic gastroenteritis
•Hepatitis
Genitourinary
•**Renal failure**
Musculoskeletal
•Myopathy, being limited to patients age >60years w/ a plasma creatinine >2mg/ dL→
  ∘Weakness &/or rhabdomyolysis
Hematologic
•Hypocalcemia
•**Myelosuppression**

Contraindications:
•**PO form**
  ∘Glomerular filtration rate–GFR <10mL/ min. or hemodialysis, as the medication is not dialyzed
•**IV form**
  ∘Hepatitis
  ∘Renal failure
  ∘Infusion extravasation mediated inflammation

Monitoring:
•Regular complete blood count for possible myelosuppression

SYSTEMIC GLUCOCORTICOID TREATMENT: Only once arthrocentesis of the joint has been performed to exclude infection

Generic	M ♀	Dose
Methylprednisolone	L ?	60mg PO/ IV q24hours X 3days
Prednisolone	L ?	60mg PO/ IV q24hours X 3days
Prednisone	L ?	60mg PO q24hours X 3days
Trimacinolone	L ?	60mg IM X 1

•Intra-articular–IA form†
  ∘Finger: 2mg IA
  ∘Knee: 40mg IA
  ∘Shoulder: 20mg IA

•Once disease control is achieved, taper to the lowest effective maintenance dose in order to minimize serious side effects, w/ the goal of discontinuation if possible, w/ attention to relapse syndrome
†Outcomes:
  •Variable & short-lasting effects. If pain relief is not achieved for several months w/ 1–2 injections, then abandon this treatment, as ≥3 intra-articular injections/ year may→
    ∘↑Tissue breakdown→
      –↑Disease severity

Glucocorticoids	Relative potencies Anti-inflammatory	Mineralocorticoid	Duration	Dose equiv.
Cortisol (physiologic†)	1	1	10hours	20mg
Cortisone (PO)	0.7	2	10hours	25mg
Hydrocortisone (PO, IM, IV)	1	2	10hours	20mg
Methylprednisolone (PO, IM, IA, IV)	5	0.5	15–35hours	5mg
Prednisone (PO)	5	0.5	15–35hours	5mg
Prednisolone (PO, IM, IV)	5	0.8	15–35hours	5mg
Triamcinolone (PO, IM)	5	~0	15–35hours	5mg
Betamethasone (PO, IM, IA)	25	~0	35–70hours	0.75mg
Dexamethasone (PO)	25	~0	35–70hours	0.75mg
Fludrocortisone (PO)	10	125	10hours	

†The physiologic rate of adrenal cortical cortisol production is 20–30mg/ 24hours

CHRONIC TREATMENT

- •To **begin 2weeks after resolution of an acute gout attack,** as plasma uric acid level fluctuations→
  - ◦Incitement or exacerbation of an acute gout attack

Target uric acid level: **<6mg/ dL**

Indications:
- •≥3 attacks in the previous year
- •Nephrolithiasis
- •Osteo−cartilagenous erosions
- •Documented state of ↑uric acid production
- •Initial attack w/ ↑recurrence risk:
  - ◦Uric acid >12mg/ dL
  - ◦Renal failure
  - ◦Necessary chronic diuretic use

ALLOPURINOL

Medication specific indications:
- •Nephrolithiasis
- •Renal failure
- •Tophi formation
- •Ineffective or intolerant to uricosuric medications

M	♀	Start	Titrate	Max
K	?	100mg PO q24hours	qweek	800mg/ 24hours†

†Doses >300mg should be divided

Dose adjustment:
- •Adjust according to renal function

Creatinine clearance	Max dose
10−20mL/ min.	200mg/ 24hours
<10mL/ min.	100mg/ 24hours

Mechanism:
- •Inhibits xanthine oxidase→
  - ◦↓**Uric acid production**
  - ◦↑Hypoxanthine & xanthine production, which are much more soluble than uric acid, & readily excreted

Side effects:

General
- •**May incite a gout attack during treatment initiation or dosage ↑**
  - Risk reduction:
    - •Concomitant administration of an anti−inflammatory drugs−NSAIDs, until the target uric acid level is reached X ≥6months

Hypersensitivity syndrome†−2% (↑w/ renal failure)
- •Dermatitis
- •Fever
- •Hepatitis
- •Renal failure
- •Vasculitis
- •Eosinophilia
- …necessitating discontinuation
  - Prognosis:
    - •20% mortality

Interactions:
- •↓Metabolism of Azathioprine, Mercaptopurine, Theophylline, Warfarin→
  - ◦↑Plasma concentration

Overdosage:

General
- •Fever

Gastrointestinal
- •Hepatitis

Genitourinary
- •Renal failure

---

†**Allopurinol desensitization**
  Indication:
- •Mild hypersensitivity syndrome

URICOSURIC MEDICATIONS

Medication specific indications:
  •Patients w/ renal uric acid underexcretion, w/ no indications for Allopurinol administration

Generic	M	♀	Start	Max
Probenecid	KL	P	250mg PO q12hours X 1week, then	
			500mg PO q12hours	1000mg q12hours
Sulfinpyrazone	K	?	100mg PO q12hours w/ meals X 1week, then	
			200mg PO q12hours	400mg q12hours

Mechanism:
  •Weak acids which compete w/ uric acid for reabsorption in the renal tubules→
    ◦↓Uric acid reabsorption→
      –↑Excretion

Limitations:
  •↓Efficacy in patients w/ renal failure, for which Allopurinol is indicated

Side effects:
  General
    •**May incite a gout attack during treatment initiation or dosage ↑**
    Risk reduction:
      •Concomitant administration of an anti–inflammatory medication until the target uric acid level
      is reached X ≥6months
  Gastrointestinal
    •Diarrhea
    •Nausea ± vomiting
  Genitourinary
    •**Nephrolithiasis (uric acid or calcium stones)**
    Risk reduction:
      •Drinking ≥1 quart of fluid/ 24hours
  Interactions
    •↓Renal secretion of Penicillins, Indomethacin, Sulfa medications→
      ◦↑Plasma concentration

Sulfinpyrazone specific:
  Cardiovascular
    •↓Platelet function

Contraindications:
  •History of nephrolithiasis
  •Renal failure

COLCHICINE

M	♀	Start
L	?	0.6mg PO q24hours

Dose adjustment:
  •Adjust according to renal function, w/ further dose↓ by 50% in patients age ≥70years

Creatinine clearance	Max dose
≥50mL/ min.	0.6mg q12hours
35–49ml/ min.	0.6mg q24hours
10–34ml/ min.	0.6mg q2–3days

CALCIUM PYROPHOSPHATE DIHYDRATE–CPPD DEPOSITION DISEASE

•Acute treatment is focused on ↓inflammation, whereas chronic treatment is focused on the diagnosis &
treatment of a possible etiologic disease, as, unlike in gout, there is no medical treatment to ↓joint
calcium pyrophosphate concentration

Acute treatment
  •As for acute gout treatment
Chronic treatment
  •Colchicine as for chronic gout treatment

Annual incidence of gout according to plasma uric acid levels:
- ≥9mg/ dL: 5%
- 8-8.9mg/ dL: 4%
- 7-7.9mg/ dL: 1%
- <7mg/ dL: 0.8%

Duration between the initial & subsequent gout flare:
- 1year–60%
- 1–2years–15%
- 2–5years–10%
- 5–10years–7%
- >10years–8%

•**A chronic, intermittently symptomatic autoimmune disease** of unknown etiology→
　◦Autoantibodies to cell membrane, cytoplasmic, & nuclear proteins→
　　−Direct damage & immune complex deposition→systemic inflammation
Statistics:
　•Affects 1/ 3000 persons in the U.S.

RISK FACTORS
•**Age:** Peak onset @ ages 20–40years, w/ rare onset @ >55years
•**Gender:** ♀ **9X** ♂
•**Skin color:** Black ♀ 4X white ♀
•**Genetics:**
　◦Family history of systemic lupus erythematosus–SLE
　　−Children of a mother w/ SLE have ↑risk (♀ 1/ 40, ♂ 1/ 250)
　◦MHC class II DR2 or DR3
　◦Complement deficiencies, esp. C4a & C4b
•**Medications:**
　◦None of the above risk factors apply to medication induced SLE as:
　　−♂=♀
　　−Whites >> blacks
　　−Age usually ≥50years
　　…w/ medications being:
　　　•Chlorpromazine
　　　•**Hydralazine**
　　　　◦10% of patients, usually @ >200mg/ 24h
　　　•Isoniazid−INH
　　　•Methyldopa
　　　•Minocycline
　　　•**Procainamide**
　　　　◦30% of patients taking for >1year
　　　•Quinidine
　　　•Sulfasalazine
　　　…w/ symptoms being reversible within 2months after discontinuation, & laboratory findings within
　　　1 year

CLASSIFICATION
•**Systemic lupus erythematosus–SLE:** Disease w/ systemic features
•**Drug induced lupus:** Disease due to medication use
•**Discoid lupus:** Disease w/ discoid cutaneous lesions only (no systemic features)
•**Neonatal lupus:** Neonatal (first 28 days of life) disease due to the transplacental passage of **anti−Ro
antibodies**→
　◦Anemia
　◦Transient dermatitis
　…usually resolving by 3–6months, w/ the rare occurrence of complete heart block

DIAGNOSIS
•Signs & symptoms worst at the initial diagnosis are usually the worst or only features of a flare, which
usually occur q1–2years during the 1st 10 years, ↓in frequency thereafter. This sequence occurs much
more commonly than either:
　◦Chronic persistent disease
　◦Sustained remission for decades
•Percentages indicate lifetime occurrence

Diagnostic criteria for Systemic lupus erythematosus–SLE:
　•≥4 of the following are required over time (need not be concomitant)
　　◦Genitourinary
　　　−Glomerulonephritis via proteinuria >0.5g/ 24h, ≥3+ dipstick proteinuria=≥200mg/ dL, or cellular
　　　casts
　　◦Mucocutaneous
　　　−Discoid lesions
　　　−Malar rash
　　　−Photosensitivity
　　　−Ulcerations (oral or nasal)
　　◦Musculoskeletal
　　　−Arthritis involving ≥2 peripheral joints

744

○Neurologic
  –Lupus encephalitis
○Serositis
  –Pericarditis
  –Pleuritis
○Hematologic
  –Cytopenia: Hemolytic anemia, leukopenia <4000/ μL, lymphopenia <1500/ μL, or thrombocytopenia <100,000/ μL
  –Positive antinuclear antibody–ANA, anti–dsDNA, anti–Sm, or antiphospholipid antibodies
  –Positive Lupus Erythematosus–LE cell prep
Outcomes:
  •Sensitivity 97%, specificity 98%

Precipitating factors:
  •?Emotional stress
  •Infections
  •Medications
    ○Echinacea
    ○Sulfa–containing medications
  •Pregnancy
  •Ultraviolet light exposure

Monitoring disease severity:
  •Complement levels, esp. C3, C4, or CH50
  •Complete blood count–CBC
  •Urinalysis
  •Creatinine
  •Quantitative assay of anti–ds DNA antibodies

General–95%
  •Inflammatory cytokines→
    ○Anorexia→
      –Cachexia
    ○Chills
    ○Fatigue–90%
    ○Fever–70%
    ○Headache
    ○Malaise
    ○Night sweats
    ○Weakness
    …which may precede the onset of other symptoms by several weeks

---

†Temperature may be normal in patients w/:
  •Chronic kidney disease, esp. w/ uremia
  •Cirrhosis
  •Heart failure
  •Severe debility
  …or those who are:
    •Intravenous drug users
    •Taking certain medications:
      ○Acetaminophen
      ○Antibiotics
      ○Glucocorticoids
      ○Nonsteroidal anti–inflammatory drugs–NSAIDs

Musculoskeletal–95%
  •Autoantibody mediated serosal inflammation of:
    ○Joints→
      –Arthritis, usually being oligoarticular (affecting <5 joints), migratory, & nonerosive

    Affected joints:
      •Small joints > large weight bearing joints, esp:
        ○Hands
        ○Wrist
        ○Feet

◦Bursae (olecranon, popliteal, subacromial, retrocalcaneal)→
　　-Bursitis
　◦Tendon sheaths→
　　-Tenosynovitis
　◦Tendons→
　　-Tendonitis
　◦Skin→
　　-Cellulitis
　...→edematous, erythematous, warm, & painful joints, bursae, tendon sheaths, &/or periarticular
　　tissue, usually **being worse in the morning, w/ deformities being reducible**
•Anti-myocyte antibodies→
　◦Myositis

Mucocutaneous-80%
•Autoantibody mediated dermal/ epidermal inflammation→
　◦**Erythematous maculopapular rash on the:**
　　-**Cheeks, w/ sparing of the nasolabial folds, being termed a malar rash or "butterfly
　　rash"-30%**
　　-Chin
　　-Forehead
　　-Chest
　　-Fingers
　　...being precipitated by sun exposure=**photosensitivity-30%**
　◦Fibrotic lesions, termed discoid on the:
　　-Scalp
　　-Face
　　-Neck
　　-Fingers
　　...which if chronic→
　　　　•↑Epidermoid cancer risk
　◦Subacute cutaneous erythematosus: Diffuse papulosquamous or annular lesions, being exquisitely
　　photosensitive
•Immune complex deposition→**dermal & subcutaneous vasculitis**→
　◦Hemorrhage→
　　-Skin &/or mucus membrane (nasal, oral, pharyngeal, &/or conjunctival) discoloration which does
　　not blanch upon pressure, termed purpura (≤3mm=petechiae or >3mm=ecchymoses) ± being
　　palpable due to tumor effect, termed palpable purpura, indicating vascular inflammaton
　　-Nailbed splinter hemorrhages
　◦Ulcerations, esp. of the oropharyngeal &/or nasal mucosa, usually being painless
　　-Necrotizing skin ulcerations w/ diffuse dermal neutrophil infiltration, termed **pyoderma
　　gangrenosum**
　◦Infarcts surrounding the nails, termed periungual infarcts
　◦Vascular stasis &/or hyalinization→
　　-Capillary & venule dilation→a net-like pattern of macular, purple-blue skin discoloration, termed
　　livedo reticularis
　◦Patchy or diffuse alopecia
　◦Focal arteriolitis→
　　-Granuloma formation w/ central necrosis, termed a **rheumatoid nodule**
　　　Rheumatod nodule locations:
　　　　•**Subcutaneous-25%**→
　　　　　◦Nodules, usually near inflamed joints or pressure-exposed areas:
　　　　　　-Achilles tendon
　　　　　　-Infrapatellar tendon
　　　　　　-Extensor surface of elbow &/or forearm
　　　　•Synovial→
　　　　　◦Intra-articular mass
　　　　　◦Bursal mass
　　　　•Other organs, esp:
　　　　　◦Lungs
　　　　　◦Myocardium
　　　　　◦Sclera

Lymphatics
•Inflammation→↑leukocyte replication→
　◦Lymphadenopathy (local or generalized)
　◦Splenomegally

746

Cardiovascular
- •Autoantibody mediated:
  - ◦Myo/ pericardial inflammation→
    - **−Myo/ pericarditis−30%**
  - ◦Endocardial inflammation→
    - **−Noninfected cardiac valve vegetations, termed Libman−Sacks endocarditis** (left sided > right sided)→valvular regurgitation
- •Immune complex deposition→focal arteriolitis→
  - ◦Myocardial ischemia ± infarction
  - ◦Myocardial rheumatoid nodules→
    - −Dysrhythmia
    - −Valvular regurgitation
- •**Antiphospholipid antibodies−50%**
  - ◦Lupus anticoagulant−7%, named due to falsely ↑coagulation studies (aPTT > INR), which paradoxically→
    - −Arterial & venous thromboembolic events→ischemia ± infarction

Gastrointestinal−45%
- •Autoantibody mediated:
  - ◦Hepatitis−40%
  - ◦Pancreatitis
- •Immune complex deposition→
  - ◦Mesenteric vasculitis−5%→
    - −Acute mesenteric ischemia ± infarction

Genitourinary~100%, w/ 50% being syndromatic (rare in drug−induced SLE)
- •Glomerular immune complex deposition ± **dsDNA deposition** & subsequent antibody attachment→
  - ◦**Glomerulonephritis** w/ 5 world health organization−WHO classes→
    - −Proteinuria
    - −Hematuria (>5 erythrocytes/ hpf)
    - −Pyuria (>5 leukocytes/ hpf)
    - −Erythrocyte casts
    - …w/ the subsequent development of:
      - •Intra−renal renal failure, w/ progression to end−stage renal disease in <5% of patients
      - •Nephrotic syndrome @ proteinuria ≥3g/ 24h→
        - ◦Albuminuria, w/ renal NaCl & H_2O retention→
          - −Edema
        - ◦Immunoglobulinuria→
          - −Immunodeficiency
        - ◦↑Hepatic protein synthesis→
          - −Hyperlipidemia via ↑lipoproteins
          - −Hypercoagulability via ↑clotting factor production
          - −↓Antithrombin 3 via urinary loss→↑renal vein thrombosis risk, occurring immediately after glomerular filtration→flank pain, ↑proteinuria, ↑hematuria, & ↓renal function

Neurologic−60%
- •Antineuronal &/or antineuroglial antibodies→
  - ◦Lupus encephalitis→
    - −Cerebrovascular accident syndrome
    - −Chronic headaches
    - −Cognitive dysfunction (ex. memory &/or concentration deficits)
    - −Depression
    - −Movement disorders
    - −Peripheral neuropathy (motor, sensory, &/or autonomic)
    - −Psychosis
    - −Seizures
    - −Transverse myelitis
    - …w/ cerebrospinal fluid showing:
      - •↑Protein (>45mg/ dL)
      - •Pleocytosis (≥5cells/ μL)−50%
      - …resembling aseptic meningitis

Pulmonary
- •Autoantibody mediated pulmonary inflammation→
  - ◦Noninfectious lung inflammation, termed pneumonitis→
    - −Pulmonary hemorrhage→hemoptysis, indicating a 50% mortality rate
  - ◦Pleuritis−35%→pleurisy, being thoracic pain exacerbated by either:
    - −Deep inhalation (including coughing & sneezing)
    - −Supine position
    - −Thoracic palpation
    - …& being relieved by leaning forward

747

◦Exudative pleural effusion
 •Immune complex deposition→pulmonary vasculitis→
  ◦Diffuse interstitial fibrosis→
   −Pulmonary hypertension
  ◦Focal arteriolitis→
   −Pulmonary rheumatoid nodules
Materno−fetal
 •**Pregnancy†→**
  ◦**↑Flare risk**
  ◦**50% chance of either:**
   −**Miscarriage**
   −**Pre−term delivery**
   ...usually during the 2nd trimester
  ◦Transplacental passage of **anti−Ro antibodies**→neonatal lupus via:
   −Anemia
   −Transient dermatitis
   ...usually resolving @ 3−6months, w/ the rare occurrence of complete heart block
 •**Antiphospholipid antibodies−50%**
  ◦Lupus anticoagulant−7% & anticardiolipin antibodies−25%→
   −Arterial & venous thromboembolic events→recurrent fetal loss, termed miscarriage, esp. during
    the 2nd trimester

---

†The best candidates for pregnancy are those whose disease is controlled for the past 6 months on
≤10mg Prednisone q24h

Hematologic
 •Chronic disease→
  ◦Splenic & hepatic macrophage mediated removal of autoantibody coated cells→
   −Normocytic, normochromic anemia−60%→fatigue
   −Leukopenia−40%→↑infection & neoplasm risk
   −Thrombocytopenia−30%→↑hemorrhage risk, esp. petechiae
  ◦Secondary amyloidosis, w/ rheumatoid arthritis being the #1 cause (osteomyelitis being #2)
 •Active disease→
  ◦Leukocytosis
  ◦↑Acute phase proteins, being useful in monitoring disease activity
   −↑Erythrocyte sedimentation rate−ESR (normal: 5mm/ decade aged + ♂ ≤10mm/h or ♀ ≤20mm/h)
   −↑C−reactive protein−CRP (normal: <2mg/ L), responding more acutely than ESR, as it rises
    within several hours & falls within 3days upon partial resolution
   −↑Fibrinogen
   −↑Platelets→thrombocytosis
 •Positive Lupus erythematosus−LE cell prep−90%
  <u>Procedure:</u>
   •In−vitro testing of plasma allows for the visualization of neutrophils w/ the formation of a round
    body composed of:
    ◦Antinuclear antibodies
    ◦Complement
    ◦Phagocytosed nucleus of another cell
 •↑Antibody production→
  ◦Polyclonal or monoclonal hypergammaglobulinemia→hypocomplementemia−60%, esp. of C3 & C4
   (not occurring in drug induced lupus)→↑infection risk via encapsulated bacteria:
   −Escherichia coli
   −Haemophilus influenzae
   −Neisseria meningitides
   −Pseudomonas aeruginosa
   −Salmonella sp.
   −Streptococcus pneumoniae

- **Antinuclear antibody–ANA production–99%** during active disease (90% during remission), being positive w/ a titer >1:160. Testing for specific antinuclear antibodies should only be ordered in ANA positive patients (except for anti–Ro as discussed below)
  - Limitations:
    - None of the antinuclear antibody titers accurately correlate w/ disease activity, except anti–dsDNA antibody levels
    - False positive:
      - ∘Other autoimmune diseases
      - ∘Certain medication reactions
      - ∘Viral infections
      - ∘General population–2%
  - Antibodies:
    - Anti–histone
    - Anti–ribonucleoprotein–RNP 40%, being rare in drug induced lupus
      - Outcomes:
        - Specificity: 90%
        - Indicates ↓**glomerulonephritis risk** in the absence of anti–dsDNA
        - Indicates ↑risk of:
          - ∘Arthritis
          - ∘Esophageal dysmotility
          - ∘Interstitial lung disease
          - ∘Mixed connective tissue disease–MCTD
          - ∘Myositis
          - ∘Raynaud's phenomenon
          - ∘Sclerodactyly
    - **Anti–dsDNA–60%** (80% w/ WHO class IV glomerulonephritis), being rare in drug induced lupus
      - Outcomes:
        - Specificity: 95%
        - **Titer correlates w/ disease activity**
        - Indicates ↑**glomerulonephritis** & vasculitis risk
    - Anti–ssDNA–80%
      - Outcomes:
        - Specificity: 50%
    - Anti–Sm (Smith)–25%, being rare in drug induced lupus
      - Outcomes:
        - Specificity: 99%
        - Indicates ↑**glomerulonephritis & central nervous system disease risk**
    - **Anti–Ro=SS–A 30%, being present in 50% of ANA negative patients**
      - Outcomes:
        - Transplacental passage→
          - ∘**Neonatal lupus–10%**
        - Indicates ↑risk of:
          - ∘Photosensitivity
          - ∘Sjogrens syndrome
          - ∘Subacute cutaneous lupus
    - Anti–La=SS–B 10%, always being associated w/ anti–Ro
      - Outcomes:
        - Indicates ↓glomerulonephritis risk
        - Indicates ↑Sjogren's syndrome risk
    - **Anti–histone–25% (95% in drug induced lupus)**
      - Outcomes:
        - Specificity: 80%

- **Antiphospholipid antibodies–50%**
  - ∘Lupus anticoagulant–7%, named due to falsely ↑coagulation studies (aPTT > INR), which paradoxically→
    - –Arterial & venous thromboembolic events→ischemia ± infarction→recurrent fetal loss, termed miscarriage, esp. during the 2nd trimester
    - –Thrombocytopenia
    - Limitations:
      - False positive:
        - ∘Other autoimmune diseases
        - ∘HIV infection
        - ∘General population
  - ∘False positive plasma VDRL or RPR test–25%

○Anticardiolipin antibody−25%
  −Indicates ↑risk of recurrent fetal loss, termed miscarriage

•**Antineuronal antibodies−60%**
•**Rheumatoid factor−20%**† production (70% of which become seropositive within 1year), being positive w/ a titer of ≥1:80
  ○Antibody towards the Fc portion of IgG, being either IgA, IgE, IgG, or IgM, w/ standard tests best at detecting IgM
  Limitations:
    •Titer does not correlate w/ disease activity
    •False negative:
      ○Other Ig types
    •False positive:
      ○Autoimmune diseases
      ○Endocarditis
      ○Interstitial pulmonary fibrosis
      ○Liver disease
      ○5−10% of healthy adults
•Positive direct antiglobulin test, termed **Coombs test−30%**, which detects IgG & complement bound to the erythrocyte cell membrane

INVASIVE PROCEDURES
•**Renal biopsy**
Indications:
  •Patients w/ suspected lupus glomerulonephritis in order to obtain:
    ○Histology
    ○Immunoflorescence or electron microscopy, as all patients w/ lupus glomerulonephritis should show antigen−antibody−complement deposition

World Health Organization−WHO Glomerulonephritis Class:
  •Class 1: Normal histology
  •Class 2: Mesangial hypercellularity−25%
  •Class 3: Focal proliferative glomerulonephritis−15%
  •Class 4: Diffuse proliferative glomerulonephritis−45%
  •Class 5: Membranous changes−15%
  •Class 6: Chronic glomerular sclerosis

TREATMENT
•Being as there is no cure, w/ sustained remissions being rare, the goal of treatment is to ↓the severity of disease flares, w/ subsequent maintenance dosing of medications so as to use the lowest dose necessary to achieve acceptable syndrome suppression

•**Avoidance of sun exposure**
Indications:
  •Photosensitivity
Methods:
  •When exposed, use:
    ○UVA & UVB sunscreen w/ a sun protection factor−SPF ≥15†
    ○Wide brim hat to shade your face, ears, & neck
    ○Long sleeved shirt & pants
•**Topical glucocorticoid preparations for dermatitides**
•**Intralesional glucocorticoid injection for discoid lesions**

---

†The sun protection factor−SPF number indicates the relative length of time skin can be exposed to UVB rays w/ little sunburn risk. Protection time is calculated as (SPF#) X (usual exposure time causing burn). However, sweating & water→
  •↓Protection time, necessitating more frequent applications

MILD DISEASE

Indications being mild:
- Fever
- Musculoskeletal disease
- Serositis

CYCLOOXYGENASE–COX 2 SELECTIVE INHIBITING NSAIDS			
Generic (Trade)	**M**	**♀**	**Dose**
Celecoxib (Celebrex)	L	U	200mg PO q12hours

Mechanism:
- Selective, reversible inhibition of the cyclooxygenase–COX 2 enzyme, being responsible for the production of inflammatory cell prostaglandins→
  - ↓Pain
  - ↓Inflammation
  - ...w/ **minimal cyclooxygenase–COX 1 mediated effects**

Background pathophysiology:
- Inflammatory cell mediated prostaglandins are released at sites of inflammation (in addition to other inflammatory cytokines)→
  - Leukocyte migration→↑inflammation via:
    - Vasodilation→↑blood flow→erythema, edema, warmth, &/or tenderness/ pain via enhanced neuronal sensitivity

In Brief:
- **Cyclooxygenase–COX1 enzymes** are found in most cells of the body, being responsible for normal physiologic processes
- **Cyclooxygenase–COX 2 enzymes** are responsible for the production of inflammatory cell prostaglandins

Cyclooxyegenase–COX 1 mediated effects	Effects of relatively ↓inhibition
Hypothalamic prostaglandin synthesis	No antipyretic effect
Platelet thromboxane A_2 synthesis	No antiplatelet effect
Gastric mucosal cell prostaglandin synthesis	↓Peptic inflammatory disease risk
Glomerular afferent arteriole prostaglandin synthesis	↓Renal failure risk

Side effects:
Cardiovascular
- Hypertension

Gastrointestinal
- Inhibition of the cyclooxygenase–COX1 enzyme→↑peptic inflammatory disease risk→↑**upper gastrointestinal hemorrhage risk** via:
  - ↓Gastric mucosal prostaglandin synthesis→
    - ↓Epithelial proliferation
    - ↓Mucosal blood flow→↓bicarbonate delivery to the mucosa
    - ↓Mucus & bicarbonate secretion from gastric mucosal cells

Genitourinary
- Patients w/ pre-existing bilateral ↓renal perfusion, not necessarily failure:
  - Heart failure
  - Bilateral renal artery stenosis
  - Hypovolemia
  - Renal failure
  - ...rely more on the compensatory production of vasodilatory prostaglandins→
    - Afferent arteriole dilation→
      - Maintained glomerular filtration rate–GFR, whereas NSAIDs→
        - ↓Prostaglandin production, which may→renal failure

Pulmonary
- Inhibition of both cyclooxygenase enzymes (COX 1 & COX2)→
  - ↑Lipoxygenase activity→
    - ↑Leukotriene synthesis→symptomatic asthma within 2hours of ingestion in 5% of asthmatics

Caution:
- Minimal inhibition of COX–1→
  - ↓Endothelial & vascular smooth muscle cell prostacyclin† production relative to platelet thromboxane‡ production→cytokine imbalance in favor of vasoconstriction→
    - Hypertension

	−↑Cerebrovascular accident syndrome risk
	−↑Myocardial ischemic syndrome risk
Contraindications:	
•Sulfa hypersensitivity due to a sulfa moiety	

NONSTEROIDAL ANTI-INFLAMMATORY DRUGS-NSAIDs

Generic	M ♀	Start	Max
Ibuprofen	L P in 1st & 2nd, U in 3rd trimester	600mg PO q8hours	3.2g/ 24hours
Indomethacin	L P in 1st & 2nd, U in 3rd trimester	50mg PO/ PR q8hours	
Naproxen	L P in 1st & 2nd, U in 3rd trimester	375mg PO q12hours	
•XR form		750mg PO q24hours	

•One cannot predict which NSAID a patient will respond to
•Attempt to eventually ↓dosage &/or limit use to exacerbations in order to ↓side effect risk

Mechanism:
•Aspirin & other anti-inflammatory medications→
  ∘Respectively to irreversible & reversible inhibition of both cyclooxygenase enzymes (COX-1 & COX-2), being responsible for the production of neural & inflammatory cell prostaglandins respectively→
    −↓Pain
    −↓Temperature (antipyretic)
    −↓Inflammation

Background pathophysiology:
•Inflammatory cell mediated prostaglandins are released at sites of inflammation (in addition to other inflammatory cytokines)→
  ∘Leukocyte migration→↑inflammation via:
    −Vasodilation→↑blood flow→erythema, edema, warmth, &/or tenderness/ pain via enhanced neuronal sensitivity
•Interleukin-IL1→
  ∘↑Hypothalamic prostaglandin production→
    −Fever

In Brief:
•**Cyclooxygenase-COX1 enzymes** are found in most cells of the body, being responsible for normal physiologic processes
•**Cyclooxygenase-COX 2 enzymes** are responsible for the production of inflammatory cell prostaglandins

Side effects:
Gastrointestinal
•Inhibition of the cyclooxygenase-COX1 enzyme→↑peptic inflammatory disease risk→↑**upper gastrointestinal hemorrhage risk** via:
  ∘↓Gastric mucosal prostaglandin synthesis→
    −↓Epithelial cell proliferation
    −↓Mucosal blood flow→↓bicarbonate delivery to the mucosa
    −↓Mucus & bicarbonate secretion from gastric mucosal cells

Indications for peptic inflammatory disease prophylaxis:
•Prophylax w/ proton pump inhibitors-PPI's, histamine 2 selective receptor blockers, or Misoprostol in patients w/ any of the following:
  ∘Age >60 years w/ a history of peptic inflammatory disease
  ∘Anticipated therapy >3 months
  ∘Concurrent glucocorticoid use
  ∘Moderate to high dose NSAID use
Note: Newer NSAIDs (Etodolac, Nabumetone, Salsalate)→
    •↓Risk of NSAID induced peptic inflammation/ ulcer

Genitourinary
•Patients w/ pre-existing bilateral ↓renal perfusion, not necessarily failure:
  ∘Heart failure
  ∘Bilateral renal artery stenosis
  ∘Hypovolemia
  ∘Renal failure
  ...rely more on the compensatory production of vasodilatory prostaglandins→

752

- •Afferent arteriole dilation→
  - ◦Maintained glomerular filtration rate–GFR, whereas NSAIDs→
    - –↓Prostaglandin production, which may→renal failure
- **Pulmonary**
  - •Inhibition of both cyclooxygenase enzymes (COX 1 & COX2)→
    - ◦↑Lipoxygenase activity→
      - –↑Leukotriene synthesis→symptomatic asthma within 2hours of ingestion in 5% of asthmatics

---

CAPSAICIN

M	♀	Dose
?	?	0.025%–0.075% applied to the affected area ≤qid, w/ prompt handwashing after application

•Continued application for 2–4 weeks is necessary to achieve benefit

Mechanism:
- •Substance P antagonism

Side effects:
- **Cutaneous**
  - •Burning pain–>30%, being ↓w/ continued use

MODERATE DISEASE ▬▬▬▬▬▬▬▬▬▬▬

Indications:
- •Fever
- •Fatigue
- •Arthritis
- •Cutaneous disease

SYSTEMIC GLUCOCORTICOID TREATMENT: Only once active infection has been excluded

Indications:
- •↓Inflammation while an immunomodulating medication is taking effect

Generic	M	♀	Dose
Methylprednisolone	L	?	30–60mg PO/ IV q24hours X 3days
Prednisolone	L	?	30–60mg PO/ IV q24hours X 3days
Prednisone	L	?	30–60mg PO q24hours X 3days
Trimacinolone	L	?	60mg IM X 1

- •Intra–articular–IA form†
  - ◦Finger: 2mg IA
  - ◦Knee: 40mg IA
  - ◦Shoulder: 20mg IA

•Once disease control is achieved, taper to the lowest effective maintenance dose in order to minimize serious side effects, w/ the goal of discontinuation if possible, w/ attention to relapse syndrome

†Outcomes:
- •Variable & short–lasting effects. If pain relief is not achieved for several months w/ 1–2 injections, then abandon this treatment, as ≥3 intra–articular injections/ year may→
  - ◦↑Tissue breakdown→
    - –↑Disease severity

Glucocorticoids	Relative potencies Anti–inflammatory	Mineralocorticoid	Duration	Dose equiv.
Cortisol (physiologic†)	1	1	10hours	20mg
Cortisone (PO)	0.7	2	10hours	25mg
Hydrocortisone (PO, IM, IV)	1	2	10hours	20mg
Methylprednisolone (PO, IM, IA, IV)	5	0.5	15–35hours	5mg
Prednisone (PO)	5	0.5	15–35hours	5mg
Prednisolone (PO, IM, IV)	5	0.8	15–35hours	5mg
Triamcinolone (PO, IM)	5	~0	15–35hours	5mg
Betamethasone (PO, IM, IA)	25	~0	35–70hours	0.75mg
Dexamethasone (PO)	25	~0	35–70hours	0.75mg
Fludrocortisone (PO)	10	125	10hours	

†The physiologic rate of adrenal cortical cortisol production is 20–30mg/ 24hours

Side effects of chronic use:
General
- Anorexia→
  - ◦Cachexia
- ↑Perspiration

Cardiovascular
- Mineralocorticoid effects→
  - ◦↑Renal tubular NaCl & water retention as well as potassium secretion→
    - –**Hypertension**
    - –**Edema**
    - –**Hypokalemia**
- Counter–regulatory=anti–insulin effects→
  - ◦↑Plasma glucose→
    - –**Secondary diabetes mellitus**, which may→ketoacidemia
  - ◦Hyperlipidemia→↑atherosclerosis→
    - –**Coronary artery disease**
    - –Cerebrovascular disease
    - –Peripheral vascular disease

Cutaneous/ subcutaneous
- ↓Fibroblast function→
  - ◦↓Intercellular matrix production→
    - –↑Bruisability→ecchymoses
    - –Poor wound healing
    - –Skin striae
- Androgenic effects→
  - ◦Acne
  - ◦↑Facial hair
  - ◦Thinning scalp hair
- Fat redistribution from the extremities to the:
  - ◦Abdomen→
    - –Truncal obesity
  - ◦Shoulders→
    - –Supraclavicular fat pads
  - ◦Upper back→
    - –Buffalo hump
  - ◦Face→
    - –Moon facies
  - …w/ concomitant thinning of the arms & legs

Endocrine
- **Adrenal failure** upon abrupt discontinuation after 2weeks

Gastrointestinal
- Inhibition of phospholipase A_2 mediated conversion of cell membrane lipids to arachidonic acid, which is the precursor for both cyclooxygenase–COX enzymes, w/ the cyclooxygenase–COX1 enzyme found in most cells of the body, responsible for normal physiologic function. Inhibition of the cyclooxygenase–COX1 enzyme→↑peptic inflammatory disease risk→↑**upper gastrointestinal hemorrhage risk** via:
  - ◦↓Gastric mucosal prostaglandin synthesis→
    - –↓Epithelial cell proliferation
    - –↓Mucosal blood flow→↓bicarbonate delivery to the mucosa
    - –↓Mucus & bicarbonate secretion from gastric mucosal cells

Musculoskeletal
- **Avascular necrosis of bone**
- **Osteoporosis**
- Proximal muscle weakness

Neurologic
- Anxiety
- Insomnia
- Psychosis

Opthalmologic
- Cataracts

754

Immunologic
- •Inhibition of phospholipase A_2 mediated conversion of cell membrane lipids to arachidonic acid, which is the precursor for both cyclooxygenase–COX enzymes (COX1 & COX2) being responsible for the production of neuronal & inflammatory cell prostaglandins respectively→
  - –↓Pain
  - –↓Temperature (antipyretic)
  - –↓**Inflammation**
- •Stabilization of lisosomal & cell membranes→
  - ○↓Cytokine & proteolytic enzyme release
- •↓Lymphocyte & eosinophil production
- ...all→
  - •**Immunosuppression**→
    - –↑**Infection** &/or neoplasm risk

Hematologic
- •↑Erythrocyte production→
  - ○Polycythemia
- •↑Neutrophil demargination→
  - ○Neutrophilia→
    - –**Leukocytosis**

IMMUNOMODULATING MEDICATIONS

•The following medications usually require 1–6 months for symptomatic improvement, making these medications not useful in the control of acute disease, but rather, useful when prolonged treatment is planned.

Generic (Trade)	M ♀	Dose
Hydroxychloroquine (Plaquenil)	K ?	400–600mg PO q24hours w/ a meal, then 200–400mg q24hours upon clnical response

•Once disease control is achieved, taper to the lowest effective maintenance dose in order to minimize serious side effects

Mechanism: Unknown

Side effects:
Gastrointestinal
- •↓Mucosal cell proliferation→
  - ○Mucosal inflammation=mucositis, including inflammation of the oral mucosa=stomatitis→
    - –Diarrhea
    - –Nausea ± vomiting

Opthalmologic
- •Accommodation defects
- •Blurred vision scotomas
- •Corneal deposits
- •Extraocular muscle weakness
- •Night blindness
- •**Retinopathy–rare**, being related to cumulative dose, which may→
  - ○Irreversible visual loss

Mucocutaneous
- •↓Hair formation→
  - ○Alopecia
- •↓Epithelial cell proliferation→
  - ○Dermatitis
- •Skin pigmentation
- •Stevens–Johnson syndrome

Musculoskeletal
- •Myopathy

Neurologic
- •Headache
- •Insomnia
- •Neuropathy
- •Tinnitus
- •Vertigo

```
┌─────────────────────────────────────────────────────────────────────────┐
│ Hematologic                                                               │
│  •Myelosuppression→                                                       │
│    ∘Macrocytic anemia→                                                    │
│      –Fatigue                                                             │
│    ∘Leukopenia→immunosuppression→                                         │
│      –↑Infection & neoplasm risk                                          │
│    ∘Thrombocytopenia→                                                     │
│      –↑Hemorrhage risk, esp. petechiae                                    │
├─────────────────────────────────────────────────────────────────────────┤
│ Monitoring:                                                               │
│  •Baseline ophthalmologic examination, then                               │
│    ∘Q6months                                                              │
└─────────────────────────────────────────────────────────────────────────┘
```

SEVERE DISEASE ▬▬▬

Indications:
- •All other manifestations
- •Syndrome refractory to the above treatments

SYSTEMIC GLUCOCORTICOID TREATMENT: Only once active infection has been excluded			
Indications:			
•↓Inflammation while an immunomodulating medication is taking effect			
Generic	M	♀	**Dose**
Methylprednisolone	L	?	1g PO/ IV pulse therapy q24hours X 3–5days, then 0.5–1mg/ kg PO/ IV q12hours
Prednisolone	L	?	1g PO/ IV pulse therapy q24hours X 3–5days, then 0.5–1mg/ kg PO/ IV q12hours
Prednisone	L	?	1g PO pulse therapy q24hours X 3–5days, then 0.5–1mg/ kg PO q12hours

- •Both the IV & PO routes have equal efficacy
- •Once disease control is achieved, taper to the lowest effective maintenance dose in order to minimize serious side effects, w/ the goal of discontinuation if possible, w/ attention to relapse syndrome

IMMUNOMODULATING MEDICATIONS				
•The following medications usually require 1–6 months for symptomatic improvement, making these medications not useful in the control of acute disease, but rather, useful when prolonged treatment is planned. Consider combination therapy in patients who have failed 1medication				
Generic (Trade)	M	♀	**Start**	**Max**
ESP. FOR MILD GLOMERULONEPHRITIS				
6-mercaptopurine	L	U	50mg PO q24hours	
Azathioprine (Imuran)†	LK	U	1mg/ kg PO q24hours	2.5mg/kg/24hours
ESP. FOR SEVERE GLOMERULONEPHRITIS OR CENTRAL NERVOUS SYSTEM DISEASE				
Cyclophosphamide (Cytoxan)			10mg/ kg IV qmonth	2.5mg/kg/24hours
ESP. FOR ARTHRITIS/ ARTHRALGIA, CUTANEOUS DISEASE, &/OR SEROSITIS				
Methotrexate (Rheumatrex)	LK	U	7.5mg PO qweek	20mg qweek

†Azathioprine's active metabolite is 6–mercaptopurine

Azathioprine/ 6–mercaptopurine mechanism:
- •Inhibition of enzymes involved in purine metabolism→
  - ∘Cytotoxicity of differentiating lymphocytes (T cell >> B cell)

Cyclophosphamide mechanism:
- •Forms reactive molecular species which alkylate nucleophilic groups on DNA bases→
  - ∘Abnormal base pairing
  - ∘Cross–linking of DNA bases
  - ∘DNA strand breakage
  - …→cytotoxicity to all proliferating cells

Methotrexate mechanism:
- •Folate analog→
  - ∘Dihydrofolate reductase inhibition→
    - –↓DNA synthesis→cytotoxicity to all proliferating cells

Side effects:
Gastrointestinal
- ↓Mucosal cell proliferation→
  - ◦Mucosal inflammation=mucositis, including inflammation of the oral mucosa=stomatitis→
    - −Diarrhea
    - −Nausea ± vomiting
Hematologic
- **Myelosuppression→**
  - ◦Macrocytic anemia→
    - −Fatigue
  - ◦Leukopenia→immunosuppression→
    - −↑Infection & neoplasm risk
  - ◦Thrombocytopenia→
    - −↑Hemorrhage risk, esp. petechiae

Azathioprine/ 6−mercaptopurine specific:
Gastrointestinal
- Hepatitis→
  - ◦Cirrhosis−rare
Mucocutaneous
- ↓Epithelial cell proliferation→
  - ◦Dermatitis
Hematologic
- Myelosuppression, esp. w/ concomitant:
  - ◦Renal failure
  - ◦Medications:
    - −Allopurinol
    - −Angiotensin converting enzyme inhibitor−ACEi

Cyclophosphamide specific:
Genitourinary
- **Hemorrhagic cystitis**
- Premature ovarian failure
- Sterility
Mucocutaneous
- ↓Hair formation→
  - ◦Alopecia

Methotrexate specific:
- Concomitant use of **folic acid** 1mg PO q24h may ↓side effects without ↓efficacy

Gastrointestinal
- Dyspepsia
- Hepatitis→
  - ◦Cirrhosis−rare
Genitourinary
- Bladder cancer
- Hemorrhagic cystitis
- Infertility
- Miscarriage
Lymphatic
- Lymphadenopathy
Mucocutaneous
- ↓Hair formation→
  - ◦Alopecia
Pulmonary
- Interstitial fibrosis→
  - ◦Pulmonary hypertension
- **Interstitial pneumonitis−2%** (noninfectious lung inflammation), not being dose related→
  - ◦Dyspnea
  - ◦Nonproductive cough
  - ◦Pulmonary hemorrhage→
    - −Hemoptysis
- Pleuritis→
  - ◦Pleuritic thoracic pain
  - ◦Exudative effusions

Azathioprine/ 6-mercaptopurine monitoring:
- •Baseline:
  - ∘Complete blood count
  - ∘Liver function tests, w/ treatment to be withdrawn @ plasma values >3 X the upper limit of normal
  - …then q2weeks X 2months, then
    - •Q2months

Cyclophosphamide monitoring:
- •Baseline:
  - ∘Complete blood count
  - ∘Liver function tests
  - ∘Renal function
  - ∘Urinalysis
  - …then:
    - •Complete blood count 1week after dose increase, then
      - ∘Q2months
- •Urinalysis w/ cytology q6months after medication is discontinued

Methotrexate monitoring:
- •Baseline:
  - ∘Complete blood count
  - ∘Liver function tests
  - ∘Albumin
  - ∘Renal function
  - ∘Hepatitis B & C serologies
  - ∘Chest x ray
  - …then q2month:
    - •Complete blood count
    - •Liver function tests, w/ treatment to be withdrawn @ plasma values >3 X the upper limit of normal
    - •Albumin
    - •Renal function

PROGNOSIS

- •Treatment→
  - ∘Immunosuppression→
    - −**Infection** (usually opportunistic), being the #1 cause of death
  - ∘Glucocorticoid use→counter-regulatory=anti-insulin effects→
    - •Hyperlipidemia→↑atherosclerosis→coronary artery disease–CAD→**myocardial ischemic syndrome**, being the #3 cause of death
- •Active disease, esp.
  - ∘**Glomerulonephritis**
  - ∘**Lupus encephalitis**
  - …being the #2 cause of death

Poor prognostic factors:
- •Indicate 50% mortality @ 10years w/ any of the following:
  - ∘Anemia
  - ∘Hypertension
  - ∘Hypoalbuminemia
  - ∘Hypocomplementemia
    - −C3 <55mg/ dL
    - −CH50 <37U/ mL
  - ∘Plasma creatinine >1.4mg/ dL
  - ∘Nephrotic syndrome

Median survival:
- •2years–95%
- •5years–85%
- •10years–75%
- •20years–70%

758

RHABDOMYOLYSIS

- •Skeletal muscle death, termed rhabdomyolysis→
  - ◦Rapid release of intracellular contents→
    - –Acute renal failure
    - –Electrolyte abnormalities

RISK FACTORS

- •**Trauma**
  - ◦Burns
  - ◦Crush injuries
  - ◦Electrocution
- •**Absolute ischemia**
  - ◦Systemic thrombo–hemorrhagic syndromes
    - –Disseminated intravascular coagulation–DIC
    - –Hemolytic–uremic syndrome–HUS
    - –Thrombotic thrombocytopenic purpura–TTP
  - ◦Lengthy coma without positional change
  - ◦Prolonged tourniquet application
  - ◦Sickle cell disease
  - ◦Vasculitis
- •**Relative ischemia**
  - ◦**Over–exercising**
  - ◦Status asthmaticus
  - ◦Seizure
- •**Electrolyte abnormalities**
  - ◦Hypocalcemia
  - ◦Hypokalemia, usually @ <2mEq/ L
  - ◦Hypophosphatemia
  - ◦Hypo or hypernatremia
- •**Endocrine**
  - ◦Hypo or hyperthyroidism
  - ◦Severe uncontrolled diabetes mellitus
    - –Diabetic ketoacidosis–DKA
    - –Hyperosmolar hyperglycemic state–HHS
- •**Hyperthermia**
  - ◦Ethanol withdrawal→
    - –Delirium tremens–DTs
  - ◦Heat stroke
    - –↑Body core temperature, usually being ≥107.6°F=42°C, being termed hyperthermia→systemic enzymatic dysfunction→cell dysfunction & death
  - ◦Malignant hyperthermia
    - –Usually in genetically predisposed persons following exposure to Halothane, Pancuronium, or Succinylcholine
  - ◦Neuroleptic malignant syndrome–NMS
    - –Idiosyncratic, life threatening complication of antipsychotic medications
  - ◦Serotonin syndrome
    - –May occur when a monoamine oxidase inhibitor–MAOI is combined w/ another serotonergic medication (any antidepressant, esp. a selective serotonin reuptake inhibitor–SSRI) or opiates (esp. Dextromethorphan, Meperidine)
- •**Hypothermia**
- •**Infectious**
  - ◦Bacteria
    - –Legionella sp.
    - –Listeria sp.
    - –Salmonella sp.
    - –Staphylococcus sp.
    - –Streptococcus sp.
  - ◦Viruses
    - –Adenovirus
    - –Coxsackievirus
    - –Cytomegalovirus–CMV
    - –Echovirus
    - –Epstein–Barr virus–EBV
    - –Herpes simplex virus–HSV
    - –Human immune deficiency virus–HIV

759

    –Influenza virus B
    –Parainfluenza virus
  ∘Sepsis
•**Genetic**
  ∘Muscular dystrophies
  ∘Primary metabolic myopathies
    –Carnitine deficiency
    –Carnitine palmitoyltransferase deficiency
    –Lactate dehydrogenase deficiency
    –Myoadenylate deaminase deficiency
    –Myophosphorylase deficiency, termed McArdle's disease
    –Phosphofructokinase deficiency
    –Phosphoglycerate mutase deficiency
    –Phosphorylase kinase deficiency
    –Short & long chain acyl–coenzyme A dehydrogenase deficiency
•**Medications**
  ∘Benzodiazepines
  ∘Barbiturates
  ∘Colchicine
  ∘Cyclosporine
  ∘Erythromycin
  ∘Glucocorticoids
  ∘**HMG Co–A Reductase Inhibitors**
    –**Myositis–3%** (being dose related & possibly sudden in onset)→muscle pain &/or weakness, which
      may→**rhabdomyolysis <0.5%** (↑risk w/ ↑age, small body frame, hypothyroidism, renal failure &
      when given concomitantly w/ fibric acid medications, bile acid sequestrants, or Niacin)
  ∘Itraconazole
  ∘Neuromuscular blocking medications
  ∘Zidovudine
•**Drugs**
  ∘3, 4–methylenedioxymethamphetamine–MDMA, termed ecstasy
  ∘**Ethanol**
  ∘Ethylene glycol
  ∘Lysergic acid diethylamide–LSD
  ∘Methanol
  ∘Opiates
    –Heroin
    –Methadone
  ∘Phencyclidine
  ∘Amphetamines→
    –↑Release of presynaptic catecholamines
  ∘Cocaine→
    –↓Presynaptic reuptake of released catecholamines
•**Other**
  ∘Dermatomyositis
  ∘Polymyositis
  ∘Hornet sting
  ∘Brown recluse spider bite
  ∘Snake bites, esp. in South America, Africa, & Asia

DIAGNOSIS

Hematologic
•**Myocyte cytoplasm release→**
  ∘↑**Creatine kinase** (>267 IU/ L)
  ∘**Myoglobinemia**
  ∘**Hyperkalemia**†, necessitating a baseline electrocardiogram–ECG, being most severe @ 10–40
    hours after injury
  ∘Hyperphosphatemia→
    –Calcium binding→hypocalcemia
  ∘↑Lactate dehydrogenase–LDH
  ∘↑Uric acid (> ~7mg/ dL)→
    –Gout syndrome
•Disseminated intravascular coagulation–DIC

---

†Also due to possible concomitant renal failure

760

Genitourinary
- •Myoglobinuria→
  - ◦**Red-brown colored urine†** @ >1g/ L
    - Urine dipstick reaction:
      - •Measure hemoglobin (both within erythrocytes & free) & myoglobin, via an orthotolidine reaction. A positive dipstick reaction for occult blood in the absence of erythrocytes on urine microscopy indicates either free hemoglobin or myoglobin in the urine
  - ◦Direct tubular toxicity→
    - –Acute tubular necrosis
  - ◦Obstructive tubular casts
- •Hyperuricemia &/or calcium phosphate→
  - ◦Intratubular crystal formation→
    - –Direct tubular toxicity→acute tubular necrosis
    - –Obstructive tubular casts
  - ...→**intra-renal renal failure-15%**

---

†Indicates the possible presence of hemoglobin (via hemolysis) &/or myoglobin (via rhabdomyolysis) w/ bedside differentiation made via the plasma, which is pink or clear based on the presence of hemoglobin or myoglobin respectively

Gastrointestinal
- •Hepatitis-25%, possibly due to proteases liberated from myocyte lysis

Musculoskeletal
- •Myositis→
  - ◦**Muscle edema, pain, & tenderness ± weakness**

Compartment syndrome
- •Muscle inflammation, termed myositis, & possible subsequent reperfusion→
  - ◦↑Intracompartmental pressure, as unyielding fascial sheaths encase muscle groups, as well as their supporting bones, blood vessels, & nerves into osteofascial compartments→
    - –Peripheral nerve compression→paresthesias, weakness, or paralysis
    - –Vascular compression (venous prior to arterial due to their relatively reduced intravascular pressure)→ischemia, w/ lack of palpable arterial pulses being a late finding
- Diagnosis: If compartment syndrome is suspected, consult an orthopedist emergently
  - •Pain upon passive flexion of the digits is the earliest & most sensitive physical finding indicative of ↑intracompartmental pressure
  - •Diagnosis is made via an indwelling needle-tipped transducer showing a compartment pressure of either:
    - ◦>30mmHg
    - ◦Within 30mmHg of the diastolic blood pressure-DBP
- Treatment:
  - •Emergent fasciotomy

TREATMENT

- •Treatment is indicated w/ either:
  - ◦Myoglobinuria
  - ◦Plasma creatine kinase-CK >5,000 IU/ L

- •**Vigorous intravenous hydration** to achieve a urine output of 100-200mL/ h→↑electrolyte, myoglobin, & uric acid excretion, w/ attention to both:
  - ◦**Intravascular volume repletion via Normal saline** (0.9% NaCl) or **lactated Ringer's solution**, as per:
    - –Vital signs
    - –Physical examination
    - –Urine output (normal being ≥0.5mL/kg/h)
    - –Blood urea nitrogen-BUN & creatinine
  - ◦**Intravascular volume maintenance via Normal saline** (0.9% NaCl) or **lactated Ringer's solution**
    - Adult maintenance fluid:
      - •Weight (kg) + 40= #mL/ hour
    - Additional febrile requirements:
      - •1L/ 24hours for every 1°F >100°F
    - Additional:
      - •Estimate loss for:
        - ◦Diaphoresis
        - ◦Diarrhea
        - ◦Polyuria
        - ◦Tachypnea

...followed by oral rehydration w/ a glucose based electrolyte solution upon both clinical stability & ability to tolerate PO

•**Treat hyperkalemia &/or hypocalcemia as necessary**

•**Urinary alkalinization**
  Mechanism:
    •↑Intravascular volume
    •Urinary alkalinization to a pH >7→
      ○↑Myoglobin and uric acid (as it is a weak acid) solubility→
        −↓Nephropathy risk
  Caution:
    •Urinary alkalinization→
      ○↑Xanthine & calcium phosphate precipitation, which may→
        −Crystal formation→tubular toxicity→acute tubular necrosis→intrarenal renal failure
        ...so avoid urinary alkalinization in patients w/ hyperphosphatemia

SODIUM BICARBONATE		
M ♀	**Dose**	
K ?	75mEq/ 1L of 1/2 normal saline IV, in order to maintain an isoosmolar solution	

±

CARBONIC ANHYDRASE INHIBITOR			
Generic (Trade)	M	♀	**Dose**
Acetazolamide (Diamox) LK	?		250mg PO q24−12hours X several days

Mechanism:
  •↓Carbonic anhydrase activity→
    ○↓Renal tubular bicarbonate ion reabsorption→
      −Bicarbonate diuresis→urinary alkalinization. However, compensatory ↓NaHCO3 renal excretion→a limited bicarbonate diuresis, lasting ≤3 days
Side effects:
  Hematologic
    •↓Renal tubular bicarbonate ion reabsorption→
      ○Hyperchloremic, non−anion gap metabolic acidemia

CARPAL TUNNEL DISEASE

•Carpal tunnel tissue edema &/or infiltration→
  ◦Median nerve compression→
    –Motor, sensory, &/or autonomic neuropathy→weakness, paresthesias, &/or autonomic dysfunction respectively

Statistics:
  •Affects 2.5% of the population→
    ◦#1 entrapment neuropathy

RISK FACTORS

•**Idiopathic**
•**Gender:** ♀ > ♂
•**Repeated minor trauma**, via occupations or vocations requiring:
  ◦↑Hand force in various wrist positions:
    –Crocheting
    –Gardening
    –Knitting
    –Painting
    –Playing musical instruments
    –Typing
    –Using certain tools
    –Upholstering
    –Waiting on tables
    –Weight lifting
    –Woodworking
  ◦Vibration exposure
•**Autoimmune disease**
  ◦Rheumatoid arthritis→
    –Synovitis
•**Endocrine**
  ◦Diabetes mellitus→
    –Endoneural edema
  ◦↑Growth hormone→
    –Acromegally
  ◦Hypothyroidism→
    –↑Interstitial fluid albumin→edema, termed myxedema
•**Infiltrative disease**
  ◦Amyloidosis
•**Medications**
  ◦Glucocorticoids
  ◦Oral contraceptive pills–OCPs
•**Trauma**
  ◦Colles' wrist fracture
  ◦Volar dislocation of the lunate bone
•**Congenital**
  ◦Congenital carpal tunnel stenosis
•**Other**
  ◦Menopause
  ◦Pregnancy, being transient

ANATOMY OF THE CARPAL TUNNEL

•A rigid compartment at the wrist, formed by the concave arch of carpal bones at the base, & roofed by the transverse carpal ligament, forming what is referred to as a tunnel, through which the median nerve & 9 digital flexor tendons pass

DIAGNOSIS

Neurologic
•**Sensory neuropathy**→
  ◦Paresthesias, esp. **pain, numbness, tingling, &/or the subjective sense of edema†** in the:
    –**Lateral 3.5 digits**, initially at the fingertips, w/ most patients reporting all 5 digits as being affected
    –Palm w/ sparing of the lateral aspect, as its sensory nerve (the palmar cutaneous branch of the median nerve) does not pass through the tunnel
    …± radiation to the forearm ± shoulder, w/ all→
      •Difficulty &/or pain upon performing certain tasks requiring wrist motion, such as:
        ◦Unscrewing bottle caps or jar lids
        ◦Turning a key

763

- °↓2 point discrimination, being a late finding
- **Motor neuropathy**→weakness of the:
  - °Abductor pollicis brevis muscle‡→
    - −**Atrophy of the thenar eminence**, being a late finding
  - °Oponens pollicis muscle°
- **Autonomic neuropathy**→
  - °Altered perspiration

Other findings:
- **Tinel's sign:** Percussion w/ a reflex hammer over the volar wrist, over the carpal tunnel, moving distally to the palmar "life line" (being the palmar crease separating the thenar eminence from the rest of the palm) & back to the wrist→
  - °Reproduction of tingling paresthesias...**think "Tinnel's tap"**
  - Outcomes:
    - •Sensitivity–65%
- **Phalen's sign:** Holding the patients wrist in passive maximal flexion, termed hyperflexion X 1min.→
  - °Reproduction of tingling paresthesias...**think "Phalen's fold"**
  - Outcomes:
    - •Sensitivity–75%

---

†Esp. @ night due to sustained wrist flexion during sleep, which may eventually cause awakening, w/ relief via:
- •Shaking or rubbing the hand
- •Hanging the arm out of bed

‡Abductor pollicis brevis muscle strength is assessed via thumb abduction at a right angle to the palm against resistance

°Opponens pollicis muscle strength is assessed via touching the base of the little finger w/ the thumb against resistance

TREATMENT

- **Treatment of possible underlying etiology**
- **Anterior wrist splinting during rest or sleep**
  - °Extending anteriorly from the proximal forearm to the metacarpophalangeal joints immobilizing the wrist in a neutral position
  - Outcomes:
    - •85% of patients experience ↓symptoms within 5 days
- **Surgical decompression, termed carpal tunnel release**
  - Indications:
    - •A fixed neurologic deficit, such as thenar atrophy
    - •Unresponsiveness or intolerance to nonsurgical treatments
  - Procedure:
    - •Flexor retinaculum division, via either an open or closed (endoscopic) procedure
  - Complications, usually being due to poor surgical technique:
    - •Adherent flexor tendons
    - •Hypertrophic scar
    - •Reflex sympathetic dystrophy
    - •Severance of median nerve branches
    - •Surgical scar tenderness within 1year after an open procedure

SECOND LINE TREATMENT

ACETAMINOPHEN

M ♀	Dose	Max
LK P	650mg PO q6hours prn	4g/ 24hours

Mechanism:
- •Reversible inhibition of the cyclooxygenase–COX 1 enzyme in the central nervous system >> peripheral tissues→
  - °Predominantly ↓central nervous system prostaglandin synthesis→
    - −↓Pain
    - −↓Temperature (antipyretic)
    - ...w/ minimal effects on inflammatory cell mediated inflammation

Background physiology:
- •Presynaptic neuronal mediated prostaglandins are released in response to afferent signals, indicating peripheral inflammation→

　　　　∘Enhanced sensitivity of pain neurons (but not direct excitement)→
　　　　　−Pain
　　　•Interleukin−IL1→
　　　　∘↑Hypothalamic prostaglandin production→
　　　　　−Fever

Side effects:
Gastrointestinal
•Hepatitis
　　Mechanism:
　　　　•90% of Acetaminophen undergoes either hepatocyte mediated:
　　　　　∘Glucoronidation→
　　　　　　−Nontoxic glucorinides
　　　　　∘Sulfation→
　　　　　　−Nontoxic sulfates
　　　　•10% of Acetaminophen undergoes hepatocyte mediated oxidation by the cytochrome P450
　　　　enzyme complex→
　　　　　∘A potentially toxic reactive electrophilic compound, which then undergoes either:
　　　　　−Conjugation w/ cellular glutathione→nontoxic compound
　　　　　−Reaction w/ cellular proteins→cellular toxicity ± death→**hepatitis**
　　　　•Normally, glutathione depletion occurs w/ ingestion of >10g of Acetaminophen. However, any
　　　　substance which ↑cytochrome P450 function (such as ethanol) causes relatively more
　　　　Acetaminophen to be diverted to the formation of the toxic compound→
　　　　　∘More rapid hepatocyte depletion of glutathione→
　　　　　−Cell toxicity at lower ingested Acetaminophen doses

Contraindications:
•Do not administer acetaminophen to chronic heavy ethanol drinkers

CYCLOOXYGENASE−COX 2 SELECTIVE INHIBITING NSAIDS

Generic (Trade)	M	♀	Dose
Celecoxib (Celebrex)	L	U	200mg PO q12hours

Mechanism:
　　•Selective, reversible inhibition of the cyclooxygenase−COX 2 enzyme, being responsible for the
　　production of inflammatory cell prostaglandins→
　　　∘↓Pain
　　　∘↓Inflammation
　　　...w/ **minimal cyclooxygenase−COX 1 mediated effects**

Background pathophysiology:
　　•Inflammatory cell mediated prostaglandins are released at sites of inflammation (in addition to other
　　inflammatory cytokines)→
　　　∘Leukocyte migration→↑inflammation via:
　　　　−Vasodilation→↑blood flow→erythema, edema, warmth, &/or tenderness/ pain via enhanced
　　　　neuronal sensitivity

In Brief:
　　•**Cyclooxygenase−COX1 enzymes** are found in most cells of the body, being responsible for
　　normal physiologic processes
　　•**Cyclooxygenase−COX 2 enzymes** are responsible for the production of inflammatory cell
　　prostaglandins

Cyclooxyegenase−COX 1 mediated effects	Effects of relatively ↓inhibition
Hypothalamic prostaglandin synthesis	No antipyretic effect
Platelet thromboxane A_2 synthesis	No antiplatelet effect
Gastric mucosal cell prostaglandin synthesis	↓Peptic inflammatory disease risk
Glomerular afferent arteriole prostaglandin synthesis	↓Renal failure risk

Side effects:
Cardiovascular
　　•Hypertension
Gastrointestinal
　　•Inhibition of the cyclooxygenase−COX1 enzyme→↑peptic inflammatory disease risk→↑**upper**
　　gastrointestinal hemorrhage risk via:
　　　∘↓Gastric mucosal prostaglandin synthesis→
　　　　−↓Epithelial proliferation
　　　　−↓Mucosal blood flow→↓bicarbonate delivery to the mucosa

765

−↓Mucus & bicarbonate secretion from gastric mucosal cells

Genitourinary
- •Patients w/ pre−existing bilateral ↓renal perfusion, not necessarily failure:
  - ◦Heart failure
  - ◦Bilateral renal artery stenosis
  - ◦Hypovolemia
  - ◦Renal failure
  - …rely more on the compensatory production of vasodilatory prostaglandins→
    - •Afferent arteriole dilation→
      - ◦Maintained glomerular filtration rate−GFR, whereas NSAIDs→
        - −↓Prostaglandin production, which may→renal failure

Pulmonary
- •Inhibition of both cyclooxygenase enzymes (COX 1 & COX2)→
  - ◦↑Lipoxygenase activity→
    - −↑Leukotriene synthesis→symptomatic asthma within 2hours of ingestion in 5% of asthmatics

Caution:
- •Minimal inhibition of COX−1→
  - ◦↓Endothelial & vascular smooth muscle cell prostacyclin† production relative to platelet thromboxane‡ production→cytokine imbalance in favor of vasoconstriction→
    - −Hypertension
    - −↑Cerebrovascular accident syndrome risk
    - −↑Myocardial ischemic syndrome risk

Contraindications:
- •Sulfa hypersensitivity due to a sulfa moiety

THIRD LINE TREATMENT ■■■■■■■■

NONSTEROIDAL ANTI-INFLAMMATORY DRUGS−NSAIDs

Generic	M ♀	Start	Max
Ibuprofen	L P in 1st & 2nd, U in 3rd trimester	600mg PO q8hours	3.2g/ 24hours
Indomethacin	L P in 1st & 2nd, U in 3rd trimester	50mg PO/ PR q8hours	
Naproxen	L P in 1st & 2nd, U in 3rd trimester	375mg PO q12hours	
•XR form		750mg PO q24hours	

- •One cannot predict which NSAID a patient will respond to
- •Attempt to eventually ↓dosage &/or limit use to exacerbations in order to ↓side effect risk

Mechanism:
- •Aspirin & other anti−inflammatory medications→
  - ◦Respectively to irreversible & reversible inhibition of both cyclooxygenase enzymes (COX−1 & COX−2), being responsible for the production of neural & inflammatory cell prostaglandins respectively→
    - −↓Pain
    - −↓Temperature (antipyretic)
    - −↓Inflammation

Background pathophysiology:
- •Inflammatory cell mediated prostaglandins are released at sites of inflammation (in addition to other inflammatory cytokines)→
  - ◦Leukocyte migration→↑inflammation via:
    - −Vasodilation→↑blood flow→erythema, edema, warmth, &/or tenderness/ pain via enhanced neuronal sensitivity
- •Interleukin−IL1→
  - ◦↑Hypothalamic prostaglandin production→
    - −Fever

In Brief:
- •**Cyclooxygenase−COX1 enzymes** are found in most cells of the body, being responsible for normal physiologic processes
- •**Cyclooxygenase−COX 2 enzymes** are responsible for the production of inflammatory cell prostaglandins

Side effects:
Gastrointestinal
- Inhibition of the cyclooxygenase−COX1 enzyme→↑peptic inflammatory disease risk→**↑upper gastrointestinal hemorrhage risk** via:
  - ∘↓Gastric mucosal prostaglandin synthesis→
    - −↓Epithelial cell proliferation
    - −↓Mucosal blood flow→↓bicarbonate delivery to the mucosa
    - −↓Mucus & bicarbonate secretion from gastric mucosal cells

Indications for peptic inflammatory disease prophylaxis:
- Prophylax w/ proton pump inhibitors−PPI's, histamine 2 selective receptor blockers, or Misoprostol in patients w/ any of the following:
  - ∘Age >60 years w/ a history of peptic inflammatory disease
  - ∘Anticipated therapy >3 months
  - ∘Concurrent glucocorticoid use
  - ∘Moderate to high dose NSAID use
Note: Newer NSAIDs (Etodolac, Nabumetone, Salsalate)→
  - •↓Risk of NSAID induced peptic inflammation/ ulcer

Genitourinary
- Patients w/ pre-existing bilateral ↓renal perfusion, not necessarily failure:
  - ∘Heart failure
  - ∘Bilateral renal artery stenosis
  - ∘Hypovolemia
  - ∘Renal failure
  - …rely more on the compensatory production of vasodilatory prostaglandins→
    - •Afferent arteriole dilation→
      - ∘Maintained glomerular filtration rate−GFR, whereas NSAIDs→
        - −↓Prostaglandin production, which may→renal failure
Pulmonary
- Inhibition of both cyclooxygenase enzymes (COX 1 & COX2)→
  - ∘↑Lipoxygenase activity→
    - −↑Leukotriene synthesis→symptomatic asthma within 2hours of ingestion in 5% of asthmatics

FOURTH LINE TREATMENT
- **Carpal tunnel glucocorticoid injection**
  Procedure:
  1. Rest the hand palm up
  2. Inject hydrocortisone acetate, 25mg intra−articular @ 90° through the distal transverse skin crease of the anterior wrist, several millimeters to the ulnar side flexor carpi radialis
  Complications:
  - Sudden pain if the needle enters the median nerve, requiring reposition
  Outcomes:
  - Variable & short-lasting effects. If pain relief is not achieved for several months w/ 1−2 injections, then abandon this treatment, as ≥3 intra−articular injections/ year→
    - ∘↑Tissue breakdown→
      - −↑Disease severity

•Caused by any disease→
  ∘↓Intracranial blood flow→
    −↓Neurologic function, being either transient or chronic

Statistics:
  •#3 cause of death in the U.S. (#1 being myocardial ischemic syndromes & #2 being cancer),
  responsible for the death of 25% of the adult population
  •>1million adults are left disabled yearly, being the #1 cause of serious long term disability in the U.S.

RISK FACTORS

•**Age:** ♂ ≥45years, ♀ ≥menopause=~50years (esp. @ ≥65years)
•**Gender:** ♂ > ♀ due to the protective effects of estrogens &/or possible atherogenic effects of androgens
•**Genetic**
  ∘Significant family history of myocardial ischemic syndrome or sudden death in a first degree relative
    −♂ **<55years**
    −♀ **<65years**
  ∘Homocystinemia
  ∘Genetic lipid diseases
•↑**Atherosclerosis**
  ∘**Endothelial stress/ damage**
    −**Cigarette smoking, being the #1 risk factor**
    −**Hypertension**
    −Homocystinemia
  ∘**Hyperlipidemia**
    −Total cholesterol ≥200mg/ dL in adults
    −Low density lipoprotein–LDL cholesterol† ≥130mg/ dL
    −Triglycerides ≥150mg/ dL
  ∘**Known peripheral or cerebrovascular disease**
  ∘↑**Hepatocyte lipoprotein formation**
    −High fat diet
    −Genetic disposition
    −Nephrotic syndrome
  ∘↓**Hepatocyte lipoprotein removal**
    −**Diabetes mellitus**
    −Estrogen containing medications (oral contraceptives–OCPs, hormone replacement therapy–HRT)
    −Genetic disposition
    −Hypothyroidism
  ∘↓**Vascular cholesterol removal**
    −↓High density lipoprotein–HDL level (<40mg/ dL)
  ∘**HIV infected patients** treated w/ combination antiretroviral regimens experience ↑**atherosclerosis** via:
    ∘HIV &/or antiretroviral mediated endothelial inflammation
    ∘HIV &/or antiretroviral mediated dyslipidemia
    ∘Antiretroviral mediated insulin resistance
•**Hematologic disease**
  ∘Hypercoagulable state
  ∘Sickle cell anemia
•**Type A aortic dissection→**
  ∘Right carotid artery ostial occlusion
•**Personality**
  ∘Poor stress management, w/ a tendency to react to various situations w/ anger &/or frustration
•**Sedentary lifestyle**
•**Illicit drug use**
  ∘Amphetamines→
    −↑Release of presynaptic catecholamines
  ∘Cocaine→
    −↓Presynaptic reuptake of released catecholamines
•**Altered vascular flow**, via thromboembolic disease
  ∘**Altered myocardial contraction**
    −**Atrial flutter or fibrillation**
    −Cardiomyopathy
    −Ischemic ± infarcted myocardial segment
    −Ventricular aneurysm

∘**Valve disease**
  −Left sided, esp. w/ mitral or aortic stenosis
  −Right sided via an atrial/ ventricular septal defect or a patent foramen ovale
•**Deep venous thromboembolism**, via an atrial/ ventricular septal defect or a patent foramen ovale
•**Cerebral vasoconstriction**
  ∘Eclampsia
  ∘Migraine headache
  ∘Subarachnoid or intraparenchymal hemorrhage
•**Mechanical prosthetic valves**, which serve as nidus for thrombus formation→
  ∘Thromboembolus
•**Myxoma**, which serves as nidus for thrombus formation→
  ∘Thromboembolus
•**Endocarditis**
  ∘Septic embolus→
  −Ischemia
  −Mycotic aneurysm formation→↑hemorrhage risk
  ∘Noninfectious=marantic endocarditis→
  −Thromboembolus
•**Inflammation**
  ∘↑**C reactive protein−CRP** (>2mg/ L), being an acute phase reactant used as a marker of systemic inflammation, being directly proportionate to severity. Elevation indicates ↑vascular disease risk via:
  −Atherosclerotic plaque mediated inflammation
  −C−reactive protein mediated compliment & endothelial cell activation, as well as tissue damage
  …↔↑atherosclerotic plaque formation & instability (a vicious cycle)
  Outcomes:
  •↑C reactive protein→
  ∘↑All cause mortality in the elderly
•**Obesity**, specifically referring to excess total body fat
  Body mass index−BMI‡ classification:
  •<18.5: Underweight
  •18.5−24.9: Normal
  •25−29.9: Overweight
  •30−34.9: Mild obesity
  •35−39.9: Moderate obesity
  •≥40: Severe, termed morbid obesity, being ≥2X the upper limit of normal body weight
  Waist circumference based obesity classification:
  •As body fat distribution affects health risks, meeting the following criteria indicate the need for weight loss regardless of BMI
  ∘**>40 inches** indicates ↑cardiovascular risk in ♂s
  ∘**>35 inches** indicates ↑cardiovascular risk in ♀s

Hemorrhagic specific risk factors:
•**Skin color/ ethnicity:** Blacks, Japanese
•**Intracranial arterial aneurysm−80%**
  ∘At the base of the brain, an anastomotic ring is formed between the vertebral & internal carotid arteries, termed the **Circle of Willis**→collateral circulation, being important if a vessel is occluded. This anastomotic ring & its bifurcations are the #1 site of intracranial aneurysms
  −**Middle cerebral artery−30%**
  −Internal carotid artery−15%
  −Anterior communicating artery−15%
  −Basilar artery−15%
  −Anterior cerebral artery−10%
  −Posterior communicating artery−6%
  −Vertebral artery−6%
  −Posterior cerebral artery−3%
•**Arteriovenous malformation−AVM−15%**
•**Other−5%**
  ∘**Coagulopathy**
  ∘**Hypertension**
  −**Putamen or thalamus−70%**
  −Cerebellum−10%
  −Cerebral white matter−10%
  −Pons−10%
  ∘**Trauma**
  ∘**Tumor**
  ∘**Vasculitis**

†LDL=total cholesterol − HDL − (triglycerides/ 5).
‡BMI= Weight (kg)   or   Weight (lbs)
         Height (m)²   Height (in)² X 703.1

•**High density lipoprotein–HDL** >60mg/ dL

CLASSIFICATION
•**Ischemic cerebrovascular accident–80%**
  Mechanism:
    •Thrombotic ± embolic mediated arterial occlusion→
      ◦Distal ischemia ± infarction→
        −**Reperfusion hemorrhage–20%**, usually occurring within 3 days postinfarction
  Thrombotic source:
    •Extraparenchymal artery disease–25%
    •Intraparenchymal artery disease–15%
  Thromboembolic source:
    •Artery–25%
    •Cardiogenic–15%
  Subclassification, based on duration of neurologic deficit(s)†:
    •**Transient ischemic attack–TIA‡**, via deficit lasting ≤24hours, usually ≤2hours
    •**Stroke**, via deficit lasting >24hours, or causing death within 24hours
      ◦Progressive ischemic stroke–20%, via deficit progression over the following several days
      ◦Minor stroke, via deficit lasting ≤3weeks
      ◦Major stroke, via deficit lasting >3weeks
      ...w/ a **lacunar stroke–20%** indicating the thrombosis or embolic enlodgement of a small
        penetrating artery, esp. the lenticulostriate arterial branches of the middle cerebral artery
        supplying the internal capsule→
        •Small area of infarcted tissue

•**Hemorrhagic cerebrovascular accident–20%**
  Mechanism:
    •Hemorrhage→
      ◦Distal ischemia ±
      −Infarction
      −Brain tissue displacement=mass effect
    •**Subarachnoid hemorrhage–10%**
    •**Intraparenchymal hemorrhage–10%** ± tissue dissection→
      ◦Subarachnoid hemorrhage
      ◦Ventricular hemorrhage

---

†**The duration criteria are now outdated as magnetic resonance imaging–MRI now allows for the
detection of infarcted cerebral tissue within min. to hours, depending on the particular modality
utilized**
‡Although thought to indicate a non–infarct ischemic event, ~50% of patients meeting the deficit duration
criteria for a transient ischemic attack have evidence of infarction via magnetic resonance imaging–MRI

PATHOPHYSIOLOGY OF ATHEROSCLEROSIS
•A disease of lipoprotein (composed of cholesterol & other lipids) deposition, being limited to arteries &
arterioles throughout the body, w/ resultant intermittent localized:
  ◦Smooth muscle cell hyperplasia, w/ concomitant intimal migration, termed neointimal hyperplasia
  ◦Fibroblast deposition of connective tissue=fibrosis
  ◦Calcium salt deposition→
    −Bone hard calcifications
  ...→atherosclerotic plaque formation→
    •Luminal bulging→
      ◦**Vascular luminal narrowing**
•The atherosclerotic plaque is considered stable unless it protrudes through the covering endothelium,
w/ **instability having little to do w/ the degree of vascular luminal narrowing, but rather w/
intermittent periods of intense biologic activity or endothelial damage**†→
  ◦Exposure of subendothelial collagen & atherosclerotic plaque→
    −Platelet adhesion & activation
    −Fibrin deposition
    ...→**thrombus formation & vasospasm**

•As the intimal atherosclerotic plaque enlarges, medial smooth muscle cells are lost→
  ◦Vascular wall weakening→dilation, **termed aneurysm**→
    −↑Rupture risk
    −Altered blood flow
    …→thrombus formation

NEURONAL EXCITOTOXICITY
•Central nervous system ischemia→
  ◦↑**Extraneuronal glutamic acid concentration**→
    −Toxic glutamic acid receptor stimulation, termed neuronal excitoxicity. Although neurons located
      deep within an ischemic focus die from O_2 deprivation, **neurons being progressively more to the
      periphery appear to die increasingly due to concomitant excessive glutamic acid
      concentrations**

DIAGNOSIS
General
•Fever–50%, due to either:
  ◦Cerebral inflammation
  ◦Concomitant infection, esp. aspiration pneumonia
  ◦Thromboembolism
Neurologic
•Central nervous system ischemia ± infarction→
  ◦Neuronal/ neuroglial dysfunction or death respectively→
    −**Sudden ↓ability to perform ≥1 nervous system mediated task(s),** based on the areas
      affected

Lesion localization:
  •**Middle cerebral artery–MCA,** supplying the:
    ◦Lateral frontal, temporal, parietal, occipital lobes
    ◦Caudate nucleus
    ◦Putamen
    ◦Internal capsule
    …→
        •Contralateral hemiparesis
        •Hemisensory loss
        •Bilateral loss of the same visual field half (nasal or temporal)=homonymous
          hemianopsia
        •↓Communication ability (expression &/or understanding)=aphasia, if the dominant
          hemisphere is affected
        •Neglect if the non–dominant hemisphere is affected
  •**Anterior cerebral artery–ACA,** supplying the:
    ◦Medial frontal & parietal lobes
    ◦Anterior corpus callosum
    …→
        •Contralateral lower extremity paresis &/or sensory loss
  •**Posterior cerebral artery–PCA** (distal territory), supplying the:
    ◦Medial temporal & occipital lobes
    ◦Corpus callosum
    …→
        •Optic tract &/or optic radiation ischemia→
          ◦Bilateral loss of the same visual field half (nasal or temporal)=homonymous
            hemianopsia
  •**Posterior cerebral artery–PCA** (proximal territory), supplying the:
    ◦Thalamus
    ◦Midbrain
    …→
        •Contralateral hemiparesis
        •Incoordination=ataxia
        •Occulomotor nerve palsy
        •Vertical gaze palsy
        •Skew deviation
        •Hemiballismus
        •Choreoathetosis
        •↓Consciousness

771

- **Vertebral artery,** branching into the **posterior inferior cerebellar artery-PICA,** supplying the:
  - Medulla
  - Lower cerebellum
  - ... →
    - Ipsilateral cerebellar ataxia
    - Difficulty speaking=dysarthria
    - Difficulty swallowing=dysphagia
    - Nystagmus
    - Spinning sensation=vertigo
    - Hiccup
    - Horner's syndrome
    - Crossed sensory loss
- **Basilar artery,** branching into the **anterior inferior cerebellar artery-AICA & superior cerebellar artery,** supplying the:
  - Lower midbrain
  - Pons
  - Mid to upper cerebellum
  - ... →
    - Hemi or quadraparesis
    - Ipsilateral cerbebellar ataxia
    - Nystagmus
    - Spinning sensation=vertigo
    - Double vision=diplopia
    - Skew deviation
    - Gaze palsies
    - Hemi or crossed sensory loss
    - Horner's syndrome
    - ↓Consciousness

- Central nervous system hemorrhage &/or edema→
  - ↑Intracranial pressure→
    - Tissue displacement=mass effect→↓function of multiple areas, distant from the area initially affected
- **Seizures-10%,** esp. focal, usually within 24hours
- Brainstem reticular activating system-RAS injury, due to either:
  - Ischemia
  - Mass effect mediated compression
  - Generalized nonconvulsive seizure
  - Postictal state
  - ...→unconsciousness

Musculoskeletal
- Motor cortex or internal capsule ischemia→either:
  - Contralateral **weakness=hemiparesis**
  - Contralateral **paralysis=hemiplegia**

ELECTRICAL STUDIES

- **Electrocardiogram-ECG**
  Indications:
  - Possible myocardial ischemic syndrome &/or dysrhythmia
  - Monitoring may be useful for suspected paroxysmal atrial fibrillation

IMAGING

- **Head computed tomographic-CT scan without contrast**
  Indications:
  - To differentiate a hemorrhagic stroke from an ischemic event
  - To document the extent of the stroke
  - To diagnose a possible space occupying lesion (tumor or abscess) mediated stroke
  Findings:
  - **A hemorrhage is viewed as a hyperdense lesion**
  - **An infarction is viewed as a hypodense lesion,** usually @ ≥12-24hours, ± reperfusion hemorrhage within 3 days
  Advantages:
  - **Superior to magnetic resonance imaging-MRI in detecting a hemorrhage within 48hours**
  Note: Subsequent encephalomalacic change over months to years→
  - ↓Tissue density & ↑cerebrospinal fluid→
    - Low density lesion

772

- **Head magnetic resonance imaging–MRI**
  - Indications:
    - •↑Ischemic stroke sensitivity
    - •↑Visualization of the posterior cranial fossa contents (cerebellum, pons, & medulla oblongata)
  - Findings:
    - **•An infarction is viewed a a hyperdense lesion**
  - Contraindications:
    - •Because the MRI uses magnetic pulses, it is contraindicated in patients w/ cardiac pacemakers, mechanical heart valves, cochlear implants, intracranial aneurism clips, intraocular metallic foreign bodies

- **Diffusion weighted imaging MRI**
  - Indications:
    - **•Allows for most infarctions to be detected within several min. of occurrence,** rather than several hours, as w/ conventional MRI
    - **•Allows differentiation of acute vs. subacute or chronic ischemic changes,** which do not appear hyperdense
  - Mechanism:
    - •Detects the random movement of water molecules, termed Brownian motion within the cerebral parenchyma. An acute infarction→
      - ∘Cell membrane Na^+/K^+ ATPase dysfunction→
        - −↑Na^+–H_2O coupled intracellular movement→cytotoxic edema→↓extracellular volume→ ↓osmosis, which can be visualized as a **hyperdense lesion**. Other cerebral lesions, such as a contusion, demyelinating diseases, infection, & tumor are not associated w/ cytotoxic edema (unless central tumor necrosis occurs) & so do not appear hyperdense

- **Carotid artery doppler ultrasound**
  - Mechanism:
    - •Visualizes the common carotid artery & proximal internal carotid artery for possible stenosis
    - •The force of compressing the ultrasound probe against the skin→
      - ∘Normal venous collapse
    - •Doppler ultrasonography uses Doppler shift to detect vessel flow velocity, allowing differentiation of veins from arteries
    - …both together are termed duplex compression ultrasonography=duplex ultrasonography

- **Transcranial Doppler ultrasound**
  - Mechanism:
    - •Visualizes the large intracranial arteries @ the base of the brain for possible stenosis

- **Magnetic resonance angiography–MRA**
  - Mechanism:
    - •Visualizes the intracranial arteries for possible stenosis, aneurysm, or arteriovenous malformation

- **Transthoracic echocardiography–TTE**
  - Indications:
    - •All patients, in order to evaluate for possible cardiogenic embolism
  - Procedure:
    - •A 2 dimensional ultrasonographic image, allowing real time visualization of:
      - ∘Ventricular wall thickness
      - ∘Cavity size (both atrial & ventricular)
      - ∘Myocardial & valve function, allowing ejection fraction–EF estimation (% of end diastolic volume ejected during ventricular systole)
      - ∘The pericardial space
    - •Doppler ultrasonography uses Doppler shift to detect vessel flow velocity→
      - ∘Valve regurgitation visualization
      - ∘Estimation of valve pressure gradients
  - Limitations:
    - •↓Visualization in obese or emphysematous patients
    - •May not allow adequate:
      - ∘Visualization of the anterior aspect of a prosthetic aortic valve
      - ∘Functional assessment of a prosthetic aortic valve
    - •Transesophageal echocardiography–TEE is more sensitive in detecting:
      - ∘Thrombotic ± infectious vegetations
      - ∘Abscesses
      - ∘Valve damage
      - …esp. in a patient w/ a prosthetic heart valve. However, transthoracic echocardiography is the

initial test of choice due to its noninvasive nature, as transesophageal echocardiography may→
•Pharyngeal swallow receptor mediated reflex:
  ◦Bradycardia
  ◦Hypotension

ACUTE TREATMENT OF ISCHEMIC CEREBROVASCULAR ACCIDENT

•**Oxygen** to maintain PaO_2 >60mmHg or SaO_2 >92%, usually accomplished via nasal cannula @ 2-4L/min.
Mechanism:
  •Oxygenation if required
  •Calming effect→
    ◦↓Autonomic sympathetic tone→
      −↓Myocardial O_2 & nutrient demand
Duration:
  •24–48hours, or longer if needed for oxygenation
•**Antipyretics** if febrile, as fever→
  ◦↑Cellular O_2 & nutrient demand
•**Hyperglycemic control** in diabetic patients, as hyperglycemia→
  ◦↑Ischemic cellular anaerobic glycolysis→
    −Cerebral lactic acidemia→neuronal dysfunction ± death
•**Cardiac monitor**, due to ↑dysrhythmia risk during the 1st 24hours
•**Swallow evaluation**, as dysphagia is a common complication
•**Hypertension management**
  ◦Hypertension is common in the early period of cerebral ischemia, & should be considered a compensatory mechanism in response to ↓cerebral autoregulation in the affected area, thus ensuring adequate perfusion. **Discontinue all antihypertensive medications** which the patient may be taking, & **lay the patient in a supine position** (or as flat as tolerated due to orthopnea) to further ↑cerebral perfusion pressure
Indications to lower the blood pressure:
  •Systolic blood pressure ≥210mmHg or diastolic blood pressure ≥120mmHg
  •Systolic blood pressure ≥180mmHg or diastolic blood pressure ≥110mmHg in either:
    ◦Symptomatic patients (other than stroke syndrome), termed hypertensive emergency
    ◦Patients to receive thrombolytic treatment

INTRACRANIAL ARTERY THROMBOSIS ± EMBOLUS

PLATELET INHIBITING MEDICATIONS
Efficacy: Glycoprotein 2b/ 3a inhibitors > thienopyridines > Aspirin

Generic	M	♀	Dose
Acetylsalicylic acid–ASA=Aspirin	K	U	325mg crushed or chewed PO X1, or PR if unable to timely administer PO, then 81mg PO q24hours lifelong

Mechanism:
  •Aspirin is the only nonsteroidal anti–inflammatory drug–NSAID→
    ◦Irreversible inhibition of both cyclooxygenase–COX enzymes (COX1 & COX2), w/ COX1 being responsible for the production of both thromboxane A_2† & prostacyclin‡→
      −**Near complete inhibition of platelet thromboxane A_2 production within 15 min.**, w/ endothelial & vascular smooth muscle cells producing new enzymes in several hours→ relatively ↑prostacyclin
  •Being that platelets lack the enzymatic machinery for protein synthesis, only newly formed platelets (platelet half life=10 days) have the functional enzyme
  …this shift in the balance of cytokine production→
    •↓**Thrombus formation**

In Brief:
  •**Cyclooxygenase–COX1 enzymes** are found in most cells of the body, being responsible for normal physiologic processes
  •**Cyclooxygenase–COX 2 enzymes** are responsible for the production of inflammatory cell prostaglandins

---

•Concomitant NSAID administration→
  ◦Competition for the cyclooxygenase–COX 1 enzyme binding site, w/:
    −Unbound Aspirin being rapidly cleared from plasma
    −Bound NSAID action being reversible & short lived
    …→↓overall antiplatelet effect, requiring either:

- •Aspirin to be taken @ ≥1hour prior to other NSAIDs
- •Switch to thienopyridine derivative for the antiplatelet effect

†Platelet mediated **thromboxane A$_2$** release at the site of vascular injury→
- •Platelet aggregation
- •Vasoconstriction
- …w/ both processes→
  - •Thrombus formation

‡Endothelial & vascular smooth muscle cell mediated **prostacyclin** release in the surrounding area→
- •Inhibition of platelet aggregation
- •Vasodilation
- …w/ both processes→
  - •↓Thrombus formation

Outcomes:
- •↓Morbidity & mortality

Side effects:
Gastrointestinal
- •Inhibition of the cyclooxygenase-COX1 enzyme→↑peptic inflammatory disease risk→↑**upper gastrointestinal hemorrhage risk** via:
  - ○↓Gastric mucosal prostaglandin synthesis→
    - −↓Epithelial cell proliferation
    - −↓Mucosal blood flow→↓bicarbonate delivery to the mucosa
    - −↓Mucus & bicarbonate secretion from gastric mucosal cells

Indications for peptic inflammatory disease prophylaxis:
- •Prophylax w/ proton pump inhibitors-PPI's, histamine 2 selective receptor blockers, or Misoprostol in patients w/ any of the following:
  - ○Age >60 years w/ a history of peptic inflammatory disease
  - ○Anticipated therapy >3 months
  - ○Concurrent glucocorticoid use
  - ○Moderate to high dose NSAID use
  - Note: Newer NSAIDs (Etodolac, Nabumetone, Salsalate)→
    - •↓Risk of NSAID induced peptic inflammation/ ulcer

Genitourinary
- •Patients w/ pre-existing bilateral ↓renal perfusion, not necessarily failure:
  - ○Heart failure
  - ○Bilateral renal artery stenosis
  - ○Hypovolemia
  - ○Renal failure
  - …rely more on the compensatory production of vasodilatory prostaglandins→
    - •Afferent arteriole dilation→
      - ○Maintained glomerular filtration rate-GFR, whereas NSAIDs→
        - −↓Prostaglandin production, which may→renal failure

Pulmonary
- •Inhibition of both cyclooxygenase enzymes (COX 1 & COX2)→
  - ○↑Lipoxygenase activity→
    - −↑Leukotriene synthesis→symptomatic asthma within 2hours of ingestion in 5% of asthmatics

Rheumatologic
- •Acetylsalicylic acid competes w/ uric acid secretion in the renal tubules→
  - ○↑Uric acid levels→
    - −↑Risk of uric acid precipitation in the tissues=gout

Pediatric
- •**Reye's syndrome**
  - ○A life threatening fulminant hepatitis→
    - −Hepatic encephalopathy in children age ≤16 years w/ a viral infection (esp. influenza or Varicella-zoster virus-VZV)

Overdose:
Pulmonary
- •Direct brainstem respiratory center mediated stimulation of pulmonary ventilation→
  - ○Hyperventilation→
    - −**Initial respiratory alkalemia, w/ the subsequent development of an anion gap metabolic acidemia**
- •Pulmonary edema

Neurologic
- Altered mental status
- Aseptic meningitis
- Depression
- Hallucinations
- Hyperactivity
- Hyperthermia
- Lightheadedness
- Seizures
- Tinnitus

Gastrointestinal
- Nausea ± vomiting

Mucocutaneous
- Pharyngitis

THIENOPYRIDINE DERIVATIVE

Indications:
- Intolerance to Aspirin

Generic (Trade)	M	♀	Dose
Clopidogrel (Plavix)	LK	P	300mg PO loading dose, then 75mg PO q24hours

Mechanism:
- Inhibits adenosine diphosphate–ADP mediated activation of the glycoprotein 2b/ 3a complex→
  - ↓Platelet activation

- A 300mg loading dose may be used, as maximal effect occurs @ 5hours rather than 5days w/ initiation of the standard 75mg dosage

Side effects:
Gastrointestinal
- Diarrhea

Mucocutaneous
- Dermatitis

Hematologic
- **Thrombotic thrombocytopenic purpura–TTP** within several weeks of initiation

LIPID LOWERING MEDICATIONS

Indications:
- All patients w/ atherosclerotic mediated mediated cerebrovascular accident syndromes should receive an HMG Co–A reductase inhibitor during hospitalization, & indefinitely regardless of baseline LDL, unless intolerant due to side effects

Relative lipid effects:
- **HMG Co–A reductase inhibitors** correct all lipids, esp. Atorvastatin, Rosuvastatin & Simvastatin

HMG Co–A REDUCTASE INHIBITORS

Generic (Trade)	M	♀	Max
Atorvastatin (Lipitor)	L	U	80mg qhs
Fluvastatin (Lescol)	L	U	80mg qhs
Lovastatin (Mevacor)	L	U	80mg qhs
Pravastatin (Pravachol)	L	U	80mg qhs
Rosuvastatin (Crestor)	L	U	40mg qhs
Simvastatin (Zocor)	L	U	80mg qhs

- These medications are maximally effective if administered in the evening, when the majority of cholesterol synthesis occurs

Mechanisms:
- Inhibit hydroxymethylglutaryl coenzyme A reductase function, being the hepatocyte rate limiting enzyme in cholesterol formation→
  - ↓Hepatic cholesterol formation→
    - Feedback ↑hepatocyte LDL receptor formation→↑**plasma LDL cholesterol removal**
- Anti–inflammatory effects→
  - ↓Atherosclerotic plaque formation, w/ ↑stability

Side effects:
Gastrointestinal
•**Hepatitis–1.5%**, usually starting within 3months of initial or ↑dose, being:
  ◦Dose related
  ◦Gradual in onset
  ◦Usually benign
•Nausea ± vomiting
Musculoskeletal
•**Myositis–3%**, being:
  ◦Dose related
  ◦Possibly sudden in onset
  ...→muscle pain &/or weakness which progress to **rhabdomyolysis <0.5%**, diagnosed via
    ↑creatine kinase–CK levels
  Risk factors:
    •↑Age
    •Hypothyroidism
    •Renal failure
    •Small body frame
    •Concomitant administration of:
      ◦Fibric acid medications
      ◦Bile acid sequestrants
      ◦Niacin
Neurologic
•Headaches
•Sleep disturbances
Ophthalmologic
•Minor lens opacities
Interactions
•**Garlic & St. Johns wort→**
  ◦↑Hepatocyte cytochrome P450 system activity→
    −↑HMG–CoA reductase inhibitor degradation→↓plasma levels (except Pravastatin)
•**Diltiazem & protease inhibitors→**
  ◦↓Hepatocyte cytochrome P450 system activity→
    −↓HMG–CoA reductase inhibitor degradation→↑plasma levels (except Pravastatin)

Monitoring:
•Baseline:
  ◦**Liver function tests,** then
    −3months after dose↑, then periodically thereafter, w/ treatment to be withdrawn @ plasma
     values >3X the upper limit of normal
  ◦**Creatine kinase** (as an asymptomatic ↑ may be present), then
    −Prior to dose↑ or adding an interacting medication, in order to compare future possible values,
     to be obtained if symptomatic, w/ treatment to be discontinued @ either plasma values >10X
     the upper limit of normal, or lower if class switching fails to relieve the syndrome

ADDITIONAL TREATMENT FOR CAROTID ARTERY THROMBOSIS ± EMBOLUS ▄▄▄▄
•**Carotid endarterectomy**
  Indications:
    •Transient ischemic attack or minor stroke due to ipsilateral **extracranial carotid artery
     atherosclerotic stenosis of ≥50 (100% occlusion being inoperable), in centers where the
     surgical risk of stroke is <6%**
  Mechanism:
    •Excision of the diseased arterial endothelium, & much or all of the media, along w/ the occluding
     atheroma→
      ◦Residual smooth lining, consisting mostly of adventitia
  Complications:
    •Bradycardia
    •Cerebrovascular accident
    •Cranial nerve injury
    •Hypotension
    •Myocardial infarction
    •Restenosis

ANTICOAGULANTS: High molecular weight

Treatment initiation:
- **Transient ischemic attack–TIA:** Promptly
- **Small ischemic infarct:** @ >48hours if repeat CT scan rules out hemorrhage
- **Large ischemic infarct:** @ >5days if repeat CT scan rules out hemorrhage

M	♀	Start
M	?	60units/ kg IV bolus (or 5000units empirically)
		12units/kg/hour infusion (or 1000units/ hour empirically)

- Titrated by 2.5units/kg/hour to achieve an activated partial thromboplastin time–aPTT of 1.5–2X control value or **50–70seconds**

aPTT (seconds)	Action	Obtain next aPTT
<40	Bolus 5000units & ↑infusion rate by 100units/ hours	6hours
40–49	↑Infusion rate by 50units/ hours	6hours
50–70 (or 1.5–2Xcontrol)	NO ACTION	**24hours**
71–85	↓Infusion rate by 50units/ hours	6hours
86–100	Hold infusion 30min., then ↓infusion rate by 100units/ hours	6hours
101–150	Hold infusion 60min., then ↓infusion rate by 150units/ hours	6hours
>150	Hold infusion 60min., then ↓infusion rate by 300units/ hours	6hours

Monitoring:
- Complete blood count q24hours to monitor for side effects

ANTICOAGULANTS: Low molecular weight Heparin

Generic (Trade)	M	♀	Start	Max
Enoxaparin (Lovenox)	KL	P	1.5mg/ kg SC q24hours or	180mg/ 24hours
			1mg/ kg SC q12hours	
Dalteparin (Fragmin)	KL	P	200 anti–factor Xa units/ kg SC q24hours or	18,000units q24hours
			100 anti–factor Xa units/ kg SC q12hours	

Dose adjustment:
- Obesity
  - Most manufacturers recommend a maximum dose of that for a 90kg patient

Monitoring:
- Monitoring of anti–Xa levels is recommended in patients w/:
  - Abnormal coagulation/ hemorrhage
  - Obesity
  - Renal failure
  - Underweight
- Check 4h after 2nd SC dose. Further monitoring is not necessary once the correct dose is established in obese patients

Administration frequency	Therapeutic anti–Xa levels
Q12hours	0.6–1 units/ mL
Q24hours	1–2 units/ mL

Mechanism:
- Heparin combines w/ plasma antithrombin 3→
  - ↑Antithrombin 3 activity in removing thrombin & activated factors 9, 10, 11,& 12→
    - –↓Coagulation→↓vascular & mural thrombus formation &/or propagation
- Heparin is metabolized by the plasma enzyme heparinase

Outcomes:
- ↓Morbidity & mortality

Side effects:
- **Cardiovascular**
  - **Hemorrhage**
  - **Heparin induced thrombocytopenia–HIT 10%**, esp. w/ high molecular weight Heparin
    Mechanism:
    - Heparin mediated platelet agglutination→
      - Monocyte/ macrophage mediated extravascular removal via the splenic trabecular network=red pulp, & hepatic sinusoids→
        - **Thrombocytopenia**
    Outcomes:
    - Benign, as it resolves spontaneously, even w/ continued exposure

- **Heparin induced thrombocytopenia ± thrombosis–HITT ≤3%,** esp. w/ high molecular weight Heparin
  - Mechanism:
    - •Heparin mediated platelet agglutination→
      - ∘Monocyte/ macrophage mediated extravascular removal via the splenic trabecular network=red pulp, & hepatic sinusoids→
        - –**Thrombocytopenia**
      - ∘Platelet release of Heparin neutralizing factor=platelet factor 4–PF4, which complexes w/ Heparin→
        - –Production of anti–complex antibodies→↑platelet activation↔↑platelet factor 4 release→ a vicious cycle of **platelet mediated arterial &/or venous thrombus formation, termed the "white clot syndrome,"** being as the clot is relatively devoid of erythrocytes
  - Outcomes:
    - •Must discontinue treatment as **20% develop thromboembolic complications.** Being that both Heparins may cross–react w/ the etiologic antibodies, their further use is contraindicated. Consider continued treatment w/ direct thrombin inhibitors
      - ∘Antibody cross–reactivity:
        - –Low molecular weight Heparins–85%
        - –Heparinoids–5%
- **Mucocutaneous**
  - •Skin necrosis–rarely occurring w/ high molecular weight Heparins, & not being associated w/ anticoagulant deficiency
- **Musculoskeletal**
  - •Osteoporosis, esp. w/ high molecular weight Heparin
    - ∘Usually @ use ≥1month
- **Hematologic**
  - •↓Aldosterone production→
    - ∘**Hyperkalemia–8%**

CHARACTERISTICS OF HEPARIN INDUCED THROMBOCYTOPENIC SYNDROMES

	HIT	HITT
Onset	<2days	4–10 days
Re-exposure	<2days	Earlier if re-exposed within 3 months
Platelet count	↓, being <150,000 or ≥50%	
Platelet median nadir	~90,000	~60,000

- •**^{14}C–Serotonin release assay**
  - Indications:
    - •Suspected HITT
  - Procedure:
    - •Normal donor platelets are radiolabeled w/ ^{14}C–serotonin. They are then washed & combined w/ patient serum & therapeutic Heparin concentrations (0.1 U/ mL). Induction of ^{14}C–serotonin release from platelets constitutes a positive test
  - Limitations:
    - •Expense, due to the use of radioactive material
  - Outcomes:
    - •Considered the gold standard in the detection of HITT
- •**Enzyme linked immunosorbent assay–ELISA**
  - Indications:
    - •Suspected HITT
  - Procedure:
    - •Heparin–PF4 complexes affixed to a plastic plate are incubated w/ the patient's serum. If the patient has produced antibodies, then the addition of enzymatically (horseradish peroxidase) labeled anti–human IgG allows for color visualization via spectrophotometer
  - Limitations:
    - •Many antibody positive patients do not develop clinical HITT
    - •30% false positive

Contraindications:
- •Active hemorrhage
- •Severe bleeding diathesis
- •Severe thrombocytopenia (platelet count ≤20,000/ μL)
- •Recent significant trauma
- •Neurosurgery, ocular surgery, or intracranial hemorrhage within 10days

Generic	M	♀	Amount IV over 10min.	Max
Protamine	P	?	1mg/ 100units of HMWH	50mg
			1mg/ 100units Dalteparin	"
			1mg/ 1mg Enoxaparin	"

Mechanism:
• Protamine combines electrostatically w/ Heparin→
  ○ Inability to bind to antithrombin 3

FOLLOWED BY

ANTICOAGULANTS

Generic	M	♀	Start

Warfarin (Coumadin) L U 5mg PO q24hours
• Because the anticoagulant proteins↓ relatively faster than the procoagulant proteins, an initial transient hypercoagulable state develops. Due to this, Warfarin is started once the patient is therapeutic on Heparin, via either:
  ○ Goal aPTT w/ high molecular weight Heparin
  ○ Evening of initiation of low molecular weight Heparin
  …requiring ~7days (corresponding to 2 half lives of factor 2, or a 75% reduction) to reach a true therapeutic level of an **international normalized ratio–INR of 2–3**

INR	Action	Obtain next INR
<1.5	↑Weekly dose by 15%	1 week
1.5–1.9	↑Weekly dose by 10%	2 weeks
2–3	NO ACTION	1 month if stable
3.1–3.9	↓Weekly dose by 10%	2 weeks
4–5	Skip 1 day, then ↓weekly dose by 15%	1 week
>5	DISCONTINUE WARFARIN	Q day until ≤3, then ↓weekly dose by 50%

Mechanism:
• Competitively inhibits hepatocyte enzymatic vitamin K reactive sites→
  ○ ↓Formation of both:
    – Procoagulant proteins 2, 7, 9, & 10
    – Anticoagulant proteins C & S
    …w/ the anticoagulant effect requiring several days, as it must await the metabolism of the pre-existing plasma procoagulant proteins, w/ normal coagulation returning within several days of discontinuation

Side effects:
Cardiovascular
• **Hemorrhage**
  ○ Fatal: 0.6%/ year
  ○ Major: 3%/ year
  ○ Minor: 7%/ year
Cutaneous
• Tissue necrosis w/ protein C or S deficiency or dysfunction

Contraindications:
• Active hemorrhage
• Severe bleeding diathesis
• Severe thrombocytopenia (platelet count ≤20,000/ mm^3)
• Recent significant trauma
• Neurosurgery, ocular surgery, or intracranial hemorrhage within 10days
• Injury risk (including falls & sports) or compliance risk via:
  ○ Alcoholism
  ○ Altered mental status
  ○ Illicit drug abuse
  ○ Orthostatic hypotension
  ○ Poor compliance
  ○ Seizure disease
  ○ Syncope
  ○ Unstable gait

Special considerations:
• **If undergoing elective surgery during treatment**
  ○ Stop warfarin 5 days prior to surgery, & begin Heparin
• **Anticoagulation during pregnancy**
  ○ Substitute low molecular weight Heparin for warfarin, followed by warfarin treatment postpartum if necessary

780

ANTIDOTES

•**Gastric lavage & activated charcoal** if recently administered; forced emesis at home.

VITAMIN K=Phytonadione

Indications:
•To correct the international normalized ration−INR or prothrombin time−PT

Dose

10mg SC/ IV slow push @ 1mg/ min. in order to ↓anaphylactoid reaction risk

Mechanism:
•Requires several hours to days for effect

Side effects:
•Avoid intramuscular administration which may→
  ◦Intramuscular hemorrhage

FRESH FROZEN PLASMA−FFP

Indications:
•To correct the international normalized ration−INR or prothrombin time−PT under the following conditions:
  ◦**INR >20**
  ◦**Severe hemorrhage**
  ◦**Other need for rapid reversal, such as an emergent procedure**

Dose†

15mL/ kg IV (w/ ~200mL FFP/ unit) q4h prn ↑INR

Mechanism:
•Contains clotting factors 2, 7, 9−13, & heat labile 5 & 7→
  ◦Immediate onset of action
•Each unit→
  ◦8% ↑coagulation factors
  ◦4% ↑blood volume

RESCUE PROCEDURES

THROMBOLYTIC MEDICATIONS

Indications:
•**Age ≥18 years** w/ both:
  ◦**Cerebral ischemic syndrome being <3hours**
                        &
  ◦**Significant neurologic deficit** not accompanied by any of the following:
    −Improvement
    −Seizure
    −Intracranial hemorrhage
    −Significant edema/ mass effect on non−contrast head computed tomographic−CT scan

Generic (trade)	M ♀	Dose	Max
Alteplase (Tissue plasminogen activator−tPA)	L ?	0.9mg/ kg	90mg
		10% via IV push	9mg
		Remainder via IV infusion over 1hour	81mg

•Do not administer antiplatelet or anticoagulant treatment until a repeat non−contrast head computed tomographic−CT scan is taken 24hours later to rule out intracranial hemorrhage
•Avoid urethral catheterization for ≥2hours

Mechanism:
•Fibrinolysis→
  ◦↑Blood flow to the ischemic neuronal areas→
    −Salvaged neurons

Complications:
Cardiovascular
•**Hemorrhage**
  ◦Most important being **intracranial hemorrhage**
    −Streptokinase−0.5%
    −Alteplase−0.7%
    −Lanetoplase, Reteplase or Tenecteplase−1%
  …→**cerebrovascular accident syndrome** having a 65% overall mortality, being 95% @ age >75years
  Risk factors:
  •Elderly
  •Hypertension
  •History of cerebrovascular accident

781

Absolute contraindications:
- Lifetime history of hemorrhagic stroke
- Ischemic stroke within 1year
- Suspected aortic dissection
- Acute pericarditis
- Active internal hemorrhage, not including menses
- Intracranial or spinal:
  - Aneurysm
  - Arteriovenous malformation–AVM
  - Neoplasm

Relative contraindications:
- ≥Severe hypertension refractory to medical treatment, via either:
  - Systolic blood pressure ≥180mmHg
  - Diastolic blood pressure ≥110mmHg
- History of ischemic stroke @ >1year
- Significant trauma or surgery within 1month
- Prolonged (>10min.) or traumatic CPR, or traumatic intubation
- Noncompressible vascular punctures
- Active peptic ulcer
- Internal hemorrhage within 1month
- Known bleeding diathesis
- Current anticoagulation treatment w/ INR ≥2
- Pregnancy
- Liver failure
- Diabetic hemorrhagic retinopathy
- Hypersensitivity reaction to Streptokinase or Anistreplase, which contains Streptokinase. Also, patients should not receive Streptokinase if it was administered within 2years

Monitoring:
- Vital signs & neurologic examination q15min. during infusion, then:
  - Q30min. X 6hours, then
    - Q1hour X 16hours

- If severe headache, acute hypertension, altered mental status, nausea, or vomiting occur, discontinue the infusion, if still running, give cryoprecipitate, & obtain an emergent non–contrast computed tomography–CT scan to rule out intracranial hemorrhage

CHRONIC TREATMENT
- **Antiplatelet or anticoagulant medication as above. NOT BOTH**
- **Smoking cessation** via smoking cessation clinic
  - Cigarette smoking contributes to 20% of deaths in the U.S., & is the #1 modifiable cause of premature death
- **Exercise**
  - An enjoyable form of aerobic exercise on a regular basis (≥3X/ week) for 20–30min., preceded by stretching
- **Emotional stress management**
  - Psychological therapy
  - Regular exercise
  - Biofeedback
  - Yoga
  - Listening to music
  - Gardening
- **Dietician consultation**
- **Glycemic control if hyperglycemic**
- **Hypertension control**
  - Systolic blood pressure <120mmHg & diastolic blood pressure <80mmHg
- **↓Sodium intake**
  - ≤100mmol sodium/ 24h=2g elemental sodium or 6g salt/ 24h, which can usually be achieved w/ a no–added salt diet. Patients w/ poorly compensated heart failure should only consume 0.5–1g elemental sodium or 1.5–3g salt/ 24h
  - →↓Renal potassium loss if taking a diuretic

- **↓Alcohol consumption**
  - ∘Only 1drink q24h (8–12 ounces of beer, 3–5 ounces of wine, or 1 ounce of liquor) in patients without a history of drug abuse
  - ∘≥2 drinks/ 24h→
    - –Hypertension
    - –Hepatitis (♀ > ♂)
    - –↑Abuse risk
  - ∘If alcohol is suspected to be causative, total abstinence is required

LIPID LOWERING MEDICATIONS
- •≥20% of Americans have a plasma lipid abnormality→
  - ∘↑Cardiovascular, cerebrovascular, & peripheral vascular disease risk

Indications:
- •↓Plasma LDL cholesterol to a goal of <70mg/ dL→
  - ∘↓Atherosclerotic disease progression, w/ some degree of regression

Note: Total & HDL cholesterol levels are more accurate in the non–fasting state, whereas triglyceride levels should only be measured in the fasting state, as they are elevated after a meal. Thus, being as ↑triglycerides→↓calculated LDL level, the LDL cholesterol level may be falsely ↓in the non–fasting state. LDL values cannot be accurately calculated w/ a triglyceride level >400mg/ dL

Relative lipid effects:
- •**HMG Co-A reductase inhibitors** correct all lipids, esp. Atorvastatin, Rosuvastatin & Simvastatin
- •**Selective cholesterol absorption inhibitors** correct all lipids to half the extent of HMG Co-A reductase inhibitors
- •**Niacin** primarily ↓triglyceride levels
- •**Fibric acid medications** primarily ↓triglyceride levels
- •**Bile acid sequestrants** primarily ↓LDL cholesterol levels
- •**Omega-3 fatty acids** primarily ↓VLDL levels
- •**Significant dietary lipid restriction** ↓total cholesterol by ~10%

HMG Co-A REDUCTASE INHIBITORS

Generic (Trade)	M	♀	Start	Max
Atorvastatin (Lipitor)	L	U	10mg PO qhs	80mg qhs
Fluvastatin (Lescol)	L	U	40mg PO qhs	80mg qhs
Lovastatin (Mevacor)	L	U	20mg PO qhs	80mg qhs
Pravastatin (Pravachol)	L	U	40mg PO qhs	80mg qhs
Rosuvastatin (Crestor)	L	U	10mg PO qhs	40mg qhs
Simvastatin (Zocor)	L	U	20mg PO qhs	80mg qhs

- •These medications are maximally effective if administered in the evening, when the majority of cholesterol synthesis occurs

Mechanisms:
- •Inhibit hydroxymethylglutaryl coenzyme A reductase function, being the hepatocyte rate limiting enzyme in cholesterol formation→
  - ∘↓Hepatic cholesterol formation→
    - –Feedback ↑hepatocyte LDL receptor formation→↑**plasma LDL cholesterol removal**
- •Anti–inflammatory effects→
  - ∘↓Atherosclerotic plaque formation, w/ ↑stability

Outcomes:
- •↓Morbidity & mortality

Side effects:
- **Gastrointestinal**
- •**Hepatitis–1.5%**, usually starting within 3months of initial or ↑dose, being:
  - ∘Dose related
  - ∘Gradual in onset
  - ∘Usually benign
- •Nausea ± vomiting

Musculoskeletal
- **Myositis-3%**, being:
  - ◦Dose related
  - ◦Possibly sudden in onset
  - …→muscle pain &/or weakness which progress to **rhabdomyolysis <0.5%**, diagnosed via
    - ↑creatine kinase–CK levels
  - Risk factors:
    - •↑Age
    - •Hypothyroidism
    - •Renal failure
    - •Small body frame
    - •Concomitant administration of:
      - ◦Fibric acid medications
      - ◦Bile acid sequestrants
      - ◦Niacin

Neurologic
- •Headaches
- •Sleep disturbances

Ophthalmologic
- •Minor lens opacities

Interactions
- •**Garlic & St. Johns wort→**
  - ◦↑Hepatocyte cytochrome P450 system activity→
    - −↑HMG–CoA reductase inhibitor degradation→↓plasma levels (except Pravastatin)
- •**Diltiazem & protease inhibitors→**
  - ◦↓Hepatocyte cytochrome P450 system activity→
    - −↓HMG–CoA reductase inhibitor degradation→↑plasma levels (except Pravastatin)

Monitoring:
- •Baseline:
  - ◦**Liver function tests**, then
    - −3months after dose↑, then periodically thereafter, w/ treatment to be withdrawn @ plasma values >3X the upper limit of normal
  - ◦**Creatine kinase** (as an asymptomatic ↑ may be present), then
    - −Prior to dose↑ or adding an interacting medication, in order to compare future possible values, to be obtained if symptomatic, w/ treatment to be discontinued @ either plasma values >10X the upper limit of normal, or lower if class switching fails to relieve the syndrome

SELECTIVE CHOLESTEROL ABSORPTION INHIBITORS: Relatively safe to use in combination w/ HMG–CoA reductase inhibitors

Generic (Trade)	M	♀	Dose
Ezetimibe (Zetia)	L	?	10mg PO q24hours

Mechanism:
- •Acts on the small intestinal brush border membrane enzymes→
  - ◦Selectively ↓cholesterol absorption↑→
    - −↓Hepatic cholesterol stores→feedback ↑hepatocyte LDL receptor formation→↑**plasma LDL cholesterol removal**

†No significant effects on lipid soluble vitamin absorption (A, D, E, K)

Side effects:
Gastrointestinal
- •Combination treatment w/ HMG Co–A reductase inhibitors→
  - ◦↑**Hepatitis** risk, but **no ↑myositis risk**, which makes it the medication of choice for combination treatment

Monitoring:
- •Liver function tests as per concomitant HMG Co–A reductase inhibitor

FIBRIC ACID MEDICATIONS

Generic (Trade)	M	♀	Start	Max
Fenofibrate (Tricor)	LK	?	67mg PO q24hours, w/ a meal	200mg q24hours
Gemfibrozil (Lopid)	LK	?	600mg PO q12hours, prior to meals	1500mg/ 24hours

Side effects:
Gastrointestinal
- •Nausea

NIACIN

Generic	M	♀	Start	Max
Niacin	K	?	50mg PO q12hours, w/ meals	6g/ 24hours
•XR form			500mg qhs w/ a low fat snack	2g qhs

Mechanism:
- •Inhibits hepatocyte VLDL synthesis & release

Side effects:
Gastrointestinal
- •Epigastric pain
- •Hepatitis, esp. w/ the XR form
- •Nausea

Mucocutaneous
- •**Cutaneous flushing reaction**, being ↓ w/ NSAID administration 30 min. prior

Neurologic
- •Headache

Hematologic
- •**Hyperglycemia**
- •↑Uric acid

BILE ACID SEQUESTRANTS

Generic (Trade)	M	♀	Start	Max
Cholestyramine (Questran)	F	?	4g PO q24hours prior to meals	12g q12hours
Colesevelam (Welchol)	F	P	3.75g=6tabs q24hours w/ a meal	5.625g=7tabs/ 24hours

Mechanism:
- •Bind to intestinal bile acids→
  - ∘↓Bile acid absorption→
    - –Feedback ↑hepatic conversion of cholesterol to bile acids→↓hepatic cholesterol stores→ feedback ↑hepatocyte LDL receptor formation→↑plasma LDL cholesterol removal

Side effects:
Gastrointestinal
- •↓Absorption of concomitantly administered medications. Other medications should be taken 1hour prior to, or 5hours after taking a bile acid sequestrant
- •Bloating
- •Constipation
- •Nausea
- •High doses→
  - ∘Lipid soluble vitamin deficiencies (A, D, E, K)
  - ∘↑Stool fat, termed Steatorrhea

COMBINATION MEDICATIONS

Generic (Trade)	M	♀	Start	Max
Lovastatin & niacin (Advicor)	LK	U	20mg/ 500mg qhs w/ a low fat snack	20mg/ 1g

DIETARY

Generic (Trade)	M	♀	Dose
Omega 3–fatty acids (Fish oil)	L	?	A combination dose of EPA + DHA†
•Cardioprotection			1g PO q24hours
•Hypertriglyceridemia			2–4g PO q24hours

†Eicosapentanoic acid–EPA & docosahexanoic acid–DHA
- •There are only 2 types of polyunsaturated fatty acids
  - ∘Omega 3–fatty acids, mainly from:
    - –**Fish or fish oils**, esp. herring, mackerel, salmon, sardines, trout, & tuna
    - –Beans, esp. soybeans
    - –Green leafy vegetables
    - –Nuts, esp. walnuts
    - –Plant seeds, esp. canola oil & flaxseed
  - ∘Omega 6–fatty acids, mainly from:
    - –Grains
    - –Meats
    - –Nuts, esp. peanuts
    - –Plant seeds, esp. borage oil, corn oil, cottonseed oil, grape seed oil, primrose oil, safflower oil, sesame oil, soybean oil, & sunflower oil
- •The Western diet is abundant in omega 6–fatty acids (which are prothrombotic & proinflammatory), w/ humans lacking the necessary enzymes to convert them to omega 3–fatty acids, which therefore need to be obtained from separate dietary sources. However, significant amounts of methylmercury

& other environmental toxins may be concentrated in certain fish species (w/ high quality fish oil supplements usually lacking contaminants):
- King Mackerel
- Shark
- Swordfish
- Tilefish, aka golden bass or golden snapper
…which are to be avoided by:
- ♀ who may become or are pregnant
- ♀ who are breastfeeding
- Young children

Mechanism:
- Vasodilation→
  ○ ↓Blood pressure, being dose dependent, w/ a minimal effect of 4/ 2 mmHg w/ doses of 3–6g q24h
- ↓Lipid, esp. triglycerides
- Anti−dysrhythmic
- Anti−inflammatory
- ↓Platelet activity

Outcomes:
- In patients w/ coronary artery disease:
  ○ ↓All cause mortality
  ○ ↓Dysrhythmia mediated sudden death

Side effects:
Cardiovascular
- ↑Bleeding time→
  ○ Excessive hemorrhage

Gastrointestinal
- Belching
- Bloating
- Fishy aftertaste
- Nausea ± vomiting

Hematologic
- Hyperglycemia

Interactions
- None known, making it safe for use in combination w/ other:
  ○ Anticoagulant medications
  ○ Antiplatelet medications
  ○ Lipid lowering medications

POTASSIUM
- **Always measure the magnesium level concomitantly**

Indications:
- Ensure a potassium of 4–5mEq/ L

Generic
- Potassium chloride−KCL
- Potassium bicarbonate
- Potassium citrate
- Potassium acetate
- Potassium gluconate
- Potassium phosphate

POTASSIUM DOSAGE ADJUSTMENT SCALE†_____

Plasma K^+ (mEq/ L)	K^+ repletion (mEq)
≥3.9	None
3.7–3.8	20
3.5–3.6	40
3.3–3.4	60
3.1–3.2	80
≤3	100

†Half all above doses @ a glomerular filtration rate−GFR ≤30mL/ min.

Outcomes:
- Anti−dysrhythmic
- ↑Cardiac contractility in heart failure
- Modest hypotensive effect in some patients
- ↓Cerebrovascular disease risk, apart from its possible blood pressure lowering effects

786

Generic (Trade)	M ♀	Dosage
Garlic (Allium sativum)	? U	600–900mg PO q24hours

Mechanism:
- ↓Blood pressure
- ↓Lipids
- ↓Platelet activity

Additional treatment for persistent neurologic deficits:
- **Periodic depression screening**, as major depression develops in 20% of stroke patients w/ persistent neurologic deficits
- **Occupational therapy**
  - To teach the patient how to better perform activities of daily living–ADLs ± assistive devices if necessary:
    - Braces, crutches, &/or walkers to ↓weight on affected joints→↓pain, ↑stability, & ↑mobility
    - Eating utensils w/ large handles
    - Nonslip rubber table & bathroom mats (including for the shower &/or bath)
    - Strategically placed rails, such as along stairwells, by the toilet, & in the bath &/or shower
- **Physical therapy**
  - For gait training
  - To teach the patient:
    - Energy conserving maneuvers
    - The therapeutic use of heat & massage, w/ heat treatment via baths, towels, electric heating pads, &/or paraffin wax baths→↓peri–articular muscle spasm→↓joint pain
  - To provide an individualized exercise program incorporating range of motion–ROM & muscle strengthening→
    - ↑Stability, ↑mobility, & ↓contracture risk
- **Decubitus ulceration** prophylaxis via:
  - Keeping the skin clean & dry
  - Padding of bony prominences
  - Frequent turning

Indications:
- In order to ↓muscle spasm→
  - ↓Pain
  - ↑Ease of activities of daily living
  - ↑Ease of caregiver mediated washing, dressing, positioning, & passive range of motion exercises
  …→↓contracture & decubitus ulceration risk

Mechanism:
- Botulinum toxin (an exotoxin formed by the bacterium Clostridium botulinum)→
  - Neuromuscular junction presynaptic cell membrane SNARE proteins (Syntaxin, Synaptobrevin, & SNAP 25) cleavage→
    - ↓Acetylcholine vesicle–cell membrane fusion→↓acetylcholine release→↓neuromuscular transmission→**localized weakness**, until new neuromuscular junctions are formed within several weeks to months

Limitations:
- Formation of anti–botulinum toxin antibody, being more likely in patients who receive ↑doses at more frequent intervals→
  - ↓Efficacy. Therefore, it is recommended that the dosage be kept as low as possible

Overdose effects:
- Although minute amounts are effective in the treatment of muscle spasm, overdose→
  - **Descending weakness & paralysis→**
    - Difficulty speaking=dysarthria
    - Difficulty swallowing=dysphagia
    - Double vision=diplopia
    - **Hypercapnic respiratory failure→death**

- **Trivalent antitoxin** (types A, B, & E): There are 8 types of toxins, w/ A, B, & E being the most common in human illness
- **3,4–Diaminopyridine**
  Mechanism:
  - ↑Acetylcholine release

787

•**35% of stroke patients die**. Of the survivors, 35% become dependent on others, whereas 65% retain or regain independence (≤80% of which retain or regain the ability to walk)

PREVENTION

•**Carotid endarterectomy**

Indications:

•**Extracranial carotid artery atherosclerotic stenosis of ≥60 (100% occlusion being inoperable), in centers where the surgical risk of stroke is <3%**

788

•Caused by any alteration of the central nervous system→
  ◦An uncontrolled, hypersynchronous, acute neuronal discharge, originating in the cerebrum, brain stem, or spinal cord, w/ variable spread→
    –Syndrome referrable to the stimulated region(s)

RISK FACTORS

•**Cerebrovascular accident**
  ◦Ischemic
  ◦Hemorrhagic
•**Hyperthermia**
•**Illicit drugs**
  ◦Alcohol withdrawal
    –50% first experienced within 24h after abrupt dose reduction
  ◦Amphetamines
  ◦Cocaine
•**Infection**
  ◦Encephalitis
  ◦Meningitis
•**Intracranial tumor**
•**Metabolic disorder**
  ◦**Hypo**calcemia
  ◦**Hypo**glycemia
  ◦**Hypo**magnesemia
  ◦**Hypo**natremia
  ◦**Hypo**xemia
  ◦**Hypo** or hyperglycemia
  ◦Hyperosmolarity
  ◦Uremia, via either:
    –Renal failure→↑creatinine, urea, & uric acid
    –Hepatic failure→↑ammonia
  ◦Porphyria
•**Post–traumatic**
  ◦Head injury
  ◦Intracranial surgery
•**Pregnancy**
  ◦Eclampsia
•**Medications**
  ◦Local anesthetics (ex. Lidocaine)
  ◦Antibiotics
    –Ciprofloxacin
    –Imipenem
    –Isoniazid–INH
    –Penicillin
  ◦Anticholinesterases
  ◦Antidepressants
  ◦Antihistamines
  ◦Antipsychotics
  ◦β receptor blockers
  ◦Cyclosporine
  ◦Hypo–osmolar parenteral solutions
  ◦Methylxanthines (ex. Theophylline)
  ◦Phencyclidine
  ◦Sympathomimetic medications
•**Withdrawal of medications**
  ◦Antiseizure medications
  ◦Barbiturates
  ◦Benzodiazepines
  ◦Opiates
•**Idiopathic**
•**Febrile convulsions of childhood**
•**Subtherapeutic plasma level of antiseizure medication**

•Postictally, the cerebrospinal fluid may contain more cells than normal, termed pleocytosis, w/ the count being ≤80cells/ µL, w/ either a polymorphonuclear or mononuclear predominance in:

789

○2% of patients after a single tonic &/or clonic seizure
○15% of patients after status epilepticus
...in the absence of infection

FOCAL SEIZURES

•Neuron depolarization→
   ○Spreading, localized reverberating circuits→synchronous, focal depolarization over adjacent grey matter regions, w/ **consciousness being either:**
     –**Preserved, termed simple focal seizures**
     –**Impaired, termed complex focal seizures**
     ...but not lost, unless secondary generalization occurs

   Potential additional features:
     •**Simple focal seizures may progress to complex focal seizures**
     •**Secondary generalization** throughout the ipsilateral & contralateral hemispheres→
      ○**Tonic–clonic seizure**
     •**Temporary paralysis**, termed **Todd's paralysis**, of affected regions, being either:
      ○Incomplete, termed paresis
      ○Complete, termed plegia
      ...for several hours to days, which may occur after any seizure type affecting the motor cortex

SIMPLE FOCAL SEIZURES

•**Motor**
   ○Focal muscle contractions
   ○Progressive, successive, motor cortex depolarization, termed a **Jacksonian seizure**→
     –March of contractions, according to the motor homunculus
•**Sensory**, indicating a **parietal lobe seizure**
   ○Somatosensory
     –Paresthesias, esp. tingling & numbness
   ○Auditory
     –Buzzing
   ○Gustatory
     –Bad taste
   ○Olfactory
     –Bad smell
   ○Vertiginous
     –Dizziness
     –Vertigo
   ○Visual
     –Flashing lights
     –Changing object size &/or distance
•**Autonomic**
   ○Vasoconstriction→
     –Pallor
   ○Vasodilation→
     –Flushing
   ○Palpitations
   ○Perspiration
•**Psychic**
   ○Anxiety
   ○Dream–like feelings of unreality
   ○Fear
   ○Recurrent perceptions, being either:
     –Familiar, termed déjà vu
     –Unfamiliar, termed jamais vu
•**Mixed**
   ○≥2 of the above

COMPLEX FOCAL SEIZURES
- **Staring** (indicating a temporal lobe seizure in 75% of patients) ± **automatisms:**
  - Blinking
  - Chewing
  - Fidgeting
  - Hand rubbing
  - Lip smacking
  - Picking movements
  - Walking

GENERALIZED SIEZURES
- Generalized neuron depolarization throughout the ipsilateral & contralateral hemispheres→
  - **Sudden loss of consciousness**

- **Absence seizure**
  - <30seconds of motionless staring ± momentary spasmodic muscle contractions, termed twitches (usually involving the head, esp. blinking), w/ subsequent regained consciousness, w/ resumption of previous activity, without post–seizure (also termed postictal) confusion or lethargy
    - Usually begins in childhood, w/ regression by age 30
    - May occur rarely or frequently throughout the day
    - May be induceable by any flickering light source &/or hyperventilation

  Potential additional features:
  - **Altered generalization** throughout the ipsilateral & contralateral hemispheres→
    - **Tonic–clonic seizure**

- **Tonic–clonic seizure**
  - **Tonic seizure** via global skeletal & smooth muscle contraction→
    - Body stiffening→fall
    - Exhalation→loud wheeze
    - Teeth clenching→tongue &/or cheek biting
    - Upward rolling of opened eyes
    - Urination
    - Defecation
  - ...followed by a **clonic seizure** via spasmodic muscle contractions→
    - Body jerking
    - Episodic exhalation→
      - Grunting
    - Teeth clenching→
      - Tongue &/or cheek biting
    - ...w/ the entire seizure lasting **several seconds to min.**, w/ post–seizure nervous system depression→
      - Confusion
      - Severe fatigue→
        - Hours of sleep

  Potential additional features:
  - **Temporary paralysis**, termed **Todd's paralysis**, of affected regions, being either:
    - Incomplete, termed paresis
    - Complete, termed plegia
    - ...for several hours to days, which may occur after any seizure type affecting the motor cortex

- **Other**
  - **Tonic seizure**
  - **Clonic seizure**
  - **Myoclonic seizure**
    - Single or repetitive bilateral rapid limb contractions, **usually w/ preserved consciousness**
  - **Atonic seizure**
    - Sudden loss of muscle tone→fall, defecation, & urination

EPILEPSY
- **Any chronic seizure disorder**
  - Tonic clonic seizures–40%
  - Complex partial seizures–40%
  - Simple partial seizures–15%

- All patients w/ epilepsy must have their condition reported to the department of motor vehicles–DMV

PSEUDOSEIZURE ▬▬▬▬▬▬▬▬▬▬▬▬▬▬▬▬▬▬▬▬▬▬▬▬▬▬▬▬▬▬▬▬▬
•Done in an attempt to:
  ◦Avoid responsibility &/or other undesired situations
  ◦Gain sympathy &/or compensation
  ...→faked seizure-like syndrome, termed malingering, usually being atypical, w/ purposeful
      movements, including:
      •Thrashing, rather than jerky limb movements
      •Pelvic thrusting
      •Opisthotonic posture
      •Deep breathing
      •Eyes held tightly shut
      •Retained consciousness→
        ◦Emotional reactions
        ◦Meaningfull speech
        ◦Response to verbal instruction

•If you suspect pseudoseizures in an unconscious patient, raise the patients arm, high over their face &
allow it to drop. A patient w/ pseudoseizures will usually not allow the arm to hit their face

STATUS EPILEPTICUS ▬▬▬▬▬▬▬▬▬▬▬▬▬▬▬▬▬▬▬▬▬▬▬▬▬▬▬▬
•**A medical emergency** of either:
  ◦**Persistent seizure**
  ◦**Recurrent seizures without intervening recovery to baseline consciousness**
  ...which may occur w/ any seizure type, though usually referring to tonic &/or clonic seizures, for which
      the following pertains:
Statistics:
  •Occurs in 60,000–160,000 persons/ year, w/ the majority occurring in the pediatric age group (esp.
    age ≤5years)
  •The #1 cause in adults is a cerebrovascular accident (ischemic &/or hemorrhagic)
  •50% of cases occur as new-onset seizures

Cardiovascular
  •↑Autonomic sympathetic tone→
    ◦**Tachycardia**
    ◦**Hypertension**
    ◦Diaphoresis
  •**Dysrhythmia** via either:
    ◦Hyperkalemia
    ◦Hyperthermia
    ◦Metabolic acidemia
Musculoskeletal
  •Continuous muscle contraction→
    ◦↑Myocyte metabolism→
      –↑Heat production→↑core temperature, termed **hyperthermia**
  •Fall &/or continuous muscle contraction→
    ◦Head &/or extremity trauma
      –Bruising
      –Lacerations
      –Fractures
Pulmonary
  •Ineffectual respiratory effort→
    ◦**Hypercapnic respiratory failure**
Hematologic
  •Stress induced neutrophil demargination→
    ◦Leukocytosis
  •Continuous muscle contraction→
    ◦↑Myocyte metabolism→
      –Lactic acidemia mediated **metabolic anion gap acidemia**
  •Skeletal muscle death, termed **rhabdomyolysis**→
    ◦Rapid release of intracellular contents→
      –Acute renal failure
      –Electrolyte abnormalities

792

•**Electroencephalography–EEG**
Indication:
•To localize & classify a seizure syndrome
Findings:
•**Focal seizures:** Focal deranged pattern
•**Absence seizures: Spike & dome wave pattern** over most or all of the cerebral cortex
•**All other generalized seizures: Spike wave pattern** over most or all of the cerebral cortex
Mechanism:
•Scalp electrodes register cortical brain electric potentials, w/ intensity & frequency determined by the level of cortical excitation, always being abnormal during & immediately after a tonic–clonic seizure
Limitations:
•Is often normal between seizures=interictally
•May miss a focal seizure, especially those occurring
    ∘In the interhemispheric fissure
    ∘Outside of the cerebral cortex

Indications:
•Identified persistent etiology
•Idiopathic w/ consent of neurology

•**Focal seizures** ± secondary generalization
    ∘First line: Carbamazepine, Phenytoin
    ∘Second line: Phenobarbitol, Primidone, Valproic acid
•**Generalized seizures**
    ∘**Tonic &/or clonic seizures**
        −First line: Valproic acid
        −Second line: Carbamazepine, Phenobarbitol, Phenytoin, Primidone
    ∘**Absence seizures**
        −First line: Ethosuxamide, Valproic acid
        −Second line: Clonazepam
    ∘**Myoclonic seizures**
        −First line: Clonazepam, Valproic acid
        −Second line: Phenobarbitol, Phenytoin

Generic (Trade)	M	♀	Dose	Max
ANTISEIZURE MEDICATIONS				
Carbamazepine (Tegretol)	LK	U		
•XR form			200mg PO q12hours, then titrate to a therapeutic plasma level of 4–12µg/ mL	1.6g q12hours
Clonazepam (Klonopin)	LK	U	0.5mg PO q8hours, then titrate to a therapeutic plasma level of 0.05–0.7µg/ mL	20mg/ 24hours
Ethosuximide (Zarontin)	LK	?	500mg PO q24hours, then titrate to a therapeutic plasma level of 40–100µg/ mL	1.5g q24hours
Phenobarbitol (Luminal)	L	U	50mg q12hours, then titrate to a therapeutic plasma level of 15–40µg/ mL	150mg q12hours
Phenytoin (Dilantin)	L	U	400mg PO, then	
			300mg PO q2hours X 2 = 1g total loading dose, then	
•XR form			300mg PO q24hours, then titrate to a therapeutic plasma level of 10–20µg/ mL†	500mg q24hours
Primidone (Mysoline)	LK	U	100mg PO qhs X 2days, then	
			1100mg PO q12hours X 2days, then	
			100mg PO q8hours X 2days, then	
			150mg PO q8hours X 2days, then	
			200mg PO q8hours X 2days, then	
			250mg PO q8hours, then titrate to a therapeutic plasma level of 5–12µg/ mL	650mg q8hours
Valproic acid (Depakote)	L	U		
•XR form			10mg/kg/24hours PO q24hours, then titrate by 5mg/kg/24hours qweek to a therapeutic plasma level of 50–150µg/ mL	60mg/kg/24hours

†Correction of measured plasma Phenytoin level for albumin:

Measured plasma Phenytoin level
(0.2 X albumin level) + 0.1

Additional Phenytoin needed if subtherapeutic:
(0.7 X wt in kg) X (desired level – actual level)
0.92

Side effects:
Neurologic
•Altered mental status
•Double vision=diplopia
•Headache
•Incoordination=ataxia
•Sedation

Overdose:
Pulmonary
•Respiratory depression

Carbemazepine specific:
•Dose related:
  ◦Diarrhea
  ◦Nausea ± vomiting
•Idiosyncratic:
  ◦Blood dyscrasias
  ◦Hepatitis

Clonazepam specific:
•Dose related:
  ◦Hypersalivation

Ethosuxamide specific:
•Dose related:
  ◦Diarrhea
  ◦Nausea ± vomiting
•Idiosyncratic:
  ◦Blood dyscrasias
  ◦Dermatitis

Phenobarbitol specific:
•Dose related:
  ◦Hyperactivity
  ◦Insomnia
•Idiosyncratic:
  ◦Blood dyscrasias
  ◦Dermatitis

Phenytoin specific:
•Dose related:
  ◦Coarse facial features, termed **leonine facies**, characterized by thickening of the subcutaneous tissue about the eyes & nose
  ◦**Gingival hyperplasia–30%**
    −Once established, may only partially regress
  ◦**Hirsutism** (5% overall, 30% of young ♀)
  ◦Vitamin D inactivation→
    −**Osteoporosis**
  ◦Polyneuropathy
  ◦Megaloblastic anemia
  ◦Teratogenic→
    −**Fetal hydantoin syndrome**

Primidone specific:
•Idiosyncratic:
  ◦Blood dyscrasias
  ◦Dermatitis

Valproic acid specific:
- •Dose related:
  - ◦↑Weight
  - ◦Tremor
  - ◦Diarrhea
  - ◦Nausea ± vomiting
  - ◦Alopecia
- •Idiosyncratic:
  - ◦Blood dyscrasias
  - ◦Dermatitis
  - ◦Thrombocytopenia
  - ◦Hepatitis–rare
  - ◦Pancreatitis–rare

•**Withdrawal** from anti–seizure medications should be done gradually in order to prevent rebound ↑seizure frequency &/or severity

Monitoring:
- •Plasma medication levels should be checked @:
  - ◦Baseline, after initiating treatment, & until therapeutic levels are reached & sustained
  - ◦Addition of a potential interacting medication
  - ◦Change in gastrointestinal, hepatic, or renal function
  - ◦Occurrence of side effects

TREATMENT OF ACTIVE SEIZURE

- •**Place the patient on a monitor**
- •**Place an oral airway, if possible, w/ 100% O$_2$ via a non–rebreather mask**
- •**Draw a finger blood glucose**
- •**Establish an IV line & draw blood** for:
  - ◦Complete blood count
  - ◦Chemistry
  - ◦Arterial blood gases
  - ◦Coagulation studies
  - ◦Toxicology screen (including ethanol level)
  - ◦Medication levels
  - ◦Other possible etiologic tests
- •**Intravenous empiric treatment**
  - ◦50mL of a 50% dextrose solution IV
  - ◦Thiamine 100mg IV†
  - ◦Naloxone 0.8mg IV
  - ◦Magnesium sulfate IV, if eclampsia is suspected
    - –4–6g IV infusion over 20min., repeated for recurrent seizures, then 2g/ hour IV infusion to be continued for ≥24hours postpartum
- •**Treat the etiologic cause** if known
- •**Seizure precautions**
  - ◦Padded bed rails
- •**If unconscious, place in the left lateral decubitus position**→
  - ◦↓Aspiration risk

†Patients should receive thiamine 100mg IV, either before or w/ the first glucose solution, in order to prevent glucose mediated thiamine reserve depletion in alcoholics→either:
- •Wernicke's encephalopathy
- •Korsakoff's syndrome

BENZODIAZEPINES

Generic (Trade)	M	♀	Dose
Lorazepam (Ativan)	LK	U	4mg IV slow push q5min. prn

Mechanism:
- •Bind to a benzodiazepine receptor site on the neuronal inhibitory gamma aminobutyric acid–GABA$_A$ chloride ion channel→
  - ◦↑Frequency of channel opening in the concomitant presence of GABA→
    - –Neuronal inhibition

Outcomes:
- •Seizure termination within 5 min. in 80% of cases

Side effects:
Cardiovascular
  •Hypotension
Gastrointestinal
  •Nausea ± vomiting
Neurologic
  •Altered mental status
  •Incoordination=ataxia
  •Double vision=diplopia
  •Headache
  •Sedation
  •Physical & psychological dependence
  •Tolerance
  •Additive central nervous system depression effects in combination w/:
    ◦Antihistamine medications
    ◦Ethanol
    ◦Sedative/ hypnotic medications
      −Barbiturates
      −Buspirone
      −Cyclic ethers
      −Meprobamate
      −Zolpidem

Overdose:
Pulmonary
  •Respiratory depression

SECOND LINE TREATMENT ▬▬▬▬▬▬▬▬

HYDANTOINS

Generic (Trade)	M	♀	Dose
Phenytoin (Dilantin)	L	U	20mg/ kg IV @ ≤50mg/ min.†, then 100mg PO/ IV q8–6hours

†In order to ↓cardiovascular depression risk

Outcomes:
  •The combination of a benzodiazepine & a hydantoin will terminate seizure activity in 90% of cases

Side effects:
Cardiovascular
  •Atrioventricular block
  •Hypotension
Hematologic
  •Being as Phenytoin does not readily dissolve in aqueous solutions, nonpolar solvents such as propylene glycol are required to keep the medication in solution, & can accumulate→
    ◦Propylene glycol toxicity→
      −Altered mental status
      −Anion gap metabolic acidemia
      −Dysrhythmias
      −Hemolysis
      −Hyperosmolarity
      −Acute tubular necrosis→renal failure
    ...→↑plasma levels & osmolar gap

Contraindications:
  •≥2nd degree heart block

OR

BENZODIAZEPINES

Indications:
  •Contraindication to Hydantoin treatment

Generic (Trade)	M	♀	Dose
Diazepam (Valium)	LK	U	10–20mg/ hour IV infusion

THIRD LINE TREATMENT
Indications:
•Seizure refractory to the above treatments–10% of patients

•**Endotracheal intubation**

&

BARBITURATES				
Generic (Trade)	**M**	♀	**Dose**	**Max**
Phenobarbital (Luminal)	L	U	500mg IV loading dose @ 50mg/ min.=10min., then 200mg IV q5min. prn until seizure termination	20mg/kg/24h
Mechanism:				

•Bind to a benzodiazepine receptor site on the neuronal inhibitory gamma aminobutyric acid–GABA$_A$ chloride ion channel→
  ○↑Duration of channel opening in the concomitant presence of GABA→
   −Neuronal inhibition

Outcomes:
•Seizure termination in 50% of refractory patients

Side effects:
Cardiovascular
 •**Hypotension**
Gastrointestinal
 •Nausea ± vomiting
Neurologic
 •Altered mental status
 •Incoordination=ataxia
 •Double vision=diplopia
 •Headache
 •Sedation
 •Physical & psychological dependence
 •Tolerance
 •Additive central nervous system depression effects in combination w/:
  ○Antihistamine medications
  ○Ethanol
  ○Sedative hypnotic medications
   −Benzodiazepines
   −Buspirone
   −Cyclic ethers
   −Meprobamate
   −Zolpidem

Overdose:
Pulmonary
 •**Respiratory depression**

FOURTH LINE TREATMENT
Indications:
•Seizure refractory to the above treatments–5% of patients

COMA INDUCING MEDICATIONS			
Generic (Trade)	**M**	♀	**Dose**
Pentobarbitol (Nembutal)	LK	U	10–15mg/ kg IV infusion over 1–2hours, then 1–1.5mg/kg/hour infusion
Inhalational anesthesia			

•Chronic, global neuronal & neuroglial dysfunction & degeneration of uncertain etiology→
  ○Dementia
•Although dementia is defined as a chronic deterioration of ≥2 cognitive=knowledge acquiring functions
in the presence of clear consciousness, the syndrome also encompasses the additional alteration of any
non-cognitive cerebral function:
  ○Behavior/ personality
  ○Mood
  ○Movement
  ○Sensation
  ...or the development of psychosis
Statistics:
  •**#1 Cause of dementia**, causing 50% of cases, affecting 10% of persons age >65years→
    ○**#4 Cause of mortality in the U.S.**

COGNITIVE FUNCTIONS

•**Memory:** Does the patient have adequate short & long term memory
•**Orientation:** Is the patient oriented to time (year, month, day, morning vs. night, season) & place
(country, state, city, current location)
•**Concentration:** Can the patient mentally focus
•**Recognition:** Does the patient recognize familiar people (including their own image via mirror or
picture), locations, & objects
•**Communication:** Can the patient communicate w/, & understand the spoken & written word, as well as
gestures & drawings
•**Abstract thought:** Can the patient decipher the underlying concept of a statement

RISK FACTORS

•**Age:** >40years, usually >65years
•**Genetic**
  ○Family history, as ≥50% are familial
  ○Mutated loci on chromosomes:
    −1, encoding the presenilin 2-PS2 protein
    −14, encoding the presenilin 1-PS1 protein†
    −21, encoding the amyloid precursor protein†
  ○1 of 3 common alleles (allele E4) on chromosome 19, encoding the apolipoprotein E (ApoE) plasma
    protein
  ○Trisomy 21, termed Down's syndrome†, as patients who live to age >40years usually develop
    Alzheimer's disease
•**?Environment:** Aluminum in water supplies &/or air
•**?Trauma:** Repeated head trauma

---

†Risk factors for early onset disease (age ≤60years)

DIAGNOSIS

•**ALWAYS** rule out possible reversible causes (see below)
•Alzheimer's disease is divided into 3 stages based on the progressive brain areas involved

1. Limbic stage, being the initial 3 years
  •**Memory**
    ○Progressive anterograde & retrograde **amnesia**→
      −New memories being progressively more difficult to form, while previous memories are
        progressively lost→confusion, frustration, &/or sadness
  •**Mood**
    ○**Depression-20%**
  •**Sensation**
    ○Progressively altered olfactory sensation→
      −↓Ability to distinguish previously familiar odors, termed odor amnesia
      −↓Sensation→loss of the sense of smell, termed **anosmia**→concomitant altered sense of taste

2. Parietal stage, beginning 3-6years after onset
  •**↓Abstract thought**
  •**Alteration of basic drives**
    ○Due to neurologic changes &/or concomitant depression
      −**Sleep**, being either ↓, termed insomnia (via difficulty initiating &/or early morning awakening) or
        ↑, termed hypersomnia
      −**Hunger**, being either ↓, termed anorexia (during nearly all wakefulness→cachexia) or ↑

- **Communication**
  - ↓Speech comprehension, w/ fluent, although increasingly erroneous, speech, termed **sensory aphasia**
- **Concentration**
  - ↓Ability to perform simple mathematics, termed **acalcula**, which may be especially difficult for people who work predominantly w/ numbers (ex. accountants, bankers, business persons, engineers, scientists, teachers)
- **Extrapyramidal effects**
  - ○Secondary Parkinson's syndrome
- **Movement**
  - ○↓Ability to perform previously learned movements, termed **apraxia**,→↓ability to:
    - −Bathe
    - −Cook
    - −Dress
    - −Groom
    - −Operate machinery (ex. car)
    - −Use eating utensils
    - −Use the toilet
    - −Write
    - …→frustration &/or sadness
- **Psychosis**
  - ○**Visual & auditory hallucinations**
  - ○**Delusions of identification** (which may in part be due to altered recognition)→
    - −Paranoia &/or hostility
- **Recognition**
  - ○↓Visual & auditory recognition, termed visual & auditory **agnosia**, respectively→misinterpretation of the environment via:
    - −Places→easily lost
    - −Sounds→easily frightened
    - −Animals→easily frightened
    - −Objects→patients may use their mouth to examine objects, termed **hyperorality**
    - −People, including family, friends, caregivers, &/or even their own image
    - …all of which seem strange→
      - •Confusion
      - •Hostility
      - •Fright
      - •Sadness
      - •Shadowing of caregivers
      - •Risk of attempting to "escape" from an unfamiliar caregiver

3. **Frontal stage**, beginning 6−9years after onset
   - **Bowel & urinary bladder incontinence**
   - **Movement**
     - ○Progressive global disturbance of movement→
       - −↓Ability to perform innate movements→↓ability to walk, talk, swallow, & eventually move at all→bedridden state→muscle wasting
       - −Spasticity: ↑Muscular tone w/ exaggeration of tendon reflexes
   - **Re−emergence of primitive reflexes**
     - ○Grasping
     - ○Sucking
   - **Seizures**

•**Folstein mini-mental state examination-MMSE**
Indications:
  •To screen for, & monitor the course of cognitive impairment

Cognitive function	Maximal score	Question
Orientation	5	•"What is the year, season, month, day of the week, & date?"
	5	•"Where are we: Country, state, city, hospital, & floor?"
Concentration	3	•Tell the patient to remember the names of 3 unrelated objects for later (ex. eraser, orange, & kite). Take 1second to say each, then ask the patient to name all 3. You may repeat the words until the patient registers them, but without credit for each repeated word
	5	•Ask the patient to subtract serial 7s from 100. Stop after 5 answers (100, 93, 86, 79, 72). If the patient refuses serial 7s, ask them to spell "'world" backwards, giving a point for every correctly positioned letter
Short term memory	3	•Ask the patient to recall the 3 objects you mentioned before
Recognition	2	•Show the patient 2 common objects (ex. pencil & cup), and ask for them to be named
Communication		
•Repetition	1	•Ask the patient to repeat "No ifs, ands, or buts."
•Comprehension	3	•Ask the patient to follow a 3-step command: "Take this paper in your right hand, fold it in half, & place it on the table."
•Reading	1	•Ask the patient to read & follow written instructions "Close your eyes"
•Writing	1	•Ask the patient to write any sentence they want ◦1pt for a subject, 1pt for a verb, 1pt if the sentence makes sense
•Visuospatial	1	•Draw interlocking pentagons, and ask the patient to copy the design ◦1pt if each figure has 5angles w/ 2angles overlapping

Total possible score	30, w/ the median score being inversely related to age, & directly related to years of schooling

Score	Severity of dementia
24-30	Normal, depending on age† and education‡
20-23	Mild
10-19	Moderate
1-9	Severe
0	Profound

•**Additional examinations**
  ◦**Asses the patients level of consciousness** along the following continuum, as patients w/ cognitive impairment & ↓consciousness have delirium
    -ALERT-DROWSY-STUPOR-COMA
  ◦**Abstract thought:** Ask the patient the meaning of any/ all of the following:
    -"There is no use crying over spilt milk."
    -"Those who live in glass houses should not throw stones."
    -"A rolling stone gathers no moss."

---

†The median score for patients age ≤24years is 29, being 27 for ages 25-79years, & 25 for age ≥80years
‡The median score for patients w/ ≥9years of education is 29, being 26 w/ 5-8years, & 22 for ≤4years

•**Electroencephalography-EEG**
Mechanism:
  •Scalp electrodes register cortical brain electric potentials, w/ intensity & frequency determined by the level of cortical excitation
Findings:
  •Progressive disease→
    ◦↓Electrical frequencies, correlating w/ cognitive decline

800

•**Brain computed tomographic–CT scan or magnetic resonance imaging–MRI**
   <u>Findings:</u>
      •Cortical atrophy→
         ◦Enlarged sulci, Sylvian fissure, suprasellar cistern, & lateral ventricles

•**Positron emission tomographic–PET scan**
   <u>Mechanism:</u>
      •Intravenous radiolabeled glucose is utilized by cells→
         ◦Visualization
   <u>Findings:</u>
      •↓Parietal & temporal blood flow & glucose metabolism, indicating neuron & neuroglial dysfunction
      ± death

•Being as there is no cure, the goal of treatment is to ↑cognitive function as measured by various
neuropsychiatric examinations (including the Folstein mini mental state examination–MMSE)

•**Occupational therapy**
   ◦To teach the patient how to better perform activities of daily living–ADLs ± assistive devices if
   necessary:
      –Braces, crutches, &/or walkers→↑stability & ↑mobility
      –Eating utensils w/ large handles
      –Strategically placed rails, such as along stairwells, by the toilet, & in the bath &/or shower
•**Physical therapy**
   ◦For gait training
   ◦To teach the patient:
      –Joint protective maneuvers
      –Energy conserving maneuvers
   ◦To provide an individualized exercise program incorporating range of motion–ROM & muscle
   strengthening
•**Home safety** evaluation to ensure:
   ◦Adequate lighting, including night lights in bedrooms, hallways, & bathrooms
   ◦Uncluttered walkways
   ◦Securely fastened stairway handrails
   ◦Bathroom grab bars in the shower/ bathtub & by the toilet
   ◦Raised toilet seats
   ◦Nonslip rubber suction mats in the shower/ bathtub & slick bathroom floors
   ◦Throw rugs are either fastened to the floor or removed
•**Daily predictability**
   ◦Tasks & life activities must be regular & predictable, w/ variations being planned w/, & explained to
   the patient, as new &/or unexpected variations ín routine (activities, places, people) may→
      –↑Confusion, fright, hostility, &/or sadness

VITAMINS			
Generic	M	♀	Dose
Vitamin E	L	S	1000 units PO q12hours

&

ACETYLCHOLINESTERASE INHIBITORS				
Generic (Trade)	M	♀	Dose	Max
Donepezil (Aricept)	LK	?	5mg PO qhs	10mg qhs
Galantamine (Reminyl)	LK	P	4mg PO q12hours w/ meals, w/ titration to 8mg q12hours @ 1month	12mg q12hours
Rivastigmine (Exelon)	K	P	1.5mg PO q12hours w/ meals, w/ titration to 3mg q12hours @ 2weeks	6mg q12hours

<u>Dose adjustments:</u>
   •**Galantamine:** Max of 8mg q12h w/ renal or hepatic disease
<u>Mechanism:</u>
   •↓Perisynaptic connective tissue acetylcholinesterase function→
      ◦↓Acetylcholine metabolism→
         –↑Synaptic cleft concentrations
<u>Side effects:</u>
   Cardiovascular
      •Bradycardia

Gastrointestinal†
- •↑Gastrointestinal smooth muscle contraction→
  - ○↑Tone & peristalsis→
    - −Abdominal discomfort
    - −Diarrhea
    - −Nausea ± vomiting

Genitourinary
- •↑Genitourinary smooth muscle contraction→
  - ○↑Tone & peristalsis→
    - −Urinary frequency

Mucocutaneous
- •↑Glandular cell secretions
  - ○↑Exocrine secretions→
    - −↑Lacrimal, mucosal, parotid, submandibular, gastric, & pancreatic secretions
  - ○↑Eccrine=merocrine secretions→
    - −↑Perspiration‡
  - ○↑Holocrine secretions→
    - −↑Sebum→oily skin

Musculoskeletal
- •Muscle cramps

Neurologic
- •Insomnia

Opthalmologic
- •↑Iris circular smooth muscle contraction→
  - ○Constricted pupil=myosis

Pulmonary
- •Bronchoconstriction

---

†↓By low starting dose, gradual titration, & continued use
- •If treatment is interrupted X several days, restart @ starting dose, w/ gradual titration

‡Perspiration is controlled by the sympathetic nervous system→
- •Postganglionic acetylcholine release, except on the palms & soles which are activated by norepinephrine

Cautionary use:
- •Severe chronic obstructive pulmonary disease−COPD, including asthma

---

GINKGO BILOBA	
♀	**Dose**
U	40mg PO q8hours of standardized extract containing 24% ginkgo flavone glycosides & 6% terpene lactones

Side effects:
Cardiovascular
- •↓Platelet activity (avoid in patients taking an anticoagulant)

Neurologic
- •**Seizures**
  - ○Avoid concomitant usage w/ medications known to ↓seizure threshold:
    - −**Acetylcholinesterase inhibitors**
    - −Antidepressants
    - −Antipsychotics
    - −Carbapenem antibiotics
    - −Decongestants
    - −Sedating antihistamines
    - −Systemic glucocorticoids

Contraindications:
- •Seizure disorder

PSYCHOSIS ▬▬▬▬▬
- •Atypical antipsychotic medications have been found to ↑mortality in elderly patients w/ dementia, & should be avoided

PROGNOSIS
- •Death usually occurs @ 8−10years, usually due to aspiration pneumonia

Findings:
- Small atrophic cerebrum & cerebellum, w/ many of the residual neurons (limbic & parietal predominance) containing:
  - **Intracellular neurofibrillary tangles**
  - **Extracellular plaques** composed of:
    - Degenerated nerve terminals
    - Apolipoprotein E4
    - An amyloid protein complex which undergoes a apple−green to yellow−orange birefringence when stained w/ Congo Red, & examined w/ a polarized light
- **Global loss of cholinergic neurons**, esp. in the cerebral cortex & nucleus basalis of Meynert

- Dementia may be caused by any disease→
  - Neuronal dysfunction &/or death, termed encephalopathy

Differential:
- **Alzheimer's disease−50%**
- **Vascular dementia−10%** via either:
  - Multi−infarct dementia
  - Binswanger's disease
- **Alcohol dementia−10%**
- **Parkinson's disease−7%**
- **Major depression→**
  - Pseudodementia−7%
- **Lewy body dementia−5%**
- **Huntington's disease−3%**
- **Intracranial neoplasia−3%**
- **Hydrocephalus−3%**

The following comprise only 2%:
- **Brain trauma**
  - Mutiple contusions→
    - Dementia pugilistica
  - Subdural hematoma
- **Central nervous system infection**
  - Any cause of encephalitis &/or chronic meningitis
    - Human immune deficiency virus−HIV & AIDS related infections
    - Treponema pallidum→neurosyphilis
- **Degenerative diseases**
  - Frontotemporal dementia
  - Pick's disease
  - Wilson's disease
- **Demyelinating diseases**
  - Multiple sclerosis
- **Electrolyte disturbance**
  - Hypercalcemia
  - Hyper or hyponatremia
- **Endocrine**
  - Cushings disease or syndrome
  - Hypothyroidism
- **Lipid storage diseases**
  - Kufs' disease
  - Tay−Sach's disease
- **Liver failure→**
  - Hepatic encephalopathy
- **Nutritional deficiency**
  - Vitamin B12=Cyanocobalamin
  - Niacin
  - Vitamin B1=Thiamine
- **Prion diseases**
  - Creutzfeldt−Jakob disease−CJD
  - Fatal familial insomnia
  - Gerstmann−Straussler−Scheinker disease
  - Kuru
- **Progressive multifocal leukoencephalopathy−PML**

803

- **Progressive supranuclear palsy**
- **Renal failure:**
  - Uremia→
    - −Encephalopathy
  - Dialysis dementia

PARKINSON'S DISEASE SYNDROMES

•Caused by any disease or substance→neuronal & neuroglial dysfunction & degeneration of the:
  ◦Basal ganglia
  ◦Substantia nigra
  …&/or their connections→
    •**Extrapyramidal movement disorder**→
      ◦Slow & stiff movement
      ◦Resting tremor
Statistics:
  •Primary Parkinson's disease affects 1% of persons age >60years

EXPLANATION OF ASSOCIATED NEURONAL ANATOMY

•The **basal ganglia** is a group of subcortical nuclei composed of the:
  ◦Caudate nucleus
  ◦Globus pallidus (not directly affected in Parkinson's disease)
  ◦Putamen
•The corticospinal tracts, termed the **pyramidal tracts** are composed of motor neurons originating in the cerebral cortex
•The **extrapyramidal tracts** are composed of motor neurons originating in the subcortical nuclei, being the:
  ◦Basal ganglia
  ◦Midbrain red nucleus
  ◦Reticular formation
  ◦Substantia nigra
  ◦Subthalamic nucleus of Luys

CLASSIFICATION/ RISK FACTORS

•**Primary Parkinson's disease–80%**
  ◦A Slow, chronically progressive movement disorder of unknown etiology→destruction of the brainstem dopaminergic nucleus, the substantia nigra→↓basal ganglia projections via the nigrostriatal tract→altered dopaminergic–cholinergic balance via:
    –**↓Basal ganglia dopamine**→relatively **↑acetylcholine**→**movement disease**
  Risk factors:
    •**Age** >40years
    •**Gender:** ♂ > ♀

•**Secondary Parkinson's disease–20%**
  ◦Due to an identifiable disease &/or substance→
    –Parkinson's disease syndrome

  Risk factors:
    •**Medications**
      ◦Dopamine receptor blockers
        –Antipsychotics
        –Metoclopramide
        …w/ effects being reversible within 1year after discontinuation
    •**Basal ganglia calcification**
      ◦Hypoparathyroidism
      ◦Idiopathic calcification
    •**Degenerative disease**
      ◦Corticobasal degeneration
      ◦Diffuse lewy body disease
      ◦Olivopontocerebellar atrophy
      ◦Progressive supranuclear palsy
      ◦Shy–Drager syndrome
      ◦Striatonigral degeneration
    •**Genetic**
      ◦Halloverden–Spatz disease
      ◦Huntington's disease
      ◦Wilson's disease
    •**Infectious**
      ◦Encephalitis
    •**Ischemic**
      ◦Multi–infarct
    •**Neoplastic**

805

- **Primary dementing illness**
  - Alzheimer's disease
  - Creutzfeldt–Jacob disease
- **Toxins**
  - Carbon disulfide
  - Carbon monoxide
  - Cyanide
  - Manganese
  - Methanol
  - 1-methyl-4-phenyl-1,2,3,6-tetrahydropyridine–MPTP
- **Trauma**
  - Head injury (ex. boxers), termed Parkinson's pugilistica

DIAGNOSIS OF PRIMARY PARKINSON'S DISEASE

Neurologic/ musculoskeletal
- Loss of dopaminergic mediated inhibition of the basal ganglia→basal ganglia overactivity→ corticospinal motor overactivity→↑contraction of the skeletal musculature (both flexor & extensor muscles)→**stiffness, termed rigidity→**
  - **Difficulty initiating purposeful body movement, termed akinesia→**
    - –↑Mental effort & anguish in initiating movement
  - **Slow movement, termed bradykinesia**
    - –**Difficulty in changing posture** (sitting, standing, rolling over in bed)
    - –**Slow, short, shuffling gait,** w/ stiff neck, trunk, knees, elbows, &/or fingers, all being predominantly flexed→**stooped posture**→forward center of gravity→involuntary, progressively rapid steps, termed **festination**
    - –↓Turning ability→whole body turning, w/ feet slowly rotating, termed **en bloc turning**
    - –↓**Arm movement while walking or talking**
    - –↓Rapid alternating movements
    - –Impaired postural righting reflex→impaired balance (esp. to rapid postural displacement such as a push)→involuntary backward shuffling, termed **retropulsion,** &/or falls
  - Facial muscle hypertonia→
    - –↓**Facial expression, termed hypomimia or mask-like facies**
    - –↓Blink rate
  - ↓Coordination of vocalization muscles→
    - –**Low, soft, & slurred monotone voice, termed hypophonia**
  - ↓Fine motor control→↓ability to:
    - –Write small, termed micrographia
    - –Apply makeup
    - –Button or fasten clothing &/or accessories
    - –Knit
    - –Shave
  - Oscillation of feedback circuits→low frequency (3–6 Hz=cycles/ second) involuntary tremor during rest, termed **resting tremor, being ↓by purposeful movement, affecting the:**
    - –Hands→flexion & extension of fingers w/ abduction & adduction of thumb→"pill-rolling" or "watch-winding" motion
    - –Head→flexion & extension→"head bobbing" motion
    - –Trunk→flexion & extension
  - Difficulty swallowing=dysphagia→
    - –Aspiration pneumonia
    - –↓Caloric intake→cachexia
    - –Saliva accumulation→drooling
- Autonomic neuropathy→
  - ↓**Sympathetic tone:**
    - –Orthostatic hypotension→falls
    - –↑Gastrointestinal tone→diarrhea
    - –↓Hypoglycemic response, termed hypoglycemic unawareness
  - ↓**Parasympathetic tone:**
    - –Fixed, resting tachycardia
    - –Impotence
    - –↓Gastrointestinal tone→abdominal distention, constipation, nausea ± vomiting
    - –Incomplete urinary bladder emptying, termed neurogenic bladder→overflow incontinence & ↑urinary tract infection risk

806

Maneuvers designed to unveil underlying disease:
- **Cogwheel rigidity:** Passive rotation or extension & flexion of a joint (ex. elbow, wrist, thumb, neck)→
  - Alternating periods of resistance & relaxation, palpated as a soft ratchety feeling
- **Glabellar tap sign:** Normally, consecutive tapping of the glabella† while standing behind the patient (so as the patient is not affected by the sight of the hand coming toward the face)→
  - Blinking several times, w/ subsequent accommodation→no further blinking, whereas Parkinson's disease patients may not make this accommodation→continuous blinking

---

†The area just above the root of the nose, between the eyebrows

Mucocutaneous
- ↑Sebaceous gland sebum production, termed seborrhea
- ↑Perspiration
- …→facial oiliness, also being due to ↓hygiene

DIFFERENTIATION OF PRIMARY & SECONDARY PARKINSON'S DISEASE		
Symptom or sign	Primary	Secondary
Age of onset	Advanced age	Young age
Tremor onset	Unilateral	Bilateral
Family history	No	Possible
Upper or lower motor neuron signs	No	Possible
Cerebellar or sensory signs	No	Possible
Impaired ocular motility	No	Possible
Medications	No	Possible
Progression	Slow	Rapidly over several years
•Dysautonomia, dysarthria, dysphagia	Late onset	Early onset
•Dementia	Late onset	Early onset
•Falling	Late onset	Early onset
Response to Levodopa	↓Syndrome	No response
Autopsy	Substantia nigra Lewy bodies† only	Widespread vs. no Lewy bodies†

†Lewy bodies are eosinophilic, intracytoplasmic inclusions

TREATMENT

- **Occupational therapy**
  - To teach the patient how to better perform activities of daily living–ADLs ± assistive devices if necessary:
    - Braces, crutches, &/or walkers→↑stability & ↑mobility
    - Eating utensils w/ large handles
    - Strategically placed rails, such as along stairwells, by the toilet, & in the bath &/or shower
- **Physical therapy**
  - For gait training
  - To teach the patient:
    - Joint protective maneuvers
    - Energy conserving maneuvers
  - To provide an individualized exercise program incorporating range of motion–ROM & muscle strengthening
- **Home safety** evaluation to ensure:
  - Adequate lighting, including night lights in bedrooms, hallways, & bathrooms
  - Uncluttered walkways
  - Securely fastened stairway handrails
  - Bathroom grab bars in the shower/ bathtub & by the toilet
  - Raised toilet seats
  - Nonslip rubber suction mats in the shower/ bathtub & slick bathroom floors
  - Throw rugs are either fastened to the floor or removed
- **Speech therapy**
  Indications:
  - Voice amplifying device

DOPAMINE REPLACEMENT TREATMENT

Generic (Trade)	M ♀	Start	Max Levodopa
Levodopa/ Carbidopa (Sinemet)	L ?	1 tab=100mg/ 25mg PO q8hours	2000mg/ 24hours
•XR form		1 tab=200mg/ 50mg PO q12hours	2000mg/ 24hours

•If the patient was not initially treated w/ Levodopa, attempt to ↓other anti−parkinsonian medications upon improvement, w/ the goal of weaning them off

Dose adjustment:
- •↓Starting dose by 50% in the elderly
- •Switching to the XR form
  - ∘Only ~70% of Levodopa is absorbed from the XR formulation, requiring that the dose be 30%↑ than that of the standard combination to achieve comparable effects

Mechanism:
- •As dopamine does not pass through the blood brain barrier, Levodopa (the immediate dopamine precursor) which does, is used→
  - ∘Intraneuronal dopa carboxylase mediated conversion to dopamine
- •In order to selectively target the central nervous system, Carbidopa (a dopa carboxylase inhibitor) is used, which does not pass through the blood brain barrier→
  - ∘Selective inhibition of peripheral dopa carboxylase (accomplished via ≥75mg q24h†)→
    - −↓Peripheral dopamine→↓peripheral side effects

†May require up to 200mg q24h to completely suppress nausea

Outcomes:
- •**The most effective treatment for symptomatic relief**
- •Eventually (~5years) the effect of Levodopa/ Carbidopa begins to:
  - ∘Wear off progressively earlier
  - ∘Cause sudden, unpredictable fluctuations between mobility & immobility, termed the "on−off effect"
    …which can be treated via ↓the dosing interval without daily dosage change or switching to the XR form

Side effects:
- •All the following side effects are **dose dependent**, w/ both peripheral (P) & central nervous system effects
- •For treatment, consider adding:
  - ∘A "wearing off effect" medication as listed below
  - ∘Switching to the XR form of the medication
    - −Due to its slower onset of action, a standard tablet may need to be taken concomitantly w/ the first dose of the day
  - ∘Crushed standard tablets mixed w/ a beverage, termed "liquid Levodopa"→
    - −Rapid absorption→rescue for "off" episodes

General
- •Anorexia (P)

Cardiovascular
- •Dysrhythmias−rare
- •Orthostatic hypotension (P)
- •Tachycardia

Gastrointestinal
- •Nausea ± vomiting (P)

Musculoskeletal
- •**Difficulty performing voluntary movements, termed dyskinesia,** usually occurring when the medication reaches peak plasma levels @ ~2hours after ingestion &/or randomly
  - ∘Dyskinesia may present in the following forms:
    - −**Chorea,** being spasmodic, nonrhythmic, involuntary muscle contractions of the facial muscles, limbs, &/or trunk
    - −**Dystonia,** being sustained muscle contraction→abnormal body postures &/or repetitive movements

Neurologic
- •Anxiety
- •Altered mental status
- •Depression
- •Narcolepsy
- •Pathologic gambling

- •Psychosis
  - ◦Delusions
  - ◦Hallucinations
- •Vivid dreams

Interactions
- •Dietary protein competes w/ the medication for intestinal absorption→
  - ◦↓Efficacy

Caution:
- •Sudden ↓dosage X several days→
  - ◦**Neuroleptic malignant syndrome–NMS** (see below)

SECOND LINE TREATMENT

DOPAMINE RECEPTOR AGONISTS: Ergot alkaloids

Generic (Trade)	M	♀	Start	Max
Bromocriptine (Parlodel)	L	P	1.25mg PO q24hours	50mg q12hours
Pergolide (Permax)	K	P	0.05mg PO q24hours	5mg/ 24hours

Bromocriptine specific mechanism:
- •Dopamine 2 receptor partial agonist

Pergolide specific mechanism:
- •Dopamine 1 & 2 receptor agonist

DOPAMINE RECEPTOR AGONISTS: Non–ergot alkaloids

Generic (Trade)	M	♀	Start	Max
Pramipexole (Mirapex)	K	?	0.125mg PO q8hours	1.5mg PO q8hours
Ropinirole (Requip)	L	?	0.25mg PO q8hours	8mg PO q8hours

Side effects: **Same as Levodopa +**
Mucocutaneous
- •Alopecia

Ergot alkaloid specific:
Cardiovascular
- •Valvular heart disease (Pergolide only)

Pulmonary
- •Pleural effusions, being rare & reversible
- •Pulmonary fibrosis
- •Retroperitoneal fibrosis

Neurologic–rare
- •Extremity:
  - ◦Digital spasms
  - ◦Edema
  - ◦A syndrome of intense burning pain & erythema of the extremities, termed erythromelalgia
  - ◦Pain

Caution:
- •Sudden ↓dosage X several days→
  - ◦**Neuroleptic malignant syndrome–NMS** (see below)

CATECHOL–O–METHYLTRANSFERASE INHIBITORS–COMTi

Indications:
- •**Only** patients experiencing a refractory Levodopa "wearing off effect", as it has no antiparkinsonian effect as monotherapy

Generic (Trade)	M	♀	Start	Max
Entacapone (Comtan)	L	?	200mg PO w/ each Levodopa/ Carbidopa dose	1600mg/ 24hours

Mechanism:
- •Catechol–O–methyl transferase is present diffusely on cell membranes→
  - ◦Catecholamine metabolism (epinephrine, norepinephrine, & dopamine), w/ inhibition→
    - –↑Synaptic cleft concentrations

Caution:
- •Sudden ↓dosage X several days→
  - ◦**Neuroleptic malignant syndrome–NMS** (see below)

ANTIVIRAL				
Generic (Trade)	M	♀	**Start**	**Max**
Amantadine (Symmetrel)	K	?	100mg PO q12hours	200mg PO q12hours

•Maximal effect noted within 2weeks, & lasting ~6months

Mechanism:
  •?↑Presynaptic dopamine synthesis, release, &/or ↓re-uptake→
    ∘↑Synaptic cleft concentrations
  •Anticholinergic effects

Side effects: **Same as Levodopa +**
  Mucocutaneous
  •Capillary & venule dilation→
    ∘A net-like pattern of macular purple-blue skin discoloration, termed livedo reticularis
  Neurologic
  •Dizziness
  •Insomnia

Caution:
  •Sudden ↓dosage X several days→
    ∘**Neuroleptic malignant syndrome-NMS** (see below)
    ∘Delirium

MONOAMINE OXIDASE B SELECTIVE INHIBITORS-MAOBi			
Generic (Trade)	M	♀	**Dose**
Selegiline=Deprenyl (Eldepryl)	LK	?	5mg PO qam & noon, due to insomnia

Mechanism:
  •Selectively inhibits the function of monoamine oxidase-MAO subtype B (an enzyme found on the outer mitochondrial membrane) which metabolizes dopamine→
    ∘↑Presynaptic vesicular dopamine concentrations→
      −↑Synaptic cleft concentrations
  •Via an unknown mechanism, the medication also slows the destruction of dopamine secreting neurons in the substantia nigra→
    ∘↓**Disease progression**

Side effects:
  Cardiovascular
  •Selegiline is metabolized to methamphetamine & amphetamine→
    ∘Insomnia

Caution:
  •Sudden ↓dosage X several days→
    ∘**Neuroleptic malignant syndrome-NMS** (see below)
Contraindications:
  •Use w/ opioids

ANTICHOLINERGIC MEDICATIONS				
Generic (Trade)	M	♀	**Start**	**Max**
Benztropine mesylate (Cogentin)	LK	?	0.5mg q24hours PO/ IM/ IV	6mg/ 24hours
Biperiden (Akineton)	LK	?	2mg PO q8hours	16mg/ 24hours
Procyclidine (Kemadrin)	LK	?	2.5mg PO q8hours	20mg/ 24hours
Trihexyphenidyl (Artane)	LK	?	1mg PO q24hours	15mg/ 24hours

•All may be divided into q8h-q6h dosing as needed
•Maximal effects noted @ 2-4weeks

Mechanism:
  •Block muscarinic receptors→
    ∘↓Acetylcholine effect

Outcomes:
  •↓Tremor, rigidity, & drooling > others

Side effects:
Mucocutaneous
- ↓Glandular cell secretions
  - ◦↓Exocrine secretions→
    - –↓Lacrimal, mucosal, parotid, submandibular, gastric, & pancreatic secretions→dry mucus membranes (including eyes)
  - ◦↓Eccrine=merocrine secretions→
    - –↓Perspiration†→dry skin→↑hyperthermia risk
  - ◦↓Holocrine secretions→
    - –↓Sebum→dry skin
  - ◦↓Apocrine secretions→
    - –↓Breast milk
    - –↓Pheromones
- Dilation of the cutaneous vasculature above the waist, being of uncertain etiology→
  - ◦Flushing, termed "atropine flush"

Opthalmologic
- ↓Ciliary smooth muscle contraction→
  - ◦Far vision, w/ near visual blurring
  - ◦Canal of Schlemm compression (a thin walled circumferential vein @ the iridocorneal junction)→
    - –↓Aqueous fluid outflow→↑anterior chamber pressure→wide=open angle glaucoma exacerbation
- ↓Iris circular smooth muscle contraction→
  - ◦Dilated pupil=mydriasis
  - ◦Compression of the drainage pathway between the cornea & the ciliary body→
    - –Narrow=closed angle glaucoma exacerbation

Neurologic
- Altered mental status
- Amnesia
- Hallucinations
- Sedation
- Seizures

Gastrointestinal/ Genitourinary
- ↓Genitourinary & gastrointestinal smooth muscle contraction→
  - ◦↓Tone & peristalsis→
    - –Urinary retention &/or constipation respectively

---

†Perspiration is controlled by the sympathetic nervous system→
- Postganglionic acetylcholine release, except on the palms & soles which are activated by norepinephrine

Contraindications:
Gastrointestinal
- Gastrointestinal obstruction

Genitourinary
- Benign prostatic hyperplasia

Opthalmologic
- Narrow angle glaucoma

THIRD LINE TREATMENT
- **Deep brain stimulation**

Procedure:
- Bilateral implanted electrode mediated, high frequency subthalamic stimulation

Outcomes:
- ↓Resting tremor
- Chronic bilateral stimulation of the subthalamic nucleus or medial globus pallidus→
  - ◦Generalized syndrome relief

Complications:
- Altered mental status
- Cognitive deficits
- Dysarthria
- Hemiparesis
- Infection
- Intracranial hemorrhage

- **Stereotactic ventrolateral thalamotomy†**
  Procedure:
  - Stereotactic mediated destruction of the ventrolateral thalamus
  Outcomes:
  - ↓Tremor, rigidity, & dystonia

- **Stereotactic medial pallidotomy†**
  Procedure:
  - Stereotactic mediated destruction of the medial globus pallidus
  Outcomes:
  - ↓Akinesia

- **Fetal tissue transplantation**
  Procedure:
  - Transplantation of substantia nigra cells from aborted fetal brains into the patient's caudate nucleus & putamen
  Outcomes:
  - At present time, the fetal cells survive for only several months
  - Has caused **uncontrollable dyskinesias**, which is why this treatment is no longer being pursued

---

†Surgery should generally be unilateral, as morbidity is ↑w/ bilateral procedures

MEDICAL TREATMENT COMPLICATION

- **Neuroleptic malignant syndrome–NMS**, being an idiosyncratic, life threatening complication of:
  ○ Antipsychotic medications
  ○ Sudden ↓dopaminergic medication dosage
    – Parkinson's disease medications
  …→↓dopamine effect→
    - Autonomic nervous system dysfunction→
      ○ Diaphoresis
      ○ Dysrhythmia
      ○ **Fever→**
        – Hyperthermia
      ○ Hypertension or hypotension
      ○ Tachycardia
    - Somatic nervous system dysfunction→
      ○ **Stiffness, termed rigidity→**
        – Difficulty initiating purposeful body movement, termed akinesia
        – Dysphagia
        – Dystonia
        – Mutism
    - Altered mental status
    - Diarrhea
    - Disseminated intravascular coagulation–DIC
    - Dyspnea
    - Renal failure
    - Seizures

PROGNOSIS

- W/ treatment, almost all patients have a normal lifespan
- 50% develop **major depression**
- 15% develop **dementia**

•A chronic autoimmune disease of unknown etiology→
  ◦Autoantibodies to neuromuscular junction end plate nicotinic acetylcholine receptors→
    −Receptor blockade & damage
    −Accelerated endocytosis
     ...→↓neuromuscular transmission→
      •Weakness→
       ◦Eventual paralysis

Statistics:
•Affects 1/ 20,000 persons in the U.S.

•**Age (Gender):** Bimodal distribution @ ages:
  ◦12–30 years (♀ > ♂)
  ◦50–70years (♂ > ♀)
•**Thymus gland abnormalities**
  ◦Thymic hyperplasia–85%
  ◦Thymoma–15%
•**Other autoimmune diseases**
  ◦Autoimmune thyroiditis
  ◦Autolmmune thrombocytopenia
  ◦Graves' disease
  ◦Lambert–Eaton myasthenic syndrome
  ◦Pemphigus
  ◦Pernicious anemia
  ◦Polymyositis
  ◦Rheumatoid arthritis
  ◦Systemic lupus erythematosus

Neuromuscular
•Because the disease affects the nicotinic M–type acetylcholine receptors, found only on the neuromuscular endplate, only the motor system is affected, thus sparing all other neurologic functions (ex. sensation, reflexes, cognition)

•**Weakness & fatigability of skeletal muscles**, esp. affecting the:
  ◦**Proximal limb musculature**
    −Deltoid muscles→difficulty abducting the arms
    −Triceps & iliopsoas muscles→difficulty rising from a seated position
  ◦**Head & neck musculature**
    −Eyelid muscles→eyelid drooping=ptosis
    −Extraocular muscles→double vision=diplopia
    −Neck extensors→head drooping
    −Facial muscles→facial "snarl"
    −Muscles of articulation→difficulty w/ speech=dysarthria
    −Muscles of phonation→altered voice production=dysphonia
    −Muscles of mastication→jaw dropping &/or difficulty chewing
    ...being exacerbated by repeated use, & improved by rest

Precipitating factors:
•**Overtreatment**, via hypercholinergic effects
•**Endocrine**
  ◦Hypo or hyperthyroidism
•**Infection**
•**Medications**
  ◦Antibiotics
    −Aminoglycosides
    −Erythromycin
    −Tetracycline
  ◦Antidysrhythmic medications
  ◦β receptor blockers
  ◦Calcium channel blockers
  ◦Lithium
  ◦Phenytoin
  ◦Quinine

- •Perimenstruaton
- •Pregnancy

Pulmonary
- •Weakness & fatiguability of the muscles of:
  - ◦Respiration→
    - −Difficulty breathing=dyspnea
  - ◦Deglutition→
    - −Difficulty swallowing=dysphagia
    - ...being **a medical emergency, termed Myasthenic crisis,** as they indicate the need for assisted ventilation or airways protection, respectively

Hematologic
- •**Anti−acetylcholine receptor antibodes−85%**

MEDICATION STUDIES			
ACETYLCHOLINESTERASE INHIBITORS			

Indications:
- •Diagnosis of Myasthenia Gravis
- •In patients w/ known myasthenia gravis, it may be used to differentiate:
  - ◦Disease progression, which will be indicated via improvement
  - ◦Overmedication mediated hypercholinergic effects, which will be indicated via worsening

Generic (Trade)	M ♀	Dose
Edrophonium† (Tensilon)	P ?	An initial test dose of 2mg IV over 15seconds, then After 1 min., administer 8mg IV over 45seconds

†An alcohol, so very short acting, w/ a duration of 5−10min.

Mechanism:
- •↓Perisynaptic connective tissue acetylcholinesterase function→
  - ◦↓Acetylcholine metabolism→
    - −↑Synaptic cleft concentrations, w/ **affected patients experiencing transiently ↑strength**

Side effects:
- **Cardiovascular**
  - •**Hypercholinergic effects→**
    - ◦Bradycardia &/or asystole. During administration, the patient should be on a cardiac monitor, w/ Atropine available

Cautionary use:
- •Severe chronic obstructive pulmonary disease−COPD, including asthma

ELECTRICAL STUDIES

- •**Electromyography−EMG**
  - Procedure:
    - •Repetitive nerve stimulation of weak or proximal muscle groups→
      - ◦Decremental ↓motor response−65%, being the electrical analog of fatigue

IMAGING STUDIES

Thoracic computed tomographic−CT scan
- Indications:
  - •All affected patients, to search for a possible thymoma

TREATMENT			
ACETYLCHOLINESTERASE INHIBITORS			
Generic (Trade)	M ♀	Dose	Max
Pyridostigmine (Mestinon, Regonal)	L ?	60mg PO q6hours	1500mg/ 24hours
•XR form		180mg PO q24−12hours	1500mg/ 24hours
•IM/ IV forms		1/30th of PO dosage q2−3hours	

- •Titrate to the lowest effective maintenance dose providing syndrome relief

Onset: 10−30min., Peak: 2hours, Duration: 3−6hours

Mechanism:
- •↓Perisynaptic connective tissue acetylcholinesterase function→
  - ◦↓Acetylcholine metabolism→
    - −↑Synaptic cleft concentrations→↑strength

Side effects:
- **Cardiovascular**
  - •Bradycardia
- **Gastrointestinal†**
  - •↑Gastrointestinal smooth muscle contraction→
    - ◦↑Tone & peristalsis→
      - −Abdominal discomfort
      - −Diarrhea
      - −Nausea ± vomiting
- **Genitourinary**
  - •↑Genitourinary smooth muscle contraction→
    - ◦↑Tone & peristalsis→
      - −Urinary frequency
- **Mucocutaneous**
  - •↑Glandular cell secretions
    - ◦↑Exocrine secretions→
      - −↑Lacrimal, mucosal, parotid, submandibular, gastric, & pancreatic secretions
    - ◦↑Eccrine=merocrine secretions→
      - −↑Perspiration‡
    - ◦↑Holocrine secretions→
      - −↑Sebum→oily skin
- **Musculoskeletal**
  - •Muscle cramps
- **Neurologic**
  - •Insomnia
- **Opthalmologic**
  - •↑Iris circular smooth muscle contraction→
    - ◦Constricted pupil=myosis
- **Pulmonary**
  - •Bronchoconstriction

---

†↓By low starting dose, gradual titration, & continued use
- •If treatment is interrupted X several days, restart @ starting dose, w/ gradual titration

‡Perspiration is controlled by the sympathetic nervous system→
- •Postganglionic acetylcholine release, except on the palms & soles which are activated by norepinephrine

Cautionary use:
- •Severe chronic obstructive pulmonary disease–COPD, including asthma

±

- **•Thymectomy**
  - Indications:
    - •Thymoma
    - •Moderate to severely generalized disease
    - •Inadequate disease control via medications to their tolerable limits
  - Procedure:
    - •The optimal technique is a maximal trans–sternal approach, designed to remove as much thymus tissue as possible. If the entire thymus cannot be removed, postoperative radiation treatment should be administered
  - Outcomes:
    - •Benefit is delayed, rarely occurring within 6months, & often requiring several years

SECOND LINE TREATMENT ▬▬▬▬▬▬

SYSTEMIC GLUCOCORTICOID TREATMENT

Indications:
- •Refractory to, or intolerant of, first line treatment
- •Control disease while an immunomodulating medication is taking effect

Generic	M	♀	Dose	Max
Methylprednisolone	L	?	10–20mg PO q24hours	1mg/kg/24hours
Prednisolone	L	?	10–20mg PO q24hours	1mg/kg/24hours
Prednisone	L	?	10–20mg PO q24hours	1mg/kg/24hours

•Once disease control is achieved X 6months, taper to the lowest effective maintenance dose in order to minimize serious side effects, w/ the goal of discontinuation if possible, w/ attention to relapse syndrome

815

Glucocorticoids	Relative potencies Anti–inflammatory	Mineralocorticoid	Duration	Dose equiv.
Cortisol (physiologic†)	1	1	10hours	20mg
Cortisone (PO)	0.7	2	10hours	25mg
Hydrocortisone (PO, IM, IV)	1	2	10hours	20mg
Methylprednisolone (PO, IM, IA, IV)	5	0.5	15–35hours	5mg
Prednisone (PO)	5	0.5	15–35hours	5mg
Prednisolone (PO, IM, IV)	5	0.8	15–35hours	5mg
Triamcinolone (PO, IM)	5	~0	15–35hours	5mg
Betamethasone (PO, IM, IA)	25	~0	35–70hours	0.75mg
Dexamethasone (PO)	25	~0	35–70hours	0.75mg
Fludrocortisone (PO)	10	125	10hours	

†The physiologic rate of adrenal cortical cortisol production is 20–30mg/ 24hours

Side effects of chronic use:

General
- Anorexia→
  - Cachexia
- ↑Perspiration

Cardiovascular
- Mineralocorticoid effects→
  - ↑Renal tubular NaCl & water retention as well as potassium secretion→
    - **Hypertension**
    - **Edema**
    - **Hypokalemia**
- Counter–regulatory=anti–insulin effects→
  - ↑Plasma glucose→
    - **Secondary diabetes mellitus**, which may→ketoacidemia
  - Hyperlipidemia→↑atherosclerosis→
    - **Coronary artery disease**
    - Cerebrovascular disease
    - Peripheral vascular disease

Cutaneous/ subcutaneous
- ↓Fibroblast function→
  - ↓Intercellular matrix production→
    - ↑Bruisability→ecchymoses
    - Poor wound healing
    - Skin striae
- Androgenic effects→
  - Acne
  - ↑Facial hair
  - Thinning scalp hair
- Fat redistribution from the extremities to the:
  - Abdomen→
    - Truncal obesity
  - Shoulders→
    - Supraclavicular fat pads
  - Upper back→
    - Buffalo hump
  - Face→
    - Moon facies
  ...w/ concomitant thinning of the arms & legs

Endocrine
- **Adrenal failure** upon abrupt discontinuation after 2weeks

Gastrointestinal
- Inhibition of phospholipase A_2 mediated conversion of cell membrane lipids to arachidonic acid, which is the precursor for both cyclooxygenase–COX enzymes, w/ the cyclooxygenase–COX1 enzyme found in most cells of the body, responsible for normal physiologic function. Inhibition of the cyclooxygenase–COX1 enzyme→↑peptic inflammatory disease risk→↑**upper gastrointestinal hemorrhage risk** via:
  - ↓Gastric mucosal prostaglandin synthesis→
    - ↓Epithelial cell proliferation
    - ↓Mucosal blood flow→↓bicarbonate delivery to the mucosa
    - ↓Mucus & bicarbonate secretion from gastric mucosal cells

Musculoskeletal
- **Avascular necrosis of bone**
- **Osteoporosis**
- Proximal muscle weakness

Neurologic
- Anxiety
- Insomnia
- Psychosis

Opthalmologic
- **Cataracts**

Immunologic
- Inhibition of phospholipase A_2 mediated conversion of cell membrane lipids to arachidonic acid, which is the precursor for both cyclooxygenase–COX enzymes (COX1 & COX2) being responsible for the production of neuronal & inflammatory cell prostaglandins respectively→
  - $-\downarrow$Pain
  - $-\downarrow$Temperature (antipyretic)
  - $-\downarrow$**Inflammation**
- Stabilization of lisosomal & cell membranes→
  - ∘$\downarrow$Cytokine & proteolytic enzyme release
- $\downarrow$Lymphocyte & eosinophil production
- ...all→
  - **Immunosuppression→**
    - $-\uparrow$**Infection** &/or neoplasm risk

Hematologic
- $\uparrow$Erythrocyte production→
  - ∘Polycythemia
- $\uparrow$Neutrophil demargination→
  - ∘Neutrophilia→
    - **Leukocytosis**

IMMUNOMODULATING MEDICATIONS
- The following medications usually require 1–6 months for symptomatic improvement, making these medications not useful in the control of acute disease, but rather, useful when prolonged treatment is planned

Generic (Trade)	M	♀	Start	Max
6–mercaptopurine	L	U	50mg PO q24hours	
Azathioprine†(Imuran)	LK	U	1mg/ kg PO q24hours	2.5mg/kg/24hours

†Azathioprine's active metabolite is 6–mercaptopurine

Mechanism:
- Inhibition of enzymes involved in purine metabolism→
  - ∘Cytotoxicity of differentiating lymphocytes (T cell >> B cell)

Side effects:
Gastrointestinal
- $\downarrow$Mucosal cell proliferation→
  - ∘Mucosal inflammation=mucositis, including inflammation of the oral mucosa=stomatitis→
    - Diarrhea
    - Nausea ± vomiting
- Hepatitis→
  - ∘Cirrhosis–rare

Mucocutaneous
- $\downarrow$Epithelial cell proliferation→
  - ∘Dermatitis

Hematologic
- Myelosuppression†→
  - ∘Macrocytic anemia→
    - Fatigue
  - ∘Leukopenia→immunosuppression→
    - $-\uparrow$Infection & neoplasm risk
  - ∘Thrombocytopenia→
    - $-\uparrow$Hemorrhage risk, esp. petechiae

817

†Esp. w/ concomitant:
- •Renal failure
- •Medications:
  - ◦Allopurinol
  - ◦Angiotensin converting enzyme inhibitor–ACEi

Monitoring:
- •Baseline:
  - ◦Complete blood count
  - ◦Liver function tests, w/ treatment to be withdrawn @ plasma values >3 X the upper limit of normal
  ...then q2weeks X 2months, then
    - •Q2months

MYASTHENIC CRISIS OR PERIOPERATIVE TREATMENT (PRE OR POST) ▬▬▬

- •For patients w/ myasthenic crisis:
  - ◦Place on a cardiac & PaO$_2$ monitor
  - ◦Consider early intubation, as this may be life saving being that respiratory arrest may occur terrifyingly fast. Anticholinesterase medications should be temporarily withdrawn in patients receiving assisted ventilation, in order to avoid both:
    - –The uncertainty of overmedication mediated cholinergic crisis
    - –Cholinergic stimulation of pulmonary secretions

INTRAVENOUS IMMUNE GLOBULIN–IVIG

Dose

1g/ kg IV q24hours X 2–5days

Mechanism:
- •Bind to macrophage IgG Fc receptors→
  - ◦Fc receptor downregulation→
    - –↓Macrophage mediated neuromuscular endplate damage
- •Bind to plasma cell IgG Fc receptors→
  - ◦Feedback inhibition mediated ↓anti–acetylcholine receptor antibody production

Side effects:
- **General**
  - •Fever ± chills
- **Cardiovascular**
  - •Flushing
  - •Hypotension
- **Gastrointestinal**
  - •Nausea ± vomiting
- **Genitourinary**
  - •Acute tubular necrosis, w/ preparations containing sucrose. If used, infuse @ ≤3mg sucrose/kg/min.
- **Neurologic**
  - •Aseptic meningitis–rare
  - •Headache
- **Pulmonary**
  - •Pulmonary failure
- **Hypersensitivity**
  - •Hypersensitivity reaction if infused rapidly
  - •**Anaphylaxis** may occur in patients w/ **IgA deficiency** due to varied amounts of IgA, w/ some products being IgA depleted

Contraindications:
- •IgA deficiency

OR

- •**Plasmapheresis**
  Procedure:
  - •Removal of blood, w/ subsequent separation of erythrocytes from the plasma. The plasma is then discarded, containing the causative anti–acetylcholine receptor antibodies, w/ the erythrocytes being reinfused w/ **fresh frozen plasma–FFP** until 1.5–2 X the plasma volume† has been exchanged q24h, until the patient is in complete remission

---

†1.5–2 X the plasma volume, being ~60–80mL/ kg, as the normal adult plasma volume is:
- •♂ 40mL/ kg
- •♀ 36mL/ kg

818

DEPRESSION

•Temporary or chronic, intermittently symptomatic ↓mood due to ↓central nervous system norepinephrine &/or serotonin production

Statistics:
- •1 in 3 patients feels depressed, of which, 1/3rd are suffering from major depression (~1 in 10 patients total)
- •Affects 8 million people in the U.S. at any time
- •80% of patients have a triggering event
- •5-10% of the population will suffer ≥1 major depressive episode(s) during their lifetime
  - ○35% suffer only 1 episode during their lifetime
  - ○65% suffer intermittent episodes of varying severity, frequency, & duration, w/ episodes lasting weeks, months, or years
- •50% do not seek treatment, & only 50% of those who do are correctly diagnosed & treated

RISK FACTORS

- •**Stressful life event**
- •**Gender:** ♀ 2X ♂
- •**Genetic:** Family history
- •**Medical disease**
  - ○**Neurologic**
    - −Cerebrovascular accident, esp. of the left frontal area
    - −Multiple sclerosis
    - −Parkinson's disease
  - ○**Endocrine**
    - −Cushing's disease or syndrome
    - −Hypothyroidism
  - ○**Neoplasia**
    - −Pancreatic cancer
- •**Medications**
  - ○Antihypertensive medications
    - −β receptor blockers
    - −Clonidine
    - −Methyldopa
    - −Reserpine
  - ○Benzodiazepines
  - ○Cyclosporine
  - ○Dapsone
  - ○Glucocorticoids
  - ○Interferon
- •**Drugs**
  - ○Alcohol
  - ○Amphetamine or cocaine withdrawal

CLASSIFICATION

- •**Major depression**
  - ○Requires **≥2weeks of a major depressive syndrome** during nearly all wakefulness, & must include either:
    - −**Depressed mood**
    - −**Loss of interest or pleasure, termed anhedonia**
    - …→significant distress &/or impairment in occupational, social, or other important areas of functioning, not being due to either:
      - •Substance use (medication or drug)
      - •Medical disease
- •**Major depression in partial remission**
  - ○Patient has a depressive syndrome not currently meeting the criteria for major depression, but having met the criteria at some previous time
- •**Major depression w/ atypical features**
  - ○Patient has a depressive syndrome w/ predominantly atypically altered basic drives:
    - −↑Sleep
    - −↑Hunger

819

•Requires ≥5 highlighted signs &/or symptoms

Neurologic
- •Brain stem
  - ∘Norepinephrine secreting neurons, esp. the locus ceruleus
  - ∘Serotonin secreting neurons, esp. the midline raphe nuclei
  - …contain limbic system axonal projections, w/ ↓function→
    - •↓Limbic system norepinephrine &/or serotonin→
      - ∘**Depressed mood** ± diurnal variation, being worse in the morning
      - ∘**Altered basic drives**
        - −**Sleep**, being ↓, termed insomnia, via difficulty initiating &/or early morning awakening.
          ↑Sleep, termed hypersomnia is atypical
        - −**Hunger**, being ↓, termed anorexia, during nearly all wakefulness→cachexia. ↑Hunger is atypical
        - −**Pleasure**, via ↓interest &/or pleasure in most activities (including ↓libido), termed anhedonia
        - −**Companionship**, via withdrawal from family, friends, &/or society in general
        - −**Self preservation**, via recurrent thoughts of death &/or suicide, termed suicidal ideation
      - ∘**Feelings of worthlessness**, w/ mistakes &/or shortcomings become sweeping self−condemnations
      - ∘**Excess or inappropriate guilt**, w/ patients falsely assuming they are responsible for some unfortunate event (may be delusional)
      - ∘**Fatigue**
      - ∘**Altered mental status→**
        - −Agitation
        - −↓Concentration
        - −Indecisiveness
        - −Reversible dementia, termed pseudodementia
      - ∘**Psychomotor retardation→**slow:
        - −Movement
        - −Speech
        - −Thought processes
      - ∘Anxiety disorders
      - ∘Failed attempts to change employment, living environment, &/or spouse, in the hope of feeling better
      - ∘Hopelessness, via seeing no relief &/or nothing to look forward to
      - ∘Change of grooming &/or appearance
      - ∘Bodily aches &/or pains (ex. headache) which worsen upon worsening depression
  - …w/ severe disease→
    - •Psychotic features
      - ∘False sensations=hallucinations
      - ∘False beliefs despite incontrovertible evidence to the contrary=delusions

•Being that the diagnosis of major depression requires the presence of either **depressed mood** or **loss of interest or pleasure**, a negative response to both the following questions rules out major depression, whereas a positive response to either requires further inquiry.
Interview questions:
  1. "During the past month, have you often been bothered by feeling down, depressed, or hopeless?"
  2. "During the past month, have you often been bothered by little interest or pleasure in doing things?"

•Being that 15% of patients w/ major depression commit suicide, w/ many more considering & attempting it, all patients w/ possible depressive syndromes should be asked about their thoughts concerning self injury & suicide, w/ questions becoming more specific as warranted
Statistics:
  •8th leading cause of death in the U.S.
Risk factors:
  •**Major depression** is the most powerful predictor of suicide, w/ risk being highest:
    ∘W/ the development of delusions
    ∘During early recovery, as patients begin to regain energy prior to an improved self attitude
  •**Previous suicide attempt**
  •**1st degree relative who committed suicide**
  •**Advanced age:** Peak occurrence @ ♂ age >45years; ♀ age >55years
  •**Skin color:** Whites > blacks

820

- **Gender:** ♂ > ♀ as:
  - ○♂ employ more lethal methods (hanging, jumping, shooting), whereas ♀ often overdose, attempt drowning, or wrist laceration
- **Severe anxiety**
- **Severe physical illness**
- **Severe stressful life event in the recent past**
- **Alcoholism or illicit drug use**
- **Personality disorder**
- **Psychotic disease**
- **Certain professions**
  - ○Dentists
  - ○Insurance agents
  - ○Law enforcement personnel
  - ○Lawyers
  - ○Musicians
  - ○Physicians
- **Unemployment**
- **High socioeconomic class**
- **Single lifestyle**

Interview questions:
1. "Sometimes when people feel depressed, they think about hurting or killing themselves. Do you ever have these kinds of thoughts?"
IF YES=SUICIDAL IDEATION ⬇
2. "Have you ever thought about how you would do it?"
IF YES=SUICIDAL PLANNING ⬇
3. **Urgent psychiatric consultation,** & ask if the patient has the means of carrying out the plan, or feels as though they will procure the means
IF YES ⬇
4. **Emergent psychiatric consult for hospitalization**
Indications:
- •Suicidal planning & delusional
- •Patient is unwilling to comply w/ a safety agreement†
- •Patient is fearful of an imminent attempt

---

†If the patient does not qualify for hospitalization, develop a safety agreement w/ the patient & family &/or close friends, w/ the patient to immediately notify the physician &/or family/ friends when suicidal thoughts progress to the point of considering an attempt

TREATMENT
- **All antidepressant medications are considered of equal efficacy,** w/ each individual medication:
  - ○Being effective in only 55% of patients
  - ○Having maximal efficacy @ ≥1month
  - ○Differing, perhaps **greatly, in their side effects profile**
- •A patient may need to try several classes of medication in order to find the one that works best for their biology, w/ the least & most tolerable side effects
- **Psychiatric referral**
  Indications:
  - •All patients, being emergent if either:
    - ○Suicidal (as above)
    - ○Psychotic, via delusions &/or hallucinations
    - ○Having profound slowing of thoughts &/or actions

Treatment duration:
- **First episode:** 1year after remission
- **Infrequent, recurrent episodes:** 1year after remission
- **Frequent, recurrent episodes:** 2years after remission to indefinitely

---

†Upon discontinuation, all medication dosages should be tapered by 25%/ week in order to avoid possible **hypercholinergic rebound symptoms** (see below), esp. w/ tricyclic antidepressants−10%. Rapid discontinuation may occur when switching to a similar antidepressant, or if toxicity develops

SELECTIVE SEROTONIN REUPTAKE INHIBITORS–SSRIs				
Generic (trade)	M	♀	Start	Max
Citalopram (Celexa)	LK	?	20mg PO q24hours	60mg q24hours
Escitalopram (Lexapro)	LK	?	10mg PO q24hours	20mg q24hours
Fluoxetine (Prozac)	L	?	20mg PO q24hours	80mg q24hours
•XR form			If effectively stabilized on 20mg PO q24hours, then may switch to the XR form @ 90mg PO qweek, after 1week off the medication	
Fluvoxamine (Luvox)	L	?	50mg PO qhs	300mg/ 24hours
Paroxetine (Paxil)	LK	?	20mg PO qam	50mg q24hours
Sertraline (Zoloft)	LK	?	50mg PO q24hours	200mg q24hours

Mechanism:
•Selectively inhibit the presynaptic reuptake of serotonin→
  ∘↑Synaptic cleft concentrations

Side effects†:
General
  •↓Weight initially, w/ subsequent ↑weight
Cardiovascular
  •Dysrhythmias
Gastrointestinal
  •Diarrhea
  •Nausea ± vomiting
  •Gastrointestinal discomfort
Mucocutaneous
  •Dermatitis
  •↑Perspiration
Neurologic
  •Anxiety
  •Headache
  •Insomnia
  •Restlessness
  •Seizures
  •Sexual dysfunction–20%
    ∘Consider adding Bupropion, which may→
      –Reversal of other antidepressant mediated sexual dysfunction
  •Tremor

Other receptor antagonism mediated side effects:
  •Anticholinergic→see below
  •Antihistamine→
    ∘Sedation
  •Anti α1→
    ∘Erectile dysfunction
    ∘Orthostatic hypotension
    ∘Sedation

†SSRIs cause less side effects than any other antidepressant

TRICYCLIC ANTIDEPRESSANTS–TCAs					
Generic (Trade)	M	♀	Start	Titrate	Max
Desipramine (Norpramine)	L	?	25mg PO qhs	q2weeks to a plasma level of 125–300ng/ mL	300mg/ 24hours
Nortriptyline (Pamelor)	L	U	25mg PO qhs	q2weeks to a plasma level of 50–150ng/ dL	150mg qhs

Mechanism:
•Inhibit the presynaptic reuptake of norepinephrine > serotonin→
  ∘↑Synaptic cleft concentrations

Side effects:
General
  •↑Appetite→
    ∘↑Weight
Cardiovascular
  •Dysrhythmias
Neurologic
  •Precipitation of manic episodes
  •Seizures

822

- **Sexual dysfunction–20%**
  - ∘Consider adding Bupropion, which may→
    - −Reversal of other antidepressant mediated sexual dysfunction
  - •Tremor

Other receptor antagonism mediated side effects:
- •**Anticholinergic**→see below
- •**Antihistamine**→
  - ∘**Sedation**
- •**Anti α1**→
  - ∘Erectile dysfunction
  - ∘**Orthostatic hypotension**
  - ∘Sedation

---

†**Cause less side effects than their parent compound tertiary amines**

Contraindications:
- •Suicidal ideation
- •Previous suicide attempt
- …as **overdose, via ingestion of ≥2 weeks supply, may be fatal**

HYPERICUM PERFORATUM (St Johns wort)

Indications:
- •Short term treatment of **mild depression**

♀	Dose
U	300mg PO q8hours, of standardized extract, w/ 0.3% hypericin

Side effects:
Mucocutaneous
- •Photosensitivity @ dose >1.8g/ 24hours

SECOND LINE TREATMENT ▬▬▬

- •If the response to first line treatment is inadequate @ 2months, add Lithium. Then, if a synergistic effect is noticed, continue both medications, otherwise discontinue both medications

LITHIUM

M ♀	Start	Titrate†	Max
K U	300mg PO q12hours	qweek by 300mg (↑plasma level by ~0.2mEq/ L) q2weeks in elderly or renal failure	1.8g/ 24hours

†Titrate to a therapeutic plasma level of 0.6−1.2 mEq/ L. Lithium toxicity may occur at therapeutic levels

Side effects:
Cardiovascular
- •Dysrhythmias

Endocrine
- •Thyroid goiter

Gastrointestinal
- •Diarrhea
- •Nausea ± vomiting
- •Gastrointestinal discomfort

Genitourinary
- •Antidiuretic hormone receptor antagonism→
  - ∘**Nephrogenic diabetes insipidus**

Mucocutaneous
- •Edema

Neurologic
- • ↓Communication ability (expression &/or understanding)=aphasia
- •Hyporeflexia
- •Incoordinaton=ataxia
- •Sedation
- •Tremor

Hematologic
- •Leukocytosis

Contraindications:
- •Pregnancy, due to congenital cardiac abnormalities

BUPROPION (Wellbutrin)

Alternative indications:
- Sexual dysfunction, as the addition of Bupropion may→
  - ∘Reversal of other antidepressant mediated sexual dysfunction

M ♀	Start	Titrate	Max
LK P	100mg PO q12hours	@ 1week to 100mg q8hours	150mg q8hours
•XR form	100mg PO qam	@ 1week to 150mg q12hours	150mg q12hours

Mechanism:
- Inhibits the presynaptic reuptake of dopamine, norepinephrine, & serotonin→
  - ∘↑Synaptic cleft concentrations

Side effects:
Cardiovascular
- Dysrhythmia

Neurologic
- Seizure–0.4%, being ↑ w/ >150mg/ dose or 450mg/ 24h

Other receptor antagonism mediated side effects:
- **Anticholinergic**→see below
- **Antihistamine**→
  - ∘**Sedation**
- **Anti α1**→
  - ∘Erectile dysfunction
  - ∘**Orthostatic hypotension**
  - ∘Sedation

Contraindications:
- **Seizure disease**

MIRTAZIPINE (Remeron)

M ♀	Start	Max
LK ?	15mg PO qhs	45mg qhs

Mechanism:
- Inhibits the presynaptic reuptake of norepinephrine > serotonin→
  - ∘↑Synaptic cleft concentrations

Side effects:
Cardiovascular
- Dysrhythmia

Neurologic
- Seizure

Hematologic
- Granulocytopenia–rare

Other receptor antagonism mediated side effects:
- **Anticholinergic**→see below
- **Antihistamine**→
  - ∘**Sedation**
  - ∘Erectile dysfunction
  - ∘**Orthostatic hypotension**
  - ∘Sedation

NEFAZODONE (Serzone)

M ♀	Start	Max
L ?	100mg PO q12hours	300mg q12hours

Mechanism:
- Selectively inhibits the presynaptic reuptake of serotonin→
  - ∘↑Synaptic cleft concentrations

Side effects:
Cardiovascular
- Dysrhythmia

Gastrointestinal
- Nausea ± vomiting

824

Neurologic
- •Headache
- •Seizure disease

Other receptor antagonism mediated side effects:
- •**Anticholinergic**→see below
- •**Antihistamine**→
  - ∘**Sedation**
- •**Anti α1**→
  - ∘Erectile dysfunction
  - ∘**Orthostatic hypotension**
  - ∘Sedation

TRAZODONE (Desyrel)		
M ♀ Start	**Max**	
L ? 25mg PO q12hours	300mg q12hours	

Mechanism:
- •Selectively inhibits the presynaptic reuptake of serotonin→
  - ∘↑Synaptic cleft concentrations

Side effects:
Cardiovascular
- •Dysrhythmia

Gastrointestinal
- •Nausea ± vomiting

Genitourinary
- •Prolonged & painful penile erection–1/ 6000, termed priapism, ± penile damage

Neurologic
- •Headache
- •Seizure disease

Other receptor antagonism mediated side effects:
- •**Anticholinergic**→see below
- •**Antihistamine**→
  - ∘**Sedation**
- •**Anti α1**→
  - ∘Erectile dysfunction
  - ∘**Orthostatic hypotension**
  - ∘Sedation

SEROTONIN–NOREPINEPHRINE REUPTAKE INHIBITOR–SNRI				
Generic (Trade)	M	♀	**Start**	**Max**
Venlafaxine (Effexor)	LK	?	37.5mg q12hours	187.5mg q12hours
•XR form			37.5mg PO q24hours	225mg q24hours

Mechanism:
- •Inhibits the presynaptic reuptake of norepinephrine & serotonin→
  - ∘↑Synaptic cleft concentrations

Side effects:
Cardiovascular
- •Diastolic hypertension
- •Dysrhythmia

Neurologic
- •Seizure

Other receptor antagonism mediated side effects:
- •**Anticholinergic**→see below
- •**Antihistamine**→
  - ∘**Sedation**
- •**Anti α1**→
  - ∘Erectile dysfunction
  - ∘**Orthostatic hypotension**
  - ∘Sedation

Monitoring:
- •Blood pressure @ 2weeks after dosage↑

FOURTH LINE TREATMENT

MONOAMINE OXIDASE INIBITORS–MAOI

Generic (Trade)	M	♀	Start	Max
Isocarboxazid (Marplan)	LK	?	10mg PO q12hours	30mg q12hours
Phenelzine (Nardil)	L	?	15mg PO q8hours	30mg q8hours
Tranylcypromine (Parnate)	L	?	10mg PO qam	30mg q12hours

Mechanism:
- Inhibit the function of monoamine oxidase–MAO†, an enzyme found on the outer mitochondrial membrane, which metabolizes catecholamines & serotonin via 2 subtypes:
  - A: Metabolizes norepinephrine & serotonin
  - B: Metabolizes dopamine
  - ...→↑presynaptic vesicular concentrations→
    - ↑Synaptic cleft concentrations

†Although these medications are considered nonselective, they appear to exert their predominant effects via inhibition of monoamine oxidase type A

Side effects:
Cardiovascular
- Dysrhythmia
- **Tyramine**, a byproduct of tyrosine metabolism in the body & in foods, is metabolized by the enzyme monoamine oxidase–MAO→
  - Suppresson of its indirect sympathomimetic effect via its causing the release of presynaptic catecholamine granules. However, patients who take an MAOI (esp. type A inhibitors) lose the ability to metabolize large amounts of ingested tyramine found in certain foods:
    - Alcoholic beverages (ale, beer, chianti, cognac, red wine, sherry, vermouth)
    - Broad & fava beans
    - Canned figs
    - Cheeses, except cottage & cream cheese
    - Chocolate
    - Fish (anchovies, herring, sardines, shrimp paste, smoked or pickled fish)
    - Liver of all types
    - Overripe fruits
    - Processed meat
    - Sauerkraut
    - Sausage
    - Soy sauce
    - Yeast
    - ...→**hypertension**

Neurologic
- Seizure
- Sexual dysfunction

Other receptor antagonism mediated side effects:
- **Anticholinergic**→see below
- **Antihistamine**→
  - **Sedation**
- **Anti α1**→
  - Erectile dysfunction
  - **Orthostatic hypotension**
  - Sedation

Contraindications:
- **Administration w/ other antidepressants**

826

- **Anticholinergic effects**
  Mucocutaneous
  - ↓Glandular cell secretions
    - ↓Exocrine secretions→
      - –↓Lacrimal, mucosal, parotid, submandibular, gastric, & pancreatic secretions→dry mucus membranes (including eyes)
    - ↓Eccrine=merocrine secretions→
      - –↓Perspiration†→dry skin→↑hyperthermia risk
    - ↓Holocrine secretions→
      - –↓Sebum→dry skin
    - ↓Apocrine secretions→
      - –↓Breast milk
      - –↓Pheromones
  - Dilation of the cutaneous vasculature above the waist, being of uncertain etiology→
    - Flushing, termed "atropine flush"

  Opthalmologic
  - ↓Ciliary smooth muscle contraction→
    - Far vision, w/ near visual blurring
    - Canal of Schlemm compression (a thin walled circumferential vein @ the iridocorneal junction)→
      - –↓Aqueous fluid outflow→↑anterior chamber pressure→wide=open angle glaucoma exacerbation
  - ↓Iris circular smooth muscle contraction→
    - Dilated pupil=mydriasis
    - Compression of the drainage pathway between the cornea & the ciliary body→
      - –Narrow=closed angle glaucoma exacerbation

  Neurologic
  - Altered mental status
  - Amnesia
  - Hallucinations
  - Sedation
  - Seizures

  Gastrointestinal/ Genitourinary
  - ↓Genitourinary & gastrointestinal smooth muscle contraction→
    - ↓Tone & peristalsis→
      - –Urinary retention &/or constipation respectively

- **Cholinergic rebound symptoms,** occurring upon abrupt discontinuation of antidepressant medications
  Cardiovascular
  - Bradycardia &/or asystole

  Gastrointestinal†
  - ↑Gastrointestinal smooth muscle contraction→
    - ↑Tone & peristalsis→
      - –Abdominal discomfort
      - –Diarrhea
      - –Nausea ± vomiting

  Genitourinary
  - ↑Genitourinary smooth muscle contraction→
    - ↑Tone & peristalsis→
      - –Urinary frequency

  Mucocutaneous
  - ↑Glandular cell secretions
    - ↑Exocrine secretions→
      - –↑Lacrimal, mucosal, parotid, submandibular, gastric, & pancreatic secretions
    - ↑Eccrine=merocrine secretions→
      - –↑Perspiration‡
    - ↑Holocrine secretions→
      - –↑Sebum→oily skin

  Musculoskeletal
  - Muscle cramps

  Neurologic
  - Insomnia

  Opthalmologic
  - ↑Iris circular smooth muscle contraction→
    - Constricted pupil=myosis

827

Pulmonary
- Bronchoconstriction

---

†Perspiration is controlled by the sympathetic nervous system→
- Postganglionic acetylcholine release, except on the palms & soles which are activated by norepinephrine

- **Serotonin syndrome**, being an idiosyncratic, life threatening complication of combining a monoamine oxidase inhibitor w/ another serotonergic medication:
  - Any other antidepressant, esp. selective serotonin reuptake inhibitors
  - Opiates, esp. Dextromethorphan & Meperidine
  - ...→
    - Autonomic nervous system dysfunction→
      - Diaphoresis
      - Dysrhythmia
      - **Fever**→
        - Hyperthermia
      - Hypertension or hypotension
      - Tachycardia
    - Somatic nervous system dysfunction
      - Hyperreflexia
      - Shivering
      - Tremor
    - Altered mental status
    - Diarrhea
    - Disseminated intravascular coagulation–DIC
    - Dyspnea
    - Renal failure
    - Seizures

Risk reduction:
- Discontinue all other antidepressant medications 2weeks prior to beginning a MAOI, & vice versa

INVASIVE PROCEDURES

- **Electroconvulsive treatment–ECT**

Indications:
- Highly effective for short term treatment when:
  - Improvement is needed urgently:
    - Severe depression
    - Suicidal
    - Postpartum depression
  - Antidepressant medications have failed, or cannot be given safely

Procedure:
1. Anesthesia is given, followed by a muscle relaxant to ↓convulsions
2. Restraints are placed in case paralysis is incomplete
3. Electrodes are typically placed unilaterally on the side of the non-dominant hemisphere:
4. An electrical current is then passed through the brain for ≤2seconds→
   - Tonic–clonic seizure lasting 20–60seconds, of which the only sign may be eyelid fluttering due to previous muscle relaxant administration
5. Vital signs are then monitored until the patient regains consciousness

Treatment duration:
- 2–3sessions/ week X 3–4weeks=6–12 sessions total

Side effects:
- Anesthesia complications
- Myalgias
- Transient headaches
- Antegrade >> retrograde **amnesia**, lasting 1–3months after the last treatment→
  - New memories being progressively more difficult to form

Risk reduction:
- Unilateral electrode placement on the side of the non-dominant hemisphere

Outcomes:
- Marked improvement in 80% of patients, lasting several weeks to 6months

- Antidepressant medical therapy→
  - **Remission in 70% of patients after ~3months of adequate dosing,** unless the patient:
    - −Meets criteria for emergent psychiatric referral
    - −Has gone untreated for ≥2 years
    - −Has causative underlying medical disease
    - ...→↓remission rate
- The year following remission is a high risk period for relapse

- Multifactorial central nervous system diseases→
  - Altered thoughts
  - Altered perceptions
    - Auditory
    - Gustatory
    - Olfactory
    - Tactile
    - Visual
  - Altered behavior
  - Altered motor functions
  ...→↓social (interpersonal relationships or self care) &/or occupational function throughout most of the illness, not being due to either:
  - Substance use (medication or drug)
  - Medical disease

Statistics:
- Schizophrenia affects 1% of the population

PATHOPHYSIOLOGY OF PSYCHOSIS

- ↑Activity of the **mesolimbic dopaminergic system** composed of neurons of the ventral tagmental nucleus of the mesencephalon, w/ projections to:
  - The medial & anterior portions of the limbic system (esp. the amygdala, hippocampus, portions of the prefrontal lobes, & anterior portions of the caudate nucleus), being behavioral control centers
  - Cortical pyramidal neurons, being movement control centers
  ...→activation of dopamine 1 & 2 receptors→
  - ↑Neuronal response to glutamate
- **Serotonergic neurons** of the dorsal raphe nucleus, having projections to the same brain centers→
  - Activation of serotonin–HT_{2A} receptors→
    - ↑Synaptic terminal glutamate release
  ...→**excessive glutaminergic neuronal excitation**→
  - **Psychosis**

CLASSIFICATION/ RISK FACTORS

- **Brief psychotic disorder**
  - ≥1 psychotic symptom(s) **lasting ≤1month**, w/ complete return to premorbid functioning

- **Schizophreniform disorder**
  - ≥1 psychotic symptom(s) **lasting 1–5months**, not meeting the criteria for delusional disorder
  Risk factors:
  - Age
    - ♂: 15–25 years
    - ♀: 25–35 years
    ...but may occur as early as age 6years, w/ severity usually being ↓in ♀ due to a possible antidopaminergic effect of estrogen
  - Low socioeconomic status
    - May be caused by **downward drift**, as people w/ psychosis drift into lower socioeconomic classes due to the disease

- **Schizophrenia**
  - ≥1 psychotic symptom(s) **lasting ≥6months**
  Risk factors:
  - Age
    - ♂: 15–25 years
    - ♀: 25–35 years
    ...but may occur as early as age 6years, w/ severity usually being ↓in ♀ due to a possible antidopaminergic effect of estrogen
  - Genetics
    - Family history of schizophrenia
      - Monozygotic twin→45% occurrence
      - Both parents→40% occurrence
      - First degree relative→10% occurrence
    - Mutation on chromosomes 1, 6, 8, 13, 15, &/or 22
  - Perinatal or childhood brain injury
  - Children of malnourished mothers
  - Children born in the winter months

830

- Children of ♀ who develop the flu during the 2nd or 3rd trimesters of pregnancy
  - Which is a reason why pregnant mothers who will be in their 2nd–3rd trimesters during the influenza season should receive the influenza vaccine
- Psychosocial stress (ex. separation from the family)
- Low socioeconomic status
  - May be caused by **downward drift**, as people w/ psychosis drift into lower socioeconomic classes due to the disease

Characteristics of schizophrenia subtypes:
- **Catatonic:**
  - Stupor
  - Bizarre posturing (waxy flexibility)
- **Disorganized**
  - Disinhibition
  - Disorganized behavior
  - Disorganized speech
  - Poor personal appearance
  - Flat or inappropriate affect
- **Paranoid**
  - Delusions of persecution or grandeur
- **Undifferentiated, being the most common**
  - Characteristics of >1 subtype
- **Residual**
  - 1 resolved schizophrenic episode, w/ residual morbidity in terms of either:
    - −Flat affect
    - −Illogical thinking
    - −Odd behavior
    - −Social withdrawal
    - …w/ an attenuated psychotic syndrome

- **Schizoaffective disorder**
  - Psychotic syndrome w/ major depression ± mania, both **being independent of each other** via the persistence of either ≥2weeks after the resolution of the other

  Risk factors:
  - Age
    - ♂: 15–25 years
    - ♀: 25–35 years
    - … w/ severity usually being ↓in ♀ due to a possible anti–dopaminergic effect of estrogen
  - Low socioeconomic status
    - May be caused by **downward drift**, as people w/ psychosis drift into lower socioeconomic classes due to the disease

- **Delusional disorder**
  - **Non–bizarre delusions** without other psychotic symptoms, lasting ≥1month

  Risk factors:
  - **Age:** >40years
  - **Gender:** ♀ > ♂

- **Shared psychotic disorder**
  - Delusion developing in the context of a close relationship w/ another person or persons who have a previously established delusion. The delusions must be similar & not due to an underlying psychotic syndrome in the secondarily affected patient

- **Postpartum psychosis**–0.2% of ♀
  - Psychotic syndrome within 2weeks postpartum, lasting ≤3months

  Risk factors:
  - Personal or family history of postpartum psychosis

Neurologic
- **Positive symptoms**, indicating the presence of unusual/ bizarre thoughts, perceptions, emotions, &/or behavior
  - ∘**Delusions:** A false belief, held w/ conviction despite incontrovertable evidence to the contrary, being unexpected given the patients cultural background
    - −**Grandeur:** False belief that they have special powers, abilities, importance, &/or wealth
    - −**Paranoid, being most common:** False belief that people are following &/or trying to hurt them
    - −**Ideas of reference:** False belief that objects or others' acts/ statements are directed toward them
    - −**Somatic:** False belief that they have a disease
    - −**Thought broadcasting:** Belief that ones thoughts are being broadcasted to others as they occur
    - −**Thought insertion:** Belief that thoughts are being placed in their minds
    - −**Thought withdrawal:** Belief that thoughts are being removed from their minds
  - ∘**Hallucinations:** Imaginary sensations (auditory > taste=gustatory, smell=olfactory, touch=tactile, visual)
  - ∘**Bizarre behavior/ affect:** Behaviors or emotions inappropriate or strange to others
  - ∘**Disorganized speech:** Illogical, nonsensical (loosening of associations), &/or incomprehensible speech
  - ∘**Altered motor function:**
    - −Catatonic via immobility
    - −Excessive, purposeless motor activity
    - −Maintenance of a rigid echolalia, being an involuntary parrot−like repetition of that just spoken by another person
- **Negative symptoms**, indicating the absence of normal social & cognitive functions
  - ∘**Lack of motivation or interest→**
    - −↓Attention→↓short term memory
  - ∘**Affective flattening:** ↓Emotional expression, being blunted/ flattened
  - ∘**Alogia:** ↓Speech or speech content
  - ∘**Asociality:** ↓Interest in interacting w/ others→
    - −Isolation

- **Brain magnetic resonance imaging−MRI**
<u>Findings:</u>
  - **Enlarged ventricles**
  - **↓Left hemispheric grey matter in either the:**
    - ∘Amygdala
    - ∘Anterior hippocampus
    - ∘Parahippocampal gyrus
    - ∘Posterior superior temporal gyrus (correlating w/ the degree of disordered thinking)

- Being that 10% of patients w/ schizophrenia commit suicide, w/ many more considering & attempting it, all patients w/ possible psychotic syndromes should be asked about their thoughts concerning self injury & suicide, w/ questions becoming more specific as warranted
<u>Statistics:</u>
- 8th leading cause of death in the U.S.
<u>Risk factors:</u>
- **Major depression** is the most powerful predictor of suicide, w/ risk being highest:
  - ∘W/ the development of delusions
  - ∘During early recovery, as patients begin to regain energy prior to an improved self attitude
- **Previous suicide attempt**
- **1st degree relative who committed suicide**
- **Advanced age:** Peak occurrence @ ♂ age >45years; ♀ age >55years
- **Skin color:** Whites > blacks
- **Gender:** ♂ > ♀ as:
  - ∘♂ employ more lethal methods (hanging, jumping, shooting), whereas ♀ often overdose, attempt drowning, or wrist laceration
- **Severe anxiety**
- **Severe physical illness**
- **Severe stressful life event in the recent past**
- **Alcoholism or illicit drug use**
- **Personality disorder**
- **Psychotic disease**

832

- **Certain professions**
  - ◦Dentists
  - ◦Insurance agents
  - ◦Law enforcement personnel
  - ◦Lawyers
  - ◦Musicians
  - ◦Physicians
- **Unemployment**
- **High socioeconomic class**
- **Single lifestyle**

Interview questions:
1. "Sometimes when people feel depressed, they think about hurting or killing themselves. Do you ever have these kinds of thoughts?"
IF YES=SUICIDAL IDEATION ⬇

2. "Have you ever thought about how you would do it?"
IF YES=SUICIDAL PLANNING ⬇

3. Urgent psychiatric consultation, & ask if the patient has the means of carrying out the plan, or feels as though they will procure the means
IF YES ⬇

4. Emergent psychiatric consult for hospitalization
Indications:
- •Suicidal planning & delusional
- •Patient is unwilling to comply w/ a safety agreement†
- •Patient is fearful of an imminent attempt

---

†If the patient does not qualify for hospitalization, develop a safety agreement w/ the patient & family &/or close friends, w/ the patient to immediately notify the physician &/or family/ friends when suicidal thoughts progress to the point of considering an attempt

TREATMENT
- •All antipsychotic medications are considered of equal efficacy for positive symptoms, w/ **atypical antipsychotics**
  - ◦**Being more effective in controlling negative symptoms**
  - ◦**Having a lower incidence of extrapyramidal symptoms**
- •A patient may need to try several classes of medication in order to find the one that works best for their biology, w/ the least & most tolerable side effects
Outcomes:
- •Syndrome improvement should occur within several days, w/ maximal effects @ 2months. Lack of improvement within 1month should prompt an increase in dose, followed by a change to another medication

- •**Stat psychiatry consult**

ATYPICAL ANTIPSYCHOTICS				
Generic (Trade)	M	♀	Start	Max
Olanzapine (Zyprexa)	L	?	5mg PO q24hours	20mg q24hours
Quetiapine (Seroquel)	LK	?	25mg PO q12hours	800mg/ 24hours
Risperidone (Risperdal)	LK	?	0.5mg PO q12hours	16mg/ 24hours
Ziprasidone (Geodon)	L	?	20mg PO q12hours w/ food	160mg/ 24hours

•Multiple medications within this class should be tried both prior to moving on to second line treatments

Mechanism:
- •Serotonin $5HT_{2A}$ & dopamine 2 receptor antagonism

Side effects:
Cardiovascular
- •↑QT interval→
  - ◦Torsades de pointes, esp. Risperidone

Gastrointestinal
- •Hepatitis
  - ◦Medication to be changed to a chemically unrelated antipsychotic @ plasma values >3 X the upper limit of normal

Mucocutaneous
- •Photosensitivity

Neurologic
- •**Seizure**
- •Serotonin receptor antagonism→
  - ∘Obsessive-compulsive disorder

Hematologic
- •Hyperlipidemia

Other receptor antagonism mediated side effects:
- •**Anti–D$_2$**→
  - ∘**Extrapyramidal dysfunction**, esp. typical antipsychotics
  - ∘Endocrine dysfunction→see below
- •**Anticholinergic**→see below
- •**Antihistamine**→
  - ∘**Sedation**
- •**Anti α1**, esp. Risperidone→
  - ∘Erectile dysfunction
  - ∘**Orthostatic hypotension**
  - ∘Sedation

SECOND LINE TREATMENT

TYPICAL ANTIPSYCHOTICS

Generic (Trade)	M	♀	Start	Max
MID–HIGH POTENCY†				
Fluphenazine (Prolixin)	LK	?		
•PO form			0.2–3mg q8hours	40mg/ 24hours
•IM form			0.5–3mg q8hours	10mg/ 24hours
•IM/ SC depot form conversion ratio:			10mg/ 24h PO=12.5mg IM/ SC q3weeks	
Haloperidol (Haldol)	LK	?		
•PO form			0.25–2.5mg q12hours	100mg q24hours
•IM form			2–5mg q8–1hours prn	
•IM depot form conversion ratio:			10mg/ 24hours PO=100–200mg IM qmonth	
Loxapine (Loxitane)	LK	?		
•PO form			10mg q12hours	250mg/ 24hours
•IM form			12.5–50mg q12–4hours prn	
Molindone (Moban)	LK	?	15–25mg PO q8hours	225mg/ 24hours
Perphenazine (Trilafon)	LK	?		
•PO form			8–16mg q12hours	64mg/ 24hours
•IM form			5–10mg q6hours	30mg/ 24hours
Thiothixene (Navane)	LK	?		
•PO form			2mg q8hours	60mg/ 24hours
•IM form			4mg q12hours	30mg/ 24hours
Trifluoperazine (Stelazine)	LK	?		
•PO form			2–5mg q12hours	80mg/ 24hours
•IM form			1–2mg q6hours prn	10mg/ 24hours
LOW POTENCY†				
Chlorpromazine (Thorazine)	LK	?		
•PO form			5–25mg q12hours	2000mg/ 24hours
•IM form			25–50mg prn	2000mg/ 24hours

†Potency refers to relative milligram dose equivalents, & should not be confused w/ efficacy

Mechanism:
- •Dopamine 2 receptor antagonism

Side effects:
- **Cardiovascular**
  - •**↑QT interval**→
    - ∘Torsades de pointes, esp. low potency
- **Gastrointestinal**
  - •Hepatitis
    - ∘Medication to be changed to a chemically unrelated antipsychotic @ plasma values >3 X the upper limit of normal
- **Mucocutaneous**
  - •Photosensitivity
- **Neurologic**
  - •**Seizure**, esp. low potency

Other receptor antagonism mediated side effects:
- **Anti−D$_2$→**
  - **Extrapyramidal dysfunction**, esp. mid to high potency
  - Endocrine dysfunction (see below)
- **Anticholinergic**, esp. low potency
- **Antihistamine**, esp. low potency→
  - **Sedation**
- **Anti α1**, esp. low potency→
  - Erectile dysfunction
  - **Orthostatic hypotension**
  - Sedation

THIRD LINE TREATMENT ▬▬▬▬
- 30% of patients will be unresponsive to the above medications

ATYPICAL ANTIPSYCHOTICS				
Generic (Trade)	M ♀	Start	Max	
Clozapine (Clozaril)	L P	12.5mg PO q24hours	900mg/ 24hours	

Mechanism:
- Serotonin 5HT$_{2A}$ & dopamine 1, 2, & **4 receptor antagonism**

Side effects:
General
- Benign hyperthermia−10%
- ↓Cigarette smoking

Cardiovascular
- Dysrhthmias
- Myocarditis−0.03%
- **↑QT interval→**
  - Torsades de pointes

Gastrointestinal
- Hepatitis
  - Medication to be changed to a chemically unrelated antipsychotic @ plasma values >3 X the upper limit of normal
- Nausea ± vomiting

Mucocutaneous
- Hypersalivation
- Photosensitivity

Neurologic
- **Seizure**
- Serotonin receptor antagonism→
  - Obsessive−compulsive disorder

Pulmonary
- **Respiratory arrest**

Opthalmologic
- Lens opacities

Hematologic
- **Agranulocytosis−1%**, usually within 2months
- Hyperlipidemia

Other receptor antagonism mediated side effects:
- **Anti−D$_2$→**
  - **Extrapyramidal dysfunction**
  - Endocrine dysfunction (see below)
- **Anticholinergic**→see below
- **Antihistamine**→
  - **Sedation**
- **Anti α1→**
  - Erectile dysfunction
  - **Orthostatic hypotension**
  - Sedation

Monitoring:
- Leukocyte count qweek X 6months, then
  - Q2weeks thereafter, including the month after discontinuation

Contraindications:
- Leukocyte count <3500 cells/ μL

LOW POTENCY† TYPICAL ANTIPSYCHOTICS				
Generic (Trade)	M	♀	Start	Max
Mesoridizine (Serentil)	LK	?	50mg PO q8hours	
Thioridazine (Mellaril)	LK	?	50mg PO q8hours	800mg/ 24hours

†Potency refers to relative milligram dose equivalents & should not be confused w/ efficacy

Mechanism:
•Dopamine 2 receptor antagonism

Side effects:
Cardiovascular
•↑QT interval→
　∘Torsades de pointes
Gastrointestinal
•Hepatitis
　∘Medication to be changed to a chemically unrelated antipsychotic @ plasma values >3 X the upper limit of normal
Mucocutaneous
•Photosensitivity
Neurologic
•Seizure

Thioridazine specific:
Opthalmologic
•Pigmentary retinopathy @ doses >800mg/ 24h

Other receptor antagonism mediated side effects:
•Anti-D_2→
　∘Extrapyramidal dysfunction
　∘Endocrine dysfunction→see below
•Anticholinergic→see below
•Antihistamine→
　∘Sedation
•Anti α1→
　∘Erectile dysfunction
　∘Orthostatic hypotension
　∘Sedation

Contraindications:
Cardiovascular
•Congenital long QT syndrome
•History of cardiac dysrhythmia
•Concomitant administration of medications which may prolong the QTc interval
　∘β receptor blockers
　∘Calcium channel blockers
　∘Digoxin
•Concomitant administration of medications which inhibit the cytochrome P450 enzyme, CYP 2D6→
　∘↓Hepatocyte metabolism→medication accumulation, for ex:
　　−Amiodarone
　　−Chloroquine, Cimetidine, Citalopram, Clomipramine
　　−Delavirdine, Diphenhydramine
　　−Fluoxetine, Fluphenazine, Fluvoxamine
　　−Haloperidol
　　−Imatinib
　　−Paroxetine, Perphenazine, Pindolol, Propafenone, Propoxyphene, Propranolol
　　−Quinacrine

ADDITIONAL TREATMENT ■━━━━━━━━━━━━━━━━━━━━━━━━━━━━
•**Shared psychotic disorder**
　∘Physical separation

•**Schizoaffective disorder**
　∘Antidepressant medication for major depression without mania
　∘Mood stabilizer if bipolar

836

•**Anticholinergic effects**
  Mucocutaneous
  •↓Glandular cell secretions
    ○↓Exocrine secretions→
      −↓Lacrimal, mucosal, parotid, submandibular, gastric, & pancreatic secretions→dry mucus
        membranes (including eyes)
    ○↓Eccrine=merocrine secretions→
      −↓Perspiration†→dry skin→↑hyperthermia risk
    ○↓Holocrine secretions→
      −↓Sebum→dry skin
    ○↓Apocrine secretions→
      −↓Breast milk
      −↓Pheromones
  •Dilation of the cutaneous vasculature above the waist, being of uncertain etiology→
    ○Flushing, termed "atropine flush"
  Opthalmologic
  •↓Ciliary smooth muscle contraction→
    ○Far vision, w/ near visual blurring
    ○Canal of Schlemm compression (a thin walled circumferential vein @ the iridocorneal
      junction)→
      −↓Aqueous fluid outflow→↑anterior chamber pressure→wide=open angle glaucoma
        exacerbation
  •↓Iris circular smooth muscle contraction→
    ○Dilated pupil=mydriasis
    ○Compression of the drainage pathway between the cornea & the ciliary body→
      −Narrow=closed angle glaucoma exacerbation
  Neurologic
  •Altered mental status
  •Amnesia
  •Hallucinations
  •Sedation
  •Seizures
  Gastrointestinal/ Genitourinary
  •↓Genitourinary & gastrointestinal smooth muscle contraction→
    ○↓Tone & peristalsis→
      −Urinary retention &/or constipation respectively

•**Endocrine dysfunction**
  ○Dopamine inhibits anterior pituitary prolactin secretion, w/ antagonism→↑prolactin secretion→
    −↑Mammary gland development & initiation of milk production→**gynecomastia in** ♂ &/or
      galactorrhea respectively
    −↓Hypothalamic gonadotropin releasing hormone−GnRH secretion→↓anterior pituitary leutinizing
      hormone & follicle stimulating hormone release→↓libido & **amenorrhea→infertility**
  ○Sedation
  ○**Weight gain**, esp. atypical antipsychotics, esp. Clozapine & Olanzapine

•**Extrapyramidal dysfunction**
  ○Loss of dopaminergic mediated inhibition of the basal ganglia→basal ganglia overactivity→
  corticospinal motor overactivity→↑contraction of the skeletal musculature (both flexor & extensor
  muscles)→
    −**Stiffness, termed rigidity→secondary Parkinson's disease**, w/ effects being reversible within
      1year after discontinuation
  Timing:
  •**Hours**
    ○**Dystonia**, being abnormal (hypo or hyper) muscle tonicity, esp. of the face, neck, & tongue
      −May be life threatening, as laryngeal dystonia→airways closure
  •**Days**
    ○**Difficulty initiating purposeful body movement, termed akinesia→**
      −↑Mental effort & anguish in initiating movement
    ○Facial muscle hypertonia→
      −↓**Facial expression, termed hypomimia or mask−like facies**
      −↓Blink rate
    ○↓Coordination of vocalization muscles→
      −**Low, soft, & slurred monotone voice, termed hypophonia**

837

- **Weeks**
  - ○Motor restlessness, termed **akathisia**→
    - −Difficulty remaining in a sitting posture
- **Months to years**
  - ○**Tardive dyskinesia−30%**, being **involuntary muscle contractions**, esp. of the face, neck, tongue, & jaw, usually being irreversible

- **Neuroleptic malignant syndrome−NMS**, being an idiosyncratic, life threatening complication of:
  - ○Antipsychotic medications
  - ○Sudden ↓dopaminergic medication dosage
    - −Parkinson's disease medications
  - ...→↓dopamine effect→
    - •Autonomic nervous system dysfunction→
      - ○Diaphoresis
      - ○Dysrhythmia
      - ○**Fever**→
        - −Hyperthermia
      - ○Hypertension or hypotension
      - ○Tachycardia
    - •Somatic nervous system dysfunction→
      - ○**Stiffness, termed rigidity**→
        - −Difficulty initiating purposeful body movement, termed akinesia
        - −Dysphagia
        - −Dystonia
        - −Mutism
    - •Altered mental status
    - •Diarrhea
    - •Disseminated intravascular coagulation−DIC
    - •Dyspnea
    - •Renal failure
    - •Seizures

- **Cholinergic rebound symptoms**, occurring upon abrupt discontinuation of antipsychotic medications
- **Cardiovascular**
  - •Bradycardia &/or asystole
- **Gastrointestinal†**
  - •↑Gastrointestinal smooth muscle contraction→
    - ○↑Tone & peristalsis→
      - −Abdominal discomfort
      - −Diarrhea
      - −Nausea ± vomiting
- **Genitourinary**
  - •↑Genitourinary smooth muscle contraction→
    - ○↑Tone & peristalsis→
      - −Urinary frequency
- **Mucocutaneous**
  - •↑Glandular cell secretions
    - ○↑Exocrine secretions→
      - −↑Lacrimal, mucosal, parotid, submandibular, gastric, & pancreatic secretions
    - ○↑Eccrine=merocrine secretions→
      - −↑Perspiration‡
    - ○↑Holocrine secretions→
      - −↑Sebum→oily skin
- **Musculoskeletal**
  - •Muscle cramps
- **Neurologic**
  - •Insomnia
- **Opthalmologic**
  - •↑Iris circular smooth muscle contraction→
    - ○Constricted pupil=myosis

- **Pulmonary**
  - •Bronchoconstriction

---

†Perspiration is controlled by the sympathetic nervous system→
  •Postganglionic acetylcholine release, except on the palms & soles which are activated by norepinephrine

•Electroconvulsive treatment–ECT

Indications:
- •Highly effective for short term treatment when:
  - ∘Improvement is needed urgently:
    - –Severe depression
    - –Suicidal
    - –Life threatening catatonia
    - –Postpartum psychosis
  - ∘Antipsychotic medications have failed, or cannot be given safely

Procedure:
1. Anesthesia is given, followed by a muscle relaxant to ↓convulsions
2. Restraints are placed in case paralysis is incomplete
3. Electrodes are typically placed unilaterally on the side of the non–dominant hemisphere:
4. An electrical current is then passed through the brain for ≤2seconds→
   - •Tonic–clonic seizure lasting 20–60seconds, of which the only sign may be eyelid fluttering due to previous muscle relaxant administration
5. Vital signs are then monitored until the patient regains consciousness

Treatment duration:
- •2–3sessions/ week X 3–4weeks=6–12 sessions total

Side effects:
- •Anesthesia complications
- •Myalgias
- •Transient headaches
- •Antegrade >> retrograde **amnesia**, lasting 1–3months after the last treatment→
  - ∘New memories being progressively more difficult to form

Risk reduction:
- •Unilateral electrode placement on the side of the non–dominant hemisphere

Outcomes:
- •Marked improvement in 80% of patients, lasting several weeks to 6months

839

ACID–BASE DISORDERS

- Any single or combination of conditions (3max)→
  - Altered H^+ &/or HCO_3 production &/or excretion, w/ a possible partial compensatory mechanism
- It is impossible to have concomitant respiratory acidemia & alkalemia, as a patient cannot hypoventilate & hyperventilate simultaneously
- Although the **normal pH ranges from 7.36–7.44**, the extreme range of altered pH compatible w/ life is ~6.75–7.90

ARTERIAL BLOOD GAS–ABG VALUES

Measurement	Normal value	Equation value	Hypoxemia	Hypercapnia
pH	7.35–7.45	7.4		
pO_2	70–100mmHg†		<60mmHg	
pCO_2	35–45mmHg	40mmHg		>45mmHg→acidemia
HCO_3	22–26mmol/ L	24mmHg		
Arterial O_2 saturation	95–98%		≤91%	
Venous O_2 saturation	60–85%			

†Age adjusted normal PaO_2 = 101 – (0.43 X age)

CLASSIFICATION/ DIAGNOSIS

- **Acidemia:** pH <7.36
- **Alkalemia:** pH >7.44

Ph MEDIATED FINDINGS

ACIDEMIA
Pulmonary
- Compensatory ↑respiratory effort→
  - Difficulty breathing=**dyspnea**→
    - Respiratory rate >16/ min.=**tachypnea**
    ...w/ severe acidemia→
      - **Kussmaul breathing**, being deep, rapid respirations reflecting major respiratory compensation
      - Accessory muscle usage (sternocleidomastoid muscles for inspiration & abdominal muscles for expiration)
      - Speech frequently interrupted by inspiration=telegraphic speech
      - Pursed lip breathing &/or grunting expirations→positive end–expiratory pressure–PEEP
      - Paradoxical abdominal motion: Negative intrathoracic pressure→fatigued diaphragm being pulled into the thorax→inspiratory inward motion of the anterior abdominal wall, rather than expected outward motion due to diaphragmatic contraction

Cardiovascular
- Altered vascular tonicity→
  - Vasodilation→**hypotension**→↓perfusion mediated organ failure, esp. involving the:
    - Central nervous system→altered mental status
    - Kidneys→renal failure
    - Lungs→respiratory failure
    ...being termed **distributive shock** if refractory to an intravenous fluid bolus

Neurologic
- Altered mental status

Hematologic
- **Hyperkalemia**, as every 0.1↓ in pH→
  - **0.5mEq/ L↑ in potassium** via the H^+/K^+ cell membrane exchange protein→
    - Potassium extracellular shift
- ↓Plasma protein–calcium binding→
  - ↑Free plasma calcium→
    - **Hypercalcemia**, w/ total plasma calcium being unaffected

ALKALEMIA
Hematologic
- **Hypokalemia**, as every 0.1↑ in pH→
  - **0.3mEq/ L↓ in potassium** via the H^+/K^+ cell membrane exchange protein→
    - Potassium intracellular shift
- ↑Plasma protein–calcium binding→
  - ↓Free plasma calcium→
    - **Hypocalcemia**, w/ total plasma calcium being unaffected

	Arterial pH	Acute primary change	Partial compensatory reaction
	↓	CO_2 retention	HCO_3 retention
Acute:	$0.008 \times \Delta PCO_2$		$0.1 \times \Delta PCO_2$
Chronic†:	$0.003 \times \Delta PCO_2$		$0.4 \times \Delta PCO_2$

†Indicates that the patient has been **hypoventilating** @ current severity long enough (≥3days) for there to be compensatory renal acid excretion→
- ↑Plasma HCO_3

HYPERCAPNIC RESPIRATORY FAILURE

- ↓**Upper airways ventilation**, w/ **oxygen clearance always being impaired** on room air, due to alveolar hypoventilation
  - Risk factors:
    - **Upper airways obstruction** (from the oropharynx to the carina)
      - ∘Bilateral vocal cord paralysis
      - ∘Epiglottitis
      - ∘Foreign body
      - ∘Inhalation injury (thermal or chemical) mediated edema
      - ∘Laryngospasm
      - ∘Laryngeal inflammation
      - ∘Tumor (including thyroid goiter)
    - **Thoracic wall abnormalities**
      - ∘Flail chest
      - ∘Kyphoscoliosis
      - ∘Massive pleural effusion
      - ∘Pneumothorax
    - **Neuromuscular abnormalities**
      - ∘Amyotrophic lateral sclerosis−AML
      - ∘**Diaphragmatic fatigue**, as occurs w/ respiratory distress
      - ∘Hypophosphatemia
      - ∘Guillain−Barre syndrome
      - ∘Muscular dystrophy
      - ∘Myasthenia gravis
      - ∘Phrenic nerve injury
      - ∘Polio
      - ∘Polymyositis
      - ∘Polyneuropathy
    - **Central nervous system mediated ↓breathing**
      - ∘Brainstem cerebrovascular accident
      - ∘Botulism
      - ∘Hypothyroidism
      - ∘Idiopathic alveolar hypoventilation
      - ∘Metabolic alkalemia
      - ∘Obstructive sleep apnea
      - ∘Sedative medication overdose
        - −Barbiturates
        - −Benzodiazepines
        - −Opiates
      - ∘Spinal cord injury @ ≥C5

- All the above are exacerbated by ↑CO_2 production via:
  - ∘Acidemia
  - ∘Carbohydrate load
  - ∘Fever
  - ∘Generalized tonic &/or clonic seizure
  - ∘Sepsis

•**Diffuse, severe parenchymal lung disease**→
  ◦Ventilation/ perfusion mismatch via:
    –↑Alveolar dead space: Alveolar ventilation through relatively underperfused capillaries
    –↑Vascular shunting†: Capillary blood flow through relatively underventilated alveoli‡. Usually
    occurring, or exacerbated via ↑venous return
  ...→↓diffusion of O_2 & CO_2→
        •Hypoxemia (SaO_2 ≤ 91% or PaO_2 ≤ 60mmHg°) on room air, w/ subsequent hypercapnia
        ($PaCO_2$ ≥45mmHg) due to either:
          ◦Respiratory muscle fatigue
          ◦Alveolar hypoventilation
        ...as CO_2 clearance is unimpaired (& may be ↑in the dyspneic patient) as long as adequate
        ventilation (including lack of diffuse severe ventilation/ perfusion mismatching) is
        maintained, as:
          •CO_2 diffuses 20X as rapidly as O_2
          •Hypercapnia→
            ◦Immediate brain stem respiratory center mediated stimulation of pulmonary
            ventilation, which may correct the hypercapnia, but not necessarily the hypoxia
Risk factors:
  •Chronic obstructive pulmonary disease–COPD, including asthma
  •Cystic fibrosis
  •Pulmonary edema

---

†Being exacerbated by the supine position→
  •↑Systemic venous return→
    ◦↑Vascular shunting→↑dyspnea, being termed:
      –**Orthopnea**, if persistent
      –**Paroxysmal nocturnal dyspnea** if intermittent
      ...causing the patient to either use multiple pillows or sleep in a chair

‡Causes of underventilated alveoli
  •↓**Upper airways ventilation**
  •**Alveolar hypoventilation** via:
    ◦**Diffuse** interstitial ± alveolar infiltration via fluid, fibrosis, &/or cells
      –Alveolar hemorrhage
      –Edema, being either cardiogenic via heart failure, or permeability via adult respiratory distress
      syndrome–ARDS or hypoalbuminemia
      –Pneumonia or pneumonitis
      –Fibrosis
    ◦Diffuse microatelectasis
    ◦Pulmonary emboli
  •↓**Alveolar–capillary O_2 diffusion**→
    ◦Interstitial infiltration via fluid, fibrosis, &/or cells

°Age adjusted normal PaO_2 = 101 − (0.43 X age)

842

RESPIRATORY ALKALEMIA		
Arterial pH	**Acute primary change**	**Partial compensatory reaction**
↑	CO_2 depletion	HCO_3 depletion
Acute:		0.2 X ΔPCO_2
Chronic†:		0.4 X ΔPCO_2

†Indicates that the patient has been **hyperventilating** @ current severity long enough (≥3days) for there
to be compensatory ↓renal acid excretion→
- ↓Plasma HCO_3

HYPOXEMIC RESPIRATORY FAILURE ▬▬▬▬▬▬▬▬▬▬▬▬▬▬▬▬▬▬▬▬
- **Diffuse, severe parenchymal lung disease→**
  ○Ventilation/ perfusion mismatch via:
   −↑Alveolar dead space: Alveolar ventilation through relatively underperfused capillaries
   −↑Vascular shunting†: Capillary blood flow through relatively underventilated alveoli‡. Usually
    occurring, or exacerbated via ↑venous return
  ...→↓diffusion of O_2 & CO_2→
    - Hypoxemia (SaO_2 ≤ 91% or PaO_2 ≤ 60mmHg) on room air, w/ subsequent hypercapnia
     ($PaCO_2$ ≥45mmHg) due to either:
      ○Respiratory muscle fatigue
      ○Alveolar hypoventilation
     ...as CO_2 clearance is unimpaired (& may be ↑in the dyspneic patient) as long as adequate
     ventilation (including lack of diffuse severe ventilation/ perfusion mismatching) is
     maintained, as:
       - CO_2 diffuses 20X as rapidly as O_2
       - Hypercapnia→
        ○Immediate brain stem respiratory center mediated stimulation of pulmonary
         ventilation, which may correct the hypercapnia, but not necessarily the hypoxia
  Risk factors:
    - Chronic obstructive pulmonary disease–COPD, including asthma
    - Cystic fibrosis
    - Pulmonary edema

- **Right to left intracardiac shunt**
  ○Eisenmenger's syndrome
- **↓Inspired O_2 concentration**
  ○High altitudes
  ○Toxic gas asphyxiation
   −Carbon monoxide–CO poisoning

†Being exacerbated by the supine position→
- ↑Systemic venous return→
  ○↑Vascular shunting→↑dyspnea, being termed:
   −**Orthopnea**, if persistent
   −**Paroxysmal nocturnal dyspnea** if intermittent
   ...causing the patient to either use multiple pillows or sleep in a chair

‡Causes of underventilated alveoli
- **↓Upper airways ventilation**
- **Alveolar hypoventilation via:**
  ○**Diffuse** interstitial ± alveolar infiltration via fluid, fibrosis, &/or cells
   −Alveolar hemorrhage
   −Edema, being either cardiogenic via heart failure, or permeability via adult respiratory distress
    syndrome–ARDS or hypoalbuminemia
   −Pneumonia or pneumonitis
   −Fibrosis
  ○Diffuse microatelectasis
  ○Pulmonary emboli
- **↓Alveolar–capillary O_2 diffusion→**
  ○Interstitial infiltration via fluid, fibrosis, &/or cells

PRIMARY HYPERVENTILATION
•**Diffuse central nervous system disease**
•**Hyperthyroidism**
•**Liver failure**
•**Pain or anxiety**
•↑**Progesterone**, as during pregnancy→
　∘↑Brainstem respiratory center CO_2 sensitivity→
　　−50% ↑min. ventilation
•**Salicylate medications**, via direct brainstem respiratory center mediated stimulation of pulmonary ventilation
•**Sepsis**
•**Vigorous ventilator treatment**

Arterial pH	Acute primary change	Partial compensatory reaction
↓	HCO_3 depletion	CO_2 depletion $1.25 \times \Delta HCO_3$ or CO_2=last 2 digits of the pH

1. Check for the presence of excess plasma anions via the plasma anion gap

Equation: $[Na^+] - ([Cl^-] + [HCO_3])$
- **Normal value: 8–12mEq/ L**
- Equation value: 12mEq/ L

Correction:
- **Hypoalbuminemia:** For each 1g/ dL ↓in albumin below 4, add 2.5 to the calculated anion gap
- **Acidemia:** Add 2 to the calculated anion gap
- **Alkalemia:** Add 4 to the calculated anion gap

Interpretation:
- A gap indicates the **presence of excess unmeasured anions**, being either:
  - Organic acids
  - Phosphates
  - Sulfates
- Causes of a low anion gap:
  - Halide (bromide, Iodide) intoxication
  - Myeloma w/ cationic IgG immunoglobulin
  - Severe hyperlipidemia, via assay error

2. If there is an anion gap, search for a concomitant metabolic disorder via the delta–delta

Equation: ΔAnion gap/ ΔHCO_3
Interpretation:
- **<1** indicates HCO_3↓ > expected→
  - Concomitant **non anion–gap metabolic acidemia**
- **1–2** indicates expected HCO_3↓→
  - A sole **anion gap metabolic acidemia**
- **>2** indicates HCO_3↓ < expected→
  - Concomitant **metabolic alkalemia**

3. Search for a concomitant respiratory disorder via Winter's formula

Equation: **Expected $PaCO_2$=1.5 (HCO_3) + 8 ± 2**
Interpretation:
- **$PaCO_2$ < expected** indicates overcompensation→
  - A concomitant **respiratory alkalemia**
- **$PaCO_2$ > expected** indicates undercompensation→
  - A concomitant **respiratory acidemia**

4. Metabolic acidemia etiologic differentiation via the urinary anion gap

Equation: **$UNa^+ + UK^+ - UCl^-$**
Interpretation:
- Being that ammonium is an unmeasured cation, this is an indirect assay for its renal excretion
  - **Negative** indicates appropriate renal compensation for acidemia via ↑ammonium excretion→
    - **–Extrarenal etiology**
  - **Positive** indicates renal under–compensation for acidemia via ↓ammonium excretion→
    - **–Renal etiology**, at least in part

5. Search for toxic ingestion mediated anion gap acidemia via the plasma osmolar gap

Equation: **Measured osmolarity – calculated osmolarity†**
- **Normal value: ≤10**

Correction:
- **Estimate ethanol's contribution to the osmolar gap: Plasma ethanol/ 4.6**
  - This result should be subtracted from the plasma osmolar gap to evaluate for the possible presence of another osmotically active toxic substance

845

<u>Interpretation:</u>
- A gap indicates the **possible presence of an osmotically active agent:**
  - ◦Chronic renal failure mediated accumulation of unidentified toxins
  - ◦Ethanol
  - ◦Ethylene glycol
  - ◦Methanol
  - ◦Mannitol
  - ◦Radiocontrast dye

---

†Calculated osmolarity: $2\,[Na^+] + (\text{blood urea nitrogen}/\,2.8) + (\text{glucose}/\,18)$
- Normal value: 280–290 mOsm/ kg H_2O

ANION GAP ▬▬▬▬▬▬
- **Antifreeze consumption**→
  - ◦Ethylene glycol→
    - –Oxalic acidemia
- **Aspirin overdose**→
  - ◦Salicylic acidemia
  <u>Mechanism:</u>
  - Direct brainstem respiratory center mediated stimulation of pulmonary ventilation→
    - ◦Hyperventilation→
      - **–Initial respiratory alkalemia, w/ the subsequent development of an anion gap metabolic acidemia**
- **Diabetes mellitus† or starvation**→
  - ◦†Acetoacetic acid & β–hydroxybutyric acid→
    - –Ketoacidemia
- **Methanol consumption**→
  - ◦Formaldehyde & formic acidemia
- **Paraldehyde**
- **Renal failure**
  - ◦@ a glomerular filtration rate <25mL/ min.→
    - –↓Excretion of sulfuric & phosphoric acids

HYPERLACTATEMIA ± ACIDEMIA_____
- **Tissue ischemia ± infarction**
  <u>Mechanism:</u>
  - ↓Cellular oxygenation→
    - ◦Cessation of aerobic metabolism via oxidative phosphorylation
    - ◦Conversion to anaerobic metabolism via the glycolysis stage of carbohydrate degradation→
      - –Cytoplasmic glucose metabolism to pyruvic acid & ATP, thus forming temporary life saving energy, being possible only as the majority of the pyruvic acid is converted to **lactic acid,** which readily diffuses out to the extracellular fluid→↓intracellular end product mediated feedback inhibition, allowing the reaction to continue for several min., until cellular death
- **Endotoxin**
  <u>Mechanism:</u>
  - ↓Mitochondrial cell membrane pyruvate dehydrogenase complex function→
    - ◦↓Pyruvic acid conversion to acetyl–CoA→
      - –↑Cytoplasmic pyruvic acid conversion to lactic acid
- **Epinephrine infusion**
  <u>Mechanism:</u>
  - ↑Cytoplasmic phosphorylase activity→
    - ◦↑Glycogen breakdown to glucose monomers, termed glycogenolysis→
      - –↑Lactic acid production
- **Hepatic failure**
  <u>Mechanism:</u>
  - ↓Hepatocyte mediated re–conversion of lactic acid to pyruvic acid→
    - ◦↑Lactic acid

846

- **Nitroprusside toxicity**
  Mechanism:
  - Cyanide accumulation→cessation of mitochondrial membrane cytochrome oxidase function, being part of the electron transport chain→
    - Cessation of aerobic metabolism via oxidative phosphorylation
    - Conversion to anaerobic metabolism via the glycolysis stage of carbohydrate degradation→
      - Cytoplasmic glucose metabolism to pyruvic acid & ATP, thus forming temporary life saving energy, being possible only as the majority of the pyruvic acid is converted to **lactic acid**, which readily diffuses out to the extracellular fluid→↓intracellular end product mediated feedback inhibition, allowing the reaction to continue for several min., until cellular death
- **Thiamine deficiency**
  Mechanism:
  - Thiamine is a co-factor for mitochondrial cell membrane pyruvate dehydrogenase complex function, w/ deficiency→
    - ↓Pyruvic acid conversion to acetyl–CoA→
      - ↑Cytoplasmic pyruvic acid conversion to lactic acid
- **Severe alkalemia**
  Mechanism:
  - ↑Glycogenolysis pathway pH dependent enzyme function→
    - ↑Lactic acid production, w/ subsequent hepatocyte metabolism, becoming evident @ a pH ≥7.6 in patients w/ normal hepatic function, being less so in those w/ hepatic disease
- **Glucose infusion during severe illness**
  Mechanism:
  - Severe illness mediated altered glucose metabolism→
    - ↑Proportion of glucose converted to lactic acid, being 5% in health, & 85% in severe illness

---

†The actual measured sodium concentration should be used to calculate the anion gap in patients w/ hyperglycemia, whereas, the corrected sodium concentration should be used to estimate the severity of dehydration. This is because the osmotic movement of water from the intracellular to the extracellular compartment equally dilutes all electrolytes, including chloride & bicarbonate, thereby not requiring a relative correction

NON–ANION GAP
- **Dilutional**
  - Rapid infusion of bicarbonate free intravenous fluid, being **all fluids, except those containing lactated Ringers solution**, which contains 27mEq of bicarbonate/ L
- **Early renal failure**
- **Exogenous acids**
  - Total parenteral nutrition–TPN
- **Gastrointestinal bicarbonate loss**
  - **Diarrhea** or equivalent, such as intestinal fistula or biliary drainage→
    - Potassium loss
    - Bicarbonate loss→**hyperchloremic, non–anion gap, metabolic acidemia**
- **Medications**
  - **Potassium sparing diuretics**
    - Amiloride & Triamterene via terminal distal convoluted tubule & collecting duct membrane sodium channel blockade→↓sodium reabsorption→↓compensatory potassium & hydrogen excretion for the maintenance of electroneutrality, regardless of the presence of aldosterone
    - Eplerenone & Spironolactone, being structurally similar to aldosterone→competetive inhibition of the intracellular aldosterone receptor in the distal convoluted tubule & collecting duct
    ...→**hyperkalemic, hypochloremic, non–anion gap, metabolic acidemia**
    - Carbonic anhydrase inhibitors→↓bicarbonate reabsorption→**hyperchloremic, non–anion gap, metabolic acidemia**
    ...w/ potassium nadir usually occurring in 7days
- **Post–hyperventilaton acidemia**
  Mechanism:
  - Respiratory alkalemia→
    - Compensatory renal bicarbonate excretion. However, rapid correction of respiratory disease→
      - Transiently ↓plasma bicarbonate until retained
- **Renal tubular acidemia**
  Mechanism:
  - Defective tubular hydrogen excretion &/or bicarbonate reabsorption
    - Type 1 involving the distal convoluted tubule
    - Type 2 involving the proximal convoluted tubule
    - Type 4

METABOLIC ALKALEMIA		
Arterial pH	Acute primary change	Partial compensatory reaction
↑	HCO_3 retention	CO_2 retention 0.75 X ΔHCO_3

1. Search for a concomitant metabolic disorder via the plasma anion gap

Equation: $[Na^+] - ([Cl^-] + [HCO_3])$
- **Normal value: 8–12mEq/ L**
- Equation value: 12mEq/ L

Correction:
- **Hypoalbuminemia:** For each 1g/ dL ↓in albumin below 4, add 2.5 to the calculated anion gap
- **Acidemia:** Add 2 to the calculated anion gap
- **Alkalemia:** Add 4 to the calculated anion gap

Interpretation:
- A gap indicates the **presence of excess unmeasured anions**, being either:
  - ○Organic acids
  - ○Phosphates
  - ○Sulfates
- Causes of a low anion gap:
  - ○Halide (bromide, Iodide) intoxication
  - ○Myeloma w/ cationic IgG immunoglobulin
  - ○Severe hyperlipidemia, via assay error

2. Search for a concomitant respiratory disorder

Equation: **Expected $PaCO_2$=0.9 (HCO_3) + 9 ± 2**

Interpretation:
- **$PaCO_2$ > expected** indicates overcompensation→
  - ○A concomitant **respiratory acidemia**
- **$PaCO_2$ < expected** indicates undercompensation→
  - ○A concomitant **respiratory alkalemia**

3. Metabolic alkalemia etiologic differentiation via urinary chloride

Interpretation:
- **<20mEq/ L** indicates chloride depletion, which indicates **saline responsiveness**
  - ○**Contraction alkalemia**
    - Mechanism:
      - •Extracellular volume contraction→
        - ○↑Bicarbonate
  - ○**Gastrointestinal hydrogen losses**
    - −Villous adenoma
    - −**Vomiting** or equivalent (nasogastric suction)→HCl loss→metabolic alkalemia
  - ○**Non−potassium sparing diuretics**
    - −Loop diuretics
    - −Thiazide diuretics
    - ...→↑hydrogen & chloride secretion→
      - •**Hypochloremic, metabolic alkalemia**
  - ○**Post−hypoventilaton alkalemia**
    - Mechanism:
      - •Respiratory acidemia→
        - ○Compensatory renal bicarbonate retention. However, rapid correction of respiratory disease→
          - −Transiently ↑plasma bicarbonate until excreted
  - ○**Severe pre−renal renal failure**

- **>20mEq/ L** indicates **saline resistance** (except w/ current diuretic use)
  - ○**Medications**
    - −Bicarbonate compounds
    - −Excessive antacid consumption
  - ○**Severe hypokalemia**
    - −Via the H^+/K^+ cell membrane exchange protein→hydrogen intracellular shift
  - ○**Hyperaldosteronism**
    - −Primary: Adrenal adenoma, adrenal cancer, adrenocortical hyperplasia
    - −Secondary, due to ↑renin secretion: Cirrhosis, coarctation of the aorta, heart failure, nephrotic syndrome, renal artery stenosis, renin secreting neoplasm

848

∘**Hypercortisolism**
  −Cushing's disease or syndrome
  −Glucocorticoid medications
  ...due to their mineralocorticoid effects†
∘**Licorice containing glycyrrhizic acid or chewing tobacco** via:
  −Inhibition of 11β−hydroxysteroid dehydrogenase, which normally prevents physiologic
   glucocorticoid renal tubule concentrations from exerting mineralocorticoid−like effects→
   ↑mineralocorticoid effect†
∘**Bartter's syndrome**
  −↓Ascending loop of Henle $Na^+/K^+/2Cl^-$ reabsorption (like loop diuretics)→**hypokalemic,
   hypochloremic, metabolic alkalemia**
∘**Gitelman's syndrome**
  −Distal convoluted tubule dysfunction (like thiazide diuretics)→**hypokalemic, hypochloremic,
   metabolic alkalemia**
∘**Liddle's syndrome**, being a rare inherited disease→
  −Distal nephron aldosterone−like hyperfunction†

---

††Mineralocorticoid action→
•Hypokalemia
•Non−anion gap metabolic alkalemia
•Hypertension
•Feedback mediated ↓aldosterone levels

•Any process→
  ◦Plasma potassium >5.0mEq/ L (normal: 3.5–5.0mEq/ L)→myocyte partial depolarization (skeletal, smooth, & cardiac)→
    –Dysfunction, which usually becomes symptomatic @ >6.5mEq/ L
Statistics:
  •Total body potassium is normally 50mEq/ L, w/ >98% being intracellular
  •Usual dietary intake is 1mEq/kg/24h, 90% of which is absorbed, w/ subsequent renal excretion

•**Hyperkalemia:** 5.1–6.9mEq/ L
•**Severe hyperkalemia:** ≥7mEq/ L, electrocardiographic changes, or symptomatic

TRANSCELLULAR SHIFT

•As <2% (~50mEq) of total body potassium is located in the extracellular fluid, even small transcellular shifts→
  ◦Significant changes in the extracellular fluid concentration, w/ an outward transcellular shift→
    –↓Renal tubule cell potassium→↓driving force for potassium secretion
•**Acidemia**→
  ◦**Hyperkalemia, as every 0.1↓ in pH→0.5mEq/ L↑ in potassium** via the H^+/K^+ cell membrane exchange protein→
    –Potassium extracellular shift
•**Release of intracellular potassium**
  ◦Burns
  ◦Crush injury
  ◦Infarction
  ◦Hemolysis
  ◦Rhabdomyolysis
  ◦Surgery
  ◦Rapidly proliferating malignancy, esp.:
    –Acute leukemias
    –Aggressive non–Hodgkin's lymphomas
    –Myeloma
  ◦Chemotherapy of either:
    –Rapidly proliferating malignancies (as above)
    –Patient w/ a large tumor burden
•**Medications**
  ◦**β2 receptor blockers**→
    –↓Cell membrane Na^+/K^+ ATPase function→potassium extracellular shift
  ◦Digoxin intoxication→
    –↓Cell membrane Na^+/K^+ ATPase function→potassium extracellular shift
  ◦Depolarizing neuromuscular blocking medications (ex.Succinylcholine)→prolonged skeletal myocyte depolarization→
    –Paralysis
    –Potassium extracellular shift, esp. in patients w/ neuromuscular disease
•**Insulin dependant diabetes mellitus,** as insulin deficiency→
  ◦↓Cell membrane Na^+/K^+ ATPase function (adipose tissue, skeletal muscle, & hepatocytes)→
    –Potassium extracellular shift
•**Massive blood transfusion,** as there is a constant outward transcellular shift of potassium in stored blood due to the dissipation of intracellular ATP→
  ◦↓Na^+/K^+ ATPase function→
    –Potassium extracellular shift
•**Hypertonicity**
    –Diabetic ketoacidosis
    –Hyperosmolar hyperglycemic state
    –Mannitol
    –High protein tube feedings
    –Glycerol
    –Radiocontrast agents
    –Sorbitol
    –↑Urea
    ...→potassium extracellular shift
•**Hyperkalemic periodic paralysis–rare**

850

- **Renal failure** via:
  - ↓Tubular secretion, occurring @ a:
    - –Glomerular filtration rate <10mL/ min.
    - –Urine output <1L/ 24h
    - ...→potassium homeostasis adaptive mechanism failure
  - Acidemia, as every **0.1↓ in pH→0.5mEq/ L↑ in potassium** via the H^+/K^+ cell membrane exchange protein→
    - –Potassium extracellular shift
  - Coagulopathy→
    - –Gastrointestinal hemorrhage→intestinal absorption
    - –Hematoma→absorption
  - Low grade, chronic hemolysis
- **Medications**
  - **Potassium sparing diuretics**
    - –Amiloride & Triamterene via terminal distal convoluted tubule & collecting duct membrane sodium channel blockade→↓sodium reabsorption→↓compensatory potassium & hydrogen excretion for the maintenance of electroneutrality, regardless of the presence of aldosterone
    - –Eplerenone & Spirinolactone, being structurally similar to aldosterone→competetive inhibition of the intracellular aldosterone receptor in the distal convoluted tubule & collecting duct
    - ...→hyperkalemic, hypochloremic, non–anion gap metabolic acidemia
  - **Trimethoprim & Pentamidine→**
    - –Terminal distal convoluted tubule & collecting duct membrane sodium channel blockade→↓sodium reabsorption→↓compensatory potassium & hydrogen excretion for the maintenance of electroneutrality, regardless of the presence of aldosterone
  - **Heparins**, both high & low molecular weight→
    - –↓Aldosterone production→hyperkalemia–8%
  - Patients w/ pre–existing bilateral ↓renal perfusion, not necessarily failure:
    - –Heart failure
    - –Bilateral renal artery stenosis
    - –Hypovolemia
    - –Renal failure
    - ...rely more on the compensatory production of angiotensin 2→
      - •Efferent arteriole constriction→
        - Maintained glomerular filtration rate–GFR, whereas either:
          - **–Angiotensin converting enzyme inhibition**
          - **–Angiotensin 2 receptor blockade**
          - ...→↓angiotensin 2 production & action respectively, which may→
            - •↓Renal tubular potassium secretion
            - •Pre–renal renal failure
- **Renal tubular dysfunction**
  - **Renal tubular damage** via:
    - –Myeloma
    - –Sickle cell disease
    - –Systemic lupus erythematosus–SLE
    - ...→unresponsiveness to aldosterone
  - **Type 4 renal tubular acidosis**

ENDOCRINE

- **Hypoaldosteronism**
  - **1° adrenocortical insufficiency, termed Addison's disease**, via:
    - –Autoimmune, hemorrhagic, infectious, or metastatic mediated adrenal cortical destruction
    - –Congenital adrenal hyperplasia, due to enzyme deficiency
  - **2° adrenocortical insufficiency**, due to:
    - –The abrupt cessation of glucocorticoid therapy of >2weeks
    - –Pituitary &/or hypothalamic tumor→↓renin secretion
  - **Pseudohypoaldosteronism–rare**, via end–organ aldosterone resistance→
    - –Feedback mediated ↑plasma renin & aldosterone levels
- **Hyporeninemic hypoaldosteronism**
  - Usually occurring in renal failure patients w/ underlying diabetes mellitus, hypertension, &/or interstitial nephritis
  - ↓Renin of unknown etiology which does not ↑within 2hours of loop diuretic administration & standing

DIETARY

- •↑**Potassium intake**
  - ○↑Potassium diet, including potassium based salt substitutes
  - ○Medications
    - −Potassium replacement treatment
    - −Potassium salts of antibiotics

PSEUDOHYPERKALEMIA

- •When either:
  - ○Blood is left standing @ room temperature too long after being drawn
  - ○Prolonged hemostasis prior to venipuncture
  - ...→hemolysis→
    - •Intracellular potassium release
- •Repeated fist clenching during phlebotomy→
  - ○Local forearm skeletal myocyte potassium release
- •Leukocytosis >100,000/ μL
- •Thrombocytosis >1X10^9
- •Laboratory error

DIAGNOSIS

Cardiovascular
- •Cardiac muscle dysfunction→
  - ○**Dysrhythmias**

Gastrointestinal
- •Smooth muscle dysfunction→
  - ○Constipation
  - ○Intestinal paralytic ileus
  - ○Nausea ± vomiting

Genitourinary
- •↓Renal ammonia production & reabsorption in the loop of Henle→
  - ○↓Acid excretion→
    - −Metabolic acidemia

Musculoskeletal
- •Skeletal muscle dysfunction→
  - ○Diffuse muscle weakness
  - ○Hyporeflexia
  - ...w/ severe hyperkalemia→
    - •Paralysis, including the respiratory muscles

Neurologic
- •Paresthesias

ELECTRICAL STUDIES

Electrocardiography–ECG
- •ECG abnormalities correlate w/ plasma potassium to some extent, unlike hypokalemia
  - Plasma potassium:
  - •>5mEq/ L→
    - ○Atrial &/or ventricular dysrhythmia
  - •≥5.5mEq/ L→
    - ○↑T wave height & duration, termed "peaked" T waves
  - •≥6mEq/ L→
    - ○Atrioventricular conduction delay→
      - −Bradycardia
    - ○↑PR interval
    - ○↑QRS duration
    - ○↓QT interval
  - •≥7mEq/ L→
    - ○P wave flattening, indicating atrial arrest
    - ○Progressive QRS widening→
      - −Merging w/ T wave, forming a sine−wave pattern
    - ○↓ST segment

1. **Measure the urine potassium via either** 24h urine collection (mEq/ 24h) or spot urine specimen (mEq/ L)
   - •<20mEq indicates a renal process   •>20mEq indicates an extrarenal process
   ↓

2. **Calculate the glomerular filtration rate**
   - •↓ Indicates renal failure
   - •**Normal** indicates either:
     - ∘Tubular dysfunction
     - ∘Hypoaldosteronism
   ↓

3. **Measure plasma renin**
   - •↓ indicates either:
     - ∘Hyporenenimic hypoaldosteronism
     - ∘Pituitary or hypothalamic disease
   - •↑: **Measure plasma aldosterone**
     - ∘↓ Indicates either:
       - −Abrupt glucocorticoid cessation
       - −Primary adrenocortical insufficiency
     - ∘↑ Indicates either:
       - −Tubular dysfunction
       - −Pseudohypoaldosteronism

SEVERE HYPERKALEMIA ▬▬▬
- •Patients must be placed on a cardiac monitor for possible dysrhythmias, w/ plasma potassium measured qhour until normalized
- •Discontinue all medications possibly associated w/ hyperkalemia

MYOCARDIAL STABILIZATION

CALCIUM		
Indications:		
•All patients, in order to stabilize myocardial cells while administering medications causing both: ∘Potassium intracellular shift ∘Total body depletion		
Generic	**Dose**	**Max**
10% Calcium chloride†	10mL (1 ampule) IV slow push over 3min. q5min. prn until electrocardiographic changes resolve	
•Continuous infusion	0.3mEq/ hour	0.7mEq/ hour
Onset: 1−2 min., Duration: 30−60 min.		
•Use cautiously in patients taking Digoxin, as hypercalcemia→ ∘Digoxin cardiotoxicity †Preferred to calcium gluconate, as it contains 3X more elemental calcium		
Mechanism: •Calcium→ ∘↑Action potential threshold→ −↓Hyperkalemia mediated membrane depolarization		
Contraindications: •Digoxin toxicity		

TRANSCELLULAR SHIFT

INSULIN	
Generic	**Dose**
Regular insulin	10units IV push q15min. prn
Onset: 10−30min., Duration: 3hours	
&	
Glucose†	25g administered as 50mL of a 50% dextrose solution (1 ampule) IV push
†Administer less to no glucose if the patient is hyperglycemic	
Mechanism: •Insulin→ ∘↑Cell membrane Na^+/K^+ ATPase action (adipose tissue, skeletal muscle, & hepatocytes)→ −Potassium intracellular shift→↓plasma potassium by 0.5−1.5mEq/ L for every 10 units administered	

853

β₂ SELECTIVE RECEPTOR AGONISTS: Short acting

Generic (Trade)	M	♀	Dose
Albuterol (Ventolin)	L	?	
•Nebulizer:			10–20mg

Onset: 15–30min., Duration: 2–4hours

Mechanism:
- •↑Cell membrane Na^+/K^+ ATPase action→
  - ∘Potassium intracellular shift→
    - −↓Plasma potassium by 0.5–1.5mEq/ L

BICARBONATE

Note: **Bicarbonate binds to calcium→**
- **•↓Calcium membrane stabilization effects, and so is best avoided**

Generic	M	♀	Dose
Sodium bicarbonate	K	?	1mEq/kg/dose IV push (1 ampule = ~50mEq)

Onset: 15–30min., Duration: 1–2hours

Mechanism:
- •Alkalemia→
  - ∘↑H^+/K^+ cell membrane exchange protein function→
    - −Potassium intracellular shift

Side effects:
- •May exacerbate volume overload due to sodium content

REMOVAL

SODIUM POLYSTYRENE SULFONATE (Kayexalate)

	Dose
PO form	60g mixed w/ 50mL of 20% Sorbitol† q6h prn
PR form‡	50g of resin mixed w/ 50mL of 20% sorbitol† in 150mL of tap water, retained for 30min. to several hours q6hours prn

Onset: 1–2hours, Duration: 4–6hours

---

†To prevent constipation
‡Subsequent irrigation w/ tap water should be performed to prevent sorbitol induced colonic necrosis

Mechanism:
- •A cation exchange resin→
  - ∘Potassium removal from the body by way of the gastrointestinal mucosa in exchange for sodium→
    - −↓Plasma potassium by 0.5–1mEq/ L for every 30–60g administered

---

LOOP DIURETICS

Generic (Trade)	M	♀	Dose
Furosemide (Lasix)	K	?	40–80mg IV push

Onset: 1hour, Duration: 6hours (La**six** lasts **six** hours)

•There is synergistic efficacy of combination treatment w/ a thiazide diuretic

Mechanism:
- •Inhibits $Na^+/K^+/2Cl^-$ reabsorption in the thick ascending limb of the loop of Henle→
  - ∘↑Potassium loss via diuresis→

Limitations:
- •↓Efficacy in patients w/ a glomerular filtration rate <10mL/ min.

Side effects:
- **Genitourinary**
  - •Acute interstitial nephritis
- **Neurologic**
  - **•Ototoxicity**
- **Hematologic**
  - •Acid base disturbances
    - ∘Hypochloremic metabolic alkalemia
  - •Dyslipidemia
    - ∘↑Cholesterol & triglycerides

•Electrolyte disturbances
∘**Hypokalemia**
∘Hypomagnesemia
∘Hyponatremia
∘Hypercalcemia
•Hyperglycemia
•Hyperuricemia
Contraindications:
•**Sulfa allergy**, as all thiazide & loop diuretics (except Ethacrynic acid) contain a sulfa component

SECOND LINE TREATMENT_____

•**Hemodialysis**
  Indications:
    •Hyperkalemia refractory to medical treatment

NON−SEVERE HYPERKALEMIA ▬▬▬▬▬▬▬▬▬▬▬▬▬▬▬▬▬▬▬▬
•The medications listed above under removal

•Any process→
  ◦Plasma potassium <3.5mEq/ L (normal: 3.5–5.0mEq/ L)→myocyte hyperpolarization (skeletal, smooth, & cardiac)→
    –Dysfunction, which usually becomes symptomatic @ <2.5mEq/ L
Statistics:
  •Total body potassium is normally 50mEq/ L, w/ >98% being intracellular
  •Usual dietary intake is 1mEq/kg/24h, 90% of which is absorbed, w/ subsequent renal excretion

CLASSIFICATION/ RISK FACTORS

•**Hypokalemia:** 2.6–3.4mEq/ L
•**Severe hyperkalemia:** ≤2.5mEq/ L, electrocardiographic changes, or symptomatic

TRANSCELLULAR SHIFT ▬▬▬▬▬▬▬▬▬▬▬▬▬▬▬▬▬▬▬▬▬▬▬▬▬▬▬▬▬▬▬▬▬

•As <2% (~50mEq) of total body potassium is located in the extracellular fluid, even small transcellular shifts→
  ◦Significant changes in the extracellular fluid concentration, w/ an inward transcellular shift→
    –↑Renal tubule cell potassium→↑driving force for potassium secretion
•**Alkalemia**→
  ◦**Hypokalemia, as every 0.1↑ in pH→0.3mEq/ L↓ in potassium** via the H^+/K^+ cell membrane exchange protein→
    –Potassium intracellular shift
•**Medications**
  ◦**β2 receptor agonists**→
    –↑Cell membrane Na^+/K^+ ATPase action→potassium intracellular shift
    –Magnesium intracellular shift
  ◦**Insulin**→
    –↑Cell membrane Na^+/K^+ ATPase function (adipose tissue, skeletal muscle, & hepatocytes)→ potassium intracellular shift
    –Magnesium intracellular shift
•**Marked anabolic states**
  ◦Rapidly proliferating malignancy, esp.:
    –Acute leukemias
    –Aggressive non–Hodgkin's lymphomas
    –Myeloma
  ◦Neutropenia treated w/ granulocyte colony stimulating factor–GCSF
  ◦Pernicious anemia treated w/ vitamin B12
•**Hypothermia**
•**Endocrine**
  ◦Hyperthyroidism–rare, esp. in Asian ♂
•**Poisoning**
  ◦Barium salt ingestion, due to contamination of table salt→
    –↓Skeletal muscle potassium efflux
  ◦Toluene
•**Hypokalemic periodic paralysis**, being a rare autosomal dominant disease→
  ◦↑Insulin secretion:
    –In response to a ↑carbohydrate meal
    –At rest after exercise
    …→hypokalemia→
      •Episodic weakness lasting ≤72hours
•**Overdose**
  ◦Treating Digoxin overdose w/ Digoxin antibody fragments (Digibind)

↑**URINARY LOSS** ▬▬▬▬▬▬▬▬▬▬▬▬▬▬▬▬▬▬▬▬▬▬▬▬▬▬▬▬▬▬▬▬▬▬▬

•All causes of volume loss→
  ◦Hypovolemia→
    –↑Aldosterone→hypokalemia & metabolic alkalemia
  ◦Extracellular volume contraction mediated ↑bicarbonate→
    –Volume contraction alkalemia→potassium intracellular shift
  ◦Concomitant magnesium loss→
    –↓Potassium tubular reabsorption

- •Medications
  - ◦Non-potassium sparing diuretics
    - –Loop diuretics
    - –Thiazide diuretics
    - …→↑hydrogen & chloride secretion→
      - •Hypochloremic, metabolic alkalemia
    - –Carbonic anhydrase inhibitors→↓bicarbonate reabsorption→hyperchloremic, non-anion gap, metabolic acidemia
    - …w/ potassium nadir usually occurring in 7days
  - ◦Antimicrobials
    - –Aminoglycosides
    - –Amphotericin B
    - …→↓ascending loop of Henle magnesium reabsorption
    - –↑Dose penicillins, which exist as sodium or potassium salts→↑sodium & water excretion, termed diuresis
  - ◦Chemotherapeutics
    - –Cisplatin
    - –Cyclosporine
    - …→↑renal tubule magnesium excretion
  - ◦Digoxin→
    - –Magnesium intracellular shift
- •Vomiting or equivalent, such as nasogastric suctioning→
  - ◦HCl loss→
    - –Metabolic alkalemia→potassium intracellular shift
- •Hypertonicity
  - –Diabetic ketoacidosis
  - –Hyperosmolar hyperglycemic state
  - –Mannitol
  - –High protein tube feedings
  - –Glycerol
  - –Radiocontrast agents
  - –Sorbitol
  - –↑Urea
  - …→osmotic diuresis
- •Renal tubule dysfunction
  - ◦Chronic obstructive nephropathy→
    - –Post-obstructive diuresis
  - ◦Diuretic phase of acute tubular necrosis
  - ◦Renal tubular acidosis–RTA via defective tubular hydrogen excretion &/or bicarbonate reabsorption, w/:
    - –Type 1 involving the distal convoluted tubule
    - –Type 2 involving the proximal convoluted tubule

GENETIC_____
- •Bartter's syndrome
  - ◦↓Ascending loop of Henle $Na^+/K^+/2Cl^-$ reabsorption (like loop diuretics)
- •Gitelman's syndrome
  - ◦Distal convoluted tubule dysfunction (like thiazide diuretics)
- •Liddle's syndrome, being a rare inherited disease→
  - ◦Distal nephron aldosterone-like hyperfunction→
    - –Hypokalemia
    - –Non-anion gap metabolic alkalemia
    - –Hypertension
    - –Feedback mediated ↓aldosterone levels

↑GASTROINTESTINAL LOSS ▬▬▬▬▬▬▬▬▬▬▬▬▬▬▬▬▬▬▬▬
- •All causes of volume loss→
  - ◦Hypovolemia→
    - –↑Aldosterone→hypokalemia & metabolic alkalemia
  - ◦Extracellular volume contraction mediated ↑bicarbonate→
    - –Volume contraction alkalemia→potassium intracellular shift
  - ◦Concomitant magnesium loss→
    - –↓Potassium tubular reabsorption

- **Diarrhea** or equivalent, such as intestinal fistula or biliary drainage→
  - ∘Potassium loss
  - ∘Bicarbonate loss→
    - −Hyperchloremic, non−anion gap metabolic acidemia
- **Medications**
  - ∘Sodium polystyrene sulfonate (Kayexalate), a potassium binding resin
- **Neoplasm**
  - ∘Villous adenoma, esp. of the rectum
  - ∘Pancreatic islet cell tumor secreting vasoactive intestinal peptide or gastrin
- **Diet**
  - ∘Clay ingestion

DIET

- **↓Intake**
  - ∘Anorexia nervosa
- **Licorice containing glycyrrhizic acid or chewing tobacco** via:
  - ∘Inhibition of 11β−hydroxysteroid dehydrogenase, which normally prevents physiologic glucocorticoid renal tubule concentrations from exerting mineralocorticoid−like effects→↑mineralocorticoid effect→
    - −Hypokalemia
    - −Non−anion gap metabolic acidemia
    - −Hypertension
    - −Feedback mediated ↓aldosterone levels

ENDOCRINE

- **Hyperaldosteronism**
  - ∘Primary
    - −Adrenal adenoma
    - −Adrenal cancer
    - −Adrenocortical hyperplasia
  - ∘Secondary, due to ↑renin secretion
    - −Cirrhosis
    - −Coarctation of the aorta
    - −Heart failure
    - −Nephrotic syndrome
    - −Renal artery stenosis
    - −Renin secreting neoplasm
- **Hypercortisolism**
  - ∘Cushing's disease or syndrome
  - ∘Glucocorticoid medications
  - …due to their mineralocorticoid effects

CUTANEOUS LOSS

- **Excessive** diaphoresis via hypovolemia→
  - ∘↑Aldosterone
  - ∘Potassium loss in sweat

PSEUDOHYPOKALEMIA

- Leukocytosis >100,000/ μL due to leukocyte mediated potassium uptake
- Laboratory error

DIAGNOSIS

Cardiovascular
- Cardiac muscle dysfunction→
  - ∘**Dysrhythmias**. However, Hypokalemia alone will not cause serious ventricular dysrhythmias unless accompanied by another pro−dysrhythmic risk factor, such as:
    - −Heart disease
    - −Magnesium depletion
    - −Digitalis
- **Endocrine**
  - ∘↓Insulin secretion & action→
    - −↓Glycemic control in diabetic patients
Gastrointestinal
- Smooth muscle dysfunction→
  - ∘Constipation
  - ∘Intestinal paralytic ileus
  - ∘Nausea ± vomiting

858

Genitourinary
- •↑Renal ammonia production which may→
  - ∘Encephalopathy in hepatic or renal failure patients
- •↓Renal tubular responsiveness to antidiuretic hormone→
  - ∘Nephrogenic diabetes insipidus

Musculoskeletal
- •Skeletal muscle dysfunction→
  - ∘Diffuse muscle weakness
  - ∘Hyporeflexia
  - …w/ severe hypokalemia→
    - •Paralysis, including the respiratory muscles
    - •Rhabdomyolysis, usually @ <2mEq/ L

Neurologic
- •Paresthesias

ELECTRICAL STUDIES

Electrocardiography–ECG
- •ECG abnormalities do not correlate w/ plasma potassium
  - Plasma potassium:
    - •<3.5mEq/ L→
      - ∘Atrial &/or ventricular dysrhythmia
      - ∘Atrioventricular conduction delay→
        - −Bradycardia
      - ∘↑PR interval
      - ∘↑QRS duration w/ ↓voltage
      - ∘↓ST segment
      - ∘↑QT interval
      - ∘↓T wave
      - ∘U waves >1mm in height

ETIOLOGIC DIFFERENTIATION

1. Measure the urine potassium via either 24hou urine collection (mEq/ 24h) or spot urine specimen (mEq/ L)

- •<20mEq indicates an extrarenal process
- •>20mEq indicates a renal process
  - ↓−Skip to step 3 if hypertensive

2. Measure plasma bicarbonate

- •↓Indicates gastrointestinal loss

- •↓Indicates either:
  - ∘Renal tubular acidosis
  - ∘Carbonic anhydrase inhibitor use
  - ∘Hypertonicity
  - ∘Magnesium depletion
- •Normal indicates profuse diaphoresis
- •↑Indicates either:
  - ∘Previous diuretic use or vomiting
  - ∘Gastric fistula
- •Normal indicates magnesium depletion
- •↑: **Measure the 24h urine chloride**
  - ∘<10mEq/ L indicates upper gastrointestinal loss
  - ∘>10mEq/ L indicates either:
    - −Loop or thiazide diuretic use
    - −Magnesium depletion
    - −Normotensive hyperaldosteronism
    - −Bartter's syndrome
    - ↓

3. Measure plasma renin
- •↑Indicates either:
  - ∘Renovascular hypertension
  - ∘Renin–secreting neoplasm
  - ∘Secondary hyperaldosteronism
- •↓: **Measure plasma aldosterone**
  - ∘↓Indicates either:
    - −Congenital adrenal hyperplasia
    - −Hypercortisolism
    - −Licorice or chewing tobacco intake
    - −Liddle's syndrome
  - •↑Indicates primary hyperaldosteronism

•For severe hypokalemia, patients must be placed on a cardiac monitor for possible dysrrhythmias, w/ plasma potassium measured qhour until normalized

---

POTASSIUM
•Always measure the magnesium level concomitantly

Indications:
•Ensure a potassium of 4–5mEq/ L

Generic

If concomitant alkalemia:
•Potassium chloride–KCL
If concomitant acidemia:
•Potassium bicarbonate
•Potassium citrate
•Potassium acetate
•Potassium gluconate
•Potassium phosphate
  ∘Preferred in diabetic ketoacidosis–DKA due to concomitant phosphate depletion
Monitoring:
•Q4hours until goal of 4–5mEq/ L X 2 consecutive readings, then q6hours

POTASSIUM DOSAGE ADJUSTMENT SCALE†_____

Plasma K^+ (mEq/ L)	K^+ repletion (mEq)
≥3.9	None
3.7–3.8	20
3.5–3.6	40
3.3–3.4	60
3.1–3.2	80
≤3	100

†Half all above doses @ a glomerular filtration rate–GFR ≤30mL/ min.

Intravenous repletion guidelines:
•Use dextrose–free solutions for the initial repletion as dextrose→
  ∘↑Insulin secretion→
    –↑Potassium transcellular shift
•The hyperosmolar infusion→
  ∘Vascular irritation/ inflammation. Add 1% Lidocaine to the bag to ↓pain
•**Do not administer >20mEq potassium IV/ hour**
  ∘≤10mEq/ hour prn via peripheral line. May give via 2 peripheral lines=20mEq/ hour total
  ∘≤20mEq/ hour prn via central line
  …as more→
    •Transient right sided heart hyperkalemia→
      ∘Dysrhythmias

Outcomes:
•Anti–dysrhythmic
•↑Cardiac contractility in heart failure
•Modest hypotensive effect in some patients
•↓Cerebrovascular disease risk, apart from its possible blood pressure lowering effects

MAGNESIUM SULFATE

M ♀	Dose
K S	Every 1g IV→0.1mEq/ L ↑in plasma magnesium

Mechanism:
•↓Magnesium→
  ∘↓Renal tubular potassium reabsorption

•Any process→
  ∘Abnormal water homeostasis→
    –Plasma sodium >145mEq/ L (normal: 135–145mEq/ L)→plasma hypertonicity (normal: 280–
    290mOsm/ L)
•This syndrome is much less common than hyponatremia, as the body's homeostatic mechanisms
against dehydration are relatively more potent. In fact, any patient w/ significant hypernatremia is
virtually sure to have been denied adequate access to water, as patients who are otherwise healthy can
↑their water intake to as much as 10L/ 24hours, which is enough to prevent even moderate
hyperosmolarity. Even in the complete absence of antidiuretic hormone secretion, patients w/ adequate
water access should have only mild hypernatremia
•Conditions potentially causing inadequate water ingestion:
  ∘**Inadequate access to water**
    –Environmental exposure
    –Illness
    –Intoxication
    –Neglect
  ∘↓**Thirst sensation** via a central nervous system disease affecting the hypothalamic thirst center
    –Cerebrovascular accident

IMPORTANT TERMS

•**Osmolarity:** The total number of dissolved solutes (in mmol/ kg) in a given solvent, which correlates
directly w/ the osmotic pressure exerted by the solution across a water permeable, solute impermeable
membrane, determined by:
  ∘Sodium
  ∘Blood urea nitrogen–BUN
  ∘Glucose
  …which cannot move freely across cell membranes, thereby inducing transcellular shifts in water
•Plasma osmolarity may be measured directly, or calculated via the following formula:
  ∘Plasma osmolarity=2 (plasma Na^+) + (plasma blood urea nitrogen/ 2.8) + (plasma glucose/ 18)

CLASSIFICATION

HYPOVOLEMIC HYPERNATREMIA ▬▬▬▬▬▬▬▬▬▬▬▬▬▬▬▬▬▬▬▬▬▬▬▬▬▬

•All causes of volume loss→
  ∘Hypovolemia→
    –↑Aldosterone→hypokalemia & metabolic alkalemia
  ∘Extracellular volume contraction mediated ↑bicarbonate→
    –Volume contraction alkalemia→potassium intracellular shift
  ∘Concomitant magnesium loss→
    –↓Potassium tubular reabsorption

•**Renal fluid volume loss**
  ∘**Neurogenic diabetes insipidus†** via either inadequate:
    –Hypothalamic production
    –Posterior pituitary secretion
    …of antidiuretic hormone. Note that the posterior pituitary is merely a storage site for antidiuretic
    hormone after its synthesis in the hypothalamus
    Risk factors:
      •Idiopathic, being the #1 cause
      •Ethanol ingestion, being transient
      •Neurologic disease
      •Medications:
        ∘Phenytoin
  ∘**Nephrogenic diabetes insipidus†** via ↓renal tubular responsiveness to antidiuretic hormone
    Risk factors:
      •Congenital
      •Medications
        ∘Amphotericin B
        ∘Demeclocycline
        ∘Foscarnet
        ∘Lithium
        ∘Methoxyflurane
      •Metabolic
        –Hypercalcemia
        –Hypokalemia

- •Renal tubular dysfunction
  - −Diuretic phase of acute tubular necrosis
  - −Amyloidosis
  - −Chronic obstructive nephropathy→post−obstructive diuresis
  - −Polycystic kidney disease
  - −Pyelonephritis
  - −Sarcoidosis
  - −Sickle cell anemia
  - −Sjogrens syndrome
  - −X−linked familial syndrome−rare
  - ◦**Medications**
    - −Thiazide diuretics→inhibition of NaCl reabsorption in the early distal convoluted tubule→ ↑urination
    - −Loop diuretics→inhibition of $Na^+/K^+/2Cl^-$ reabsorption in the thick ascending limb of the loop of Henle→↑urination
    - ...→↑chloride & hydrogen secretion→
      - •Hypochloremic, metabolic alkalemia
    - −Carbonic anhydrase inhibitors→↓bicarbonate reabsorption→hyperchloremic, non−anion gap, metabolic acidemia
    - ...w/ potassium nadir usually occurring in 7days
  - ◦**Osmotic diuresis**
    - −Diabetic ketoacidosis
    - −Hyperosmolar hyperglycemic state
    - −Mannitol
    - −High protein tube feedings
    - −Glycerol
    - −Sorbitol
    - −↑Urea

- •**Gastrointestinal fluid volume loss**
  - ◦**Diarrhea** or equivalent, such as intestinal fistula or biliary drainage→
    - −Potassium loss
    - −Bicarbonate loss→hyperchloremic, non−anion gap metabolic acidemia
  - ◦**Medications**
    - −Lactulose
    - −Sodium polystyrene sulfonate (Kayexalate), a potassium binding resin
  - ◦**Neoplasm**
    - −Villous adenoma, esp. of the rectum
    - −Pancreatic islet cell tumor secreting vasoactive intestinal peptide or gastrin

- •**Cutaneous fluid volume loss**
  - ◦Severe burn
  - ◦Diaphoresis

HYPERVOLEMIC HYPERNATREMIA
- •**Extrarenal sodium gain**
  - ◦**Exogenous sodium infusion**
    - −Hypertonic NaCl infusion
    - −Hypertonic $NaHCO_3^-$ infusion
    - −Hypertonic saline enemas
    - −Hypertonic feeding preparations
    - −Hypertonic dialysis
    - −Intrauterine injection of hypertonic saline
    - −NaCl ingestion
    - −Sea water ingestion
    - −NaCl rich emetics
- •**Renal sodium gain**
  - ◦**Hyperaldosteronism**
    - −Primary: Adrenal adenoma, adrenal cancer, adrenocortical hyperplasia
    - −Secondary, due to ↑renin secretion: Cirrhosis, coarctation of the aorta, heart failure, nephrotic syndrome, renal artery stenosis, renin secreting neoplasm
  - ◦**Hypercortisolism**
    - −Cushing's disease or syndrome
    - −Glucocorticoid medications, being due to their mineralocorticoid effects

862

EUVOLEMIC HYPERNATREMIA ▬▬▬▬▬▬▬▬▬▬▬▬▬▬▬▬▬▬▬▬▬▬▬▬▬
- **Diabetes insipidus** (neurogenic or nephrogenic) patients may also be euvolemic w/ mild hypernatremia
- **Reset osmostat** via reset antidiuretic physiology to regulate ↑plasma sodium

PSEUDOHYPERNATREMIA–rare ▬▬▬▬▬▬▬▬▬▬▬▬▬▬▬▬▬▬▬▬▬▬▬▬▬
- Being isotonic or hypotonic, due to:
  - ○Hypoproteinemia
  - ○Hypotriglyceridemia ·
  - ○Laboratory error

DIAGNOSIS
General
- •Anorexia
- •Fatigue
- •Malaise

Gastrointestinal
- •Nausea ± vomiting

Neurologic
- •Hypernatremia→
  - ○Osmosis of water from the intracellular to the extracellular compartment, including the central nervous system→neuronal & neuroglial dehydration→dysfunction. If sodium rises by ≥9mEq/L/24h, a demyelination syndrome occurs, termed **central pontine myelinosis**→neuronal & neuroglial dysfunction, injury, &/or death→
    - **–Altered mental status**
    - –Seizures
    - –Death

ETIOLOGIC DIFFERENTIATION
1. **Measure plasma osmolarity**

•> **295mOsm/ L** indicates hypertonic hypernatremia   •<**295mOsm/ L** indicates pseudohypernatremia
⬇
2. **Assess extracellular fluid volume status**

HYPOVOLEMIC
⬇
3. **Measure urine sodium & osmolarity**
- •Na⁺<20mEq/ L indicates extrarenal volume loss
- •Na⁺>20mEq/ L indicates renal volume loss, w/ diabetes insipidus diagnosed via either:
  - ○Administration of antidiuretic hormone, w/ subsequent **re–measurement of urine osmolarity**
    - –>**50%**↑ indicates neurogenic diabetes insipidus
    - **–Unchanged** indicates nephrogenic diabetes insipidus
  - ○**Water deprivation** test, in which fluids & food are withheld beginning in the morning in order to avoid severe nocturnal dehydration. Urine & plasma osmolarity are then measured qhour, w/ failure of the urine osmolarity to ↑by >30mOsm/ kg within several hours, being diagnostic of diabetes insipidus

---

•The defect in urine concentrating ability is more severe in neurogenic relative to nephrogenic diabetes insipidus
  - ○Urine osmolarity w/ no antidiuretic hormone activity: 60mOsm/ L
  - ○Urine osmolarity w/ maximal antidiuretic hormone activity: 1200mOsm/ L

TREATMENT
<u>Caution:</u> In chronic hypernatremia, cells retain osmoles in order to minimize intracellular dehydration. Subsequent aggressive restoration of a normal plasma sodium→
- •↓Extracellular osmolarity relative to cellular→
  - ○Rapid osmosis of water from the extracellular to the intracellular compartment, including the central nervous system→**cerebral edema**→neuronal & neuroglial dysfunction, injury, &/or death→
    - **–Altered mental status**
    - –Seizures
    - –Death

•**Intravenous fluid**
  ○↓**Plasma sodium @ a rate of ≤0.5mEq/L/hour†** (max 8mEq/L/24h) in order to gradually ↓plasma osmolarity to <295mOsmol/ kg
  ○The following formula shows the effect of 1L of any infusate on plasma sodium:

$$\text{Plasma Na}^+ \Delta= \frac{(\text{infusate Na}^+ + \text{infusate K}^+) - \text{plasma Na}^+}{0.55 \text{ (weight in kg)}}$$

Infusate	Na$^+$ (mEq/L)	K$^+$ (mEq/L)	Extracellular fluid dist.
5% NaCl in water=hypertonic saline†	855	0	100%
3% NaCl in water=hypertonic saline†	513	0	100%
0.9% NaCl in water=normal saline	154	0	100%
0.45% NaCl in water=1/2 normal saline	77	0	73%
0.2% NaCl in 5% dextrose in water=hypotonic saline	34	0	55%
Ringers lactate solution	130	4	97%
5% dextrose in water=free water	0	0	40%

†Hypertonic solutions must be administered via a central venous line. In addition to their complete distribution in the extracellular compartment, this infusate→
  •Osmosis of water from the intracellular to the extracellular compartment

Neurogenic diabetes insipidus:
  •**Brain magnetic resonance imaging–MRI** to view the hypothalamic & pituitary regions

&

ANTI-DIURETIC HORMONE ANALOGUE: Long acting				
Generic (Trade)	M ♀	Start	Max	
Desmopressin (DDAVP)	LK P			
•PO form		0.05mg PO q24hours	1.2mg/ 24hours	
•SC/ IV forms		1µg q12hours	2µg q12hours	
•Intranasal form		10µg q24hours	40µg q8hours	

Nephrogenic diabetes insipidus:
  •**Treat the underlying cause**
  •**Protein restriction**
  •↓**Sodium intake**
    ○0.5–1g elemental sodium or 1.5–3g salt/ 24hours

864

HYPONATREMIA

•Any process→
  ◦Abnormal water homeostasis→
    –Plasma sodium <135mEq/ L (normal: 135–145mEq/ L)→plasma hypotonicity (normal: 280–290mOsm/ L)

IMPORTANT TERMS

•**Osmolarity:** The total number of dissolved solutes (in mmol/ kg) in a given solvent, which correlates directly w/ the osmotic pressure exerted by the solution across a water permeable, solute impermeable membrane, determined by:
  ◦Sodium
  ◦Blood urea nitrogen–BUN
  ◦Glucose
  …which cannot move freely across cell membranes, thereby inducing transcellular shifts in water
•Plasma osmolarity may be measured directly, or calculated via the following formula:
  ◦Plasma osmolarity=2 (plasma Na^+) + (plasma blood urea nitrogen/ 2.8) + (plasma glucose/ 18)

CLASSIFICATION

HYPOVOLEMIC HYPONATREMIA ▬▬▬▬▬▬▬

•All causes of volume loss→
  ◦Hypovolemia→
    –↑Aldosterone→hypokalemia & metabolic alkalemia
  ◦Extracellular volume contraction mediated ↑bicarbonate→
    –Volume contraction alkalemia→potassium intracellular shift
  ◦Concomitant magnesium loss→
    –↓Potassium tubular reabsorption

•**Renal fluid volume loss**
  ◦**Neurogenic diabetes insipidus**† via either inadequate:
    –Hypothalamic production
    –Posterior pituitary secretion
    …of antidiuretic hormone. Note that the posterior pituitary is merely a storage site for antidiuretic hormone after its synthesis in the hypothalamus
    Risk factors:
      •Idiopathic, being the #1 cause
      •Ethanol ingestion, being transient
      •Neurologic disease
      •Medications:
        ◦Phenytoin
  ◦**Nephrogenic diabetes insipidus**† via ↓renal tubular responsiveness to antidiuretic hormone
    Risk factors:
      •Congenital
      •Medications
        ◦Amphotericin B
        ◦Demeclocycline
        ◦Foscarnet
        ◦Lithium
        ◦Methoxyflurane
      •Metabolic
        –Hypercalcemia
        –Hypokalemia
      •Renal tubular dysfunction
        –Diuretic phase of acute tubular necrosis
        –Amyloidosis
        –Chronic obstructive nephropathy→post–obstructive diuresis
        –Polycystic kidney disease
        –Pyelonephritis
        –Sarcoidosis
        –Sickle cell anemia
        –Sjogrens syndrome
        –X–linked familial syndrome–rare

- **Medications**
  - Thiazide diuretics→inhibition of NaCl reabsorption in the early distal convoluted tubule→ ↑urination
  - Loop diuretics→inhibition of $Na^+/K^+/2Cl^-$ reabsorption in the thick ascending limb of the loop of Henle→↑urination
  - ...→↑chloride & hydrogen secretion→
    - •Hypochloremic, metabolic alkalemia
  - Carbonic anhydrase inhibitors→↓bicarbonate reabsorption→hyperchloremic, non-anion gap, metabolic acidemia
  - ...w/ potassium nadir usually occurring in 7days
- **Osmotic diuresis**
  - Diabetic ketoacidosis
  - Hyperosmolar hyperglycemic state
  - Mannitol
  - High protein tube feedings
  - Glycerol
  - Sorbitol
  - ↑Urea
- **•Gastrointestinal fluid volume loss**
  - **Diarrhea** or equivalent, such as intestinal fistula or biliary drainage→
    - Potassium loss
    - Bicarbonate loss→hyperchloremic, non-anion gap metabolic acidemia
  - **Medications**
    - Lactulose
    - Sodium polystyrene sulfonate (Kayexalate), a potassium binding resin
  - **Neoplasm**
    - Villous adenoma, esp. of the rectum
    - Pancreatic islet cell tumor secreting vasoactive intestinal peptide or gastrin
- **•Cutaneous fluid volume loss**
  - Severe burn
  - Diaphoresis

HYPERVOLEMIC HYPONATREMIA
- **•Renal fluid volume gain**
  - Advanced renal failure

- **•Extrarenal fluid volume gain**
  - Cirrhosis
  - Heart failure
  - Nephrotic syndrome

EUVOLEMIC HYPONATREMIA
- **•Syndrome of inappropriate secretion of antidiuretic hormone-SIADH,** being the #1 cause of hyponatremia
  - Risk factors:
    - •Neurologic disease
    - •Thoracic disease
    - •Endocrine disease
      - Adrenal failure
      - Hypothyroidism
    - •Medications
      - ↑Antidiuretic hormone release
        - Carbamazepine
        - Nicotine
        - Phenothiazines
        - Tricyclic antidepressants
        - Selective serotonin reuptake inhibitors-SSRIs
      - Direct renal effects
        - Desmopressin
        - Oxytocin
        - Prostaglandin synthesis inhibitors: Nonsteroidal anti-inflammatory drugs-NSAIDS, glucocorticoids

866

- ○Other
  - −Barbiturates
  - −Chlorpropamide
  - −Clofibrate
  - −Cyclophosphamide
  - −Opiate derivatives
  - −Oral hypoglycemics
  - −Vincristine
- •Other
  - ○Human immune deficiency virus−HIV infection
  - ○Nausea
  - ○Pain
  - ○Postoperative state

- **•Endocrine**
  - ○Adrenal failure
  - ○Glucocorticoid deficiency
  - ○Hypothyroidism
  - …as mineralocorticoids, glucocorticoids, & thyroid hormones are essential for normal renal tubular function
- **•Hypokalemia**
- **•↓Solute intake**
  - ○↑Beer intake, termed beer potomonia
  - ○Predominantly tea & toast diet, as may be seen in the elderly
- **•↑Water intake**
  - ○Psychogenic polydipsia, usually in psychiatric patients, requiring the intake of >12−20L/ 24h
  - ○Accidental ingestion of large amounts of water, as during swimming lessons
  - ○Multiple tap water enemas, w/ the resultant hyponatremia being either:
    - −Hypotonic w/ an irrigant containing 1.5% glycine or 3.3% mannitol
    - −Isotonic w/ an irrigant containing 5% mannitol
  - ○Absorption of sodium free irrigant solutions†, used in:
    - −Hysteroscopy
    - −Laparoscopy
    - −Transurethral resection of the prostate−TURP
- **•Reset osmostat** via reset antidiuretic physiology to regulate ↓plasma sodium

PSEUDOHYPONATREMIA ▬▬▬▬▬▬▬▬▬▬▬

Isotonic:
- •Hyperproteinemia
  - ○Myeloma
  - Correction formula:
    - •[Plasma protein level (g/ dL) − 8] X 0.025 = mEq/ L ↓plasma sodium
- •Hypertriglyceridemia
  - ○Uncontrolled diabetes mellitus
  - Correction formula:
    - •Plasma triglyceride level (g/ L) X 0.002 = mEq/ L ↓plasma sodium
- •Laboratory error

Hypertonic:
- •↑Levels of molecules which cannot move freely across cell membranes→
  - ○Hypertonic extracellular fluid→
    - −Osmosis of water from the intracellular to the extracellular compartment→dilutional effect→ ↓measured plasma sodium
- •**Hyperglycemia**, being the #1 cause of pseudohyponatremia, as every 100mg ↑plasma glucose above a baseline of 100mg/ dL→
  - ○Falsely measured ↓sodium by 1.6mEq/ L. However, the actual measured sodium concentration should be used to calculate the anion gap in patients with hyperglycemia†, whereas, the corrected sodium concentration should be used to estimate the severity of dehydration
- •Hypertonic substances
  - ○Glycine
  - ○Mannitol
  - ○Radiocontrast agents
- •Methanol or ethylene glycol ingestion

---

†This is because the osmotic movement of water from the intracellular to the extracellular compartment equally dilutes all electrolytes, including chloride & bicarbonate, thereby not requiring a relative correction

•Symptomatic hyponatremia usually occurs w/ a plasma sodium <125mEq/ L, or rapid ↓ (within hours), w/ premenopausal ♀ being more sensitive to rapid fluxes in plasma sodium than are ♂ or postmenopausal ♀

General
•Anorexia
•Fatigue
•Malaise
Gastrointestinal
•Ileus
•Nausea ± vomiting
Musculoskeletal
•Muscle cramps
Neurologic
•Hyponatremia→
 ○Osmosis of water from the extracellular to the intracellular compartment, including the central nervous system→**cerebral edema**→neuronal & neuroglial dysfunction, injury, &/or death→
  –**Altered mental status**
  –Seizures
  –Death

1. Measure plasma osmolarity
 •< 280mOsm/ L indicates hypotonic hyponatremia

2. Assess extracellular fluid volume status

   HYPOVOLEMIC or HYPERVOLEMIC

3. Measure the urine sodium
 •<20mEq/ L indicates extrarenal fluid volume loss or gain
 •>20mEq/ L indicates renal fluid volume loss or gain

   EUVOLEMIC
 ↓
3. Measure both the urine sodium & osmolarity†
 •**Na <20mEq/ L** & **osmolarity <100mOsm/ L** indicates psychogenic polydipsia
 •**Na >20mEq/ L** & **osmolarity >100mOsm/ L** indicates SIADH‡

---

†Normal urine concentrating ability is:
 •Urine osmolarity w/ no antidiuretic hormone activity: 60mOsm/ L
 •Urine osmolarity w/ maximal antidiuretic hormone activity: 1200mOsm/ L
‡Although the diagnosis ultimately rests upon an ↑ or inappropriately normal plasma antidiuretic hormone level in the face of concomitant hypotonicity, empiric treatment need not await the assay result

Caution: In chronic hyponatremia, cells secrete osmoles in order to minimize intracellular swelling. Subsequent aggressive restoration of a normal plasma sodium→
 •↑Extracellular osmolarity relative to cellular→
 ○Osmosis of water from the intracellular to the extracellular compartment, including the central nervous system→neuronal & neuroglial dehydration→dysfunction. If sodium rises by ≥9mEq/L/24h, a demyelination syndrome occurs, termed **central pontine myelinosis**→neuronal & neuroglial dysfunction, injury, &/or death→
  –**Altered mental status**
  –Seizures
  –Death

HYPOVOLEMIC HYPONATREMIA ▬▬▬▬▬
•**Intravenous fluid**
 ◦↑**Plasma sodium @ a rate of ≤0.5mEq/L/hour**† (max 8mEq/L/24hours) in order to gradually
 ↑plasma osmolarity to >295mOsmol/ kg
 ◦The following formula shows the effect of 1L of any infusate on plasma sodium:

$$\text{Plasma Na}^+ \, \Delta = \frac{(\text{infusate Na}^+ + \text{infusate K}^+) - \text{plasma Na}^+}{0.55 \, (\text{weight in kg})}$$

Infusate	Na$^+$ (mEq/L)	K$^+$ (mEq/L)	Extracellular fluid dist.
5% NaCl in water=hypertonic saline†	855	0	100%
3% NaCl in water=hypertonic saline†	513	0	100%
0.9% NaCl in water=normal saline	154	0	100%
0.45% NaCl in water=1/2 normal saline	77	0	73%
0.2% NaCl in 5% dextrose in water=hypotonic saline	34	0	55%
Ringers lactate solution	130	4	97%
5% dextrose in water=free water	0	0	40%

†Hypertonic solutions must be administered via a central venous line. In addition to their complete
distribution in the extracellular compartment, this infusate→
 •Osmosis of water from the intracellular to the extracellular compartment

HYPERVOLEMIC HYPONATREMIA ▬▬▬▬▬
•**Fluid restriction**
 ◦Restrict fluid intake to ≤1.5L/ 24hour (~6 cups)
  Guide:
   •1oz = 30mL
   •1cup = 8oz = 240mL
   •4cups = 32oz = ~1L
•↓**Sodium intake**
 ◦0.5–1g elemental sodium or 1.5–3g salt/ 24hours

LOOP DIURETICS				
Generic (Trade)	**M**	♀	**Start**	**Max**
Furosemide (Lasix)	K	?	20mg q24–12hours PO/ IM/ IV	600mg/ 24hour
•IV infusion†:			0.05mg/kg/hour	160mg/ hour
Onset: 1hour, Duration: 6hours (La**six** lasts **six** hours)				

•There is synergistic efficacy of combination treatment w/ a thiazide diuretic
•Intravenous administration may be preferred, as intestinal edema→
 ◦↓Absorption
•Administer 2nd dose in the mid–afternoon to avoid nocturia
†Furosemide→
 •↑Juxtaglomerular cell renin secretion→
  −↑Angiotensin 2 & aldosterone levels→vasoconstriction→↑afterload→↓cardiac output, which
   may→clinical deterioration during acute decompensated heart failure. Being that the diuretic
   effect is related predominantly to its renal tubular secretion rate (as it is not filtered by the
   glomerulus), while its vasoconstricting effects are related to its plasma concentration, some
   advocate the **administration of continuous intravenous Furosemide** when >80mg IV is
   needed for adequate diuresis, thus providing a means for ↑diuretic effectiveness

Dose adjustment:
 •For patients currently on chronic loop diuretic treatment, starting dose=current dose + above
  starting dose
 •Once organ edema has resolved, consider maintenance dosing @ same dose q24h w/ titration

Conversion equivalents
40mg PO = 20mg IV

Limitations:
 •↓Efficacy in patients w/ a glomerular filtration rate <10mL/ min.

Side effects:
 Genitourinary
  •Acute interstitial nephritis
 Neurologic
  •Ototoxicity

Hematologic
- Acid base disturbances
  - Hypochloremic metabolic alkalemia
- Dyslipidemia
  - ↑Cholesterol & triglycerides
- Electrolyte disturbances
  - **Hypokalemia**
  - Hypomagnesemia
  - Hyponatremia
  - Hypercalcemia
- Hyperglycemia
- Hyperuricemia

Contraindications:
- **Sulfa allergy**, as all thiazide & loop diuretics (except Ethacrynic acid) contain a sulfa component

EUVOLEMIC HYPONATREMIA
- **Fluid restriction**
  - Restrict fluid intake to ≤1.5L/ 24hours (~6 cups)
    Guide:
    - 1oz = 30mL
    - 1cup = 8oz = 240mL
    - 4cups = 32oz = ~1L

±

LOOP DIURETICS

Generic (Trade)	M	♀	Start	Max
Furosemide (Lasix)	K	?	20mg q24–12hours PO/ IM/ IV	600mg/ 24hour
• IV infusion†:			0.05mg/kg/hour	160mg/ hour

Onset: 1hour, Duration: 6hours (La**six** lasts **six** hours)

- There is synergistic efficacy of combination treatment w/ a thiazide diuretic
- Intravenous administration may be preferred, as intestinal edema→
  - ↓Absorption
- Administer 2nd dose in the mid−afternoon to avoid nocturia
- †Furosemide→
  - ↑Juxtaglomerular cell renin secretion→
    - −↑Angiotensin 2 & aldosterone levels→vasoconstriction→↑afterload→↓cardiac output, which may→clinical deterioration during acute decompensated heart failure. Being that the diuretic effect is related predominantly to its renal tubular secretion rate (as it is not filtered by the glomerulus), while its vasoconstricting effects are related to its plasma concentration, some advocate the **administration of continuous intravenous furosemide** when >80mg IV is needed for adequate diuresis, thus providing a means for ↑diuretic effectiveness

Dose adjustment:
- For patients currently on chronic loop diuretic treatment, starting dose=current dose + above starting dose
- Once organ edema has resolved, consider maintenance dosing @ same dose q24h w/ titration

Conversion equivalents
40mg PO = 20mg IV

Limitations:
- ↓Efficacy in patients w/ a glomerular filtration rate <10mL/ min.

Syndrome of inappropriate secretion of antidiuretic hormone−SIADH:

DEMECLOCYCLINE (Declomycin)

Indications:
- Severe or chronic SIADH

M	♀	Dose
KF	U	300mg PO q8−q6hours

Onset: Within 2weeks

Mechanism:
- Inhibits antidiuretic hormone action on the late distal renal tubule & collecting duct→
  - Reversible nephrogenic diabetes insipidus

870

OBESITY

- A chronic disease due to **altered feeding regulatory mechanisms**→
  - ◦Energy intake (in the form of food) > energy expenditure→
    - −An excess of total body fat
- The % of body fat ↑steadily w/ age in both ♂ & ♀

<u>Statistics:</u>
- •60% of adult ♂ & 50% of adult ♀ are ≥overweight

RISK FACTORS

PRIMARY OBESITY ━━
- **Dietary**
  - ◦↑Fat diet, w/ infrequent exercise
- **Maternal smoking**
  - ◦Children whose mother smoked during pregnancy
- **Psychological factors**
  - ◦A coping mechanism in times of stress
  - ◦Learned behavior that one must "clean their plate" or "feel full" prior to stopping
- **Smoking cessation**
  - ◦2−4 lbs within 1month
  - ◦6−10 lbs within 6months
  - …w/ the average weight gain being 10 lbs, w/ the potential to be much greater
- **Genetic**
  - ◦Altered hypothalamic feeding centers† endocrine &/or neurotransmitter function
  - ◦Altered adipose cell function

Obese biologic parents	Probability of child developing obesity (%)
0	10%
1	40%
Both	90%

†Arcuate, dorsomedial, lateral, paraventricular, & ventromedial nuclei

SECONDARY OBESITY ━━━
- **Endocrine**
  - ◦Cushing's syndrome or disease→
    - −Hypercortisolemia
  - ◦Insulinoma→
    - −Hyperinsulinemia
  - ◦Pituitary destruction→
    - −↓Growth hormone
- **Medications**
  - ◦Antipsychotic medications, esp. atypical antipsychotics, esp. Clozapine & Olanzapine
  - ◦Antiseizure medications
    - −Carbamazepine
    - −Gabapentin
    - −Valproic acid
  - ◦Glucocorticoids
  - ◦Hypoglycemic medications
    - −Insulin
    - −Sulfonylureas
    - −Thiazolinediones
  - ◦Oral contraceptive medications
- **Polycystic ovary syndrome**
- **Psychiatric**
  - ◦Bulimia nervosa
- **Hypothalamic disease, being rare**
  - ◦Inflammation
  - ◦Neoplasm

•**Obesity**, specifically referring to excess total body fat
Body mass index—BMI‡ classification:
  •<18.5: Underweight
  •18.5–24.9: Normal
  •25–29.9: Overweight
  •30–34.9: Mild obesity
  •35–39.9: Moderate obesity
  •≥40: Severe, termed morbid obesity, being ≥2X the upper limit of normal body weight

Waist circumference based obesity classification:
  •As body fat distribution affects health risks, meeting the following criteria indicate the need for weight loss regardless of BMI
    ○**>40 inches** indicates ↑cardiovascular risk in ♂
    ○**>35 inches** indicates ↑cardiovascular risk in ♀

---

†LDL=total cholesterol − HDL − (triglycerides/ 5).
‡BMI= $\dfrac{\text{Weight (kg)}}{\text{Height (m)}^2}$ or $\dfrac{\text{Weight (lbs)}}{\text{Height (in)}^2}$ X 703.1

Cardiovascular
•**Atherosclerosis** mediated macrovascular disease, via:
  ○↑Autonomic sympathetic tone & ↓autonomic parasympathetic tone→hypertension
  ○Dyslipidemia
  ○Direct endothelial effects
  …→
      •**Coronary artery disease**→
        ○Myocardial ischemic syndromes
      •**Cerebrovascular disease**→
        ○Cerebrovascular accident syndromes
      •**Peripheral vascular disease**→
        ○Renal artery stenosis, intermittent claudication, & thromboembolic disease
•↑Cardiac work to pump blood against the ↑systemic vascular resistance, termed the afterload→
    −Myocardial hypertrophy, termed **secondary hypertrophic cardiomyopathy** ± **heart failure‡**→
      ↑Myocardial O_2 & nutrient demand, w/ concomitant ↓relative myocardial vascularity→myocardial ischemia→eventual **dilated cardiomyopathy** ± **heart failure**
•Varicose veins
Cutaneous
•Juxtaposed skin surfaces, termed intertriginous areas (ex. abdominal folds, buttocks, thigh–scrotum interface, breast–underskin interface)→
  ○Friction, sweat, warmth, & moisture→
    −Local microorganism overgrowth
    −Irritant dermatitis, termed intertrigo
    …→↑bacterial &/or fungal infection risk
Endocrine
•Cellular insulin resistance (adipose, hepatic, & skeletal muscle cells)→
  ○Hyperglycemia→
    −**Diabetes mellitus type 2**
Gastrointestinal
•Cholelithiasis (cholesterol gallstones)
Genitourinary
•Adipocyte aromatase mediated androgen conversion (testosterone & androstendione→β estradiol & estrone respectively)→
  ○↑Estrogenic effects→
    −Altered menstrual hemorrhage, being either ↑ or ↓
    −Gynecomastia, being the ↑development of male mammary glands
Musculoskeletal
•↓Ambulation→
  ○↑Venous thromboembolic syndrome risk
•↑Weight bearing joint stress→
  ○**Osteoarthritis**
Psychiatric
•↓Self esteem→
  ○Depression

Pulmonary
- •↑Peri–oropharyngeal pressure→
  - ∘**Obstructive sleep apnea–OSA**

Hematologic
- •Dyslipidemia
  - ∘Hypercholesterolemia (↑VLDL, ↑LDL, &/or ↓HDL)
  - ∘Hypertriglyceridemia
- •↑Uric acid→
  - ∘Gout

Neoplastic
- •♂:
  - ∘Colorectal cancer
  - ∘Prostate cancer
- •♀:
  - ∘Biliary tract cancer
  - ∘Breast cancer
  - ∘Endometrial cancer

Surgical
- •↑Perioperative complications→
  - ∘↑Morbidity, & mortality via:
    - −Infections
    - −Surgical wound dehiscence
    - −Venous thromboembolic syndrome
  - ∘↑Recovery time

Materno–fetal
- •↑Pregnancy morbidity & mortality

---

†Also occurring as a direct consequence of obesity
‡Heart failure occurrence doubles in obese patients relative to persons w/ a normal BMI

TREATMENT

- •Weight loss of even 5–10% may substantially improve:
  - ∘Blood pressure
  - ∘Diabetes mellitus
  - ∘Dyslipidemia
  - ∘Hypertension

- •**Exercise**
  - ∘An enjoyable form of aerobic exercise on a regular basis (≥3X/ week) for 20–30min., preceded by stretching
- •**Dietician consultation**
- •**Glycemic control if hyperglycemic**
- •**Weight loss if overweight/ obese†, via goal daily caloric requirement**
  - ∘The caloric total needed to reach & maintain a goal weight depends on physical activity level
  - ∘10 calories/ lb of goal weight +
    - −33% if sedentary
    - −50% if moderately physically active
    - −75% if very physically active
  - ∘3500 calories are roughly equivalent to 1 lb of body fat
    - −Consuming 500calories less/ day X 1week→1 lb weight loss
    - −Exercising 500calories/ day X 1week→1 lb weight loss
  - …w/ the average human body being able to lose 3.5 lbs/ week maximum, aside from a diuretic effect

Caloric content:
- •**1g Fat:** 9
- •**1g Alcohol:** 7
- •**1g Carbohydrate:** 4
- •**1g Protein:** 4
- •**1g Undigestable carbohydrate, termed fiber:** 0

- •**Hypertension control**
  - ∘Systolic blood pressure <120mmHg & diastolic blood pressure <80mmHg
- •↓**Sodium intake**
  - ∘≤100mmol sodium/ 24h=2g elemental sodium or 6g salt/ 24h, which can usually be achieved w/ a no–added salt diet. Patients w/ poorly compensated heart failure should only consume 0.5–1g elemental sodium or 1.5–3g salt/ 24h
  - ∘→↓Renal potassium loss if taking a diuretic

- •↓**Alcohol consumption**
  - ◦Only 1drink q24hours (8–12 ounces of beer, 3–5 ounces of wine, or 1 ounce of liquor) in patients without a history of drug abuse
  - ◦≥2 drinks/ 24hours→
    - −Hypertension
    - −Hepatitis (♀ > ♂)
    - −↑Abuse risk
  - ◦If alcohol is suspected to be causative, total abstinence is required
- •↓**Saturated & total fat consumption**
- •↑**Fruit & vegetable consumption**
  - ◦Eating fiber rich food (fruits, vegetables, whole grains)→
    - −Satiety w/ ↓caloric intake
- •↓**Concentrated sweet consumption** such as candy, ice cream, & regular sodas
- •↓**Artificial sweetener consumption** as a substitute for sugar in beverages & sodas
  - ◦Aspartame
  - ◦Saccharin
- •**Fat substitutes**, such as Olestra, an undigestable fat substitute, is approved for use as a food additive
  Outcomes:
  - •No clinical controlled trials have proven its efficacy in terms of weight loss

MEDICAL TREATMENT

Indications:
- •**BMI ≥27 who suffer from sequelae & have failed dietary treatment X 6months†**
- •**Mild obesity who have failed dietary treatment X 6months†**

†Dietary failure is defined as losing <1 lb/ month

AMPHETAMINE–LIKE				
Generic (Trade)	M	♀	Start	Max
Phentermine (Adipex-P)	KL	?	15mg PO qam	37.5mg qam

- •Take at least 1hour prior to, or after meals
- •Intended for use ≤3months, as continued use→
  - ◦Tolerance→
    - −Ineffectiveness
    - −↑Dependence & abuse risk

Mechanism:
- •↑Release of presynaptic catecholamines

Side effects:
Cardiovascular
- •Hypertension
- •Palpitations
- •Tachycardia

Gastrointestinal
- •Constipation
- •Dry mouth

Neurologic
- •Abuse potential
- •Anxiety
- •Euphoria
- •Insomnia

Contraindications:
- •Coronary artery disease
- •Glaucoma
- •Severe hypertension
- •History of drug abuse
- •≤2weeks of MAOI administration

SEROTONIN–NOREPINEPHRINE–DOPAMINE REUPTAKE INHIBITORS–SNRI				
Generic (Trade)	M	♀	Start	Max
Sibutramine (Meridia)	KL	?	10mg PO qam	15mg qam

Mechanism:
- •Inhibit the presynaptic reuptake of norepinephrine & serotonin > dopamine→
  - ◦↑Hyopthalamic synaptic cleft serotonin concentrations→
    - −↓Appetite

874

Side effects:
Cardiovascular
- Hypertension, usually being mild
- Tachycardia, usually being mild
Gastrointestinal
- Constipation
- Dry mouth
Neurologic
- Headache
- Insomnia

Contraindications:
- Coronary artery disease
- Severe hypertension
- ≤2weeks of MAOI administration

PANCREATIC LIPASE INHIBITOR			
Generic (Trade)	M	♀	Dose
Orlistat (Xenical)	Gut	P	120mg PO tid w/ or within 1hour after meals, w/ a multivitamin q24hours taken ≥2hours prior to or after the dose

Mechanism:
- ↓Lipid absorption→
  ○ 30% of ingested fat passed in the stool

Side effects:
Gastrointestinal
- ↓Fat absorption→
  ○ ↑Stool fat, termed steatorrhea (esp. w/ a ↑fat diet)→
    – Diarrhea
    – Foul smelling, floating stools
    – Oily residue on toilet after flushing
    – Oily spotting on underwear
  ○ Fecal urgency
  ○ Flatulence ± discharge
  ○ Mildly ↓fat soluble vitamin (A, D, E, K) absorption

Medications removed from the U.S. market:
- **Phenylpropanolamine:** An amphetamine–like medication previously available as an over the counter weight loss medication, was removed from the U.S. market due to an association w/ **hemorrhagic cerebrovascular accidents in ♀**
- **Fenfluramine** & its derivative **Dexfenfluramine:** Serotonin reuptake inhibitors &/or presynaptic releasing agents were removed from the U.S. market in 1997 as their use for ≥3months→
  ○ 23 fold ↑risk of **primary pulmonary hypertension**
- **Fenfluramine in combination w/ Phentermine (Fen-Phen)→**
  ○ **Cardiac valve lesions**

SURGICAL TREATMENT
Indications:
- Surgery is considered an option for highly motivated, psychologically stable patients w/ the following:
  ○ **Moderate obesity who suffer from sequelae & have repeatedly failed diet & medical treatment**
  ○ **Severe obesity who have repeatedly failed diet & medical treatment**
Generalized complication:
- **Soft calorie syndrome:** Patients may "outeat" the procedure via frequent, small, high–calorie feedings (ex. liquid or semisolid foods such as shakes)

- **Roux-en-y gastric bypass surgery**
  Procedure:
  - The proximal 10% of the stomach is converted into a 15–30mL communicating pouch, being closed off by staples, w/ a 1cm anastomosis to the jejunum, thereby bypassing 90% of the stomach (as well as the duodenum & the first 15–20cm of the jejunum) which→
    ○ Rapid gastric filling & slow emptying→
      – Earlier & longer lasting satiety→↓food consumption
  Perioperative mortality: <1%

875

Side effects:
- •Duodenal ulceration
- •Gastrojejunostomy stoma ulceration
- •Vomiting, w/ progressively ↓frequency–70%
- •↓Functional parietal cells→
  - ○↓Hydrogen & intrinsic factor secretion→
    - –↓Non–heme iron & vitamin B12 absorption respectively
- •↓Calcium & vitamin D absorption

Complications:
- •Anastomotic obstruction
- •**Dumping syndrome**
  - Early phase:
    - •Gastric pouch distention due to rapid filling of food→
      - ○Epigastric fullness, pain, &/or nausea ± vomiting
    - •↑Osmotic load being "dumped" into the jejunum→
      - ○Rapid jejunal fluid shift→
        - –↓Intravascular volume→↑autonomic sympathetic tone→diaphoresis, tachycardia, & palpitations
  - Late phase:
    - •Rapid entry of food into the jejunum→
      - ○↑Plasma glucose levels→
        - –↑Insulin secretion→hypoglycemia @ 1–2h after the meal
  - Treatment:
    - •Small frequent meals (including small liquid volumes) containing ↑protein & ↓carbohydrate

Outcomes:
- •Average weight loss of 30%, lasting >5years

- •**Vertical banded gastropathy**

Procedure:
- •The proximal 10% of the stomach is converted into a 10–20mL communicating pouch via stapling, w/ external banding of the stomach in order to reduce the opening from the pouch to the distal stomach to 1cm in diameter→
  - ○Rapid gastric filling & slow emptying→
    - –Earlier & longer lasting satiety→↓food consumption

Perioperative mortality: <1%

Side effects:
- •Vomiting, w/ progressively ↓frequency
- •Gastroesophageal reflux–GERD
- •Outlet stenosis

Complications:
- •18% of patients require a second operation due to either:
  - ○Outlet stenosis
  - ○Severe gastrointestinal reflux disease–GERD
- •Band erosion into the stomach
- •Rupture of the staple line

Outcomes:
- •Average weight loss of 30% in the initial postoperative period, w/ many patients regaining much of the lost weight over the following 5–10years

- •**Gastric banding**

Procedure:
- •The proximal 10% of the stomach is converted into a 10–20mL communicating pouch via a band that can be inflated w/ saline or silicone from a subcutaneous reservoir→
  - ○Rapid gastric filling & slow emptying→
    - –Earlier & longer lasting satiety→↓food consumption

Side effects:
- •Vomiting, w/ progressively ↓frequency
- •Gastroesophageal reflux–GERD

Complications:
- •Reservoir deterioration tending to occur in the long term, requiring reoperation

Outcomes:
- •Average weight loss of ~20% in the initial postoperative period

876

•**Fad diets,** being based on only 2 possible nutrient arrangements, mirroring what an excess consumption of 1 nutrient will cause to the amount of the other nutrients in the body. None are recommended due to their side effect profiles & because they do not result in sustained weight loss, as patients eventually will go off the diet & drift back to their former eating habits. This may set the stage for repeated cycles of weight loss & gain, termed "yo–yo dieting"→
  ○↑Cardiovascular disease risk relative to that of remaining at a stable mildly ↑weight
•**Total fast** (w/ fluid, electrolyte, vitamin, & mineral supplementation) may be utilized for severely obese patients on an inpatient basis only, monitored by a physician experienced w/ the technique. It is typically used to induce short–term (pre–surgical) weight loss

Diet type side effects:
  •↑**Carbohydrate w/ ↓protein & fat**
    Gastrointestinal
      •↑Fiber content→
        ○Flatulence & gastric distress
    Mucocutaneous
      •Dry skin
    Hematologic
      •Vitamin & mineral deficiencies (calcium, iron, vitamin B12)
  •↓**Carbohydrate w/ ↑protein & fat**
    General
      •Anorexia
      •Ketonemia
    Gastrointestinal
      •Constipation
      •Halitosis
    Genitourinary
      •Diuresis→
        ○Dehydration
        ○Hypokalemia
        ○Hyponatremia
      •Nephrolithiasis
    Musculoskeletal
      •Osteopenia/ osteoporosis
    Hematologic
      •Dyslipidemia
      •↑Uric acid
      •Vitamin & mineral deficiencies (calcium, folic acid, iron, riboflavin, thiamine, vitamins A & C)
  •**Modified fast,** consuming ≤1000 cal/ 24h
    Neurologic
      •↓Cognitive function (altered reaction time, ↓memory)
      •Depression
      •Irritability
    Hematologic
      •Dyslipidemia during rapid weight loss

877

ETHANOL INTOXICATION SYNDROMES

•Alcoholic beverages contain ethanol, which is completely absorbed by the gastrointestinal tract→
  ∘Peak blood concentrations @30–90min.→**central nervous system depression** via:
    –↑Gamma aminobutyric acid–GABA mediated synaptic transmission
    –Altered cell membrane fluidity
    –Altered cellular enzyme function
    ...the degree of which depends on both the plasma & tolerance level of the patient
Statistics:
  •#1 used psychoactive drug in the world→
    ∘100,000 deaths/ year, w/:
      –50% of Americans age >12years drinking ethanol on a regular basis
      –10% of adult Americans being current or recovering alcoholics
      –An annual economic cost of $100 billion in the U.S.

COMMONLY USED TERMS

•Persons consume ethanol for a wide range of reasons, from religious or cultural ceremonies to social gatherings &/or therapeutically, as a method of coping w/ life's stresses as it functions as a:
  ∘**Sedative**→
    –**Relaxation**
  ∘**Hypnotic**→
    –**Sleep**
  ...at mild doses, much like its medication counterparts benzodiazepines & barbiturates, which also ↑gamma aminobutyric acid–GABA mediated synaptic transmission
•However, chronic use→
  ∘The development of **tolerance** to its effects, as the dosage previously sufficient to produce effects, progressively fails to do so, as both the central nervous system & liver adapt their homeostatic mechanisms to the chronic presence of a substance by altering:
    –Neuronal membrane constituents
    –Neurotransmitter release & re–uptake
    –Hepatic clearance
    ...which set the stage for the vicious cycle of **alcoholism, defined as the dependence & craving for ever ↑amounts of alcohol, regardless of the professional, social, or health risks**, w/ prolonged abstinence→
      •**Withdrawal syndrome** lasting days to weeks, ranging in severity from mild to severe, as the organ systems re–adjust their homeostatic mechanisms→
        ∘**Dependence** on access to the substance at any time in order to avoid the withdrawal syndrome for which the altered neuronal function causes the experience of a voracious craving for the substance much like water, food, or sex
•It is a combination of:
  ∘The fear of withdrawal symptoms
  ∘Intense cravings
  ∘The continued presence of the substances' initiating factors
  ...which cause many to continue ingesting the substance regardless of the potential harm, which allows the organ systems to continually become more adaptive to the substances presence, leading to a vicious cycle of ↑tolerance→↑dependence→↑need for access to the substance at shorter time intervals→
    •Hiding or "stashing" the alcohol
    •Ingesting alcohol prior to attending an event where alcohol might be limited, termed "pre–drinking."
•Eventually, the manner & timing of the ingestion becomes increasingly stereotyped, as the person begins to ingest the same amount of the same substance at the same times of day, every day, as a way to methodically control both their cravings & avoid withdrawal symptoms. They become preoccupied w/ drug seeking, turning to the substance over other activities that were previously more important, ranging from career, to family obligations, to personal health maintenance. Basically, alcohol acquisition & ingestion overwhelm the majority of other thoughts & activities.

RISK FACTORS

•**Gender:** ♂ 3X ♀
•**Genetic**
  ∘Alcoholism is 4X more prevalent in children (sons > daughters) of alcoholics, regardless of who raises them
•**Ethnicity**
  ∘American Indians & Eskimos > others
•**Environment**
  ∘Homeless
  ∘Prison inmate

878

THE CAGE ALCOHOLISM SCREENING QUESTIONNAIRE	
Question	Features being sought
Have you ever felt a need to Cut down on your drinking?	Inability to control drinking urge
Have people Annoyed you by criticizing your drinking?	Drinking causing domestic problems
Have you ever felt bad or Guilty about your drinking?	Bad feelings regarding consequences
Have you ever had a drink first thing in the morning (Eye-opener) to steady your nerves or get rid of a hangover?	Dependence

Outcomes:
- •Sensitivity: 80% w/ a positive response to ≥1 question(s)
- •Specificity: 85% w/ a negative response to all 4 questions

Hematology
- •↑Mean corpuscular volume–MCV
- •↑γ–glutamyl transpeptidase–GGT

WITHDRAWAL SYNDROMES

- •**Withdrawal syndromes** occur following an abrupt reduction in alcohol consumption, even if the patient is still drinking
  - ∘May be experienced in reformed alcoholics after only several days of resumed heavy drinking if they subsequently reduce the amount
- •The syndrome experienced is likely to recur in future withdrawals
- •The severity of the withdrawal syndrome is proportional to:
  - ∘The amount & duration of drinking
  - ∘Current co–morbidities
  - ∘Number & dosage of medications being taken
  - …w/ **major syndromes capable of occurring independently of minor syndromes**

MINOR WITHDRAWAL SYNDROMES–80%
- •↑**Central nervous system tone**
  - ∘Agitation
  - ∘Anxiety
  - ∘Craving for alcohol
  - ∘Disturbed sleep
  - ∘Dysphoria
  - ∘Fever
  - ∘Hyperacusis
  - ∘Hyperreflexia
  - ∘Irritability
  - ∘Morning gagging ± retching, causing patients to skip breakfast &/or avoid brushing their teeth
  - ∘Muscle cramps
  - ∘Tinnitus
- •↑**Autonomic sympathetic tone**, which may persist ≤2 weeks after other withdrawal symptoms have abated
  - ∘Anorexia
  - ∘Diaphoresis
  - ∘Hypertension
  - ∘Hypervigilance
  - ∘Palpitations
  - ∘Pupil dilation, termed mydriasis
  - ∘Tachycardia
  - ∘**Tremulousness**

Timing:
- •**8hours after abrupt dose reduction, w/ peak severity @ 24–36hours**

MAJOR WITHDRAWAL SYNDROMES
- •**Alcoholic hallucinosis–20%**
  - ∘**Visual, being the most common**, usually of people, insects, or small animals
  - ∘Auditory, usually threatening or derogatory
  - ∘Tactile, usually of insects crawling on or under the skin, termed formication

  Timing:
  - •**24hours after abrupt dose reduction, w/ resolution within 72hours**
    - ∘However, auditory hallucinations may persist for several weeks to months after other withdrawal symptoms have abated

879

- **Tonic-clonic seizures-25%**, being ↑in patients w/ pre-existing seizure disease
  - ∘Usually self-limited, w/ 1seizure >> multiple seizures
  - ∘20% first experienced while still drinking an abruptly reduced dose
  - ∘50% first experienced within 24hours after abrupt dose reduction
  - ...w/ 3% progressing to status epilepticus
  - Timing:
    - **•8hours after abrupt dose reduction, w/ peak @24hours**
  - Associations:
    - **•35% will develop delirium tremens**

- **Delirium tremens-DTs 5%**
  - ∘↓of >1 cognitive function, w/ episodes of altered level of consciousness, usually separated by episodes of lucidity, termed delirium
  - Timing:
    - **•2-14days (usually 2-5days) after abrupt dose reduction, w/ usual resolution within 72hours,** but may last several weeks
  - Outcomes:
    - •Mortality:
      - ∘1% treated
      - ∘15% untreated
      - ...due to:
        - •Dysrhythmia
        - •Fluid & electrolyte abnormality
        - •Hypertensive emergency
        - •Hyperthermia
        - •Infection, esp. aspiration pneumonia
        - •Suicide
  - Associations:
    - **•35% will develop tonic-clonic seizures**

<hr>

DIAGNOSIS OF ALCOHOL INTOXICATION

- •Ethanol is toxic to all organ systems, w/ its acute effects being clinically apparent on the central nervous system→
  - ∘Progressive neuronal & neuroglial dysfunction ± death, beginning in the higher brain centers, eventually affecting the brainstem, & being directly proportional to the **blood alcohol level-BAL**

Blood alcohol level-BAL† (mg/ dL):
- •0 being normal
- •**25-50**→
  - ∘Diuresis‡
  - ∘Relaxation
- •**50-100**→cerebral cortex dysfunction→
  - ∘A feeling of well-being, termed euphoria
  - ∘Warmth°
  - ∘Loud conversation
  - ∘↓Reaction time
  - ∘↓Social inhibitions
  - ∘↑Sexual desire
  - ∘↓Erection
  - ...w/ most states defining **legal intoxication as >80mg/ dL**
- •**100-200**→limbic system & cerebellar dysfunction→
  - ∘↓Attention span
  - ∘↓Coordination
  - ∘Dysarthria→
    - -Slurred speech
  - ∘↓Fine motor control
  - ∘↓Judgement
  - ∘↓Memory
  - ∘↓Mentation
  - ∘↓Sensitivity to pain
  - ∘Variable & labile mood, being:
    - -Belligerent ± violent
    - -Obnoxious
    - -Overly friendly
    - -Sad
    - ...depending on their personality, social setting, & mood at the time

880

- **200–300**→reticular activating system dysfunction→
  - ○↓↓Coordination
  - ○Irritability
  - ○Lethargy
  - ○Marked slurred speech
  - ○Nausea ± vomiting
  - ○Sleep
  - ○Obtundation
  - ○Tremor
- **300–400**→
  - ○Coma
  - ○Amnesia, termed "blackouts"
- **>400**→medulla oblongata dysfunction→
  - ○Respiratory failure

---

†Although most clinical laboratories report the blood alcohol level–BAL in mg/ dL, you may see it reported as a percentage, indicating grams of ethanol per 100mL of blood. Thus, a BAL of 150mg/ dL may be reported as 0.15%

‡Ethanol→
- •↓Posterior pituitary antidiuretic hormone release→
  - ○Diuresis→
    - −Dehydration→orthostatic hypotension
- °Ethanol & acetaldehyde→
- •Peripheral vasodilation→
  - ○Sensation of warmth, although core body temperature is ↓, w/ **ethanol intoxication being the #1 cause of hypothermia in the U.S.**, as patients may inadequately dress for the cold weather &/or allow prolonged exposure due to either the warm sensation or inebriation→
    - −↓Core temperature

Factors causing slowed ethanol absorption:
- •↓Concentration of alcohol in the ingested substance
- •↓Rate of consumption
- •Presence of food in the stomach, esp. fatty foods
- •↑Rate of alcohol metabolism based on tolerance

MEDICAL SEQUELAE

- •♀ are at ↑risk via:
  - ○Relatively ↓gastric mucosal absorption→
    - −↑Intestinal absorption→↑hepatic exposure via first pass metabolism
  - ○Relatively ↑body fat→
    - −↓Total body water→↑body fluid ethanol concentration, as it distributes preferentially into total body water

General
- •Ethanol intoxication→
  - ○↑**Accidents**, such as burns, car accidents, drownings, & falls
  - ○↑**Acts of aggression**, such as fighting, rape, homicide, & suicide
  - ○**Unintentioned affection**→
    - −↑Sexually transmitted disease risk
- •Alcoholism, including consequent malnutrition→
  - ○Immunosuppression→
    - −↑**Infection** &/or neoplasm risk
- •**Nutritional deficiencies** develop as heavy drinkers consume largely nutritionally devoid alcohol, containing 7calories/ g rather than eating. Alcohol also→
  - ○↓B vitamin absorption, metabolism, & storage
    - −Vitamin B1=Thiamine
    - −Vitamin B2=Riboflavin
    - −Vitamin B3=Niacin
    - −Vitamin B6=Pyridoxine
    - −Vitamin B9=Folic acid
  - ○↓Mineral absorption, metabolism, & storage
    - −Calcium
    - −Magnesium
    - −Zinc

Cardiovascular
- >2 alcoholic drinks/ 24h→
  - **Hypertension,** causing 8% of hypertension in ♂
- Ethanol & acetaldehyde→
  - Myocyte toxicity→
    - Myocarditis→**dilated cardiomyopathy**

Pulmonary
- Inebriation→altered mental status→
  - ↓Cough reflex→
    - ↑Aspiration risk→↑**aspiration pneumonia** & choking risk

Endocrine
- Ethanol→
  - ↓Hepatic gluconeogenesis→**hypoglycemia,** esp. w/ concomitant ↓hepatocyte glycogen storage due to starvation & liver disease
    - Fasting hypoglycemia being most common, occurring @10–20hours after after patients stop eating & drinking
    - Postprandial hypoglycemia @ 2–6h after drinking alcohol w/ a meal
  - ↑Estrogen concentration→
    - ↑**Breast & ovarian cancer risk**

Musculoskeletal
- Ethanol & acetaldehyde→
  - Myocyte toxicity→
    - Skeletal muscle myopathy→**myositis**→muscle pain &/or weakness which may→ **rhabdomyolysis**
  - ↓Renal excretion of uric acid→
    - Gout

Genitourinary
- Ethanol→
  - Sertoli cell & interstitial cell of Leydig toxicity→↓**sperm & testosterone production** respectively→ hypogonadism→
    - Impotence, being the inability to achieve &/or maintain an erection
    - Gynecomastia, being the ↑development of male mammary glands
  - Ovarian toxicity→altered menstrual function→
    - ↓Vaginal lubrication
    - Infertility
    - Spontaneous abortion
  - ↓Posterior pituitary antidiuretic hormone release→diuresis→
    - Dehydration→orthostatic hypotension
    - Hypokalemia
    - Hypomagnesemia

Gastrointestinal
- Ethanol→
  - Hepatocyte toxicity (>2drinks/ 24h in ♂ or >1 drink/ 24h in ♀)→hepatocyte triglyceride accumulation→fat infiltration of the liver, termed **hepatic steatosis**†, occurring in 40% of chronic heavy drinkers→hepatomegally→liver capsule (Glisson's capsule) distention→continuous right upper quadrant abdominal pain ±
    - Tenderness to palpation, which may be worsened by bending, sleeping on the right side, &/or eating
    - Radiation to the right scapular area
    ...w/ abstinence usually→
      - Complete recovery, whereas continued use→
        - **Hepatitis–20%**‡, requiring years of chronic heavy drinking→
          - **Cirrhosis–80%** (occurring in 20% of patients who abstain during hepatitis)→ **hepatocellular cancer**
  - ↑Gastric mucosal HCl & pepsin secretion, as well as direct gastroduodenal mucosa toxicity→
    - Gastritis→**peptic ulcer disease**→upper gastrointestinal hemorrhage
  - Reverse gastroesophageal peristaltic movements→persistent vomiting &/or retching, esp. after an alcoholic binge→
    - ↑Intra-abdominal pressure→↑intra-gastric pressure→gastroesophageal junction mucosal horizontal tear, termed **Mallory Weiss tear**→upper gastrointestinal hemorrhage
  - Pancreatic toxicity→**pancreatitis,** w/ ethanol being:
    - The #2 cause of acute pancreatitis (#1 being a biliary tract gallstone, termed choledocholithiasis), accounting for 35% of all cases. However, it only occurs in 5% of alcoholics, & rarely in casual drinkers
    - The **#1 cause of chronic relapsing pancreatitis, accounting for 90% of cases**
  - Esophageal & gastric toxicity→
    - ↑**Esophageal & gastric cancer risk** respectively

882

∘↓Lower esophageal sphincter–LES tone→
　–Gastroesophageal reflux disease

---

†Other causes of hepatic steatosis:
•Cushing's disease or syndrome
•Diabetes mellitus
•Dyslipidemia
•Obesity
‡30% of patients w/ alcoholic hepatitis are infected w/ the hepatitis C virus

Neurologic
•Ethanol→
　∘Neuronal & neuroglial toxicity→
　　–**Dementia**, which is diagnosed only if cognitive deficits persist >1month after cessation, w/ exclusion of other possible causes. Cognitive deficits occur in 70% of actively drinking chronic alcoholics via psychological testing, w/ 10% of those being clinically symptomatic
　　–Segmental axonal demyelination→nerve disease=**neuropathy**, over years
　∘↓**Thiamine**=vitamin B1→
　　–Beriberi
　　–Dementia
　　–Optic neuritis
　　–Peripheral neuropathy
　　–**Korsakoff's syndrome**
　　–**Wernicke's encephalopathy**
　∘↓**Pyridoxine**=vitamin B6→
　　–Peripheral neuropathy
•Although ethanol induces sleep, the effect is short lived→
　∘Withdrawal syndrome→
　　–↑Autonomic sympathetic tone→insomnia

Peripheral symmetrical polyneuropathy (sensory >> motor)
•**Abnormal sensations, termed paresthesias** (numbness, pain, &/or tingling), beginning in the hands & feet (as longer neurons have ↑myelination, & so are affected sooner), w/ proximal progression
　∘Numbness→
　　–↑**Unrecognized foot trauma** (cut, blister)→↑infection risk
Diagnosis:
•**A nylon monofilament** designated 5.07 is pressed against the skin to the point of buckling. A patients inability to feel the buckled monofilament indicates neuropathy

Autonomic neuropathy
•↓**Sympathetic tone:**
　∘Orthostatic hypotension→
　　–Falls
　∘↑Gastrointestinal tone→
　　–Diarrhea
　∘↓Hypoglycemic response, termed hypoglycemic unawareness
•↓**Parasympathetic tone:**
　∘Fixed, resting tachycardia
　∘Impotence
　∘↓Gastrointestinal tone→
　　–Abdominal distention
　　–Constipation
　　–Nausea ± vomiting
　∘Incomplete urinary bladder emptying, termed neurogenic bladder→
　　–Overflow incontinence
　　–↑Urinary tract infection risk

883

- **Korsakoff's syndrome** via damage to the thalamic dorsomedial nucleus & mammillary bodies→
  - ○**Memory impairment, esp. short term**, being out of proportion to other cognitive deficits, in the absence of dementia or delirium→
    - −The filling of memory gaps w/ manufactured material, termed **confabulation**
- **Wernicke's encephalopathy**, being the triad of:
  - ○**Altered mental status**
  - ○**Cerebellar ataxia**→
    - −Incoordination
  - ○**Ocular dysfunction**→either:
    - −Nystagmus
    - −Opthalmoplegia
  ...being reversible w/ early thiamine treatment, & potentially permanent w/ delayed treatment

Hematologic
- Ethanol substitution for food &/or repeated vomiting→
  - ○Starvation→
    - −↑Activation of adipose cell lipase→↑triglyceride breakdown→↑plasma free fatty acids
    - −↑Fatty acid oxidation→**hepatocyte ketone formation** (acetoacetic acid, β hydroxybutyric acid, & acetone) w/ acetoacetic acid being used by peripheral cells for energy (except neurons & neuroglia). Unregulated fatty acid oxidation→ketone accumulation in excess of the body's ability to metabolize or excrete them→**ketoacidemia→widened anion gap↑ metabolic acidemia**
- **Alcoholic hepatitis**→
  - ○↑Aminotransferases, w/ **aspartate aminotransferase−AST 2−3 X alanine aminotransferase−ALT**, (normal being 1:1) w/ the AST usually <500 U/ L
- **Myelosuppression**→
  - ○Anemia ± macrocytosis (mean corpuscular volume−MCV ≥100fL), regardless of folic acid deficiency
  - ○Leukopenia→
    - −↑Infection & neoplasm risk
  - ○Thrombocytopenia
    - −↑Hemorrhage risk, esp. petechiae

Materno−fetal
- Alcohol is a **teratogen**, w/ 35% of ♀ who chronically drink alcohol (even 1drink/ 24h) during pregnancy→
  - ○**Fetal alcohol syndrome**, occurring in 1/ 2000 live births, characterized by:
    - −↓Growth→↓birth weight
    - −Congenital physical anamolies, including cardiac defects & mild facial hypoplasia characterized by a short nose w/ anteverted nares, a poorly developed long philtrum, & narrow palpebral fissures
    - −↓Development
    - −Cognitive impairment, ranging from hyperactivity to retardation
- ↓Folic acid→
  - ○↑Neural tube defect risk

---

†Plasma anion gap= $[Na^+] - ([Cl^-] + [HCO_3])$
- **Normal value: 8−12mEq/ L**
- Equation value: 12mEq/ L

Correction:
- **Hypoalbuminemia:** For each 1g/ dL ↓in albumin below 4, add 2.5 to the calculated anion gap
- **Acidemia:** Add 2 to the calculated anion gap
- **Alkalemia:** Add 4 to the calculated anion gap

Interpretation:
- A gap indicates the **presence of excess unmeasured anions**, being either:
  - ○Organic acids
  - ○Phosphates
  - ○Sulfates
- Causes of a low anion gap:
  - ○Halide (bromide, Iodide) intoxication
  - ○Myeloma w/ cationic IgG immunoglobulin
  - ○Severe hyperlipidemia, via assay error

QUANTITATIVE TESTS
- Ethanol is excreted via the liver >> kidneys & lungs, being measured via:
  - ○**Plasma ethanol level**, w/ whole blood ethanol concentration being 15% less
  - ○**Breath ethanol level**
  - ○**Urine ethanol level**

•**Abdominal ultrasound**
   Findings:
    •Hepatic steatosis→
     ○↑Hepatic echogenicity

COMPLICATIONS
ACETAMINOPHEN MEDIATED HEPATITIS ▬▬▬▬▬▬▬▬
•**Do not administer Acetaminophen to chronic, heavy ethanol drinkers**
Mechanism:
  •90% of Acetaminophen undergoes either hepatocyte mediated:
   ○Glucoronidation→
    −Nontoxic glucorinides
   ○Sulfation→
    −Nontoxic sulfates
  •10% of Acetaminophen undergoes hepatocyte mediated oxidation by the cytochrome P450
   enzyme complex→
   ○A potentially toxic reactive electrophilic compound, which then undergoes either:
    −Conjugation w/ cellular glutathione→nontoxic compound
    −Reaction w/ cellular proteins→cellular toxicity ± death→**hepatitis**
  •Normally, glutathione depletion occurs w/ ingestion of >10g of Acetaminophen. However, any
   substance which ↑cytochrome P450 function (such as ethanol) causes relatively more
   Acetaminophen to be diverted to the formation of the toxic compound→
   ○More rapid hepatocyte depletion of glutathione→
    −Cell toxicity at lower ingested Acetaminophen doses

Plasma levels associated w/ hepatotoxicity

Hours after ingestion†	Acetaminophen plasma concentration (µg/ mL)
4	150
8	75
12	32
16	16
20	8
24	4

Treatment:
•**Gastric lavage**

&
CHARCOAL		
M ♀	**Dose**	
Ø P	1g/ kg or 10X the amount of poison ingested, PO q4hours prn	

&
OSMOTIC LAXATIVE		
Generic M ♀	**Dose**	
Sorbitol NA P	50mL of a 70% solution PO given w/ the 1st charcoal dose	

Mechanism:
  •Given w/ charcoal in order to:
   ○↑Gastrointestinal transit time
   ○Improved taste over charcoal alone

&
N−ACETYLCYSTEINE	
M ♀	**Dose**
L P	140mg/ kg PO loading dose, then 70mg/ kg q4hours X 17doses

Mechanism:
  •Replenishes glutathione stores
Side effects:
  General
   •Being that the medication tastes & smells like rotten eggs, consider:
    ○Having the patient pinch their nostrils closed
    ○Administering an antiemetic
    ○Placing a nasogastric tube
    ...as the patient may vomit the medication

ACETALDEHYDE INTOXICATION SYNDROME ▬▬▬▬▬▬▬▬▬▬▬▬▬▬▬▬▬▬▬▬▬
<u>Mechanism:</u>
- •Ethanol is metabolized by the hepatocyte enzymes:
  - ∘Alcohol dehydrogenase
  - ∘The microsomal ethanol oxidizing system–MEOS, which ↑in activity w/ chronic exposure to central nervous system depressant substances
    - –Ethanol
    - –Barbiturates
    - –Benzodiazepines
  - …to the potentially **toxic acetaldehyde**, which is then metabolized by **aldehyde dehydrogenase**, being a mitochondrial enzyme found in cells throughout the body→
    - •Acetic acid
- •Certain medications (Chlorpropamide, Isosorbide dinitrate, **Metronidazole**†, & Tolbutamide)→
  - ∘↓Aldehyde dehydrogenase function→
    - –↑Acetaldehyde formation→
    - **General**
      - •Diaphoresis
      - •Headache, characterized by throbbing head & neck pain
      - •Thirst
    - **Gastrointestinal**
      - •Nausea ± vomiting
    - **Cardiovascular**
      - •Chest pain
      - •Vasodilation→
        - ∘Flushing
        - ∘Hypotension→
          - –Distributive shock
    - **Pulmonary**
      - •Dyspnea
    - **Neurologic**
      - •Altered mental status
    - **Opthalmologic**
      - •Blurred vision

- •Most Asians (Chinese, Pacific islanders, Japanese, & Koreans) have weak aldehyde dehydrogenase activity, w/ ethanol consumption→
  - ∘↑Acetaldehyde→
    - –Characteristic flushing reaction & poor tolerance of alcohol→↓prevalence of alcoholism
- •A form of alcoholism treatment is based on the acetaldehyde effect, using the medication Disulfuram which irreversibly inactivates aldehyde dehydrogenase→
  - ∘Symptoms upon ethanol ingestion
- †Ethanol should be avoided during, & 3days after Metronidazole treatment

REFEEDING SYNDROME ▬▬▬▬▬▬▬▬▬▬▬▬▬▬▬▬▬▬
- •Refeeding of a chronically malnourished patient→
  - ∘The patient switching from lipid to carbohydrate as an energy source→↑insulin secretion→ intercellular shift of:
    - –Glucose→hypoglycemia
    - –Magnesium→hypomagnesemia
    - –Phosphorous→hypophosphatemia→dysrhythmias, encephalopathy, cardiac & skeletal myopathy, seizures, erythrocyte & leukocyte dysfunction
    - –Potassium→hypokalemia→dysrhythmia, cardiac & skeletal myopathy
  - ∘↓Renal excretion of NaCl & water
  - ∘Significant fluid third spacing→
    - –Edema
- <u>Timing:</u>
  - •Within 3weeks of refeeding

- **Alcohol cessation**
- **Electrolyte replacement prn**, esp. potassium & magnesium
- **Intravenous fluid,** w/ attention to both:
  - ○**Intravascular volume repletion†** via **Normal saline** (0.9% NaCl) or **lactated Ringer's solution,** as per:
    - −Vital signs
    - −Physical examination
    - −Urine output (normal being ≥0.5mL/kg/h)
    - −Blood urea nitrogen−BUN & creatinine
  - ○**Intravascular volume maintenance via ½ Normal saline** (0.45% NaCl), w/ **5% dextrose added**
    - Adult maintenance fluid:
      - •Weight (kg) + 40= #mL/ hour
    - Additional febrile requirements:
      - •1L/ 24hours for every 1°F >100°F
    - Additional:
      - •Estimate loss for:
        - ○Diaphoresis
        - ○Diarrhea
        - ○Polyuria
        - ○Tachypnea

VITAMINS & MINERALS

Generic	M	♀	Dose
Folic acid=vitamin B9	K	S	1mg PO q24hours
Thiamine†=vitamin B1	K	S	100mg PO q24hours X 3days‡
Multivitamin	LK	P	1 tab PO q24hours
Vitamin K=Phytonadione	L	?	5−10mg PO/ SC q24hours X 3days°
Indications:			
•INR >1.3			

†All heavy drinkers should receive thiamine 100mg IV, either before, or w/ the 1st glucose solution (if used) or meal, as **glucose→**
  - •**Thiamine reserve depletion→**
    - ○**Korsakoff's syndrome**
    - ○**Wernicke's encephalopathy**
‡After which, the multivitamin dose should suffice
°Requires several hours to days for effect
Note: A 5% dextrose−water solution is available, premixed w/ thiamine & other vitamins & minerals, being referred to as a "banana bag" as the fluid has a yellow color

BENZODIAZEPINES

Indications:
  - •Alcohol withdrawal prophylaxis & treatment

Generic (Trade)	M	♀	Dose	Max	Half−life
Chlordiazepoxide (Librium)	LK	U	25−100mg PO/ IM/ IV q6hours	300mg/ 24hours	5−30hours
Diazepam (Valium)	LK	U	5−20mg PO/ IM/ IV q6hours		20−80hours
Lorazepam†(Ativan)	LK	U	1−2mg PO/ IM/ IV q4hours	4mg/ dose	10−20hours
Oxazepam†(Serax)	LK	U	15−30mg PO q4hours		8hours

†Lorazepam & Oxazepam are preferred in patients w/ severe liver disease, as they have no active metabolites

Dose adjustment:
  - •For breakthrough syndrome, all the above medications & dosages may be given q2hours prn, w/ standing times as listed. If breakthrough medication is needed, ↑the standing dosage
  - •Once the patient has been stable X 24hours, taper the benzodiazepine dose by 25% q2days

Mechanism:
  - •Bind to a benzodiazepine receptor site on the neuronal inhibitory gamma aminobutyric acid− $GABA_A$ chloride ion channel→
    - ○↑Frequency of channel opening in the concomitant presence of GABA→
      - −Neuronal inhibition

Side effects:
Cardiovascular
•Hypotension
Gastrointestinal
•Nausea ± vomiting
Neurologic
•Altered mental status
•Incoordination=ataxia
•Double vision=diplopia
•Headache
•Sedation
•Physical & psychological dependence
•Tolerance
•Additive central nervous system depression effects in combination w/:
  ◦Antihistamine medications
  ◦Ethanol
  ◦Sedative hypnotic medications
    −Barbiturates
    −Buspirone
    −Cyclic ethers
    −Meprobamate
    −Zolpidem

Overdose→
•Respiratory depression

•**Withdrawal** should be done gradually, in order to prevent an ethanol−like withdrawal syndrome

ANTIDOTE				
Generic (Trade)	**M**	♀	**Dose**	**Max**
Flumazenil (Romazicon)	LK	?	0.2mg IV push, then	
			0.5mg q30seconds prn	3mg total

Mechanism:
•A benzodiazepine analogue→
  ◦Competitive inhibition of benzodiazepine receptor site binding

Side effects:
Cardiovascular
•Extravasation→
  ◦Local irritation
Neurologic
•Sudden reversal may→
  ◦**Seizures**

Contraindications:
•Chronic benzodiazepine use
•Acute overdose w/ tricyclic antidepressants
…due to seizure risk

HIGH DOSE THIAMINE=Vitamin B1			

Indications:
•Korsakoff's syndrome or Wernicke's encephalopathy

M	♀	Dose
K	S	100mg IV stat, then
		100mg IV q24hours

TYPICAL ANTIPSYCHOTICS			

Indications:
•Combative behavior
•Psychosis

Generic (Trade)	**M**	♀	**Start**
Mid to high potency:			
Haloperidol (Haldol)	LK	?	5−10mg IM/ IV prn

†Potency refers to relative milligram dose equivalents, & should not be confused w/ efficacy

Mechanism:
•Dopamine 2 receptor antagonism

888

Side effects:
Cardiovascular
- •↑QT interval→
  - ◦Torsades de pointes, esp. low potency

Gastrointestinal
- •Hepatitis
  - ◦Medication to be changed to a chemically unrelated antipsychotic @ plasma values >3 X the upper limit of normal

Mucocutaneous
- •Photosensitivity

Neurologic
- •**Seizure**, esp. low potency

Other receptor antagonism mediated side effects:
- •**Anti−D$_2$→**
  - ◦**Extrapyramidal dysfunction**, esp. mid to high potency
  - ◦Endocrine dysfunction (see psychotic syndromes)
- •**Anticholinergic**, esp. low potency (see psychotic syndromes)
- •**Antihistamine**, esp. low potency→
  - ◦**Sedation**
- •**Anti α1**, esp. low potency→
  - ◦Erectile dysfunction
  - ◦**Orthostatic hypotension**
  - ◦Sedation

HIGH DOSE BENZODIAZEPINES

Indications:
- •Seizure
- •Delirium tremens

Generic (Trade)	M	♀	Dose
Lorazepam (Ativan)	LK	U	4mg IV slow push q5min. prn

- •Achieve relaxation in patients w/ delirium tremens

Outcomes:
- •Seizure termination within 5 min. in 80% of cases

ANTISEIZURE MEDICATIONS

Indications:
- •Any prior history of seizure disease (withdrawal or otherwise)

Generic (Trade)	M	♀	Dose
Phenytoin (Dilantin)	L	U	1g IV loading dose, then 100mg PO q8hours X 5days

Dose adjustment:
- •The standard therapeutic plasma range trough level (just prior to the upcoming dose) is 10–20µg/ mL. However levels ≥3µg/ mL have been therapeutic in withdrawal seizure prophylaxis, indicating ↑responsiveness of withdrawal seizures to Phenytoin

Correction of measured plasma Phenytoin level for albumin:

Measured plasma Phenytoin level
(0.2 X albumin level) + 0.1

Side effects:
Mucocutaneous
- •Coarse facial features, termed **leonine facies**, characterized by thickening of the subcutaneous tissue about the eyes & nose
- •**Gingival hyperplasia−30%**
  - ◦Once established, may only partially regress
- •**Hirsutism** (5% overall, 30% of young ♀)

Musculoskeletal
- •Vitamin D inactivation→
  - ◦**Osteoporosis**

Neurologic
- •Altered mental status
- •Incoordination=ataxia
- •Double vision=diplopia
- •Headache
- •Polyneuropathy
- •Sedation

Hematologic
- •Megaloblastic anemia

Materno–fetal
- •Teratogenic→
  - ◦**Fetal hydantoin syndrome**

Overdose→
- •Respiratory depression

NONSELECTIVE PHOSPHODIESTERASE INHIBITOR

Indications:
- •Severe alcoholic hepatitis via:
  - ◦Discriminate function score >32†
  - ◦Encephalopathy, without concomitant gastrointestinal hemorrhage or infection
  - …as either indicates a 35% mortality within 6 months

†Discriminate function = 4.6 (prothrombin time − control) + total bilirubin (mg/ dL)

Generic (Trade)	M	♀	Dose
Pentoxifylline (Trental)	L	?	400mg PO q8hours X 1month

Mechanism:
- •↑Intracellular cAMP & cGMP→
  - ◦↓Inflammatory cytokine production
  - ◦↓Endothelial adhesion molecule display
  - ◦↓Fibroblast mediated interstitial tissue formation

Outcomes:
- •40%↓ mortality
- •65%↓ new onset hepatorenal syndrome
  - ◦70%↓ mortality from hepatorenal syndrome

CHRONIC TREATMENT AFTER DETOXIFICATION

- •**Treatment goal is to achieve complete abstinence**
- •Alcohol detoxification can usually be accomplished as an outpatient–90% (esp. via **Alcoholics anonymous–AA**). Admission for inpatient detoxification is based on the patients comorbidities & previous or current withdrawal syndrome severity.
- •Although there is some thought that alcoholics can learn controlled drinking habits, this approach has been shown to be unrealistic for the majority of alcoholics, & should be avoided.
- •Relapse is an integral & expected part of treatment, requiring urgent intervention (within days) in order to abort the full re–instatement of dependence. Relapse indicates possible:
  - ◦Incomplete or ineffective treatment
  - ◦Unanticipated contingency

890

•Caused by heat exposure→
  ◦↑Body core temperature→↑systemic metabolism, w/ eventual diffuse cellular dysfunction→
  –↓**Hypothalamic ability to regulate body temperature**

RISK FACTORS

•**Heat exposure**
◦**Altered mental status**
  –Alcohol
  –Cerebrovascular accident syndrome
  –Central nervous system inflammation (encephalitis, meningitis)
  –Delirium
  –Dementia
  –Electrolyte or acid–base abnormalities
  –Glycemic abnormalities (hypo or hyperglycemia)
  –Head trauma
  –Illicit drugs
  –**Infection**, esp. in the elderly or neonates
  –Mental retardation
  –Psychosis
  ...all of which→
    •↓Perception of environmental discomfort &/or danger
◦**Immobility**, being unable to escape the threatening environment, typically occurring in:
  –Children
  –Elderly
  –Handicapped

•**Other**
◦**Endocrine**
  –Hyperthyroidism→mild hyperthermia

CLASSIFICATION

•**Heat cramps**
  ◦A mild syndrome of cramps developing in large, heavily used muscle groups (ex. calves) over **several days** of heat exposure w/ concomitant dehydration

•**Heat exhaustion**
  ◦A mild syndrome w/ a core temperature ranging from normal to 100.4°F, developing over **several days**, resulting from heat exposure w/ concomitant dehydration

HEAT STROKE ▬▬▬▬▬▬
•↑**Body core temperature, usually being ≥107.6°F=42°C**, being termed **hyperthermia**→systemic enzymatic dysfunction→cell dysfunction & death→
  ◦Organ system failure, including cerebral failure→
    –**Altered mental status**
    –Seizures

Subsyndromes:
  •**Exertional:** Usually develops **suddenly** in patients who perform physically strenuous activities in excessive heat &/or humidity
  •**Non–exertional:** Usually develops over **several days** of heat exposure, in which the patient cannot either:
    ◦Drink adequate fluids
    ◦Escape to a cooler place

DIAGNOSIS

General
  •Anorexia
  •↑**Core body (rectal) temperature**, not occurring w/ heat cramps
  •Fatigue
  •Headache
  •Malaise
  •Muscle cramps
  •Thirst
  •Weakness

Cardiovascular
- Dehydration→↓intravascular volume→
  - ≥10% blood volume loss→
    - ↑Autonomic sympathetic tone→↑pulse
  - ≥20% blood volume loss→
    - Orthostatic hypotension (supine to standing→↑20 pulse, ↓20 SBP, &/or ↓10 DBP)→ lightheadedness upon standing
    - Urine output 20–30mL/ hour (normal being >30mL/ hour)
  - ≥30% blood volume loss→
    - Recumbent hypotension &/or tachycardia
  - ≥40% blood volume loss→
    - Altered mental status &/or urine output <20mL/ hour
    - Hypovolemic shock, being hypotension + organ failure, unresponsive to fluid resuscitation

Genitourinary
- Dehydration→
  - **Pre–renal renal failure**

Mucocutaneous
- Dehydration→
  - Dry mucous membranes
  - Dry skin→
    - ↓Skin turgor→skin tenting

Hematologic
- Check the creatinine & blood urea nitrogen–BUN for possible pre–renal renal failure

Heat stroke specific syndromes:
Cardiovascular
- A core body temperature of >104°F=40°C→
  - ↓Cardiac contractility→hypotension

Gastrointestinal
- **Hepatitis**

Musculoskeletal
- **Rhabdomyolysis**

Hematologic
- Tissue damage→
  - Tissue factor release→
    - **Disseminated intravascular coagulation–DIC**

TREATMENT

- **Heat cramps**
  - Passive stretching of the involved muscle groups
  - Intravenous or oral fluid resuscitation

- **Heat exhaustion**
  - Rest in a cool place
  - Intravenous or oral fluid resuscitation

HEAT STROKE
- ↓Core body temperature
  - Spray cool water† onto the undressed patient, while fans blow air over the skin, in order to rapidly cool the patient. Active cooling should be stopped when the core body temperature falls to ~101°F = 38°C, w/ subsequent monitoring, as hyperthermia may recur several hours after cooling is stopped, w/ **thermoregulatory mechanisms being unstable for possibly several weeks**

- **Intravenous fluid**, w/ attention to both:
  - **Intravascular volume repletion via Normal saline** (0.9% NaCl) or **lactated Ringer's solution**, as per:
    - Vital signs
    - Physical examination
    - Urine output (normal being ≥0.5mL/kg/h)
    - Blood urea nitrogen–BUN & creatinine
  - **Intravascular volume maintenance via Normal saline** (0.9% NaCl) or **lactated Ringer's solution**
    Adult maintenance fluid:
    - Weight (kg) + 40= #mL/ hour
    Additional febrile requirements:
    - 1L/ 24hours for every 1°F >100°F

892

<u>Additional:</u>
- •Estimate loss for:
  - ∘Diaphoresis
  - ∘Diarrhea
  - ∘Polyuria
  - ∘Tachypnea
  …followed by oral rehydration w/ a glucose based electrolyte solution upon both clinical stability & ability to tolerate PO

- •**Oxygen** to maintain PaO_2 >60mmHg or SaO_2 >92%, usually accomplished via nasal cannula @ 2−4L/ min.
  <u>Mechanism:</u>
  - •Oxygenation if required
  - •Calming effect→
    - ∘↓Autonomic sympathetic tone→
      - −↓Myocardial O_2 demand
  <u>Duration:</u>
  - •24−48hours or longer if needed for oxygenation

- •**Consider empiric antibiotics**, esp. in:
  - ∘Elderly
  - ∘Neonates
  - ∘Immunosuppressed

- •**Admit to an intensive care unit** for continuous monitoring of:
  - ∘Vital signs, including the core temperature
  - ∘Electrocardiograph−ECG
  - ∘Urinary output, via urinary catheter
  …X ≥2 days as:
    - •Acute renal failure
    - •Recurrent hyperthermia
    - •Rhabdomyolysis
    …can be late sequelae

---

†This is preferred to cool water baths or cooling blanket treatment, as it allows easy access to the patient in terms of monitoring devices & intravenous lines

893

•Caused by
　◦Cold exposure→
　　−↓Local tissue temperature ± cellular freezing
　◦Cold exposure, endocrinopathy, or severe malnutrition→↓core body temperature→↓systemic
　　metabolism, w/ eventual diffuse cellular dysfunction→
　　−↓**Hypothalamic ability to regulate body temperature**

•**Cold exposure**
　◦**Wet skin**
　　−Rain
　　−Snow
　　−Water immersion
　　...→↑evaporation
　◦**Altered mental status**
　　−Alcohol, w/ **ethanol intoxication being the #1 cause of hypothermia in the U.S.**, as patients may
　　　inadequately dress for the cold weather &/or allow prolonged exposure due to either inebriation or
　　　the peripheral vasodilation mediated warm sensation→↓core temperature
　　−Cerebrovascular accident syndrome
　　−Central nervous system inflammation (encephalitis, meningitis)
　　−Delirium
　　−Dementia
　　−Electrolyte or acid−base abnormalities
　　−Glycemic abnormalities (hypo or hyperglycemia)
　　−Head trauma
　　−Illicit drugs
　　−**Infection**, esp. in the elderly or neonates
　　−Mental retardation
　　−Psychosis
　　...all of which→
　　　•↓Perception of environmental discomfort &/or danger
　◦**Immobility**, being unable to escape the threatening environment, typically occurring in:
　　−Children
　　−Elderly
　　−Handicapped

•**Other**
　◦**Endocrine**
　　−Hypothyroidism→mild hypothermia or myxedema coma, being hypothermia & altered mental
　　　status, w/ actual coma being uncommon
　◦**Severe malnutrition**
　　−Anorexia nervosa

•**Pre−frostbite**
　◦Local cold exposure (usually affecting the ears, fingers, nose, &/or toes)→vasoconstriction→
　　ischemia→
　　−**Pain**
　　−↓Neuronal metabolism→↓neuronal transmission→**numbness**
　　...w/ rewarming→
　　　•Chilblain, being erythema, itching, &/or pain

•**Frostbite**
　◦Local cold exposure→
　　−Freezing of an extremity, w/ **ice crystal formation**→tissue destruction
　　...w/ rewarming→
　　　•**Gangrene**, w/ degree indicative of frostbite severity
　　　　◦Mild frostbite: Minimal gangrene upon rewarming
　　　　◦Severe frostbite: Extensive gangrene upon rewarming
　　　•**Severe pain**, as previously & newly formed inflammatory cytokines→
　　　　◦Pain neuron depolarization if proper function is regained

HYPOTHERMIA ▬▬▬▬

- **Mild: Core body (rectal) temperature of 90-95°F** = 32°-35°C
- **Severe: Core body (rectal) temperature <90°F** = <32°C

Hypothermia specific syndromes:

Cardiovascular
- •↓Myocardial metabolism→
  - ∘**Sinus bradycardia**
  - ∘↓Contractile strength
  - ...→↓cardiac output→
    - •Generalized relative ischemia, as the metabolic demands of the peripheral tissues remain relatively higher than those of the myocardium→↑lactic acid production→**anion gap metabolic acidemia**
- •Acidemia &/or hypo or hyperkalemia→
  - ∘Myocardial dysfunction→
    - −**Dysrhythmia**, w/ death usually being the result of ventricular fibrillation or asystole

Pulmonary
- •↓Brainstem respiratory center metabolism→
  - ∘↓Respiratory rate→
    - −**Hypercapnic respiratory failure**→acidemia

Neurologic
- •↓Central nervous system metabolism→
  - ∘**Altered mental status**→
    - −Death

Hematologic
- •**Hypokalemia**
- •Acidemia ± cell death→
  - ∘**Hyperkalemia**, via the cellular membrane H^+/ K^+ transport protein & cellular release, respectively
- •Tissue damage→
  - ∘Tissue factor release→
    - −**Disseminated intravascular coagulation−DIC**

- •Unconsciousness (sleep, coma)→
  - ∘Further ↓central nervous system heat regulating mechanisms, including the prevention of shivering

ELECTRICAL STUDIES

- •**Electrocardiogram−ECG**

Findings:
- •↓Atrioventricular conduction→
  - ∘↑PR interval (>0.2seconds = 1big block)
- •↑QT interval (>0.5 RR' interval)
- •↑QRS complex duration (>0.12seconds = 3small blocks)
- •**Osborn−J wave**, being an altered terminal QRS complex w/ an upward wave immediately after the S wave

TREATMENT

- •**Frostbite**
  - ∘**Rapid rewarming** of the frostbitten area in a water bath w/ a temp of 107-111°F=42-44°C
    - −Vasoconstriction in the frostbitten area may persist, thus requiring angiography w/ intra-arterial infusion of vasodilating medications ± surgical sympathectomy
  - ∘**Intravenous analgesia**, as the pain that is experienced upon rewarming is often severe
  - ∘**Amputation** of the gangrenous extremity in severe frostbite, in order to prevent infection

HYPOTHERMIA ▬▬▬▬

- •**Avoid precipitating a dysrhythmia** via unnecessary body manipulation
  - ∘Only essential procedures should be done, if necessary, such as cardiopulmonary resuscitation. **Once cardiopulmonary resuscitation is initiated, it may be continued for several hours, w/ subsequent full neurologic recovery.** Remember that a patient is not to be considered dead unless they are normothermic
  - ∘Bag-mask ventilation prior to intubation→↓hypoxemia risk→↓intubation mediated dysrhythmia risk
  - ∘Anti-dysrhythmic medications are usually ineffective in patients w/ a core body temperature <86°F= 30°C
- •**Prevent further ↓core body temperature**
  - ∘Cover the patient
  - ∘Maintain ambient temperature @ >72°F

- **Treat possible hypoglycemia**
  - ∘Bolus 50mL of 50% dextrose in a water solution
- **Treat possible narcotic overdose**
  - ∘Naloxone hydrochloride 2mg IV q2min. prn
- •↑**Core body temperature** only after the patient is removed from the cold environment
  - <u>Rewarming tempo</u>
    - •Rapid rewarming if the patient was rapidly cooled over a brief time period, as via brief ice water immersion
    - •Gradual rewarming otherwise, in order to prevent extremity warming prior to core body temperature warming→
      - ∘Peripheral vasodilation→
        - −Hypotension†→distributive shock
  - <u>Rewarming methods</u>
    - •Active rewarming via:
      - ∘**Heated (113°F=45°C) & humidified O$_2$**, w/ an FiO$_2$ of ≥50%
      - ∘**Heated (113°F=45°C) 5% dextrose in a saline solution**, initially @ 250−500mL/ hour, w/ 100mg intravenous thiamine for possible thiamine deficiency
    - •Passive rewarming via:
      - ∘**Warming blanket**
      - ∘Mildly hypothermic patients may be passively rewarmed w/ blankets & warm oral fluids

- **Consider empiric antibiotics**, esp. in:
  - ∘Elderly
  - ∘Neonates
  - ∘Immunosuppressed
- **Admit to an intensive care unit** for continuous monitoring of:
  - ∘Vital signs, including the core temperature
  - ∘Electrocardiograph−ECG
  - ∘Urinary output, via urinary catheter

---

†The first sign of too rapid rewarming, being treated by allowing the patient to cool down slightly.

•Caused by the psychoactive compound **9–tetrahydrocannabinol–THC**, found in the hemp plant, Cannibis sativa, which is:
  ◦Smoked via cigarette, pipe, or water pipe
  ◦Eaten (ex. in brownies)
  ...via:
    •Dried plant leaves, termed marijuana
    •Resin from the flowering tops (esp. of the ♀ plants), termed hashish, in which THC is 5–10X more concentrated than marijuana
•All nonprescription forms are **ILLEGAL in the U.S.**
Statistics:
  •The most commonly used illicit drug in the world, w/ ~10 million Americans being current users, & 70 million having used during their lifetime
Mechanism:
  •Tetrahydrocannabinol–THC binds to cerebral cannabinoid 1 & peripheral cannabinoid 2 receptors for the endogenous ligand anandamide. THC is lipophilic→
    ◦Adipose cell distribution, accumulation, & slow release
Slang:
  •Marijuana="chronic", "dope", "grass", "indo", "kush", "mary–jane", "pot", "reefer", "stress", or "weed"
  •Marijuana cigarette="doobie", "joint", or "stogie"
  •Water–pipe= "bong"

ACUTE EFFECTS ━━
•Usually lasting from 2–6hours
•1st time users often have no syndrome

Neurologic
  •Relaxation
  •Mild euphoria
  •Distorted time perception, as time seems long
  •↓Logical thinking, short term memory, & ability to perform complex tasks (ex. drive a car)
  •↑Appetite, termed "the munchies"
  •↑Sensory awareness
  •↑Tendency to laughter &/or silliness
Cardiovascular
  •Tachycardia
Mucocutaneous
  •Dry mouth
  •Dry eyes (noted mainly by contact lens wearers)→
    ◦Conjunctival inflammation→
      –Erythema, termed conjunctival injection

Complications†:
  •**Overdose**→
    ◦Auditory &/or visual hallucinations‡
    ◦Catatonia–like immobility
    ◦Disorientation
    ◦Dream–like state, termed depersonalization
    ◦Heavy sedation
    ◦Perceptual distortions
    ◦Severe anxiety ± paranoid ideation‡

---

†When eaten, gastrointestinal absorption→
  •Slower onset & longer lasting effects→
    ◦User (esp. inexperienced) continuing to eat until effects are felt→↑overdose risk
‡A familiar pleasant environment→
  •↓Risk of anxiety &/or frightening hallucinations &/or delusions

CHRONIC EFFECTS ■■■■■■■■■■
•Moderate tolerance develops

Endocrine
•↓♂ plasma testosterone levels, although the average level remains within normal limits
Genitourinary
•Anovulation
•Shortened pregnancies
Neurologic
•**Amotivational syndrome:** Impaired memory w/ ↓energy, mental drive, & interest→
　◦Impairment in initiating & sustaining tasks, which may continue for weeks to months after smoking
　　cessation
Pulmonary
•Respiratory tract inflammation & ↓respiratory mucosal ciliary function→
　◦↓Mucus clearance→
　　–Cough, usually being nonproductive
　　–↑Respiratory tract infection risk
　　–Chronic obstructive pulmonary disease–COPD (chronic bronchitis &/or emphysema)

Minor withdrawal syndrome:
•Anxiety
•↓Appetite
•↓Concentration
•Depression
•Headaches
•Irritability
•Restlessness
•Sleep disturbance

DRUG TESTING
•**Tetrahydrocannabinol–THC &/or metabolite detection testing** requires informed voluntary consent
of either:
　◦A patient age ≥18years
　◦Parent or legal guardian of a patient age <18years
　◦Medical emergency
　◦Employers may require drug testing

Detection time:
•**Urine analysis:**
　◦Occasional use: 2weeks
　◦Chronic use: 2months
•**Hair follicle analysis**
　◦Hair grows 0.5 inches/ month

†Efavirenz, a nonnucleoside reverse transcriptase inhibitor–NNRTI used in HIV/ AIDS patients may→
•False positive THC testing for marijuana

TREATMENT
•**Chronic use:** Drug–free environment & participation in Alcoholics Anonymous or Narcotics Anonymous
± psychological counseling

POTENTIAL MEDICAL USES OF MARIJUANA

Disease	Action
Cerebral disease† mediated spastic paralysis	↓Muscle contraction
Chemotherapy induced nausea ± vomiting	Anti–emetic
Chronic disease mediated anorexia	↑Appetite
Glaucoma	↓Intraocular pressure
Mild to moderate aches & pains	Likely due to shifting concentration

†Stroke, cerebral palsy, multiple sclerosis

898

DRONABINOL (MI, ♀?)		
FDA approved indication	**Dose**	**Max**
AIDS mediated anorexia	2.5mg PO pre-lunch & dinner	20mg/ 24hours
Chemotherapy induced nausea ± vomiting	5mg/ m^2 1-3hours pre-chemo & q2-4hours post-chemo X 5doses/ 24hours	15mg/ m^2
Mechanism: •Synthetic THC-like compound		

899

Plasma component	Units
5′ nucleotidase	2–15 IU/ L

α1–antiprotease	110–270
α–fetoprotein	<20ng/ mL
ACTH	20–100pg/ mL
Alanine aminotransferase–ALT	<35 U/ L
Albumin	3.5–5.0g/ dL
Aldolase	1.0–7.5 U/ L
Aldosterone	10–160ng/ L
Alkaline phosphatase	40–135 IU/ L
Aluminum	4–10µg/ L
Anion gap	**8–12mEq/ L**
Ammonia	20–60µg/ dL
Amylase	20–110 U/ L
Angiotensin converting enzyme–ACE	10–35 U/ L
Antinuclear antibody–ANA	<1:80 titer
Antithrombin 3	20–40mg/ dL
Aspartate aminotransferase–AST	<35 IU/ L

β–human chorionic gonadotropin–HCG	<2mIU/ mL in ♂ & nonpregnant ♀
β–type natriuretic peptide–BNP	<50pg/mL
Bicarbonate	**22–26mmol/ L**
Bilirubin, total ▌ direct/ conjugated	0.1–1.2mg/ dL ▌ 0.1–0.5mg/ dL
Bleeding time	2–10min
Blood urea nitrogen–BUN	**8–20mg/ dL**

C–peptide	0.8–4ng/ mL
C–reactive protein–CRP	0–2mg/dL
Calcitonin ♂ ▌ ♀	<90pg/ mL ▌ <70pg/ mL
Calcium, total ▌ ionized ▌ urine	8.5–10.5mg/ dL ▌ 4.5–5.5mg/ dL ▌ 100–300mg/ 24h
Carbon dioxide, partial pressure–pCO$_2$	**35–45mmHg**
Carboxyhemoglobin–HbCO	<9%
Carcinoembryonic antigen–CEA	<2.5ng/ mL
Ceruloplasmin	20–35mg/ dL
Chloride	98–110mmol/ L
Cholesterol, total ▌ LDL ▌ HDL ▌ Chol:LDL	<200mg/ dL ▌ <130mg/ dL ▌ >40mg/ dL ▌ <6
Complement C3 ▌ C4 ▌ CH50	65–165mg/ dL ▌ 15–45mg/ dL ▌ 20–40 U/ mL
Copper	70–160µg/ dL
Cortisol, morning ▌ urine	5–20µg/ dL ▌ 10–110µg/ 24h
Creatinine	**0.6–1.2mg/ dL**
Creatine kinase–CK ▌ MB	30–270 IU/ L ▌ <5% of total CK

Erythrocyte count ♂ ▌ ♀	4.5–5.5 X 10^6/ µL ▌ 4–5 X10^6/ µL
•Reticulocyte count	0.5–1.5% of erythrocytes; 35,000–135,000/ µL
Erythrocyte sedimentation rate–ESR	5mm/ decade aged + ♂ ≤10mm/ h; ♀ ≤20mm/ h
Erythropoietin	5–20mIU/ mL
Ethanol	0mg/ dL

Ferritin ♂ ▌ ♀	15–300ng/ mL ▌ 5–160ng/ mL
Fibrin degradation products=Fibrin d–dimers	<0.5µg/ mL
Fibrinogen	150–450mg/ dL
Fibrinogen degradation products	≤10mg/ dL
Folate plasma ▌ erthrocyte	3–12.5ng/ mL ▌ 165–760ng/ mL
Follicle stimulating hormone–FSH	
•♀, follicular ▌ luteal	4–15mIU/ L ▌ 2–15mIU/ L
midcycle ▌ postmenopausal	5–25mIU/ L ▌ 20–140mIU/ L

Gamma glutamyl transpeptidase–GGT	10–85 U/ L
Gastrin	<100pg/ mL
Glucose, fasting	60–115mg/ dL
Glucose–6–phosphate dehydrogenase	5–15units/ gHb
Growth hormone–GH, fasting, ♂ ▌ ♀	<5ng/ mL ▌ <10ng/ mL

900

Plasma component	Units
Haptoglobin	45–315mg/ dL
Hematocrit ♂ ▌♀	**40–50% ▌35–45%**
Hemoglobin ♂ ▌♀	**14–17g/ dL ▌ 12–16g/ dL**
Hemoglobin A1c	4–6%
Homocysteine	3–15μmol/L

Insulin, fasting	≤20mU/ L
International normalized ratio–INR	1–1.3
Iron	50–180μg/ dL
Iron binding capacity, total–TIBC	250–450 μg/ dL

Lactate dehydrogenase–LDH	90–230 U/ L
Lactic acid	0.5–2meq/ L
Leukocyte count	**4,000–10,000/ μL**
•Neutrophils ▌ **Band cells**	50–70% ▌**3–5%**
•Lymphocytes ▌ monocytes	20–40% ▌2–8%
•Eosinophils ▌ basophils	1–4% ▌0–1%
Leutinizing hormone–LH, ♂	2–12 IU/ L
•♀, follicular ▌ luteal	1–20mIU/ L ▌ ≤20mIU/ L
midcycle ▌ postmenopausal	25–105mIU/ L ▌ 15–60mIU/ L
Lipase	<160 U/ L

Magnesium	1.5–3mg/ dL
Mean corpuscular hemoglobin–MCH	25–35pg
Mean corpuscular volume–MCV	**80–100fL**

Osmolarity serum ▌ urine	**275–295mosm/ kg H_2O ▌ 100–900mosm/ kg H_2O**
Oxygen, partial pressure–pO_2	**70–100mmHg**

Parathyroid hormone–PTH	10–55pg/ mL
Partial thromboplastin time–PTT	25–35seconds
pH arterial ▌ venous	**7.35–7.45 ▌7.30–7.40**
Phosphorous	2.5–4.5mg/ dL
Platelet count	**150,000–450,000/ μL**
Potassium	**3.5–5meq/ L**
Progesterone, ♂	<0.5ng/ mL
•♀, follicular phase	0.1–1.5ng/ mL
luteal phase	2.5–30ng/ mL
1st trimester ▌ 3rd trimester	10–50ng/ mL ▌ 55–255ng/ mL
postmenopausal	<0.5ng/ mL
Prolactin	<20ng/ mL
Prostate specific antigen–PSA	<4ng/ mL
Protein, total	6–8g/ dL
Protein C	70–175%
Protein S	75–180%
Prothrombin time–PT	11–15seconds

Renin	1–3ng/mL/h

Sodium	**135–145meq/ L**

T4 index	1.5–4.5
Testosterone, total, ♂ ▌ ♀	270–1070ng/ dL ▌ 5–85ng/ dL
Testosterone, free, ♂ ▌ ♀	10–30ng/ dL ▌ 0.1–2ng/ dL
Thrombin time	6.5–11seconds
Thyroid stimulating hormone–TSH	0.4–6μU/ mL
Thyroxine–T4, total ▌ free	5–11μg/ dL ▌ 0.8–2.7ng/ dL
Total iron binding capacity–TIBC	250–450μg/ dL
Transferrin saturation	20–40%
Triglycerides, fasting	<165mg/ dL
Triiodothyronine–T3, total	95–190ng/ dL
Troponin I	<0.1ng/ mL

Uric acid ♂ ▌ ♀	2.5–7mg/ dL ▌ 1.5–6mg/ dL

Plasma component	Units
Vanillylmandelic acid–VMA, urine	2–7mg/ 24h
Vitamin B12	150–800pg/ mL
Vitamin D3, 25 hydroxycholecalciferol	10–50ng/ mL
25 dihydroxycholecalciferol	20–75pg/ mL